FIFTH EDITION

RAPID REVIEW

PATHOLOGY

EDWARD F. GOLJAN, MD

Retired Professor
Department of Pathology
Oklahoma State University Center for Health Sciences
College of Osteopathic Medicine
Tulsa, Oklahoma

ELSEVIER

ELSEVIER

1600 John F. Kennedy Blvd.
Ste 1800
Philadelphia, PA 19103-2899

RAPID REVIEW PATHOLOGY, FIFTH EDITION

ISBN: 978-0-323-47668-3

Notices

Knowledge and best practice in this field are constantly changing. As new research and experience broaden our understanding, changes in research methods, professional practices, or medical treatment may become necessary.

Practitioners and researchers must always rely on their own experience and knowledge in evaluating and using any information, methods, compounds, or experiments described herein. In using such information or methods they should be mindful of their own safety and the safety of others, including parties for whom they have a professional responsibility.

With respect to any drug or pharmaceutical products identified, readers are advised to check the most current information provided (i) on procedures featured or (ii) by the manufacturer of each product to be administered, to verify the recommended dose or formula, the method and duration of administration, and contraindications. It is the responsibility of practitioners, relying on their own experience and knowledge of their patients, to make diagnoses, to determine dosages and the best treatment for each individual patient, and to take all appropriate safety precautions.

To the fullest extent of the law, neither the Publisher nor the authors, contributors, or editors, assume any liability for any injury and/or damage to persons or property as a matter of products liability, negligence or otherwise, or from any use or operation of any methods, products, instructions, or ideas contained in the material herein.

Previous editions copyright © 2014, 2011, 2007, 2004.

Library of Congress Cataloging-in-Publication Data

Names: Goljan, Edward F., author.
Title: Rapid review pathology / Edward F. Goljan.
Other titles: Rapid review series.
Description: Fifth edition. | Philadelphia, PA : Elsevier, Inc., [2019] |
Series: Rapid review series | Includes bibliographical references and index.
Identifiers: LCCN 2017056975 | ISBN 9780323476683 (hardcover : alk. paper)
Subjects: | MESH: Pathology | Examination Questions | Outlines
Classification: LCC RB120 | NLM QZ 18.2 | DDC 617.1/07–dc23 LC record available at
https://lccn.loc.gov/2017056975

Executive Content Strategist: James Merritt
Senior Content Development Specialist: Joan Ryan
Publishing Services Manager: Catherine Jackson
Project Manager: Kate Mannix
Design Direction: Amy Buxton
Illustrations Manager: Nichole Beard

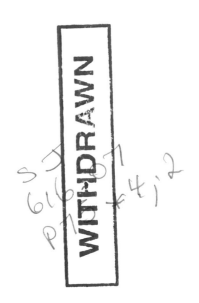

Printed in Canada

Last digit is the print number: 9   8   7   6   5   4   3   2   1

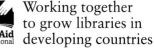

Working together
to grow libraries in
developing countries

www.elsevier.com • www.bookaid.org

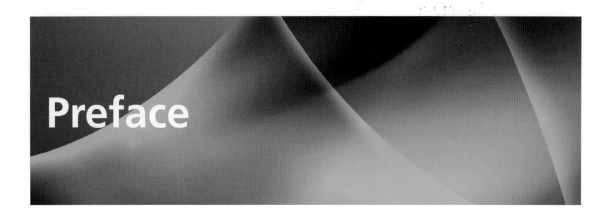

Preface

Writing a new edition of a book provides an opportunity to update information about disease processes and to improve upon previous editions based on feedback from colleagues and medical students. In addition to updating information on all disease processes, in this edition I summarize important anatomy, histology, and/or embryology in an overview section at the beginning of Chapters 18 to 23, 25, and 26. Because integration is important in understanding disease processes, physical diagnosis, epidemiology, pathophysiology, clinical findings, laboratory tests, and radiographic findings are discussed for the clinical disorders in the systemic pathology part of the book. Infectious diseases for each system are thoroughly discussed in extensive tables. This provides students with a "big picture" of each clinical disorder. Pediatric and geriatric disorders are also discussed throughout the book. An up-to-date *Ferri's Clinical Advisor* is recommended for treatment of the various clinical disorders.

Because quality pictures and schematics of disease processes are important for understanding and passing board examinations (Steps 1 and 2), there are more than 1100 figures in the text. Arrows and circles are used extensively to show exactly where the pathology is located in the photograph. Many of the photographs are grouped together in collages or as separate photographs at the top of the page. Because figures take up a considerable amount of space, an additional 1800+ figures can be found as Links, located on Student Consult. In electronic versions of the text, clicking on a Link will bring the reader to the figure. In hardcopy versions of the book, students must access Student Consult to see the Links. Thousands of Margin Notes that briefly summarize important facts have been added to this new edition. These are excellent for a quick overview of key facts in the chapter. Five hundred board-quality questions and discussions covering all pertinent subjects throughout the book are also available on Student Consult. To activate your Student Consult version, see the PIN page on the inside front cover of the book and follow the instructions to activate your PIN. Access to this site is required for locating corrections in the book, questions, and other activities.

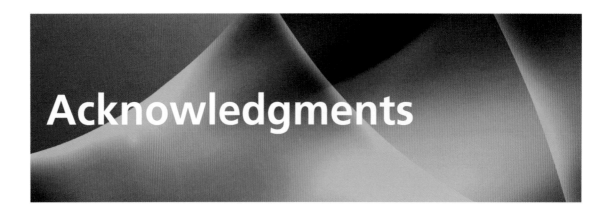

Acknowledgments

The fifth edition of *Rapid Review Pathology* has been extensively revised to provide students with even more high-yield information and photographs than in previous editions. As in previous editions, I especially want to thank my good friend Ivan Damjanov, MD, PhD, whose many excellent photographs and schematics have been utilized throughout this book and in previous editions. I highly recommend his book *Pathophysiology* as a companion text to *Rapid Review Pathology*, fifth edition, for providing students an even greater understanding of pathophysiologic processes in disease.

Special thanks to Margaret Nelson, Joan Ryan, Nicole DiCicco, Kate Mannix, and Ryan Pettit, who kept track of all the major changes of this new edition. I especially want to thank Jim Merritt, who is an excellent friend and the inspiration and primary energy for not only this book but all the books in the *Rapid Review* series. Thanks, Jim, for being my spokesperson in getting this new edition completed. Thanks also to the myriad of medical students who have read previous editions of the book and recommended the book to their friends. Special thanks to my precious wife Joyce, who has stood by me for the past 53 years!

Edward F. Goljan, **MD** (**"Poppie"**)

Contents

I. Purposes of Laboratory Tests

- Screen for disease, confirm disease, monitor disease

  Screen, confirm, monitor disease

A. Screen for disease

1. General criteria for screening
   a. Effective therapy that is safe and inexpensive must be available.
   b. Disease must have a high enough prevalence to justify the expense.
   c. Disease should be detectable *before* symptoms arise.
   d. Test must *not* have many false positives (people misclassified as having disease).
   e. Test must have extremely high sensitivity.

   ↑Sensitivity/specificity/prevalence; cost-effective; treatable

2. Screening for disease is an example of secondary prevention (identify latent disease).
   a. **Definition:** Primary prevention refers to the prevention of disease or injury (e.g., regular physical activity to reduce the risk of developing cardiovascular disease and stroke).

   1° prevention: prevention of disease/injury

   b. **Definition:** Secondary prevention refers to detection of a disease process in its earliest stage, *before* symptoms appear, and initiation of interventions in order to prevent progression of a disease (i.e., "catch it early").

   2° prevention: identify latent disease ("catch it early")

   c. **Definition:** Tertiary prevention refers to the reduction of disability and the promotion or rehabilitation from disease (e.g., cardiac or stroke rehabilitation programs).

   3° prevention: reduction of disability; promotion of rehabilitation from disease

3. Examples of screening tests
   a. Newborn screening for inborn errors of metabolism. Examples: phenylketonuria (PKU), galactosemia, congenital hypothyroidism, maple syrup urine disease

   PKU, galactosemia, hypothyroidism, maple syrup urine disease

   b. Adult screening tests
      (1) Mammography for breast cancer

      Mammography for breast cancer

      (2) Cervical Papanicolaou (Pap) smear for cervical cancer

      Overall best screening test for cancer

      (3) Screen for human papillomavirus (HPV) DNA

      HPV DNA screen

      (4) Colonoscopy to detect/remove precancerous polyps

      Colonoscopy

      (5) Fecal occult blood test (FOBT) to detect colon cancer

      FOBT

      (6) Bone densitometry scans to detect osteoporosis in women

      Bone densitometry

      (7) Fasting lipid profiles (measuring high-density lipoprotein + cholesterol [HDL-CH], low-density lipoprotein + cholesterol [LDL-CH]) to evaluate coronary artery disease (CAD) risk

      Fasting HDL-CH, LDL-CH: evaluate CAD risk

      (8) Fasting blood glucose or 2-hour oral glucose tolerance (OGT) test to screen for diabetes mellitus (DM)

      Fasting glucose or 2-hr OGT test for DM

   c. Screening for individuals in high-risk populations
      (1) Abdominal ultrasound (US) for identifying an abdominal aortic aneurysm (AAA) in current or previous male smokers 65 to 75 years of age (5%–9% have an AAA).

      US AAA male smokers 65–75 yrs old

      (2) Gonorrhea screen for individuals with high-risk sexual behavior (e.g., HIV-positive individuals).

      Gonorrhea screen

      (3) Syphilis screen (rapid plasma reagin [RPR] or venereal disease research lab [VDRL]) for individuals with high-risk sexual behavior (e.g., HIV-positive individuals).

      Syphilis screen

(4) Hepatitis C (HCV) test for individuals born between 1945 and 1965 or those with a history of intravenous drug abuse (IVDA).

(5) Purified protein derivative (PPD) for specific immigrant groups coming from countries with a high risk for developing tuberculosis; prisoners; HIV-positive patients.

(6) Low-dose computed tomography (CT) scan for lung cancer in smokers with at least a 30 pack-year smoking history; current smokers or those who quit smoking within the past 15 years.

(7) Screen for depression by asking the following questions:

    (a) In the past 2 weeks, have you felt hopeless, depressed, or down?

    (b) In the past 2 weeks, have you lost interest or pleasure in doing things that you normally enjoyed?

  d. Screening people with symptoms of a disease. Example: serum antinuclear antibody (ANA) test to rule out autoimmune disease (e.g., systemic lupus erythematosus [SLE])

B. Confirm disease; examples:

1. Anti-Smith (Sm) and double-stranded (ds) DNA antibodies to confirm SLE.
2. Chest x-ray to confirm pneumonia.
3. Urine culture to confirm a bacterial urinary tract infection (UTI).
4. Serum troponins I and T to confirm an acute myocardial infarction (AMI).
5. Tissue biopsy (Bx) to confirm cancer.
6. Fluorescent treponemal antibody absorption (FTA-ABS) test to confirm syphilis.

C. Monitor disease status; examples:

1. Hemoglobin (Hb) A_{Ic} to evaluate long-term glycemic control in diabetics.
2. International normalized ratio (INR) to monitor warfarin therapy (anticoagulation).
3. Therapeutic drug monitoring (TDM) to ensure drug levels are in the optimal range.
4. Pulse oximeter to monitor oxygen saturation during anesthesia or asthmatic attacks.

II. Operating Characteristics of Laboratory Tests

  A. Terms for test results for people *with* a specific disease (Fig. 1-1)

    1. True positive (TP)

      • **Definition:** A true positive is where a diagnostic test *correctly* determines the positive state (diseased state) of the tested individual.

    2. False negative (FN)

      • **Definition**: A false negative is where a diagnostic test *incorrectly* classified a positive state (person with disease) as negative for disease.

  B. Terms for test results for people *without* disease (Fig. 1-1)

    1. True negative (TN)

      • **Definition:** A true negative is where a diagnostic test *correctly* determines the negative state (nondiseased state) of the tested individual.

    2. False positive (FP)

      • **Definition:** A false positive is where a diagnostic test *incorrectly* classified a positive state in a person *without* disease.

  C. Sensitivity of a test

    1. **Definition:** Sensitivity is the likelihood that a person with a specific disease will correctly be identified with a positive test result ("positivity in disease").

    2. Determined by performing the test on people who are known to have the specific disease for which the test is intended (e.g., serum antinuclear antibody [ANA] test in people with SLE).

    3. Formula for calculating sensitivity is TP ÷ (TP + FN). False negative (FN) percentage determines the test's sensitivity.

Test result	Specific disease	No disease
+ Test	True positive(TP)	False positive (FP)
− Test	False negative (FN)	True negative (TN)

1-1: People with a specific disease either have true positive (TP) or false negative (FN) test results. People without disease either have true negative (TN) or false positive (FP) test results.

4. Usefulness of a test with 100% sensitivity (no false negatives)
   a. Normal test result *excludes* disease (must be a true negative).
   b. Positive test result *includes* all people with disease.
      (1) Positive test result does *not* confirm disease.
      (2) Positive test result could be a true positive or a false positive.
   c. Tests with 100% sensitivity are primarily used to screen for disease.

D. Specificity of a test
   1. **Definition:** Specificity is the likelihood that a person *without* disease will have a negative test result ("negative in health").
   2. Specificity of a test is obtained by performing the test on people who do *not* have the specific disease for which the test is intended.
   3. Formula for calculating specificity is TN ÷ (TN + FP). False positive rate determines the test's specificity.
   4. Usefulness for a test with 100% specificity (no false positives)
      a. Positive test result *confirms* disease (must be a true positive).
      b. Negative test result does *not* exclude disease, because a test result could be a true negative or a false negative.

E. Comments on using tests with high sensitivity and specificity
   1. When a test with 100% sensitivity (or close to it) returns negative (normal) on a patient on one or more occasion, the disease is *excluded* from the differential list.
      - For example, if the serum antinuclear antibody (ANA) test returns negative on more than one occasion, the diagnosis of SLE is excluded.
   2. When a test with 100% sensitivity returns positive on a patient, a test with 100% specificity (or close to it) should be used to decide if the test result is a true positive or a false positive.
      a. For example, if the serum ANA returns positive in a patient who is suspected of having SLE, the serum anti-Smith (Sm) and anti–double-stranded DNA test should be used because they both have extremely high specificity for diagnosing SLE.
      b. If either test or both tests return positive, the patient has SLE.
      c. If both tests consistently return negative, the patient most likely does *not* have SLE but some other closely related disease (e.g., systemic sclerosis).

F. Use of multiple tests to improve sensitivity or specificity of a test
   1. Parallel testing involves performing a series of tests simultaneously.
      a. **Definition:** In parallel testing, if any one test is positive, the entire series is considered positive. Test A and Test B → Test A positive, Test B negative → entire series is considered positive
      b. This type of testing improves the overall net sensitivity of the test (fewer false negatives [FNs]); however, it markedly reduces the test's specificity.
         (1) Very useful when a rapid diagnosis (Dx) is necessary.
         (2) Parallel testing is commonly used in the emergency room (ER).
      c. Example: in the emergency room, when a patient presents with chest pain, multiple tests are performed.
         - If any one of the tests returns positive (e.g., ST elevation in an electrocardiogram [ECG], plus increased level of serum troponin or increased level of serum creatine kinase isoenzyme MB [CK-MB]), the patient is admitted to the hospital as having an AMI and is treated accordingly.
   2. Serial testing involves performing a series of tests.
      a. **Definition:** In serial testing, all of the tests must be positive for the test to be considered positive.
         - Test A positive → Test B positive = positive test
         - Test A positive → Test B negative = negative test
      b. This improves the overall net specificity of the test (fewer false positives [FPs]); however, it markedly reduces the test's sensitivity.
         (1) This is very useful when false positives (FPs) are undesirable.
         (2) Example: oncologists commonly use serial testing because treatment involves the use of very toxic drugs and radical surgical procedures.
      c. Example: if a FOBT is positive, additional tests are performed (e.g., colonoscopy to identify a lesion and a biopsy [Bx] to prove cancer is present) *before* the colon is resected.

G. "Gold standard" test
   1. **Definition:** A "gold standard" test is the benchmark with which to compare the results of a new test or the definitive test for any disease state or condition.

Normal test result excludes disease; + test result TP or FP

"Negative in health"

TN ÷ (TN + FP); FP rate determines specificity

+ Test must be TP (confirms disease); – test TN or FN

Exclude disease if test returns normal

Test with 100% specificity: distinguish TP from FP test

Any one test is +, entire series considered +

Improves net test sensitivity (fewer FNs); markedly reduces test specificity

Useful when rapid Dx necessary; commonly used in ER

Patient with chest pain → ECG with ST elevation, + serum troponin or CK-MB

Test A and B positive = positive test

Test A positive, B negative = negative test

Improves test specificity (fewer FPs); ↓ test sensitivity

Useful when FPs are undesirable

Commonly used by oncologists

+FOBT → colonoscopy and Bx must be positive → colectomy

Benchmark to compare new test results; definitive test

TABLE 1-1 Examples of the Sensitivity and Specificity of a Few Common Tests and Physical Diagnosis Findings

DISEASE	SENSITIVITY %	SPECIFICITY %	COMMENTS
Serial testing for CK isoenzyme MB at increasing time intervals for the diagnosis of an AMI	95	95	This is an excellent test with very few false positive tests (e.g., myocarditis, chest trauma). It begins to increase within 4 to 8 hours. Cardiac troponins appear to have a slightly greater sensitivity and specificity than CK-MB (see Chapter 11).
12-lead ECG post admission for an AMI	28	97	In the early stages of an AMI (first few hours), the ECG is not a good initial screen, but when the ECG shows new Q waves, ST elevation, and inverted T waves, it confirms an AMI.
Serum ANA test for diagnosing SLE	≈100%	80%	The serum ANA test is an excellent screen for SLE. However, it has a low specificity, because patients with other autoimmune diseases (e.g., systemic sclerosis, dermatomyositis) can have positive ANA test results.
Physical exam for detecting hepatomegaly by palpating the liver edge in the right upper quadrant	67	73	Physical exam is not very good in detecting hepatomegaly regardless of the expertise of the clinician. However, it is an important physical finding because, when detected, it is always an important indicator of a disease process (e.g., hepatitis, metastasis).
Ventilation (V)/perfusion (Q) scan for detection of a PE	77	98	Because of the low sensitivity of the V/Q scan as an initial test for diagnosing a PE, the CT pulmonary angiogram is frequently used as the initial test for detecting pulmonary embolism. It has a sensitivity of 89% and a specificity of 95%.

AMI, Acute myocardial infarction; *ANA,* antinuclear antibody; *CK,* creatine kinase; *CT,* computed tomography; *ECG,* electrocardiogram; *PE,* pulmonary embolus; *SLE,* systemic lupus erythematosus.

2. Examples include: throat culture for group A beta-hemolytic *Streptococcus pyogenes*; a chest x-ray for pneumonia; a tissue biopsy to rule out cancer or a specific disease; cardiac catheterization to rule out coronary artery stenosis.
3. A "gold standard" test is *not* routinely used because it may be expensive, invasive, dangerous, or all of these.

  H. **Examples of sensitivity and specificity of common tests** (Table 1-1)
III. **Predictive Value of Positive and Negative Test Results Likelihood Ratio**
  A. **Predictive value of a negative test result (PV−)**

Likelihood that negative test result TN rather than FN

PV− = TN ÷ (TN + FN)

Best reflects the true FN rate of a test

Sensitivity 100% → PV− always 100% → excludes disease

Likelihood positive test result TP rather than FP

Best reflects true FP rate of test

Specificity 100% → PV+ 100% → *confirms* disease

Total # people with disease in population under study

People with/without specific disease

Prevalence: (TP + FN) ÷ (TP + FN + TN + FP)

Low prevalence disease: ambulatory population

↓Prevalence of disease: ↑PV−, ↓PV+ (more FPs)

  1. **Definition:** A predictive value of a negative test result is the likelihood that a negative test result is a true negative (TN) rather than a false negative (FN).
  2. Formula for calculating PV− is TN ÷ (TN + FN). Predictive value of a negative test result (PV−) best reflects the true false negative (FN) rate of a test.
  3. Tests with 100% sensitivity (no FNs) always have a PV− of 100% (disease is *excluded* from the differential list).
  B. **Predictive value of a positive test result (PV+)**
  1. **Definition:** A predictive value of a positive test result is the likelihood that a positive test result is a true positive rather than a false positive.
  2. Formula for calculating PV+ is TP ÷ (TP + FP). Predictive value of a positive test result best reflects the true false positive (FP) rate of a test.
  3. Tests with 100% specificity (no false positives) always have a positive predictive value of 100% (disease is *confirmed*).
  C. **Effect of prevalence on PV− and PV+**
  1. **Definition:** Prevalence refers to the total number of people with disease in the population that is under study. Population selected includes people *with* disease and people *without* disease.
  2. To calculate prevalence, people with disease are in the numerator (TP + FN) and people *with* disease (TP + FN) and *without* disease (TN + FP) are in the denominator.

$$\text{Prevalence} = (TP + FN) \div (TP + FN + TN + FP)$$

Disease   Disease No disease

  3. Low prevalence of disease (e.g., ambulatory population) (Fig. 1-2)
    a. Negative predictive value (PV−) *increases* because more true negatives (TNs) are present than false negatives (FNs).
    b. Positive predictive value (PV+) *decreases* because more false positives (FPs) are present than true positives (TPs).

Prevalence of a specific disease	PV–	PV+
Low prevalence of a specific disease	Increases (TN > FN)	Decreases (FP > TP)
High prevalence of a specific disease	Decreases (FN > TN)	Increases (TP > FP)

1-2: Effect of low prevalence and high prevalence of systemic lupus erythematosus on the PV– and PV+.

TABLE 1-2   Diagnostic Value of Tests Defined by Sensitivity, Specificity, Predictive Value, and Efficiency

RESULTS OF A DIAGNOSTIC TEST		
Patient	*Test Positive*	*Test Negative*
Disease present	True positive (TP)	False negative (FN)
Disease absent	False positive (FP)	True negative (TN)
Sensitivity (%)	$= TP / (TP + FN) \times 100$	
Specificity (%)	$= TN / (FP + TN) \times 100$	
Positive predictive value (%)	$= TP / (TP + FP) \times 100$	
Negative predictive value (%)	$= TN / (FN + TN) \times 100$	

Modified from Adkison LR: *Elsevier's Integrated Review Genetics*, 2nd ed, Philadelphia, Saunders Elsevier, 2012, p 226, Table 13-3.

4. High prevalence of disease (e.g., cardiology clinic) (Fig. 1-2)
    a. Negative predictive value (PV–) *decreases* because more false negatives (FNs) are present than true negatives (TNs).
    b. Positive predictive value (PV+) *increases* because more true positives (TPs) are present than false positives (FPs).

↑Prevalence of disease: ↓PV–, ↑PV+

5. Table 1-2 summarizes the diagnostic value of tests defined by sensitivity, specificity, and predictive value.
6. Link 1-1 shows a calculation of the effect of a change in prevalence in SLE on the negative predictive value (PV–) and positive predictive value (PV+).

D. Likelihood ratio (LR)
1. **Definition:** Likelihood ratios are an expression of the degree to which a positive or negative test influences the likelihood of the disease after the test.

Degree to which a + or – test influences odds of disease after the test

   a. LR tells clinicians how much they should shift their suspicion for a particular test result, whether it is positive or negative.
   b. LR is *not* influenced by the prevalence of disease.

Not influenced by prevalence of disease

   c. Positive LR (LR+) tells the clinician how much to increase the likelihood of disease (ruling-in disease) if the test is positive.
      • Calculation is: LR+ = Sensitivity ÷ (1 − Specificity)
      • Stated another way: LR+ = Likelihood that an individual **with** disease has a positive test ÷ (Likelihood that an individual **without** disease has a positive test)

LR+ = Sensitivity ÷ (1 − Specificity)

   d. Negative LR (LR–) tells the clinician how much to decrease the likelihood of disease (ruling-out disease) if the test is negative.
      • Calculation is: LR– = (1 − Sensitivity) ÷ Specificity
      • Stated another way: LR– = (1 − Likelihood that an individual **with** disease has a negative test) ÷ Likelihood that an individual **without** disease has a negative test

LR– = (1 − Sensitivity) ÷ Specificity

2. Interpretation of LR results (Table 1-3)
    a. Note that an LR+ > 1 increases the likelihood that disease is present, while an LR– < 1 decreases the likelihood that disease is present.
    b. Note that any LR+ > 10 markedly increases the likelihood of disease.
    c. Note that any LR– < 0.1 markedly decreases the likelihood of disease.
    d. Note that, an LR = 1 means that the test result does *not* change the likelihood of disease at all; hence, the test is *not* worth doing.
      • Similar to flipping a coin and calling "heads" an abnormal result

LR+ > 1: likelihood of disease rises

LR+ > 10 markedly ↑ likelihood of disease

LR– close to 0: lowers likelihood of disease

LR = 1: test not worth doing

3. Example: a test for an autoimmune disease has a sensitivity of 95% and a specificity of 90%. Calculate the LR+ and the LR–.

TABLE 1-3   **Interpretation of Likelihood Ratios in Disease**

LIKELIHOOD RATIO	INTERPRETATION
>10	Large and often conclusive increase in the likelihood of disease
5–10	Moderate increase in the likelihood of disease
2–5	Small increase in the likelihood of disease
1–2	Minimal increase in the likelihood of disease
1	No change in the likelihood of disease (worthless test)
0.5–1.0	Minimal decrease in the likelihood of disease
0.2–0.5	Small decrease in the likelihood of disease
0.1–0.2	Moderate decrease in the likelihood of disease
<0.1	Large and often conclusive decrease in the likelihood of disease

Modified from Wikipedia, The Free Encyclopedia: Likelihood ratios in diagnostic testing. www.wikipedia.org/wiki/Likelihood_ratios_in _diagnostic_testing.

$$LR+ = .95 \div (1 - .90) = 9.5$$

$$LR- = (1 - .95) \div .90 = 0.06 \,(\text{rounded off})$$

Interpretation: the LR+ is 9.5 (between 5 and 10), indicating a moderate increase in the likelihood of autoimmune disease when the test returns positive. The LR− is 0.06 (<0.1), indicating a large decrease in the likelihood of autoimmune disease when the test returns negative.

4. Example: The rapid antigen test for diagnosing *Streptococcus pyogenes* pharyngitis has a sensitivity of 80% and a specificity of 95%. Calculate the LR+ and the LR−.

$$LR+ = .80 \div (1 - .95) = 16$$

$$LR- = (1 - .80) \div .95 = 0.71$$

Interpretation: the LR+ is 16 indicating a conclusive increase in the likelihood of streptococcal pharyngitis when the rapid antigen test is positive. The LR− is 0.71, indicating a minimal decrease in the likelihood of streptococcal pharyngitis when the test returns negative. If the suspicion is still high that streptococcal pharyngitis is present, then a culture should be ordered.

5. Example: The serum antinuclear antibody test (ANA) has a sensitivity of 41% and specificity of 56% in diagnosing rheumatoid arthritis. Calculate the LR+ and LR−.

$$LR+ = .41 \div (1 - .56) = 0.93$$

$$LR- = .56 \div (1 - .41) = 1.05$$

Interpretation: Since both are close to 1, the test is *not* useful for either ruling in or ruling out rheumatoid arthritis.

IV. **Precision and Accuracy of Test Results**

  A. **Precision**

    1. **Definition:** Precision refers to the ability to produce the same test result consistently.

      a. *High precision* if there is a close grouping of test results with repeated measurements (Figs. 1-3 A, B). Does *not* mean that the test result is accurate (see the following).

      b. *Low precision* if there is *not* a close grouping of test results with repeated measurements (Fig. 1-3 C).

    2. Test result deviations usually have a random distribution.

      a. Standard deviation (SD) of a test

        (1) **Definition:** Standard deviation is the variation from the mean value of a test performed in a normal population.

        (2) **Definition:** Standard deviation reflects the precision of a test.

      b. Normal random (Gaussian) distribution curve (Fig. 1-4)

        (1) One standard deviation encompasses 68% of the normal population. Therefore, 32% of normal people are outside of this range.

        (2) Two standard deviations encompass 95% of the normal population. Therefore, 5% of normal people are outside of this range.

Produce same test result consistently

Close grouping test results

No close grouping test results

Best reflects precision of test

2 SD encompasses 95% population; 5% normal people outside this range

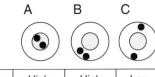

	A	B	C
Precision	High	High	Low
Accuracy	High	Low	Low

1-3: Precision and accuracy of a test. Using a target as an example, the bull's-eye is the true value of the test. Test A has both accuracy and precision. Test B has precision but is not accurate. Test C has neither precision nor accuracy. *(From Goljan E, Sloka K: Rapid Review Laboratory Testing in Clinical Medicine, St. Louis, Mosby Elsevier, 2008, p 3, Fig. 1-2)*

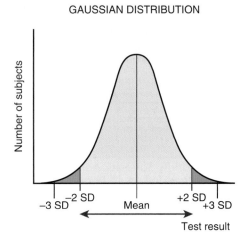

GAUSSIAN DISTRIBUTION

Number of subjects

−3 SD −2 SD   Mean   +2 SD +3 SD

Test result

1-4: Using ± 2 standard deviations (SD) from the mean as the reference interval (normal value; red arrow) for a test, 5% of the normal population is outside the normal range and have a FP test result. Repeating the test usually produces a normal result (TN). The usual reference interval for a test uses ± 2 SD from the mean of the test. The SD of a test is an excellent indicator of precision of a test. The smaller the SD is, the greater the precision will be; the greater the SD is, the less the precision of the test will be. *(From Marshall W, Bangert S: Clinical Chemistry, 6th ed, Philadelphia, Elsevier, 2007. As redrawn in O'Connell TX, Pedigo RA, Blair TE: Crush Step I: The Ultimate USMLE Step I Review, Philadelphia, Saunders Elsevier, 2014, p 2, Fig. 1-2.)*

     (3) Three standard deviations encompass 99.7% of the normal population. Therefore, 0.3% of normal people are outside of this range.

   c. Tests with high precision have a low standard deviation. Example: serum potassium.

   d. Tests with low precision have a high standard deviation. Example: serum enzymes.

   e. Figure 1-4 shows the relationship of standard deviation and the precision of a test.

B. Accuracy

  1. **Definition:** Accuracy is the ability to produce a test result that is very close to the accepted standard (i.e., true value of the test; Fig. 1-3 A).

  2. Evaluating the accuracy of a test

   • Laboratory measurement of control samples with known assay values is the basis of quality control in the laboratory. It evaluates the accuracy of the laboratory's performance of the test.

V. Normal Range of a Test

  A. Establishing the normal range (reference interval) of a test using a Gaussian distribution (Fig. 1-4)

  1. Normal range is established by adding and subtracting 2 standard deviations (SD) from the mean of the test.

   a. Adding 2 SD to the mean establishes the upper cutoff point of a test.

   b. Subtracting 2 SD from the mean establishes the lower cutoff point of a test.

   c. Example:

    (1) 2 SD = 10 mg/dL, mean = 100 mg/dL, normal range = 90–110 mg/dL

    (2) The high cutoff is 110 mg/dL and the low cutoff is 90 mg/dL for the test.

  2. Out of normal range test results (outliers) occur in 5% of normal people.

   a. Using ±2 SD, the normal range encompasses 95% of the normal population.

   b. Remaining 5% of the normal population are called outliers (false positives [FPs]).

    (1) Often, if the test is repeated on the same or a different sample, the outlier will end up within the normal range.

    (2) If there is any doubt about the outlier being a false positive, order a different test that has a high specificity.

  3. Likelihood of an outlier (FP test) increases as the number of tests ordered increases.

   a. Calculation for establishing the likelihood of an outlier is as follows:

   • $100 - (0.95^n \times 100)$, where n is the number of tests ordered

   b. Example of the likelihood of an outlier if six tests are ordered:

   • $100 - (0.95^6 \times 100) = \approx 27\%$ that one of the tests will be outside the normal range.

  B. General methods of reporting laboratory test results

  1. Quantitative test

   a. **Definition:** A quantitative test gives a numeric value with specific units and not just a number result.

   b. Examples: serum cholesterol (CH) is reported in mEq/L; serum albumin is reported in g/dL; serum CK is reported in units per liter (U/L); arterial partial pressure of CO_2 ($PaCO_2$) is reported in millimeters of mercury (mm Hg).

Margin notes:

Tests with high precision → low SD

Tests with low precision → high SD

Accuracy: Test result very close to accepted standard (true value) of test

Adding 2 SD to mean → upper cutoff point of test; subtracting 2 SD establishes lower cutoff point

Normal range: ±2 SD from mean

±2 SD from mean 95% normal population; 5% normal people

Using ±2 SD from mean, 5% normal population are outliers (FPs)

Number outliers increases as number tests ordered increases

Numeric value with specific units

Serum CH reported in mEq/L

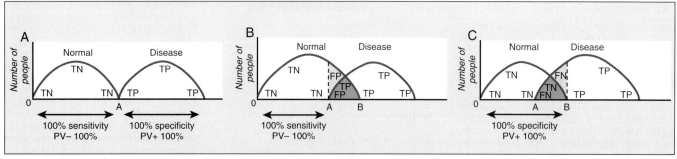

1-5: Establishing tests with 100% sensitivity and specificity. Schematic **A** shows an ideal test with 100% sensitivity (100% PV−) and 100% specificity (100% PV+) when the normal range is 0 to A. Test results below the A cutoff point are all true negative (TN), whereas those beyond the A cutoff point are all true positive (TP). Schematic **B** shows a test with 100% sensitivity (100% PV−) when the upper cutoff point is at A. Note that as sensitivity increases, the specificity and PV+ decrease because of an increase in false positive (FP) results. Schematic **C** shows a test with 100% specificity (100% PV+) when the upper cutoff point is at B. Note that as specificity increases, the sensitivity and PV− decrease because of an increase in false negatives (FNs). *PV−,* Predictive value of a negative test result; *PV+,* predictive value of a positive test result. *(From Goljan E, Sloka K: Rapid Review Laboratory Testing in Clinical Medicine, St. Louis, Mosby Elsevier, 2008, p 5, Fig. 1-3.)*

2. Semiquantitative test

    a. **Definition:** A semiquantitative test gives results as a number.

Gives results as a number

    b. Example of urine red blood cells (RBCs): urine RBCs 10 RBC/hpf (normal ≤2 RBCs/hpf)

Urine RBCs (normal ≤RBCs/hpf)

       • hpf is one high-power field as viewed under the microscope.

3. Semiqualitative tests

    a. **Definition:** A semiqualitative test reports a test as positive/negative; yes or no; detected or not detected, or equivocal (neither positive nor negative).

Yes/no; detected, not detected, or equivocal

FOBT reported as negative or positive

    b. Example: FOBT is reported as negative or positive.

VI. Creating Highly Sensitive and Specific Tests

  A. Ideal test (Fig. 1-5 A)

    1. **Definition:** The ideal test has 100% sensitivity (PV− 100%) and 100% specificity (PV+ 100%).

100% sensitivity (PV− 100%), 100% specificity (PV+ 100%)

    2. Note in the schematic that there are no false negatives (FNs) or false positives (FPs), because there is *no overlap* between the normal and disease population.

    3. An ideal test is nonexistent; however, there are some tests that have very high sensitivity and specificity that come close to being the ideal test (e.g., serum levels of troponins I and T or CK-MB in diagnosing an AMI).

Serum troponins/CK-MB: ↑sensitivity/specificity; screen/confirm AMI

    4. Most normal ranges (reference intervals) do *not* distinguish the normal from the disease population (Fig. 1-5 B, C). Note that there is an overlap between the normal and the disease population in parts B and C of Figure 1-5.

  B. Establishing a test with 100% sensitivity and 100% PV− (Fig. 1-5 B and Link 1-2)

    1. To establish a test with 100% sensitivity and a negative predictive value (PV−) of 100%, set the cutoff point for the reference interval at the *beginning* of the disease curve (point A).

      a. Note that this creates a test with 100% sensitivity and 100% negative predictive value (PV−), because there are no false negatives (FNs) within the newly established reference interval (0 to point A). This is a good screening test.

Put cutoff point at beginning of disease curve; no FNs

    2. Note that by increasing sensitivity there is *always* a corresponding decrease in the specificity and positive predictive value (PV+) of the test due to a greater number of false positives (FPs) (Fig. 1-5 B).

  C. Establishing a test with 100% specificity and PV+ (Fig. 1-5 C and Link 1-2)

    1. To establish a test with 100% specificity and 100% positive predictive value (PV+), set the upper cutoff point for the reference interval at the *end* of the normal curve (point B).

      a. Note that this creates a test with 100% specificity and 100% positive predictive value (PV+), because there are no false positives (FPs) outside the reference interval (0 to point B). Good test to confirm disease.

Cutoff point at end of normal curve; no FPs

    2. Note that by increasing specificity there is *always* a corresponding decrease in sensitivity and the negative predictive value (PV−), due to a greater number of false negatives (FNs).

  D. Critical values ("panic or "alert" values) for a test

    • **Definition:** A critical value refers to any test result that may require rapid clinical attention by the caregiver in order to prevent significant patient morbidity and mortality. Critical values are usually established by the laboratory and/or clinicians.

Any test result that requires rapid clinical attention by caregiver

VII. Variables Affecting Selected Laboratory Tests (Preanalytic Variables)

  A. Age

    1. Newborns (NBs)

      a. **Definition:** The newborn period begins at birth (regardless of gestational age) and includes the first month of life.

      b. In the fetus, hemoglobin F (HbF; $2\alpha/2\gamma$ globin chains) is the predominant hemoglobin (Hb).

        (1) Conversion of HbF to HbA (adult Hb; $2\alpha/2\beta$ globin chains) begins to occur at about 32 weeks of gestation.

        (2) HbF ($2\alpha/2\gamma$ globin chains) leftward shifts oxygen dissociation curve (ODC) (see Fig. 2-4; less release of oxygen [O_2] to tissue) causing the synthesis and release of erythropoietin (EPO) by the kidneys.

          (a) Erythropoietin causes an increase in the hemoglobin (Hb), hematocrit (Hct), and the red blood cell (RBC) count.

          (b) Hematocrit (Hct) is the proportion of a blood sample that is RBCs (packed RBCs), measured as a percent of whole blood.

        (3) At birth, about 70% of the Hb is HbF; by 6 to 12 months only a trace is present.

        (4) Newborns have higher normal ranges for Hb, Hct, and RBC counts than do infants and children owing to the effect of increased EPO in response to a leftward shift of the oxygen dissociation curve (ODC) by HbF.

        (5) Full-term newborns have a drop in Hb from a normal Hb of 16.8 g/dL (range 14–20 g/dL) to 9–11 g/dL over the next 2 to 3 months, while preterm infants during this same time period have a drop to 7–10 g/dL.

          (a) This drop is called *physiologic anemia* and is due to splenic macrophage removal of HbF–containing cells and bone marrow synthesis of RBCs containing HbA (>97%), HbA_2 (2.0%), and HbF (1%). Physiologic anemia is the most common "anemia" at this age.

          (b) Drop in levels of HbF causes the oxygen dissociation curve (ODC) to shift back to normal, hence improving O_2 exchange in tissue (see Chapter 2).

        (6) Nonphysiologic anemia in both preterm (<37 weeks gestation) and full-term newborns is defined as a Hb < 13 g/dL or a Hct < 45%.

        (7) Hemoglobin value below which children are considered to be anemic is as follows: 3 months: 9.5 g/dL; 1 to 3 years: 11.0 g/dL; 4 to 12 years: 11.5 g/dL; 12 to 16 years: 12.0 g/dL

      c. Sequential bilirubin changes in newborns

        (1) All newborns experience a progressive increase in unconjugated (indirect; UCB) bilirubin at birth (called physiologic jaundice).

        (2) Average umbilical cord blood unconjugated (indirect) bilirubin is 1–3 mg/dL and rises at a rate of <5 mg/dL/24 hr.

        (3) Jaundice becomes visible on the 2nd to 3rd day, usually peaking between the 2nd and 4th days at 5–6 mg/dL.

          • This normal increase in bilirubin is called physiologic jaundice and is due to the normal breakdown of fetal RBCs containing HbF by splenic macrophages as well as inability of the immature fetal liver to convert unconjugated bilirubin (UCB) to conjugated (direct) bilirubin.

        (4) Bilirubin then decreases to <2 mg/dL by the 5th to 7th day after birth.

        (5) Approximately 6% to 7% of full-term newborns have unconjugated bilirubin levels >13 mg/dL and less than 3% have levels >15 mg/dL. Factors that determine this greater increase in unconjugated bilirubin (UCB) than usual include breast-feeding, transient decreases in the liver conjugating enzyme glucuronyltransferase in the liver, maternal age, race (Chinese, Japanese, Korean, Native Americans), maternal diabetes, and prematurity, to name a few.

      d. Immunoglobulin (Ig) synthesis in newborns

        (1) Synthesis of IgM begins shortly *after* birth.

        (2) Newborns normally *lack* IgM isohemagglutinins (natural antibodies against blood groups) in their plasma. For example, blood group A newborns normally lack anti-B IgM isohemagglutinin in their plasma (see Chapter 16).

Margin notes:

Begins at birth and includes 1st month of life

Production HbF ($2\alpha/2\gamma$ globin chains) is predominant

Conversion HbF to adult HbA ($2\alpha/2\beta$ globin chains) begins 32 wks gestation

HbF leftward shifts ODC → ↑EPO

EPO: ↑Hb, Hct, RBC count

Hct packed RBCs measured as % whole blood

NBs: ↑HbF

↑HbF → leftward shift ODC → ↑EPO → ↑Hb, Hct, and RBC production

Hb drops after birth; drop greater in preterm than full-term NBs

RBCs contain HbA (97%), HbA_2 (2%), HbF (1%)

Physiologic anemia: MC anemia early infancy

Preterm/full-term anemia: Hb < 13 g/dL

Progressive ↑ UCB at birth; physiologic jaundice

Jaundice visible by 2nd to 3rd day life

Physiologic jaundice

Macrophage breakdown HbF RBCs → ↑UCB

Normal levels by 5–7 days after birth

Small % normal NBs have high UCB levels

Breast-feeding, ↓liver conjugating enzyme, race, maternal DM

IgM synthesis begins shortly after birth

NBs lack IgM blood group antibodies at birth

Lack IgM *at* birth; ↑cord blood IgM may indicate congenital infection

---

Clinical correlation: Newborns with an increase in cord blood IgM that is greater than normal may have an underlying congenital infection (e.g., cytomegalovirus, rubella). Immunoglobulin M is the first immunoglobulin (Ig) to increase in an infection. The newborn blood should be screened for antibodies against the common congenital infections.

IgG absent at birth maternal origin; IgM/IgA cannot pass through placenta

IgG synthesis 2–3 months *after* birth

(3) All IgG antibodies (abs) in newborns are of *maternal* origin.
  (a) Maternal IgG antibodies pass through the placenta (transplacental) to the fetus. IgM and IgA antibodies *cannot* pass through the placenta.
  (b) Newborns *begin* synthesizing IgG 2 to 3 months *after* birth.
  (c) Adult levels of IgG are achieved by 6 to 10 years of age.

Clinical correlation: A mother with a positive test for human immunodeficiency virus (e.g., IgG antibodies against the glycoprotein gp120) transplacentally transfers maternal IgG antibodies to the fetus. This does *not* mean that the child is infected by the virus.

Childhood: time between 1 month of age and 18 years of age

ALP ≫ in children than adults (↑bone growth)

Children have ≫ serum phosphorus than adults

Phosphorus drives calcium into bone

Children *lower* Hb levels than adults; anemia < 11.5 gm/dL

Children ↑↑ 2,3 BPG → right shift ODC → ↑↑ O_2 release RBCs to tissue

Anemia in women is < 12.5 g/dL

Menstrual blood/iron loss (↓serum iron/ferritin)

Women < testosterone than men

↑Estrogen/LH proliferative phase; ↑progesterone secretory phase

T stimulates erythropoiesis

Anemia in men is < 13.5 g/dL

↓GFR, CCr; danger drug nephrotoxicity

↑Serum ALP: bone origin; OA

2. Children
  a. **Definition:** Childhood includes the period of time from 1 month of age to 18 years of age.
  b. When compared to an adult, children have *higher* serum alkaline phosphatase (ALP) levels.
    (1) Due to *increased* bone growth in children and release of the enzyme alkaline phosphatase (ALP) from osteoblasts in growing bone.
    (2) Function of alkaline phosphatase is to remove the phosphate from pyrophosphate, which normally *inhibits* bone mineralization.
    (3) Compared to an adult, children have *higher* serum phosphorus levels. For normal mineralization of bone to occur, phosphorus is required to drive calcium into growing bone; hence, the need for higher phosphorus levels in children.
  c. Compared to an adult, children have a *lower* hemoglobin (Hb) concentration (11.5 g/dL; anemia < 11.5 g/dL).
    (1) Most likely related to the increased serum phosphorus levels in children. A proportionately greater amount of 2,3-bisphosphoglycerate (2,3-BPG) is synthesized because of the availability of phosphorus.
    (2) Increasing 2,3-BPG synthesis causes a greater RBC release of O_2 to tissue (shifts the O_2 dissociation curve to the right; see Chapter 2); hence, an 11.5 g/dL Hb concentration in a child delivers as much O_2 to tissue as a 13.5 g/dL Hb concentration does in an adult.
3. Adults
  a. Compared to men, women have slightly *lower* levels of serum iron, ferritin (marker of iron storage), and hemoglobin (Hb; 12.5 g/dL; anemia <12.5 g/dL), which is attributed to the following:
    (1) Monthly menstrual flow. The loss of blood and iron decreases serum iron and ferritin.
    (2) Lower testosterone levels than men.
  b. When compared to men, women have varying blood levels of estrogen and progesterone because of the menstrual cycle.
    (1) In the initial proliferative phase of the menstrual cycle, estrogen is the key hormone and is responsible for endometrial gland proliferation and stimulation of luteinizing hormone (LH) release, which initiates ovulation (see Chapter 22).
    (2) In the secretory phase of the cycle after ovulation has occurred, progesterone is the key hormone and increases endometrial gland tortuosity and secretion.
  c. Men have higher testosterone levels than women.
    (1) Testosterone (T) stimulates erythropoiesis, thus the higher hemoglobin (Hb) level in men (13.5 g/dL) than women.
    (2) Anemia in men is a hemoglobin (Hb) < 13.5 g/dL.
4. Advanced age (see Chapter 6)
  a. Normal *decrease* in the glomerular filtration rate (GFR) and creatinine clearance (CCr) in advanced age. This is potentially harmful to the proximal kidney tubules if nephrotoxic drugs (e.g., aminoglycosides) are *not* dose-adjusted to the age and glomerular filtration rate (GFR) of the elderly person (see Chapter 20).
  b. *Increase* in serum alkaline phosphatase (ALP)
    (1) Increase in serum ALP is of bone origin and relates to degeneration of articular cartilage in the weight-bearing joints (osteoarthritis [OA]), a condition that invariably occurs in the elderly (see Chapter 24).

(2) In osteoarthritis, reactive bone formation (called osteophytes) occurs at the margins of the joints, leading to the slight increase in serum alkaline phosphatase.

Serum ALP ≫ young adults; due to osteophytes in OA

c. When compared to young adult males, there is a slight *decrease* in the Hb concentration in elderly males.

(1) Hb drops into the range of a normal adult woman (12.5 g/dL) and should *not* be misinterpreted as anemia.

(2) Anemia in advanced age is defined as a Hb < 12.5 g/dL.

(3) Decrease in Hb parallels the normal decrease in testosterone associated with aging. Testosterone (T) normally stimulates erythropoiesis.

Slight decline male Hb levels (12.5 g/dL); anemia < 12.5 g/dL

↓Hb in males parallels ↓T

T stimulates erythropoiesis

d. In advanced age, there is often a *loss* of blood group isohemagglutinins (e.g., anti-B IgM in a group A individual) because of a *decrease* in antibody synthesis.

Advanced age loss isohemagglutinins

Clinical correlation: Loss of isohemagglutinins explains why some elderly individuals transfused with the wrong type of blood do *not* develop a hemolytic transfusion reaction. For example, a blood group A individual inadvertently transfused with group B blood may *not* hemolyze the group B RBCs, because they do *not* have anti-B IgM antibodies. This is *not* to say that elderly people can safely be given any blood group for transfusion. They should always receive blood group and Rh type specific blood.

e. *Decrease* in cell-mediated immunity (CMI; see Chapter 4). For example, a PPD test for tuberculosis is weakly reactive in elderly patients who have previously been exposed to tuberculosis.

↓ Antibody synthesis/CMI

B. Pregnancy (see Chapter 22)

1. There is a normal *increase* in plasma volume (↑↑PV) and RBC production (↑RBC mass; total number of RBCs) in pregnancy.

Normal ↑↑PV and ↑RBC mass (total number of RBCs)

2. A proportionally greater increase in plasma volume (PV) than RBC mass produces a dilutional effect that slightly *decreases* the hemoglobin (Hb) concentration.

a. This accounts for the normally lower Hb levels seen in pregnancy (11 g/dL).

b. Anemia in pregnancy is a Hb < 11 g/dL.

Dilutional effect of ↑↑PV causes Hb to drop to 11 g/dL in pregnancy

Hb < 11 g/dL

c. Other effects of an *increase* in plasma volume (PV):

(1) *Increased* glomerular filtration rate (GFR) and creatinine clearance (CCr)

(2) *Increased* renal clearance of blood urea nitrogen (BUN), creatinine, and uric acid (UA), with corresponding *decreased* levels in the serum

(3) *Increased* uterine blood flow, which allows more oxygen containing RBCs to deliver oxygen to the developing fetus

↑GFR, CCr

↓Serum BUN, creatinine, UA

↑Uterine blood flow → more O₂ to fetus

3. *Increase* in serum alkaline phosphatase (ALP) is of placental origin.

4. *Increase* in serum human placental lactogen (HPL).

↑Serum ALP (placental origin)

a. Human placental lactogen is normally synthesized by syncytiotrophoblasts lining the chorionic villi in the placenta.

b. Human placental lactogen normally inhibits the sensitivity of peripheral tissue to insulin. This produces the normal *glucose intolerance* in pregnancy.

c. Human placental lactogen *increases* the β-oxidation of fatty acids (FAs) in the liver. Excess acetyl CoA is produced, leading to increased liver synthesis of ketone bodies and the normal *ketonemia/ketonuria* that occurs in pregnancy.

HPL synthesized by syncytiotrophoblasts

↓Insulin sensitivity → mild glucose intolerance

↑ β-oxidation FAs

↑Acetyl CoA→ ↑synthesis ketone bodies → ketonemia/ ketonuria

5. Mild respiratory alkalosis (RAlk) in pregnancy.

a. This is due to stimulation of the respiratory center by progesterone (PG).

b. Increased alveolar ventilation (tidal volume) is responsible for the respiratory alkalosis (↓PaCO₂ [arterial partial pressure]); *not* accompanied an increase in the respiratory rate, which is the usual cause of respiratory alkalosis (see Chapter 5).

RAlk due to PG stimulation respiratory center

Respiratory alkalosis (↓PaCO₂)

• Decrease in PaCO₂ causes a corresponding *increase* in PaO₂ in maternal blood, which *increases* the amount of oxygen that is available to the developing fetus. PaO₂ is usually >100 mm Hg in pregnancy.

↓PaCO₂ → ↑PaO₂

PaO₂ > 100 mm Hg

6. *Increase* in the total serum thyroxine (T₄) and cortisol (see Chapter 23).

a. Normal measurement of total serum T₄ and cortisol includes bound and free fractions of the hormone.

b. Estrogen increases liver synthesis of the *binding proteins* for T₄ (thyroid binding globulin) and cortisol (transcortin); however, the free hormone levels (metabolically active) are unaffected. Because the free hormone levels are normal, the serum thyroid-stimulating hormone (TSH) and adrenocorticotropic hormone (ACTH) levels are also normal.

↑Total serum T₄/cortisol → ↑ binding proteins; free hormone levels normal

C. Diet

↑Glucose, TG after eating

1. Both serum glucose and serum triglyceride (TG) are increased after eating.
2. Serum total bilirubin (TB) levels may slightly increase 48 hours after fasting.

↑TB (unconjugated fraction) 48 hrs after fasting ↑UCB

   a. Total serum bilirubin includes unconjugated bilirubin (bilirubin bound to albumin) and conjugated bilirubin (free bilirubin).
   b. Unconjugated bilirubin (UCB; formerly called "indirect bilirubin") fraction of the total serum bilirubin is normally slightly increased after fasting.

↓Serum glucose in women; ↑TG and FFA in men

3. In healthy women, fasting for 3 days decreases the serum glucose to as low as 45 mg/dL, while in men, there is an increase in plasma triglyceride (TG) and free fatty acids (FFAs) *without* an increase in CH.

Tests requiring fasting state: glucose, TG, lipid profile

4. The following common lab tests should be drawn in the fasting state (≈12 hrs after the last ingestion of food): glucose, triglyceride (TG), or any lipid profile that includes triglyceride.

Most detect heme via detection of peroxidase

FP FOBT peroxidase in meat, fish, iron, horseradish

5. Standard FOBT that detects heme via detection of peroxidase may have a false positive test result due to the presence of peroxidase in meat, fish, iron, and horseradish.

↓VLDL, ↓TG, ↓LDL, ↓vitamin B$_{12}$

6. Long-term vegetarian diets lead to a decrease in very-low-density lipoprotein (VLDL; triglyceride [TG] is the primary lipid), low-density lipoprotein (LDL; main vehicle for carrying CH), and vitamin B$_{12}$ (only present in animal products).

↑Serum uric acid, ammonia, BUN

7. High meat and or protein-rich diet increase the serum levels of uric acid (UA), ammonia, and blood urea nitrogen (BUN).

↑Serum lactate, UA, TG

8. Ethanol ingestion increases serum lactate, uric acid (UA), and triglyceride (TG) levels (this increases VLDL levels).

D. Other variables

1. Hemolyzed blood specimen related to venipuncture
   a. Potassium is the major intracellular cation; therefore, a hemolyzed blood sample *falsely increases* serum potassium (FP).
   b. RBCs primarily use anaerobic glycolysis as a source of ATP; therefore, lactate dehydrogenase (LDH), which normally converts pyruvate to lactate, is also *falsely increased* (FP).

↑Serum K$^+$, LDH

2. Posture during phlebotomy
   a. Upright position increases the plasma hydrostatic pressure, which normally pushes a protein-poor fluid through the thin-walled venules and capillaries into the interstitial space (see Chapter 5).
   b. Slightly reduces the plasma volume (PV) leading to a slight increase in the concentration of plasma albumin, which, in turn, increases the total serum protein (albumin + globulins) as well.

↓PV→ ↑serum albumin, total serum protein (↑albumin + globulin)

   c. Variation would *not* be present if the patient was supine (lying face upward).

3. Diurnal variations

PRA, ACTH, aldosterone, insulin lower at night

   a. The following analytes are lower at night: plasma renin activity (PRA), adrenocorticotropic hormone (ACTH), aldosterone, and insulin.

Peaks 4–6 AM, lowest 8 PM–12 AM, 50% lower at 8 PM than 8 AM

   b. Cortisol peaks between 4 and 6 AM; lowest between 8 PM and 12 AM; 50% lower at 8 PM than at 8 AM. Stress at any time increases cortisol as well as ACTH.

Iron peaks early/late morning; ↓ up to 30% during day

   c. Iron peaks early to late morning and decreases up to 30% during the day. The best time to draw blood or a serum iron is in the late morning, because if decreased during this time the patient is truly iron deficient.

GH higher in afternoon/ evening

   d. Growth hormone (GH) is higher in the afternoon and evening. The best time to draw blood when you suspect growth hormone (GH) deficiency is in the afternoon or evening, because if decreased level at this time increases the likelihood of growth hormone deficiency.

↑Serum enzymes, proteins, protein-bound substances

4. Prolonged tourniquet application causes hemoconcentration of certain analytes as water leaves the vein because of backpressure. Analytes that increase include serum enzymes, proteins, and protein-bound substances.

Reduces Hb levels

5. Hospitalization frequently reduces hemoglobin (Hb) levels.

Frequent phlebotomy ↓Hb

   a. Frequent phlebotomy plays a significant role in producing anemia in premature newborns, full-term newborns, children, and adults.
   b. During hospitalization, the patient is supine most of the time.

↑PV produces drop Hb/Hct (dilutional effect)

      (1) This increases plasma volume (PV), hence producing a mild hemodilutional effect causing a drop in the hemoglobin (Hb) and hematocrit (Hct), which is *not* pathologic.
      (2) This is best understood by understanding the relationship between RBC count and RBC mass and plasma volume (PV).

(a) RBC count = RBC mass/PV; therefore, if plasma volume (PV) is increased the RBC count is decreased (note: RBC mass is the total number of RBCs in the peripheral blood in mL/kg body weight).

$$\downarrow RBC\ count = RBC\ mass/\uparrow PV$$

(b) Decline in RBC count causes a decrease in hemoglobin (Hb) and should *not* be misinterpreted as representing anemia.
   - Since RBCs carry hemoglobin (Hb), if RBCs are truly decreased, hemoglobin (Hb) will also be decreased.

6. Stress
   a. Mental and physical stress lead to an increase in adrenocorticotropic hormone (ACTH), cortisol, and catecholamines (e.g., epinephrine).
   b. Serum CH may increase with stress, while HDL-CH may decrease by as much as 15%.
   c. Hyperventilation (rapid breathing) from stress produces respiratory alkalosis (RA) (decrease in arterial $PaCO_2$), a drop in the serum ionized calcium leading to tetany (thumb adduction into the palm, perioral numbness and tingling; see Chapter 23), an increase in the white blood cell (WBC) count, and an increase in serum lactate (anaerobic glycolysis).

7. Exercise
   a. Transient effects of exercise
      (1) Initial decrease and then increase in free fatty acids (FFA; hydrolysis of triglyceride [TG] from the adipose by cortisol)
      (2) 300% increase in serum lactate (from anaerobic glycolysis)
      (3) Increase in skeletal muscle enzymes (serum CK, aldolase, aspartate aminotransferase [AST], and lactate dehydrogenase [LDH]) from minor damage to skeletal muscle
      (4) Activation of the coagulation system, fibrinolytic system, and platelets
   b. Long-term effects of exercise
      (1) Smaller increases of the previously mentioned enzymes
      (2) Decreased levels of serum gonadotropins (applies to long-distance running; possible loss of menses in women). There is a correlation between excessive loss of body fat and weight with decreased secretion of gonadotropin releasing hormone (GnRH) from the hypothalamus and a corresponding decrease in serum gonadotropins.

8. Differences in tests performed on venous, arterial, capillary blood
   a. Blood gas results are different in venous (blood returning to the heart) and arterial blood (blood leaving the heart). Example: the PO_2 (partial pressure of oxygen dissolved in blood) in venous blood is 28 to 48 mm Hg, while the PO_2 in arterial blood is 80 to 90 mm Hg, because of oxygenation in the lungs.
   b. Capillary blood (fingerstick) glucose levels may differ significantly from venous and arterial blood.

Margin notes:

$\downarrow RBC\ count = RBC\ mass/\uparrow PV$

$\downarrow RBC$ count automatically $\downarrow Hb$ concentration

$\uparrow ACTH$, cortisol, catecholamines

$\uparrow Serum\ CH$, $\downarrow HDL$

Hyperventilation $\rightarrow$ $\downarrow PaCO_2$ (RA)

RA $\rightarrow$ $\downarrow$serum ionized calcium $\rightarrow$ tetany (thumb adducts into palm)

Initial $\uparrow FFA$ from hydrolysis TG

$\uparrow$Lactic acid (anaerobic glycolysis)

Skeletal muscle injury $\rightarrow$ $\uparrow AST$, aldolase, LDH enzymes

Less increase in enzymes

Long-distance running: $\downarrow$serum GnRH $\rightarrow$ loss menses

Blood gas PO_2 different in venous vs arterial blood

Glucose levels differ significantly from venous/arterial blood

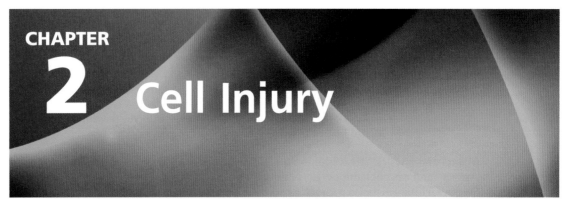

CHAPTER 2 Cell Injury

ABBREVIATIONS

MC most common   MCC most common cause   Rx treatment

I. **Overview of Cell Injury**
  • Major Causes of Cell Injury (Table 2-1)
II. **Tissue Hypoxia**
  A. **Hypoxia**

Inadequate oxygenation tissue

Complete lack tissue oxygenation

  1. **Definition:** Hypoxia is inadequate oxygenation of tissue.
    • Anoxia is an extreme form of hypoxia wherein there is a complete lack of oxygen (O_2) supply to the body or to a specific organ (e.g., high altitude; cardiac arrest; respiratory failure).
  2. Factors contributing to the total amount of O_2 carried in blood
    a. Normally, O_2 diffuses down a gradient from the atmosphere to the alveoli, to plasma, and into the red blood cells (RBCs), where it attaches to heme groups (Table 2-2; Link 2-1).

PAO_2 partial pressure alveolar O_2

PaO_2 partial pressure arterial O_2

O_2 attached heme groups Hb → SaO_2

O_2 atmosphere → ↑PAO_2 → ↑PaO_2 → ↑SaO_2

      (1) In the alveoli, O_2 increases the partial pressure of O_2 (PAO_2).
      (2) In the plasma of the pulmonary capillaries, dissolved O_2 increases the partial pressure of arterial O_2 (PaO_2).
      (3) In the RBC, O_2 attaches to heme groups on hemoglobin (Hb) and increases the arterial O_2 saturation (SaO_2). If the PaO_2 is decreased, less O_2 is available to diffuse into the RBCs, and SaO_2 must decrease (Link 2-2).
    b. PaO_2 and SaO_2 are reported in arterial blood gas analyses.
    c. **Definition:** O_2 content is a measure of the total amount of O_2 carried in blood and includes the Hb concentration as well as the PaO_2 and SaO_2.

O_2 content = (Hb g/dL × 1.34) × SaO_2 + PaO_2 × 0.003

↓O_2 content→ ↑EPO renal synthesis

↓ATP synthesis by oxidation phosphorylation

Falsely ↑SaO_2 in metHb/COHb; Co-oximeter measures ↓SaO_2 in metHb/COHb

      • O_2 content = (Hb g/dL × 1.34) × SaO_2 + PaO_2 × 0.003. A decrease in O_2 content, due to a decrease in Hb, PaO_2, or SaO_2, causes an increase in erythropoietin (EPO) synthesis in the kidneys.
  3. In hypoxia, there is decreased synthesis of adenosine triphosphate (ATP).
    a. ATP synthesis occurs in the inner mitochondrial membrane by the process of oxidative phosphorylation (see later).
    b. O_2 is an electron acceptor located at the end of the electron transport chain (ETC) in complex IV of the oxidative pathway.
    c. Lack of O_2 and/or a defect in oxidative phosphorylation culminates in a decrease in ATP synthesis.

Definition: Pulse oximetry (Fig. 2-1 A) is a noninvasive test for measuring SaO_2. It utilizes a probe that is usually clipped over a patient's finger. A pulse oximeter emits light at specified wavelengths that identify oxyhemoglobin (over the range of 100% to ≈75%) and deoxyhemoglobin, respectively. The wavelengths emitted by a pulse oximeter *cannot* identify dyshemoglobins such as methemoglobin (metHb; heme group has +3 valence) and carboxyhemoglobin (i.e., carbon monoxide bound to Hb [COHb]), which normally decrease the SaO_2 (see later). In the presence of these dyshemoglobins, the oximeter calculates a falsely high SaO_2 (Fig. 2-1 B). However, unlike the standard oximeter, a co-oximeter emits multiple wavelengths and identifies metHb and COHb as well as oxyhemoglobin and deoxyhemoglobin. Hence, in the presence of these dyshemoglobins, the SaO_2 will be decreased. Pulse oximeters are very useful in following patients with respiratory failure, severe asthma, obstructive sleep apnea, and those under general anesthesia. Most clinicians consider pulse oximeters to be inaccurate when SaO_2 values are less than 70%.

TABLE 2-1 Mechanisms of Cell Injury

TYPE OF INJURY	CLINICAL EXAMPLES	CHAPTER (S)
Aging	Decreased replicative capacity of cells	Chapters 2, 6
Anoxia (complete lack of oxygen), hypoxia (inadequate oxygen)	It is most commonly due to circulatory (e.g., myocardial infarction) or respiratory dysfunction (e.g., chronic obstructive pulmonary disease)	Chapter 2
Chemicals	Alcohol, polycyclic hydrocarbons (e.g., cigarette smoke), heavy metals (e.g., mercury), drugs (e.g., acetaminophen), drugs of abuse (e.g., cocaine)	Chapter 7
Free radicals	Acetaminophen poisoning, iron overload diseases (e.g., hemochromatosis)	Chapters 2, 19, respectively
Genetic and metabolic disorders	Phenylketonuria, diabetes mellitus	Chapters 6, 23, respectively
Inflammation and immune reactions	Abscess/cellulitis, autoimmune diseases	Chapters 3, 4, respectively
Intracellular accumulations	Endogenous (e.g., bilirubin, triglyceride), exogenous (e.g., anthracotic pigment, lead)	Chapters 2, 6, 7, 12, 17, 19
Microbes	Infections by viruses, bacteria, fungi, parasites	Chapters 10 through 26
Nutritional deficiencies	Protein deficiency (e.g., kwashiorkor), vitamin deficiency (e.g., scurvy)	Chapter 8
Physical agents	Skin wounds, burns, frostbite, radiation	Chapter 7

TABLE 2-2 Terminology Associated With Oxygen Transport and Hypoxia

TERM	DEFINITION	CONTRIBUTING FACTORS	SIGNIFICANCE
O_2 content	The total amount of O_2 carried in blood. O_2 content = (Hb g/dL × 1.34) × SaO_2 + PaO_2 × 0.003. ↑O_2 content causes ↓EPO. ↓O_2 content causes ↑EPO.	Hb concentration in RBCs is the most important of the three components in O_2 content. PaO_2 SaO_2	• Hb is the most important carrier of O_2. • The Hb concentration determines the total amount of O_2 delivered to tissue. In anemia, less O_2 is delivered to tissue. • O_2 content is decreased in hypoxemia, anemia, CO poisoning, and methemoglobinemia. • In cyanide poisoning, the venous O_2 content is greater than the arterial O_2 content, because there is no extraction of O_2 by the tissue. In addition, the MVO_2 content is essentially the same as the O_2 content of arterial blood, because no O_2 was extracted from the venous blood.
PaO_2	It is the pressure that is keeping O_2 dissolved in the plasma of arterial blood (PaO_2 × 0.003).	Percentage of O_2 in inspired air Atmospheric pressure PAO_2 concentration in the lungs Normal O_2 exchange in the lungs across the alveolar-capillary membrane	• PaO_2 is decreased in hypoxemia. • PaO_2 is the driving force for the diffusion of O_2 from the capillaries, where there is a higher concentration of O_2, into tissue, where there is a lower concentration of O_2. If PaO_2 is decreased, there is less diffusion of O_2 into tissue.
SaO_2	The average percentage of O_2 bound to each of the four heme groups in Hb in the RBCs.	Same factors listed previously for PaO_2. The normal valence of heme iron in each of the four heme groups in RBCs is Fe^{2+} (reduced, ferrous), which is the only valence of iron that can bind to O_2. For example, a valence of Fe^{3+} (oxidized, ferric) in heme iron *cannot* bind to O_2.	• An SaO_2 < 80% produces cyanosis (bluish discoloration) of the skin and mucous membranes.

EPO, Erythropoietin; Fe^{2+}, ferrous iron; Fe^{3+}, ferric iron; *Hb*, hemoglobin; O_2, oxygen; PAO_2, partial pressure of alveolar PO_2; PaO_2, partial pressure of arterial oxygen; SaO_2, arterial oxygen saturation.

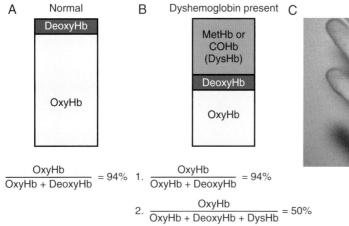

$$\frac{OxyHb}{OxyHb + DeoxyHb} = 94\%$$

1. $\dfrac{OxyHb}{OxyHb + DeoxyHb} = 94\%$

2. $\dfrac{OxyHb}{OxyHb + DeoxyHb + DysHb} = 50\%$

2-1: **A,** Pulse oximetry is a noninvasive alternative for measuring Sao₂. It utilizes a probe that is usually clipped over a patient's finger. The oximeter emits red and infrared light at specified wavelengths that identify oxyhemoglobin (oxyHb) and deoxyhemoglobin (deoxyHb), respectively. The oximeter calculates the Sao₂ using the following equation: oxyHb/oxyHb + deoxyHb. The wavelengths emitted by a pulse oximeter cannot identify dyshemoglobins such as methemoglobin (metHb) and carboxyhemoglobin (i.e., carbon monoxide bound to Hb [COHb]), which normally decrease the Sao₂. In the presence of these dyshemoglobins, the oximeter calculates a normal Sao₂, because metHb or COHb are *not* included in the calculation of Sao₂ in equation 1 in figure part B. **B,** However, a co-oximeter, which emits multiple wavelengths, calculates the decrease in Sao₂ because it identifies metHb and COHb and includes them in the calculation of Sao₂: oxyHb/oxyHb + deoxyHb + metHb or COHb (equation 2 in B). **C,** Hand of a child with tetralogy of Fallot, a congenital heart disease associated with cyanosis. Note the blue discoloration beneath the nails and the duskiness of the skin when compared to the hand of a normal adult. *(**A** and **B** from Goljan E, Sloka K:* Rapid Review Laboratory Testing in Clinical Medicine, *Philadelphia, Mosby Elsevier, 2008, p 78, Fig. 3-6;* **C** *from Taylor S, Raffles A:* Diagnosis in Color Pediatrics, *London, Mosby-Wolfe, 1997, p 91, Fig. 3.6.)*

Cyanosis bluish skin discoloration → hypoxia

4. Clinical findings
   a. Cyanosis (bluish discoloration of skin and mucous membranes) (Fig. 2-1 C)
   b. Confusion, anxiety, lethargy, tachycardia (increased heart rate), tachypnea (increased respiratory rate), seizures, coma, and even death

B. **Causes of tissue hypoxia**

1. Ischemia

↓Arterial flow *to* tissue/↓venous outflow *from* tissue

Coronary artery atherosclerosis, ↓cardiac output, thrombosis SMV

   a. **Definition:** Ischemia is decreased arterial blood flow to tissue or decreased venous outflow of blood from tissue.
   b. Examples: coronary artery atherosclerosis, decreased cardiac output, thrombosis of the superior mesenteric vein (SMV)
   c. Consequences

Atrophy, infarction, organ dysfunction

   (1) Atrophy (reduction in cell/tissue mass; discussed later)
   (2) Infarction of tissue (localized area of tissue necrosis; discussed later)
   (3) Organ dysfunction (inability to perform normal metabolic functions)

2. Hypoxemia

↓Pao₂

   a. **Definition:** Hypoxemia is a decrease in Pao₂ measured in an arterial blood gas.

Pao₂: %O₂ inspired air, V̇, Q̇, diffusion

   b. Normal Pao₂ depends on the percentage of O₂ in inspired air, ventilation (V̇; breathing), perfusion (Q̇; blood flow to lungs), and diffusion of O₂ from the alveoli into the pulmonary capillaries (Fig. 2-2 A).

Pio₂ 150 mm Hg, Pico₂ 0 mm Hg

   (1) Note in the schematic (Fig. 2-2 A) that the normal partial pressure of O₂ (Po₂) in inspired air (Pio₂) is 150 mm Hg and the normal partial pressure of carbon dioxide (Pico₂) is 0, due to the absence of CO₂ in the atmosphere.
   (2) In the alveoli, O₂ diffuses into the pulmonary capillary; hence, the alveolar PAo₂ drops to 100 mm Hg.

MVO₂ 40 mm Hg returning *from* tissue

Pao₂ 100 mm Hg *leaving* lungs

       (a) Note that mixed venous blood O₂ (MVO₂) returning from tissue to the lungs normally has a partial pressure of O₂ of 40 mm Hg due to the normal diffusion of O₂ derived from RBCs into tissue. However, after O₂ from the alveoli diffuses into pulmonary capillaries, the systemic arterial Po₂, or Pao₂, increases to 100 mm Hg.

MVPCO₂ 46 mm Hg from tissue → Paco₂ 40 mm Hg leaving lungs

       (b) Note that mixed venous blood (MVPCO₂) returning from tissue to the lungs normally has a partial pressure of CO₂ of 46 mm, due to the diffusion of CO₂ from tissue into the venous blood returning to the lungs. However, after CO₂ from mixed venous blood diffuses into the alveoli for elimination, the systemic arterial Pco₂ (Paco₂) drops to 40 mm Hg.

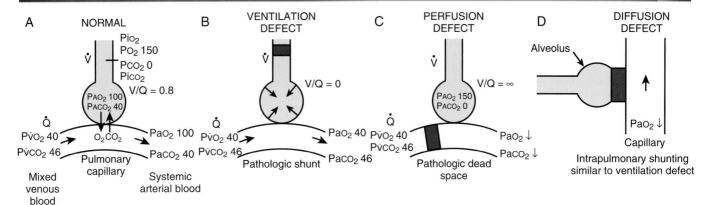

2-2: Ventilation ($\dot{V}$)-perfusion ($\dot{Q}$) defects. **A,** Schematic of normal ventilation and perfusion. **B,** Schematic of a ventilation defect. The schematic shows collapse of the alveoli *(arrows)* due to a lack of surfactant *(arrows)*. See the text for further discussion. **C,** Schematic of a perfusion defect showing blockage of perfusion but normal ventilation. **D,** Schematic of a diffusion defect showing blockage of diffusion of O_2 through the alveolar-capillary interface into the pulmonary capillaries. See the text for further discussion. $Paco_2$, Partial pressure of arterial carbon dioxide; Pao_2, partial pressure of arterial oxygen; Pco_2, partial pressure of carbon dioxide; Po_2, partial pressure of oxygen; $Pvco_2$, partial pressure of carbon dioxide in mixed venous blood; Pvo_2, partial pressure of oxygen in mixed venous blood. *(Modified from Goljan E, Sloka K:* Rapid Review Laboratory Testing in Clinical Medicine, *Philadelphia, Mosby Elsevier, 2008, p 76, Fig. 3-5.)*

  c. Causes of hypoxemia ($\downarrow Pao_2$)
   (1) Respiratory acidosis
    (a) **Definition:** Respiratory acidosis is defined as retention of CO_2 in the lungs (hypoventilation) causing an increase in $Paco_2$ (see Chapter 5) and a corresponding decrease in Pao_2 (see the following).

    > Hypoventilation $\rightarrow \uparrow Paco_2$, $\downarrow Pao_2$

    (b) A partial list of causes of respiratory acidosis includes depression of the medullary respiratory center (e.g., barbiturates), paralysis of the diaphragm (e.g., amyotrophic lateral sclerosis), and chronic bronchitis.
    (c) Carbon dioxide (CO_2) retention in the alveoli ($\uparrow$alveolar Pco_2) *always* produces a corresponding decrease in alveolar Po_2 ($\downarrow PAo_2$), which, in turn, decreases both Pao_2 in the blood and Sao_2 in the RBCs (see the following).

    > $\uparrow$Alveolar $Pco_2 \rightarrow \downarrow PAo_2$ $\rightarrow \downarrow Pao_2$ (blood) $\rightarrow \downarrow Sao_2$ (RBCs)

    (d) Because of the equal effect CO_2 retention has on both alveolar PAo_2 and arterial Pao_2, the alveolar-arterial (A-a) gradient (difference in mm Hg of the Po_2 levels in alveoli and arterial blood) remains normal. The A-a gradient is fully discussed in Chapter 17.

    > A-a gradient normal

> The sum of the partial pressures of O_2, CO_2, and nitrogen in alveoli of the lungs must equal 760 mm Hg at sea level. Assuming that the partial pressure of nitrogen is a constant, an increase in $PAco_2$ must be accompanied by a decrease in PAo_2 in order for the sum of the partial pressures to equal 760 mm Hg. This leads to a decrease in Pao_2 and Sao_2. The reverse is also true. If the $PAco_2$ is decreased (respiratory alkalosis; hyperventilation [breathing faster]), then PAo_2 must increase, which should increase Pao_2 and Sao_2 if ventilation, perfusion, and diffusion are normal in the lungs.

   (2) Decreased Pio_2
    • Examples: breathing at high altitude and breathing reduced %O_2 mist. The A-a gradient is normal (no damage to the lungs).

    > $\downarrow PAco_2 = \uparrow$alveolar $PAo_2 = $ $\uparrow Pao_2 = \uparrow Sao_2$; A-a gradient normal; $\uparrow PAco_2 = $ $\downarrow PAo_2 = \downarrow Pao_2 = \downarrow Sao_2$; A-a gradient normal

> The **ventilation-perfusion ratio** is the ratio of alveolar ventilation ($\dot{V}$ in liters/min) to pulmonary blood flow ($\dot{Q}$ in liters/min). The normal $\dot{V}/\dot{Q}$ ratio = 4 liters/min/5 liters/min = 0.8. The term *normal* in this context means that breathing frequency, tidal volume (volume of air moved into or out of the lungs during quiet breathing), and cardiac output are all normal.

    > $\downarrow Pio_2$ causes hypoxemia; A-a gradient normal

   (3) Ventilation/perfusion ($\dot{V}/\dot{Q}$) defects
    (a) Fig. 2-2 B shows a ventilation defect.
     • **Definition:** In a ventilation defect, alveoli are perfused; however, there is impaired O_2 delivery to the alveoli ($\dot{V}$ decreased).

     > Alveoli perfused but *not* ventilated

     • Diffuse ventilation defects produce intrapulmonary shunting of blood (a pathologic shunt) characterized by pulmonary capillary blood having the same Po_2 and Pco_2 as venous blood returning from tissue.

     > Intrapulmonary shunting blood (pathologic shunt)
     > $\dot{V}/\dot{Q} = 0$; $\uparrow$A-a gradient

     • Note that the $\dot{V}/\dot{Q}$ in a large ventilation defect is 0.
     • Because a great disparity between PAo_2 and Pao_2 is present, the A-a gradient is increased (see Chapter 17).

     > RDS/CF diffuse ventilation defects (intrapulmonary shunting)

The respiratory distress syndrome (RDS; see Chapter 17) is an example of a diffuse ventilation defect (intrapulmonary shunting of blood). In RDS, there is a lack of surfactant (lubricant in the alveoli that decreases surface tension allowing them to remain expanded) that causes collapse of the distal airways (called atelectasis) in both lungs (note the arrows in Fig. 2-2 B). Another example of a diffuse ventilation defect and intrapulmonary shunting of blood is cystic fibrosis (CF) where thick mucus plugs block the airways (blue rectangle in airway) and there is distal resorption of air from the alveoli (called atelectasis).

$\dot{V}$ normal, $\dot{Q}$ decreased

PE, fat embolism

$\dot{Q}$ defect → ↑pathologic dead space → no O_2/CO_2 exchange

Physiologic dead space nose/mouth to respiratory bronchioles

Perfusion defect $\dot{V}/\dot{Q} = \infty$ (infinity)

Perfusion defect → ↑A-a gradient

↑FiO_2 → ↑PaO_2
↓O_2 diffusion across alveolar-capillary interface

↓PaO_2 > ↓PAO_2 → ↑A-a gradient

Interstitial fibrosis, pulmonary edema

Cyanotic CHD → venous into arterial blood (right-to-left shunt); ↓PaO_2; ↑A-a gradient

- Increasing the fraction of inspired oxygen (FiO_2) does *not* significantly increase the PaO_2 in diffuse ventilation defects involving both lungs (e.g., RDS).
  - Smaller ventilation defects are usually compensated for in the normally ventilated lung.
  (b) Fig. 2-2 C shows a perfusion defect.
  - **Definition:** In a perfusion defect, alveoli are ventilated ($\dot{V}$ normal), but there is *no* perfusion of the alveoli ($\dot{Q}$ decreased).
  - Examples: pulmonary embolus (PE; see Chapters 5 and 17) and fat embolism (see Chapter 5)
  - Perfusion defects produce an increase in pathologic dead space (no O_2/CO_2 exchange).
  - Normal dead space (physiologic dead space) includes the nose/mouth to the beginning of the respiratory bronchioles.
  - Note that both the PaO_2 and $PaCO_2$ are decreased.
  - PaO_2 is decreased, because there is no O2 exchange in the nonperfused lung.
  - $PaCO_2$ is decreased, because patients breathe faster, causing the loss of CO_2 into the atmosphere.
  - In a perfusion defect the $\dot{V}/\dot{Q} = \infty$ (infinity).
  - Because of the great disparity between PAO_2 and PaO_2, the A-a gradient is increased in perfusion defects.
  - Increasing the FiO_2 increases the PaO_2 in perfusion defects, because they tend to be less extensive than ventilation defects. Other portions of the lung, which are normally ventilated and perfused, will have normal gas exchange, thus compensating for most perfusion defects (e.g., pulmonary embolus).
  (4) Diffusion defects
  (a) **Definition:** In a diffusion defect, there is decreased diffusion of O_2 across the alveolar-capillary interface into the pulmonary capillaries.
  (b) Equilibration of O_2 is impaired; hence, the decrease in PaO_2 is greater than the decrease in PAO_2, causing the A-a gradient to be increased.
  (c) Examples of a diffusion defect include interstitial fibrosis and pulmonary edema.
  (5) Anatomic right-to-left shunt (e.g., cyanotic congenital heart disease [CHD]; e.g., tetralogy of Fallot; see Chapter 11)
  - In tetralogy of Fallot, there is shunting of venous blood in the right ventricle into the left ventricle (right-to-left shunt) causing a drop in the PaO_2 that is much greater than the decrease in PAO_2, causing an ↑A-a gradient.
  (6) High altitude

At **high altitude** (Link 2-3), the atmospheric pressure is decreased; however, the percentage of O_2 in the atmosphere remains the same (i.e., 21%). This produces hypoxemia (↓PaO_2), which stimulates peripheral chemoreceptors (e.g., carotid and aortic bodies), causing an increase in the respiratory rate (hyperventilation) leading to respiratory alkalosis (↓arterial pH, ↓$PaCO_2$). The A-a gradient is normal because there is an equal effect on both the PAO_2 and the PaO_2. Respiratory alkalosis, in turn, increases intracellular pH, which activates phosphofructokinase (PFK), the rate-limiting enzyme in glycolysis. An increase in glycolysis leads to increased production of 1,3-bisphosphoglycerate (BPG), which is converted to 2,3-BPG by a mutase reaction. 2,3-BPG rightward shifts the O_2-dissociation curve (ODC), causing an increased release of O_2 from RBCs into the tissue. Hypoxic vasoconstriction of the smooth muscles in the pulmonary arteries eventually increases pulmonary artery resistance to blood flow, which, in turn, increases the pulmonary artery pressure (called pulmonary artery hypertension [PH]). Over long periods of time, PH produces right ventricular hypertrophy (RVH; thickening of the muscle). The combination of PH and RVH is called cor pulmonale (see Chapter 17).

↓Atmospheric pressure; normal % atmospheric O_2—Hypoxemia/respiratory alkalosis; ↓PAO_2/PaO_2; normal A-a gradient—↑2,3-BPG; rightward shift ODC—PH + RVH → cor pulmonale

3. Hemoglobin (Hb)-related abnormalities
   a. Anemia (see Chapter 12)
      (1) **Definition:** Anemia is a decrease in the hemoglobin concentration in the peripheral blood. O_2 content is always decreased in anemia; thus there is a lack of O_2 available to the tissue.

      $\downarrow$Hb concentration; $\downarrow O_2$ content

      (2) Causes (see Chapter 12):
         (a) Decreased production of hemoglobin (e.g., iron deficiency), increased destruction of RBCs (e.g., hereditary spherocytosis)
         (b) Decreased production of RBCs (e.g., aplastic anemia), increased sequestration (trapping) of RBCs (e.g., splenomegaly)

      $\downarrow$Production Hb/RBCs; $\uparrow$destruction/sequestration RBCs

      (3) Pao_2 and Sao_2 are normal in anemia.
         (a) Even though the Pao_2 and Sao_2 are normal in anemia, the total amount of O_2 delivered to tissue is decreased ($\downarrow O_2$ content). Anemia has no effect on oxygenation of blood in the lungs.
         (b) A-a gradient is normal, because the Pao_2 is normal.

      Normal Pao_2/Sao_2; $\downarrow O_2$ content; A-a gradient normal

   b. Methemoglobinemia
      (1) **Definition:** Methemoglobin (metHb) is hemoglobin with oxidized heme groups (Fe^{3+} rather than Fe^{2+}; Fig. 2-3 A).

      MetHb = heme Fe^{3+}; cannot attach to O_2

Methemoglobin (Fe^{3+}) is converted to the ferrous state (Fe^{2+}) by the reduced nicotinamide adenine dinucleotide (NADH) reductase system located off of the glycolytic pathway in RBCs (see reactions, later). Electrons from NADH are transferred to cytochrome b5 and then to metHb by cytochrome b5 reductase to produce ferrous hemoglobin. Newborns are particularly at risk of developing methemoglobinemia after oxidant stresses (see later). This is because they have decreased levels of cytochrome b5 reductase until at least 4 months of age.

Newborns $\downarrow$cytochrome b5 reductase

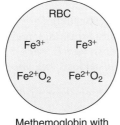

Methemoglobin with an SaO_2 50% normal PaO_2

A

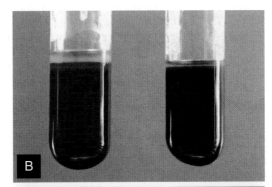

B

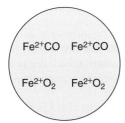

Carboxyhemoglobin with and SaO_2 of 50% normal PaO_2

C

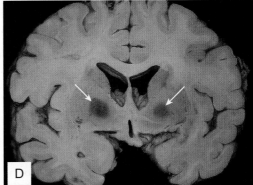

D

2-3: **A,** Methemoglobin (metHb) is Hb in the oxidized Fe^{3+} state. It decreases Sao_2 but has no effect on the Pao_2. MetHb prevents normal Hb in the reduced state from releasing O_2 to the tissue, causing the O_2 dissociation curve (ODC) to be left-shifted. **B,** Arterial whole blood *(left)* versus arterial whole blood with an increased concentration of metHb *(right)*. The arterial blood is bright red because of increased amount of oxyhemoglobin, whereas the arterial blood with increased metHb has the characteristic chocolate brown color due to an increase in deoxyhemoglobin (correlates with a decreased arterial O_2 saturation). **C,** RBC with carboxyhemoglobin ($Fe^{2+}CO$). Similar to metHb, it decreases Sao_2 but has no effect on the Pao_2. Similar to metHb, it prevents normal Hb in the reduced state from releasing O_2 to the tissue causing the O_2 dissociation curve (ODC) to be left-shifted. **D,** Carbon monoxide poisoning. Hemorrhagic discoloration *(arrows)* of the pallidum in acute carbon monoxide poisoning. The dorsal part of the nucleus is most severely affected. *(**A, C** courtesy of Edward Goljan. **B** from Kliegman R: Nelson Textbook of Pediatrics, 20th ed, Philadelphia, Saunders Elsevier, 2016, p 2348, Fig. 462-6; protocol based on personal communication with Dr. Ali Mansouri, December 2002. **D** from Ellison D, Love S, et al: Neuropathology: A Reference Text of CNS Pathology, 3rd ed, St. Louis, Mosby Elsevier, 2013, p 532, Fig. 25.12a.)*

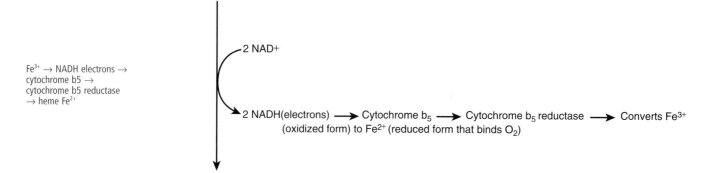

Glyceraldehyde 3-P

2 NAD+

Fe^{3+} → NADH electrons → cytochrome b5 → cytochrome b5 reductase → heme Fe^{2+}

2 NADH(electrons) ⟶ Cytochrome b$_5$ ⟶ Cytochrome b$_5$ reductase ⟶ Converts Fe^{3+} (oxidized form) to Fe^{2+} (reduced form that binds O$_2$)

1, 3-Bisphosphoglycerate

Oxidant stresses (nitro/sulfur drugs, sepsis)

Normal Pao$_2$, ↓Sao$_2$; ↓O$_2$ content; normal A-a gradient

EPO synthesis kidney interstitial cells

Impaired cooperativity (↓ unloading O$_2$ from RBCs)

Leftward shift ODC; lactic acidosis

Cyanosis

Headache, anxiety, dyspnea, tachycardia

Confusion, lethargy, lactic acidosis

Anaerobic glycolysis → lactic acidosis

(2) Causes: oxidant stresses. Examples: nitrite- and/or sulfur-containing drugs, nitrates (fertilizing agents), and sepsis
Pathogenesis of hypoxia in methemoglobinemia
(a) Fe^{3+} *cannot* bind O$_2$; therefore, the Pao$_2$ is normal and A-a gradient normal, but the Sao$_2$ is decreased. A decrease in Sao$_2$ decreases the O$_2$ content, which stimulates the synthesis of EPO in the renal cortex by interstitial cells in the peritubular capillary bed. The A-a gradient is normal, because the Pao$_2$ is normal.
(b) Ferric heme groups impair unloading of O$_2$ by oxygenated ferrous heme in the RBCs (impairs cooperativity). Normally, when the first O$_2$ binds to Fe^{2+}, it makes it easier for the second O$_2$ to bind to Fe^{2+}, and the process repeats itself until all ferrous groups are occupied by O$_2$. This is called cooperativity.
(c) MetHb leftward shifts the ODC (see later).
(4) Clinical findings
(a) Cyanosis at low levels of metHb (levels <20%)
(b) Headache, anxiety, dyspnea (difficulty breathing), and tachycardia (levels >20%)
(c) Confusion, lethargy, and lactic acidosis (levels >40%). Lack of O$_2$ causes a shift to anaerobic glycolysis leading to lactic acidosis (see later).

Patients with **methemoglobinemia** have chocolate-colored blood (increased concentration of deoxyhemoglobin; Fig. 2-3 B) and cyanosis. Clinically evident cyanosis occurs at metHb levels >1.5 g/dL. Skin color does *not* return to normal after administration of O$_2$. Treatment is intravenous methylene blue, which accelerates the enzymatic reduction of metHb by NADPH-metHb reductase located in the pentose phosphate shunt. This shunt is *not* normally operational in reducing metHb. Exchange transfusion and hyperbaric oxygen treatment are second-line options for patients with severe methemoglobinemia whose condition does *not* respond to intravenous methylene blue or who cannot be treated with methylene blue (e.g., those with glucose-6-phosphate dehydrogenase [G6PD] deficiency).

Cyanosis unresponsive to O$_2$ administration—IV methylene blue; accelerates NADPH-metHb reductase

Colorless/odorless gas; incomplete combustion carbon-containing compounds

Leading cause of death due to poisoning

MCC car exhaust

High affinity for heme groups (COHb)

↓Sao$_2$ normal Pao$_2$

Inhibits cytochrome oxidase ETC

Cytochrome oxidase: CO$_2$ → water

ETC shuts down → disrupts O$_2$ diffusion gradient

Impairs cooperativity (unloading O$_2$)

CO leftward shifts ODC

↓Sao$_2$ → O$_2$ content → ↑EPO

c. Carbon monoxide (CO) poisoning (see Chapter 7)
(1) **Definition:** Carbon monoxide is a colorless, odorless gas that is produced by incomplete combustion of carbon-containing compounds.
(2) Leading cause of death due to poisoning
(3) Causes of CO poisoning: automobile exhaust (MCC), smoke inhalation, wood stoves, indoor gasoline-powered generators (fall and winter months in cold climates), and clogged vents for home heating units (e.g., methane gas)
(4) Pathogenesis of hypoxia in CO poisoning
(a) CO has a high affinity for heme groups and competes with O$_2$ for binding sites on hemoglobin (COHb). Sao$_2$ is decreased (if blood is measured with a co-oximeter) *without* affecting the Pao$_2$.
(b) CO also inhibits cytochrome oxidase in complex IV of the ETC (see later).
  • Cytochrome oxidase normally converts O$_2$ into water. Inhibition of the enzyme prevents O$_2$ consumption, shuts down the ETC, and disrupts the diffusion gradient that is required for O$_2$ to diffuse from the blood into the tissue.
(c) Similar to metHb, CO attached to heme groups impairs unloading of O$_2$ from oxygenated ferrous heme in RBCs into tissue (impairs cooperativity; Fig. 2-3 C). CO shifts the ODC (see later) to the left.
(d) A ↓Sao$_2$ decreases the O$_2$ content causing an increase in EPO.

(5) Pathologic findings

    (a) In the first few hours the brain is swollen, congested, and cherry red.

    (b) After 24 hours, pinpoint areas of hemorrhage (called petechial hemorrhage) occur in the white matter and larger areas of hemorrhage may occur into the globus pallidum (Fig. 2-3 D). Globus pallidus (GP) lesions become necrotic and cavitate in several days/weeks, if the patient survives.

(6) Clinical findings

    (a) Cherry red discoloration of the skin and blood (usually a postmortem finding)

    (b) Headache (first symptom at levels of 10%–20%); dyspnea, dizziness (levels of 20%–30%); seizures, coma (levels of 50%–60%)

    (c) Other findings: atraumatic rhabdomyolysis (breakdown of muscle tissue; myoglobin binds CO preventing normal muscle function) and delayed neurologic deficits in 14% to 40% of patients (e.g., memory deficits, apathy)

      • Neurologic toxicity is due to the combination of hypoxia and intracellular actions of CO involving activation of an inflammatory cascade resulting in oxidative damage and brain lipid peroxidation (free radical [FR] damage; discussed later).

      • Brain magnetic resonance imaging (MRI) and computed tomography (CT) reveal damage primarily in the GP and white matter.

(7) CO effect in pregnant women

      • Signs of fetal distress occur if carboxyhemoglobin (COHb) is >20% in the pregnant woman. Fetal distress occurs because fetal hemoglobin (hemoglobin F; $2\alpha2\gamma$) has a higher affinity for CO than adult hemoglobin.

(8) Laboratory findings

    (a) ↑COHb levels in arterial blood when measured with a co-oximeter

    (b) Lactic acidosis (shift to anaerobic glycolysis; see later)

    (c) ↓Sao$_2$ (if measured with a co-oximeter) and a normal Pao$_2$

d. Factors that cause a leftward shift to the oxygen dissociated curve (ODC; Fig. 2-4)

  (1) Decreased 2,3-BPG.

    (a) Recall that 2,3-BPG is an intermediate of glycolysis in RBCs and is formed by the conversion of 1,3-BPG to 2,3-BPG. 2,3 BPG stabilizes the taut form of hemoglobin, which decreases O$_2$ affinity to hemoglobin and allows O$_2$ to diffuse into tissue.

  (2) CO, alkalosis (↑arterial pH), metHb, fetal hemoglobin, and hypothermia

Margin notes:

Brain initially swollen + cherry red color

Petechial hemorrhages
GP hemorrhage/cavitation

Cherry red color skin/blood at postmortem

Headache 1st symptom

Seizures, coma

Rhabdomyolysis; delayed neurologic deficits

Hypoxia + FR damage

MRI/CT show damage GP + white matter

Fetal distress

Fetal Hb > affinity for CO than adult Hb

↑COHb arterial blood (co-oximeter)

Lactic acidosis (hypoxia), normal Pao$_2$, ↓Sao$_2$

2,3-BPG glycolysis intermediate

CO, alkalosis, metHb, fetal Hb, hypothermia

All factors that shift the ODC to the left increase the affinity of hemoglobin for O$_2$ with less release of O$_2$ to tissue. For example, at the capillary PO$_2$ concentration in tissue, a right-shifted ODC (↑2,3-BPG, acidosis, fever) has released most of its O$_2$ to tissue (80% to tissue), whereas a left-shifted ODC still has most of its O$_2$ attached to heme groups (only 20% goes to tissue; Fig. 2-4).

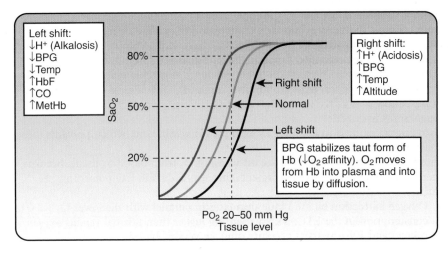

2-4: Oxygen-dissociation curve (ODC). Note that at the Po$_2$ in tissue (range, 20–50 mm Hg) a left-shifted ODC still has an O$_2$ saturation (Sao$_2$) of 80% (only released 20% of its O$_2$ to tissue), a normal-shifted ODC has an Sao$_2$ of 50% (only released 50% of its O$_2$ to tissue), and a right-shifted curve has an Sao$_2$ of 20% (released 80% of its O$_2$ to tissue). 2,3-Bisphosphoglycerate (2,3-BPG) improves O$_2$ delivery to tissue by stabilizing the hemoglobin (Hb) in the taut form, which decreases O$_2$ affinity, hence facilitating the movement of O$_2$ from Hb into tissue by diffusion (high concentration to low concentration). *CO,* carbon monoxide; *H$^+$,* hydrogen ions; *HbF,* fetal hemoglobin; *metHb,* methemoglobin.

Figure labels:

Left shift:
↓H$^+$ (Alkalosis)
↓BPG
↓Temp
↑HbF
↑CO
↑MetHb

Right shift:
↑H$^+$ (Acidosis)
↑BPG
↑Temp
↑Altitude

← Right shift
← Normal
← Left shift

BPG stabilizes taut form of Hb (↓O$_2$ affinity). O$_2$ moves from Hb into plasma and into tissue by diffusion.

80% 50% 20%

Sao$_2$

Po$_2$ 20–50 mm Hg
Tissue level

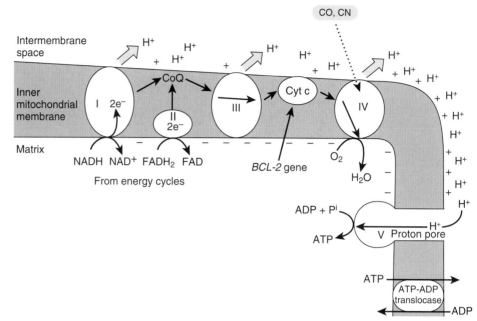

2-5: Oxidative phosphorylation. The inner mitochondria membrane is the primary site for ATP synthesis. The *BCL-2* gene proteins maintain mitochondrial membrane integrity by preventing cytochrome c from leaving the mitochondria. Refer to the text for additional discussion. *ADP,* Adenosine diphosphate; *ATP,* adenosine triphosphate; *CN,* cyanide; *CO,* carbon monoxide; *Cyt c,* cytochrome; *e⁻,* electrons; *FAD,* oxidized flavin adenine dinucleotide; *FADH₂,* reduced flavin adenine dinucleotide; *NAD⁺,* oxidized form of nicotinamide adenine dinucleotide; *NADH,* reduced form of nicotinamide adenine dinucleotide; *Pⁱ,* inorganic phosphorus. *(Modified from Pelley J, Goljan E: Rapid Review Biochemistry, 3rd ed, Philadelphia, Mosby Elsevier, 2011, p 59, Fig. 5-8.)*

C. Mitochondrial causes of ATP depletion
1. Enzyme inhibition of oxidative phosphorylation (Fig. 2-5)

Oxidative phosphorylation occurs in the mitochondria. The **oxidative part of the pathway** in the inner mitochondrial (mt) membrane transfers donated electrons from NADH and reduced flavin adenine dinucleotide (FADH₂) derived from the energy cycles to complex I and II, respectively, in the ETC. The electrons move through electron transport complexes to O_2, which is a strong electron acceptor located at the end of the chain on complex IV, and O_2 is converted to water. The transfer of electrons is coupled with the transport of protons (H^+) across the inner mt membrane into the intermembranous space, which establishes both a proton and a pH gradient. The *BCL-2* gene prevents cytochrome c in the ETC from leaving the mt by maintaining the integrity of the mt membrane. Should cytochrome c enter the cytoplasm, caspases are activated, resulting in apoptosis of the cell (programmed cell death; see later). The **phosphorylation part of the pathway** in the mitochondria involves the synthesis of ATP. A certain amount of heat is required to synthesize ATP. ATP synthesis occurs when the protons on the cytoplasmic side of the inner mt membrane enter small channels (proton pores) within the ATP synthase molecule (complex V) and reenter the mt matrix, where ATP is synthesized. The inner mt membrane is normally impermeable to protons except through the channel in the ATP synthase molecule. This relationship is critical to the maintenance of the proton gradient. If enzymatic reactions in electron transport are inhibited (e.g., cytochrome oxidase), the formation of protons and the proton gradient are disrupted as well, leading to a decrease in ATP synthesis.

BCL-2 gene: prevents cytochrome c from leaving mitochondria by maintaining integrity of mt membrane—Oxidative pathway: transfer electrons from NADH, FADH₂—Phosphorylation pathway: synthesis of ATP

Enzyme inhibition shuts down ETC

CO + CN: inhibit cytochrome oxidase; ETC shuts down (↓ATP synthesis)

Ion/salt containing CN⁻ anion

House fires → CO + CN poisoning
Excessive use nitroprusside; amygdalin; suicide

a. Enzyme inhibition at any level of oxidative phosphorylation decreases ATP synthesis and completely shuts down the ETC.
b. CO and cyanide (CN) specifically inhibit cytochrome oxidase in complex IV of the ETC, hence reducing the synthesis of ATP.
c. CN poisoning (see Chapter 7)
   (1) **Definition:** Cyanide is any ion or salt containing a CN⁻ anion.
   (2) Poisoning is most frequently caused by combustion of synthetic products in house fires (CO poisoning as well).
   (3) Other causes include prolonged exposure to nitroprusside (used in treating hypertensive emergencies), ingestion of amygdalin (cyanogenic glucoside found in the seeds of apricot, peach, plums, and bitter almond), and suicidal consumption of CN compounds.
   (4) Pathogenesis of hypoxia

Shutdown ETC prevents diffusion O_2 from blood to tissue

   (a) Cytochrome oxidase in complex IV of the ETC is inhibited, which prevents the consumption of O_2.
   (b) Shutdown of the ETC prevents the diffusion of O_2 from blood to tissue, because there is a loss of the diffusion gradient (this also occurs in CO poisoning; see earlier).
      • Oxygen extraction by the tissue decreases in parallel with the lower O_2 consumption in the ETC, with a resulting *higher* than normal *venous oxygen content* and PVo₂ (partial pressure of O_2 in venous blood).

TABLE 2-3 Comparison of Anemia, Methemoglobinemia, Carbon Monoxide Poisoning, and Cyanide Poisoning

	PaO$_2$	SaO$_2$	O$_2$-DISSOCIATION CURVE (ODC)	CYTOCHROME OXIDASE
Anemia	Normal	Normal	Normal	Normal
Carbon monoxide poisoning	Normal	Decreased (less O$_2$ is available to tissue)	Leftward shift	Inhibited
Methemoglobinemia	Normal	Decreased (less O$_2$ is available to tissue)	Leftward shift	Normal
Cyanide poisoning	Normal	Normal (however, O$_2$ *cannot* diffuse into tissue; see cyanide discussion)	Normal	Inhibited

- Although normally lower due to tissue extraction of O$_2$, in CN poisoning, the MVO$_2$ content is essentially the same as the O$_2$ content of arterial blood. This is a useful clue to diagnosing CN poisoning.

    (c) CN poisoning most adversely affects the heart and the central nervous system (CNS).

  (5) Clinical findings: bitter almond smell of the breath, seizures, coma, arrhythmias, and cardiovascular collapse

  (6) Laboratory findings

    (a) Increased anion gap metabolic acidosis (see Chapter 5), due to increased serum lactate levels from anaerobic glycolysis. Inhibition of cytochrome oxidase in the ETC causes a shift to anaerobic glycolysis for production of ATP.

    (b) Increased mixed venous O$_2$ content (MVO$_2$; normally should be decreased denoting tissue extraction of O$_2$) when compared to the arterial O$_2$ content (no extraction of O$_2$ in tissue).

  (7) Table 2-3 compares anemia, CO poisoning, methemoglobinemia, and CN poisoning.

2. Uncoupling of oxidative phosphorylation

  a. Uncoupling proteins carry protons in the intermembranous space through the inner mt membrane into the mt matrix *without* damaging the membrane.

    (1) Since uncouplers bypass ATP synthase in complex V, ATP synthesis is decreased.

    (2) Examples of uncouplers

      (a) Thermogenin, a natural uncoupler in the brown fat of newborns

      (b) Dinitrophenol used in synthesizing trinitrotoluene

  b. If dinitrophenol is involved, the heat normally used to synthesize ATP is redirected into raising the core body temperature, leading to hyperthermia (increased core body temperature).

  c. If thermogenin is involved, the heat normally used to synthesize ATP is used to stabilize the normally erratic body temperature in newborns and is *not* harmful to newborns.

Agents such as **alcohol** and **salicylates** are mt toxins and act as "uncouplers." They damage the inner mt membrane, causing protons to move into the mt matrix. This may result in hyperthermia.

D. Tissues susceptible to hypoxia

1. Watershed areas between terminal branches of major arterial blood supplies are susceptible to hypoxic injury.

  a. **Definition:** A watershed area is an area where the blood supply from two arteries do *not* overlap.

  b. Examples of watershed areas

    (1) Area between the distribution of the anterior and middle cerebral arteries (ACA and MCA). Global hypoxia (e.g., shock) may result in a watershed infarction (see later) at the junction of these two overlapping blood supplies (Fig. 2-6 A; see Chapter 26).

    (2) Area between the distribution of the superior and inferior mesenteric arteries (SMA and IMA; i.e., splenic flexure area, see Fig. 18-24 A). Decreased blood supply to either of the previously mentioned vessels (e.g., thrombosis overlying an atherosclerotic plaque) produces a watershed infarction (called ischemic colitis; see Chapter 18) at the junction of these two overlapping blood supplies, which is the splenic flexure of the colon which is located in the left upper quadrant (LUQ).

2. Hepatocytes located around the central venules (Fig. 2-6 B)

Side notes:

MVO$_2$ content similar to arterial O$_2$ content

Most adversely affects heart/CNS

Bitter almond smell; seizures/coma/arrhythmias/ cardiovascular collapse

↑Anion gap metabolic acidosis (lactic acidosis)

Lactic acidosis due to hypoxia

↑MVO$_2$

Uncouplers bypass ATP synthase → ↓ATP synthesis

Thermogenin (brown fat), dinitrophenol

Danger hyperthermia

Thermogenin stabilizes body temp in newborns

mt toxins: alcohol, salicylates; act as "uncouplers"

Blood supply from two arterial blood vessels do *not* overlap

Distribution ACA/MCA

Watershed infarction in brain complication global hypoxia

SMA and IMA; splenic flexure area

Ischemic colitis: splenic flexure (junction SMA/IMA in LUQ)

Hepatocytes around central venules

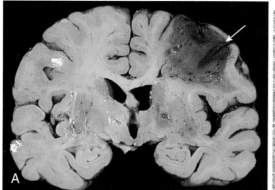
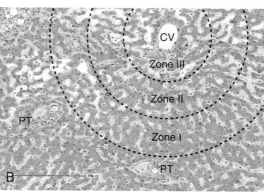

2-6: Watershed infarction in the brain showing a wedge-shaped hemorrhagic infarction at the junction of the distribution of the anterior and middle cerebral arteries *(white arrow).* **B,** Schematic of a hepatic lobule with central venule *(CV)* and portal triads *(PT).* Refer to the text for discussion of zones I, II, and III. *(A from my friend Ivan Damjanov MD, PhD, Linder J: Anderson's Pathology, 10th ed, St. Louis, Mosby, 1996, p 375, Fig. 17-16; B courtesy of my friend William Meek PhD, Professor of Anatomy and Cell Biology, Oklahoma State University, Center for Health Sciences, Tulsa, OK.)*

In the **portal triads,** hepatic artery tributaries carrying oxygenated blood and portal vein tributaries carrying unoxygenated blood empty blood into the liver sinusoids (mixed oxygenated and unoxygenated blood). The sinusoids, in turn, drain blood into the central venules. The central venules eventually become the hepatic vein, which empties into the inferior vena cava. Hepatocytes closest to the portal triads (zone I) receive the most oxygen and nutrients, whereas those furthest from the portal triads (zone III around the central venules) receive the least amount of oxygen and nutrients. Production of free radicals from drugs (e.g., acetaminophen, see later), tissue hypoxia (e.g., shock, CO poisoning), and alcohol-related fatty change of the liver (see later) initially damage zone III hepatocytes, which, owing to their relative lack of O_2, are more susceptible to injury. Depending on the severity of the injury, the other liver zones may also become involved.

Zone III hepatocytes (around central venules) most susceptible to hypoxia

3. Subendocardial tissue. Coronary vessels penetrate the epicardial surface; therefore the subendocardial tissue receives the *least* amount of O_2.

Factors decreasing coronary artery blood flow (e.g., coronary artery atherosclerosis) produce subendocardial ischemia, which is manifested by chest pain (i.e., angina) and ST-segment depression in an electrocardiogram (ECG). Increased thickness of the left ventricle (i.e., hypertrophy associated with aortic stenosis or hypertension) in the presence of increased myocardial demand for O_2 (e.g., exercise) also produces subendocardial ischemia and the possibility of infarction (discussed later).

Subendocardial tissue subject to hypoxic injury

ST-segment depression ECG: subendocardial ischemia/infarction—

Subendocardial ischemia: coronary artery atherosclerosis; cardiac hypertrophy

Susceptible to hypoxia: portal triads in cortex; TAL cells in medulla

CNS neurons most adversely affected cells in tissue hypoxia

4. Renal cortex and medulla
   a. Straight portion of the proximal tubule in the cortex is most susceptible to hypoxia. Primary site for reclaiming bicarbonate and reabsorbing sodium (see Chapter 5).
   b. Thick ascending limb (TAL) cells of the medulla are also susceptible to hypoxia (location of the $Na^+/K^+/2Cl^-$ symporter). Primary site for regenerating free water, which is necessary for normal dilution and concentration of urine (see Chapter 5).
5. Neurons in the CNS
   a. Examples of neurons: Purkinje cells in the cerebellum (Link 2-4) and neurons in the cerebral cortex (Link 2-5).
   b. Irreversible damage occurs ≈5 minutes after global hypoxia (e.g., shock). Neurons and Purkinje cells are the most adversely affected cells in tissue hypoxia.
E. **Consequences of hypoxic cell injury**
   1. Reversible changes in the cells
      a. Decreased synthesis of ATP in the mitochondria causes the cells to shift to anaerobic glycolysis for ATP synthesis.
         (1) Low citrate levels and increased adenosine monophosphate (AMP) activate PFK, the rate-limiting enzyme of glycolysis.
         (2) Results in a net gain of (2) ATP (see following schematic; phosphoenolpyruvate [PEP]).

↓mt synthesis ATP → shift anaerobic glycolysis for ATP synthesis

↓Citrate + ↑AMP → activate PFK (rate-limiting enzyme glycolysis)

Anaerobic glycolysis: 1° ATP source in hypoxia; lactic acidosis

Glucose ┈┈┈> (2) PEP → (2) Pyruvate ──→ (2) Lactate

2 NADH   2 NAD

2 ADP   2 ATP   Lactate dehydrogenase

(3) Pyruvate is converted to lactate, which decreases intracellular pH (lactic acidosis).

    (a) Lactic acid increases in the blood, producing an increased anion gap metabolic acidosis (see Chapter 5). Lactic acid may be a sign of tissue hypoxia.

    (b) Intracellular lactic acid denatures structural and enzyme proteins. Ultimately, this may result in coagulation necrosis in the cell (see later).

(4) Na^+/K^+-ATPase pump is impaired from a lack of ATP.

    (a) Normally, this pump keeps Na^+ and H_2O out of the cell and K^+ in the cell (Link 2-6).

    (b) Diffusion of Na^+ and H_2O into cells causes cellular swelling (called hydropic degeneration), which is the first visible sign of tissue hypoxia detected by the light microscope (Link 2-7, Link 2-8).

    (c) Cellular swelling is potentially reversible with restoration of O_2.

(5) Hydrolysis of glycogen leads to decreased glycogen stores.

  b. Protein synthesis is decreased due to detachment of ribosomes from the rough endoplasmic reticulum (RER) (Link 2-9).

2. Irreversible changes in the cell

Calcium plays a key role in irreversible damage to the cell. Normal sequestered calcium stores include mitochondria and the endoplasmic reticulum lumen. Calcium is pumped into the extracellular space and is bound to binding proteins (e.g., albumin).

  a. Calcium (Ca^{2+})-ATPase pump is impaired because of insufficient ATP. Normal function of the pump is to pump Ca^{2+} out of the cytoplasm.

  b. Increased cytoplasmic Ca^{2+} has many lethal effects (Link 2-10).

(1) Cytoplasmic Ca^{2+} activates enzymes.

    (a) Activated phospholipase damages plasma and lysosomal membranes, causing a loss of cell components and release of lysosomal enzymes.

    (b) Activated proteases (e.g., calpain) damage the cytoskeleton. Calpain is a calcium-dependent, nonlysosomal cysteine protease.

    (c) Activated endonuclease causes nuclear condensation (pyknosis), fragmentation of the nucleus (karyorrhexis) followed by fading of the nuclear chromatin (karyolysis). (Link 2-11)

    (d) Activated ATPase* leads to ↓ATP.

    (e) Activated protein kinases causes phosphorylation of proteins.

    (f) Cytoplasmic Ca^{2+} directly activates caspases, causing apoptosis of the cell (individual cell death; see later).

(2) Cytoplasmic Ca^{2+} enters the mitochondria (mT).

    (a) mt membrane permeability is increased. Cytochrome c in the ETC is released into the cytoplasm, where it activates the caspases, causing apoptosis (programmed cell death; see later).

    (b) mt conductance channels (pores) are opened leading to loss of H^+ ions and membrane potential; therefore, oxidative phosphorylation (OP) cannot occur, leading to a decrease in ATP synthesis.

III. Free Radical Cell Injury

A. Overview of free radicals (FRs)

1. **Definition:** FRs refer to any unstable chemical species that has a single unpaired electron in the outer orbital.

2. Radicals attack a molecule and "steal" its electron, causing that molecule to become an FR, the net result of which is a chain of reactions that ultimately leads to cell death.

3. Biologic FRs are generated predominantly from oxygen metabolism (Link 2-12).

4. FRs primarily target nucleic acids and cell membranes (CMs).

  a. In the nucleus, FRs produce DNA fragmentation and dissolution of chromatin.

  b. In the cell and mt membranes, FRs produce fatty acid (FA) FRs that react with molecular O_2 to produce peroxyl–FA FRs (called lipid peroxidation).

(1) FR damage to CMs causes increased permeability leading to an increased concentration of Ca^{2+} in the cytoplasm (see earlier discussion).

(2) FR damage to mt membranes allows cytochrome c in the ETC to escape into the cytoplasm and activate caspases leading to apoptosis (cell death; see later).

  c. FRs produce protein fragmentation and cross-linking.

  d. FRs produce ion pump damage.

Margin notes:

Lactic acidosis → ↑anion gap metabolic acidosis; possible sign tissue hypoxia

Acid pH denatures structural/enzymatic proteins

Impaired Na^+/K^+-ATPase pump → intracellular swelling (↑Na^+/H_2O; hydropic degeneration)

Intracellular swelling potentially reversible if O_2 restored

↓Glycogens stores

↓Protein synthesis: ribosomes detach from RER (reversible change)

Calcium key role in irreversible cell damage

Ca^{2+}-ATPase pump impaired (irreversible): cannot pump Ca^{2+} out of cytoplasm

↑Cytoplasmic Ca^{2+} activates enzymes

Phospholipase → damage plasma/lysosomal membranes

Proteases → damages cytoskeleton

Endonuclease → pyknosis → karyorrhexis (fragmentation) → karyolysis

ATPase → ↓ATP

Caspases → apoptosis

↑Ca^{2+} in mitochondria: ↑membrane permeability to cytochrome c → apoptosis

Mitochondria pores open → loss H^+ ions/membrane potential → loss OP → loss of ATP synthesis

Unstable chemical species; single unpaired electron outer orbital

"Steal" electrons from molecules→ become FRs → cell death

Target nucleic acids/CMs

FRs → cell/mt membranes → FA FRs + O_2 → lipid peroxidation

Damage CMs

Damage mt membranes→ cytochrome c activates caspases → apoptosis

Protein fragmentation/cross-linking
Ion pump damage

Cumulative; part of aging process

Microbial killing by leukocytes

AMI reperfusion injury

5. FR damage is cumulative and is part of the normal aging process (see Chapter 6).
6. FRs are important in microbial killing by neutrophils and monocytes (see later and see Chapter 3).
7. FRs are important in the reperfusion injury associated with fibrinolytic therapy in an acute myocardial infarction (AMI; see Chapter 11).

B. Production and types of FRs
1. Reactive oxygen species
   a. **Definition:** Reactive oxygen species include superoxide, hydrogen peroxide (H_2O_2), and hydroxyl FRs.
      (1) H_2O_2 is technically *not* an FR; however, it is classified as a reactive oxygen species owing to its production of hydroxyl FRs by reacting with transition metals (Fe^{2+}, Cu^+) via the Fenton reaction (see later).
      (2) Hydroxyl FRs have the distinction of being the most destructive of all the FRs.
         (a) Administration of high concentrations of oxygen produces superoxide FRs (e.g., oxygen therapy in respiratory distress syndrome [RDS]).
         (b) Ionizing radiation splits water in tissue into hydroxyl and hydrogen FRs.
         (c) Nicotinamide adenine dinucleotide phosphate hydrogen (NADPH) oxidase reaction generates superoxide FRs in neutrophils and monocytes in phagolysosomes (see Chapter 3).
         (d) Xanthine oxidase (XO) acting on xanthine (a degradation product of ATP) produces superoxide FRs that are important in the reperfusion injury that may follow an AMI (see Chapter 11).
2. Other examples of FRs
   a. Drugs: acetaminophen (*N*-acetyl-*p*-benzoquinone imine [NAPQI]; see later).
   b. Chemicals: carbon tetrachloride (CCl_4; see later)
   c. Nitric oxide (NO)
      (1) NO is an FR gas produced by NO synthase in macrophages and endothelial cells.
      (2) NO reacts with superoxide FRs to form the potent FR called peroxynitrite that has bacteriocidal properties (kills bacteria; see Chapter 3). Peroxynitrite is an unstable structural isomer of nitrate, NO_3^-.
   d. Low-density lipoprotein (LDL)
      (1) Small, dense subtypes of LDL enter the intima of arteries and are oxidized by FRs produced by macrophages, smooth muscle cells, and endothelial cells.
      (2) Oxidized LDL contributes to the formation of fatty streaks, which are progenitors of fibrous caps, the pathognomonic lesion of atherosclerosis (see Chapter 10).

C. Neutralization of FRs
1. Superoxide dismutase (SOD). SOD converts superoxide FRs into H_2O_2.
2. Glutathione peroxidase (enhances glutathione [GSH])
   a. GSH is an enzyme in the pentose phosphate pathway (PPP).
   b. GSH neutralizes H_2O_2, hydroxyl, and NAPQI (toxic intermediate of acetaminophen) FRs.
3. Catalase in peroxisomes degrades peroxide into water and oxygen (O_2).
4. Vitamins C and E act as antioxidants.
   a. Antioxidants neutralize FRs by donating one of their own electrons.
      (1) Providing an electron stops the "electron stealing" of FRs.
      (2) Antioxidants remain stable and do *not* become FRs.
   b. Vitamin E (fat-soluble vitamin; see Chapter 8)
      (1) Vitamin E prevents lipid peroxidation in CMs (see earlier).
      (2) Vitamin E neutralizes oxidized LDL (see earlier).
   c. Vitamin C (water-soluble vitamin; ascorbic acid; see Chapter 8)
      (1) Vitamin C neutralizes FRs produced by pollutants and cigarette smoke.
         Smokers have decreased levels of vitamin C, because they are used up in neutralizing FRs derived from cigarette smoke.
      (2) Vitamin C is the best neutralizer of hydroxyl FRs and also regenerates vitamin E.

D. Clinical examples of FR injury
1. Acetaminophen poisoning
   a. In normal doses, acetaminophen is glucuronidated (combined with glucuronic acid) or sulfated (combined with sulfo groups) by the cytochrome P450 system in the smooth endoplasmic reticulum of the liver into a harmless metabolite that is excreted by the kidney.
   b. In toxic doses, acetaminophen causes diffuse chemical hepatitis due to its conversion by a cytochrome P450 isoenzyme into a toxic intermediate called NAPQI (a drug FR).

Iron, copper: generate hydroxyl FRs

Hydroxyl FR most destructive

Superoxide FRs: high O_2 concentration

Ionizing radiation

NADPH oxidase: superoxide FRs in neutrophils/monocytes in phagolysosomes

XO: generates superoxide FRs; reperfusion injury

Acetaminophen → NAPQI

CCl_4

NO FR gas: macrophages/endothelial cells; cigarettes

Oxidized LDL: FR important in atherosclerosis

SOD neutralizes superoxide FRs

GSH in PPP

GSH neutralizes H_2O_2, hydroxyl, NAPQI

Peroxisomes: catalase degrades H_2O_2 into water/O_2

Vitamins C/E neutralize FRs

Prevents FR injury CMs

Neutralizes oxidized LDL

Neutralizes FRs produced by pollutants/cigarette smoke

Smokers ↓vitamin C levels

Best neutralizer hydroxyl FRs

Rendered into harmless metabolite in cytochrome P450 system

Diffuse chemical hepatitis due to NAPQI

(1) Cytochrome P450 isoenzyme responsible for this conversion is called CYP2E1 (cytochrome P), which is part of the microsomal ethanol-oxidizing system located in the liver.

(2) Liver cell necrosis *initially* occurs around the central venules (zone III; see Fig. 2-6 B).

(3) Liver cell necrosis may occur at *nontoxic* levels in alcoholics. Alcohol induces the synthesis of CYP2E1 isoenzyme, causing a higher percentage of acetaminophen to be converted to NAPQI.

  c. *N*-acetylcysteine is used to treat acetaminophen poisoning.

    (1) *N*-acetylcysteine is a cysteine donor for the synthesis of GSH.

    (2) GSH reduces levels of NAPQI and increases its excretion in the kidneys.

  d. Acetaminophen in association with nonsteroidal antiinflammatory agents (NSAIDs) may cause renal papillary necrosis (RPN; see Chapter 20).

2. Carbon tetrachloride (CCl_4) FRs

  a. CCl_4 is used as a solvent in the dry cleaning industry.

  b. Cytochrome P450 system in the SER converts CCl_4 into an FR.

  c. CCl_4-derived FRs produce liver cell necrosis with fatty change (discussed later).

3. Ischemia/reperfusion injury in AMI (see Chapter 11 for complete discussion; Link 2-13). Superoxide FRs are involved in reperfusion injury (reestablishment of blood flow), along with cytoplasmic Ca^{2+}, and neutrophils (white blood cells [WBCs]).

4. Retinopathy of prematurity (ROP). Blindness due to destruction of retinal cells by superoxide FRs may occur in the treatment of RDS with a concentration of O_2 >50%.

5. Iron overload disorders (hemochromatosis, hemosiderosis; see Chapter 19)

  a. Intracellular iron produces hydroxyl FRs that damage the parenchymal cells.

    (1) Hydroxyl (OH·) FRs are produced via the nonenzymatic Fenton reaction using H_2O_2.

    (2) $Fe^{2+} + H_2O_2 \rightarrow Fe^{3+} + OH· + OH^-$

  b. Consequences of FR injury from iron overload disorders include cirrhosis and exocrine/endocrine dysfunction of the pancreas.

6. Copper overload (Wilson disease; see Chapters 19 and 26)

  a. **Definition:** Wilson disease is an autosomal recessive disorder characterized by the inability to excrete copper in bile.

  b. Copper excess in hepatocytes increases the production of hydroxyl FRs.

    (1) Hydroxyl FRs are produced via the nonenzymatic Fenton reaction using H_2O_2 (similar to the reaction with iron shown earlier).

    (2) Consequences of FR injury in Wilson disease include damage to hepatocytes leading to cirrhosis and damage to the lenticular nuclei and cortex in the brain.

IV. Injury to Cellular Organelles (overview Fig. 2-7)

A. Mitochondria

- Salicylates and alcohol are mt toxins that produce megamitochondria (large mitochondria) with destruction of the cristae (Fig. 2-8).

B. Smooth endoplasmic reticulum (SER)

1. Liver cytochrome P450 system (cyto P450) enzymes are embedded in the phospholipid bilayer of the SER membrane with a portion exposed to the cytoplasm.

2. Drug induction (increased synthesis) of liver cytochrome P450 system enzymes occurs in the smooth endoplasmic reticulum.

  a. Induction of the SER enzymes may be caused by a variety of drugs (e.g., alcohol, barbiturates, and phenytoin [PHT]).

  b. Alcohol increases the synthesis of CYP2E1 isoenzyme in the cytochrome P450 system.

    (1) Isoenzyme increases the metabolism of alcohol. Alcohol is converted to acetaldehyde by alcohol dehydrogenase, and acetaldehyde to acetate by acetaldehyde dehydrogenase.

    (2) With alcohol excess, acetaldehyde conversion to acetate by acetaldehyde dehydrogenase is *not* fast enough; therefore, the acetaldehyde level may increase and damage hepatocytes.

  c. Phenobarbital (PBT) increases the synthesis of CYP2B2 isoenzyme, which converts PBT into an *inactive* metabolite. Alcohol inactivates the PBT-oxidizing cytochrome P450 system; therefore, if both alcohol and PBT are consumed in large amounts, PBT toxicity will occur.

  d. PHT increases the synthesis of CYP3A4, which accelerates the metabolism of PHT.

Margin notes:

CPY2E1 (cytochrome P)

Necrosis initially around central venules (zone III)

Alcohol induces synthesis CYP2E1 isoenzyme; more acetaminophen converted to NAPQI

GSH ↓ levels NAPQI

Acetaminophen + NSAIDs: FR injury of kidneys; RPN

Solvent dry cleaning

Cytochrome P450 converts into FR

Liver necrosis + fatty change

Superoxide FRs + ↑cytoplasmic Ca^{2+} + WBCs

ROP: ↑superoxide FRs from O_2 Rx

Iron produces hydroxyl FRs

Fenton reaction uses H_2O_2

Iron overload: cirrhosis, pancreas exocrine/endocrine dysfunction

Autosomal recessive disease; inability to excrete copper in bile

FRs hepatotoxic/neurotoxic

Salicylates, alcohol damage mitochondria; megamitochondria in hepatocytes

Phospholipid bilayer SER membrane

Alcohol: ↑CYP2E1 synthesis → ↑metabolism of alcohol

PBT ↑CYP2B2 synthesis → converts PBT to inactive metabolite

Alcohol enhances PBT toxicity

PHT: ↑CYP3A4 synthesis in cyto P450 system → ↑PHT metabolism

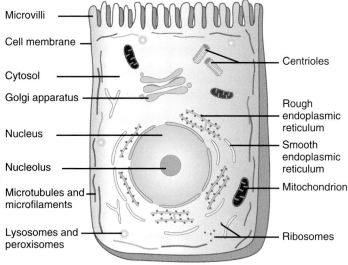

Labels for figure 2-7:
Microvilli
Cell membrane
Cytosol
Golgi apparatus
Nucleus
Nucleolus
Microtubules and microfilaments
Lysosomes and peroxisomes
Centrioles
Rough endoplasmic reticulum
Smooth endoplasmic reticulum
Mitochondrion
Ribosomes

2-7: Organelles present in an epithelial cell. *(From Carroll RG:* Elsevier's Integrated Physiology, *St. Louis, Mosby Elsevier, 2007, p 28, Fig. 4-1.)*

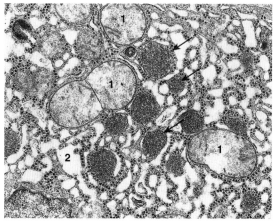

2-8: Electron micrograph showing damaged mitochondria *(1)* (megamitochondria) and hyperplasia of the smooth endoplasmic reticulum *(2)* in alcoholic liver disease. Dark circular areas represent peroxisomes *(red arrows). (From MacSween R, Burt A, Portmann B, Ishak K, Scheuer P, Anthony P:* Pathology of the Liver, *4th ed, London, Churchill Livingstone, 2002, p 288, Fig. 6-20.)*

Induction cyto P450 → SER hyperplasia

SER hyperplasia → ↑drug metabolism → ↓drug effectiveness

Cytochrome enzyme inhibitors: proton/histamine H₂-receptor blockers

Cytochrome enzyme inhibition → ↓drug metabolism → drug toxicity

Cytoplasmic organelles with lytic enzymes (acid hydrolases)

Acid hydrolases synthesized RER → PTM in Golgi apparatus

Golgi apparatus phosphotransferase attaches phosphate to mannose residues on enzymes → M6P

M6P on lysosomal enzyme attaches to receptors on Golgi apparatus membrane

1° lysosomes: vesicles that pinch off Golgi apparatus membrane

1° lysosomes: fuse with each other → ↑hydrolytic enzymes

2° lysosomes: heterophagosomes, autophagosomes

Fusion of pinocytic vacuoles, phagosomes, 1° lysosome

Pinocytosis → incorporation fluids into cell by invagination CM

Neutrophil/macrophage engulfs solid particles (bacteria) → phagosome

e. Induction of enzyme synthesis in the cytochrome P450 system produces SER hyperplasia (more SER are present in the cytoplasm; Fig. 2-8). Increased drug metabolism by SER hyperplasia causes *lower than expected* therapeutic drug levels.

3. Inhibition of enzymes of the cytochrome P450 system
  a. Causes of the inhibition of cytochrome enzymes
    (1) Proton receptor blockers (e.g., omeprazole)
    (2) Histamine H₂-receptor blockers (e.g., cimetidine)
  b. Decreased drug metabolism leads to *higher than expected* therapeutic drug levels. Example: cimetidine inhibits the metabolism of PHT leading to high serum levels of PHT.

C. Lysosomes
1. **Definition:** Lysosomes are membrane-bound digestive cytoplasmic organelles that contain lytic enzymes (acid hydrolases) that degrade exogenous materials taken up by the cell by phagocytosis and also degrade worn-out cell constituents (e.g., CMs, organelles).
  a. Acid hydrolases that are present in the lysosomes are active at an acidic pH of 5.0.
  b. Hydrolases break down proteins, nucleic acids, carbohydrates, lipids, and cellular debris.
2. Lysosome enzyme synthesis and the formation of primary lysosomes
  a. Acid hydrolases synthesized by the RER are transported to the Golgi apparatus for posttranslational modification (PTM; Fig. 2-9).
  b. In the Golgi apparatus, enzyme modification occurs by attaching phosphate (via phosphotransferase) to mannose residues on the enzymes to produce mannose 6-phosphate (M6P).
  c. Modified lysosomal enzymes then attach to specific M6P receptors located on the Golgi apparatus membranes.
  d. Vesicles that pinch off the Golgi apparatus membrane are called primary (1°) lysosomes and contain the modified enzymes located on the Golgi membranes (Fig. 2-9). Fusion of primary lysosomes with each other (*not shown* in Fig. 2-9) further increases the content of hydrolytic enzymes in the primary lysosomes.
3. Secondary (2°) lysosomes are called heterophagosomes and autophagosomes (Link 2-14, Link 2-15; Fig. 2-9).
  a. **Definition:** Heterophagosomes are vacuoles that are derived from the fusion of pinocytic vacuoles, phagosomes, and primary lysosomes containing lysosomal enzymes.
    (1) Pinocytosis refers to the incorporation of fluids into a cell by invagination of the CM, followed by formation of pinocytic absorptive vesicles.
    (2) Phagocytosis is the process by which a cell (e.g., neutrophil, macrophage) engulfs solid particles (e.g., bacteria, foreign material) to form an internal vesicle known as a phagosome.

b. **Definition:** Autophagosomes are vacuoles that contain fragments of worn-out cellular components (e.g., mitochondria) and lysosomal enzymes derived from primary lysosomes.

Vacuoles with worn-out cellular components + 1° lysosomal enzymes

c. Residual bodies (RBs) and lipofuscin granules (LFGs; discussed later) are remnants remaining in secondary lysosomes (heterophagosomes, autophagosomes) after digestion by acid hydrolases (see Link 2-14, Link 2-15; Fig. 2-9). RBs with LFGs are extruded from the cell by a process called exocytosis.

RBs/LFGs in 2° lysosomes

RBs/LFGs removed by exocytosis

4. Lysosomal functions
   a. Fusion of 1° lysosomes with phagocytic vacuoles located in neutrophils, monocytes, and macrophages containing bacteria; phagocytic vacuoles are called *phagolysosomes*

Phagolysosomes neutrophils/monocytes/ macrophages kill bacteria

   b. Destruction of worn-out cell organelles (autophagy; discussed later)

Destruction of worn-out organelles (autophagy)

   c. Degradation of complex substrates (e.g., sphingolipids, glycosaminoglycans)

Degrade complex substrates

5. Selected lysosomal disorders
   a. Inclusion (I)-cell disease

Definition: Inclusion (I)-cell disease is a rare inherited condition in which there is a defect in PTM of lysosomal enzymes in the Golgi apparatus. Mannose residues on newly synthesized lysosomal enzymes coming from the RER are *not* phosphorylated because of a *deficiency* of phosphotransferase. Without M6P to direct the enzymes to the M6P receptors on the walls of the Golgi apparatus, the vesicles that pinch off the Golgi to form primary lysosomes are empty and the unmarked (nonphosphorylated) enzymes are extruded into the extracellular space where they are degraded in the bloodstream. Undigested substrates (e.g., carbohydrates, lipids, and proteins) that lysosomes would normally degrade accumulate as large inclusions in the lysosomes, hence the term *inclusion cell disease*. Symptoms include psychomotor retardation and early death.

M6P, mannose 6-phosphate

b. Deficiency of lysosomal enzymes involved in degradation of complex substrates characterize the *lysosomal storage diseases* (see Chapter 6).

c. Chédiak-Higashi syndrome

Defect PTM lysosomal enzymes; ↓phosphotransferase

Lysosomal storage diseases: ↓lysosomal enzymes; accumulation complex substrates

Chédiak-Higashi syndrome is an autosomal recessive disease with a defect in a lysosomal transport protein that affects the synthesis and/or maintenance of secretory granule storage in various cells (e.g., lysosomes in leukocytes, azurophilic granules in neutrophils, dense bodies in platelets). Granules in these cells tend to fuse together (fusion defect) to become megagranules that do *not* function properly (Fig. 2-10). In addition, there is a defect in microtubule function in neutrophils and monocytes that prevents the fusion of lysosomes with phagosomes to produce phagolysosomes. This produces a bactericidal defect. In particular, there is increased susceptibility to developing *Staphylococcus aureus* infections. Microtubule dysfunction also produces defects in chemotaxis (directed migration; see Chapter 3), which further exacerbates the susceptibility to infection.

Autosomal recessive disease; giant lysosomal granules (fusion defect); defect formation phagolysosomes

D. **Cytoskeleton**
   1. Normal functions of the cytoskeleton
      a. **Definition:** The cytoskeleton is a network of protein filaments in the cell. Protein filaments maintain the shape of the cell and, in some cases, are involved in the motility of the cell.

Network cell protein filaments

Maintain shape/motility

      b. Three types of protein filaments are recognized and include microtubules, actin filaments, and intermediate filaments.

Microtubules, actin filaments, intermediate filaments

         (1) **Definition:** Microtubules are polymers composed of the protein tubulin.

Polymers of tubulin

         (2) **Definition:** Actin thick and thin filaments are involved in the contractile process.

Actin thick/thin filaments: contractile process

         (3) **Definition:** Intermediate filaments are important in the integration of cell organelles.

Integration cell organelles

            (a) Anchored to transmembrane proteins on the CM (e.g., desmosomes), intermediate filaments spread tensile forces evenly throughout tissue, hence limiting damage to individual cells.

Spread out tensile forces in tissue → limit damage to individual cells

            (b) Intermediate filaments include keratins (in epithelial cells; e.g., squamous cells), vimentin (in mesenchymal cells; e.g., fibroblasts), desmin (e.g., muscle), neurofilaments (e.g., nerve tissue), glial fibrillary protein (e.g., glial cells)

Keratin, vimentin, desmin, neurofilaments, glial fibrillary protein

   2. Factors causing defects in the synthesis of tubulin
      a. **Definition:** Tubulin is required for the synthesis of microtubules in the mitotic spindle (MS). Tubulin also plays a role in cell motion and intracellular organelle transport.

Synthesis microtubules in MS

      b. Synthesis of tubulin occurs in the G_2 phase of the cell cycle (see Chapter 3). Tubulin is composed of α- and β-tubulin.

Synthesized G_2 phase

      c. Etoposide, bleomycin produce G_2 phase defects by decreasing tubulin synthesis.

Etoposide, bleomycin produce G_2 phase defects → ↓tubulin synthesis

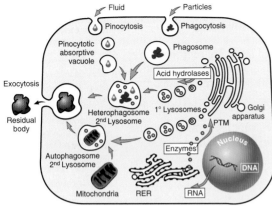

2-9: Lysosomes. Note the lysosomal enzymes (golden brown granules) are produced by the rough endoplasmic reticulum *(RER)* and are then transported to the Golgi apparatus, where they undergo posttranslational modification *(PTM)*. Primary *(1°)* lysosomes originate as small vesicles budding off the lateral sides of the Golgi apparatus, give rise to heterophagosomes and autophagosomes. Undigested material in phagosomes is extruded from the cell or remains in the cytoplasm as lipofuscin-rich residual bodies. *(From my friend Ivan Damjanov MD, PhD: Pathology for the Health Professions, 4th ed, Philadelphia, Saunders Elsevier, 2012, p 5, Fig. 1-3.)*

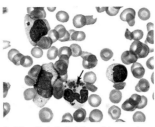

2-10: Chédiak-Higashi neutrophil *(arrow)* and lymphocytes with giant granules (megagranules). See the text for discussion. *(From McPherson R, Pincus M: Henry's Clinical Diagnosis and Management by Laboratory Methods, 21st ed, Philadelphia, Saunders, 2007, p 551, Fig. 32-7.)*

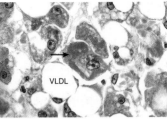

2-11: Mallory bodies in alcoholic liver disease. Hyaline (eosinophilic) inclusions *(arrow)* are present in the cytosol of hepatocytes. Many of the hepatocytes have vacuoles containing triglyceride, which is packaged in very-low-density lipoprotein *(VLDL)*. *(From Kumar V, Fausto N, Abbas A: Robbins and Cotran's Pathologic Basis of Disease, 7th ed, Philadelphia, Saunders, 2004, p 34, Fig. 1-34A.)*

MS synthesized M phase cell cycle

Vinca alkaloids/colchicine interfere with assembly MS

Paclitaxel interferes with disassembly MS

Stress protein that binds to damaged intermediate filaments

Ubiquinated intermediate filaments degraded in proteasomes/lysosomes

Mallory bodies ubiquinated cytokeratin

Eosinophilic inclusion in hepatocytes alcoholic liver disease

Protein aggregates α-synuclein + ubiquitin; IPD

Eosinophilic cytoplasmic inclusions SNN

Cytoplasmic accumulation TG liver cells; alcohol MCC

VLDL: liver-synthesized TGs

DHAP: three-carbon intermediate of glycolysis; converted to G3P

G3P carbohydrate substrate for TG synthesis

G3P + 3 FAs → TG

3. Factors causing MS defects
   a. MS is synthesized in the M (mitotic) phase of the cell cycle.
   b. Vinca alkaloids (chemotherapy agents) and colchicine (used in the treatment of gout) bind to tubulin in microtubules, thus interfering with MS assembly.
   c. Paclitaxel (chemotherapy agent) enhances tubulin polymerization, which interferes with disassembly of the MS.
4. Ubiquitin and damage to intermediate microfilaments
   a. **Definition:** Ubiquitin, a stress protein, binds to damaged intermediate filaments (Link 2-16). Ubiquitin binding marks these damaged ("ubiquinated") intermediate filaments for degradation in proteasomes (a cytoplasmic protease) and lysosomes in the cytoplasm.
   b. Mallory bodies
      (1) **Definition:** Mallory bodies are ubiquinated cytokeratin intermediate filaments in hepatocytes associated with alcoholic liver disease (Fig. 2-11).
      (2) Mallory bodies appear as eosinophilic inclusion bodies in the cytoplasm of hepatocytes.
   c. Lewy bodies
      (1) **Definition:** Lewy bodies are aggregates of protein-containing α-synuclein and ubiquitin that are located in substantia nigra neurons (SNNs) in idiopathic Parkinson disease (IPD; see Chapter 26).
      (2) Lewy bodies appear as eosinophilic cytoplasmic inclusions in degenerating SNNs (see Link 26-122).

V. **Intracellular Accumulations**
   A. **Types of accumulations** (Table 2-4)
   B. **Fatty change in the liver**
      1. **Definition:** Fatty change is cytoplasmic accumulation of triglycerides (TGs) in hepatocytes. Alcohol is the most common cause of fatty change.
      2. Epidemiology
         a. Liver-synthesized TGs are packaged in the very-low-density lipoprotein (VLDL) fraction, which normally circulates in plasma (see Chapter 10).
         b. Normal synthesis of TGs in the liver
            (1) Synthesis of TGs in hepatocytes begins with conversion of dihydroxyacetone phosphate (DHAP), a three-carbon intermediate of glycolysis, to glycerol 3-phosphate (G3P; see following diagram).
            (2) G3P is the carbohydrate substrate for synthesizing TG.
            (3) Addition of three FAs to G3P produces TGs.

TABLE 2-4 Selected Intracellular Accumulations

SUBSTANCE	CLINICAL SIGNIFICANCE
Endogenous Accumulations	
Bilirubin	Kernicterus (see Fig. 16-6): Free, unbound lipid-soluble unconjugated bilirubin,* derived from macrophage destruction of RBCs in Rh hemolytic disease of the newborn, enters the basal ganglia nuclei of the brain, causing permanent damage.
Cholesterol	Xanthelasma (see Fig. 10-4 B): It is a yellow plaque on the eyelid due to cholesterol accumulated within macrophages (foam cells) in the interstitial tissue. Atherosclerosis (see Link 10-11): Cholesterol-laden smooth muscle cells and macrophages (i.e., foam cells) are the early components of atherosclerotic plaque formation before they further progress into fibrous plaques, the pathognomonic lesion of atherosclerosis. See Chapter 10.
Glycogen	Diabetes mellitus: In diabetes mellitus, there is increased glycogen synthesis in the proximal renal tubule cells, due to increased uptake of glucose via glucose transporters in the proximal tubule. The increased glucose is then converted into glucose 6-phosphate, which is a substrate that is used to synthesize glycogen. See Chapter 23. Von Gierke glycogenosis: This deficiency of glucose-6-phosphatase (a gluconeogenic enzyme) leads to an increase in glucose 6-phosphate, a substrate for glycogen synthesis. Glycogen excess primarily occurs in hepatocytes and renal tubular cells (hepatorenomegaly), because these are the primary sites that have this enzyme for gluconeogenesis. See Chapter 6.
Hematin	Melena: When blood is exposed to gastric acid, Hb is converted into a black pigment called hematin. Hematin is the pigment responsible for the black, tarry stools called melena. Melena is a sign of an upper gastrointestinal bleed (bleed above the ligament of Treitz where the duodenum joins the jejunum). Gastric and duodenal ulcers are the most common causes of melena. See Chapter 18.
Hemosiderin and ferritin	Iron overload disorders (e.g., hemochromatosis; see Fig. 19-7 G, H): In these disorders, excess hemosiderin (a lysosome breakdown product of ferritin) deposition in parenchymal cells, leading to increased free radical damage (via the Fenton reaction) and eventual organ dysfunction (e.g., cirrhosis). Serum ferritin is increased. See Chapter 19. Pulmonary congestion: In left-sided heart failure, there is pulmonary hemorrhage with phagocytosis of RBCs by alveolar macrophages. Within the macrophage, iron is bound to ferritin, a soluble iron-binding protein, which is then degraded into hemosiderin, a brown pigment. Alveolar macrophages containing hemosiderin are called "heart failure" cells (see Links 11-10, 11-11). When these cells are coughed up, the sputum has a rusty brown color. See Chapter 11. Anemia of chronic disease: Hepcidin, a protein released from the liver in inflammation, blocks the release of iron from bone marrow macrophages, causing a decrease in heme synthesis, with a corresponding decrease in hemoglobin synthesis. This causes anemia and an increase in serum ferritin as well as an increase of hemosiderin within bone marrow macrophages. See Chapter 12. Other associations: Bleeding into tissue allows macrophages to phagocytose RBCs and eventually convert the iron to ferritin and then to hemosiderin (Link 2-17).
Melanin	Skin color: Melanin is normally responsible for skin color. It is also normally present in substantia nigra neurons (Link 2-18). Refer to Chapters 25 and 26, respectively. Addison disease (see Fig. 23-15 A): In this disease, there is autoimmune destruction of the adrenal cortex that leads to hypocortisolism. Hypocortisolism causes a corresponding increase in ACTH via a negative feedback relationship between the pituitary gland and the adrenal cortex. ACTH has melanocyte-stimulating properties that cause hyperpigmentation of the skin and mucous membranes due to increased synthesis of melanin. See Chapter 23.
Amyloid	Amyloid (see Figs. 4-20 B, C): Amyloid is a misfolded protein (incorrectly shaped) that derives from various precursor proteins (e.g., light chains, amyloid precursor protein). Amyloid stains red with Congo red but exhibits an apple green birefringence under polarized light. Amyloid is deposited in the interstitium of tissue in various organs causing pressure atrophy of adjacent cells, potentially leading to organ dysfunction. For example, if deposited in the heart, it decreases ventricular compliance (ability of the heart to fill up with blood) causing heart failure and death. See Chapter 4.
Triglyceride	Fatty liver (Figs. 2-12 A, B): Excess triglyceride synthesis in hepatocytes pushes the nucleus to the periphery causing enlargement and dysfunction of the liver. See Chapter 19.
Exogenous Accumulations	
Anthracotic pigment	Coal worker's pneumoconiosis (see Fig. 17-12 A): Phagocytosis of black anthracotic pigment (coal dust) by alveolar macrophages produces a black discoloration of the lung and sputum containing black, pigmented alveolar macrophages called "dust cells." Inhalation of coal dust causes increased deposition of collagen in the interstitial tissue of the lungs, ultimately causing a lack of compliance (alveoli cannot fill up with air) and eventual respiratory failure. See Chapter 17.
Lead	Lead poisoning: Lead deposited in the nuclei of proximal renal tubular cells (acid-fast inclusion) leads to dysfunction of the proximal tubules (proximal renal tubular acidosis). Lead (Pb) also deposits in the epiphyses of bone in children, causing growth retardation. Radiographs show increased density in the epiphyses (see Fig. 12-14 C).

*Unconjugated bilirubin, insoluble bilirubin, because it is bound to albumin.
ACTH, Adrenocorticotropic hormone; *RBCs,* red blood cells.

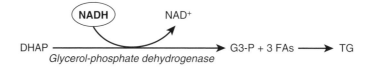

(4) Once TGs are synthesized, the VLDL fraction is produced (see Chapter 10).
 (a) Lipoproteins have hydrophilic (water-loving) groups of phospholipids, cholesterol (CH), and proteins that are directed outward.
 (b) Protein component in VLDL, and other lipoproteins, renders the lipoprotein water-soluble in the sodium-containing water comprising 90% of the plasma in blood.
  • Apoprotein B (apoB)-100 is the protein component of VLDL that renders it soluble in water. An additional function of apoB-100 is to enhance the secretion of VLDL into the blood.
c. Fatty change in the liver is most often caused by increased hepatic synthesis of TGs. A less common etiology involves disordered packaging of TGs into VLDL or its secretion into blood (see Chapter 10).
 (1) Increased synthesis of TGs is caused by increased conversion of DHAP to G3P.
 (2) Examples include kwashiorkor (see Chapter 8) and excessive alcohol consumption (see Chapter 19).
 (3) In kwashiorkor, there is increased intake of carbohydrates and little to no intake of proteins (see Chapter 8). Increased carbohydrate intake increases the amount of DHAP produced during glycolysis, which in turn provides more substrate for synthesizing TGs.
 (4) In alcohol excess, increased production of the reduced form of nicotinamide adenine dinucleotide (NADH) from alcohol metabolism (see following reactions) accelerates conversion of DHAP to G3P (see previous reaction), which, when combined with FAs, produces TG (G3P + FA → TG).

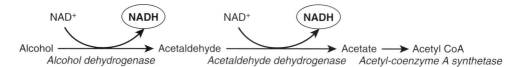

  (a) An additional factor enhancing TG synthesis in alcohol excess is increased availability of FAs to combine with G3P to form TGs. Recall that acetyl CoA is used to synthesize FAs. Since acetyl CoA is the end-product of alcohol metabolism (see previous reactions), more is available to synthesize additional FAs.
  (b) Alcohol activates hormone-sensitive lipase, which converts TG in VLDL into FAs and glycerol. Glycerol is converted into G3P, which combines with FAs to produce TG.
  (c) Alcohol inhibits the release of VLDL from the liver.
  (d) Alcohol inhibits β-oxidation of FAs in the mitochondria; hence, more FAs are available for liver synthesis of TG.
 (5) Another cause of fatty change in the liver is decreased synthesis of apoB-100.
  (a) This decreases packaging of TG into VLDL and decreases the secretion of VLDL into the blood.
  (b) In kwashiorkor, because of decreased protein intake, apoB-100 synthesis is decreased. Therefore, TGs that are synthesized in the hepatocyte remain in the hepatocyte producing fatty change.
d. Morphology
 (1) Liver is of normal size or enlarged with yellowish discoloration (Fig. 2-12 A). Painful on palpation.
 (2) Under the light microscope, hepatocytes have a clear space pushing the nucleus to the periphery (Fig. 2-12 B).
C. Iron accumulation (see Table 2-4)
 1. Ferritin (see Chapter 12)
  a. **Definition:** Ferritin is a soluble iron-binding protein that stores iron in macrophages.
  b. Primarily synthesized and stored in macrophages (bone marrow is the most common site) and hepatocytes (second most common site).

Margin notes (left column):

Lipoproteins: phospholipids + CH + proteins

ApoB-100 allows VLDL to be soluble in plasma
ApoB-100 helps secretion of VLDL into blood

↑Synthesis TG MCC fatty change

Kwashiorkor: ↑carbohydrate → ↑DHAP → ↑G3P → ↑TG synthesis

Alcohol ↑NADH → ↑conversion DHAP to G3P → ↑synthesis TG

Alcohol ↑acetyl CoA → ↑synthesis FAs in liver
Alcohol activates hormone sensitive lipase → converts TG into FAs + glycerol
Glycerol → G3P; G3P + FAs → TG
Alcohol inhibits release of VLDL from liver
Alcohol inhibits β-oxidation FAs in mitochondria → more FAs for TG synthesis
Fatty change: ↓synthesis apoB-100

Kwashiorkor: ↓protein intake → ↓apoB-100 → ↓packaging/secretion VLDL

Normal/large; yellow discoloration; painful on palpation

Soluble iron-binding protein stored in macrophages

Synthesized macrophages/hepatocytes

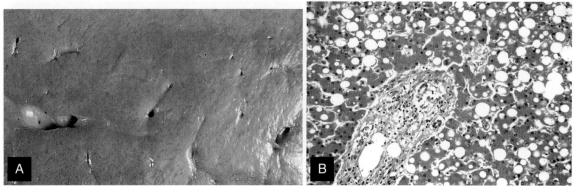

2-12: **A,** Bulging cut surface of a liver with diffuse fatty change giving it a yellow appearance. **B,** Fatty change of the liver. The microscopic slide shows clear vacuoles containing triglycerides in most of the hepatocytes. The nucleus of the cells is displaced to the periphery. (**A** from my friend Ivan Damjanov, MD, PhD, Linder J: *Pathology: A Color Atlas*, St. Louis, Mosby, 2000, p 153, Fig. 8-37; **B** from Kumar V, Fausto N, Abbas A: *Robbins and Cotran's Pathologic Basis of Disease*, 7th ed, Philadelphia, Saunders, 2004, p 36, Fig. 1-36B.)

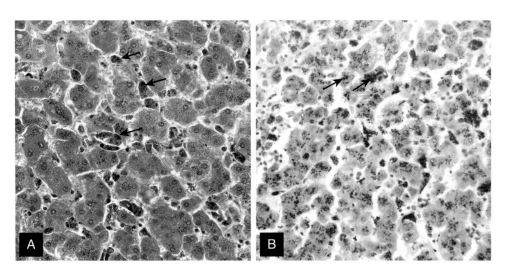

2-13: Hereditary hemochromatosis. **A,** The disease is characterized by an accumulation of hemosiderin, an iron-rich golden brown pigment in liver and Kupffer cells (*black arrows*; hematoxylin and eosin [H&E] stain). **B,** The Prussian blue reaction in the same slide gives hemosiderin a blue color *(black arrows)*. *(From my friend Ivan Damjanov MD, PhD:* Pathology for the Health Professions, *4th ed, Saunders Elsevier 2012, p 15, Fig. 1-18.)*

   c. Small amounts of ferritin circulate in the serum.
     (1) Serum levels directly correlate with the bone marrow iron stores.
     (2) Decrease in serum ferritin is the first sign of iron deficiency even before anemia occurs (see Chapter 12).

↓Serum ferritin 1st sign iron deficiency

  2. Hemosiderin
    a. **Definition:** Hemosiderin is an insoluble product of ferritin degradation in lysosomes.
    b. Unlike ferritin, it does *not* circulate in serum. Appears as golden brown granules in hematoxylin-eosin (H&E) stained tissue (Fig. 2-13 A; Link 2-17) or as blue granules when stained with Prussian blue (Fig. 2-13 B).

Ferritin degradation product; +Prussian blue

Golden brown; blue with Prussian blue stain

D. Pathologic calcification
  1. Dystrophic calcification
    a. **Definition:** Dystrophic calcification refers to the deposition of calcium phosphate in necrotic (damaged) tissue.
    b. Calcium deposition in tissue is *unrelated* to the serum calcium and phosphate levels, whether they are normal, increased, or decreased.
    c. Mechanism of dystrophic calcification
     (1) Calcium enters the necrotic cells and binds to phosphate (released from damaged membranes by phosphatase) to produce calcium phosphate.
     (2) Calcium phosphate is basophilic (blue staining) in H&E stained tissue.
    d. Examples
     (1) Calcification in chronic pancreatitis (Fig. 2-14 A)
     (2) Calcified atherosclerotic plaques (see Link 10-11)
     (3) Periventricular calcification in congenital cytomegalovirus infection (see Fig. 26-14 A)
     (4) Calcium in psammoma bodies in papillary carcinoma of the thyroid (see Fig. 23-9)

Calcification damaged tissue

Serum calcium/phosphate normal

Calcium binds phosphate

Basophilic in H&E stained tissue

Chronic pancreatitis

Atherosclerotic plaques

Periventricular congenital cytomegalovirus

Psammoma bodies papillary thyroid cancer

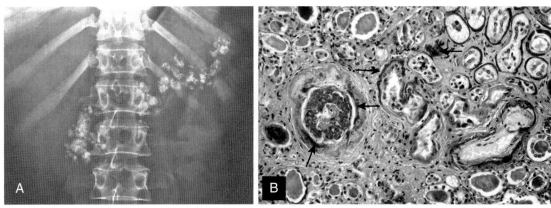

2-14: A, The radiograph shows multiple dystrophic calcifications in the pancreas in a patient with chronic pancreatitis. **B,** Kidney biopsy with nephrocalcinosis. Calcification is present in the interstitium and outlines the tubular basement membranes of renal tubules *(arrows)*. Calcium stains blue with the H&E stain. *(**A** from Katz D, Math K, Groskin S: Radiology Secrets, Philadelphia, Hanley & Belfus, 1998, p 155, Fig. 4. **B** from Fogo AB, Kashgarian M: Atlas of Renal Pathology, 2nd ed, Philadelphia, Elsevier, 2012, p 455, Fig. 3.118.)*

Calcification normal tissue; ↑serum calcium and/or phosphate

1° HPTH, malignancy-induced hypercalcemia

Renal failure, 1° hypoparathyroidism

Excess phosphate drives calcium into normal tissue

Nephrocalcinosis: metastatic calcification collecting ducts

Produces NDI

Lung calcification

↓Size/number/weight tissue/organ

↓Hormone: hypopituitarism; atrophy target organs

↓Innervation: skeletal muscle atrophy

↓Blood flow: cerebral atrophy

↓Nutrients: marasmus
↑Luminal pressure

Hydronephrosis → atrophy cortex/medulla

Thick duct secretions CF → atrophy exocrine glands

Chronic pancreatitis: ↓exocrine/endocrine function

Cell loss by apoptosis

    2. Metastatic calcification

      a. **Definition:** Metastatic calcification refers to the deposition of calcium phosphate in the interstitium of normal tissue due to an increase in serum levels of calcium and/or phosphate.

      b. Unlike dystrophic calcification, it is due to increased serum levels of calcium and/or phosphate.

        (1) Common causes of hypercalcemia include primary hyperparathyroidism (HPTH) and malignancy-induced hypercalcemia (see Chapter 23).

        (2) Common causes of hyperphosphatemia include chronic renal failure and primary hypoparathyroidism. Excess phosphate in blood drives calcium into normal tissue.

        (3) Examples

          (a) Calcification of renal tubular basement membranes in the collecting ducts (called nephrocalcinosis; Fig. 2-14 B). Produces nephrogenic diabetes insipidus (NDI; tubules are resistant to stimulation by antidiuretic hormone [ADH]) and renal failure.

          (b) Calcification in the lungs, which may cause respiratory problems

VI. Adaptation to Cell Injury: Growth Alterations

  A. Atrophy

    1. **Definition:** Atrophy refers to a decrease in size, number of cells, and weight of a tissue or organ. (Link 2-19)

      • An interesting feature of atrophy that directly affects patient survival is its propensity to be greater in nonessential tissues, such as adipose tissue, than in higher functional tissue, such as that found in the brain.

    2. Causes

      a. Decreased hormone stimulation. Example: hypopituitarism causing atrophy of target organs, such as the thyroid and adrenal cortex

      b. Decreased innervation. Example: skeletal muscle atrophy following loss of lower motor neurons in amyotrophic lateral sclerosis (Link 2-20)

      c. Decreased blood flow. Example: cerebral atrophy due to a reduction in blood flow associated with atherosclerosis of the carotid artery (Fig. 2-15 A; Link 2-21)

      d. Decreased nutrients. Example: total calorie deprivation in marasmus (see Fig. 8-1 A, **right photo**)

      e. Increased luminal pressure

        (1) Example: atrophy of the renal cortex and medulla in hydronephrosis (see Fig. 20-8 A). Increased luminal pressure of backed-up urine compresses vessels in the cortex and medulla leading to atrophy.

        (2) Example: thick pancreatic duct secretions in CF occlude the duct lumens, causing increased luminal back pressure and compression atrophy of the exocrine glands (Fig. 2-15 B).

          • Atrophy of exocrine glands in the pancreas causes malabsorption of proteins and fats (amylase from the salivary glands is enough to digest carbohydrates). Eventually, the entire pancreas is damaged (chronic pancreatitis), including the islet cells, leading to type 1 diabetes mellitus.

      f. Loss of cells by apoptosis (programmed cell death, see later)

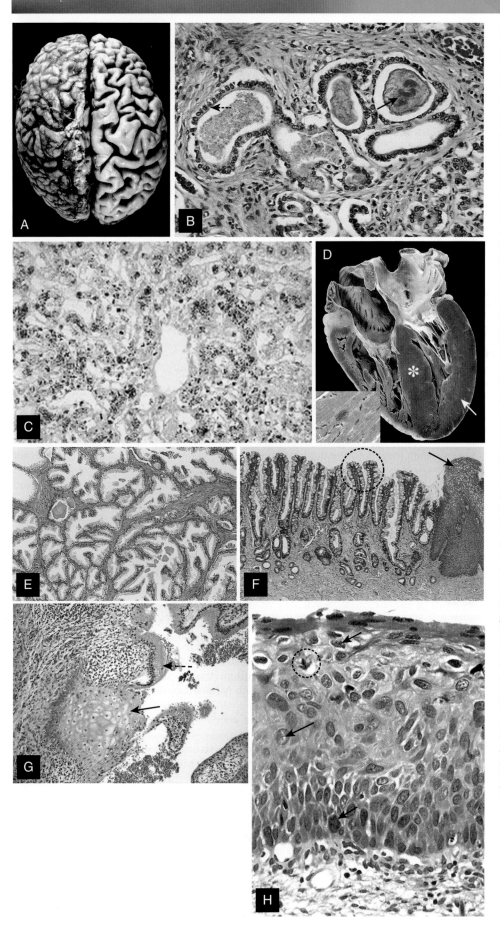

2-15: A, Atrophy of the brain. The meninges have been stripped from the right half of the brain. Note the narrow gyri and widened sulci. **B,** Pancreas in a patient with cystic fibrosis showing dilated ducts filled with thickened eosinophilic material *(arrow).* The duct epithelial cells are flattened and the ducts are surrounded with fibrous tissue. **C,** Liver showing hepatocytes with yellow-brown granules representing lipofuscin (polymer of protein + undigested lipid). **D,** Left ventricular hypertrophy, showing the thickened free left ventricular wall (right side; *white arrow)* and the thickened interventricular septum *(white asterisk).* The right ventricle wall (left side) is of normal thickness. The **insert** shows hypertrophy of cardiac myocytes. Note the increased fiber diameter and nuclear enlargement from increased DNA synthesis. **E,** Benign prostatic hyperplasia. The prostatic glands show infolding of the mucosa into the glandular spaces. **F,** Barrett esophagus showing an extensive area of glandular (intestinal) metaplasia with numerous goblet cells *(interrupted circle).* A small section of squamous epithelium remains on the right *(arrow).* **G,** Section of the transitional zone of the uterine cervix showing squamous metaplasia *(solid arrow)* replacing the normal glandular, mucus-secreting endocervical cells *(interrupted arrow).* **H,** Squamous dysplasia of the cervix. Squamous dysplasia is a precursor of squamous cell carcinoma. There is a lack of orientation of the squamous cells throughout the upper two thirds of the epithelium. Many of the nuclei are enlarged *(arrows),* are hyperchromatic, and have irregular nuclear margins. An abnormal mitotic spindle is present in one of the cells *(interrupted circle).* *(A from Kumar V, Abbas A, Fausto N, Mitchell, R: Robbins Basic Pathology, 8th ed, Philadelphia, Saunders, 2007, p. 5, Fig. 1-4.* **B, E, F** *from my friend Ivan Damjanov MD, PhD, Linder J: Pathology: A Color Atlas, St. Louis, Mosby, 2000, pp 169, 249, 111, Figs. 9-6, 12-32, 6-26, respectively.* **C** *from my friend Ivan Damjanov MD, PhD, Linder J: Anderson's Pathology, 10th ed, St. Louis, Mosby, 1996, p 371, Fig. 17-7.* **D insert, G** *from King TS: Elsevier's Integrated Pathology, St. Louis, Mosby Elsevier, 2007, pp 9, 11, Figs. 1-10, 1-13, respectively.* **D, H** *from Kumar V, Fausto N, Abbas A: Robbins and Cotran's Pathologic Basis of Disease, 7th ed, Philadelphia, Saunders, 2004, pp 561, 1075, Figs 12-3A, 12-19C, respectively.)*

Cell shrinkage

Catabolic pathway degrade/recycle cellular components

Autophagic vacuoles fuse with 1° lysosomes → autophagosomes

RBs: undigested lipids from FR lipid peroxidation CMs

Lipofuscin: brown "wear and tear" pigment

Brown atrophy: ↑lipofuscin

↓Protein synthesis; ↑protein degradation

Ubiquitin-proteasome pathway

↑Cell size → ↑organ size/weight

Cardiac muscle hypertrophy: ↑preload; ↑afterload

ΔWall stress → Δgene expression → sarcomere duplication → thicker or longer muscle

↑Cytoplasm, # organelles, DNA content

Skeletal muscle weight training

Remaining kidney postnephrectomy → compensatory hypertrophy

Cytomegalovirus cell hypertrophy

↑Number normal cells

↑Estrogen → endometrial hyperplasia

↑Hormone sensitivity DHT → prostate hyperplasia

Scratching → skin hyperplasia (eczema)

Smoker/asthmatic → mucous gland hyperplasia

Alcohol excess → regenerative nodules (cirrhosis)

↓Serum Ca^{2+} → parathyroid gland hyperplasia

3. Cellular and metabolic changes
   a. Shrinkage of cells. Related to increased catabolism of cell organelles (e.g., mitochondria) and reduction in the cytoplasm.
   b. Organelles and cytoplasm form autophagic vacuoles (Link 2-22).
      (1) **Definition:** Autophagy is a catabolic pathway that is used to degrade or recycle cellular components.
         (a) Controlled by a group of genes that control each of the steps of autophagy.
         (b) Dysregulation of autophagy contributes to the process of aging, liver disease, cancer, and inflammation.
      (2) Autophagic vacuoles fuse with primary lysosomes (currently called autophagosomes) for enzymatic degradation.
      (3) Undigested lipids derived from FR lipid peroxidation of CMs in primary lysosomes are stored as RBs.
         (a) Polymers of undigested lipids plus protein in RBs are called lipofuscin (sometimes called "wear and tear" pigment).
         (b) Excessive accumulation of lipofuscin imparts a brown color to tissue. In the setting of atrophy, it is called brown atrophy (Fig. 2-15 C).
         (c) Brown atrophy is commonly seen in the elderly population and is considered a normal age-related finding (see Chapter 6).
   c. Protein synthesis is decreased and protein degradation is increased. Increased protein degradation is handled by the ubiquitin-proteasome pathway (Link 2-16).

B. **Hypertrophy**
   1. **Definition:** Hypertrophy is an increase in cell size causing an increase in organ size and weight.
   2. Hypertrophy in muscle tissue is caused by increased workload.
      a. Left ventricular hypertrophy occurs in response to an increase in afterload (resistance to overcome) or preload (volume to expel) (Fig. 2-15 D; Link 2-23).
         (1) In ventricular hypertrophy, the changes (Δ) in wall stress produce changes in gene expression leading to the duplication of sarcomeres causing the muscles to be thicker or longer (see Fig. 11-1).
         (2) In addition, there is an increase in cytoplasm, number of cytoplasmic organelles, and DNA content in each hypertrophied cell.
      b. Skeletal muscle hypertrophy occurs in response to weight training (Link 2-24).
   3. Surgical removal of one kidney produces compensatory hypertrophy (some degree of hyperplasia) of the remaining kidney.
   4. Cell enlargement occurs in cytomegalovirus infections (see Fig. 17-6 B). Cytomegaly occurs because the virus increases the uptake of iron into the cytoplasm, which increases the growth of the cell.

C. **Hyperplasia**
   1. **Definition:** Hyperplasia is an increase in the number of normal cells.
   2. Causes
      a. Increased hormone stimulation
         (1) Endometrial gland hyperplasia, which is caused by an increase in estrogen (see Fig. 22-11 D); increased risk of developing endometrial cancer
         (2) Benign prostatic hyperplasia (BPH), which is caused by an increase in sensitivity to dihydrotestosterone (DHT; Fig. 2-15 E)
            (a) Unlike endometrial gland hyperplasia, there is *no* increased risk of developing cancer.
            (b) BPH is frequently complicated by obstructive uropathy (blockage of urine flow) with thickening of the bladder wall by smooth muscle, which exhibits both hyperplasia and hypertrophy (see Fig. 21-4 B).
      b. Chronic irritation
         (1) Constant scratching of itchy skin; can produce thickening (hyperplasia) of the epidermis (eczema; see Fig. 25-12 C)
         (2) Bronchial mucous gland hyperplasia; common in smokers and asthmatics
         (3) Regenerative nodules in cirrhosis of the liver; may occur in response to alcohol excess (see Fig. 19-7 B)
      c. Chemical imbalance
         (1) Hypocalcemia (decreased serum calcium); stimulates parathyroid gland hyperplasia (secondary hyperparathyroidism) to bring serum calcium levels back toward the normal range

(2) Iodine deficiency; produces thyroid enlargement (goiter; see Fig. 23-8 A) as the gland works harder to increase thyroid hormone synthesis. Both hypertrophy and hyperplasia are operative in producing goiters.

d. Stimulating antibodies. Hyperthyroidism in Graves disease is due to thyroid-stimulating antibodies (TSAs) IgG directed against thyroid hormone receptors, which cause the gland to synthesize excess thyroid hormone (see Chapter 23, Link 22 B).

e. Viral infections

  (1) Skin infection by the human papillomavirus (HPV) produces epidermal hyperplasia or the common wart (see Fig. 25-5 A).

  (2) Viral genes produce growth factors causing epidermal hyperplasia.

3. Mechanisms of hyperplasia

  a. Hyperplasia depends on the regenerative capacity of different cell types (see Chapter 3).

  b. Labile cells (stem cells)

   (1) **Definition:** Labile cells divide continuously. Stem cells are located in the bone marrow, crypts of Lieberkühn, and the basal cell layer of the epidermis.

   (2) Labile cells may undergo hyperplasia as an adaptation to cell injury.

  c. Stable cells (resting cells)

   (1) **Definition:** Stable cells divide infrequently because they are normally in the G_0 (resting) phase of the cell cycle.

   (2) Examples include hepatocytes, astrocytes, and smooth muscle cells.

   (3) Stable cells must be stimulated (e.g., growth factors, hormones, absence of tissue) to enter the cell cycle.

   (4) Depending on the cell type, stable cells may undergo hyperplasia and/or hypertrophy as an adaptation to cell injury.

  d. Permanent cells (nonreplicating cells)

   (1) **Definition:** Permanent cells are highly specialized cells that *cannot* replicate.

   (2) Examples include neurons and skeletal and cardiac muscle cells.

   (3) Of the permanent cells, only skeletal and cardiac muscle undergo hypertrophy (not hyperplasia) as an adaptation to injury.

4. Increased risk for progressing into cancer, in some types of hyperplasia

  a. Endometrial hyperplasia may progress into cancer (endometrial adenocarcinoma).

  b. Regenerative nodules in cirrhosis may progress into cancer (hepatocellular carcinoma).

D. Metaplasia

1. **Definition:** Metaplasia is the replacement of one fully differentiated cell type by another fully differentiated cell.

  a. Substituted cells are less sensitive to a particular stress. Change in phenotype of differentiated cells allows cells to better withstand stress.

  b. For example, mucus-secreting glandular epithelium is more likely to protect itself from acid injury than is squamous epithelium.

2. Types of metaplasia

  a. Metaplasia from squamous to glandular epithelium

   (1) Example of this type of metaplasia occurs when there is acid reflux from the stomach into the distal esophagus.

   (2) Distal esophageal mucosa, which is normally comprised of squamous epithelium, is converted into an epithelium comprised of goblet cells and mucus-secreting cells. This allows protection against acid injury (Fig. 2-15 F; see Chapter 18).

   (3) This condition is called Barrett esophagus.

    (a) Note that the cell types involved in this metaplasia are normally present in the intestine (e.g., goblet cells), hence the term *intestinal metaplasia* (see Fig. 18-13 B).

    (b) There is an increased risk of developing cancer (distal adenocarcinoma).

  b. Metaplasia from glandular to other types of glandular epithelium

   (1) Occurs in the pylorus and antrum epithelium in the stomach when there is a chronic infection (chronic gastritis) caused by *Helicobacter pylori* (see Chapter 18).

   (2) Inflammatory cytokines, which are released by the pathogen, produce a chronic gastritis that is characterized by the synthesis of goblet cells and Paneth cells; these cell types are normally present in intestinal epithelium (intestinal metaplasia).

   (3) There is an increased risk of developing a gastric cancer in the pylorus or antrum.

  c. Metaplasia from glandular to squamous epithelium

   (1) Occurs in the mainstem bronchus mucosa when pseudostratified columnar epithelium is replaced by squamous epithelium in response to irritants in cigarette

---

↓Iodine → goiter (hyperplasia/hypertrophy)

TSAs → Graves disease

HPV → epidermal hyperplasia (common wart)

Cell must enter cell cycle

Continuously divide; bone marrow stem cells

Resting cells G_0 phase cell cycle

Hepatocytes/smooth muscle cells

Stimulated to enter cell cycle

Hyperplasia and/or hypertrophy

Cannot replicate

Neurons/cardiac muscle

Skeletal/cardiac muscle → hypertrophy

Endometrial hyperplasia → endometrial adenocarcinoma

Regenerative nodules → hepatocellular carcinoma

One adult cell type replaces another

Substituted cells less stress sensitive

Squamous to glandular epithelium

Acid reflux

Squamous to glandular: acid reflux distal esophagus (Barrett esophagus)

↑Risk adenocarcinoma

Glandular to other glandular epithelium

H. pylori chronic gastritis

Intestinal metaplasia → goblet cells/Paneth cells

H. pylori chronic gastritis → gastric cancer

Glandular to squamous epithelium

Pseudostratified columnar → squamous → chronic bronchitis

smoke (chronic bronchitis). Associated with an increased risk of developing a squamous cell cancer (SCC) of the mainstem bronchus.

(2) Mucus-secreting endocervical cells (ECCs) encountering the acid pH of the vagina undergo squamous metaplasia (Fig. 2-15 G). Metaplasia can progress to dysplasia (see later) and cancer.

   d. Metaplasia from transitional to squamous epithelium

      (1) Occurs in a *Schistosoma haematobium* infection in the urinary bladder, which causes transitional epithelium to undergo squamous metaplasia

      (2) Increased risk of developing squamous cancer of the urinary bladder

   e. Mesenchymal metaplasia involving connective tissue

      (1) Occurs when bone tissue develops in an area of muscle trauma (osseous metaplasia)

      (2) *No* risk of developing cancer (e.g., osteosarcoma)

  3. Mechanisms of metaplasia

   a. Stem cells normally have an array of progeny cells that have different patterns of gene expression. Under normal physiologic conditions, differentiation of these progeny cells is restricted.

   b. However, under stressful conditions, metaplasia may result from reprogramming stem cells to utilize progeny cells with a different pattern of gene expression.

   c. Signals that may initiate this change include hormones (e.g., estrogen), vitamins (e.g., retinoic acid), and chemical irritants (e.g., cigarette smoke).

   d. Metaplasia is sometimes reversible if the irritant is removed.

E. Dysplasia

  1. **Definition:** Dysplasia is disordered cell growth that is a potential precursor to cancer if the irritant is *not* removed.

  2. Risk factors

   a. Some types of hyperplasia (e.g., endometrial gland hyperplasia; see earlier)

   b. Some types of metaplasia (e.g., Barrett esophagus; see earlier discussion)

   c. Infection. Example: HPV types 16 and 18 causing squamous dysplasia of the cervix

   d. Chemicals. Example: irritants in cigarette smoke, may cause squamous metaplasia to progress to squamous dysplasia in the mainstem bronchus (see earlier discussion)

   e. Ultraviolet (UV) light. Example: solar damage of the skin, may cause squamous dysplasia (see Fig. 25-11 A)

   f. Chronic irritation of skin. Example: skin in a full-thickness (third-degree) burn may develop squamous dysplasia

  3. Microscopic features of dysplasia (Fig. 2-15 H)

   a. May involve squamous, glandular, or transitional epithelium

   b. Nuclear features of dysplasia: increased mitotic activity, with *normal* MSs and increased nuclear size and chromatin

   c. Disorderly proliferation of cells: occurs with loss of cell maturation as the cells progress to the surface

   d. Sometimes reversible if the irritant is removed

VII. Cell Death

Cell death occurs when cells or tissues are unable to adapt to injury.

  A. Necrosis

   1. **Definition:** Necrosis is the death of groups of cells often accompanied by an acute inflammatory infiltrate containing neutrophils.

   2. Coagulation necrosis

    a. **Definition:** Coagulation necrosis is the temporary preservation of the structural outline of groups of dead cells.

    b. Mechanism

      (1) Denaturation of enzymes and structural proteins. May be due to intracellular accumulation of lactate (most common), ingestion of heavy metals (e.g., lead, mercury), or exposure of cells to ionizing radiation (e.g., cancer treatment).

      (2) Inactivation of intracellular enzymes (including those in the lysosomes due to lactic acid) prevents dissolution (autolysis) of the cell. Neutrophils and macrophages coming in from normal tissue surrounding the area of coagulation necrosis will liquefy and remove the dead tissue.

    c. Microscopic features (Fig. 2-16 A; Links 2-25, 2-26)

      (1) Indistinct outlines of cells are present within the dead tissue.

      (2) Nuclei are either absent or undergoing karyolysis (fading of nuclear chromatin).

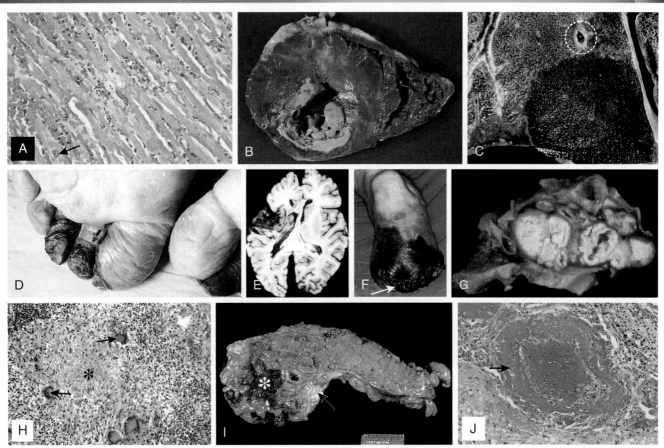

2-16: **A,** Acute myocardial infarction (MI) showing coagulation necrosis. This section of myocardial tissue is from a 3-day-old acute MI. The outlines of the myocardial fibers are still intact; however, most of the fibers lack nuclei and cross-striations. Those dead cells with persistent nuclei show fading of the nuclear chromatin *(arrow).* A neutrophilic infiltrate is present between some of the dead fibers. **B,** Acute MI showing a pale infarction of the posterior wall of the left ventricle *(bottom left).* **C,** Hemorrhagic infarction of the lung. There is a roughly wedge-shaped area of hemorrhage extending to the pleural surface of the lung. The arrow shows an embolus in one of the pulmonary artery tributaries. **D,** Dry gangrene involves the first four toes and one of the toes of the other foot. The dark black areas of gangrene are bordered by light-colored, parchment-like skin. **E,** Cerebral infarction with hemorrhage showing liquefactive necrosis of the cerebral cortex leaving a large cystic cavity. **F,** Wet gangrene of the leg. Note the pus *(arrow)* at the closing edges of the below-the-knee amputation site. **G,** Caseous necrosis in the hilar lymph nodes. Note the friable, cheesy material completely replacing the lymph nodes and cavitation in the central portion of the nodes. **H,** Caseous granuloma showing a central area of acellular, necrotic material *(asterisk)* surrounded by activated macrophages (epithelioid cells), lymphocytes, and multiple multinucleated Langhans-type giant cells. **I,** Enzymatic fat necrosis in acute pancreatitis. Dark areas of hemorrhage are present in the head of the pancreas *(asterisk),* and focal areas of pale fat necrosis *(arrow)* are present in the peripancreatic fat. **J,** Fibrinoid necrosis of a parenchymal arteriole. Note effacement of the normal arteriolar structures. The vessel wall has been replaced by deeply eosinophilic hyaline material *(arrow)* and is surrounded by acute hemorrhage. *(A and B from my friend Ivan Damjanov MD, PhD, Linder J: Pathology: A Color Atlas, St. Louis, Mosby, 2000, p 375, Figs. 17-15, 17-13. C, E, H, I from Kumar V, Fausto N, Abbas A: Robbins and Cotran's Pathologic Basis of Disease, 7th ed, Philadelphia, Saunders, 2004, pp 138, 1385, 83, 943, respectively. D, G from Ivan Damjanov MD, PhD: Pathology for the Health-Related Professions, 2nd ed, Philadelphia, Saunders, 2000, p 18, Fig. 1-24. F from Grieg JD: Color Atlas of Surgical Diagnosis, London, Mosby-Wolfe, 1996, p 6, Fig. 2-2. J from Ellison D, Love S, et al: Neuropathology: A Reference Text of CNS Pathology, 3rd ed, St. Louis, Mosby Elsevier, 2013, p 248, Fig. 10.32.)*

d. Infarction
  (1) **Definition:** Infarction is a *gross* (visible to the naked eye) manifestation of coagulation necrosis that is secondary to the sudden occlusion of a vessel. An *exception* to this is a cerebral infarction, which is a gross manifestation of liquefactive necrosis, *not* coagulation necrosis (discussed later).

  Gross manifestation coagulation necrosis due to sudden vessel occlusion

  (2) Grossly, infarctions are usually wedge-shaped if dichotomously branching vessels (e.g., pulmonary artery) are occluded.

  Usually wedge-shaped

  (3) There are two types of infarction: pale (ischemic) and hemorrhagic (red).

  Pale/hemorrhagic types

  (4) Pale (ischemic) types of infarctions (Links 2-27, 2-28, and 2-29). Increased density of tissue (e.g., heart, kidney, spleen) prevents RBCs released from damaged vessels from diffusing through the necrotic tissue; therefore, the tissue has an overall pale appearance (Fig. 2-16 B).

  Pale infarctions: dense tissue; heart, kidney, spleen

  (5) Hemorrhagic (red) types of infarctions. Loose-textured tissue (e.g., lungs, small bowel, testicle) allows RBCs released from damaged vessels to diffuse through the necrotic tissue; therefore, the tissue has a hemorrhagic appearance (Fig. 2-16 C; Link 2-30).

  Hemorrhagic infarctions: loose tissue; lung, bowel, testicle

Dry gangrene of the toes in individuals with diabetes mellitus is a form of infarction that results from ischemia. Coagulation necrosis is the primary type of necrosis that is present in the dead tissue (Fig. 2-16 D).

e. Factors influencing whether an infarction will occur in tissue

(1) Infarction is likely if a thrombus overlies an atherosclerotic plaque in a coronary artery or cerebral artery, because it takes time for fibrinolysis of the thrombus to occur and reestablish blood flow.

(a) Explains why it is important to implement fibrinolytic therapy to patients with an acute coronary artery thrombosis as soon as possible (e.g., <3 hours) in order to prevent an infarction from occurring or at least to limit the size of the infarction.

(b) Concept also applies to prevention of ischemic strokes due to atherosclerosis (see Chapter 26).

(2) Presence of a dual blood supply

(a) Infarction is *less* likely to occur if a dual blood supply is present
- Pulmonary and bronchial arteries in the lungs; hepatic artery and portal vein in the liver
- Radial and ulnar arteries supplying the hand/forearm; arcade system between the SMA and IMA in the bowel

(b) Renal and splenic arteries are end arteries with an inadequate network of anastomosing vessels beyond potential points of obstruction; hence infarction is *more likely* to occur in these tissues.

(3) Sudden onset of ischemia in the lungs will more likely produce an infarction if there is *preexisting* disease in the lungs (decreased blood flow through pulmonary arteries; e.g., chronic obstructive pulmonary disease) or the heart (decreased blood flow through the bronchial arteries, a branch of the aorta; e.g., congestive heart failure with decreased cardiac output).

(4) Rate of occlusion of a vessel

(a) If there is a slow rate of occlusion of vessel, there may be enough time for the tissue to develop a collateral circulation and prevent infarction.

(b) Example: slow occlusion of a coronary artery by atherosclerosis may allow time for the development of collateral pathways with other coronary vessels to occur, hence, preventing an infarction. However, if multiple coronary arteries already have significant reduction in blood flow from atherosclerosis, an infarction will likely occur.

(5) Tissues with a high O_2 requirement (e.g., brain, heart) are *more likely* to infarct than those that require less O_2 (e.g., skin, muscle, and cartilage).

3. Liquefactive necrosis

a. **Definition:** Liquefactive necrosis is necrotic degradation of tissue that softens and becomes liquefied.

b. Mechanism. Release of lysosomal enzymes by necrotic cells and/or the release of hydrolytic enzymes by neutrophils entering the tissue cause the tissue to liquefy.

c. Examples

(1) CNS infarction. Autocatalytic effect of hydrolytic enzymes released by neuroglial cells produces a cystic space in the brain (Fig. 2-16 E; Link 2-31).

(2) Abscess in a bacterial infection. Hydrolytic enzymes released by neutrophils liquefy the dead tissue, producing a cavity filled with purulent material, which is called an abscess (see Fig. 3-8 A).

Dry gangrene of the toes with a superimposed anaerobic infection (e.g., *Clostridium perfringens*) leads to acute inflammation, in which liquefactive necrosis is the primary type of necrosis. This condition is called **wet gangrene** (Fig. 2-16 F).

4. Caseous necrosis

a. **Definition:** Caseous necrosis is an acellular variant of coagulation necrosis. Acellular, cheese-like (caseous) material is present on gross examination of the tissue (Fig. 2-16 G).

b. Mechanism

(1) Caseous material is most often present in granulomas (any small nodular delimited aggregation of mononuclear cells (monocytes, macrophages). Discussed more thoroughly in Chapter 3.

(a) Caseous necrosis is an acellular material that is produced by the release of lipid from the cell walls of *Mycobacterium tuberculosis* (also some atypical

---

Margin notes (left column):

Predominantly coagulation necrosis

Thrombus overlies plaque

Dual blood supply beneficial

Pulmonary/bronchial arteries

Hepatic artery/portal vein

Radial/ulnar arteries hand/forearm

Arcade system SMA/IMA

Renal/splenic end arteries; infarction more likely

Lung infarct likely if preexisting lung and/or heart disease

Slow rate vessel occlusion → chance collateral vessels to develop

High O_2 requirement (brain, heart) more likely to infarct

Necrotic degradation of tissue that liquefies

Lysosomal enzyme destruction tissue by neutrophils

Cerebral infarction: liquefactive *not* coagulation necrosis

Bacterial abscess: liquefactive necrosis

Wet gangrene predominantly liquefactive necrosis

Acellular variant coagulation necrosis

Nodular aggregation monocytes/macrophages

Cheesy appearance lipid cell wall *Mycobacterium*/systemic fungi

Mycobacteria) and systemic fungi (e.g., *Histoplasma*) after immune destruction by macrophages in the granulomas.

    (b) Tuberculosis is the most common cause of granulomas with caseous necrosis.

        (1) Other diseases associated with granuloma formation do *not* exhibit caseation (noncaseating), because the granulomas are *not* associated with destruction of pathogens.

        (2) Examples: Crohn disease, sarcoidosis, and reaction to foreign bodies (FBs)

  c. Microscopic features of caseous necrosis in a granuloma

    (1) Caseous material is acellular and granular in appearance and is usually located in the center of a granuloma.

    (2) Caseous material is surrounded by activated macrophages, CD4 helper T cells, and multinucleated giant cells (MGCs; Fig. 2-16 H; see Chapter 3).

5. Gummatous necrosis

  a. **Definition:** Gummatous necrosis is a variant of coagulation necrosis associated with spirochetal diseases (e.g., tertiary syphilis). It is located within the center of a gumma, which is a small, rubbery granuloma with a fibrous capsule and necrotic center.

  b. Mechanism. Gummatous necrosis is thought to be a hypersensitivity reaction (exaggerated immune response) directed against spirochetes.

  c. Locations for gummas include the skin and bone (most common sites). Other sites for gummas include the liver (called hepar lobatum), testicle, and soft tissue.

  d. Gross and microscopic appearance of gummas

    (1) **Definition:** Gummas are firm and rubbery, unlike a caseous granuloma, which is soft and friable.

    (2) Histologically, they do *not* have complete obliteration of cellular architecture unlike caseous necrosis where there is no definable architecture.

        (a) Gummas are surrounded by a rim of fibroblasts, macrophages, lymphocytes, plasma cells, and occasional MGCs.

        (b) Treponemes are *rarely* identified in the tissue.

6. Enzymatic fat necrosis

  a. **Definition:** Enzymatic fat necrosis is an enzyme-mediated necrosis that is peculiar to adipose tissue located around an acutely inflamed pancreas.

  b. Mechanism in the pancreas

    (a) Activation of pancreatic lipase and phospholipase (e.g., excess alcohol consumption) causes hydrolysis of TGs in fat cells with the release of FAs.

    (b) Calcium combines with the FAs to produce soap (saponification). Dystrophic calcification commonly occurs in areas of saponification.

  c. Gross appearance. Chalky yellow-white deposits are primarily located in peripancreatic and omental adipose tissue (Fig. 2-16 I; Link 2-32).

  d. Microscopic appearance. Pale outlines of fat cells with a granular pink appearance and absence of nuclei with or without basophilic staining areas representing dystrophic calcification (Link 2-33).

7. Traumatic fat necrosis

  a. **Definition:** Traumatic fat necrosis is a non-enzyme-mediated necrosis that occurs in fatty tissue (e.g., female breast tissue, abdomen) as a result of blunt trauma or surgery.

  b. Recall that pancreatic fat necrosis is enzyme-mediated.

8. Fibrinoid necrosis (Fig. 2-16 J)

  a. **Definition:** Fibrinoid necrosis is an acellular type of necrosis that may occur in small muscular arteries, arterioles, venules, glomerular capillaries, valve leaflets, myocardium, and subcutaneous tissue.

  b. Mechanism. Fibrinoid necrosis refers to the deposition of pink-staining proteinaceous material that is present in damaged vascular tissue (Link 2-34).

  c. Examples: immune vasculitis (e.g., Henoch-Schönlein purpura [HSP]), malignant hypertension, and rheumatic fever (endocarditis, myocarditis, Aschoff bodies).

B. Apoptosis

1. **Definition:** Apoptosis is a programmed, enzyme-mediated cell death that may occur as a response to developmental or environmental triggers or as a response to functional damage detected by the cell's internal surveillance system.

2. Normal and pathologic processes associated with apoptosis

  a. Normal destruction of cells during embryogenesis

    (1) In a male fetus, Sertoli cells in the testicles synthesize müllerian inhibitory substance (MIS), which results in the loss of müllerian structures (normally develop female organs) in a male fetus.

Margin notes:

TB MCC granuloma with caseous necrosis

Noncaseating granulomas: Crohn disease, sarcoidosis, FB reaction

Granuloma: rim activated macrophages, CD4 T cells, MGCs with central caseous necrosis

Variant coagulation necrosis associated with spirochetal disease (e.g., syphilis)

Skin, bone MC sites
Liver (hepar lobatum) testicle, soft tissue other sites

Gummas: firm/rubbery

Cellular architecture *not* completely obliterated

Gummas: treponemes rarely identified

Enzyme-mediated necrosis adipose tissue; acute pancreatitis

Activation pancreatic lipase/phospholipase → hydrolysis TGs in adipose cells → release FAs

Saponification: calcium + FAs; dystrophic calcification

Chalky-white deposits in pancreatic fat

Pale outlines fat cells; no nuclei; with/without dystrophic calcification

Non-enzyme-mediated fat necrosis from trauma/surgery

Vascular acellular necrosis in immune-mediated disease

Pink-staining material in vessel wall

HSP, rheumatic fever, malignant hypertension

Programmed cell death in response to various triggers

Embryogenesis: MIS → apoptosis müllerian structures male fetus

Lost tissue between fingers/toes; shaping inner ear; cardiac morphogenesis

Drop in estrogen/progesterone → menses

↓Stimulating hormones → apoptosis-induced atrophy target tissue

Involution of thymus

Apoptosis B cells in germinal centers

Death tumor cells/virus infected cells by cytotoxic CD8 T cells

Corticosteroid destruction B/T cells

Removal acute inflammatory cells in AI

Removal cells with DNA damage due to radiation, FRs, toxins

Incorrectly folded inactive protein

Amyloid, β-amyloid protein, proteins in prion-related disease

Defects in apoptosis lead to exposure to nuclear antigens in necrotic material

Sepsis, AMI, neurodegenerative disease, diabetes mellitus

Death receptor (extrinsic) pathway activation

TNFR1 death receptor activated by TNF-α

Macrophages (main source); endothelial/cardiac cells, neurons

TNFR1 binding with TNF-α activates initiator caspases 8/10

Initiator caspases activate effector caspases (proteases, endonucleases)

Intrinsic mt pathway activation most important pathway initiating apoptosis

mt pathway → release sensors → leakage mt protein cytochrome c → activation caspases

Antiapoptotic genes (*BCL-2* gene)/proapoptotic genes (*BAX, BAK* genes)

Antiapoptosis gene; proteins maintains mt membrane integrity; prevent leakage cyto c

(2) Other examples include normal removal of tissue between fingers and toes in the fetus (Link 2-35); shaping of the inner ear; and, cardiac morphogenesis.
   b. Shrinkage of hormone-dependent tissue after withdrawal of the hormone
      (1) Sudden withdrawal of estrogen and progesterone in the menstrual cycle is the signal for apoptosis of endometrial gland cells leading to menses.
      (2) Removal of stimulating hormones (e.g., thyroid-stimulating hormone [TSH], adrenocorticotropic hormone [ACTH], follicle-stimulating hormone [FSH]) causes apoptosis-induced atrophy of the target tissue (e.g., thyroid, adrenal cortex, and ovarian follicles).
   c. Normal involution of the thymus with increasing age
   d. Apoptosis of lymph node germinal centers with apoptosis of individual B cells undergoing antigen selection (Link 2-36).
   e. Death of tumor cells and virus-infected cells by cytotoxic CD8 T cells (e.g., hepatitis B)
   f. Corticosteroid destruction of lymphocytes (B and T cells).
   g. Removal of acute inflammatory cells (e.g., neutrophils) from healing sites in acute inflammation (AI)
   h. Removal of cells with damage to DNA by radiation, FRs, and toxins
   i. Removal of misfolded proteins in various diseases
      (1) **Definition:** A misfolded protein is an incorrectly shaped (folded) protein that is usually inactive.
      (2) Examples of misfolded proteins include amyloid, β-amyloid protein (Alzheimer disease), and proteins in prion-related disease (Creutzfeldt-Jakob disease).
   j. In systemic lupus erythematosus, defective apoptosis may lead to exposure of nuclear antigens (normally sequestered) in necrotic material. These antigens may then be targeted by lymphocytes, resulting in the production of antibodies directed against nuclear antigens.
   k. Excessive apoptosis contributes to injury associated with several diseases, including sepsis, AMI, ischemia, neurodegenerative diseases, and diabetes mellitus.
3. Mechanisms (Fig. 2-17)
   a. Death receptor (extrinsic) pathway activation
      (1) Death receptors are cell surface receptors that transmit signals for apoptosis when they are bound by specific ligands.
      (2) Tumor necrosis factor receptor 1 (TNFR1) is the best known death receptor and is activated by TNF-α.
      (3) TNF-α is an important cytokine that is involved in systemic inflammation, autoimmune disease, and wasting (cachexia) in cancer.
      (4) TNF-α is primarily produced by macrophages; however, it can also be produced by T cells, mast cells, endothelial cells, cardiac cells, and neurons, which explains its multiple disease associations.
      (5) Activation of TNFR1 by TNF-α directly activates *initiator* caspases (caspase-8 and caspase-10) in the cytoplasm.
      (6) Initiator caspases, in turn, activate *effector* caspases (proteases and endonucleases), which mediate the execution phase of apoptosis leading to death of a cell (see later). Proteases destroy the cytoskeleton. Endonucleases act on the nucleus of the cell, causing pyknosis (nuclear condensation) and fragmentation.
   b. Intrinsic (mt) pathway activation
      (1) The intrinsic (mt) pathway is the most important pathway for initiating apoptosis.
      (2) Unlike the death receptor (extrinsic) pathway of apoptosis, the mt pathway involves the release of sensors that lead to leakage of mt proteins (cytochrome c) followed by activation of the caspases.
      (3) In order to understand the previous cascade of events, an understanding of the *BCL* family of genes is important.
         (a) *BCL* gene family contains genes that are antiapoptotic (*BCL-2* gene) and genes that are proapoptotic (*BAX* and *BAK* genes).
         (b) *BCL-2* gene is located on chromosome 18, and its protein product resides in the inner mt membrane. BCL-2 proteins maintain mt membrane integrity and prevent the leakage of mt proteins that can trigger apoptosis (e.g., cytochrome c).
         (c) Damage to DNA, misfolded proteins, FR damage, viral infections, and other injurious events activate sensor genes in the *BCL-2* gene family. Activation of these genes then cause the release of proteins that activate the proapoptotic genes (*BAX* and *BAK*).

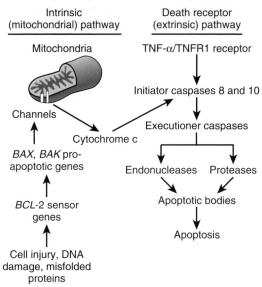

Intrinsic (mitochondrial) pathway / Death receptor (extrinsic) pathway

2-17: Simplified schematic of apoptosis. Refer to the text for discussion. *TNF,* Tumor necrosis factor; *TNFR,* tumor necrosis factor receptor.

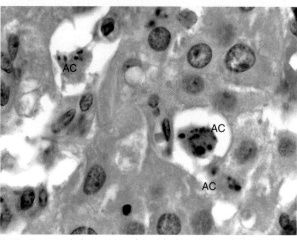

2-18: Apoptosis in a normal involuting corpus luteum in an ovary. In this micrograph several apoptotic cells *(AC)* can be identified by their condensed fragmented nuclei and deeply eosinophilic cytoplasm. Note that the cells are detached from other cells and surrounded by a clear space. *(From Young B, O'Dowd G, Woodford P: Wheater's Functional Histology: A Text and Colour Atlas, 6th ed, Philadelphia, Churchill Livingstone Elsevier, 2014, p 42, Fig. 2.7a.)*

- Activation of *BAX* and *BAK* genes produces protein products that form channels in the mt membrane. These channels cause leakage of cytochrome c into the cytosol.
- Cytochrome c complexes with another protein leading to activation of an initiator caspase (caspase-9), which in turn activates effector caspases (proteases, endonucleases) that mediate the execution phase of apoptosis.
  - d. Execution phase of apoptosis
    - (1) Proteases destroy the cytoskeleton (cytoskel) of the cell and endonucleases destroy the nucleus of the cell.
    - (2) Cytoplasmic buds begin to form on the CM. Buds contain nuclear fragments, mitochondria, and other organelles.
    - (3) Cytoplasmic buds break off and form apoptotic bodies.
    - (4) Apoptotic bodies are phagocytosed by neighboring cells or macrophages.
  - 4. Microscopic appearance
    - a. Apoptotic cell detaches from neighboring cells.
    - b. Apoptotic cells have deeply eosinophilic-staining cytoplasm with the H&E stain (Fig. 2-18; Link 2-37).
    - c. Nucleus is pyknotic, fragmented, or absent.
    - d. Inflammatory infiltrate is absent or minimal.
  - 5. Table 2-5 and Link 2-38 compare cell necrosis with apoptosis.
- **C. Pyroptosis**
  - 1. **Definition:** Pyroptosis is a proinflammatory programmed cell death that involves caspase-1, which differs from the caspases that are active in apoptosis.

BAX/BAK activation: mt channels leak cytochrome c into cytoplasm → triggers apoptosis

Cytochrome c → activates cytoplasm caspases → apoptosis

Destruction cytoskel, destruction nucleus

Contain nuclear/mt/organelle fragments

Form apoptotic bodies

Apoptotic bodies → phagocytosed by cells/macrophages

Detaches from neighboring cells

Deeply eosinophilic cytoplasm

Pyknotic, fragmented, absent nucleus

Minimal/absent inflammation

Proinflammatory cell death using caspase-1

TABLE 2-5   Cell Necrosis Compared With Apoptosis

FEATURE	CELL NECROSIS	APOPTOSIS
General	Death of groups of cells is usually accompanied by an inflammatory infiltrate.	Programmed, enzyme-mediated individual cell death does *not* have an inflammatory infiltrate.
Size of cell	Intracellular swelling is due to sodium-containing water entering the cell (dysfunctional Na^+/K^+ ATPase pump).	Shrunken cells are present due to loss of cytoplasm from cytoplasmic buds that pinch off and become apoptotic bodies.
Enzymes involved	Phospholipase, protease, endonuclease	Initiator caspases, executioner caspases (protease, endonuclease)
Genes involved	None	*BCL-2* (antiapoptotic), *BAX* (proapoptotic), *BAK* (proapoptotic)
Role	Usually associated with a pathologic process	Physiologic functions (e.g., embryology, thymus involution); pathologic function (e.g., removal misfolded proteins, removal of neutrophils in acute inflammation)

BOX 2-1 Clinical Enzymology

Enzymes are protein catalysts of biological origin that increase the rate of chemical reactions without being consumed or structurally altered. **Isoenzymes** (isozymes) are multiple forms of the same enzyme that differ in stereotypical, biochemical, and immunological properties (e.g., lactate dehydrogenase isoenzymes L_1–L_5; creatine kinase isoenzymes MM, MB, and BB). Measurement of individual isoenzymes is frequently more specific in identifying a disease than is total enzyme activity (e.g., CK-MB isoenzyme in identifying an acute myocardial infarction [AMI]). **Isoforms** are subtypes of the individual isoenzymes (e.g., CK-MM isoforms).

Enzymes distribute in cell membranes (e.g., alkaline phosphatase), endoplasmic reticulum (e.g., γ-glutamyltransferase), lysosomes (e.g., muramidase), zymogen (e.g., amylase), cytoplasm (e.g., alanine aminotransferase, a transaminase), and mitochondria (e.g., aspartate aminotransferase, a transaminase).

Factors influencing the release of enzymes into body fluids include disruption or damage to the cell membrane (e.g., alanine aminotransferase, CK), increased synthesis owing to regeneration of injured cells (e.g., alkaline phosphatase), and enzyme induction in the smooth endoplasmic reticulum by drugs (e.g., alcohol and its effect on increasing γ-glutamyltransferase synthesis).

The amount of enzyme released into body fluids depends on the amount of tissue injury, the rate of diffusion out of the damaged cell, and the overall rate of catabolism or clearance of the enzyme. The following table lists important serum enzymes that are increased in tissue injury. These enzymes are further discussed in reference to organ system pathology.

Enzyme	Diagnostic Use
Aspartate aminotransferase (AST)	Marker of diffuse liver cell necrosis (e.g., viral hepatitis); also increased in an AMI. A mitochondrial enzyme that is preferentially increased in alcohol-induced liver disease.
Alanine aminotransferase (ALT)	A marker of diffuse liver cell necrosis (e.g., viral hepatitis). More specific for liver cell necrosis than AST.
Alkaline phosphatase (ALP)	ALP is present in many tissues (e.g., bone [in osteoblasts], liver [synthesized in bile ducts], and placenta). Increased in a normal child due to increased bone growth. Increased in a normal pregnancy, because it is derived from the placenta. An excellent marker of bile duct obstruction in obstructive jaundice. Increased in a bone fracture during the phase of bone repair with increased osteoblastic activity. Increased in osteoblastic metastasis, because tumors secrete factors that enhance osteoblastic activity (e.g., prostate cancer and breast cancer metastatic to bone).
Creatine kinase MB (CK-MB)	Isoenzyme is increased in AMI or myocarditis; therefore, it is *not* a specific enzyme for diagnosing AMI.
Amylase and lipase	They are marker enzymes for acute pancreatitis; however, they are less useful for diagnosing chronic pancreatitis. Lipase is more specific than amylase for diagnosing acute or chronic pancreatitis. Amylase is also increased in salivary gland inflammation (e.g., mumps); therefore, it is *not* a specific enzyme for diagnosing pancreatitis.
Gamma glutamyltransferase (GGT)	Located in the smooth endoplasmic reticulum (SER) in hepatocytes. Increased in drug or chemical induction of the cytochrome P450 system (e.g., alcohol; see previous discussion). It is an excellent marker for alcohol ingestion and is used clinically in this regard. Increased in obstructive jaundice (conditions that block bile ducts within the liver [intrahepatic] or the common bile duct [extrahepatic]). This is called cholestasis. Used in differentiating the source of an increased alkaline phosphatase (ALP). Both enzymes are increased in either intrahepatic or extrahepatic obstruction. A normal GGT in the presence of an increased ALP indicates that the ALP is *not* of liver origin (e.g., bone metastasis with increased osteoblastic activity).
Lactate dehydrogenase (LDH)	LDH is a nonspecific marker of tissue breakdown. Elevated levels can be associated with tumor cell necrosis (e.g., leukemia, malignant lymphoma) in which case the degree of elevation may correlate with the size of the tumor mass.
Serum immunoreactive trypsin	Trypsin is specific for the pancreas, unlike AST and ALT. Very sensitive for the diagnosis of acute pancreatitis (95%–100%). In addition, it is an excellent newborn screen for cystic fibrosis, which damages the pancreas by blocking tubular lumens with thick secretions.

Host defense

2. Important role in the host defense system for fighting off microbial pathogens.
   a. Occurs in monocytes, macrophages, and dendritic cells infected with certain types of microbial pathogens.

Mono/macro/dendritic cell destruction *Salmonella, Shigella, Legionella*

   b. Microbial pathogens that may be killed by pyroptosis include *Salmonella typhimurium, Shigella flexneri, Legionella pneumophila, Pseudomonas aeruginosa, Candida albicans,* adenovirus, and influenza virus.
3. Overwhelming activation of caspase-1 has also been implicated in the pathogenesis of several diseases that are *not* related to infectious stimuli, including myocardial infarction (MI), neurodegenerative diseases (NDDs), inflammatory bowel disease (IBD), cerebral ischemia, and endotoxic shock.

MI, NDDs, IBD, cerebral ischemia, endotoxic shock

   D. Enzyme markers of cell death (Box 2-1)

ABBREVIATIONS

MC most common	MCC most common cause	Rx treatment

I. Acute Inflammation (AI)
  A. Overview of AI

    1. **Definition:** Acute inflammation is a transient and early response to injury that is characterized by the release of numerous chemical mediators and leads to stereotypic small vessel and leukocyte (white blood cell [WBC]) responses.

    2. Characterized by the release of numerous chemical mediators. Leads to stereotypic small vessel and leukocyte (WBC) responses. *Not* a synonym for infection.

  B. Cardinal signs of AI (Fig. 3-1)

    1. Redness and heat. Both signs are due to histamine-mediated vasodilation of the precapillary sphincters in arterioles, which leads to flooding of the capillary network and dilation of capillaries and postcapillary venules (Link 3-1).

    2. Swelling of tissue (synonymous with edema). Due to a histamine-mediated increase in venule permeability.

      • Edema refers to increased fluid in the interstitial space (space between the extracellular fluid compartment and the intracellular fluid compartment).

    3. Pain. Prostaglandin E_2 (PGE_2) sensitizes specialized nerve endings to the effects of bradykinin and other pain mediators.

  C. Stimuli for AI

    1. Infections (e.g., bacterial or viral), immune reactions (e.g., reaction to a bee sting)

    2. Other stimuli: tissue necrosis (e.g., acute myocardial infarction), trauma, radiation, burns, and foreign bodies (e.g., glass, splinter)

  D. Sequential vascular events in AI

    1. Vasoconstriction of arterioles. First vascular event in AI and is due to a neurogenic reflex lasting only a few seconds.

    2. Vasodilation of arterioles

      a. Arterioles are impermeable small arteries that have a few elastic fibers and only one to three smooth muscle layers in their tunica media.

      b. Histamine and other vasodilators (e.g., nitric oxide [NO]) relax the vascular smooth muscle in arterioles, causing increased blood flow. Histamine is released from mast cells located in interstitial tissue around the small vessels (Fig. 3-2).

      c. Increased blood flow, due to vasodilation of arterioles, increases the hydrostatic pressure (pressure generated by fluid) within the lumens of venules.

    3. Increased permeability of venules

      a. Venules are permeable, collect blood from capillary networks, have only one or two layers of muscle fibers, and gradually merge to form veins.

      b. Histamine and other mediators contract endothelial cells (ECs) in venules, producing endothelial gaps that expose a bare basement membrane. Tight junctions are simpler in venules than in arterioles; therefore, they are easier to contract.

Transient/early response to injury

Chemical, vascular, cellular responses

Rubor (redness)/calor (heat): histamine-mediated vasodilation

Histamine-mediated ↑venular permeability

Edema ↑fluid interstitial space

Mediated by PGE_2/bradykinin

Infections, immune reactions

Tissue necrosis, trauma, radiation, foreign bodies

Vasoconstriction first vascular event in AI; neurogenic reflex

Impermeable small arteries

Vasodilation arterioles: histamine, NO

Mast cells release preformed histamine

Venules collect blood from capillaries

Histamine contracts venule ECs; endothelial gaps expose basement membrane

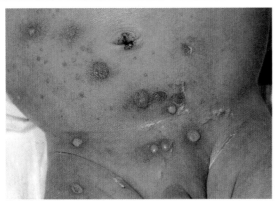

3-1: Signs of acute inflammation (AI). This neonate has the scalded child syndrome caused by *Staphylococcus aureus*. Signs of AI that are present in the photograph include redness (rubor) and swelling (tumor). The infection is also associated with warm skin (calor) and pain (dolor). The yellow, raised areas are pustules filled with neutrophils. *(From Bouloux, P: Self-Assessment Picture Tests Medicine, Vol 3, London, Mosby-Wolfe, 1997, plate 75, Fig. 148.)*

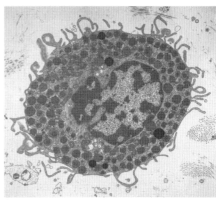

3-2: Electron micrograph of a tissue mast cell. The cytoplasmic granules contain histamine, eosinophil chemotactic factor, and other preformed inflammatory mediators. *(Electron micrograph courtesy of my friend William Meek, PhD, Professor of Anatomy and Cell Biology, Oklahoma State University, Center for Health Sciences, Tulsa, Oklahoma.)*

↑Venule hydrostatic pressure → transudate in interstitial tissue

Swelling tissue → cardinal sign AI

Reduced blood flow

Neutrophils 1° leukocytes AI

Circulating/marginating pool

Blacks lower WBC count than whites

WBC distribution altered by activating/inactivating adhesion molecules

RBCs "stacks of coins"

Neutrophils pushed to periphery venule lumens

Adhere-release-adhere-release

Selectin adhesion molecules neutrophils/venular ECs

L-Selectin leukocytes, E-/P-selectin venular ECs

    c. Because of increased intraluminal hydrostatic pressure (pressure exerted by fluid in the venule lumen), a transudate (fluid low in proteins and cells) moves through the intact venular basement membrane into the interstitial tissue.

4. Swelling of tissue. Tissue swelling (edema; "tumor" old term) occurs when the net outflow of fluid from venules surpasses the capacity of lymphatics to remove the fluid (i.e., AI). It is a cardinal sign of AI.

5. Reduced blood flow eventually occurs because of the leakage of fluid into the interstitial tissue and increased uptake of the fluid by the lymphatics.

E. Sequential cellular events in AI

- Events described in the following section will emphasize the neutrophil component of AI using a bacterial infection (e.g., *Staphylococcus aureus*) as an example.

1. **Definition:** Neutrophils are the primary leukocytes in AI (Fig. 3-3).

    a. Peripheral blood neutrophils are subdivided into a circulating pool and a marginating pool (those that are adherent to ECs).

    b. In the white population, ≈50% of neutrophils are in the circulating pool and ≈50% in the marginating pool, whereas in the black population, more neutrophils are in the marginating pool than the circulating pool. The complete blood count measures only the circulating pool of WBCs. This explains why blacks have a slightly lower WBC count than whites.

       (1) The circulating pool is located in the central axial stream of blood flowing through small blood vessels (Link 3-2).

       (2) Evaluation of the WBC differential count may be made either by a blood analyzer or manually with a peripheral blood smear.

    c. Neutrophil distribution in these pools is altered by activating or inactivating neutrophil adhesion molecules (see later discussion).

2. Margination of neutrophils (Fig. 3-4)

    a. In AI, red blood cells (RBCs) aggregate into rouleaux ("stacks of coins") in the venules (see Fig. 3-4). Rouleaux is caused by fibrinogen, an acute phase reactant (APR) protein (discussed later) that is synthesized and released by the liver.

    b. Rouleau mechanically forces neutrophils out of the central axial stream and pushes them to the periphery of the venules (called margination; Link 3-3). **Caution:** margination of neutrophils is *not* the same as the marginating pool of neutrophils.

3. Rolling of neutrophils (see Fig. 3-4)

    a. Rolling occurs in venules and is due to expression of selectin adhesion molecules on neutrophils and venular ECs. Neutrophils adhere to the endothelium and then release, adhere and then release as they circulate through the venules.

    b. Selectins are carbohydrate-binding adhesion molecules.

    c. L-Selectin is located on leukocytes (e.g., neutrophils), whereas E-selectin and P-selectin are located on the surface of venular ECs (*not* shown in the schematic).

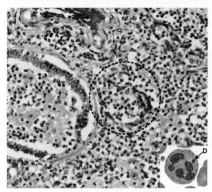

3-3: Acute inflammation (AI). Histologic section of lung in bronchopneumonia showing sheets of neutrophils with multilobed nuclei *(interrupted circle)*. The pink staining material in between the neutrophils is an exudate, which is protein- and cell-rich fluid that is characteristic of AI. The insert shows a neutrophil. *D,* Döhle body. *(From my friend Ivan Damjanov, MD, PhD:* Pathology for the Health-Related Professions, *2nd ed, Philadelphia, Saunders, 2000, p 182, Fig. 8-8. Insert from Young B, O'Dowd G, Woodford P:* Wheater's Functional Histology: A Colour Text and Atlas, *6th ed, Churchill Livingstone Elsevier, 2014, p 55, Fig. 3.9d.)*

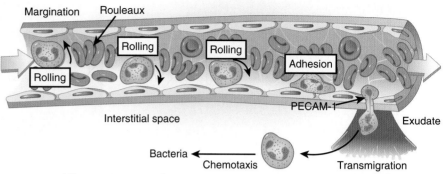

3-4: Neutrophil events in acute inflammation. Rolling is due to activation of selectin adhesion molecules on the surface of neutrophils, whereas firm adhesion is due to activation of β_2-integrin (CD11a:CD18) adhesion molecules on the surface of neutrophils (not shown). Ligands (attachment sites) for selectin and β_2-integrin are located on the surface of endothelial cells (not shown). Neutrophil transmigration through the basement membrane mainly occurs in venules. Neutrophils dissolve the exposed venular basement membrane and transmigrate into the interstitial tissue. This leads to an outpouring of protein-rich fluid (called exudate) along with neutrophils. Once in the interstitial space, chemotactic factors direct the neutrophils to the site of inflammation. *(From Goljan E:* Rapid Review Pathology, *4th ed, Saunders Elsevier, 2014, p 37, Fig. 3-3.)*

    (1) P-selectin is produced in the Weibel-Palade bodies in venular ECs.

    (2) Weibel-Palade bodies are the "glue factory" of ECs because they synthesize P-selectin, an adhesion molecule for leukocytes, and von Willebrand factor (vWF), the adhesion molecule of the platelet (see Chapter 15).

  d. Interleukin-1 (IL-1) and tumor necrosis factor (TNF) stimulate the expression of selectin ligands on the surface of neutrophils (L-selectin) and the expression of selectin molecules on the surface of venular ECs (E-selectin, P-selectin).

  e. Binding of circulating neutrophils to E-selectin and P-selectin on venular ECs is weak and transient, causing them to "roll" (bind–detach, bind–detach) along the surface.

4. Firm adhesion in venules is due to neutrophil expression of β_2-integrins and venular EC expression of integrin adhesion molecules.

  a. Activation of neutrophil β_2-integrin (CD11a:CD18) adhesion molecules

    (1) β_2-Integrins are located on neutrophils and interact with corresponding ligands on venular ECs.

    (2) β_2-Integrins on neutrophils are activated by C5a and leukotriene B_4 (LTB_4).

    (3) Catecholamines and corticosteroids *inhibit* activation of these neutrophil adhesion molecules.

      (a) Inhibition of neutrophil β_2-integrins, leads to an increase in the peripheral blood neutrophil count (called neutrophilic leukocytosis).

      (b) Occurs because the normal marginating pool becomes part of the circulating pool because they can no longer adhere to venular endothelium.

    (4) Endotoxins enhance activation of neutrophil β_2-integrins.

      (a) Enhanced activation of neutrophil β_2-integrins causes the total circulating neutrophil count to decrease (called neutropenia).

      (b) Occurs because the normal circulating neutrophil pool becomes part of the marginating neutrophil pool.

  b. Activation of *endothelial cell* integrin adhesion molecules (ligands)

    (1) IL-1 and TNF activate intercellular adhesion molecule (ICAM) and vascular cell adhesion molecule (VCAM) on venular ECs.

    (2) Activated (A*) ICAM ligands bind to activated β_2-integrins on neutrophils/macrophages causing them to *firmly* adhere to venular endothelium.

    (3) Activated (A*) VCAM ligands bind to activated β_1-integrins on eosinophils, monocytes, and lymphocytes, which then firmly bind to ECs.

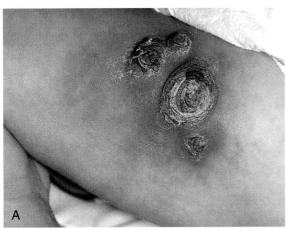 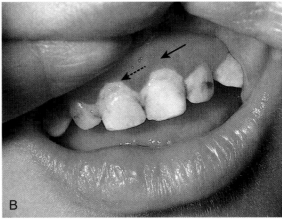

3-5: **A,** Skin infection in a patient with leukocyte adhesion deficiency type 1 (LAD-1). Note the lack of pus in this wound, inability to demarcate the skin debris, and the limited amount of signs of acute inflammation. **B,** Note the gingivitis *(solid arrow)* and periodontitis *(interrupted arrow),* which are hallmarks of LAD-1. *(From Rich RR: Clinical Immunology Principles and Practices, ed 4, Philadelphia, 2013, Saunders, Fig. 21-3, 21-2, respectively, p 273.)*

LAD disorders

Autosomal recessive inheritance

LAD-1: deficiency β₂-integrin

CD: cluster designation

LAD-2: deficiency EC selectin that binds neutrophils

Delayed separation umbilical cord

Poor wound healing, gingivitis, leukocytosis

Movement neutrophils from venules into interstitial space

Neutrophils dissolve venular basement membrane with collagenase

PECAM-1 mediates neutrophil transmigration

Protein/cell-rich fluid (pus)

Dilutes bacterial toxins; opsonins (assist phagocytosis)

Directed migration neutrophils; follow chemical gradient

Follow chemical gradient

Chemotactic mediators bind neutrophils

C5a, LTB₄, bacterial products, IL-8

Binding ↑neutrophil motility

Neutrophil phagocytosis: opsonization → ingestion → killing

c. Leukocyte adhesion deficiency (LAD) disorders
   (1) Autosomal recessive inheritance pattern (see Chapter 6).
   (2) LAD type 1 (LAD-1) is a deficiency of β_2-integrin (CD11a:CD18) on neutrophils.
      • CD stands for cluster of designation.
   (3) LAD type 2 (LAD-2) is a deficiency of an EC selectin that normally binds neutrophils.
   (4) Clinical findings in LAD disorders
      (a) First manifestation (either type) is delayed separation of the umbilical cord, which usually separates and sloughs by the end of the second postnatal week. Neutrophil enzymes are important in cord separation; therefore, in a histologic section of the surgically removed umbilical cord, no neutrophils would be seen adhering to venular endothelium or within the interstitial tissue.
      (b) Additional clinical findings include poor wound healing (Fig. 3-5 A), severe gingivitis (Fig. 3-5 B), and peripheral blood neutrophilic leukocytosis (loss of marginating pool).
5. Transmigration (diapedesis) of neutrophils into the interstitial space (Links 3-4 and 3-5; see Fig. 3-4)
   a. Neutrophils moving along the venular endothelium enter gaps produced by histamine-mediated EC contraction. In this location, neutrophils release type IV collagenase, which dissolves the basement membrane allowing neutrophils to enter (transmigrate) into the interstitial tissue.
   b. Platelet-endothelial cell adhesion molecule-1 (PECAM-1; CD31) is expressed on the surface of platelets, neutrophils, and ECs. PECAM-1 mediates the transmigration of neutrophils between ECs and the interstitial tissue.
   c. Plasma-derived fluid rich in proteins and cells (called exudate or pus) accumulates in the interstitial tissue (Link 3-6).
   d. Functions of exudate
      • Dilutes bacterial toxins, if present. Provides opsonins (immunoglobulin G [IgG], C3b) to assist in phagocytosis by neutrophils, macrophages, and dendritic cells (see later).
6. Chemotaxis of neutrophils
   a. **Definition:** Chemotaxis is a directed migration of neutrophils.
   b. Neutrophils follow chemical gradients that lead to the infection site (see Fig. 3-4).
   c. Chemotactic mediators bind to neutrophil receptors. Mediators include C5a, LTB₄, bacterial products, and interleukin-8 (IL-8).
   d. Binding causes the release of calcium, which increases neutrophil motility.
7. Neutrophil phagocytosis and killing of bacteria
   a. Neutrophil phagocytosis is a multistep process, consisting of opsonization, ingestion, and killing.
   b. Neutrophil opsonization (Links 3-7 and 3-8)

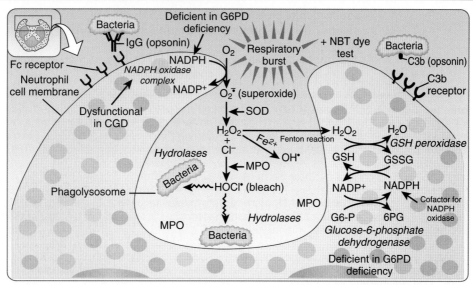

3-6: O_2-dependent myeloperoxidase system. A series of biochemical reactions occurs in the phagolysosome, resulting in the production of hypochlorous free radicals (bleach [HOCl·]) that destroy bacteria. Conversion of H_2O_2 to $OH^·$ using reduced Fe^{2+} as a source of electrons is called the Fenton reaction. NADPH produced by the pentose phosphate shunt is a cofactor for NADPH oxidase, which is deficient in CGD. A decrease in the cofactor NADPH (i.e., glucose-6-phosphate dehydrogenase [G6PD] deficiency) also interferes with the normal functioning of the O_2-dependent MPO system. IgG and C3b are opsonins that facilitate the actions of phagocytic leukocytes (neutrophils, monocytes). A newer test for the presence of a respiratory burst is the oxidation of dihydrorhodamine to fluorescent rhodamine. *CGD,* Chronic granulomatous disease; *Fe²⁺,* reduced iron; *GSH,* reduced glutathione; *GSSG,* oxidized glutathione; *H_2O_2,* hydrogen peroxide; *MPO,* myeloperoxidase; *NADP,* oxidized form of nicotinamide adenine dinucleotide phosphate; *NADPH,* reduced nicotinamide adenine dinucleotide phosphate; *NBT,* nitroblue tetrazolium; *OH·,* hydroxyl free radical; *6PG,* 6-phosphogluconate; *SOD,* superoxide dismutase.

(1) Opsonins attach to bacteria (or foreign bodies).
  (a) Opsonins include IgG, the C3b fragment of complement, and other proteins (e.g., C-reactive protein [CRP]).
  (b) Neutrophils have membrane receptors for IgG and C3b.
(2) Opsonization enhances neutrophil recognition and attachment to bacteria (and foreign bodies).
(3) Bruton agammaglobulinemia is an opsonization defect (see Chapter 4). Pre–B cells *cannot* mature to B cells; therefore plasma cells, which are derived from B cells, *cannot* synthesize immunoglobulins (i.e., IgG).
  c. Neutrophil ingestion
(1) Neutrophils engulf (phagocytose) and then trap bacteria/fungi in phagocytic vacuoles (phagosomes).
(2) Primary lysosomes in neutrophils empty hydrolytic enzymes into phagocytic vacuoles producing phagolysosomes. In Chédiak-Higashi syndrome (see Chapter 2), there is a defect in microtubule function, which prevents lysosomes from fusing with phagosomes to produce a phagolysosome.
  d. Neutrophil killing of bacteria/fungi by the oxygen (O_2)-dependent myeloperoxidase (MPO) system; Fig. 3-6).
(1) **Definition:** The O_2-dependent MPO system in neutrophils and monocytes uses the reduced nicotinamide adenine dinucleotide phosphate (NADPH) oxidase enzyme complex to convert molecular O_2 to superoxide free radicals (FRs) to kill bacteria and fungi.
(2) O_2-dependent MPO system is only present in neutrophils and monocytes (*not* macrophages).
  • MPO is a neutrophil/monocyte lysosomal enzyme.
(3) MPO system is the most potent microbicidal system available to neutrophils and monocytes.
(4) Production of superoxide FRs. NADPH oxidase enzyme complex converts molecular O_2 to superoxide FRs, which releases energy called the respiratory, or oxidative, burst.
(5) Production of hydrogen peroxide (H_2O_2)
  (a) Superoxide dismutase (SOD) converts $O_2^{·-}$ to H_2O_2.
  (b) Some H_2O_2 is converted to hydroxyl FRs by iron via the Fenton reaction (see Chapter 2).

Opsonins attach to bacteria, foreign bodies

IgG, C3b, CRP

Neutrophils: IgG/C3b receptors

IgG/C3b enhance neutrophil recognition/attachment of bacteria

Bruton agammaglobulinemia: opsonization defect (lack IgG)

Phagocytose → trap bacteria/fungi in phagosomes

1° lysosomes enzymes → phagocytic vacuole → phagolysosome

Chédiak-Higashi: defect microtubule function; cannot produce phagolysosomes

O_2-dependent MPO system

NADPH oxidase enzyme complex → O_2 to superoxide FRs

Neutrophils/monocytes *not* macrophages

MPO neutrophil/monocyte lysosomal enzyme

Most potent microbicidal system

Converts molecular O_2 to superoxide FRs

Converts $O_2^{·-}$ to H_2O_2

End-product bleach
(hypochlorous acid)

(6) Production of bleach (HOCl·). MPO in the phagolysosome combines H_2O_2 with chloride (Cl^-) to form hypochlorous FRs (HOCl·), which kill bacteria and some fungi.

(7) Chronic granulomatous disease and MPO deficiency are examples of diseases that have a defect in the O_2-dependent MPO system.

Definition: Chronic granulomatous disease (CGD) is an X-linked recessive disorder (XR; 65% of cases) or autosomal recessive disorder (30% of cases). The X-linked type is characterized by a mutation in the *CYBB* gene that encodes for a component of the NADPH oxidase enzyme complex (PHOX system) rendering the complex dysfunctional. The reduced production of $O_2^{\bullet-}$ results in an absent respiratory (oxidative) burst. Catalase-positive organisms that produce H_2O_2 (e.g., *Staphylococcus aureus, Nocardia asteroides, Serratia marcescens, Aspergillus* species, and *Candida* species) are ingested but *not* killed, because the catalase degrades the H_2O_2 produced by these pathogens. Myeloperoxidase is present, but HOCl· is *not* synthesized because of the absence of H_2O_2. However, catalase-negative organisms (e.g., *Streptococcus* species) that produce H_2O_2 are ingested and can be killed when MPO combines H_2O_2 (derived from the bacteria) with Cl^- to form HOCl·. Granulomatous inflammation occurs in tissue, because the neutrophils, which can phagocytose bacteria but *not* kill most of them, are eventually replaced by chronic inflammatory cells, mainly lymphocytes and macrophages. Macrophages fuse to form multinucleated giant cells, which is a characteristic feature of granulomatous inflammation. Patients with CGD have severe infections involving the lungs (pneumonia is the most common presentation), skin, visceral organs, and bones. The classic screening test for CGD is the nitroblue tetrazolium (NBT) dye test. In this test, leukocytes in a test tube are incubated with the NBT dye, which turns blue if superoxide FRs are present, indicating that the respiratory (oxidative) burst is intact (considered to be a positive test). The NBT dye test is negative in the X-linked type of CGD (NBT dye is *not* converted to a blue dye), because the NADPH oxidase enzyme complex is dysfunctional. Because of its lack of sensitivity, however, the NBT dye test has been replaced by a more sensitive test involving the oxidation of dihydrorhodamine to fluorescent rhodamine. This test is abnormal in both variants of CGD.

Definition: MPO deficiency is an autosomal recessive disorder that differs from CGD in that both $O_2^{\bullet-}$ and H_2O_2 are produced (normal respiratory burst). However, the absence of MPO prevents the synthesis of HOCl·.

CGD/MPO deficiency defect
in the O_2-dependent MPO
system

↓NADPH → ↓NADPH
oxidase complex →
microbiocidal defect/
hemolytic anemia

Lack NADPH interferes with
normal function of
O_2-dependent MPO system

(8) Deficiency of NADPH (e.g., glucose-6-phosphate dehydrogenase [G6PD] deficiency) produces a microbicidal defect.

(a) NADPH is a cofactor for the NADPH oxidase complex; therefore, absence of NADPH in G6PD deficiency, a cause of hemolytic anemia (see Chapter 12), renders the enzyme nonfunctional. Hemolytic anemia is characterized by disruption of the RBC membrane with release of hemoglobin into the plasma.

(b) Patients with G6PD deficiency are very susceptible to bacterial and certain fungal infections, because the O_2-dependent MPO system is dysfunctional. Infection is usually responsible for precipitating the hemolytic anemia.

(9) Table 3-1 compares CGD and MPO deficiency.

e. Neutrophil killing of bacteria by O_2-independent microbial systems

(1) Oxygen-independent systems for killing bacteria are through the release of lethal substances from leukocyte granules.

Lactoferrin (neutrophils),
MBP (eosinophils)

Phagocytosis depletes
neutrophil glycogen →
neutrophil dies

Histamine: important
mediator of AI

(2) Lethal substances include *lactoferrin* (present in neutrophil granules), which binds iron that is necessary for normal bacterial growth and reproduction and *major basic protein* (MBP), an eosinophil product that is cytotoxic to helminths (parasitic worms).

f. Process of phagocytosis depletes neutrophil glycogen reserves, ultimately leading to the demise of the neutrophil.

F. **Chemical mediators in AI** (Table 3-2)

1. Chemical mediators derive from plasma, leukocytes, local tissue, and bacterial products. Example: histamine (most important mediator of AI) is released from mast cells;

TABLE 3-1   Comparison of Chronic Granulomatous Disease and Myeloperoxidase Deficiency

	CHRONIC GRANULOMATOUS DISEASE	MYELOPEROXIDASE DEFICIENCY
Inheritance pattern	X-linked recessive	Autosomal recessive
NADPH oxidase	Dysfunctional	Present
Myeloperoxidase	Present	Absent
Respiratory burst	Absent	Present
Peroxide (H_2O_2)	Absent	Present
Bleach (HOCl)	Absent	Absent

TABLE 3-2   Sources and Functions of Chemical Mediators (Also Useful for Chapter 4)

MEDIATOR	PRINCIPAL SOURCE(S)	FUNCTION(S)
Arachidonic Acid Metabolites		
Prostaglandins (PGs)	Macrophages, endothelial cells, platelets PGH_2: major precursor of PGs and thromboxanes	• PGE_2: vasodilation, pain, fever • PGI_2: vasodilation; inhibition of platelet aggregation
Thromboxane A_2	Platelets Converted from PGH_2 by thromboxane synthase	• Vasoconstriction, platelet aggregation
Leukotrienes (LTs)	Leukocytes Converted from arachidonic acid by lipoxygenase mediated hydroxylation	• LTB_4: chemotaxis and activation of neutrophil adhesion molecules • LTC_4, LTD_4, LTE_4: vasoconstriction, increased venular permeability, bronchoconstriction • Zileuton inhibits 5-lipoxygenase: ↓synthesis LTB_4, LTC_4, LTD_4, LTE_4 • Montelukast is a LT receptor antagonist: ↓activity of LTC_4, LTD_4, LTE_4
Bradykinin	Product of kinin system activation by activated factor XII	• Vasodilation, increased venular permeability, pain
Chemokines	Leukocytes, endothelial cells	• Activate neutrophils and stimulate their migration through the endothelium to the site of infection (chemotaxis; see Fig. 3-4)
Complement	Synthesized in liver (acute phase reactant [APR])	• C3a, C5a (anaphylatoxins): stimulate mast cell release of histamine • C3b: opsonization • C5a: activation of neutrophil adhesion molecules, chemotaxis • C5–C9 (membrane attack complex): cell lysis
Cytokines		
IL-1, TNF (cachectin)	IL-1: Macrophages (main source), endothelial cells, some epithelial cells	**IL-1 functions:** • Hypothalamus: stimulate secretion of corticotropin-releasing hormone; anterior pituitary: stimulate secretion of ACTH; adrenal zona fasciculata: stimulate secretion of glucocorticoid (cortisol) • Initiate PGE_2 synthesis in the anterior hypothalamus, leading to production of fever • Liver: synthesis APRs • Activate endothelial cell adhesion molecules • T cells: T_H17 differentiation (see Chapter 4)
	TNF: macrophages, T cells	**TNF functions:** • Promoter of apoptosis of many cell types (see Chapter 2) • Endothelial cell activation • Neutrophil activation • Cachexia (muscle wasting)
IL-2	Helper T (T_H) cells	• B cells: proliferation, in vitro antibody synthesis • T cells: proliferation/differentiation into memory cells and effector cells • NK cells: activation, proliferation
IL-3	T cells	• Stimulates maturation of all hematopoietic lineages in the bone marrow
IL-4	CD4 T_H2 cells, mast cells	• B cells: isotype switching to IgE • T cells: T_H2 differentiation, proliferation (see Chapter 4)
IL-5	CD4 T_H2 cells	• B cells: proliferation • Enhances class type switching to IgE • Increased production of eosinophils
IL-6	Macrophages, endothelial cells, T cells	• Primary cytokine responsible for increased liver synthesis of APRs (e.g., C-reactive protein) • T cells: T_H17 differentiation (see Chapter 4) • B cells: proliferation of B cells
IL-8	Macrophages, epithelial cells, endothelial cells, airway smooth muscle cells	• Neutrophil chemotaxis and respiratory burst • Stimulates neutrophil release of granule-derived mediators (exocytosis)

IL-10	T cells	• Inhibitor of activated macrophages and dendritic cells involved in the control of innate immunity and cell-mediated immunity by
		  • inhibiting production of IL-12 by activated macrophages/dendritic cells
		  • inhibiting expression of costimulators and class II MHC molecules on macrophages/dendritic cells

Continued

TABLE 3-2 Sources and Functions of Chemical Mediators (Also Useful for Chapter 4)—cont'd

MEDIATOR	PRINCIPAL SOURCE(S)	FUNCTION(S)
IL-12	Macrophages, dendritic cells	• T cell: TH1 differentiation • Stimulates interferon (IFN)-γ production by NK cells and T cells • Enhances NK cell and cytotoxic T cell mediated cytotoxicity
Histamine	Mast cells (primary cell), platelets, enterochromaffin cells	• Vasodilation, increased venular permeability
Nitric oxide (NO)	Macrophages, endothelial cells FR gas released during conversion of arginine to citrulline by NO synthase	• Vasodilation, bactericidal

ACTH, Adrenocorticotropic hormone; *FR,* free radical; *IL,* interleukin; *MHC,* major histocompatibility complex; *NK,* natural killer cell; *TNF,* tumor necrosis factor.

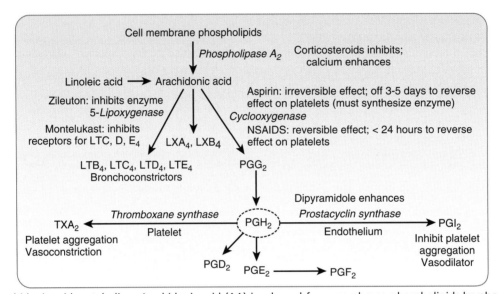

3-7: Simplified arachidonic acid metabolism. Arachidonic acid (AA) is released from membrane phospholipids by phospholipase A_2. The enzyme is inhibited by corticosteroids and enhanced by calcium. Linoleic acid is an ω-6 essential fatty acid that is used to synthesize AA. AA is converted by cyclooxygenase in one pathway into prostaglandins (PGs). Note the effect of aspirin and NSAIDS on platelet cyclooxygenase. The COX-1 isoform (not depicted) is constitutively expressed in various tissues, whereas the COX-2 isoform (not depicted) is induced by various growth factors and proinflammatory cytokines. PGH_2 is a precursor PG that is converted to thromboxane A_2 (TXA_2) in platelets by thromboxane synthase and to PGI_2 in endothelial cells by prostacyclin synthase. Note that dipyramidole enhances the enzyme. Also note that TXA_2 and PGI_2 have opposing actions in the platelets. PGH_2 is also converted into PGD, E, and F_2. In another pathway, 5-lipoxygenase converts AA into leukotrienes (LTs). 5-Lipoxygenase is inhibited by zileuton, while the receptors for LTC_4, LTD_4, LTE_4 are inhibited by montelukast. Note that AA is also converted to lipoxin A_4 (LXA_4) and lipoxin B_4 (LXB_4). See text and Table 3-2 for further discussion. *NSAIDs,* Nonsteroidal antiinflammatory drugs; *PGI$_2$,* prostacyclin.

Plasma, leukocytes, local tissue, bacteria

Histamine most important chemical mediator of AI

Local/systemic effects; e.g., histamine

LTC_4, LTD_4, LTE_4; LT (leukotriene)

Histamine, NO, PGI_2, PGE_2, PGD_2

TXA_2

Histamine, bradykinin, LTC4/D4/E4, C3a, C5a, PGE_2/D_2

PGE_2, bradykinin

PGE_2, IL-1, TNF

C5a, LTB_4, IL-8, LXA_4, LXB_4

LXA_4, LXB_4

LXA_4, LXB_4

APRs

arachidonic acid mediators are released from membrane phospholipids in macrophages, ECs, and platelets (Fig. 3-7). They have short half-lives (e.g., seconds to minutes).

2. Local and systemic effects. Example: histamine may produce local signs of itching or systemic signs of anaphylaxis.
3. Mediators have diverse functions.
   a. Bronchoconstriction (wheezing, difficulty breathing). Examples: LTC_4, LTD_4, LTE_4.
   b. Vasodilation. Examples: histamine, NO, PGI_2, PGE_2, PGD_2.
   c. Vasoconstriction. Example: thromboxane A_2 (TXA_2).
   d. Increasing venular permeability. Examples: histamine, bradykinin, LTC_4, LTD_4, LTE_4, C3a, and C5a (anaphylatoxins), PGE_2, PGD_2.
   e. Producing pain. Examples: PGE_2, bradykinin.
   f. Producing fever. Examples: PGE_2, IL-1, TNF.
   g. Neutrophil chemotaxis. Examples: C5a, LTB_4, IL-8, lipoxygenase A_4 (LXA_4), LXB_4.
   h. Neutrophil adhesion. Examples: LXA_4, LXB_4.
   i. Inhibit inflammation. Examples: LXA_4, LXB_4.
   j. Liver synthesis of APRs (see the following).

5. APRs
   a. **Definition:** Acute phase reactants are proteins whose serum concentrations either increase or decrease by at least 25% during an inflammatory state. All APRs are synthesized by the liver.

   Proteins ↑/↓ during inflammation; liver synthesis

   b. Interleukin-6 (IL-6) is the major cytokine inducer of most APRs.

   IL-6 major inducer APRs

   (1) Other cytokine inducers include IL-1, TNF-α, interferon (IFN)-γ.

   IL-1β, TNF-α, and IFN-γ.

   (2) These cytokines also suppress liver synthesis of albumin, which provides more amino acids for synthesis of these inducers.

   Suppress liver synthesis of albumin

   c. APRs synthesized by the liver that are *increased*
   (1) Ceruloplasmin, a binding protein for copper that also reduces swelling in inflammation

   Ceruloplasmin

   (2) Lactoferrin, an iron-binding protein in neutrophil granules

   Lactoferrin

   (3) Various complement components for chemotaxis and opsonization

   Complement

   (4) Fibrinogen (wound healing)

   Fibrinogen

   (5) CRP (discussed later)

   CRP

   (6) Serum amyloid A (SAA; marker of inflammation like CRP)

   SAA

   (7) α₁ Antitrypsin (AAT; antioxidant)

   AAT

   (8) Haptoglobin (antioxidant; important in wound repair)

   Haptoglobin

   (9) IL-1 receptor (R) antagonist.

   IL-1 R antagonist

   (10) Hepcidin (decreases iron reabsorption and macrophage release of iron required for bacteria reproduction)

   Hepcidin

   (11) Ferritin (iron storage protein)

   Ferritin

   d. Proteins that are synthesized by the liver that are *decreased* include albumin (amino acids used to synthesize APRs), transferrin (protein that binds to iron), and transthyretin (also called prealbumin).

   Albumin, transferrin, transthyretin

   e. APRs are *not* always beneficial; harmful effects include muscle wasting (cachexia), anorexia (suppression of appetite), impaired growth in children.

   Cachexia (wasting), anorexia, impaired growth in children

G. **Types of AI**
   1. Location, cause, and duration of inflammation determine the morphology of an inflammatory reaction.
   2. Purulent (suppurative) inflammation
      a. **Definition:** Purulent inflammation is a localized proliferation of pus-forming organisms, such as *Staphylococcus aureus* (e.g., skin abscess; Fig. 3-8 A).

      Localized proliferation pus-producing pathogens (e.g., S. aureus)

      b. *Staphylococcus aureus* contains coagulase, which cleaves fibrinogen into fibrin and traps bacteria and neutrophils, thereby keeping the infection localized.

      Coagulase cleaves fibrinogen → fibrin: localizes infection

   3. Cellulitis
      a. **Definition:** Cellulitis is a spreading type of bacterial infection of subcutaneous tissue that usually follows some type of skin trauma (Fig. 3-8 B).

      Spreading bacterial infection of subcutaneous tissue

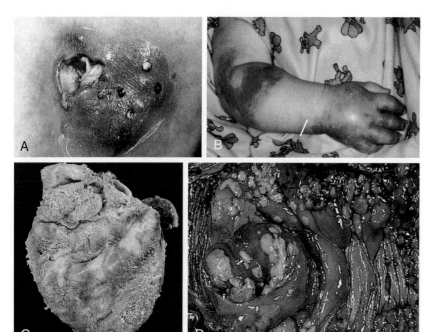

3-8: **A,** Purulent (suppurative) inflammation. The photograph shows a skin abscess (furuncle) caused by *Staphylococcus aureus*. Abscesses are pus-filled nodules located in the dermis. Note the multiple draining sinus tracts filled with pus. **B,** Cellulitis. Note the erythematous patches and plaques with edema, involving the arm of this 18-month-old male. Note the multifocal nature of the infection and the sharp borders. Most cases are caused by *Staphylococcus aureus* and group A β-hemolytic streptococcus. **C,** Fibrinous inflammation. The surface of the heart is covered by a shaggy, fibrinous exudate. **D,** Pseudomembranous inflammation. There is necrosis and a yellow-colored exudate covering the mucosal surface of the colon as a result of a toxin produced by *Clostridium difficile*. (*A from Bouloux P: Self-Assessment Picture Tests Medicine, Vol 1, London, Mosby-Wolfe, 1997, p 33, Fig. 66; B from Paller AS, Mancini AJ: Hurwitz Clinical Pediatric Dermatology, 4th ed, Philadelphia, Saunders Elsevier, 2011, p 327, Fig. 14.15; C from my friend Ivan Damjanov, MD, PhD, Linder J: Pathology: A Color Atlas, St. Louis, Mosby, 2000, p 25, Fig. 1-59; D from Grieg J: Color Atlas of Surgical Diagnosis, London, Mosby-Wolfe, 1996, p 202, Fig. 26-10.)*

Streptococcus pyogenes;
hyaluronidase → spread
through tissue

Fever, redness, tenderness,
swelling, painful
lymphadenopathy

Fatigue, shaking or chills,
sweating

Fibrin exudate covering
serosal surfaces (heart,
lungs, peritoneum)

Friction rub: pericarditis

Friction rub: pleuritis

Small bowel adhesions

Thin watery exudate

Blisters 2nd-degree burns,
viral pleuritis

Bacterial toxin-induced
mucosal injury → necrotic
membrane

Diphtheria;
pseudomembranous colitis
(*Clostridium difficile*)

Inflammation loss of
epithelial lining

Peptic ulcer; Herpes
genitalis/gingivitis

IL-1, TNF →
thermoregulatory centers
hypothalamus → synthesize
PGE$_2$

b. Group A streptococcus (e.g., *Streptococcus pyogenes*) is a common pathogen causing cellulitis. Hyaluronidase produced by the pathogen allows it to spread through tissue.

c. Signs (what the clinician observes) of cellulitis include fever, an expanding area of redness, tenderness, swelling, painful lymphadenopathy in areas of drainage, and red streaks, representing lymphatic spread of the infection.

d. Symptoms (what the patient complains about) of cellulitis include fatigue, shaking or chills, and sweating.

4. Fibrinous inflammation
   a. **Definition:** Fibrinous inflammation is inflammation that is due to increased vessel permeability, with deposition of a fibrin-rich exudate on the surface of the tissue (Fig. 3-8 C).
   b. Common locations include the serosal lining of the pericardium, peritoneum, or pleura.
   c. Clinical signs of fibrinous inflammation
      (1) Friction rub may be heard over the precordium in fibrinous pericarditis associated with a myocardial infarction or rheumatic fever (see Chapter 11).
      (2) Friction rub may be heard over the precordium or lungs in fibrinous pleuritis secondary to a pulmonary infarction or pneumonia (see Chapter 17).
      (3) Small bowel obstruction from serosal adhesions between other loops of bowel may occur from peritoneal irritation related to previous abdominal surgery (see Chapter 18). Adhesions frequently cause small bowel obstruction.

5. Serous inflammation
   a. **Definition:** Serous inflammation refers to inflammation associated with a thin, watery exudate that has an insufficient amount of fibrinogen to produce fibrin.
   b. Examples of serous inflammation include blisters in second-degree burns (Link 3-9) and viral pleuritis (inflammation of the pleura).

6. Pseudomembranous inflammation
   a. **Definition:** Pseudomembranous inflammation refers to a type of bacterial toxin-induced mucosal injury with a resulting shaggy membrane comprised of necrotic tissue.
   b. Examples include pseudomembranes associated with
      (1) *Clostridium difficile,* in pseudomembranous colitis (Fig. 3-8 D)
      (2) *Corynebacterium diphtheriae,* which produces a toxin resulting in a pseudomembrane formation involving the pharynx and trachea (see Fig. 17-5 D).

7. Ulcerative inflammation
   a. **Definition:** Ulcerative inflammation refers to inflammation that is associated with a loss of epithelial lining that may extend into the deeper connective tissues.
   b. Examples of ulcerative inflammation include peptic ulcer in the stomach (Fig. 3-9), ulcerative colitis, and an ulcer on the skin or mucous membranes (e.g., Herpes genitalis or gingivitis).

8. Granulomatous inflammation: discussed later

H. Pathogenesis and role of fever in AI
   1. Pathogenesis of fever. IL-1 and TNF stimulate the release of endogenous pyrogens from leukocytes and/or macrophages during inflammation that act on thermoregulatory centers in the hypothalamus to synthesize PGE$_2$ (vasodilator), leading to the production of fever (Link 3-10).

3-9: Ulcerative inflammation: peptic ulcer in the stomach. An ulcer represents a defect of the epithelial lining. Note the bleeding at the base of the ulcer. *(From my friend Ivan Damjanov, MD, PhD: Pathology for the Health Professions, 4th ed, Philadelphia, Saunders Elsevier, 2012, p 33, Fig. 2-16.)*

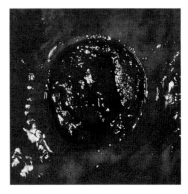

2. Beneficial effects of fever
    a. O_2-dissociation curve (ODC; see Chapter 2) is rightward shifted. More O_2 is available for the O_2-dependent MPO system.
    b. Provides a hostile environment for bacterial and viral reproduction.
3. Fever in children
    a. Most commonly caused by viral and bacterial infections.
    b. Common viral infections include common colds (MCC), croup, bronchiolitis, and gastroenteritis.
    c. Common bacterial infections include otitis media (MCC) and lower urinary tract infections (UTIs, urethritis, cystitis; usually females).
4. Fever in adults is most commonly due to viral upper respiratory infections (URIs; runny nose, sore throat, nonproductive cough) or viral gastrointestinal (GI) infections (nausea, vomiting, diarrhea).
5. Fever in hospitalized patients, is most commonly due to bacterial infections targeting the respiratory tract, urinary tract, or skin and soft tissue.
6. Fever in travelers recently in the tropics. Overall most common causes of fever in travelers recently returned from the tropics include malaria, typhoid fever, viral hepatitis, and dengue fever.
7. Fever of unknown origin (FUO)
    a. **Definition:** Fever of unknown origin is an illness characterized by temperatures > 38.3°C (101°F) on several occasions for >3 weeks with no known cause despite an extensive workup.
    b. Epidemiology
        (1) In descending order, the most common causes of an FUO are noninfectious inflammatory disease (22%; e.g., vasculitis, adult Still's disease), infection (17%; e.g., tuberculosis [TB], HIV, bacterial endocarditis), malignancy (7%; e.g., malignant lymphoma [especially non-Hodgkin lymphoma]), drug-induced fever (e.g., procainamide, penicillins, methyldopa, phenytoin), pulmonary embolus, alcoholic hepatitis, and other causes (e.g., inflammatory bowel disease, Crohn disease, ulcerative colitis).
        (2) Table 3-3 provides a summary of definitions and major features of four subtypes of FUO.

I. Termination of AI
1. AI mediators have a short half-life.
2. Lipoxins (LXA_4, LXB_4; antiinflammatory mediators) are synthesized from arachidonic acid metabolites.

Margin notes:
ODC rightward shift
↓Bacterial/viral reproduction
MCC viral/bacterial infections
Common cold (MCC), croup, bronchiolitis, gastroenteritis
Otitis media, UTIs (females)
URIs, GI viral infections
Respiratory, urinary, skin/soft tissue
Malaria, viral hepatitis, typhoid, dengue fever
Temp > 38.3°C (101°F) > 3 weeks, no known cause
Noninfectious inflammatory > infection > malignancy > other
Mediators short half-life
Lipoxins

TABLE 3-3 Major Features of Four Subtypes of Fever of Unknown Origin

FEATURE	CLASSIC	HEALTH CARE–ASSOCIATED (HCA)	IMMUNODEFICIENCY	HIV-RELATED
Definition	>38°C for >3 wks	>38°C for >1 wk; not present on admission	>38°C for >1 wk; negative cultures after 48 hrs	>38°C for >3 wks (outpatient) >1 wk (inpatient); HIV infection confirmed
Patient location	Community, clinic, hospital	Acute care hospital	Clinic, hospital	Community, clinic, hospital
Leading causes	Cancer, infections, inflammatory conditions	HCAI, postoperative complications, drug fever	Majority due to infections (documented only in 40%–60%)	HIV (primary infection), mycobacteria (typical/atypical), CMV, *Cryptococcus*, lymphoma, toxoplasmosis
Physical exam emphasis	Fundus, oropharynx, temporal artery, abdomen, lymph nodes, spleen, joints, skin, nails, genitalia, rectum, prostate, deep veins legs	Wounds, drains, devices, sinuses, urine	Skin folds, IV sites, lungs, perianal	Mouth, sinuses, skin, lymph nodes, eyes, lungs, perianal area
Investigation emphasis	Imaging, biopsies, ESR/CRP, skin tests	Imaging, bacterial cultures	CXR, bacterial cultures	Blood/lymphocyte count, serologic tests, CXR, stool exam, biopsies (marrow, lung, liver for culture/cytologic tests), brain imaging

CMV, Cytomegalovirus; *CRP,* C-reactive protein; *CXR,* chest x-ray; *ESR,* erythrocyte sedimentation rate; *FUO,* fever of unknown origin; *HCAI,* health care-associated infection; *HIV,* human immunodeficiency virus; *IV,* intravenous.
Modified from Ferri FF: *2014 Ferri's Clinical Advisor,* Philadelphia, Mosby Elsevier, 2017, p 472, Table F1-5.

a. Inhibit transmigration and chemotaxis of neutrophils.

b. Signal macrophages to phagocytose apoptotic bodies (see later).

3. Resolvins are synthesized from ω-3 fatty acids. Inhibit production and recruitment of inflammatory cells to the site of AI. Results in increased clearance of neutrophils by apoptosis (see later).

J. Consequences of AI

1. Complete resolution of AI. Occurs with mild injury to cells that have the capacity to enter the cell cycle (e.g., labile and stable cells). Examples: first-degree burn, bee sting.

2. Tissue destruction and scar formation. Destruction of tissue and scar tissue formation occurs with extensive injury or damage to permanent cells. Examples: third-degree burn, acute myocardial infarction

3. Abscess formation. An abscess is a localized collection of neutrophils with liquefactive necrosis. Example: a lung abscess may develop in bacterial pneumonias.

4. Fistula formation. A fistula refers to an open lumen connecting two hollow spaces. Examples: fistula between loops of bowel or between the vagina and rectum.

5. Progression of AI to chronic inflammation.

6. Fig. 3-10 summarizes clinical findings in AI.

II. Chronic Inflammation (CI)

A. Definition of CI

- Chronic inflammation refers to prolonged inflammation (weeks to years) that most often results from persistence of an injury-causing agent.

B. Causes of CI

1. Infection is the most common cause of CI. Examples: TB, leprosy.

2. Autoimmune disease. Examples: rheumatoid arthritis (RA), systemic lupus erythematosus (SLE).

Inhibit transmigration/chemotaxis

Enhance apoptosis

Inhibit recruitment inflammatory cells

Complete resolution AI

1st-degree burn, bee sting

Tissue destruction, scar formation

3rd-degree burn, acute myocardial infarction

Collection liquefied material (pus); lung abscess

Open lumen connecting two hollow spaces

Progression to chronic inflammation

Prolonged inflammation; persistence injury-causing agent

Infection MCC CI

TB, leprosy

Autoimmune disease: SLE, RA

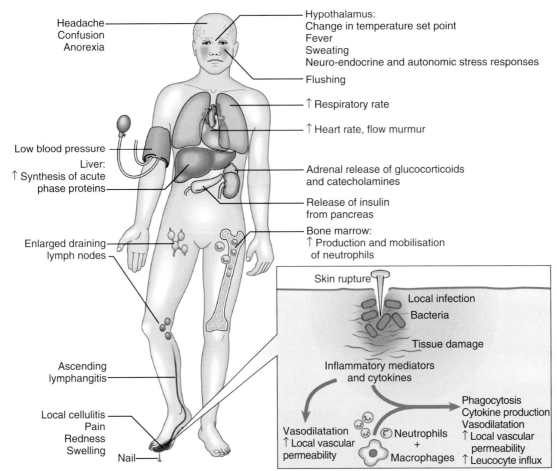

3-10: Summary slide of the clinical findings in acute inflammation using a penetrating injury as an example. *(From Walker BR, Colledge NR, Ralston SH, Penman ID: Davidson's Principles and Practice of Medicine, 22nd ed, Churchill Livingstone Elsevier, 2014, p 83, Fig. 4.8.)*

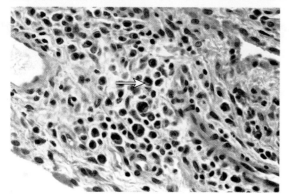

3-11: Chronic inflammation. This tissue shows an infiltrate of predominantly lymphocytes and occasional plasma cells (cells with eccentric nuclei and perinuclear clearing, *white arrow*). *(From my friend Ivan Damjanov, MD, PhD, Linder J: Anderson's Pathology, 10th ed, St. Louis, Mosby, 1996, p 390, Fig. 18-7B.)*

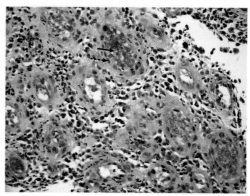

3-12: Granulation tissue. Note the mixture of acute (neutrophils) and chronic inflammatory cells (lymphocytes, plasma cells, macrophages) intermixed with dilated, newly formed blood vessels *(solid arrow)* filled with red blood cells. Numerous, plump endothelial cells *(interrupted arrow)* are also present. In normal tissue, these cells are usually inconspicuous. *(From King TS: Elsevier's Integrated Pathology, St. Louis, Mosby Elsevier, 2007, p 24, Fig. 2-4.)*

3. Inflammatory reaction to sterile agents. Examples: silica (silicosis in the lungs), uric acid (gout), silicone in breast implants, suture material.

> Silicosis, gout, silicone breast implants, suture material

C. **Morphology of CI**
   1. Cell types that define CI
      a. Monocytes and macrophages are the key cells. Other cells include lymphocytes, plasma cells, and eosinophils (Fig. 3-11; Link 3-11).

> Monocytes and/or macrophages: 1° leukocytes CI

      b. Transforming growth factor (TGF)-β is chemotactic for macrophages, lymphocytes, and fibroblasts.
   2. Destruction of parenchyma. With loss of parenchyma, there is loss of functional tissue, with repair by fibrosis.

> Loss parenchyma → loss functional tissue → repair by fibrosis

   3. Formation of granulation tissue
      a. **Definition:** Granulation tissue is a type of highly vascular tissue that is composed of blood vessels and activated fibroblasts (Fig. 3-12; Links 3-12 and 3-13).

> Vascular tissue composed blood vessels/fibroblasts

         (1) Blood vessels derive from preexisting blood vessels and de novo from EC precursors recruited from the bone marrow (i.e., angiogenesis). Important growth factors in angiogenesis include vascular endothelial cell growth factor (VEGF), fibroblast growth factor (FGF), epidermal growth factor (EGF), platelet-derived growth factor (PDGF), and TGF-β (see Table 3-5).

> Preexisting vessels/EC precursors from bone marrow
> VEGF, FGF, EGF, TGF-β

         (2) Vascularization is essential for normal wound healing.

> Vascularization essential

         (3) Granulation tissue is the precursor of scar tissue.

> Precursor of scar tissue

      b. Fibronectin is required for granulation tissue formation.

> Fibronectin required

         (1) **Definition:** Fibronectin is a cell adhesion glycoprotein located in the extracellular matrix (ECM) that binds to collagen, fibrin, and cell surface receptors (e.g., integrins).

> Adhesion glycoprotein ECM

         (2) Chemotactic factor that attracts fibroblasts (synthesize collagen) and ECs (form new blood vessels, angiogenesis).

> Chemotactic factor for fibroblasts/ECs

   4. Table 3-4 compares features of AI and CI.
   5. Granulomatous inflammation
      a. **Definition:** Granulomatous inflammation is a specialized type of CI characterized by the formation of granulomas.

> Specialized CI forming granulomas

      b. Causes of granulomatous inflammation
         (1) Infections
            • Examples: TB and systemic fungal infection (e.g., histoplasmosis). Infections caused by TB and systemic fungi are usually associated with caseous necrosis (i.e., soft granulomas; see Chapter 2). Caseous ("cheese-like") material is due to lipid released from the cell walls of dead pathogens.

> TB, systemic fungi (e.g., histoplasmosis)

         (2) Noninfectious causes of granulomatous inflammation
            • Examples: sarcoidosis and Crohn disease. Sarcoidosis and Crohn disease have noncaseating granulomas (i.e., hard granulomas), with no central areas of necrosis.

> Sarcoidosis, Crohn disease

      c. Morphology of a granuloma
         (1) **Definition:** A granuloma is a pale, white nodule composed of activated macrophages (epithelioid cells) with or without a central area of caseation.

> Nodule composed of epithelioid cells with/without central caseation

TABLE 3-4 Comparison of Acute and Chronic Inflammation

FEATURE	ACUTE INFLAMMATION	CHRONIC INFLAMMATION
Pathogenesis	Microbial pathogens, trauma, burns	Persistent AI, foreign bodies (e.g., silicone, glass), autoimmune disease, certain types of infection (e.g., TB, leprosy)
Primary cells involved	Neutrophils	Monocytes/macrophages (key cells), B and T lymphocytes, plasma cells, fibroblasts
Primary mediators	Histamine (key mediator), prostaglandins, leukotrienes	Cytokines (e.g., IL-1), growth factors
Necrosis	Present	Less prominent
Scar tissue	Absent	Present
Onset	Immediate	Delayed
Duration	Few days	Weeks, months, years
Outcome	Complete resolution, progression to chronic inflammation, abscess formation	Scar tissue formation, disability, amyloidosis (see Chapter 4)
Main immunoglobulin (Ig)	IgM	IgG
SPE effect	Mild hypoalbuminemia	Polyclonal gammopathy; greater degree of hypoalbuminemia
Peripheral blood leukocyte response	Neutrophilic leukocytosis	Monocytosis

AI, Acute inflammation; *IL,* interleukin; *SPE,* serum protein electrophoresis; *TB,* tuberculosis.

Well-circumscribed

Epithelioid cells, CD4T$_H$1 cells, multinucleated giant cells

TNF-α/IFN-γ formation/ maintenance granulomas

TNF-α inhibitors: dissemination disease (TB)

Parenchymal cell regeneration/repair by fibrosis

Labile cells (stem cells)/ stable cells (fibroblasts, smooth muscle cells) can replicate

Permanent cells *cannot* regenerate (cardiac/striated muscle)

Depends on parenchymal cell regeneration/migration

G$_0$: Resting phase of stable cells

G$_1$: Growth phase

G$_1$: Most variable phase

G$_1$: Synthesis RNA, protein, organelles (mitochondria, ribosomes), cyclin D

S: Synthesis of DNA, RNA, protein

G$_2$: Synthesis tubulin for mitotic spindle

M: Two daughter cells produced

G$_1$ to S: Most critical phase

(2) Usually well-circumscribed in tissue (see Fig. 2-16 G, H).

(3) Cell types in an infectious granuloma (e.g., TB) include epithelioid cells (activated macrophages), CD4T$_H$1 cells, and multinucleated giant cells (fusion of the nuclei of epithelioid cells into one giant cell) (Links 3-14 and 3-15).

(4) TNF-α is important in the formation and maintenance of granulomas seen in TB and systemic fungal infections. TNF-α and IFN-γ recruit cells for granuloma formation. TNF-α inhibitors (e.g., infliximab, a monoclonal antibody against TNF-α) cause the breakdown of granulomas, which may result in dissemination of disease (e.g., disseminated TB).

(5) Specifics concerning the sequence of events in the formation of a granuloma are fully discussed in Chapter 4 under type IV hypersensitivity reactions.

III. **Tissue Repair**

A. **Factors involved in tissue repair include** parenchymal cell regeneration and repair by connective tissue (fibrosis).

B. **Parenchymal cell regeneration**

1. Cell regeneration depends on the ability of cells to replicate (divide; see Chapter 2).

   a. Labile cells (e.g., stem cells in epidermis) and stable cells (e.g., fibroblasts, smooth muscle cells) can replicate.

   b. Permanent cells (e.g., cardiac muscle and striated muscle) *cannot* regenerate. When damaged, cardiac and striated muscle are replaced by scar tissue (fibrosis).

2. Cell regeneration depends on factors that stimulate parenchymal cell division and migration. Stimulatory factors include loss of tissue and production of growth factors (Table 3-5).

3. Cell cycle (simplified; Fig. 3-13)

   a. Phases of the cell cycle

      (1) **Definition:** G$_0$ phase is the resting phase of stable parenchymal cells.

      (2) **Definition:** G$_1$ phase is the growth phase of the cell cycle. Most variable phase in the cell cycle. There is synthesis of RNA, protein, organelles (e.g., mitochondria, ribosomes), and cyclin D.

      (3) S (synthesis) phase. **Definition:** Phase where there is synthesis of DNA, RNA, and protein.

      (4) G$_2$ phase. **Definition:** Phase where there is synthesis of tubulin, which is required to produce microtubules in the mitotic spindle.

      (5) M (mitotic) phase. **Definition:** Phase where two daughter cells are produced.

   b. Regulation of the G$_1$ checkpoint (G$_1$ to S phase)

      (1) Most critical phase of the cell cycle. Mutations in genes that enter the S phase are copied, hence the risk for cancer.

TABLE 3-5   Factors Involved in Tissue Repair

FACTOR	FUNCTIONS
Growth Factors	
Vascular endothelial cell growth factor (VEGF)	• Stimulates angiogenesis (embryonic angiogenesis, particularly in the heart), repair of tissue, cancer angiogenesis (stimulates from preexisting vessels) • Stimulation factors: TNF released by macrophages, hypoxia via hypoxia-inducible factor released by cells
Fibroblast growth factor (FGF)	• Chemotactic for fibroblasts; stimulates keratinocyte migration, angiogenesis, wound contraction
Epidermal growth factor (EGF)	• Stimulates keratinocyte migration, granulation tissue formation
Platelet-derived growth factor (PDGF)	• Chemotactic for neutrophils, macrophages, fibroblasts, endothelial cells (angiogenesis), smooth muscle cells (angiogenesis)
Transforming growth factor-β (TGF-β)	• Chemotactic for macrophages, lymphocytes, fibroblasts, smooth muscle cells (angiogenesis)
Interleukins (ILs), Cytokines	
IL-1	• Stimulates synthesis of metalloproteinases (i.e., enzymes containing trace metals; e.g., zinc) • Stimulates synthesis and release of acute phase reactants (APRs) from the liver
Tumor necrosis factor (TNF)	• Activates macrophages; stimulates release of APRs

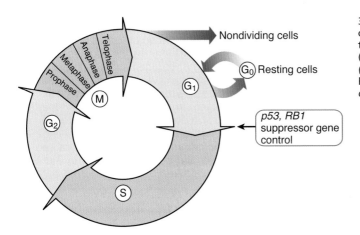

3-13: Cell cycle. The G_1 to S phase is the most critical phase of the cell cycle and is controlled by the *p53* and *RB1* suppressor genes. (See more detailed discussion in the text.) *(Modified from Burns E, Cave D:* Rapid Review: Histology and Cell Biology, *Philadelphia, Mosby, 2004, p 36, Fig. 3-5.)*

(2) Control proteins include cyclin-dependent kinase 4 (Cdk4) and cyclin D.
  (a) Growth factors activate nuclear transcribing proto-oncogenes (see Chapter 9) to produce cyclin D and Cdk4.
  (b) Cyclin D binds to Cdk4, forming a complex causing the cell to enter the S phase.
(3) Role of the *RB1* (retinoblastoma) suppressor gene in the cell cycle
  (a) RB1 protein product arrests the cell in the G_1 phase.
  (b) Cdk4 phosphorylates the RB1 protein, causing the cell to enter S phase. If the *RB1* protein is *not* phosphorylated, the cell remains in the G_1 phase.
(4) Role of the *p53* suppressor gene in the cell cycle
  (a) p53 protein product arrests the cell in G_1 phase by inhibiting Cdk4. Inhibition of Cdk4 prevents RB1 protein phosphorylation, which provides time for repair of damaged DNA in the cell.
  (b) In the event that there is excessive DNA damage, the *p53* suppressor gene produces protein products that inhibit the translation of the *BCL-2* antiapoptosis genes, which leads to apoptosis of the cell, or inhibits the translation of growth-promoting genes (e.g., *MYC* proto-oncogene; see Chapter 9), leading to growth arrest.
  (c) Absence of the *p53* gene product allows the cell to enter the S phase of the cell cycle.
  (d) Approximately 70% of human cancers are associated with a mutation causing loss of *p53* gene activity.
  c. Sites of action in the cell cycle of various chemotherapeutic agents (Link 3-16)

Cdk4, cyclin D

RB1 product arrests cell G_1 phase

Cdk4 phosphorylates *RB1* protein→ cell enter S phase

p53 protein product → inhibits Cdk4 (cell arrested G_1 phase)

p53 protein products → initiates apoptosis, initiates growth arrest

Absence of *p53* gene product → allows cell to enter S phase

≈70% human cancers loss *p53* gene activity

4. Restoration to normal
   a. Restoration to normal requires preservation of the basement membrane and a relatively intact ECM (e.g., collagen, adhesive proteins).
   b. Laminin, the key adhesion protein in the basement membrane, interacts with type IV collagen, cell surface receptors, and components in the ECM.

C. **Repair by connective tissue (fibrosis)**
   1. Repair by connective tissue occurs when injury is severe or persistent. Tissue in a third-degree burn *cannot* be restored to normal, owing to loss of skin, basement membrane, and connective tissue infrastructure.
   2. Steps in normal connective tissue repair
      a. Repair requires neutrophil transmigration (see previous discussion) to liquefy injured tissue and then macrophages to remove the debris.
      b. Repair requires formation of granulation tissue, the precursor of scar tissue (see earlier discussion). Granulation tissue accumulates in the ECM and eventually produces dense fibrotic tissue (scar).
      c. Repair requires the initial production of type III collagen. Type III collagen has poor tensile strength; hence, the wound can easily be reopened.

> **Definition: Collagen** is the major fibrous component of connective tissue. Tropocollagen, the structural unit of collagen, is a triple helix of α-chains. Tropocollagen undergoes extensive posttranslational modification. Hydroxylation reactions in the rough endoplasmic reticulum convert proline to hydroxyproline and lysine to hydroxylysine. **Ascorbic acid** is required in these hydroxylation reactions. Hydroxyproline residues produce bonds that stabilize the triple helix in the tropocollagen molecule. Hydroxylysine residues are oxidized to form an aldehyde residue that produces covalent cross-links at staggered intervals between adjacent tropocollagen molecules. Lysyl oxidase is a metalloproteinase enzyme containing copper that mediates the cross-linking of tropocollagen molecules. Cross-linking increases the overall tensile strength of collagen (also elastic tissue). Type I collagen in skin, bone, and tendons has the greatest tensile strength, whereas type III collagen, the initial collagen in wound repair, has poor tensile strength (fewer cross-links than type I collagen). Cross-linking of collagen and elastic tissue increases with age; thus there is decreased elasticity of skin, joints, and blood vessels in older individuals. The decreased elasticity of blood vessels results in vessel instability and rupture with minor trauma (e.g., senile purpura; see Chapter 15). Decreased cross-linking (e.g., vitamin C deficiency) reduces the tensile strength of collagen. In vitamin C deficiency, the structurally weakened collagen is responsible for a bleeding diathesis (e.g., bleeding into skin and joints) and poor wound healing (see Chapter 7). **Ehlers-Danlos syndrome** is a group of mendelian disorders characterized by defects of type I and type III collagen synthesis and structure. Clinical findings include hypermobile joints, aortic dissection (most common cause of death), mitral valve prolapse, bleeding into the skin (ecchymoses), rupture of the bowel, and poor wound healing (Fig. 3-14; Link 3-17).

      d. Dense scar tissue produced from granulation tissue contains type III collagen (weak collagen) that must be remodeled.
         (1) Remodeling increases the tensile strength of scar tissue.
         (2) Metalloproteinases (collagenases containing zinc) replace type III collagen with type I collagen (strong collagen), which increases the tensile strength of the wound to ≈70% to 80% of the original after ≈3 months. Scar tissue after 3 months is primarily composed of acellular connective tissue that is devoid of inflammatory cells and adnexal structures and is surfaced by an intact epidermis.
   3. Primary, secondary, and tertiary intention wound healing (Box 3-1)
      a. Healing by primary intention (Fig. 3-15 top; Link 3-18)
         • **Definition:** Wound healing by primary intention refers to approximation of the wound edges by simple suturing, skin graft replacement, or flap closure. Reserved for the healing of clean surgical wounds.
      b. Healing by secondary (spontaneous) intention wound healing (Fig. 3-15 bottom; Link 3-19)
         • **Definition:** Wound healing by secondary intention refers to leaving the wound open and allowing it to close by reepithelialization, which results in contraction and eventual closure of the wound. Reserved for highly contaminated wounds.
      c. Healing by tertiary intention (delayed primary closure)
         • **Definition:** Wound healing by tertiary intention refers to a contaminated wound that is initially treated (Rx) with repeated débridement and topical or systemic antibiotics for several days to control infection. Once the wound is considered ready for closure, surgical intervention (i.e., suturing, skin graft replacement, flap) is performed.

D. **Factors that impair wound healing**
   1. Persistent infection
      a. Most common cause of impaired wound healing.
      b. *Staphylococcus aureus* is the most common pathogen.

Margin notes (left column):

Intact basement membrane; intact ECM

Laminin: key adhesion glycoprotein in basement membrane

3rd-degree burn → tissue *cannot* be restored to normal

Neutrophil transmigration → liquefy debris; macrophages → remove debris

Granulation tissue essential normal connective tissue repair

Granulation tissue → scar tissue

Type III collagen in early wound repair; poor tensile strength

Remodeling ↑ tensile strength scar tissue

Metalloproteinases replace type III with type I collagen; 80% tensile strength

Acellular; lacks inflammatory cells/adnexal structures; intact epidermis

Clean wound approximated by suturing

Contaminated wound left open for reepithelialization

Delayed primary closure

Contaminated wound débrided

Infection MCC impaired wound healing

S. aureus MC pathogen causing wound infection

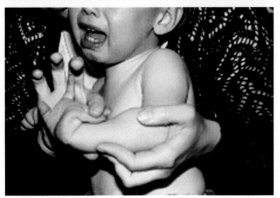

3-14: Ehlers-Danlos syndrome. In this child, note the hyperextension of the fingers so that they are parallel to the extensor surface of the forearm. This is a classic sign of Ehlers-Danlos syndrome. (From Taylor S, Raffles A: Diagnosis in Color Pediatrics, London, Mosby-Wolfe, 1997, p 257, Fig. 10-4.)

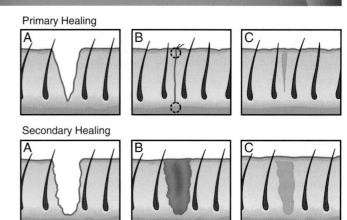

3-15: Wound closure types. Top, Primary (or first) intention closure. A clean incision is made in the tissue (A) and the wound edges are reapproximated (B) with sutures, staples, or adhesive strips. Minimal scarring is the end result (C). Bottom, Healing by secondary intention. The wound is left open to heal (A, B) by a combination of contraction, granulation, and epithelialization. A large scar results (C). (From Townsend C: Sabiston Textbook of Surgery, 18th ed, Philadelphia, Saunders Elsevier, 2008, p 192, Fig. 8-1.)

BOX 3-1   Wound Healing by Primary, Secondary, Tertiary Intention

Primary Intention
Day 1: Fibrin clot (hematoma) develops. Neutrophils infiltrate the wound margins (PDGF chemotactic to neutrophils); increased mitotic activity of basal cells of squamous epithelium in the opposing wound margins (FGF, EGF involved in keratinocyte migration).
Day 2: Squamous cells from apposing basal cell layers migrate under the fibrin clot and seal off the wound after 48 hours. Macrophages migrate into the wound (PDGF, TGF-β chemotactic to macrophages).
Day 3: Granulation tissue begins to form (FGF, EGF, PDGF, TGF-β all involved in angiogenesis). Initial deposition of type III collagen by fibroblasts begins but does *not* bridge the incision site (FGF, PDGF, TGF-β chemotactic to fibroblasts). Macrophages replace neutrophils.
Days 4–6: Granulation tissue formation peaks; collagen bridges the incision site.
Week 2: Collagen compresses blood vessels in fibrous tissue, resulting in reduced blood flow. Tensile strength is ≈10%.
Month 1: Collagenase remodeling of the wound occurs (breaks peptide bonds), with degradation of type III collagen and replacement by type I collagen. Tensile strength increases, reaching ≈80% within 3 months. Scar tissue is devoid of adnexal structures (e.g., hair, sweat glands) and inflammatory cells.

Secondary Intention
Typically, these wounds heal differently from primary intention:
- More intense inflammatory reaction than primary healing
- Increased amount of granulation tissue formation than in primary healing
- Wound contraction caused by increased numbers of myofibroblasts

Tertiary Intention
Contaminated wound is initially treated with débridement and antibiotics followed by surgical wound closure (suture, skin graft replacement, flap).

EGF, Epidermal growth factor; *FGF,* fibroblast growth factor; *PDGF,* platelet-derived growth factor; *TGF,* transforming growth factor.

c. Nosocomial and community-acquired methicillin-resistant *S. aureus* (MRSA) wound infections are increasing.
  (1) MRSA strains are resistant to β-lactam antibiotics (e.g., penicillin, cephalosporin).
  (2) Disruption of skin and malnutrition are the greatest risk factors for wound infections.
  (3) Key to preventing wound infections is proper hand washing. Approximately 20% to 40% of people are carriers of MRSA in their anterior nares.
  (4) Majority of community-acquired MRSA (CA-MRSA) infections produce the Panton-Valentine leukocidin.
    (a) Accelerates apoptosis of neutrophils, hence decreasing the number of neutrophils available in the wounds to phagocytose and destroy the bacteria
    (b) Causes the infection to progress to necrotizing fasciitis (see Chapter 24)

MSRA: methicillin-resistant *S. aureus*

Skin disruption/malnutrition ↑↑ risk wound infection

Proper hand washing

20%–40% people carry MRSA in anterior nares

Produce Panton-Valentine leukocidin

Accelerates neutrophil apoptosis

Danger for developing necrotizing fasciitis

Susceptibility to infection: ↓blood flow, ↑tissue glucose levels

2. Diabetes mellitus. Increases susceptibility to infection by decreasing blood flow to tissue and by increasing tissue levels of glucose.

3. Nutritional deficiencies that impair wound healing

Malnutrition

a. Protein deficiency (e.g., malnutrition)

Vitamin C deficiency

b. Vitamin C deficiency (see earlier discussion)

Trace metal deficiency

c. Trace metal deficiency (see Chapter 8)

↓Copper: ↓cross-linking of collagen

(1) Copper deficiency leads to decreased cross-linking in collagen (also in elastic tissue).

↓Zinc: ↑type III collagen; ↓tensile strength

(2) Zinc deficiency leads to defects in removal of type III collagen in wound remodeling. Type III collagen has decreased tensile strength, which impairs wound healing.

4. Glucocorticoids

↓Collagen formation, ↓tensile strength

a. Interfere with collagen formation and decrease tensile strength

Prevent excessive scar formation

b. Clinically useful in preventing excessive scar formation

(1) Dexamethasone is used along with antibiotics to prevent scar formation in bacterial meningitis.

(2) Plastic surgeons inject high-potency steroids into wounds to prevent excessive scar tissue formation.

c. Other effects of glucocorticoids

↓ Production of IL-1, IL-6, TNF, prostaglandins, histamine

(1) Inhibit production of cytokines (including IL-1, IL-6, and TNF) and other inflammatory mediators (e.g., histamine, prostaglandins).

Dexamethasone reduces the amount of cytokines (e.g., TNF-α and IL-1 in the cerebrospinal fluid) and has been associated with decreased inflammation, decreased cerebral edema, and lower rates of hearing loss.

↓Cytokines; ↓cerebral edema/hearing loss

(2) Reduce vasodilation in response to inflammatory mediators, which reduces the accumulation of cells and fluid in the interstitial space (reduces swelling).

Apoptosis of lymphocytes

(3) Reduce the immune cell response by inducing apoptosis of lymphocytes.

5. Keloids and hypertrophic scars

Raised scars extending beyond borders of original wound

a. **Definition:** Keloids are raised scars that grow *beyond* the borders of the original wound (Fig. 3-16; Link 3-20).

• Develop in 15% to 20% of African Americans, Asians, and Hispanics, suggesting a genetic predisposition. Often refractory to medical and surgical intervention.

Raised scar remaining in confines of original wound; frequently regress spontaneously

b. **Definition:** Hypertrophic scars are raised scars that remain *within* the confines of the original wound. Frequently regress spontaneously.

c. Normal scars have collagen bundles that are randomly arrayed (not all in the same direction), whereas keloids and hypertrophic scars have stretched collagen bundles arranged in the *same plane* as the epidermis.

E. **Repair in other tissues** (Link 3-21)

1. Liver

a. Mild injury (e.g., hepatitis A). Regeneration of hepatocytes with restoration to normal is possible if the cytoarchitecture is intact.

b. Severe or persistent injury (e.g., hepatitis C)

Regenerative nodules/ fibrosis; danger of cirrhosis

(1) Regenerative nodules develop that show twinning of liver cell plates (two cells thick). Double line of hepatocytes is present and nuclei seem to run in parallel (Fig. 3-17).

Twinning liver cell plates (two cells thick)

(2) Portal triads are *not* present in regenerative nodules.

Absence portal triads

Increased fibrosis → cirrhosis

(3) Increased fibrosis occurs around the regenerative nodules, which leads to cirrhosis of the liver if the injurious agent is not removed (see Chapter 19).

2. Lung

Type II pneumocyte repair cell; synthesizes surfactant

• Type II pneumocytes are the key repair cells of the lung and also synthesize surfactant (keeps alveoli from collapsing). Type II pneumocytes also replace damaged type I and type II pneumocytes.

3. Brain

Proliferation astrocytes (gliosis)/microglial cells

a. Astrocytes proliferate in response to an injury (e.g., brain infarction). Proliferation of astrocytes is called gliosis.

Microglial cells (macrophages) remove debris

b. Microglial cells (macrophages) are scavenger cells that remove debris (e.g., myelin).

4. Peripheral nerve transection (Link 3-22)

a. Without innervation, muscle atrophies in ≈15 days.

Distal degeneration axon/ myelin sheath

b. After nerve transection, there is distal degeneration of the axon and myelin sheath (wallerian degeneration) and proximal axonal degeneration up to the next node of Ranvier.

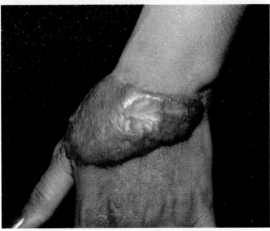

3-16: Keloid formation. Note the raised, thickened scar over the dorsum of the hand. Unlike a hypertrophic scar, keloids grow beyond the borders of the original wound and are refractive to medical and surgical therapy. *(From Lookingbill D, Marks J:* Principles of Dermatology, *3rd ed, Philadelphia, Saunders, 2000, p 115, Fig. 8-5A.)*

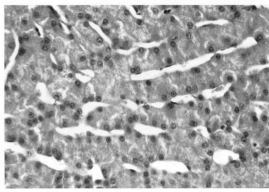

3-17: Regenerative nodule in liver injury. Note the twinning of cell plates. The plates are thicker than normal, owing to division of hepatocytes. A double row of nuclei along each hepatocyte plate is evident. Portal triads are not present in regenerative nodules. *(From MacSween R, Burt A, Portmann B, Ishak K, Scheuer P, Anthony P:* Pathology of the Liver, *4th ed, London, Churchill Livingstone, 2002, p 590, Fig. 13.6.)*

(1) Macrophages and Schwann cells phagocytose axonal/myelin debris.
(2) Nerve cell body undergoes central chromatolysis.
   (a) Nerve cell body swells.
   (b) Nissl bodies (composed of rough endoplasmic reticulum and free ribosomes) disappear centrally, and the nucleus moves to the periphery.

> Nerve body swells; Nissl bodies disappear; nucleus moves peripherally

(3) Schwann cells proliferate in the distal stump and are the key cell in establishing reinnervation.

> Schwann cell key in reinnervation

(4) Axonal sprouts develop in the proximal stump and extend distally using the Schwann cells for guidance.
(5) Regenerated axon grows 2 to 3 mm/day.
(6) Axon becomes remyelinated.
(7) Muscle is eventually reinnervated.

  5. Heart
    a. Cardiac muscle is permanent tissue.

> Permanent tissue

    b. Damaged muscle is replaced by noncontractile scar tissue.

> Repair by fibrosis

  6. Skeletal muscle after exercise
    a. After exercise, there is damage to the sarcomeres in the skeletal muscle.
      Sarcomere is the basic unit of a skeletal muscle and gives skeletal muscle its striated appearance.

> Damage to sarcomeres in skeletal muscle

> Sarcomere basic unit of muscle

    b. Satellite cells are stem cells that repair and form new myofibers in sarcomeres that have been damaged by mechanical strain.

> Satellite cells: stem cells repair/form new myofibers

IV. Laboratory Findings Associated with Inflammation
  A. Leukocyte and plasma alterations
    1. AI (e.g., bacterial infection)
      a. Absolute neutrophilic leukocytosis (Fig. 3-18)
        (1) Absolute means that the actual number of neutrophils increases in the bone marrow and the peripheral blood (discussed more extensively in Chapter 13).

> Total # neutrophils increased

        (2) Various cytokines (e.g., IL-1) release the postmitotic pool of neutrophils (metamyelocytes, band neutrophils, segmented neutrophils) from the bone marrow causing an absolute neutrophilic leukocytosis.

> IL-1 releases postmitotic pool neutrophils from bone marrow

        (3) Presence of increased numbers of band neutrophils (usually >10%) and occasional metamyelocytes is called a left-shifted smear.

> ↑Band neutrophils (>10%)

      b. Toxic granulation is present.
        (1) **Definition:** Toxic granulation refers to the presence of dark blue to purple primary granules in metamyelocytes, bands, and segmented neutrophils (see Fig. 3-18). Primary granules begin forming in the promyelocyte stage of neutrophil development.

> Dark blue/purple 1° granules in neutrophils

> Abnormality in maturation 1° granule

        (2) Toxic granulation is due to an abnormality in the maturation of the primary granules. Occurs in severe inflammatory conditions (infectious and noninfectious).

> Sign severe inflammatory condition

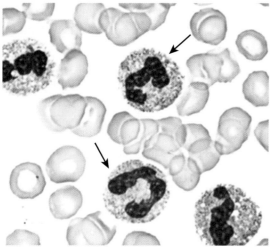

3-18: Absolute leukocytosis with left shift. Arrows point to band (stab) neutrophils, which exhibit prominence of the azurophilic granules (toxic granulation). Vacuoles in the cytoplasm represent phagolysosomes. A left shift is due to accelerated release of post-mitotic neutrophils from the bone marrow and is defined as >10% band neutrophils or the presence of earlier precursors (e.g., meta-myelocytes). *(From Hoffbrand I, Pettit J, Vyas P: Color Atlas of Clinical Hematology, 4th ed, Philadelphia, Mosby Elsevier, 2010, p 162, Fig. 10-13A.)*

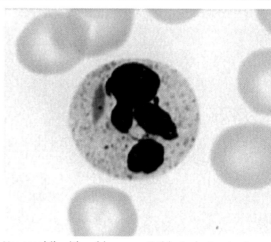

3-19: Neutrophil with a blue-gray Döhle inclusion body and toxic granulation in the cytosol. *(From Naeim, F: Atlas of Bone Marrow and Blood Pathology, Philadelphia, Saunders, 2001, p 28, Fig. 2-23G.)*

Gray-blue inclusions in neutrophils

Stacks of rough endoplasmic reticulum

IgM predominant immunoglobulin in AI

Isotype switching; IgM becomes IgG

CI: absolute monocytosis

CI: ↑serum IgG

Corticosteroid therapy: neutrophilic leukocytosis

Marginating pool → circulating pool

Bone marrow release postmitotic pool

↓B/T lymphocytes, monocytes, eosinophils by apoptosis

APR: opsonin enhances neutrophil phagocytosis

CRP: marker of necrosis in AI

↑Inflammatory plaques; bacterial/fungal infections

Excellent monitor disease activity (e.g., RA)

c. Döhle bodies are present in neutrophils (Fig. 3-19).
   (1) **Definition:** Döhle bodies are round to oval, pale, grayish blue inclusions that are found in the cytoplasm of neutrophils. Electron microscopy shows that they consist of stacks of rough endoplasmic reticulum.
   (2) Commonly seen in conjunction with toxic granulation.
d. Serum IgM is increased.
   (1) In AI, serum IgM peaks in 7 to 10 days. Predominant immunoglobulin in AI.
   (2) Isotype switching (immunoglobulin class change) occurs in plasma cells, leading to replacement of IgM by IgG in 12 to 14 days. In isotype switching, plasma cells replace the μ heavy chains in IgM with γ heavy chains to produce IgG.
2. Chronic inflammation (CI; e.g., TB, RA)
   a. Absolute monocytosis is the primary leukocyte finding in CI.
   b. Increased serum IgG is the key finding in CI.
3. Table 3-6 summarizes the types of cells involved in inflammation (Fig. 3-20 A–D).
4. Peripheral blood findings associated with corticosteroid therapy
   a. Neutrophilic leukocytosis (increase in total number of neutrophils)
      (1) Corticosteroids inhibit activation of neutrophil adhesion molecules (see previous discussion); therefore, the marginating pool (neutrophils attached to ECs; see Table 3-6) becomes part of the circulating pool.
      (2) Corticosteroids increase the bone marrow release of neutrophils from the postmitotic pool (metamyelocytes, band neutrophils [stabs], neutrophils; see Table 3-6).
   b. Decrease in the number of B and T cells, eosinophils, and monocytes in the peripheral blood. Corticosteroids are a signal for apoptosis of these cells.
B. **C-reactive protein (CRP)**
   1. **Definition:** CRP is an APR that acts as an opsonin by attaching to bacteria, thereby enhancing neutrophil phagocytosis.
   2. Measurement of serum CRP is clinically useful.
      a. CRP is a very sensitive indicator of necrosis associated with AI.
         (1) Levels of CRP increase within 6 hours of an inflammatory stimulus and levels fall promptly when the stimulus is removed.
         (2) CRP is increased in inflammatory (disrupted) atherosclerotic plaques (useful tool in cardiology) and in bacterial and fungal infections.
         (3) CRP is *not* significantly increased in AI due to SLE, systemic sclerosis, ulcerative colitis, leukemia and viral infections (exception for upper respiratory infections due to influenza, adenovirus, or rhinovirus).
      b. CRP is an excellent monitor of disease activity (e.g., rheumatoid arthritis [RA]).

TABLE 3-6 Summary of Leukocytes (Also Useful for Chapter 4)

CELL	CELL CHARACTERISTICS

Neutrophil (see Fig. 3-18)	Key cell in acute inflammation
	Receptors for IgG and C3b: important in phagocytosis of opsonized bacteria
	Primary or azurophilic granules contain myeloperoxidase, bactericidal/permeability-increasing (BPI) protein, defensins, and the serine proteases neutrophil elastase and cathepsin G
	Secondary granules contain lysozyme, collagenase, lactoferrin, alkaline phosphatase, NADPH oxidase, and cathelicidin (group of antimicrobial peptides)
	Bone marrow neutrophil pools
	  Mitotic pool: myeloblasts, promyelocytes, myelocytes
	  Postmitotic pool: metamyelocytes, band neutrophils (stabs), segmented neutrophils
	Peripheral blood neutrophil pools
	  Marginating pool: adherent to the endothelium; account for ≈50% of peripheral blood pool (higher percentage in black population)
	  Circulating pool: measured in complete blood cell count; account for ≈50% of peripheral blood pool (lower percentage in black population)
	Causes of neutrophilic leukocytosis
	  Infections (e.g., acute appendicitis)
	  Sterile inflammation with necrosis (e.g., acute myocardial infarction)
	  Drugs inhibiting neutrophil adhesion molecules: corticosteroids, catecholamines

Monocytes and macrophages (see Figs. 3-20A and 13-2D)	Key cells in chronic inflammation
	Receptors for IgG and C3b
	Monocytes become macrophages: fixed (e.g., macrophages in red pulp of spleen), wandering (e.g., alveolar macrophages)
	Functions: phagocytosis, process antigen, enhance host immunologic response (secrete cytokines like IL-1, TNF)
	Causes of monocytosis
	  Chronic inflammation
	  Autoimmune disease
	  Malignancy

Plasma cells (see Figs. 3-11 and 3-20B, C)	Antibody producing cells derived from B cells (see Fig. 3-20B) Morphology: well-developed rough endoplasmic reticulum (site of protein synthesis; see Fig. 3-20 C). Bright blue cytoplasmic staining with Wright-Giemsa. Nucleus eccentrically located and has perinuclear clearing.
Mast cells and basophils (see Fig. 3-2)	Release mediators in acute inflammation and allergic reactions (type I HSR)Receptors for IgE Early release reaction: release of preformed mediators (i.e., histamine, chemotactic factors, proteases) Late phase reaction: new synthesis and release of prostaglandins and leukotrienes, which enhance and prolong the acute inflammatory process

Eosinophils (see Figs. 3-20D and 13-2 A)	Receptors for IgE
	Red granules contain crystalline material. Become Charcot-Leyden crystals in the sputum of asthmatics.
	Preformed chemical mediators in granules
	  Major basic protein (MBP) kills invasive helminths.
	  Histaminase neutralizes histamine.
	  Arylsulfatase neutralizes leukotrienes.
	Functions of eosinophils
	  Modulate type I HSRs by neutralizing histamine and leukotrienes
	  Destruction of invasive helminths: IgE receptors interact with IgE coating the surface of invasive helminths → antibody dependent cytotoxicity reaction (type II hypersensitivity reaction) causes the release of MBP → kills helminths
	Causes of eosinophilia
	  Type I HSRs: allergic rhinitis, bronchial asthma.
	  Invasive helminthic infections *excluding* pinworms and adult worms in ascariasis, which are not invasive
	  Dientamoeba fragilis: only protozoan that produces eosinophilia

Ig, Immunoglobulin; *HSR,* hypersensitivity reaction; *IL,* interleukin; *MBP,* major basic protein; *NADPH,* reduced nicotinamide adenine dinucleotide phosphate; *TNF,* tumor necrosis factor.

  C. Erythrocyte sedimentation rate

    1. **Definition:** The erythrocyte sedimentation rate (ESR) is the rate (in mm/hr) of settling of RBCs in a vertical tube containing anticoagulated blood. Unlike CRP, the ESR is an indirect measure of inflammation.

        ESR: rate settling RBCs vertical tube mm/hr

    2. RBCs have negatively charged cell membranes, which prevent them from sticking to each other in the circulation; hence, their rate of sedimentation in a vertical tube containing an anticoagulant is minimal (normal ESR) in a normal hematologic state. Sedimentation refers to the settling of particles (e.g., RBCs) in a fluid (e.g., plasma).

        RBCs negatively charged membranes → repel each other

    3. Plasma proteins (e.g., fibrinogen [FG], immunoglobulins [Igs]) have a positive charge; however, in a normal hematologic state, it is *not* great enough to overcome the normal sedimentation of negatively charged RBCs.

        FG, Igs: + charge
        Fewer RBCs (anemia) → less impedance to settle → ↑ESR

    4. RBC disorders that increase the ESR. In anemia, where there is a decrease in the total number of RBCs, there is less impedance to prevent their settling in a vertical tube.

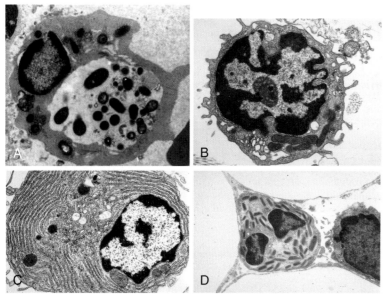

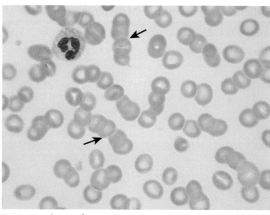

3-21: Rouleaux formation. The arrows show red blood cells stacked like coins. This is due to an increase in fibrinogen and/or immunoglobulins. *(From Goldman L, Schafer AI: Goldman-Cecil Medicine, 25th ed, Philadelphia, Saunders, 2016, p 1055, Fig. 157-18.)*

3-20: A, Macrophage. Note the phagocytic debris in the cytosol. **B,** Lymphocyte. Note the large nucleus and scant cytoplasm. **C,** Plasma cell. Note the extensive rough endoplasmic reticulum and dark globules of immunoglobulin in the cytosol. **D,** Eosinophil. Note the crystalline material in the cytosol that becomes Charcot-Leyden crystals in sputum of asthmatics. *(A–D courtesy of my friend William Meek, PhD, Professor and Vice Chairman of Anatomy and Cell Biology, Oklahoma State University, Center for Health Sciences, Tulsa, Oklahoma.)*

Abnormally shaped RBCs (sickle cells, spherocytes) ↓ESR

Polycythemia inhibits RBCs from clumping → ↓ESR (usually zero)

Rouleaux: stack-of-coins appearance

Plasma proteins (fibrinogen; Igs) → + charges neutralize negative charge RBCs → rouleaux

AI/CI, multiple myeloma

↑APRs in acute bacterial/fungal infections

History/physical exam most important evaluation

ESR > 100 mm/hr: significant disease

AI: ↓albumin; no alteration in γ-globulin peak

---

5. RBC disorders that *decrease* the ESR
   a. Abnormally shaped RBCs prevent sedimentation (e.g., sickle cells, spherocytes [loss of the normal biconcave disk]); therefore, the ESR is decreased.
   b. Marked *increase* in RBCs (e.g., polycythemia) overrides any increase in plasma proteins (fibrinogen, immunoglobulins); hence, the ESR is usually zero.
6. Plasma factors that promote RBC rouleaux formation (stack-of-coins appearance) increase the ESR by increasing particle size (Fig. 3-21).
   a. Increase in plasma proteins (e.g., fibrinogen and/or immunoglobulins [Igs]) overrides the negative surface charge of RBCs, causing rouleaux.
   b. Examples of causes of an increase in plasma proteins include AI and CI and multiple myeloma, a malignancy of plasma cells that causes an increase in production of immunoglobulins.
7. Most common cause of an increased ESR is an increase in APRs due to acute bacterial and fungal infections (viral infections are less likely to increase the ESR).
8. Evaluating an unexplained increase in ESR
   a. Perform a thorough history and physical exam. Most important evaluation!
   b. ESR > 100 mm/hr usually indicates significant disease is present.
   c. CRP is very useful in evaluating an unexplained increase in the ESR.
   D. Serum protein electrophoresis in inflammation

Proteins in serum are separated into individual fractions by serum protein electrophoresis (SPE; Fig. 3-22). Charged proteins placed in a buffered electrolyte solution will migrate toward one or the other electrode when a current is passed through the solution. Proteins with the most negative charges (e.g., albumin) migrate to the positive pole, or anode, and those with the most positive charges (e.g., γ-globulins) remain at the negatively charged pole, or cathode. Beginning at the anode, proteins separate into five major peaks on cellulose acetate—albumin, followed by α_1-, α_2-, β-, and γ-globulins. The γ-globulins in decreasing order of concentration are IgG, IgA, and IgM (IgD and IgE are in very low concentration).

1. AI (Fig. 3-23 A)
   a. Slight decrease in serum albumin
      (1) Decrease in albumin is a catabolic effect of inflammation.
      (2) Amino acids designated for the synthesis of albumin are used by the liver to synthesize APRs (e.g., fibrinogen).

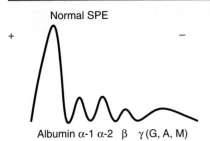

3-22: Normal serum protein electrophoresis (SPE). See text for discussion. *(From Goljan E: Rapid Review Pathology, 4th ed, Philadelphia, Saunders Elsevier, 2014, p 55, Fig. 3-20.)*

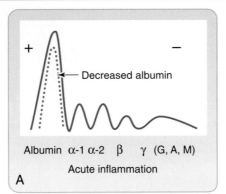

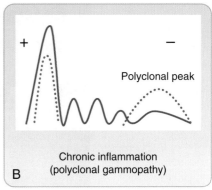

3-23: Serum protein electrophoresis (SPE) in acute inflammation **(A)** and chronic inflammation **(B)**. Albumin is decreased because of increased synthesis of acute phase reactants in the liver. The primary difference between acute versus chronic inflammation is the marked increase in IgG antibody production in chronic inflammation producing a diffusely enlarged γ-globulin peak (polyclonal gammopathy). Refer to Fig. 3-22 and the text for discussion of each of the components of the SPE. *(From Goljan E: Rapid Review Pathology, 4th ed, Philadelphia, Saunders Elsevier, 2014, p 55, Fig. 3-21.)*

  b. Normal γ-globulin peak. Serum IgM level is increased in AI; however, it does *not* reach a high enough concentration to alter the configuration of the γ-globulin peak.

2. CI (Fig. 3-23 B)

  a. Greater decrease in serum albumin occurs with CI than with AI, due to the use of amino acids for prolonged synthesis of APRs by the liver.

  b. Increase in γ-globulins is due to the marked increase in the synthesis of IgG in CI. Diffuse increase in the γ-globulin peak in CI is due to many clones of benign plasma cells producing IgG, hence the term *polyclonal gammopathy.*

AI: normal γ-globulin peak

CI: ↓serum albumin; amino acids diverted to APR synthesis

↑ γ-Globulin (IgG)

Polyclonal gammopathy; many clones plasma cells synthesizing IgG

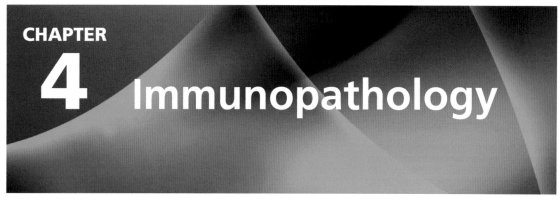

ABBREVIATIONS

Bx biopsy
COD cause of death

MC most common

MCC most common cause

I. Cells of the Immune System

A. Innate (natural) immunity (Link 4-1)

1. **Definition**: Innate immunity is a nonadaptive immune response to microbial pathogens as well as nonmicrobial antigens that have been released during cell death or injury.

   a. Includes anatomic barriers (e.g., skin), phagocytic cells, complement, and acute phase reactants (APRs)

   b. Recognizes microbial structures on nonmammalian tissue and can be deployed within minutes

2. Types of effector cells in innate immunity (Table 4-1)

   a. Phagocytic cells (e.g., neutrophils, macrophages, monocytes); natural killer (NK) cells (large granular lymphocytes) and dendritic cells (DCs) (Links 4-2 and 4-3)

   b. Microglial cells (macrophage of the central nervous system [CNS]); Kupffer cells (macrophage of the liver)

   c. Eosinophils (blood granulocytes with enzymes harmful to parasites); mast cells (present in skin and mucosal epithelium)

   d. Mucosal cells (barrier against microbial invasion; gastrointestinal, respiratory, genitourinary, conjunctiva); endothelial cells (detect foreign pathogens and lipopolysaccharide in the cell wall of gram-negative bacteria)

3. Toll-like receptors (TLRs) in innate immunity

   a. **Definition:** TLRs are proteins expressed on activated effector cells (listed earlier).

   b. TLRs recognize nonself antigens (molecules) commonly shared by pathogens (pathogen-associated molecular patterns [PAMPs]). Examples of PAMPs include endotoxin in gram-negative (G−) bacteria and peptidoglycan in gram-positive (G+) bacteria.

   c. PAMPs are *not* present on normal host effector cells.

   d. Interaction of TLRs with PAMPs on effector cells.

      (1) Interaction initiates intracellular transmission of activating signals to nuclear transcription factors (NFs), one of the most important being NF-κB.

         (a) NF-κB is the "master switch" to the nucleus for induction of inflammation.

         (b) NF-κB stands for <u>n</u>uclear <u>f</u>actor <u>k</u>appa-light-chain-enhancer of activated <u>B</u> cells and plays a key role in regulating the immune response to infection.

      (2) Examples of innate immunity mediators (see Chapter 3)

         (a) Nitric oxide (NO); cytokines (e.g., tumor necrosis factor [TNF], interleukin-1 [IL-1])

         (b) Adhesion molecules for neutrophils and monocytes (e.g., selectin)

         (c) Reactive oxygen species (e.g., peroxide); antimicrobial peptides (e.g., defensins)

Margin notes (left column):

Nonadaptive immune response microbial/nonmicrobial pathogens

Anatomic barriers, phagocytes, complement, APRs

Recognizes microbial structures

Phagocytic, NK/DCs

Microglial/Kupffer cells

Eosinophils, mast cells

Mucosal, endothelial cells

Proteins expressed on activated effector cells

PAMPs: pathogen-associated molecular patterns

Endotoxin (G−), peptidoglycan (G+)

NF-κB: "master switch" to nucleus for induction inflammation

NO; cytokines

Selectin

Reactive oxygen species; antimicrobial peptides

TABLE 4-1   Types of Effector Cells (Neutrophils, Monocytes, Mast Cells Discussed in Table 3-6)

CELL TYPE	DERIVATION	LOCATION	FUNCTION
Natural killer (NK) cells	• Bone marrow stem cells	• Peripheral blood (large granular lymphocytes 10%–15%)	• Recognize class I MHC proteins • Markers: Fc receptors for IgG and KIR • When activated, can release TNF-α and IFN-γ, which have direct antiviral and antitumor effects • Activated by binding antigen-antibody immunocomplexes to surface receptors (ADCC) • Activate macrophage destruction of microbes via release of IFN-γ • Kill virus-infected and neoplastic cells via attachment to altered class I proteins or binding to IgG-coated target cells (ADCC; type II HSR) • Kill cells by using pore-forming proteins (e.g., perforin) that induce direct cell lysis; release granzymes, which are proteolytic enzymes that stimulate apoptosis
Macrophages	• Conversion of monocytes into macrophages in connective tissue	• Connective tissue • Organs (e.g., alveoli, lymph node sinuses, spleen and liver, bone marrow)	• Markers: large granular cells that have Fc and C3b receptors • Activated by INF-γ and TNF • Involved in phagocytosis and cytokine production • Act as APCs to T cells • Kill intracellular microbes (*Mycobacteria*, systemic fungi) after activation by IFN-γ released by activated CD4 helper T cells Microbial killing through oxidative and nonoxidative mechanisms • Initiate and amplify the inflammatory response by stimulation of acute phase response; activation of vascular endothelium; stimulate neutrophil maturation/monocyte chemotaxis • Involved in clearance, resolution, and repair by removing necrotic debris and apoptotic cells; tissue remodeling using elastase, collagenase, and matrix proteins; wound healing and scar formation via production of IL-1, PDGF, and FGF • Link between innate and adaptive immunity
Dendritic cells	• Bone marrow stem cells	• Skin (Langerhans cells), sinuses of lymph nodes	• Most potent APC; initiates and determines the nature of T-cell response in the paracortex of lymph nodes and B cells in the germinal follicles • Produce interferons and antiviral cytokines that inhibit infection and reproduction • Interact with T cells and B cells to initiate and shape the adaptive immune response

ADCC, Antibody-dependent cell-mediated cytotoxicity; *APC,* antigen-presenting cell; *FGF,* fibroblast growth factor; *HSR,* hypersensitivity reaction; *IFN,* interferon; *IL,* interleukin; *KIR,* killer cell immunoglobulin-like receptors; *MHC,* major histocompatibility complex; *PDGF,* platelet-derived growth factor; *TNF,* tumor necrosis factor.

(d) Chemokines (activate neutrophil and monocyte chemotaxis); complement proteins and complement regulatory proteins (e.g., decay accelerating factor [DAF])

Chemokines

Complement; DAF

e. TLRs also react with nonself antigens (molecules) released from damaged tissue, which are called damage-associated molecular patterns (DAMPs) or cell death–associated molecules.

DAMPs: damage-associated molecular patterns

(1) Many DAMPs are derived from the plasma membrane, nucleus, endoplasmic reticulum, mitochondria, and cytosol. Examples of DAMPs include heat shock protein (HSP), which is expressed in response to stresses such as heat, hypoxia, and toxic compounds; chromatin-associated high-mobility group box 1 (HMGB1), which is a major mediator of endotoxic shock; and purine metabolites (adenosine triphosphate, adenosine, uric acid).

Derived from cell components

HSP, HMGB1, purine metabolites (e.g., uric acid)

(2) DAMPs are recognized by TLRs; causes the release of proinflammatory cytokines and chemokines.

TLRs → ↑proinflammatory cytokines/chemokines

4. Nucleotide-binding oligomerization domain (NOD)-like receptors (NLRs)

a. **Definition:** NLRs are cytosolic receptors expressed predominantly in DCs, monocytes, and macrophages that are important in recognizing PAMPs and DAMPs. NLRs function in concert with TLRs.

Cytosolic receptors monocytes/macrophages, DCs

Function in concert with TLRs

b. Pathogens that activate NLRs include *Salmonella typhimurium, Shigella flexneri, Pseudomonas aeruginosa, Legionella pneumophila, Candida albicans,* and certain viruses (e.g., hepatitis C, adenovirus, influenza virus).

c. DAMPs that activate NLRs are listed earlier [IV.C.3.e.(1)].

d. When NLRs are activated, they form multiprotein inflammasome complexes that facilitate activation of caspase-1 (see Chapter 2, discussion of pyroptosis), which in turn increases secretion of IL-1β and IL-18.

Activated NLRs → multiprotein inflammasome complexes → activate caspase-1

e. Overwhelming overproduction of IL-1β and IL-18 has been implicated in the pathogenesis of several diseases, including autoimmune disease (e.g., rheumatoid arthritis, multiple sclerosis [MS]), Crohn disease, gout, Alzheimer disease, metabolic syndrome, and atherosclerosis.

f. Antagonists of the IL-1β receptor (e.g., anakinra, a recombinant homolog of the human IL-1 receptor) have been used in treating some of the diseases just mentioned.

5. Examples of noncellular innate immunity responses to infections

   a. Sequestration of iron in the liver and macrophages by hepcidin (see Chapter 12)

     (1) Iron is essential for bacterial growth and reproduction.

     (2) IL-6 increases the synthesis and release of hepcidin by the liver. Hepcidin decreases iron absorption in the duodenum and also prevents iron release from macrophages in the bone marrow (BM) and other sites, hence sequestering iron from bacteria.

   b. Synthesis and release of APRs (see Chapter 3) by the liver

     (1) IL-6 is the most important cytokine that increases liver synthesis and release of APRs.

     (2) Some APRs inhibit or destroy microbial pathogens. For example, C-reactive protein (CRP) enhances opsonization (see Chapter 3); complement component C3b enhances opsonization; complement component C5a is chemotactic to neutrophils and mast cells; and ferritin is a soluble iron-binding protein within macrophages that keeps iron away from bacteria.

   c. Protective bacteria in the colon. For example, protective bacteria limit the dominance of pathogenic microbes (e.g., *Clostridium difficile, Clostridium botulinum*) in the colon. They compete for nutrients, thus limiting the amount of nutrients available for pathogenic microbes in the colon. They also activate host defenses in the colon.

   d. Human β-defensins. **Definition**: Defensins are antimicrobial peptides that are produced by mucosal epithelial cells. They are constitutive (continually transcribed) or inducible by TNF-α. Functions of human β-defensins include attraction of neutrophils and resistance to colonization of microbes to mucosal surfaces.

   e. Epithelial barriers (e.g., skin and mucous membranes)

   f. Physiologic barriers (e.g., fever inhibits viral and bacterial reproduction; acid gastric pH inhibits bacterial growth)

   g. Chemical barriers (see Chapter 3); examples include chemotactic factors (e.g., C5a, leukotriene B₄), opsonization factors (e.g., C3b, immunoglobulin G [IgG], CRP), and the oxygen-dependent myeloperoxidase (MPO) system

6. Examples of human diseases associated with mutations or dysfunction of TLRs include invasive meningococcal disease and recurrent invasive *Streptococcus pneumoniae* infection, gram-negative bacterial sepsis, and *Staphylococcus aureus* sepsis.

B. Adaptive (acquired) immunity

1. **Definition:** Adaptive immunity refers to protection from an infectious agent by B and T lymphocytes following their exposure to specific antigens produced by microbial pathogens.

2. Rather than recognizing PAMPs, as in innate immunity, antigens produced by microbial pathogens are recognized by B and T lymphocytes, which then eliminate the microbial agents.

3. B lymphocytes produce antibodies (i.e., humoral immune response) (Link 4-4).

   a. Antibodies are primarily directed against extracellular microbial pathogens.

   b. Naïve mature B cells begin to produce IgM and IgD at birth.

     (1) Antigen-stimulated B cells may differentiate into IgM antibody–secreting cells, or via class (isotype) switching, may produce IgG (beginning at 3 months of age), IgE, or IgA.

     (2) Isotype switching to other Ig classes involves changes in the heavy chain locus in the constant region of the gene.

     (3) Isotype switching is induced by a combination of CD40 ligand-mediated signals and cytokines (e.g., IFN-γ for IgG, IL-4 for IgE, and transforming growth factor [TGF] in mucosal tissues for IgA). CD4 helper T (CD4 T$_H$) cells contribute to isotype switching.

   c. Table 4-2 summarizes key information concerning B cells.

4. T cells are primarily involved in cell-mediated immunity (CMI).

   a. T cells are subdivided into CD4 T$_H$ cells and CD8 cytotoxic T cells.

   b. Activated T cells eliminate intracellular microbial pathogens. Recall that extracellular pathogens are eliminated by antibodies produced by B cells.

   c. Functions of T cells are summarized in Table 4-2.

5. Fig. 4-1 depicts humoral immunity and CMI.

TABLE 4-2   Overview of B and T Cells

CELL TYPE	DERIVATION	LOCATION	FUNCTION
T cells CD4 (helper) CD8 (cytotoxic)	• Derive from bone marrow lymphocyte stem cells but mature in the thymus	• Peripheral blood (60%–70%) and bone marrow, thymus, paracortex of lymph nodes, Peyer patches	**CD4 cell types:** • Naïve (unstimulated) CD4 T cells • CD4 T$_H$1 subset cells: memory T cells; produced via release of IL-12 from activated macrophages in DRH • CD4 T$_H$2 subset cells: produced via release of IL-4 from APCs, causing naïve CD4 T cells to differentiate into this subset • CD4 T$_H$17 subset cells: CD4 helper T cells stimulated by IL-6 + TGF-β • **CD4 T-cell functions:** • Recognize antigens in association with class II MHC proteins • Help macrophages kill intracellular pathogens via release of IFN-γ • Help produce clonal expansion of CD4 T cells in DRH via release of IL-2 • Help activate CD8 cytotoxic T cells via release of IL-2 • Activate B cells to produce antibodies against microbes and toxins • CD4 T$_H$1 subset cells: critical reservoir for HIV in the latency phase of the disease • CD4 T$_H$2 subset cells via release of IL-4, stimulate B cells to differentiate into IgE-secreting plasma cells • CD4 T$_H$2 subset cells via release of IL-5, activate eosinophils (useful in killing helminths) • CD4 T$_H$2 subset cells via release of IL-13, enhance IgE production and mucus secretion by epithelial cells (important in asthma) • CD4 T$_H$17 subset cells: release proinflammatory cytokines that activate epithelium and neutrophils and also promote cell-mediated autoimmune responses (e.g., rheumatoid arthritis) **CD8 cytotoxic T-cell types:** • Naïve (unstimulated) CD8 cytotoxic T cells • CD8 cytotoxic subset memory cells • **CD8 cytotoxic T-cell functions:** • Recognize antigens in association with class I MHC proteins • Kill virus-infected, neoplastic, and donor graft cells via release of perforins and granzymes
B cells	• Bone marrow stem cells	• Peripheral blood (10%–20%) and bone marrow, germinal follicles in lymph nodes, Peyer patches in small intestine	**B-cell functions:** • Differentiate into plasma cells that produce immunoglobulins to kill encapsulated, extracellular bacteria (e.g., *Streptococcus pneumoniae*) • Antigen-presenting cell

DRH, Delayed-type hypersensitivity; *IFN,* interferon; *IgE,* immunoglobulin E; *IL,* interleukin; *MHC,* major histocompatibility complex; *TGF-β,* transforming growth factor-β.

II. Major Histocompatibility Complex (MHC)
A. Overview of the MHC
1. **Definition:** The MHC is a genetic focus located on chromosome 6 that contains genes that encode for proteins located on the surface membrane of all body cells and mark them as "self." MHC is very important in organ transplantation.
2. MHC proteins are also known as human leukocyte antigens (HLAs), which are expressed on the surface of *all* nucleated cells with the *exception* of nucleated red blood cells (RBCs).
   a. *HLA* genes and their subtypes are transmitted from parents to their children.
   b. Each individual has a unique set of *HLA* genes. Only identical twins have the same set of *HLA* genes.
3. Genes of the HLA locus encode for two classes of cell surface molecules called class I and class II molecules (Link 4-5).
   a. Class I molecules are located on three closely linked loci that are designated HLA-A, HLA-B, and HLA-C.
      (1) Class I molecules interact with CD8 T cells and NK cells.
      (2) For example, class I molecules that are bound to the surface of peptides on virus-infected cells or neoplastic cells are destroyed by CD8 T cells and/or NK cells.
      (3) **Rule of 8:** CD8 T cells recognize class I molecules ($8 \times 1 = 8$).
   b. Class II molecules are encoded in the HLA-D region, which is subdivided into HLA-DP, HLA-DQ, and HLA-DR subregions.

Mark all body cells as "self"

Important in transplantation

Human leukocyte antigens (HLAs)

Leukocytes; all nucleated cells except nucleated RBCs

Parents to children

Unique to each individual

Identical twins same set *HLA* genes

HLA-A, HLA-B, HLA-C gene loci

Interact with CD8 T/NK cells

Altered antigens → destroyed by CD8 T cells/NK cells

CD8 T cells recognize class I molecules ($8 \times 1 = 8$)

Encoded in HLA-D region (DP-DQ-DR subregions)

4-1: Types of adaptive immunity. In humoral immunity, B lymphocytes secrete antibodies that primarily target extracellular microbes. In cell-mediated immunity, T lymphocytes either activate macrophages to destroy phagocytosed microbes or kill infected cells. *(From Abbas A, Lichtman A: Basic Immunology: Function and Disorders of the Immune System, 3rd ed, Philadelphia, Saunders Elsevier, 2011, p 5, Fig. 1-4.)*

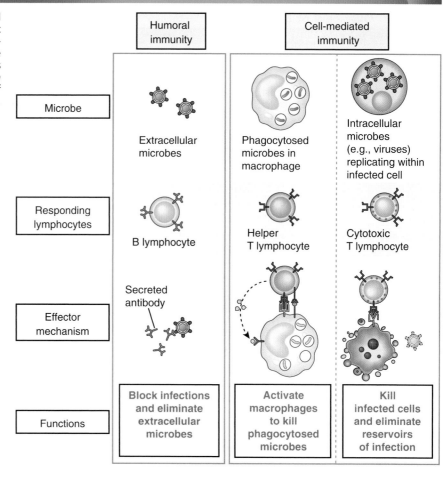

Class II proteins → CD4 T_H cells

APCs: B cells, macrophages, DCs

Rule of 8: CD4 T_H cells recognize class II molecules ($4 \times 2 = 8$)

Code for complement, HSP, TNF

Transplantation workup

Disease risk

Pregnancy

Fetal-maternal hemorrhage → maternal anti-HLA antibodies

Blow to abdomen, MVA, abruptio placenta, amniocentesis

Mother develops anti-HLA antibodies against fetal HLA antigens on leukocytes/platelets

(1) Class II proteins interact with CD4 TH cells.
  Antigen-presenting cells (APCs) include B cells, macrophages, and DCs.
(2) Example: extracellular microbes that are phagocytosed by macrophages (APCs) are digested in lysosomes and the peptides released from the lysosomes associate with class II molecules that eventually are transported in vesicles to the surface of the macrophage, where they interact with CD4 TH cells.
(3) **Rule of 8:** CD4 TH cells recognize class II molecules ($4 \times 2 = 8$).
B. **Class III molecules**
  • **Definition:** Class III *MHC* genes code for proteins involved in the inflammatory process (e.g., complement components, HSP, TNF).
C. **HLA associations with disease** (Table 4-3)
D. **Applications of HLA testing**
  1. Transplantation workup (discussed later). Close matches of HLA class I (A, B) typing and HLA class II (DR) typing between the patient and each potential donor increase the chance of graft survival.
  2. Determining disease risk. Example: individuals positive for HLA-B27 have an increased risk of developing ankylosing spondylitis (90-fold relative risk).
E. **Developing antibodies against HLA antigens**
  1. Pregnancy
    a. Developing antibodies against HLA antigens in pregnancy is most often caused by a fetal-maternal hemorrhage. Fetal-maternal hemorrhage refers to the passage of fetal blood into the maternal circulation and is most often due to a breach in the integrity of the placental circulation.
    b. Causative factors include a direct blow to the abdomen, motor vehicle accident (MVA), abruptio placenta (premature separation of the placenta due to a retroplacental clot; see Chapter 22), or amniocentesis (sampling of amniotic fluid using a needle inserted into the uterus).
    c. Fetal HLA antigens on leukocytes/platelets that are foreign to the mother will result in the development of anti-HLA antibodies in the mother (see Chapter 16).

TABLE 4-3 Clinically Important Hla Associations With Disease

HLA ANTIGEN	DISEASE ASSOCIATION
HLA-A3	Hemochromatosis
HLA-B27	Ankylosing spondylitis, Reiter syndrome, postinfectious arthritis
HLA-BW47	21-Hydroxylase deficiency (also lack HLA-B8)
HLA-DR2	Multiple sclerosis
HLA-DR3	Graves disease, systemic lupus erythematosus
HLA-DR4	Rheumatoid arthritis
HLA-DR3/DR4	Type 1 diabetes mellitus
HLA-DR5	Hashimoto thyroiditis
HLA-DQ2	Celiac disease
HLA-DQB1	Guillain-Barré syndrome

2. Blood transfusion. Antibodies develop against HLA antigens on platelets and leukocytes in transfused blood that are foreign to the recipient.

> Recipient develops antibodies against foreign HLA antigens in donor leukocytes/platelets

3. Transplanted organs. Antibodies develop against HLA antigens present on the transplanted organ that are foreign to the recipient.

> Recipient develops antibodies against foreign HLA antigens in donor organ

III. **Hypersensitivity Reactions (HSRs)**
   A. **Type I (immediate) HSR** (Table 4-4)
      1. **Definition:** A type I (immediate) HSR is an IgE antibody–mediated activation of mast cells and/or basophils (effector cells) that is followed by a localized and/or generalized acute inflammatory reaction.

> IgE activation mast cells/basophils (effector cells)

      2. IgE antibody production (sensitization; Fig. 4-2)
         a. Allergens (e.g., pollen, drugs) are first processed by APCs (macrophages or DCs). This is not shown in Fig. 4-2.

> Allergens first processed by APCs (macrophages/DCs)

         b. APCs then release IL-4, which induces naïve (unstimulated) CD4 T cells to become CD4 TH2 cells (subset of CD4 cells) that produce IL-4 and IL-5.

> IL-4 → naïve CD4 T$_H$2 cells → CD4 T$_H$2 cells → produce IL-4/IL-5.

            (1) IL-4 causes plasma cells to switch from IgM to allergen-specific IgE antibody synthesis.

> IL-4 → switch from IgM to IgE allergen-specific antibodies

            (2) IL-5 stimulates the production and activation of eosinophils. This is *not* shown in Fig. 4-2.

> IL-5: stimulates production/activation eosinophils

      3. Mast cell activation (re-exposure to allergen; see Fig. 4-2)
         a. Allergen-specific IgE antibodies bind to the surface of mast cells/basophils.

> Allergen-specific IgE antibodies → bind to surface mast cells/basophils

         b. Allergens cross-link to allergen-specific IgE antibodies that are already located on the mast cell membranes (also basophils) from the first exposure to the allergen.

> Allergens cross-link allergen-specific IgE antibodies

         c. Cross-linking of allergens to IgE antibodies results in an *early phase reaction* or immediate hypersensitivity that is characterized by mast cell/basophil release of *preformed* mediators (released within minutes after re-exposure of allergen).

> Early phase reaction: mast cell release *preformed* histamine, ECF, serotonin

            (1) Preformed chemicals include histamine, eosinophil chemotactic factor (ECF), and serotonin.

> Histamine → vasodilation → ↑capillary permeability

               (a) Histamine increases smooth muscle contraction, produces vasodilation, and increases capillary permeability.

> Eosinophils neutralize histamine/leukotrienes

               (b) Eosinophils release histaminase to neutralize histamine and arylsulfatase to neutralize histamine and leukotrienes.

> Serotonin → vasodilation, ↑capillary permeability, constrict smooth muscle

               (c) Serotonin produces vasodilation, increases capillary permeability, and constricts smooth muscle.

            (2) Early phase chemicals released by mast cells produce tissue swelling and constriction of bronchi and terminal bronchioles (wheezing, cough).

> Mast cells release preformed chemicals → tissue swelling; constriction bronchi, terminal bronchioles

         d. Late phase reaction
            (1) Mast cells synthesize (de novo) and release prostaglandins (PGs), leukotrienes, and platelet-activating factor (PAF) 6 to 24 hours after repeat exposure to the allergen.

> Late phase reaction: mast cells synthesize/release chemicals

            (2) Inflammatory mediators prolong the acute inflammatory reaction initiated by the early phase chemical mediators.

> Chemical mediators prolong acute inflammatory reaction

               (a) Leukotrienes increase vascular permeability, cause bronchospasm (contract smooth muscle cells), and recruit neutrophils, eosinophils, and monocytes.

> Leukotrienes: ↑vessel permeability; recruit neutrophils, eosinophils, monocytes

TABLE 4-4 Overview of Hypersensitivity Reactions

REACTION	PATHOGENESIS	CLINICAL EXAMPLES
Type I	IgE-dependent activation of mast cells/basophils	**Atopic hypersensitivity:** usually has a strong familial predisposition; occurs in 40% of people in the United States; exposure to allergens Environmental allergens: dust (dust mite), food (eggs, peanuts, shellfish, citrus foods), pollens (trees: spring, grass: spring/summer, weeds: summer/fall); insect envenomations (bees, wasps, hornets, fire ants) **Drug hypersensitivity:** e.g., penicillin; usually a metabolic intermediate rather than the intact drug causes the reaction **Transfusion reaction in IgA immunodeficiency:** some cases are associated with IgE antibodies directed against IgA from previous exposure to IgA in blood products; antigen-specific IgE antibodies are located on mast cells and presence of IgA causes mast cell release of histamine; most cases of anaphylaxis have unknown mechanism **Clinical findings in type I hypersensitivity reaction:** Overview of clinical findings (Link 4-6) **Allergic shiner** (Link 4-7): dark circles beneath the eye due to backup of venous blood from decreased drainage of blood into the veins of the inflamed nasal mucosa **Nasal crease** across the lower third of the nose (Link 4-8): caused by chronic upward rubbing of the itchy nose with the hand (allergic salute) **Rhinitis:** due to swelling of the nasal mucosa; responsible for snoring at night and difficulty with breathing through the nose in the AM and PM; produces a postnasal drip (mucus accumulation in the throat or back of the nose) and cobblestoning of the posterior nasopharynx (Link 4-9) **Allergic cobblestoning of the conjunctiva** (Link 4-10): granular appearance of the mucosa of the eyelid due to edema and hyperplasia of the papillae **Asthma:** wheezing due to inflammation of segmental bronchi and small airways (bronchioles) **Dermatitis:** eczema (see Fig. 25-12 B,C); hives (urticaria; see Fig. 25-12 P) **Vomiting** and **diarrhea:** various foods **Systemic anaphylaxis:** shock, widespread edema, hives, wheezing (from bronchospasm), inspiratory stridor if laryngeal edema is present; serious reactions most likely to be associated with bee envenomation, penicillin, and peanuts
Type II	Antibody-dependent reactions	**Complement-dependent antibody reactions** **Cell lysis (IgM mediated):** • Example: *anti-I cold antibodies (IgM)* in immune hemolytic anemia due to *Mycoplasma pneumoniae* (see Chapter 12) • Example: *incompatible RBC transfusion,* i.e., transfusion of group A blood (contains anti-B-IgM antibodies) into a group B individual (see Chapter 16; Link 4-11) **Cell lysis (IgG mediated):** IgG attaches to the basement membrane/matrix → activates complement system → C5a is produced (chemotactic factor) → recruitment of neutrophils/monocytes to activation site → enzymes, reactive oxygen species released → tissue is damaged (see Fig. 4-4) • Example: *Goodpasture syndrome* with IgG antibodies directed against pulmonary and glomerular capillary basement membranes (see Chapter 20; Link 4-12) • Example: *pernicious anemia,* in which IgG antibodies are directed against the proton pump in parietal cells (see Chapter 12) • Example: *acute rheumatic fever,* in which IgG antibodies similar to those present in the M protein of certain strains of Group A *Streptococcus pyogenes* are directed against antigens in the human heart, skin, brain, subcutaneous tissue, and joints (see Chapter 11) **Phagocytosis** (see Fig. 4-5 A): • Example: *warm (IgG) immune hemolytic anemia,* in which RBCs coated by IgG and/or C3b are phagocytosed and destroyed by splenic macrophages see Chapter 12) • Example: *ABO hemolytic disease of the newborn,* in which a Group O mother has anti-A,B-IgG antibodies that cross the placenta and attach to fetal blood group A or B RBCs that are phagocytosed by splenic macrophages (have receptors for IgG) and destroyed (see Chapter 16) • Example: *penicillin attaches to RBCs* → IgG antibodies are made against penicillin → splenic macrophages phagocytose the RBCs (see Chapter 12) • Example: *idiopathic thrombocytopenic purpura,* in which platelets have IgG antibodies directed against their GpIIb:IIIa fibrinogen receptors and are removed by splenic macrophages (see Chapter 15) **Complement-independent antibody reactions** **Antibody (IgG)-dependent cell-mediated cytotoxicity:** • Example: natural killer cell destruction of antibody-coated neoplastic and virus-infected cells (Link 4-13) **Antibody (IgE)-dependent cell-mediated cytotoxicity:** • Example: *helminth in tissue* is coated by IgE antibodies → eosinophil IgE receptors attach to the IgE → eosinophils release major basic protein, which kills the helminth. (Link 4-14) **Antibodies directed against cell surface receptors:** • Example: in *Graves disease* (see Fig. 4-5 B schematic on left), IgG antibodies directed against thyroid hormone receptors stimulate the gland to synthesize excessive amounts of thyroid hormone (refer to Chapter 23) • Example: in *myasthenia gravis* (see Fig. 4-5 B schematic on the right), IgG autoantibodies directed against acetylcholine receptors impair the function of the receptor (see Chapter 24)

TABLE 4-4 Overview of Hypersensitivity Reactions—cont'd

REACTION	PATHOGENESIS	CLINICAL EXAMPLES
Type III	Deposition of antigen-antibody complexes (Link 4-15)	• Example: *systemic lupus erythematosus* (DNA–anti-DNA immunocomplexes; discussed later in the chapter) • Example: *Arthus reaction* (Link 4-16): farmer's lung, involving thermophilic actinomycetes in moldy hay • Example: *serum sickness* (Link 4-17): systemic immune-complex disease caused by injection of a foreign serum (e.g., horse antithymocyte globulin), chronic exposure to an antigen (e.g., hepatitis B surface antigen) leading to polyarteritis nodosa [see Chapter 10]), drugs (e.g., penicillin); clinical findings include fever, rash (urticaria, maculopapular), arthralgia, painful lymphadenopathy, splenomegaly, and eosinophilia a few days or weeks after exposure to antigen • Example: *glomerulopathies:* poststreptococcal glomerulonephritis, type IV diffuse proliferative glomerulonephritis in SLE, IgA glomerulopathy, membranous glomerulopathy (see Chapter 20) • Example: *polyarteritis nodosa* (see Chapter 10) • Example: *subacute bacterial endocarditis* (see Chapter 11)
Type IV	Antibody-independent T cell–mediated reactions	**CD4 helper T cell mediated:** *Granulomas* associated with systemic fungal infections (e.g., *Histoplasma, Coccidioides*) and mycobacterial infections (*Mycobacterium tuberculosis,* MAI, *Mycobacterium leprae*) (Link 4-18) *Tuberculin skin reaction* *Chronic asthma* (eosinophil-mediated) *Multiple sclerosis* *Rheumatoid arthritis* *Type 1 diabetes mellitus* *Allergic contact dermatitis:* poison ivy/oak/sumac (see Fig. 25-12 D; Link 4-19), chemicals (e.g., nickel [Fig. 4-7 E], formaldehyde, laundry detergent [Link 4-20]), topical antibiotics (e.g., neomycin, sulfonamides), rubber gloves *Graft rejection* **CD8 T cell mediated:** destruction of virus-infected, neoplastic, or donor graft cells

DM, Diabetes mellitus; *Gp,* glycoprotein; *Ig,* immunoglobulin; *MAI, Mycobacterium avium-intracellulare* complex; *RBC,* red blood cell; *SLE,* systemic lupus erythematosus.

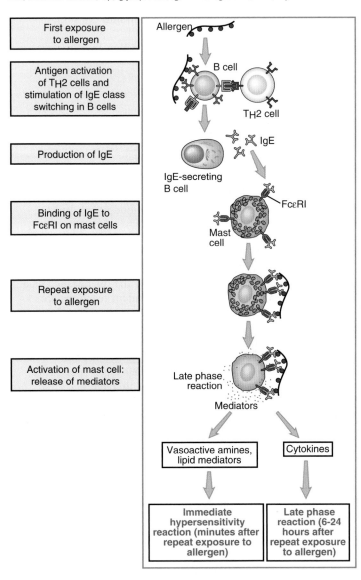

First exposure to allergen

Antigen activation of T$_H$2 cells and stimulation of IgE class switching in B cells

Production of IgE

Binding of IgE to FcεRI on mast cells

Repeat exposure to allergen

Activation of mast cell: release of mediators

Allergen / B cell / T$_H$2 cell / IgE / IgE-secreting B cell / FcεRI / Mast cell / Late phase reaction / Mediators / Vasoactive amines, lipid mediators / Cytokines / Immediate hypersensitivity reaction (minutes after repeat exposure to allergen) / Late phase reaction (6-24 hours after repeat exposure to allergen)

4-2: The sequence of events in type I (immediate) hypersensitivity reactions (HSRs). Type I HSRs are initiated by the introduction of an allergen, which stimulates CD4 T$_H$2 reactions and immunoglobulin E (IgE) production. IgE binds to Fc receptors on mast cells, and subsequent exposure to the allergen leads to cross-linking of subjacent IgE antibodies, causing activation of the mast cells and the release of preformed mediators (e.g., histamine) that produce an inflammatory reaction. Not shown in the schematic is the late phase reaction, in which the mast cells synthesize and release prostaglandins, leukotrienes, and platelet-activating factor, which prolong the inflammatory response. *(From Abbas A, Lichtman A: Basic Immunology: Function and Disorders of the Immune System, 3rd ed, Philadelphia, Saunders Elsevier, 2011, p 208, Fig. 11-2.)*

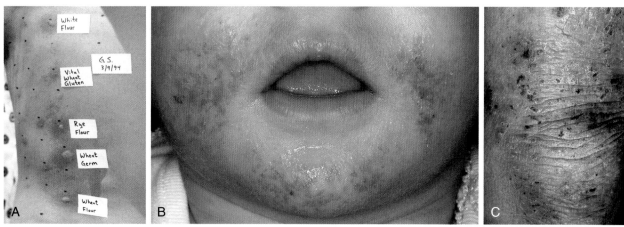

4-3: **A,** Scratch (prick) test showing a classic wheal and flare reaction against antigens in flour and wheat. The patient was a baker. **B,** Atopic dermatitis with eczematous plaques that are moist and oozing serum. **C,** Chronic atopic dermatitis of the knee with lichenification and hemorrhage from excessive scratching. *(A from Fitzpatrick JE, Morelli JG: Dermatology Secrets Plus, 4th ed, Philadelphia, Mosby Elsevier, 2011, p 65; **B, C** from Habif TB: Clinical Dermatology: A Color Guide to Diagnosis and Therapy, 6th ed, Elsevier, 2016, p 155, Figs. 5-8 B, 5-3, respectively.)*

PGD$_2$: ↑mucus, bronchospasm

Late phase reactions: PGs, leukotrienes, PAF

Scratch test → wheal/flare post allergen

RAST test: detects IgE specific allergens

Serum levels IgE

    (b) PGD$_2$ increases mucus production and produces bronchospasm.
    (c) PAF has similar functions as leukotrienes and PGs and also causes platelet aggregation.
  4. Laboratory tests for type I hypersensitivity
    a. Scratch (prick) test (best overall sensitivity). Positive response is a histamine-mediated wheal and flare reaction after introduction of an allergen into the skin (Fig. 4-3).
    b. Radioallergosorbent test (RAST). Detects IgE antibodies in serum that are directed against specific allergens.
    c. Serum levels of IgE.
  5. Clinical examples (see Table 4-4; Links 4-6, 4-7, 4-8, 4-9, and 4-10)

Desensitization therapy in atopic individuals involves repeated injections of increasingly greater amounts of allergen, resulting in production of IgG antibodies that attach to allergens and prevent them from binding to mast cells.

Desensitization → individual produces IgG antibodies against allergens

IgM/G/E antibodies directed against cell surface/ECM antigens

Cell lysis IgM-mediated

IgM activates MAC

Cell lysis: IgG-mediated

Goodpasture syndrome, acute rheumatic fever

Fixed macrophages (spleen/liver) → phagocytose RBCs (IgG antibodies, C3b coated)

ABO hemolytic disease of newborn

C-independent reactions

ADCC

NK attaching to IgG in virally infected cell/cancer cell

Eosinophil destruction IgE-coated helminth

B. Type II (cytotoxic) HSR (see Table 4-4; Links 4-11, 4-12, 4-13, and 4-14)
  1. **Definition:** A type II (cytotoxic) HSR is where IgM, IgG, or IgE antibodies are directed against cell surface or extracellular matrix (ECM) antigens.
  2. Complement-dependent reactions
    a. Cell lysis (IgM-mediated)
      • **Definition:** An IgM antibody directed against an antigen on the cell membrane activates the complement system, leading to lysis of the cell by the membrane attack complex (MAC; C5-C9). Clinical examples of cytotoxic-dependent reactions are discussed in Table 4-4.
    b. Cell lysis (IgG-mediated) (Fig. 4-4)
      • **Definition:** IgG attaches to the basement membrane/matrix → activates the complement system → C5a is produced (chemotactic factor) → neutrophils/monocytes recruited to activation site → enzymes and reactive oxygen species are released → tissue is damaged. Clinical examples are discussed in Table 4-4.
    c. Phagocytosis (Fig. 4-5 A)
      (1) **Definition:** Fixed macrophages (e.g., in spleen or liver) phagocytose hematopoietic cells (e.g., RBCs) coated by IgG antibodies and/or complement (C3b).
      (2) Clinical examples are discussed in Table 4-4.
  3. Complement-independent reactions
    a. Antibody (IgG)-dependent cell-mediated cytotoxicity (ADCC)
      • **Definition:** Cells are coated by IgG → leukocytes (neutrophils, monocytes, NK cells) bind to IgG → activated cells release inflammatory mediators that cause cell lysis. Clinical examples are discussed in Table 4-4.
    b. Clinical examples of ADCC discussed in Table 4-4

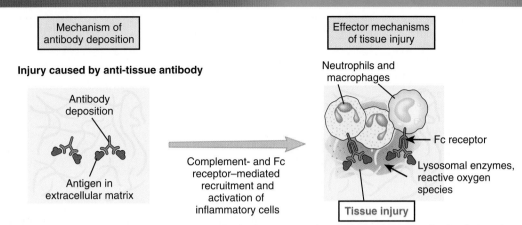

| Mechanism of antibody deposition | Effector mechanisms of tissue injury |

Injury caused by anti-tissue antibody

4-4: Type II hypersensitivity with complement-mediated antibody destruction of antigens in tissue. Antibodies (other than immunoglobulin E [IgE]) may cause tissue injury and disease by binding directly to their target antigens on cells and extracellular matrix. An example of this mechanism occurs in Goodpasture syndrome, in which IgG antibodies are directed against antigens in collagen within the basement membrane of pulmonary and glomerular capillaries. *(Modified from Abbas A, Lichtman A: Basic Immunology: Function and Disorders of the Immune System, 4th ed, Philadelphia, Saunders Elsevier, 2014, p 215, Fig. 11-7 A.)*

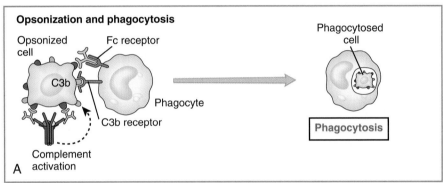

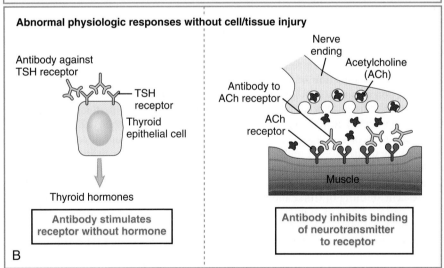

4-5: Type II hypersensitivity reactions. Antibodies may cause disease by opsonizing cells (e.g., RBCs) for phagocytosis **(A)**. In addition, they may produce disease by interfering with normal cellular functions, such as hormone receptor signaling **(B)**. In Graves disease, stimulatory IgG antibodies against the TSH receptor cause increased function. In myasthenia gravis, blocking antibodies prevent acetylcholine binding to acetylcholine receptors. *TSH,* Thyroid-stimulating hormone. *(Modified from Abbas A, Lichtman A: Basic Immunology: Function and Disorders of the Immune System, 3rd ed, Philadelphia, Saunders Elsevier, 2014, p 217, Fig. 11-8 B, C.)*

   c. Antibody directed against cell surface receptors (Fig. 4-5 B)
- IgG autoantibodies directed against cell surface receptors either impair the function of the receptor or stimulate the function of the receptor. Clinical examples are discussed in Table 4-4.

4. Tests used to evaluate type II hypersensitivity disease
   a. Direct Coombs test detects IgG and/or C3b or C3d (degradation product of C3b) attached to the surface of RBCs (see Fig. 12-27 A).
   b. Indirect Coombs test detects antibodies in serum that are directed against antigens on the surface of RBCs (e.g., anti-D directed against D antigen; see Fig. 12-27 B).

Ab against cell surface receptors

Impair or stimulate receptor function

Myasthenia gravis

Direct Coombs test

Indirect Coombs test

4-6: Type III hypersensitivity. Immunocomplexes in the lumen of the blood vessel attach to the vessel wall. They locally activate the complement system, leading to recruitment of inflammatory cells (e.g., neutrophils) that damage the tissue. The result is small vessel vasculitis. *(Modified from Abbas A, Lichtman A: Basic Immunology: Function and Disorders of the Immune System, 3rd ed, Philadelphia, Saunders Elsevier, 2011, p 214, Fig. 11-7.)*

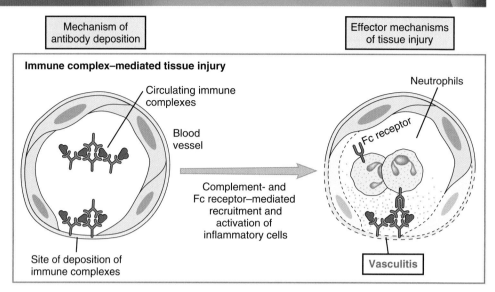

C. **Type III (immunocomplex [IC]) HSR** (Table 4-4; Links 4-15, 4-16, and 4-17)

1. **Definition:** A type III (IC) HSR is when circulating antigen-antibody complexes (e.g., DNA [antigen]-anti-DNA [antibody]) produce acute inflammation with damage to tissue at the site of their deposition.

2. IC formation and their mechanism of tissue damage (Fig. 4-6)
   a. *First exposure* to antigen leads to the synthesis of antibodies.
   b. *Second exposure* leads to formation of antigen-antibody complexes (ICs) that circulate in the blood and deposit on the endothelial surface of small blood vessels or, less commonly, within extravascular sites (e.g., joints, basement membrane of skin). In normal circumstances, ICs are cleared from the blood by the reticuloendothelial system, but occasionally they persist and deposit in tissues.
   c. When ICs deposit in tissue, they activate the complement system and produce C5a, which attracts neutrophils. These neutrophils are ultimately what is causing the tissue damage.

3. Arthus reaction
   a. **Definition:** An Arthus reaction refers to the formation of ICs (type III HSR) at a localized site after an injection of antigen into the skin of a previously sensitized animal.
   b. Example: injection of an antigen into the skin of a previously sensitized animal (i.e., the animal had circulating antibodies against that antigen) leads to rapid attachment of antibody to the injected antigen, resulting in IC formation, which then are deposited in the wall of small arteries at the injection site. The ICs attract neutrophils to the injection site. Neutrophilic infiltration of the vessels and fibrinoid necrosis result in vessel thrombosis and ischemic ulceration.

4. Other clinical examples: see Table 4-4

5. Immunofluorescent staining of tissue biopsies identifies IC deposition (e.g., ICs deposited in glomeruli in certain types of glomerulonephritis; see Chapter 20)

D. **Type IV HSR** (Table 4-4; Links 4-18, 4-19, and 4-20)

1. **Definition:** A type IV HSR is an antibody-independent, T cell–mediated type of immunity (CMI) reaction. They are often delayed reactions.
   • Initiated by antigen activation of CD4 and/or CD8 T cells. Inflammatory response is sometimes "delayed" (hours or days; delayed-type hypersensitivity reaction).

2. Functions of CMI
   • CMI controls infections caused by viruses, fungi, helminths, mycobacteria, and intracellular bacterial pathogens. Important in certain types of graft rejection and in tumor surveillance.

3. Types of cell-mediated immunity
   a. **Definition:** Delayed reaction hypersensitivity (DRH) is a type of CMI that primarily involves CD4 T_H1 cells (killing *Mycobacterium tuberculosis* will be used as an example) (Fig. 4-7 A).
      (1) First phase of DRH involves processing of antigen (tubercle bacilli in this case) by APCs, which, in this case, are alveolar macrophages.

Circulating antigen-antibody complexes damage tissue

1st exposure: synthesis antibodies

2nd exposure: antigen-antibody complexes (ICs)

ICs activate C → C5a attracts neutrophils → tissue damage

Type III HSR; ICs formed at localized site

Immunofluorescent staining of biopsies identifies IC location

Summary antibody-mediated HSRs: types I, II, III

Antibody-independent T-cell CMI

Antigen activation CD4 and/or CD8 T cells

Delayed reaction hypersensitivity

Infection control all pathogens (e.g., tuberculosis [TB])

Graft rejections, tumor surveillance

DRH: macrophages (APCs), CD4 T_H1 cells

Processing antigen in alveolar macrophages

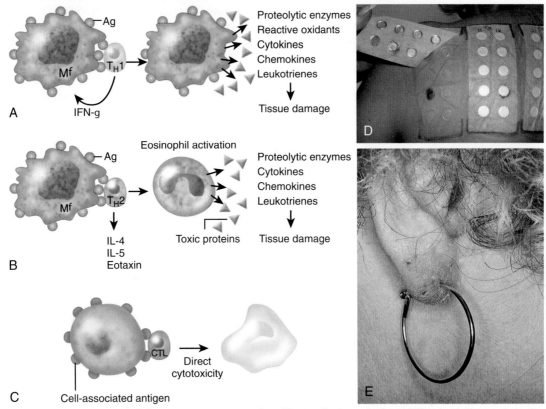

4-7: Type IV hypersensitivity reaction (HSR). Type IV HSRs are mediated by T cells through three different pathways. **A,** In the first pathway, CD4 T$_H$1 subset cells recognize soluble antigens and release interferon-γ (IFN-γ) to activate effector cells, in this case macrophages (Mψ), and cause tissue injury. **B,** In the second pathway, eosinophils predominate in T$_H$2-mediated responses. CD4 T$_H$2 cells produce cytokines to recruit and activate eosinophils, leading to their degranulation and tissue injury. **C,** In the third pathway, damage is caused directly by CD8 T cells, which interact with altered class I antigens on neoplastic, virus-infected, or donor graft cells. The activated CD8 T cells release chemicals that lyse the cells. **D,** Patch test for allergens in contact dermatitis (type IV HSR). Unlike patch tests for immediate (allergic) type I HSRs, these require more than 48 hours and a final inspection after 3 or 4 days. **E,** Nickel allergy to earring. It is a contact dermatitis (type IV HSR). *IL,* Interleukin. *(A–C modified from Goldman L, Schafer AI: Cecil's Medicine, 24th ed, Philadelphia, Saunders Elsevier, 2012, p 230, Fig. 46-4; D from Marks JG, Miller JJ:* Lookingbill and Marks' Principles of Dermatology, *Saunders Elsevier, 5th ed, 2013, p 38, Fig. 4.13; E from Habif TB:* Clinical Dermatology: A Color Guide to Diagnosis and Therapy, *ed 6, Elsevier, 2016, p 139, Fig. 4-20.)*

(2) After processing the tubercle bacilli, alveolar macrophages interact with class II antigen sites on naïve (unstimulated) CD4 T cells located in lymph nodes, causing the CD4 T cells to secrete IL-2, which stimulates proliferation of the CD4 T cells.

Alveolar macrophages interact via class II antigen sites with naïve CD4 T cells

(3) Activated alveolar macrophages secrete IL-12, causing the naïve CD4 T cells to differentiate into CD4 T$_H$1 subset cells, or memory cells.

Activated macrophages secrete IL-12; causes naïve CD4 cell → CD4 T$_H$1 memory cells

(4) CD4 T$_H$1 cells produce interferon (IFN)-γ, which further amplifies the conversion of naïve T cells to CD4 T$_H$1 memory T cells.

Activated CD4 T$_H$1 cells → produce interferon (IFN)-γ (more memory T cells)

(5) Some of these memory cells remain in lymph nodes, whereas others enter the circulation where they remain in the memory pool for long periods of time.

Some remain in nodes

(6) If the CD4 T$_H$1 cells are reexposed to the tubercle bacilli at a later date via interaction with macrophages, they release IFN-γ, which activates the macrophages, thus enhancing their ability to phagocytose and kill the bacteria.

Activated with reexposure (e.g., TB)

  (a) Activated alveolar macrophages change their appearance becoming *epithelioid cells* because they resemble epithelial cells when stained with hematoxylin-eosin.

Activated macrophages → epithelioid cells

  (b) With the help of TNF, the epithelioid cells aggregate and are surrounded by a collar of CD4 T$_H$1 cells producing a granuloma. Activated alveolar macrophages frequently fuse to form multinucleated giant cells (MGCs; see Fig. 2-16 H).

TNF → epithelioid cells aggregate/collar CD4 T$_H$1 cells → granuloma → MGCs

  (c) Because cell walls of tubercle bacilli (also systemic fungi) have a high lipid content, the central portion of the granulomas are composed of granular material representing caseous necrosis (Fig. 2-16 H).

Granuloma: central caseous necrosis

(7) Tuberculin skin reaction is another example of DRH involving CD4 T$_H$1 cells.

PPD reaction: DRH

  (a) Purified protein derivative (PPD) containing antigen of the tubercle bacillus is injected intradermally.

PPD injected intradermally

  (b) Langerhans cells in skin (DC in the skin) phagocytose and process the PPD.

Skin Langerhans cells; phagocytoses PPD

Langerhans cells + CD4T$_H$1 cells → release cytokines → inflammatory reaction

PPD reaction dependent on CMI competency

CMI diminished in older and AIDS patients

DRH: naïve CD4 T cells → CD4 T$_H$17

    (c) Langerhans cells, via their class II antigen sites, react with CD4 T$_H$1 subset memory cells, causing activation of both cells and the release of cytokines that produce the inflammatory reaction, which reaches its peak in 24 to 72 hours.

    (d) CMI is diminished in older adults; hence the degree of skin induration is less than in a younger individual. Another example is a person with AIDS, in which CMI is markedly diminished due to the loss of CD4 T cells.

  b. In DRH, if the APCs release IL-1, IL-6, and IL-23 along with TGF-β, naïve CD4 T cells differentiate into T$_H$17 subset cells (see the following).

CD4 T$_H$17 subset: cytokines recruit neutrophils/monocytes → neutrophils react against extracellular bacterial pathogens; neutrophils + monocytes react against fungi; important in immune-mediated chronic inflammatory reactions in autoimmune diseases.

Macrophages process antigen → interact CD4 T$_H$2 cells → release eotaxin, IL-4/5

IL-5/eotaxin → activate eosinophils → release MBP

Epithelial cell damage → bronchoconstriction → irreversible airway disease

DRH: allergic contact dermatitis

Poison ivy, topical drugs, rubber, chemicals

Induction phase

Allergens bind to Langerhans cells

Langerhans cells process antigen

Processed antigen presented to nodal CD4 T cells

CD4 T$_H$1 memory cells/ effector memory cells in nodes

Effector cytotoxic CD8 memory T cells in circulation

Elicitation phase (re-exposure of antigen)

Effector CD8T lymphocytes → release cytokines → contact dermatitis

Pruritus, erythema, edema, vesicles

T cells interact with altered class I antigen sites

Lysis neoplastic, virus-infected, donor graft cells

Patch test: confirm allergic contact dermatitis

Nickel allergen

Quantitative T cell count; mitogenic assays

  c. DRH involving macrophages, CD4 T$_H$2 subset cells, and eosinophils (in chronic asthma) (Fig. 4-7 B)

    (1) In the lungs, macrophages process antigen, and via their class II antigen sites they interact with CD4 T$_H$2 subset cells, causing the release of eotaxin, IL-4, and IL-5.

    (2) IL-5 and eotaxin recruit and activate eosinophils (effector cells), which release major basic protein (MBP), cationic protein, and leukotrienes.

    (3) Inflammatory reaction results in epithelial cell damage in the lungs, bronchoconstriction, and the potential for chronic, irreversible airway disease (see Chapter 17).

  d. DRH in allergic contact dermatitis

    (1) Allergic contact dermatitis occurs after sensitization to plant materials (e.g., poison ivy, poison oak, poison sumac; see Chapter 25), topically applied drugs (e.g., neomycin, benzocaine, sulfonamides), rubber gloves, or chemicals (e.g., nickel, formaldehyde).

    (2) Pathophysiology of contact dermatitis involves induction (i.e., sensitization) and elicitation phases.

      (a) In the *induction phase*, small molecules (usually <500 daltons) of the allergen enter the skin and bind to carrier proteins located on Langerhans cells in the suprabasilar area of skin.

      (b) Langerhans cells take up and process the antigen.

      (c) Processed antigen is presented to CD4 T cells, which differentiate in regional lymph nodes into CD4 T$_H$1 subset memory cells, whereas others become effector cytotoxic CD8 T memory lymphocytes (effector memory cells) that enter into the circulation.

      (d) In the *elicitation phase,* re-exposure to the antigen leads to penetration of the skin, uptake and processing by Langerhans cells, and presentation of processed antigen to the circulating effector CD8 T memory lymphocytes.

      (e) Activation of these lymphocytes causes the release of cytokines that mediate the characteristic inflammatory response of allergic contact dermatitis, usually within hours of reexposure.

      (f) Key clinical findings include pruritus, erythema, edema, and the formation of vesicles containing clear fluid.

  e. CD8 T cell–mediated cytotoxicity

    (1) CD8 cytotoxic T cells interact with altered class I antigens on neoplastic, virus-infected, or donor graft cells, causing cell lysis (Fig. 4-7 C).

    (2) Activated cytotoxic CD8 T cells lyse the cells by releasing preformed perforins and granzymes that are normally stored in granules in the cells.

4. Tests used to evaluate type IV hypersensitivity disorders

  a. Patch test: used to confirm allergic contact dermatitis (Fig. 4-7 D)

    Example: a suspected allergen (e.g., nickel) is placed on an adhesive patch and is applied to the skin to determine whether a skin reaction occurs.

  b. Tests used to evaluate whether CMI is intact

    (1) Quantitative count of T cells; mitogenic assays (functional test of T lymphocytes)

    (2) Intradermal injection of *Candida* antigen: normal skin reaction is development of an erythematous rash at injection site.

Candida intradermal injection → rash (intact CMI)

      c. Anergy: lack of a response to mitogenic assays and/or lack of a skin response to *Candida*

   5. Additional clinical examples of CMI are listed in Table 4-4.

IV. Transplantation Immunology

A. Factors that enhance graft viability

   1. Must be ABO blood group compatibility between recipients and donors

      a. Most important requirement

      b. Using a kidney transplantation as an example (see Chapter 16)

         (1) Blood group AB patients can receive a kidney of any blood type, because they lack anti-A and anti-B antibodies in their serum that could potentially attack A or B antigens in a donor kidney.

         (2) Blood group A patients can get a kidney from someone with an O (no A or B antigens) or A blood type.

         (3) Blood group B patients can get a kidney from someone with an O (no A or B antigens) or B blood type.

         (4) Blood group O patients can get a kidney only from someone with the O blood type, because blood group O patients have anti-A and anti-B antibodies in their serum.

   2. Must be an absence of preformed anti-HLA cytotoxic antibodies in graft recipients; must have had previous exposure to human blood products to develop anti-HLA cytotoxic antibodies

   3. Must be close matches of HLA-A, HLA-B, HLA-C (minor importance), and HLA-DR loci between recipients and donors

B. Types of grafts

   1. Autograft. **Definition:** Graft from self to self. Autografts have the best survival rate. Example: skin graft from one part of the body to another part of the body.

   2. Syngeneic graft (isograft). **Definition:** Graft between identical twins.

   3. Allograft. **Definition:** Graft between genetically different individuals of the same species.

   4. Xenograft. **Definition:** A xenograft is a graft between two different species. Example: transplant of a pig's heart valve into a human.

C. Types of rejection (Link 4-21)

   1. Transplantation rejection involves a humoral and/or cell-mediated host response against MHC antigens in the donor graft.

   2. Hyperacute rejection (Fig. 4-8 A)

      a. **Definition:** A hyperacute reaction is an *irreversible* reaction that occurs within minutes or hours after transplantation.

      b. Pathogenesis

         (1) Type II HSR involving immunoglobulin and complement that targets the endothelium of small vessels (e.g., arterioles, capillaries). This immunologic reaction results in a neutrophilic infiltrate with fibrinoid necrosis (see Chapter 2) and vessel thrombosis, leading to infarction. Because the reaction is irreversible, the organ must be removed.

         (2) Causes

            (a) ABO incompatibility (e.g., a blood group A person inadvertently receives a kidney from a blood group B person)

            (b) Reaction between preformed anti-HLA antibodies in the recipient directed against similar donor HLA antigens located in the vascular endothelium of a donor graft

         (3) Hyperacute rejections are uncommon because of pretransplantation screening (see later).

   3. Acute rejection

      a. **Definition:** An acute rejection is a *reversible* reaction that occurs usually within days or weeks after transplantation.

      b. Most common transplant rejection

         (1) Combination of a type II and a type IV HSR

         (2) Dendritic cells in the donor organ (e.g., kidney) have high levels of both class I and class II MHC molecules (key cell).

Margin notes

Anergy: no mitogenic and/or skin response to *Candida*

ABO compatibility most important

AB: kidney any blood group

A: kidney group O/A

B: kidney group O/B

O: kidney only O

Graft recipient: absence preformed anti-HLA antibodies important

Anti-HLA cytotoxic antibodies present → previous exposure human blood products

Close matches HLA-A, HLA-B, HLA–DR loci

Autograft: self to self; best survival rate

Syngeneic graft: graft between identical twins

Allograft: graft genetically different individuals; same species

Xenograft: graft between two different species

Humoral and/or cell-mediated host response against MHC antigens donor graft

Irreversible reaction; mins/hrs

Type II HSR

Small vessel vasculitis; neutrophils, fibrinoid necrosis, thrombosis

ABO mismatch; A person receives B blood

Preformed anti-HLA antibodies

Reversible reaction occurring days/wks after transplantation

MC rejection

Combination type II/IV HSR

DCs have class I/II MHC molecules; key cell

4-8: Mechanisms of graft rejection. A, In **hyperacute rejection,** preformed antibodies (e.g., ABO, HLA) react with alloantigens on the vascular endothelium of the graft, activate complement, and trigger rapid intravascular thrombosis and necrosis of the vessel wall. **B,** In **acute rejection,** CD8+ T lymphocytes reactive with alloantigens (foreign antigen) on graft endothelial cells and parenchymal cells cause damage to these cell types. Inflammation of the endothelium is called endothelialitis. Alloreactive antibodies also may contribute to vascular injury. **C,** In **chronic rejection,** there is vessel atherosclerosis and cytokine-induced proliferation of smooth muscle cells, leading to luminal occlusion. Not shown in the figure is cytokine stimulation of fibroblasts leading to interstitial fibrosis. This type of rejection is most likely a chronic delayed reaction hypersensitivity *(DRH)* reaction to alloantigens in the vessel wall. *APC,* Antigen-presenting cell. *(From Abbas A, Lichtman A:* Basic Immunology: Function and Disorders of the Immune System, *3rd ed, Philadelphia, Saunders Elsevier, 2011, p 201, Fig. 10-9.)*

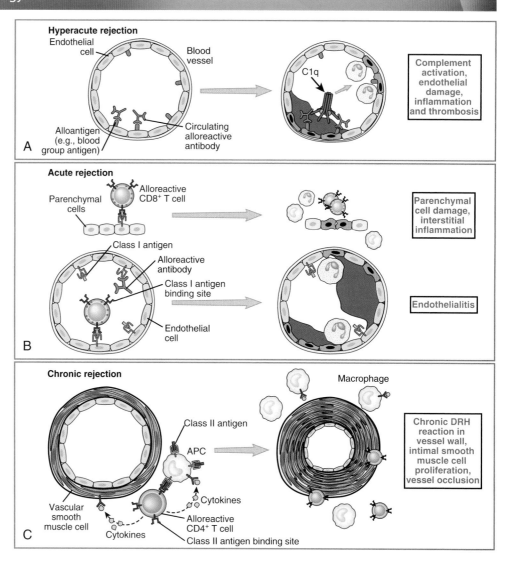

"Endothelialitis," interstitial tissue inflammation; type IV HSR

Type IV CD8-mediated cytotoxicity HSR; type IV

Alloreactive antibodies recipient → vasculitis in donor organ (type II HSR)

Key cells rejected donor organ: CD4/CD8 T cells, macrophages

Recipient has preexisting anti-HLA antibodies against donor HLA antigens

Endothelialitis

Necrotizing vasculitis → vessel thrombosis

(a) Recipient CD4 T cells react against the class II MHC molecules on the donor DCs and differentiate into subset T_H1 memory cells and, in some cases, T_H17 effector cells. Cytokines (e.g., IFN-γ) released from subset T_H1 memory cells in the *recipient* activate macrophages in the *donor transplant.* The activated macrophages in the donor transplant attack both the vessels ("endothelialitis") and the parenchymal cells, leading to extensive tissue damage and rejection of the transplant (type IV DRH reaction).

(b) Recipient CD8 T cells react against class I MHC molecules on the donor DCs and also attack class I MHC molecules (Fig. 4-8 B) in parenchymal cells and endothelial cells (type IV CD8-mediated cytotoxicity HSR; see Table 4-4 under Type IV antibody-independent T cell–mediated reaction). Alloreactive antibodies (see following discussion [IV.C.3.b.(3)]) also contribute to vascular damage (type II HSR).

(c) Histologic sections of the donor organ reveal large numbers of mononuclear cells (CD4 and CD8 T cells, macrophages) in the interstitium.

(3) Antibody-mediated type II HSR component of an acute rejection is caused by the recipient having preexisting alloreactive antibodies (e.g., anti-HLA antibodies) against donor HLA antigens.

(a) Alloreactive antibodies are antibodies from one individual that will recognize antigens on cells or tissues of another, genetically nonidentical individual.

(b) Antibodies activate complement, leading to small vessel damage ("endothelialitis"; shown in Fig. 4-8 B).

(c) Small vessel damage is characterized by a necrotizing vasculitis with neutrophils, fibrinoid necrosis, and vessel thrombosis.

(d) Presence of complement component C4d (degradation product of C4 activation) in the inflammatory tissue indicates that the complement system has been activated and is an important marker that there is a humoral component in the rejection.

    (4) If the vasculitis is less acute or the graft is rejected months or years later, the vessels are more likely to show intimal thickening with proliferation of smooth muscle cells reminiscent of atherosclerosis.

  c. Acute rejection is potentially reversible with immunosuppressive therapy (e.g., cyclosporine). Immunosuppressive therapy is associated with an increased risk of squamous cell carcinoma (SCC) of the cervix, malignant lymphoma, and SCC of the skin (most common cancer).

4. Chronic rejection (Fig. 4-8 C)
  a. **Definition:** Chronic rejection is an *irreversible* reaction involving host CD4 T cells that occurs over months to years, usually in patients who have survived acute rejection due to immunosuppression therapy.
  b. Pathogenesis. Most likely due to a chronic DRH reaction involving host CD4 T cells (type IV HSR).
  c. Main pathologic findings are related to the release of cytokines by CD4 T cells in the recipient (*not* the donor graft); the findings in the donor graft include the following:
    (1) Atherosclerosis of vascular endothelium related to proliferation of intimal smooth muscle cells (see Chapter 10) leading to obliteration of vascular lumens
    (2) Proliferation of fibroblasts leading to interstitial fibrosis with atrophy of epithelial tissue (*not* shown in Fig. 4-8 C; e.g., renal tubular cell atrophy, glomerular sclerosis)
    (3) Interstitial infiltrate of plasma cells and eosinophils

5. Infections associated with transplantation
  a. Cytomegalovirus (CMV) is the most common infection in transplant recipients.
  b. CD8 T cells are important in preventing latent CMV infections from recurring.
  c. In solid organ transplantation, *Candida* is the most common infection, followed by *Aspergillus.*
  d. In bone marrow (BM) transplantation, *Aspergillus* is the most common infection, followed by *Candida.*

6. Transplantation screening tests
  a. Blood type testing of recipient and donor
    (1) ABO blood group type (i.e., A, B, AB, O; see Chapter 16)
    (2) Recipient and donor must have either the same blood type or compatible blood types.
    (3) Rh type (+ or −) is *not* a factor in donor matching.
  b. Identification of tissue histocompatibility antigens and genes of recipients and potential donors to assess the degree of match between them; the closer the HLA antigens match between the donor and the recipient, the less the chance of an immune reaction
  c. Detection and characterization of HLA-specific antibodies in recipients
  d. Crossmatch (CX) testing, which determines if the recipient has developed HLA antibodies that will attack donor cells

D. Graft-versus-host (GVH) reaction
1. **Definition:** A GVH reaction is where immunocompetent T cells in the donor graft recognize recipient antigens as foreign and react against them.
2. Key prerequisites for GVH reaction
  • Donor graft must contain immunocompetent T cells; recipient must be immunocompromised; and recipient must have MHC antigens that are foreign to donor T lymphocytes.
3. Causes of a GVH reaction
  a. A GVH reaction is a potential complication in BM transplants (85% of cases), liver transplants, and blood transfusion given to patients with a T-cell immunodeficiency (e.g., DiGeorge syndrome) or normal newborns.
  b. Removing T cells from a BM transplant markedly reduces the incidence of a GVH reaction.
  c. When newborns receive RBC transfusions, blood is irradiated to destroy donor T lymphocytes in the transfusion that may produce a GVH reaction.
4. Acute GVH reaction (Fig. 4-9)
  a. **Definition:** Donor CD8 cytotoxic T cells recognize the host tissue as foreign, proliferate in the host tissue, and produce severe organ damage. Type IV cytotoxic T-cell HSR (see Table 4-4).

C4d indicates humoral (antibodies) component present

Less severe/late onset: vessels thicker; intima similar to atherosclerosis

Potentially reversible with immunosuppressive Rx

Danger cervical/skin SCC, malignant lymphoma

Irreversible; mos/yrs; previous acute rejection immunosuppression

Chronic type IV HSR

Cytokine release CD4T cells recipient against donor graft

Atherosclerosis; occlusion vascular lumens

Fibroblast proliferation → interstitial fibrosis (atrophy epithelial tissue)

Infiltrate plasma cells/eosinophils

CMV MC infection

CD8T cells prevent latent CMV recurrence

Solid organ: *Candida* MC infection

BM: *Aspergillus* MC infection

ABO blood group: recipient/donor must be compatible

Rh type (+ or −) *not* a factor in donor matching

Identify HLA antigens/genes recipients and potential donors

Detect/characterize HLA-specific antibodies in recipients

CX testing: detects HLA antibodies in recipient

T cells donor graft recognize recipient antigens as foreign

Donor graft has T cells; recipient immunocompromised; recipient MHC antigens foreign to donor T cells

BM and liver transplants; blood transfusion T-cell immunodeficiency; normal newborns

Remove T cells from BM transplant

Newborns: irradiate blood to remove T cells

Donor CD8 cells recognize host tissue as foreign → type IV HSR

4-9: Acute graft-versus-host (GVH) reaction. In GVH, donor T cells attack host major histocompatibility complex antigens located in the skin, bile duct epithelium, and mucosa of the gastrointestinal tract. *(Modified from Actor JK: Elsevier's Integrated Immunology and Microbiology, Philadelphia, Mosby, 2007, p 68, Fig. 8-4.)*

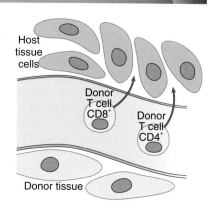

TABLE 4-5   Some Types of Transplants

TYPE OF TRANSPLANT	COMMENTS
Cornea	Best allograft survival rate Danger of transmission of Creutzfeldt-Jakob disease
Kidney	Better survival with kidney from living donor than from cadaver
Bone marrow	Graft contains pluripotential cells that repopulate host stem cells Host assumes donor ABO group Danger of graft-versus-host reaction and cytomegalovirus infection

b. Clinical findings
   (1) Bile duct necrosis, leading to jaundice
   (2) Gastrointestinal mucosa ulceration, leading to bloody diarrhea
   (3) Generalized skin rash, sometimes leading to desquamation
   (4) Hepatosplenomegaly
E. **Types of grafts** (Table 4-5)
V. **Autoimmune Disease**
   A. **Definition of autoimmune disease**
      1. Autoimmune disease refers to the loss of self-tolerance, resulting in immune reactions that are directed against host tissue (self-antigens).
      2. Self-antigens include class I and II MHC antigens, nuclear antigens, and cytoplasmic antigens.
   B. **Mechanisms of autoimmune disease**
      1. Strong association with certain HLA types and autoimmune disease (e.g., class I and class II genes; see earlier discussion)
         a. In general, class I–related diseases (e.g., ankylosing spondylitis [HLA-B27]) are more common in men than in women.
         b. In general, class II–related diseases (e.g., rheumatoid arthritis [HLA-DR4]) are more common in women than men.
         c. Having an HLA type that is associated with an autoimmune disease (e.g., HLA-B27) does *not* guarantee that the person will develop that disease.
         d. Various environmental triggers are required to initiate the autoimmune disease in genetically susceptible individuals.
      2. Infection as an environmental trigger for autoimmune disease
         a. Mechanisms
            (1) Upregulation of co-stimulators on APCs (they have class I and class II HLA antigens) leads to the formation of self-reactive CD4 T cells and CD8 cytotoxic T cells that damage tissue.
               Self-reactive lymphocytes means that they release IL-2, causing clonal proliferation of the CD4 and CD8 T cells.
            (2) Sharing of antigens between the host and pathogen (molecular mimicry). Example: in rheumatic fever, certain strains of *Streptococcus pyogenes* producing pharyngitis have antigens in their M proteins that are similar to antigens in the human heart, joints, and other tissues.
            (3) Polyclonal activation of B lymphocytes. Results in the formation of autoantibodies against host tissue. Polyclonal activators include Epstein-Barr virus (EBV), human immunodeficiency virus (HIV), and CMV.

Jaundice, diarrhea, dermatitis, hepatosplenomegaly

Loss self-tolerance; host tissue considered foreign

Self-antigens: class I/II MHC, nuclear/cytoplasmic

Class I–related (HLA-B27) men > women

Class II–related (HLA-DR4) women > men

Disease not inevitable

Genetic predisposition involving HLA system + environmental trigger

Upregulation co-stimulators on APCs (class I/II antigens)

Self-reactive lymphocytes release IL-2 → clonal proliferation CD4/CD8 T cells

Sharing antigens between host and pathogen: S. pyogenes–rheumatic fever

Autoantibodies against host tissue

EBV, HIV, CMV; produce autoantibodies

b. Viruses implicated in triggering autoimmune disease
    (1) Coxsackievirus: myocarditis (B3), type 1 diabetes mellitus (B4)
    (2) Measles virus: allergic encephalitis; CMV: systemic sclerosis
    (3) EBV: hepatitis B, systemic lupus erythematosus (SLE), rheumatoid arthritis
    (4) Human herpesvirus type 6 (HHV-6), influenza A virus: multiple sclerosis
c. Bacteria implicated in triggering autoimmune disease
    (1) *Streptococcus pyogenes*: rheumatic fever; *Chlamydia trachomatis*: reactive arthritis
    (2) Enteric *Klebsiella pneumoniae*, *Shigella* species: ankylosing spondylitis
    (3) *Mycoplasma pneumoniae*, *Campylobacter jejuni*: Guillain-Barré syndrome (GBS)
3. Drugs as an environmental trigger for autoimmune disease
  a. Procainamide and hydralazine
    (1) Drugs bind to histones, causing them to become immunogenic.
    (2) Autoantibodies develop against histones, producing a lupus-like syndrome.
  b. Methyldopa
    (1) Alters Rh antigens on the surface of RBCs.
    (2) IgG autoantibodies develop against the altered Rh antigens on RBCs.
    (3) Splenic macrophages with receptors for IgG phagocytose and destroy the RBCs, producing and autoimmune normocytic hemolytic anemia (AIHA; type II HSR; see Chapter 12).
4. Hormones as a trigger for autoimmune disease
  a. Approximately 90% of all autoimmune diseases occur in women.
  b. It is possible that estrogen triggers B cells to produce antibodies against DNA. (RBCs in the BM are nucleated and contain DNA.)
5. Release of sequestered antigens (antigens that are *not* normally exposed to the immune system) act as a trigger for autoimmune disease.
  a. Tissues with sequestered antigens include the testicles (sperm is antigenic), lens in the eye, uveal tract in the eyes, and the CNS. Damage to these tissues may result in autoimmune disease (e.g., azoospermia, cataracts, endophthalmitis [inflammatory condition of the aqueous and/or vitreous humor], encephalitis [inflammation of the brain]).
  b. Intracellular antigens like DNA and histones are *not* normally exposed to the immune system.
    (1) SLE, genetic, immunologic, and environmental factors damage cells leading to the formation of autoantibodies against double-stranded DNA (dsDNA).
    (2) Second exposure to the release of DNA results in IC formation (type III HSR; DNA–anti-DNA ICs), leading to various manifestations of the disease (e.g., diffuse proliferative glomerulonephritis; see following discussion).
  c. Defects in apoptosis may also lead to exposure of nuclear antigens in necrotic material that may be targeted by lymphocytes to produce autoantibodies.
6. Ultraviolet (UV) radiation is a trigger for autoimmune disease.
  a. UV radiation is important in producing the characteristic malar rash that is present in SLE.
  b. UV radiation induces apoptosis of keratinocytes, releasing sequestered intracellular nuclear antigens.
    (1) Leads to formation of autoantibodies that combine with the nuclear antigens to form ICs (autoantibody–nuclear antigen IC).
    (2) ICs produce a vasculitis (leads to vessel rupture), which is responsible for the erythematous rash in SLE.
7. T-cell theories implicated in autoimmune disease
  a. Theories include defects in the thymus, decreased CD8 T cell function, and altered CD4 T-cell function.
  b. Thymus is responsible for exposing developing T cells to self-proteins either produced in the thymus or delivered to the thymus.
    (1) If self-proteins are *not* exposed to developing T cells, then they are recognized as foreign and are subsequently attacked.
    (2) Autoimmune diseases associated with this inability to recognize self-proteins tend to be generalized (e.g., SLE).
8. Non-*MHC* genes associated with autoimmune disease
  a. **Definition:** Non-*MHC* genes are a group of genes that interfere with normal immune regulation and self-tolerance.
  b. *PTPN-22* gene (protein tyrosine phosphatase, nonreceptor gene) encodes for a functionally defective protein tyrosine phosphatase that *cannot* control tyrosine kinase activity, which is an important enzyme in normal lymphocyte responses.

Coxsackievirus

Measles

EBV

HHV-6, influenza virus

Streptococcus pyogenes (rheumatic fever), *Chlamydia trachomatis* (reactive arthritis)

K. pneumoniae, Shigella: ankylosing spondylitis

M. pneumoniae, C. jejuni: GBS

Procainamide, hydralazine

Bind histones → autoantibodies against histones; lupus-like syndrome

Methyldopa

Alters RBC Rh antigens

IgG antibodies against RBC Rh antigens

Splenic macrophages destroy RBCs; AIHA; type II HSR

Autoimmune disease women > men

Possible that estrogen triggers B-cell production antibodies against DNA

Release of sequestered antigens

Sequestered antigens: sperm, lens, uveal tract, CNS

Intracellular DNA, histone antigens *not* normally exposed

SLE, genetic, immunologic, environmental factor: damage cells → autoantibodies

Autoantibodies develop against dsDNA

2nd exposure: release DNA results in IC formation (type III HSR)

Defects apoptosis: exposure of nuclear antigens

UV light malar rash in SLE

Apoptosis keratinocytes releases intracellular nuclear autoantibodies

Autoantibodies combine with nuclear antigens → ICs

ICs produce vasculitis → erythematous rash of SLE

Defects thymus; CD8 T cell function; CD4 T-cell function

Thymus exposes developing T cells to self-proteins (from/delivered to thymus)

Self-proteins *not* exposed → recognized as foreign → destroyed

SLE: e.g., inability to recognize self-antigens

Non-*MHC* genes: interfere with immune regulation/self-tolerance

PTPN-22 gene: functionally defective protein tyrosine phosphatase

Rheumatoid arthritis, type 1 diabetes mellitus

NOD-2 gene: implicated in Crohn disease

IRF5: interferes with IFN activity

IFNs important defense against microbial pathogens, tumor cells

STAT4 important in lymphocyte activation

Immune destruction adrenal cortex

Pernicious anemia: vitamin B$_{12}$ deficiency

Immune destruction parietal cells → no intrinsic factor → no B$_{12}$ reabsorption

Neurologic problems

Immune destruction thyroid → hypothyroidism

SLE, rheumatoid arthritis, systemic sclerosis

Most useful screening test for autoimmune disease

Antibodies directed against nuclear antigens

Anti-dsDNA: SLE with glomerulonephritis

Basic pH proteins in chromatin

Antihistone antibodies: drug-induced lupus

Acid nuclear protein

Anti-Smith: SLE

Anti-RNP: systemic sclerosis

Anti-nucleolar: systemic sclerosis

Fluorescent antibody test; pattern/titer

Speckled, homogeneous, nucleolar, rim

SLE: Rim pattern + anti-dsDNA + renal disease

Serum ANA titers: follow disease activity

Specific antibody tests: antibodies against proton pump in pernicious anemia

Chronic multisystem autoimmune disease

Women childbearing age (20–45 yrs)

More common in African Americans, Asians, Hispanics than Caucasians

DR2, DR3; ↓C1q, C2, C4

c. Functionally defective tyrosine phosphatase is most frequently implicated in producing autoimmune diseases (e.g., type 1 diabetes mellitus, rheumatoid arthritis).
d. *NOD-2* gene has been implicated in Crohn disease.
Allows intestinal bacteria to enter the bowel and produce chronic inflammation.

C. Markers of autoimmune disease
1. Interferon regulatory factor 5 (IRF5) increases IFN activity. IFNs are signaling proteins made and released by host cells in response to the presence of pathogenic viruses, bacteria, and parasites as well as tumor cells.
2. STAT4 (signal transducer and activator of transcription) is a signaling molecule that is important in lymphocyte activation.

D. Classification of autoimmune disorders
1. Organ-specific disorders
   a. Addison disease: caused by immune destruction of the adrenal cortex. This leads to hypocortisolism (see Chapter 23).
   b. Pernicious anemia: causes vitamin B$_{12}$ deficiency. In pernicious anemia, there is immune destruction of parietal cells in the stomach, which produce intrinsic factor, a factor that is required to bind with vitamin B$_{12}$ in order for it be absorbed in the terminal ileum (see Chapter 18).
   This leads to a severe macrocytic anemia (large RBCs) and neurologic problems (e.g., dementia, demyelination of the spinal cord, and peripheral neuropathy).
   c. Hashimoto thyroiditis: caused by immune destruction of the thyroid due to the formation of autoantibodies, which leads to underactivity of the thyroid gland (hypothyroidism; see Chapter 23).
2. Systemic disorders: examples include SLE, rheumatoid arthritis, and systemic sclerosis (see Chapter 24).

E. Laboratory evaluation of autoimmune disease
1. Serum antinuclear antibody (ANA) test
   a. Serum ANA is the most useful screening test for autoimmune disease.
   b. **Definition:** ANAs are directed against various nuclear antigens.
      (1) DNA: Antibodies against dsDNA are present in patients with SLE who have renal disease (e.g., glomerulonephritis).
      (2) Histones. **Definition:** Histones are basic pH proteins in chromatin (a combination of DNA and protein) in the cell nucleus. Antihistone antibodies are present in drug-induced lupus.
      (3) Ribonucleoprotein (RNP)
         (a) **Definition:** RNP is an acidic nuclear protein that contains RNA (ribonucleic acid).
         (b) Two antibodies against RNP include anti-Smith antibodies in SLE and anti-RNP antibodies in systemic sclerosis (most common) and SLE.
      (4) Nucleolar antigens. Anti-nucleolar antibodies are present in systemic sclerosis.
   c. Serum ANA is a fluorescent antibody test.
      (1) Patterns of immunofluorescence are useful in making specific diagnoses (Link 4-22).
         (a) Patterns include speckled, homogeneous, nucleolar, and rim.
         (b) Rim pattern correlates with anti-dsDNA antibodies and the presence of renal disease in SLE.
      (2) Titer of ANA can be periodically measured to follow disease activity.
2. Specific antibody tests document organ-specific autoimmune diseases. Example: antibodies directed against the proton pump in parietal cells are diagnostic of pernicious anemia.
3. Table 4-6 summarizes autoantibodies that are involved in various autoimmune diseases.

F. Systemic lupus erythematosus (SLE)
1. **Definition:** SLE is a chronic, multisystem, autoimmune disease that is characterized by production of autoantibodies that deposit in tissues (e.g., skin, kidneys) and fix complement leading to systemic inflammation.
2. Epidemiology
   a. Primarily affects women of childbearing age (female/male ratio 9:1; >90% of cases). Women are usually in the childbearing age between 20 and 45 years old. More common in African Americans, Asians, and Hispanics than in Caucasians.
3. Etiology and pathogenesis
   a. Genetic factors
      (1) Certain HLA associations are more common in people with SLE than in the general population (e.g., HLA-DR2, HLA-DR3).
      (2) Inherited deficiencies of certain complement components increase the risk for developing SLE (e.g., C1q, C2, C4 deficiency).

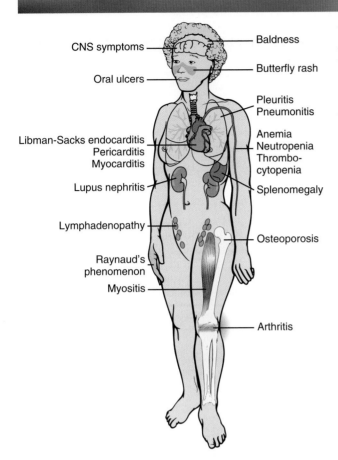

CNS symptoms — Baldness
Oral ulcers — Butterfly rash
— Pleuritis
Pneumonitis
Libman-Sacks endocarditis
Pericarditis — Anemia
Myocarditis — Neutropenia
Thrombo-
cytopenia
Lupus nephritis — Splenomegaly
Lymphadenopathy — Osteoporosis
Raynaud's
phenomenon
Myositis — Arthritis

4-10: Clinical and pathologic features of systemic lupus erythematosus. The disease affects most frequently the skin, joints, kidneys, and the liver, whereas other organs are affected less often. *CNS,* Central nervous system. *(From my friend Ivan Damjanov, MD, PhD:* Pathology for the Health Professions, *Saunders Elsevier, 4th ed, 2012, p 60, Fig. 3-18.)*

  b. Environmental triggers are important in exacerbating SLE or triggering its initial onset; examples include infectious agents (EBV), UV light (see earlier), estrogen (see earlier), and medications (e.g., procainamide, hydralazine).

  c. Defects in apoptosis or in the clearance of apoptotic fragments are frequently present. Exposure of nuclear antigens (normally sequestered antigens) in necrotic debris on the cell surface leads to polyclonal B- and T-cell activation and autoantibody production.

  d. Mechanisms of injury
    (1) ICs (e.g., DNA–anti-DNA) are most important in producing inflammation in the skin, glomeruli/tubules, joints, and small vessels. All are examples of a type III HSR.
    (2) Autoantibodies are important in the pathogenesis of various cytopenias involving RBCs, neutrophils, lymphocytes, and platelets. All of these cytopenias are type II HSRs.

  4. Clinical findings (Fig. 4-10)
    a. Classic presentation in most cases of SLE is a triad of fever, joint pain, and rash in a woman of childbearing age.
    b. Constitutional symptoms include fatigue (most common), fever, arthralgia, and weight loss (occur 90%–95% of cases).
    c. Hematologic findings (15%–20% for each finding)
      (1) Autoimmune hemolytic anemia, thrombocytopenia, leukopenia (neutropenia and lymphopenia
      (2) Lymphopenia is a good guide to disease activity (bad sign).
    d. Lymphatic findings include generalized painful lymphadenopathy and splenomegaly.
    e. Musculoskeletal findings (80%–90%)
      (1) Arthralgia (joint pain; *not* inflammation) is one of the most common initial complaints.
      Morning stiffness in the hands is particularly common.
      (2) Arthritis (inflammatory joint disease)
        (a) Most common sites are the proximal interphalangeal (PIP) and metacarpophalangeal joints (MCP) in both hands and the wrists.
        (b) Usually symmetric, nonerosive, and nondeforming, unlike rheumatoid arthritis, which is deforming
      (3) Other findings that may occur include avascular (aseptic) necrosis, osteoporosis (loss of organic bone matrix and mineralized bone) from long-term corticosteroid therapy, and myositis (muscle inflammation) (see Chapter 24).

EBV, UV light, estrogen
Procainamide, hydralazine

Apoptosis defects

ICs
Skin, glomeruli/tubules, joints, small vessels
Autoantibodies
Cytopenias: RBCs, neutrophils, lymphocytes, platelets
Fever, joint pain, rash woman childbearing age
Fatigue (MC), fever, arthralgia, weight loss

Autoimmune anemia, neutro/lympho/ thrombocytopenia
Generalized painful lymphadenopathy, splenomegaly

Arthralgia (joint pain)
Morning hand stiffness
Arthritis

PIP/MCP hands/wrists

Symmetric; nonerosive/ deforming

Avascular necrosis, osteoporosis, myositis

TABLE 4-6 Autoantibodies in Autoimmune Disease

AUTOANTIBODIES	DISEASES	TEST SENSITIVITY %
Anti-acetylcholine receptor	Myasthenia gravis	>85
Anti–basement membrane	Goodpasture syndrome	>90
Anticentromere	CREST syndrome	82–96
Anti-DNA topoisomerase	Systemic sclerosis (scleroderma)	30–70
Anti-dsDNA	SLE	70–98
Anti-ssDNA	SLE	60–70
Antiendomysial IgA	Celiac disease	95
Antigliadin IgA	Celiac disease	80
Antihistone	Drug-induced lupus Procainamide Penicillamine, isoniazid, methyldopa	 96 100
Anti-insulin	SLE Type 1 diabetes	50–70 50
Anti–intrinsic factor	Pernicious anemia	60
Anti–islet cell	Type 1 diabetes	75–80
Anti–Jo-1 (transfer RNA synthetase)	Polymyositis	25–30
Antimicrosomal	Hashimoto thyroiditis Chronic active hepatitis	97 60–80
Antimitochondrial	Primary biliary cirrhosis Cryptogenic cirrhosis	90–100 30
Antimyeloperoxidase	Microscopic polyangiitis	80 (p-ANCA)
Antinucleosome	SLE	61–85
Antinuclear	SLE Systemic sclerosis CREST syndrome Dermatomyositis Mixed connective tissue disease Polymyositis	98 60–80 98% <30 95–99 33%
Antinuclear cytoplasmic antibodies (c-ANCA)	Wegener granulomatosis (GPA) Microscopic polyangiitis Churg-Strauss syndrome	>90
Antinuclear cytoplasmic antibodies (p-ANCA		>80 70
Antinucleosome	SLE	61–85
Anti–parietal cell	Pernicious anemia	90
Antiphospholipid (APL)	SLE	30–40
Anti-PM-1	Polymyositis or polymyositis/ systemic sclerosis overlap syndrome MCTD Primary biliary cirrhosis Wegener granulomatosis	60–90 95–99 50 >90 (c-ANCA)
Anti–rheumatoid arthritis nuclear antigen (RANA)	Sjögren syndrome with rheumatoid arthritis	60–76
Anti-ribonucleoprotein (U1-RNP) Antiribosomal	MCTD SLE SLE	≈100 5–12 30–40
Anti-Smith	SLE	20 (white) 30–40 (black, Asian)
Anti–smooth muscle	Chronic active hepatitis	60–91
Anti–soluble nucleoprotein (sNP)	SLE	50

TABLE 4-6   Autoantibodies in Autoimmune Disease—cont'd

AUTOANTIBODIES	DISEASES	TEST SENSITIVITY %
Anti–SS-A (Ro)	Sjögren syndrome without rheumatoid arthritis	60–70
	SLE	26–50
	Neonatal SLE	>95
	SLE	30
	Primary biliary cirrhosis	15–19
Anti–SS-B (La)	Sjögren syndrome without rheumatoid arthritis	40–60
	Sjögren syndrome with rheumatoid arthritis	5
	SLE	5–15
	Systemic sclerosis	15–43
Antithyroglobulin	SLE	10–15
	Hashimoto thyroiditis	85
Anti–tissue transglutaminase IgA	Celiac disease	98
Anti–TSH receptor	Graves disease	85

Anti-dsDNA, Anti–double-stranded DNA; *anti-ssDNA,* anti–single-stranded DNA; *c-ANCA,* cytoplasmic antineutrophil cytoplasmic antibody; *CREST,* calcinosis, Raynaud phenomenon, esophageal dysfunction, sclerodactyly, telangiectasia; *GPA,* granulomatosis with polyangiitis; *MCTD,* mixed connective tissue disease; *p-ANCA,* perinuclear antineutrophilic cytoplasmic antibody; *SLE,* systemic lupus erythematosus; *TSH,* thyroid-stimulating hormone.

 f. Skin and mucocutaneous findings (80%–90%)
  (1) Butterfly-shaped malar rash over the cheeks and bridge of the nose with sparing of the nasolabial folds is a very characteristic sign of SLE and it subtypes (Fig. 4-11 A).

> Butterfly malar rash, photosensitive

   (a) Erythematous lesions also commonly involve the dorsum of the hands and fingers and also the skin *between* the joints rather than over the joints.

> Dorsum hands/fingers; skin *between* joints

   (b) UV light exposure either initiates or exacerbates the rash.

> UV light exacerbates

   (c) Immunofluorescence (IF) studies show IC deposition along the basement membrane in both involved and uninvolved areas of skin (Link 4-23).

> Linear IF basement membrane skin; involved/uninvolved skin

  (2) Discoid lupus (≈25%)
   (a) **Definition:** Discoid lupus is a chronic, plaque-like rash that often develops in sun-exposed areas.

> Chronic plaque-like rash sun-exposed areas

   (b) Plaque is defined as a solid, raised, flat-topped lesion that is greater than 1 cm in diameter.
  (3) Oral ulcers (15%–45%); locations include the hard palate, buccal mucosa, tongue, and nose.

> Oral ulcers hard palate, buccal mucosa, tongue/nose

  (4) Alopecia (partial or complete loss of hair)

> Partial/complete loss hair (alopecia)

 g. Renal findings (40%–60%)
  (1) Kidney is the most common visceral organ involved in SLE.

> Kidney MC visceral organ involved

  (2) Diffuse proliferative glomerulonephritis is the most common and severe glomerular disease. Presents with a nephritic syndrome (hematuria, RBC casts in the urine, proteinuria, hypertension; see Chapter 20).

> Diffuse proliferative glomerulonephritis (nephritic)

  (3) Diffuse membranous glomerulonephritis presenting with the nephrotic syndrome (massive proteinuria) is less common (see Chapter 20).

> Diffuse membranous glomerulonephritis (nephrotic)

  (4) Other types of glomerulonephritis include focal proliferative glomerulosclerosis, mesangial proliferative glomerulonephritis, and advanced sclerosing glomerulonephritis.
  (5) Chronic renal failure is a common cause of death.

> Chronic renal failure common COD

 h. Cardiovascular findings
  (1) Fibrinous pericarditis (serositis) with or without effusion is the most common cardiac finding (50%–70%; see Chapter 11).

> Fibrinous pericarditis MC

  (2) Libman-Sacks endocarditis (LSE; see Chapter 11). Sterile fibrin containing vegetations involving the mitral valve surface produce valve deformity and mitral valve regurgitation.

> LSE: sterile vegetations mitral valve

  (3) Myocarditis can present with chest pain and heart failure (left- and/or right-sided).

> Myocarditis

  (4) Digital vasculitis is associated with Raynaud phenomenon (see Chapter 10).

> Digital vasculitis: Raynaud

 i. Respiratory findings
  (1) Pleuritic chest pain (serositis; sharp pain on inspiration) with or without a pleural effusion is the most common respiratory finding (50%–70%).

> Pleuritis (serositis) with/without effusion MC lung finding

   (a) Most common acute pulmonary finding in SLE

> MC lung finding

   (b) Inflammation of the pleural membrane (serositis) is a key finding in SLE.

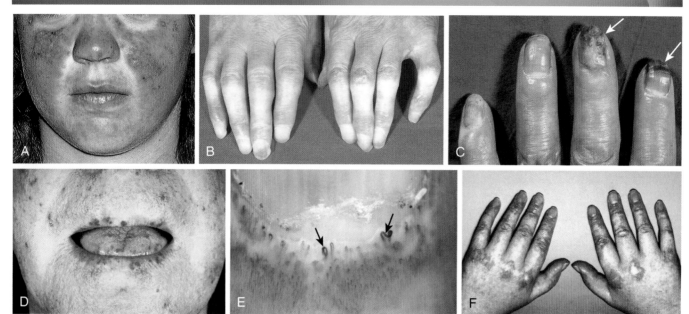

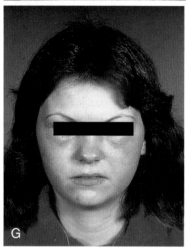

4-11: **A,** Malar rash in systemic lupus erythematosus showing the butterfly-wing distribution. **B,** Raynaud phenomenon, one of the first signs of systemic sclerosis, is due to a digital vasculitis. The usual color changes are white (this patient) to blue to red. **C,** Systemic sclerosis. The skin is erythematous and tightly bound. The fingertips are tapered (called sclerodactyly) and have digital infarcts *(arrows)* due to fibrosis of the digital vessels. **D,** Systemic sclerosis and CREST syndrome. Note the thinned lips and characteristic radial furrowing around the mouth, giving a pursed-lip appearance. This is due to increased deposition of collagen in the subcutaneous tissue. There are also dilatations of small vessels (telangiectasia) on the face and oral mucosa. **E,** Nail fold capillary microscopy in systemic sclerosis. Note the abnormal capillary loops *(arrows).* **F,** Dermatomyositis. Note the characteristic purple papules overlying the knuckles and proximal and distal interphalangeal joints (Gottron patches). **G,** Dermatomyositis. Note the characteristic swelling and red-mauve discoloration below the eyes. *(A from Marx J:* Rosen's Emergency Medicine Concepts and Clinical Practice, *7th ed, Philadelphia, Mosby Elsevier, 2010, p 1498, Fig. 116.1; taken from Habif TP:* Clinical Dermatology, *4th ed, New York, Mosby, 2004, pp 592-606; B from Savin JA, Hunter JAA, Hepburn NC:* Diagnosis in Color: Skin Signs in Clinical Medicine, *London, Mosby-Wolfe, 1997, p 205, Fig. 8.43; C, D, and G courtesy RA Marsden, MD, St. George's Hospital, London; E from Habif TB:* Clinical Dermatology, *6th ed, Philadelphia, Elsevier, 2016, Fig. 17-36; F courtesy of Carol M. Ziminski, MD, from Ashar BH, Miller RG, Sisso SD:* The Johns Hopkins Internal Medicine Board Review, *4th ed, Elsevier, 2012, p 384, Fig. 45-8.)*

Interstitial fibrosis: RLD, PH

Headache (MC), psychosis, seizures, chorea

APL syndrome (stroke)

CHB in newborns: IgG anti-Ro antibodies

Recurrent spontaneous abortions (placental vessel thrombosis; APL)

Procainamide MC drug in drug-induced lupus

Serositis, arthralgia, fever

Antihistone antibodies; *no* antibodies against DNA

No ↓ serum C; ↓ incidence renal/CNS disease

Disappearance symptoms/ lab abnormalities D/C drug

(2) Interstitial fibrosis may occur, leading to restrictive lung disease (RLD) and pulmonary hypertension (PH; see Chapter 17).
j. CNS findings (40%–60%)
(1) Headache (most common), psychosis, visual hallucinations, seizures, chorea (movement disorder), and strokes.
(2) Vessel thrombosis causing strokes is most often associated with the antiphospholipid (APL) syndrome (see Chapter 15).
k. Pregnancy-related findings
(1) Complete heart block (CHB) in newborns may occur. Caused by IgG anti–Sjögren syndrome (SS)-A (Ro) antibodies crossing the placenta and attacking the newborn's cardiac conduction system. IgM antibodies cannot cross placenta.
(2) Recurrent spontaneous abortions commonly occur. Complication of thrombosis from APL antibodies (see Chapter 15).
l. Revised American Rheumatism Association criteria are available online for SLE.
5. Drug-induced lupus erythematosus
a. Procainamide (most common) and hydralazine
b. Clinical findings: serositis (inflammation pleura, pericardium), arthralgia, and fever
c. Features that distinguish drug-induced lupus from SLE
(1) Presence of antihistone antibodies; *no* antibodies against native DNA
(2) *No* decrease in serum complement (C) levels; *low* incidence of renal and CNS involvement
(3) Disappearance of symptoms and laboratory test results when the drug is discontinued

6. Laboratory testing in SLE
   a. Serum ANA (see Table 4-6)
      (1) Best test for screening for SLE (sensitivity 98%)
         (a) False negative test results are uncommon (see Chapter 1).
         (b) Antibodies are frequently present *before* clinical findings occur.
         (c) High titers are generally more specific for SLE (>1:160) than other autoimmune diseases.
      (2) Specificity of serum antinuclear antibodies in diagnosing SLE is 80%. Other autoimmune diseases have an increase in serum ANA; hence, the low specificity.
   b. Anti-dsDNA antibodies
      (1) Most often used to *confirm* the diagnosis of SLE (95% specificity). If positive, it usually indicates that renal disease is present.
      (2) Sensitivity of the test for diagnosing SLE is 70% to 98%.
   c. Anti-Smith antibodies
      (1) Used to *confirm* the diagnosis of SLE (99% specificity; rare false positives)
      (2) Decreased sensitivity (20% in the white population and 30% to 40% in the black and Asian population). *Not* a good screening test.
   d. Anti-Ro (SS-A) antibodies and anti-La (SS-B) antibodies have a low sensitivity (26%–50% and 5%–15%, respectively) and a low specificity. Anti-Ro (SS-A) has a sensitivity of >95% in diagnosing neonatal heart block.
   e. APL antibodies (sensitivity 30%–40%; see Chapter 15)
   f. Antihistone antibodies
      (1) Sensitivity is 96% for procainamide.
      (2) Sensitivity is 100% for penicillamine, isoniazid, and methyldopa.
   g. Lupus erythematosus cell. **Definition:** Refers to a neutrophil that contains phagocytosed altered DNA. No longer available for the diagnosis of SLE because it is a time-consuming test.
   h. Serum complement: usually decreased because of activation of the complement system by ICs.
   i. Erythrocyte sedimentation rate (ESR) is increased in active SLE.
   j. CRP is often normal in active SLE *except* if coexisting serositis or infection is present.
   k. IF testing
      (1) Identifies ICs in a band-like distribution along the dermal-epidermal junction of involved and uninvolved skin (called *band test*; Link 4-23).
      (2) IF studies of kidney biopsies are used to identify different types of glomerulonephritis.
7. Prognosis
   a. Overall 10-year survival is 85% to 90%. Improved survival due to advances in diagnosis and treatment.
   b. Most common (MC) causes of death (COD) in SLE
      (1) Cardiovascular disease (30%–40%)
      (2) Lupus glomerulonephritis, CNS lupus, vasculitis, and pneumonitis—most lethal conditions (35%)
      (3) Infection due to immunosuppression therapy (25% of all deaths)
      (4) Malignancy (5%–10%; human papilloma virus–related [cervical cancer], and malignant lymphoma)

G. Systemic sclerosis
1. **Definition:** Systemic sclerosis is a multisystem disease characterized by vascular dysfunction and excessive production of normal collagen that primarily targets the skin (scleroderma) and internal organs. Two major forms of systemic sclerosis include systemic scleroderma and CREST syndrome.
2. Epidemiology
   a. Female dominant disorder (female/male 4:1) usually presenting between the ages of 35 and 64 years
   b. Increased incidence in the black female population and female Choctaw Native Americans (Oklahoma; highest reported prevalence in the United States)
   c. Etiology and pathogenesis
      (1) Increase in CD4 T_H2 cells in the skin reacting against an unknown antigen; T cells release cytokines (IL-13 and TGF-β) that activate inflammatory cells and fibroblasts.
      (2) Increase in autoantibody production, particularly against DNA topoisomerase I (old term anti–Scl-70) and centromeres

---

Serum ANA

Best screen: sensitivity 98%

ANAs present *before* clinical findings

↑ANA titers more specific for SLE

Specificity serum ANA 80%

Confirm SLE; specificity 95%

Renal disease present

Sensitivity 70%–98%

High specificity (99%); confirm SLE

Decreased sensitivity

+Anti-Ro neonatal heart block

APL; strokes, recurrent abortions

Antihistone antibodies

Procainamide: antihistone antibodies (96% sensitivity)

Penicillamine, isoniazid, methyldopa (100% sensitivity)

Lupus erythematosus cell: neutrophil containing phagocytosed altered DNA

↓Serum C: C consumed forming ICs

↑ESR active SLE

↑CRP serositis/infection present

IF along dermal-epidermal junction from ICs

IF studies identify types glomerulonephritis

Overall 10-year survival 85%–90%

Cardiovascular disease MC COD

Vascular dysfunction, fibrosis skin/visceral organs

Diffuse/limited systemic sclerosis

Female dominant

Black females, female Choctaw Native Americans

↑CD4 T_H2 cells against unknown antigen

↑Antibodies against DNA-topoisomerase, centromeres

ED earliest manifestation

Vasculitis digital vessels

ED: ↓NO, PGI$_2$; ↑endothelin

Mechanism perivascular fibrosis ↑PDGF, TGF-β

↑Exposure to silica dust (fibrogenic)

Progressive fibrosis: PDGF, TGF-β

Raynaud phenomenon digital vessels

White to blue to red

MC initial sign Sjögren syndrome

Sclerodactyly, digital infarcts

Skin MC target organ

Swollen fingers/hands

Thickened skin from subcutaneous fibrosis

Dystrophic calcification, radial furrowing

Telangiectasia

Nail fold abnormal capillary loops

Gastrointestinal tract commonly involved

Dysphagia sign esophageal motility disorder

Manometry → absent peristalsis (collagen deposition)

Esophageal ulceration, strictures

Dysfunction LES → GA reflux → Barrett esophagus

Stomach: dysmotility/bloating

Small intestine

Loss villi → malabsorption

Small intestine dysmotility

Wide-mouthed diverticula

Large intestine: dysmotility, constipation

Respiratory

Interstitial fibrosis → RLD → hypoxemia

Respiratory failure MC COD

Dyspnea, cough

(3) Endothelial dysfunction (ED): earliest manifestation of the disease
   (a) Vascular injury, particularly involving the digital vessels, is most likely related to cytokines released by CD4 T$_H$2 cells and other unknown factors.
   (b) Digital vessels have a decrease in vasodilators (NO, PGI$_2$) and an increase in vasoconstrictors (endothelin).
   (c) Damaged endothelial cells release platelet-derived growth factor (PDGF) and TGF-β. Growth factors attract fibroblasts causing perivascular fibrosis, with narrowing of vessel lumens leading to ischemic injury (see later).
(4) Environmental factor: increased exposure to silica dust (very fibrogenic; see Chapter 17)
(5) Progressive fibrosis in the skin and visceral organs: primarily due to PDGF and TGF-β

4. Clinical findings
   a. Raynaud phenomenon occurs in digital vessels.
      (1) Sequential color changes (white to blue to red) are caused by digital vessel vasculitis/thrombosis and perivascular fibrosis (Fig. 4-11 B, C; Link 4-24; also see Chapter 10). Raynaud phenomenon is the most common initial complaint in Sjögren syndrome (eventually occurring in all cases).
      (2) Fingers are tapered and claw-like (called sclerodactyly) and often have digital infarcts (Fig. 4-11 C; Link 4-25).
   b. Cutaneous findings
      (1) Skin is the most common overall target organ.
      (2) Cutaneous changes begin with edema manifested as swollen fingers and swollen hands.
      (3) Edema is followed by the development of firm, thickened skin, beginning in the fingers and extending proximally to involve the upper arms, shoulders, trunk, neck, and face. Thickened skin is present in 100% of cases and is due to subcutaneous fibrosis.
      (4) Dystrophic calcification may be present in the subcutaneous tissue (5% of cases; Link 4-26). Facial skin has a tightened appearance, and radial furrowing occurs around the mouth, giving the mouth a mouse-like appearance (Fig. 4-11 D; Link 4-27). Telangiectasia (dilated venules, capillaries, arterioles) are commonly present on the face (Link 4-28).
      (5) Nail fold capillary microscopy shows abnormal capillary loops (arrows; Fig. 4-11 E).
   c. Gastrointestinal tract findings
      (1) Gastrointestinal tract is involved in approximately 90% of cases.
      (2) Esophageal findings in diffuse systemic sclerosis
         (a) Dysphagia (difficulty in swallowing) occurs for *both* solids and liquids. It is a sign of an esophageal motility disorder (see Chapter 18).
         (b) Esophageal manometry reveals the absence of peristalsis in the lower two-thirds of the esophagus because of extensive collagen deposition in the lamina propria and submucosa. Esophageal manometry measures the rhythmic muscle contractions that occur in the esophagus when swallowing.
         (c) Esophageal mucosa is thin and often has areas of ulceration. Esophageal strictures are common.
         (d) Dysfunction of the lower esophageal sphincter (LES) leads to reflux of gastric acid (GA) and glandular metaplasia (Barrett esophagus; see Chapters 2 and 18).
      (3) Stomach findings: collagen deposition in the wall of the stomach produces dysmotility and postprandial (after eating) bloating.
      (4) Small intestine findings
         (a) Loss of villi produces malabsorption of carbohydrates, fats, and protein.
         (b) Small intestine dysmotility produces cramps and bloating.
         (c) Diverticula (usually wide-mouthed) may develop.
      (5) Large intestine findings: colonic hypomotility produces constipation.
   d. Respiratory findings
      (1) Interstitial fibrosis produces RLD and hypoxemia (>50 of cases; Link 4-29). Respiratory failure is the most common cause of death in systemic sclerosis.
      (2) Dyspnea and nonproductive cough are *early* findings of lung involvement.

(3) PH (see Chapter 17) may occur due to endothelial cell dysfunction similar to what was previously discussed in the digital vessels. PH produces right ventricular hypertrophy (RVH) and right-sided heart failure (RHF, called cor pulmonale; see Chapters 11 and 17).

PH → RVH → cor pulmonale (RHF)

  e. Renal findings

    (1) Renal disease occurs in the majority of cases (>60% of cases).

Renal disease common

    (2) Vasculitis involving afferent and efferent arterioles is characterized by fibrinoid necrosis and smooth muscle cell proliferation (called "onion skinning" or hyperplastic arteriolosclerosis; see Fig. 20-7 B).

Hyperplastic arteriolosclerosis afferent/efferent arterioles

      (a) Vasculitis causes thrombosis and infarction in the kidneys.

Thrombosis, infarction

      (b) Malignant hypertension may occur (sudden increase in systolic and diastolic blood pressure, renal failure, and cerebral edema).

Malignant hypertension → renal failure, cerebral edema

5. Clinical findings in CREST syndrome: C–calcification; E–esophageal dysmotility; S–sclerodactyly (i.e., tapered, claw-like fingers); T–telangiectasias (i.e., multiple punctate blood vessel dilations)

Calcification

Raynaud

Esophageal dysmotility

Sclerodactyly

Telangiectasia

6. Laboratory findings in systemic sclerosis and CREST syndrome

  a. Serum ANA test is positive in 70% to 90% of cases in systemic sclerosis.

+Serum ANA systemic sclerosis

  b. Anti–DNA topoisomerase antibody is positive in 30% to 70% of cases of systemic sclerosis and 10% to 20% of cases in CREST syndrome.

Anti–DNA topoisomerase systemic sclerosis/CREST

  c. Anticentromere antibodies are present in 82% to 96% in CREST syndrome.

Anticentromere CREST

7. Prognosis: overall 10-year survival is approximately 80%.

H. Noninfectious inflammatory myopathies

Immune-mediated myopathies

1. **Definition:** Group of immune-mediated disorders with symmetric muscle involvement and involvement of other organ systems. Disorders include polymyositis and dermatomyositis. Less common disorders such as juvenile dermatomyositis and sporadic inclusion body myositis are not discussed here.

Polymyositis, dermatomyositis

2. Polymyositis

  a. **Definition:** Polymyositis is an idiopathic inflammatory myopathy associated with symmetric, proximal muscle weakness, elevated skeletal muscle enzyme levels (e.g., serum creatine kinase), and characteristic electromyography (EMG) and muscle biopsy findings.

Polymyositis: inflammatory myopathy

  b. Epidemiology

    (1) Female dominant disease with an increased incidence in the African American population. Female/male ratio is 2:1.

Female dominant

    (2) Primarily occurs in persons aged 40 to 60 years

40–60 yrs old

    (3) Increased risk of malignant neoplasms (15%–20% of cases), particularly lung and bladder cancer, and non-Hodgkin lymphoma (NHL)

↑Risk malignancies (lung, bladder, NHL)

    (4) Cytotoxic CD8 T cell (predominant cell) mediated process directed against unknown skeletal muscle antigens

Cytotoxic CD8 T cells against skeletal muscle antigens

      (a) Triggers for the T-cell response may be associated with viruses, including human retroviruses (HIV), human T-cell lymphotropic virus type 1 (HTLV-1), and coxsackievirus B.

Triggers: HIV, HTLV-1, coxsackievirus B

      (b) Viruses just mentioned damage skeletal muscle, leading to altered class I and II MHC antigens.

Viruses damage skeletal muscle

    (5) Autoantibodies are directed against transfer RNA synthetases (synthesize RNA) and other nuclear and cytoplasmic antigens in skeletal muscle.

Autoantibodies against nuclear/cytoplasmic antigens skeletal muscle

  c. Clinical findings

    (1) Constitutional signs in polymyositis include fever, muscle pain, morning stiffness, fatigue, and weight loss.

Fever, muscle pain, morning stiffness

    (2) Symmetric, proximal muscle weakness (with or without pain) occurs in the upper and lower extremities as well as the trunk, shoulders, and hips.

Muscle weakness upper/lower extremity

    (3) Dysphagia (difficulty with swallowing) for solids and liquids occurs in the oropharynx and upper esophagus, areas that contain skeletal muscle rather than smooth muscle.

Oropharyngeal/upper esophagus dysphagia solids/liquids

    (4) Respiratory difficulties are related to interstitial lung disease (ILD; see Chapter 17).

ILD → respiratory difficulties

  d. Laboratory findings

    (1) Serum creatine kinase, aldolase, and myoglobin are markedly increased.

↑↑Creatine kinase, aldolase, myoglobin

    (2) Antibody findings in polymyositis

      (a) Serum ANA is increased in 33% of cases.

+/– Serum ANA

      (b) Anti–transfer RNA synthetase (Jo-1) antibodies are increased in 25% to 30% of cases.

↑Anti–Jo-1

    (3) ESR and CRP are increased in 50% of patients (see Chapter 3).

↑ESR/CRP

EMG abnormal

Bx: necrosis/lymphocyte/ macrophage

Atrophy *not* prominent

Inflammatory myopathy with skin manifestations

Female dominant; ↑malignancy risk

CD4 T cells target skeletal muscle capillaries

Cutaneous findings key distinction from polymyositis

Gottron papules knuckles/ PIP joints

Heliotrope eyes

Erythematous rash shoulder area

Muscle Bx: lymphocyte infiltrate

Muscle atrophy prominent unlike polymyositis

Mixture SLE, systemic sclerosis, polymyositis findings

Female dominant

Young people; renal disease uncommon

B/T cell activation; antibodies against RNP (U1-RNP)

Raynaud phenomenon, sclerodactyly, swollen hands

Ulceration, calcification

Myositis, arthralgia/arthritis hands

Esophageal dysmotility

PH, pleuritis

APL antibodies if PH present

Pericarditis

Trigeminal neuralgia

Leukopenia

+ANA

U1-RNP antibodies 100% cases

(4) EMG shows muscle dysfunction. Muscle biopsies show necrotic and regenerating muscle with a lymphocyte and macrophage infiltrate. Muscle atrophy is *not* a prominent feature.

   e. Prognosis: majority respond well to therapy (>80% 5-year survival).

3. Dermatomyositis

   a. **Definition:** Dermatomyositis is an idiopathic, inflammatory myopathy associated with characteristic dermatologic manifestations.

   b. Epidemiology

      (1) Female/male ratio is 2:1; increased risk for malignancies

      (2) Pathogenesis

         (a) Activated CD4 T cells primarily target the capillaries in skeletal muscle.

         (b) Antibodies and complement are involved in the capillary damage.

         (c) Foci of myofiber injury accompany microvascular changes.

   c. Clinical findings

      (1) Muscle complaints are similar to those in polymyositis.

      (2) Cutaneous findings are key to distinguishing dermatomyositis from polymyositis.

         (a) Reddish purple papules called Gottron papules are noted over the knuckles and PIP joints on both hands (Fig. 4-11 F).

         (b) Purple-red eyelid discoloration occurs (called heliotrope eyelids or "raccoon eyes"; Fig. 4-11 G).

      (3) Erythematous skin rash appears in the shoulder area ("shawl" sign; Link 4-30).

   d. Laboratory findings

      (1) Similar to those described for polymyositis.

      (2) Muscle biopsies show an inflammatory reaction (primarily lymphocytic).

      (3) Unlike polymyositis, atrophy of muscle fibers is a prominent feature. Damage to the capillaries in the muscle leads to ischemia and atrophy of the muscle fibers.

   e. Prognosis: most patients with dermatomyositis survive unless it is associated with respiratory disease or cancer.

H. Mixed connective tissue disease

1. **Definition:** Mixed connective tissue disease is an idiopathic, inflammatory myopathy associated with characteristic dermatologic manifestations and signs and symptoms similar to SLE, systemic sclerosis, and polymyositis along with the presence of a distinctive antibody against U1-RNP.

2. Epidemiology

   a. Female/male ratio is 4:1.

   b. Occurs in persons aged 15 to 25 years. Renal disease is uncommon.

   c. Pathogenesis

      (1) Involves the activation of T cells and B cells, the latter producing antibodies against U1-ribonucleoprotein (U1-RNP).

      (2) Vascular endothelial proliferation and an infiltrate of B and T cells occur in involved tissues.

3. Clinical findings

   a. Vascular and digital findings in mixed connective tissue disease include Raynaud phenomenon (>95% of cases); sclerodactyly (50% of cases), similar to systemic sclerosis; and swollen hands (65%).

   b. Skin findings: cutaneous ulceration occurs due to subcutaneous dystrophic calcification similar to systemic sclerosis.

   c. Musculoskeletal findings include myositis (50%) and arthralgia (pain) and arthritis (pain, joint swelling, tenderness and warmth; signs of inflammation) involving the hands (>95% of cases).

   d. Gastrointestinal findings include esophageal dysmotility similar to that seen in systemic sclerosis (65%).

   e. Respiratory findings include PH (20%) and pleuritis (40% of cases) and a high association with APL antibodies if PH is present.

   f. Cardiovascular findings: pericarditis occurs in 40% of cases.

   g. CNS findings: trigeminal neuralgia is common.

   h. Hematologic findings: leukopenia (decreased leukocyte count) occurs in 50% of patients.

4. Laboratory findings

   a. Positive serum ANA (95%–99% of cases)

   b. Anti-RNP antibodies (U1-RNP; ≈100% of cases)

   c. Other antibodies such as APL antibodies, rheumatoid factor, anti–dsDNA (similar to SLE), and anti–DNA topoisomerase (similar to systemic sclerosis)

5. Prognosis is variable, with one-third going into remission, one-third progressing to severe disease (the most important of which is PH), and the remaining one-third having moderately severe disease. PH is the most common cause of death.

PH MC COD

J. Rheumatoid arthritis and Sjögren syndrome (discussed in Chapter 24)

VI. Immunodeficiency Disorders

A. Definition
- Immunodeficiency disorders are either primary (usually genetically determined) or secondary disorders that involve defects in B cells, T cells, NK cells, complement, mannose binding lectin, or phagocytic cells.

Primary or secondary

B. Risk factors: prematurity, autoimmune disease (e.g., SLE), lymphoproliferative disorders (e.g., malignant lymphoma), infections (e.g., HIV), and immunosuppressive drugs (e.g., corticosteroids)

Prematurity, autoimmune disease, lymphoproliferative disorders

Infections; immunosuppressive drugs

C. B-cell tests
1. Ig quantitation (IgG, IgM, IgA, IgE, and IgG subclasses)

Ig quantitation

2. Functional B-cell tests

Functional B-cell tests

   a. Measuring natural antibodies for blood groups A, B, and O individuals (see Chapter 16)

Blood group natural antibodies

      (1) Blood group O people should have anti-A and anti-B IgM antibodies.

O: anti-A, anti-B

      (2) Blood group A people should have anti-B IgM antibodies.

A: anti-B

      (3) Blood group B people should have anti-A IgM antibodies.

B: anti-A

      (4) Blood group AB people do have any natural antibodies, so other functional tests must be performed (see the following).

AB: no natural antibodies

   b. Measuring serum antibody titers after diphtheria and tetanus booster immunization (IZ)

Antibody titers post diphtheria/tetanus/ pneumococcus IZ

      (1) Serum antibody titers are assayed *before* and 3 weeks after the immunizations.

      (2) Test assesses the capacity of an individual to synthesize IgG antibodies against protein antigens in the vaccines.

      (3) Absence of IgG antibodies indicates that a B cell immunodeficiency is present.

Antibody titers post pneumococcal vaccine

   c. Measuring serum antibody titers after administering pneumococcal vaccine
      (1) Similar to the immunizations mentioned previously, in that serum antibodies are assayed *before* and 3 weeks after the immunization.

      (2) Assesses the immune system's capacity to synthesize antibodies against polysaccharide antigens in the cell wall of the bacteria.

No IgG = B cell immunodeficiency

      (3) Absence of IgG antibodies indicates a B cell immunodeficiency is present.

3. In vitro B-cell tests

In vitro B-cell tests

   a. Total B-cell count in the peripheral blood of the individual

Total B-cell count in peripheral blood

   b. Determining B-cell subsets (e.g., class switched vs. nonswitched memory B cells) in the individual

Determine B-cell subsets

   c. In vitro Ig synthesis (e.g., stimulate peripheral blood mononuclear cells collected in a test tube with pokeweed mitogen)

Pokeweed mitogen Ig response

   d. Genetic testing (mutation analysis)

Mutation analysis

D. T-cell tests
1. Absolute lymphocyte count: test measures the total white blood cell (WBC) count and the percentage of lymphocytes that are present in the peripheral blood.

Total WBC count + %lymphocytes

2. In vivo functional tests. *Candida* skin test is performed to examine the degree of induration of the skin reaction after 48 to 72 hours. *No* skin reaction to *Candida* indicates the presence of T-cell dysfunction.

***Candida* skin test**

3. Skin testing for delayed reaction hypersensitivity (DRH), if the *Candida* skin test is negative. Antigens that are used include PPD, *Trichophyton*, mumps, and tetanus or diphtheria toxoid. No skin reaction to the previously mentioned tests indicates the presence of T-cell dysfunction.

DRH skin testing fusing PPD + other antigens

4. In vitro T-cell tests are performed.

In vitro T-cell tests

   a. Quantitation of total T, NK, CD4$^+$ and CD8$^+$ subset T cells

#T, NK, CD4$^+$/CD8$^+$ subset T cells

   b. Lymphocyte blastic transformation (LBT)

LBT

      (1) Test assesses the ability of T cells to take up radiolabeled thymidine after stimulation with PHA (e.g., phytohemagglutin) or *Candida*.

      (2) Absence of lymphocyte blast transformation (no takeup of the radiolabeled thymidine after PHA or *Candida* stimulation) indicates a lack of T-cell function.

E. Summary of primary immunodeficiency disorders (Table 4-7)

F. Acquired immunodeficiency syndrome (AIDS)
1. **Definition:** AIDS is caused by <u>h</u>uman <u>i</u>mmunodeficiency <u>v</u>irus (HIV), which is a retrovirus.

Cause: HIV (retrovirus)

2. Epidemiology

   a. HIV is the most common cause of death due to infection worldwide.

MCC death due to infection worldwide

   b. Globally, sub-Saharan Africa has the greatest number of people with AIDS.

MC in sub-Saharan Africa

TABLE 4-7   Congenital Immunodeficiency Disorders

DISEASE	DEFECT(S)	CLINICAL FEATURES
B-CELL DISORDERS		
Bruton agammaglobulinemia	• XR disorder • Failure of pre–B cells to become mature B cells • Mutated tyrosine kinase (*BTK*) gene (important in signal transduction involved in rearrangement of Ig-light chain genes required for B-cell maturation)	• SP infections • Sepsis due to bacteria requiring opsonization (IgG) and phagocytosis (*Streptococcus pneumoniae, Staphylococcus aureus, Haemophilus influenzae*) • Chronic meningitis due to enteroviruses (echovirus, poliovirus, coxsackievirus) that require neutralizing antibodies to keep them in check • *Giardia lamblia* infection in the small bowel (diarrhea and malabsorption of fat) due to decrease in secretory IgA production, which normally protects the bowel from these infections; maternal antibodies protective from birth to age 6 months • Paradoxical increase in incidence of autoimmune disease (e.g., arthritis, dermatomyositis) • All immunoglobulins markedly decreased
IgA deficiency	• Failure of IgA B cells to mature into plasma cells	• Most common primary immunodeficiency disease • More common in blacks than whites • May be asymptomatic (80% of cases) or develop SP infections (most common infection) and/or giardiasis • Increased risk for autoimmune disease (rheumatoid arthritis, SLE, PA, ITP, celiac disease, ulcerative colitis), atopic (IgE) disorders (asthma, rhinitis, food allergies, dermatitis, conjunctivitis) • Anaphylaxis may occur if exposed to blood products that contain IgA • ↓Serum IgA and secretory IgA
Common variable immunodeficiency	• Defect in B-cell maturation to plasma cells • Adult immunodeficiency disorder	• SP infections (90%–100% of cases) • GI infections (e.g., *Giardia, Salmonella, Shigella, Campylobacter*) • Pneumonia • Increased risk for autoimmune disease (ITP, AIHA) and malignancy (malignant lymphoma, gastric cancer) • Viral infections: recurrent *Herpes* infection; enterovirus infections leading to meningitis • Common pathogens: *Actinomyces israeli, Streptococcus pneumoniae, Haemophilus influenzae*; chronic infections—*Staphylococcus aureus, Pseudomonas aeruginosa* • ↓Serum immunoglobulins
T-CELL DISORDER		
DiGeorge syndrome (thymic hypoplasia)	• Chromosome 22 deletion syndrome • Failure of third and fourth pharyngeal pouches to develop • Thymus (site for T-cell synthesis) and parathyroid glands fail to develop	• Bacterial sepsis • Viral infections: CMV, EBV, varicella (chickenpox) • *Candida* infections • *Pneumocystis jiroveci* pneumonia • Hypoparathyroidism (tetany): hypocalcemia with seizures occurs in newborns • Absent thymic shadow on radiograph • Defective CMI • Danger of GVH reaction • Increased incidence cleft lip and congenital heart defects (≈80% of cases; most common defects include tetralogy of Fallot, truncus arteriosus, defects in the aortic arch)
COMBINED B- AND T-CELL DISORDERS		
Hyper-IgM syndrome	• XR (70% of cases) • Mutation in a gene encoding for CD40 ligand in CD4 T cells • CD40 ligand normally reacts with CD40 on the surface of B cells to allow for Ig class switching; defect in ligand results in failure of B cells to switch from IgM to other classes of Ig	• Recurrent pyogenic infections (decreased IgG for proper opsonization) • Pneumonia due to *P. jiroveci* (defect in CD4 T cells adversely affects CMI)

TABLE 4-7   Congenital Immunodeficiency Disorders—cont'd

DISEASE	DEFECT(S)	CLINICAL FEATURES
Severe combined immunodeficiency (SCID)	• XR type MCC (50%–60% of cases) • Mutation in the IL-2 receptor on T cells resulting in a lack of γ-chain, which is necessary for the development of T cells • Various autosomal recessive forms have gene defects in coding for kinases involved in signal transduction • **Adenosine deaminase deficiency** (15% of cases): autosomal recessive disorder; lack of the enzyme causes an increase in deoxyadenosine, which is toxic to B and T cells	• Defective CMI due to lack of T cells • ↓Serum immunoglobulins • Thymic shadow absent on radiograph • Rx: gene therapy (for adenosine deaminase deficiency), bone marrow transplant (patients with SCID do *not* reject allografts)
Wiskott-Aldrich syndrome	• XR disorder: mutation in a gene that encodes for a protein involved in assembly of actin filaments in the cytoskeleton of all hematopoietic cells; actin defect causes problems in cell migration, signal transduction, and other cell functions • Inability to elicit an IgM response to capsular polysaccharides of bacteria • Progressive deletion of B and T cells	• Symptom triad: atopic eczema, thrombocytopenia, SP infections • Increased risk for malignancy (malignant lymphoma and leukemia) • Prone to infections caused by encapsulated organisms (*Streptococcus pneumoniae*), *Pneumocystis jiroveci*, and viral infections • Defective CMI • Immunoglobulins: ↓IgM, normal IgG, ↑IgA and IgE • Bone marrow transplantation essential for survival
Ataxia-telangiectasia	• Autosomal recessive disorder • Mutation in a gene that encodes for DNA repair enzymes • Thymic hypoplasia	• Cerebellar ataxia, telangiectasia (dilated vessels) in the eyes and skin • ↑Risk for malignancy: malignant lymphoma and/or leukemia, adenocarcinoma (e.g., stomach, breast) • ↑Serum α-fetoprotein and carcinoembryonic antigen • Defective CMI: ↓total lymphocyte count; defective T-cell function • Deficient antibody production to viral or bacterial antigens • Immunoglobulins: ↓IgA 50%–80%; ↓IgE; normal to ↑IgM; ↓IgG2/IgG4; normal to ↓total IgG

AIHA, Autoimmune hemolytic anemia; *CMI,* cell-mediated immunity; *CMV,* cytomegalovirus; *EBV,* Epstein-Barr virus; *GI,* gastrointestinal; *GVH,* graft-versus-host; *Ig,* immunoglobulin; *ITP,* idiopathic thrombocytopenic purpura; *MCC,* most common cause; *PA,* pernicious anemia; *Rx,* treatment; *SLE,* systemic lupus erythematosus; *SP,* sinopulmonary; *XR,* sex-linked recessive.

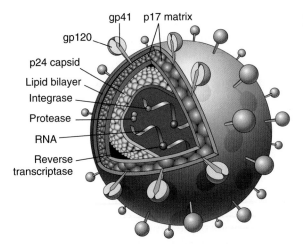

4-12: The structure of the human immunodeficiency virus (HIV)-1 virion. See text for discussion. *(From Kumar V, Fausto N, Abbas A, Aster J: Robbins and Cotran Pathologic Basis of Disease, 8th ed, Philadelphia, Saunders Elsevier, 2010, p 237, Fig. 6.43.)*

c. Virus characteristics

(1) HIV is the retrovirus that causes AIDS (Fig. 4-12). A key feature of retroviruses is the enzyme reverse transcriptase (RT), which converts viral RNA into proviral dsDNA.

(2) HIV-1 is the most common cause of AIDS in the United States and worldwide.

(3) HIV-2 is more restricted, being most prevalent in West Africa.

(4) Virus *cannot* penetrate intact skin or mucosa. Ulceration of skin or mucosa must be present for the virus to enter CD4 T cells or DCs in tissue.

RT: converts viral RNA into proviral dsDNA

HIV-1 MCC AIDS U.S./world

HIV-2 most prevalent in West Africa

Cannot penetrate intact skin/mucosa

Ulceration required

3 Retroviral genes: *gag, env, pol*

gag gene: p24 core antigen

env gene: gp120

pol gene: RT, integrase, protease

Sexual transmission MC cause AIDS

Man-to-man anal intercourse MCC U.S.

Heterosexual transmission: MCC AIDS developing countries

STDs ↑risk for HIV

IVDA 2nd MCC AIDS

Vertical transmission

Transplacental, blood contamination during delivery, breast-feeding

Pediatric AIDS: MC vertical transmission

Accidental needlestick

Common cause HIV health care workers

Transfusion blood products

Reduced risk HIV from blood bank p24 antigen screening

Mucous membrane exposure risk 0.1%

Ulcers/cuts ↑↑risk

↑↑Volume blood, prolonged contact

Repeated sexual encounters

Unprotected anal intercourse

Intermediate risk vaginal intercourse

Blood, semen/vaginal secretions, breast milk

Saliva inhibits HIV

Defect in CMI

Key infected cells: CD4 T cells, macrophages, DCs

HIV cytotoxic to CD4 T cells (↓with progression)

Macrophages ↑↑viral particles in vacuoles

Macrophages resistant to virus cytolytic effect

Macrophages most important virus reservoir

DCs reservoirs for HIV

HIV entry via interrupted mucosal surfaces (genital/anus)

After viral entry → infects CD4 T cells/DCs

Cells drain viral particles into lymph nodes/spleen

Follicular DCs: important reservoir for HIV during latency

(5) HIV contains three retroviral genes.
  (a) The *gag* gene directs synthesis for inner structural proteins (e.g., p24 core antigen).
  (b) The *env* gene directs synthesis for the viral envelope with outer structural proteins that give cell-type specificity (e.g., glycoprotein [gp]120 binds the virus to the host CD4 T cell).
  (c) The *pol* gene directs synthesis for RT, integrase, and protease.
d. Modes of transmission of HIV
  (1) Sexual transmission (≈80% of cases)
    (a) Man-to-man transmission by anal intercourse (≈50% of cases). Most common cause in the United States.
    (b) Heterosexual transmission (30% of cases). Most common cause of AIDS in developing countries.
    (c) Prior or current sexually transmitted diseases (STDs) increase the risk of HIV infection. STDs that increase the risk for HIV infection include gonorrhea and chlamydia (threefold risk), syphilis (sevenfold risk), and herpes genitalis (25-fold risk).
  (2) Intravenous drug abuse (IVDA; ≈20% of cases): rate of HIV infection is markedly increasing in female sex partners of male IV drug abusers.
  (3) Other modes of transmission of HIV
    (a) Vertical transmission refers to transmission via the transplacental route, blood contamination during delivery, and breastfeeding (women should be counseled *not* to breastfeed). Most pediatric cases of AIDS are due to transmission of the virus from mother to child.
    (b) Accidental needlestick: common mode of HIV infection in health care workers. There is a 0.3% to 0.45% seroconversion risk with an accidental needlestick.
    (c) Transfusion of blood products: risk of contracting an HIV infection is estimated to be 1 in more than 2 million units of blood transfused. Current marked reduction in risk of transfusion-associated HIV infection in the United States is the result of blood bank testing for the p24 antigen.
    (d) Mucous membrane exposure (e.g., genitals, anus, rectum): risk is estimated to be 0.1%. Greater risk if the integrity of the membrane is visibly compromised (e.g., ulcers, cuts). Greater risk if a large volume of blood is involved and if there is prolonged contact with the membrane surface.
    (e) Repeated sexual encounters. Risk is highest with unprotected receptive anal intercourse (50 per 10,000 exposures). Intermediate risk with receptive vaginal intercourse (10 per 10,000 exposures; greater risk if a genital ulcer is present or another STD is present)
e. Body fluids containing HIV include blood, semen, vaginal secretions, and breast milk. Saliva inhibits HIV; hence, human bites are a rare cause of HIV infection.
3. Pathogenesis
  a. Overall, HIV is a defect in CMI. Major cells that are infected by HIV-1 are CD4 T cells, macrophages, DCs, astrocytes, retinal cells, BM stem cells, cervical cells, and enterochromaffin cells in the duodenum, colon, and rectum.
    (1) HIV is cytotoxic to CD4 T cells; hence, the number of these cells decreases with disease progression.
    (2) Macrophages contain large numbers of viral particles in cytoplasmic vacuoles; however, unlike CD4 T cells, they are resistant to the cytolytic effects of the virus. Macrophages are the most important reservoirs of the virus.
    (3) Similar to macrophages, DCs also contain large numbers of the virus and are important reservoirs of the virus.
  b. Primary infection due to HIV occurs via entry of the virus through interrupted mucosal surfaces in the genital tract or anus where it infects CD4 T cells and DCs in the underlying tissue.
    (1) These cells, which are filled with viral particles, drain into lymph nodes and spleen where the virus is held in check by the patient's immune system.
    (2) Follicular DCs in the germinal centers of the lymph nodes are an important reservoir of the virus during the early latent stages of the disease *before* the virus is released into the blood and produces the acute retroviral syndrome (see later).

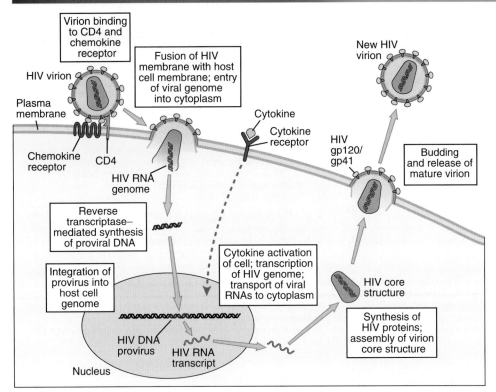

4-13: The life cycle of human immunodeficiency virus type 1 (HIV-1). The sequential steps in HIV reproduction are shown, from initial infection of a host cell to release of a new virus particle (virion). For the sake of clarity, the production and release of only one new virion are shown. An infected cell actually produces many virions, each capable of infecting nearby cells, which spreads the infection. (From Abbas A, Lichtman A: Basic Immunology: Function and Disorders of the Immune System, 3rd ed, Philadelphia, Saunders Elsevier, 2011, p 233, Fig. 12-8.)

c. Life cycle of HIV-1 (Fig. 4-13)
- (1) Gp120 in the viral envelope binds to CD4 and various chemokine co-receptors.
- (2) Viral membrane fuses with the host cell membrane and gains entry into the cytoplasm. Gp41 helps with fusion of the virus to the host cell membrane.
- (3) Viral protease uncoats the virus, which results in release of viral RNA.
- (4) RT converts viral RNA into dsDNA.
- (5) Integrase inserts the viral DNA into the host cell's DNA where it becomes a provirus. Provirus may be latent for months or years (latent infection).
- (6) Activation of the host cell by an extrinsic stimulus (e.g., microbial infection) leads to upregulation of transcription factors (e.g., NF-κB), which stimulates transcription of genes encoding for cytokines (e.g., IL-2 and its receptor). Cytokines also stimulate gene transcription of the HIV genome, causing the release of viral RNA into the cytoplasm.
- (7) Synthesis of HIV proteins produces an HIV core structure containing the RNA.
- (8) HIV core structures migrate to the cell membrane, acquire a lipid bilayer, and form buds containing infectious viral particles that detach from the membrane.
- (9) Mature, infectious viral particles are able to infect other cells.

3. Laboratory tests for HIV (Table 4-8)
4. Natural history of HIV infection (Fig. 4-14; Link 4-31)
- a. Acute phase of HIV
  - (1) Approximately 1 to 6 weeks (usually 2 to 3 weeks) after infection, individuals experience fever, malaise, pharyngitis, generalized rash, myalgia/arthralgia, and generalized painful lymphadenopathy, which usually subsides without treatment within 1 to 2 weeks.
  - (2) Greatest risk for contracting HIV is the first few weeks of infection. Range is 1 in 5 to 1 in 250 chance per coital act.
- b. Asymptomatic carrier phase of HIV
  - (1) Lasts 2 to 10 years after contracting the infection.
  - (2) CD4 T-cell count is >500 cells/mm³.
  - (3) Viral replication occurs in latently infected resting CD4 T cells in lymph nodes. Cytotoxic T cells control but do not clear HIV reservoirs.
- c. Early symptomatic phase of HIV
  - (1) CD4 T-cell count is 200 to 500 cells/mm³.
  - (2) Characterized by generalized painful lymphadenopathy.

Gp120 in viral envelope: binds to CD4/chemokine co-receptors

Fusion virus with host cell membrane; Gp41

Viral protease: release viral RNA

RT: converts viral RNA → dsDNA

Integrase: inserts viral DNA into host DNA; provirus

Upregulation NF-κB → ↑transcription genes for cytokines

Cytokines stimulate gene transcription → release viral RNA into cytoplasm
HIV core structure (contain viral RNA)
HIV core structure → detaches as infective viral particle
Infectious viral particles infect other cells
≈1 to 6 wks after infection
Fever, malaise, pharyngitis
Rash, myalgia/arthralgia
Generalized lymphadenopathy
Subsides without Rx
↑↑Risk contracting infection 1st few wks
Asymptomatic carrier phase
Lasts 2–10 years
CD4 T-cell count >500 cells/mm³
Viral replication latently infected resting CD4 T cells in nodes
Early symptomatic phase
CD4 T-cell count 200–500 cells/mm³
Generalized painful adenopathy

TABLE 4-8   Laboratory Tests Used in HIV and AIDS

TEST	USE	COMMENTS
ELISA	Screening test Newer more sensitive screening tests	• Detects anti-gp120 antibodies • Sensitivity ≈100% • Positive within 3–5 weeks; all are positive in 3 months • Detect antibodies for HIV-1, HIV-2, and p24 antigen (see later)
Western blot and nucleic acid assays	Confirmatory tests	• Western blot used if ELISA is positive or indeterminate • Positive test: presence of p24 antigen and gp41 antibodies, and either gp120 or gp160 antibodies • Test misses significant number of people with HIV who have indeterminate test results • HIV-1 RNA in vitro nucleic acid assays now replacing the Western blot as confirmatory test • Specificity ≈100%
p24 antigen	Indicator of active viral replication Present *before* anti-gp120 antibodies	• Positive *before* seroconversion and when AIDS is diagnosed (two distinct peaks) • Test used by blood banks to screen for HIV; has markedly decreased chance for contracting HIV by blood transfusion
CD4 T-cell count	Monitor of immune status	• Useful in determining when to initiate HIV treatment and when to administer prophylaxis against opportunistic infections
HIV viral load	Detection of actively dividing virus Marker of disease progression	• Most sensitive test for diagnosis of acute HIV *before* seroconversion • Recommended at least one time per year in patients with HIV

AIDS, Acquired immunodeficiency syndrome; *ELISA,* enzyme-linked immunosorbent assay; *HIV,* human immunodeficiency virus.

4-14: **Natural history of HIV.** Infection of CD4⁺ lymphocytes (and other cell types) leads to virus production and cytolysis or long-term latent infection that progresses from primary infection through late symptomatic infection (AIDS). Accompanying this process are profound defects in T_H and cytotoxic cell activity, with concomitant development of opportunistic infections. *(Actor JK:* Elsevier's Integrated Immunology and Microbiology, *Philadelphia, Mosby, 2007, p 134, Fig. 14-4.)*

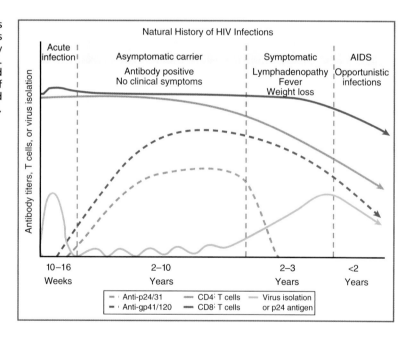

NAD: hairy leukoplakia (EBV), oral candidiasis

Fever, weight loss, diarrhea

CD4 T-cell count ≤200 cells/ mm³ and/or AIDS-defining lesion

MC AIDS-defining infections: *P. jiroveci* pneumonia, systemic candidiasis

AIDS-defining malignancies

Kaposi, Burkitt lymphoma, 1° CNS lymphoma, cervical carcinoma

Disseminated infection (CMV, MAI)

(3) Non–AIDS-defining (NAD) infections include hairy leukoplakia (glossitis caused by EBV [see Fig. 18-3 B]) and oral candidiasis (see Fig. 18-3 J).

(4) During this phase, there is fever, weight loss, and diarrhea.

d. Organ systems affected by AIDS (Table 4-9; Fig. 4-15)

(1) Criteria for defining AIDS is to be HIV-positive with a CD4 T-cell count ≤200 cells/ mm³ and/or an AIDS-defining condition.

(2) Most common AIDS-defining infections are *Pneumocystis jiroveci* pneumonia (Fig. 4-16 A) and systemic candidiasis.

(3) AIDS-defining malignancies include Kaposi sarcoma (see Fig. 4-16 B-D), Burkitt lymphoma (EBV), primary CNS lymphoma (EBV), and cervical carcinoma (human papilloma virus).

(4) Common causes of death in AIDS include disseminated infections due to CMV and *Mycobacterium avium-intracellulare* [MAI] complex).

TABLE 4-9   Organ Systems Affected by AIDS

ORGAN SYSTEM	CONDITION	COMMENTS
Cardiovascular system	Increased risk for atherosclerotic coronary artery disease	• Major cause of death in AIDS patients
Central nervous system (CNS) and special senses	AIDS dementia complex (see Fig. 26-14 C)	• Caused by HIV (↑risk if CD4 count < 200 cells/mm³) • Multinucleated microglial cells are reservoir of virus in the CNS
	CMV retinitis	• Retinitis: most common end-organ complication of CMV; may cause blindness
	Primary CNS malignant lymphoma	• Caused by EBV; CNS most common extranodal site (not in a lymph node) for malignant lymphoma
	Cryptococcosis (see Fig. 26-16 A)	• Most common cause of CNS fungal infection; usually occurs when CD4 count < 50 cells/mm³
	Toxoplasmosis (see Fig. 26-16 E)	• Most common cause of space-occupying lesion (toxoplasmosis abscess) in the brain; occurs when CD4 count < 100 cells/mm³
	CMV retinitis (see Fig. 26-26 M)	• Most common cause of blindness in AIDS; occurs when CD4 count < 50 cells/mm³
Gastrointestinal system	Mouth	• Oral hairy leukoplakia: caused by EBV when CD4 count < 400 cells/mm³ • Oral thrush: caused by *Candida* when CD4 count < 400 cells/mm³
	Esophagitis	• *Candida* most commonly causes esophagitis when CD4 count < 400 cells/mm³; *Candida* is most common cause of odynophagia (painful swallowing) in AIDS • Herpesvirus most commonly causes esophagitis when CD4 count < 200 cells/mm³ • CMV most commonly causes esophagitis when CD4 count < 50 cells/mm³
	Diarrhea (see Fig. 18-20)	• CMV most commonly produces diarrhea when CD4 count < 50 cells/mm³ • *Salmonella* sp. most commonly produces diarrhea when CD4 count < 400 cells/mm³ • *Shigella* sp. most commonly produces diarrhea when CD4 count < 400 cells/mm³ • MAI most commonly produces diarrhea when CD4 count < 50 cells/mm³ • *Cryptosporidium* most commonly produces diarrhea when CD4 count < 200 cells/mm³ • *Microsporidium* most commonly produces diarrhea when CD4 count < 50 cells/mm³ • *Isospora* most commonly produces diarrhea when CD4 count < 200 cells/mm³ • *Giardia lamblia* most commonly produces diarrhea when CD4 count < 200 cells/mm³
	Perianal	• Herpes simplex virus
Hepatobiliary system	Biliary tract infection	• CMV is most common cause
Renal system	Focal segmental glomerulosclerosis	• Occurs at any CD4 count level but usually occurs when CD4 count < 200 cells/mm³; causes hypertension and nephrotic syndrome; overall most common cause of nephrotic syndrome (see Chapter 20); renal failure occurs in 1 to 4 months
Respiratory system	Pneumonia	• CMV most commonly produces pneumonia when CD4 count < 50 cells/mm³ • *Streptococcus pneumonia* may produce pneumonia regardless of CD4 count • MAI most commonly produces pneumonia when CD4 count < 50 cells/mm³ • *Mycobacterium tuberculosis* most commonly produces pneumonia when CD4 count < 400 cells/mm³ • *Pneumocystis jiroveci* most commonly produces pneumonia when CD4 count < 200 cells/mm³ (Fig. 4-16 A) • *Histoplasma capsulatum* most commonly produces pneumonia when CD4 count < 100 cells/mm³ • *Coccidioides immitis* most commonly produces pneumonia when CD4 count < 200 cells/mm³)

Continued

TABLE 4-9 Organ Systems Affected by AIDS—cont'd

ORGAN SYSTEM	CONDITION	COMMENTS
Reticuloendothelial system	Lymphadenopathy or splenomegaly	• MAC: most common cause of lymphadenopathy or splenomegaly when CD4 count < 50 cells/mm³ • EBV: most common cause of lymphadenopathy or when CD4 count < 50 cells/mm³
	Non-Hodgkin lymphoma (NHL)	• NHL usually occurs when CD4 count < 200 cells/mm³; majority of NHLs are B-cell derived; intermediate or high-grade NHLs are AIDs defining; extranodal locations (e.g., gastrointestinal tract) are common sites for these lymphomas
	Immune reconstitution syndrome (IRSS)	• IRSS: paradoxical clinical worsening due to new ability to initiate inflammatory response against underlying (subclinical) opportunistic infection; may occur 2–12 wks after initiating therapy for AIDs; usually occurs when CD4 count < 100 cells/mm³ with rapid decline in HIV viral load
Skin	Kaposi sarcoma (see Fig. 4-16 B–D).	• Caused by HHV-8; most common malignancy in HIV/AIDS; predominantly seen in men
	Bacillary angiomatosis (see Fig. 10-14 A)	• Caused by Bartonella henselae
	Shingles (see Fig. 25-5 J)	• Caused by Herpes zoster; occurs when CD4 count < 400 cells/mm³

CMV, Cytomegalovirus; *EBV,* Epstein-Barr virus; *HHV-8,* human herpesvirus type 8; *HIV,* human immunodeficiency virus; *MAC,* membrane attack complex; *MAI, Mycobacterium avium-intracellulare* complex.

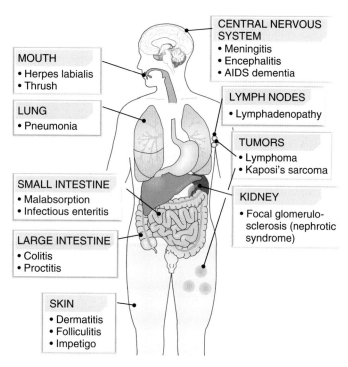

4-15: Pathologic changes and clinical findings associated with AIDS. *(From my friend Ivan Damjanov, MD, PhD: Pathophysiology, Philadelphia, Saunders Elsevier, 2009, p 82, Fig. 3-16.)*

CENTRAL NERVOUS SYSTEM
• Meningitis
• Encephalitis
• AIDS dementia

MOUTH
• Herpes labialis
• Thrush

LUNG
• Pneumonia

LYMPH NODES
• Lymphadenopathy

TUMORS
• Lymphoma
• Kaposi's sarcoma

SMALL INTESTINE
• Malabsorption
• Infectious enteritis

KIDNEY
• Focal glomerulo-sclerosis (nephrotic syndrome)

LARGE INTESTINE
• Colitis
• Proctitis

SKIN
• Dermatitis
• Folliculitis
• Impetigo

e. Immunologic abnormalities in AIDS

(1) Lymphopenia, due to a low CD4 T-cell count

(2) Cutaneous anergy, due to a defect in CMI from decreased CD4 T cells. Persons with cutaneous anergy have diminished ability to exhibit a delayed T-cell HSR on the skin to injected antigens because of a defect in CMI.

(3) Hypergammaglobulinemia, due to polyclonal B cell stimulation by EBV and CMV (see Chapter 3)

(4) CD4:CD8 ratio <1: Normally, the ratio is >2, but lysis of CD4 T cells cause the ratio to decrease.

(5) NK cell cytotoxicity function is decreased.

f. CD4 count and the risk for certain diseases in AIDS

(1) 700 to 1500: normal

Lymphopenia

Cutaneous anergy

Hypergammaglobulinemia (EBV/CMV)

CD4/CD8 ratio <1

↓NK cytotoxicity function

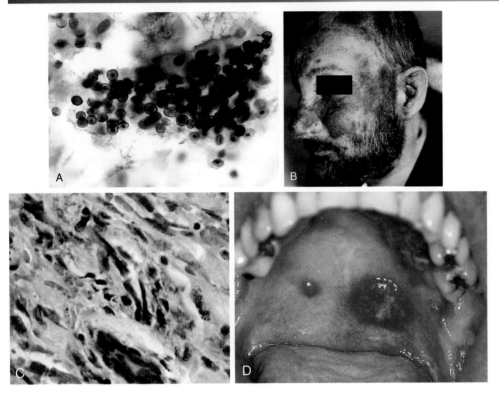

4-16: **A,** *Pneumocystis jiroveci* pneumonia. This silver-impregnated cytologic smear prepared from bronchial washings in an HIV-positive patient contains numerous *P. jiroveci* cysts with central dots representing spores. Some cysts look like crushed ping-pong balls. **B,** Kaposi sarcoma. Note the large confluent, raised, erythematous plaques on the face. **C,** Histology of Kaposi sarcoma. High-power magnification showing neoplastic vessels, multiple abnormal slit-like vascular spaces, marked cytologic atypia, and extravasated erythrocytes. **D,** Oral Kaposi sarcoma in an HIV-positive patient. (*A from my friend Ivan Damjanov, MD, PhD, Linder J:* Pathology: A Color Atlas, *St. Louis, Mosby, 2000, p 56, Fig. 4-22 B;* **B** *from Cohen J, Opal SM, Powderly WG:* Infectious Diseases, *3rd ed, London, Mosby Elsevier, 2010, p 990, Fig. 94.1;* **C** *from Morse SA, Holmes KK, Ballard RC, Moreland AA:* Atlas of Sexually Transmitted Diseases and AIDS, *Saunders Elsevier, 4th ed, 2010, p 261, Fig. 15.16 C;* **D** *from Walker BR, Colledge NR, Ralston SH, Penman ID:* Davidson's Principles and Practice of Medicine, *Churchill Livingstone Elsevier, 22nd ed, 2014, p 398, Fig. 14.6.*)

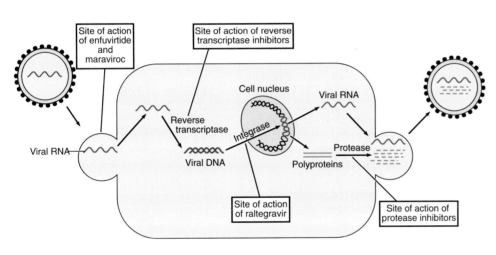

4-17: Sites of action of antiretroviral therapy. (*From Brenner G, Stevens C:* Pharmacology, *3rd ed, Philadelphia, Saunders Elsevier, 2010, p 474, Fig. 43.2.*)

(2) 200 to 500: risk for oral candidiasis, herpes zoster (shingles), hairy leukoplakia, community-acquired pneumonia, pulmonary TB, malignant lymphoma, Kaposi sarcoma, and cervical intraepithelial neoplasia

(3) 100 to 200: risk for *P. jiroveci* pneumonia, AIDS dementia, disseminated histoplasmosis, extrapulmonary TB, and cachexia (wasting)

(4) Below 100: risk for toxoplasmosis, cryptococcosis, cryptosporidiosis, and primary CNS lymphoma (due to EBV)

(5) Below 50: risk for CMV retinitis, disseminated CMV, MAI complex, and progressive multifocal leukoencephalopathy

5. Pregnant women with AIDS
   • Treatment with an RT inhibitor reduces transmission to newborns to <8%.

6. Immunization in HIV patients
   a. Indicated immunizations include hepatitis A and B, *Pneumococcus*, influenza, and tetanus-diphtheria.
   b. Contraindicated immunizations (live virus vaccines) include varicella, measles-mumps-rubella, Bacille Calmette-Guérin (BCG), and smallpox.

7. Sites of action of antiretroviral therapy (Fig. 4-17)

Rx RT inhibitors ↓newborns transmission <8%

Live vaccines contraindicated

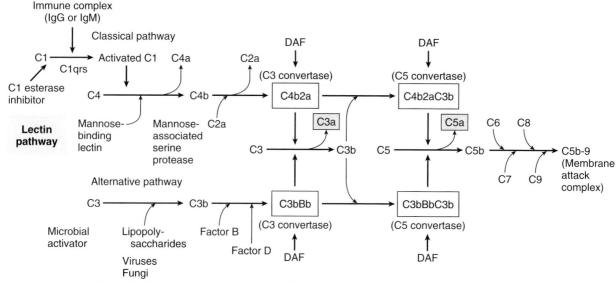

4-18: Complement cascade. Activation of complement through the classical pathway (via immunocomplexes; e.g., systemic lupus erythematosus), the alternative pathway (via endotoxins [lipopolysaccharides]), or the lectin pathway (via pathogens with mannose on the cell wall; e.g., *Salmonella*, *Candida*) promote activation of C3 and C5, leading to formation of the membrane attack complex (C5b-C9). Decay accelerating factor *(DAF)* degrades C3 convertase and C5 convertase in both classical and alternative pathways. The functions of C3a, C3b, C5a, and C5b-C9 are described in the text. *(Modified from Actor JK:* Elsevier's Integrated Immunology and Microbiology, *2nd ed, Philadelphia, Mosby, 2011, Fig. 6-6.)*

E. **Complement system disorders**
   1. Overview of the complement system
      a. Complement is synthesized in the liver.
      b. **Definition**: Complement is part of the innate immune defense and is one of the APRs released in inflammation (see Chapter 3).
      c. Complement circulates as an inactive protein.
         (1) Complement is activated by IgM, IgG-antigen complexes, and endotoxin.
         (2) Only complement cleavage products are functional.
      d. Functions of complement cleavage products
         (1) C3a, C5a (anaphylatoxins): stimulate mast cell release of histamine
         (2) C3b: opsonization (enhances phagocytosis)
         (3) C5a: activates neutrophil adhesion molecules and involved in neutrophil chemotaxis
         (4) C5b-C9 (MAC): involved in cell lysis
   2. Complement pathways (cascades) (Fig. 4-18)
      a. Classical pathway
         (1) Activated by ICs that contain antibodies bound to an antigen
         (2) Contains complement components C1, C4, and C2
         (3) Requires antibody to activate the pathway
         (4) C1 esterase inhibitor
            (a) Inactivates the protease activity of C1: C1 normally cleaves C2 and C4 to produce the C4b2a complex (called C3 convertase)
            (b) Deficient in hereditary angioedema (discussed later)
      b. Alternative pathway
         (1) Activated by lipopolysaccharides (endotoxin from gram-negative bacteria), viruses, and fungi
         (2) Contains complement components factor B, properdin (stabilizes the alternative pathway convertases), and factor D
         (3) Does *not* require antibodies for its activation
      c. Lectin pathway
         (1) Very important for the destruction of microbial pathogens (bacteria, fungi, viruses, and protozoa)
         (2) Mannose-binding lectin: structurally similar to the C1 complex. Lectin complexes with mannose-associated serine protease.
         (3) Lectin attaches to mannose and other carbohydrate molecules on the wall of gram-negative pathogens (e.g., *Salmonella, Neisseria, Listeria*), fungi (e.g., *Candida*,

Margin notes (left column):

Synthesized in liver

Important in innate immunity

Activation: IgM, IgG-antigen complexes, endotoxin

Cleavage factors functional

C3a, C5a

Mast cell release histamine

C3b: opsonization

C5a: activate neutrophil adhesion molecules, chemotaxis

C5b-C9: cell lysis

Classical pathway

ICs activate

C1, C4, C2

Requires antibody for activation

Inactivates protease activity of C1

Deficient in hereditary angioedema

Activated lipopolysaccharides, endotoxins

Factor B, properdin, factor D

Antibodies *not* required for activation

Lectin: destruction bacteria, fungi, viruses

TABLE 4-10   Complement Disorders

DISORDER	COMMENTS
Hereditary angioedema (Fig. 4-19 A–C)	• Autosomal dominant disorder with deficiency of C1 esterase inhibitor, which normally inactivates the protease activity of C1. Activated C1 normally cleaves C2 and C4 to produce C4b2a complex (C3 convertase). Hereditary angioedema is associated with episodic attacks of edema formation that can sometimes be life-threatening if it involves the larynx. Nonpitting edema involving the face, extremities, upper airways, and gastrointestinal tract (abdominal pain, diarrhea, vomiting) develops suddenly. The edema is thought to be due to increased levels of C2-derived kinins produced by excessive amounts of activated C1. These kinins increase vessel permeability and are primarily responsible for the swelling of tissue in hereditary angioedema. Episodes of swelling are usually self-limited and usually resolve in 48 hrs. It usually first presents in adolescence. A family history is present in 80% of causes (recall that in autosomal dominant disease, patients who are homozygous or heterozygous express the disease). Hereditary angioedema is *not* associated with allergic diseases and is *not* associated with urticaria (a characteristic finding in allergic skin diseases). Acute episodes are accompanied by low levels of C4 (best screen) and C2, because of excessive activation by C1 (see Fig. 4-18), and the diagnosis is confirmed by low C1 inhibitor levels. C3 levels are normal because C3 is in the alternative pathway, which does not require C1 esterase inhibitor.
C2 deficiency	• Most common complement deficiency • Associated with septicemia (usually *Streptococcus pneumoniae*) and SLE
C6-C9 deficiency	• Increased susceptibility for disseminated *Neisseria gonorrhoeae* or *Neisseria meningitidis* infections
Paroxysmal nocturnal hemoglobinuria (PNH) (see Chapter 12)	• Acquired stem cell disease with a mutation in the PIG (phosphatidyl inositol glycan) complementation group A gene in a myeloid stem cell clone. This results in a defect in the anchoring of inhibitors of complement (CD55 [decay accelerating factor] and CD59) on the surface of RBCs, neutrophils, and platelets. In *normal people*, these inhibitors *degrade* C3 and C5 convertase on hematopoietic cell membranes so that RBCs, neutrophils, and platelets are *not* destroyed. • This is an example of complement-mediated intravascular lysis of RBCs (hemoglobinuria), platelets, and neutrophils that leads to pancytopenia (all hematopoietic cell lines destroyed). • The diagnosis is made with flow cytometry which detects the clones.

Cryptococcus), viruses (e.g., HIV, respiratory syncytial virus, influenza A), and protozoa (e.g., *Leishmania*).

    (4) Does *not* require antibodies for its activation

   d. Membrane attack complex (C5b-C9): final common pathway for the classical, alternative, and lectin pathways

   e. DAF

    (1) Present on cell membranes of hematopoietic cells and other cells in the body

    (2) Enhances the degradation of C3 convertase and C5 convertase in the classical and alternative pathways

    (3) Deficient in paroxysmal nocturnal hemoglobinuria (PNH; Table 4-10; see Chapter 12), a hemolytic anemia

  3. Epidemiology and clinical findings in complement disorders

   a. Complement deficiencies are uncommon.

   b. Complement deficiencies predispose to infections via the following mechanisms:

    (1) Ineffective opsonization, due to a lack of C3b (see Chapter 3)

    (2) Defects in cell lysis, due to a lack of MAC components

   c. Opsonization defects are usually present with recurrent pyogenic infections due to encapsulated bacteria (e.g., *Streptococcus pneumoniae*). Infections are more likely to occur at an early age (few months to a few years of age).

   d. Patients with deficiencies in early classical pathway components (i.e., C1, C4, C2) do *not* have recurrent infections but are more often predisposed to developing autoimmune disease, particularly SLE.

   e. Adults with deficiencies in the formation of MAC have a high risk for developing recurrent infection with *Neisseria gonorrhoeae* and/or *Neisseria meningitidis*. Children and neonates with deficiency of MAC are more likely to have severe pyogenic infections and sepsis.

   f. Summary of complement disorders (see Table 4-10; Fig. 4-19 A-C)

  4. Testing of the complement system

   a. Total hemolytic complement assay (CH50) tests the functional ability of both complement systems (classical and alternative).

   b. Test results that indicate activation of the classical system include decreased C4 and C3 and a normal factor B.

   c. Test results that indicate activation of the *alternative system* include decreased factor B and C3 and a normal C4.

Margin notes:

Antibodies *not* required for activation

C5-C9; final common pathway

DAF: cell membranes hematopoietic cells

↑Degradation C3/C5 convertases classical/alternative

Deficient in PNH: hemolytic anemia

Deficiencies uncommon

Predispose to infections

Ineffective opsonization

Defects cell lysis

↓Opsonization: recurrent pyogenic infections; encapsulated bacteria

C1, C4, C2 → autoimmune disease (SLE)

MAC defects: recurrent infection *N. gonorrhoeae/ meningitidis*

CH50: tests functional ability both C systems

Activation classical pathway: ↓C4, C3; normal factor B

Activation alternative pathway: ↓factor B, C3; normal C4

4-19: A, Hereditary angioedema. Note the swollen fingers in this child. **B,** Normal appearance before an attack. **C,** Angioedema during an acute attack. *(A from Marks JG, Miller JJ: Lookingbill and Marks' Principles of Dermatology, 5th ed, Philadelphia, Saunders, 2013, p214, Fig. 16.16 modified; B, C from Helbert M: Flesh and Bones of Immunology, Edinburgh, Churchill Livingstone, 2006.)*

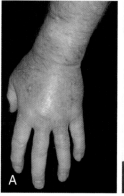
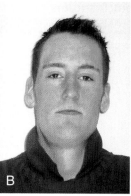
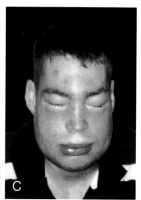

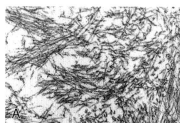
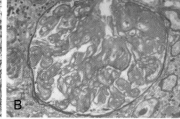
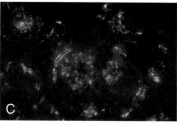

4-20: A, Electron micrograph showing linear, nonbranching fibrils of amyloid. **B,** Amyloidosis. Hematoxylin-eosin–stained slide of a glomerulus shows eosinophilic acellular amyloid material in the glomerular tuft, mesangium, and capillary walls. **C,** Amyloidosis. Congo red–stained section of glomerulus and tubules reveals apple-green birefringence under polarized light in areas with amyloid deposition. *(A from my friend Ivan Damjanov, MD, PhD, Linder J: Anderson's Pathology, 10th ed, St. Louis, Mosby, 1996, p 453, Fig. 20.4; B, C from Kern WF, Silva FG, Laszik ZG, et al: Atlas of Renal Pathology, Philadelphia, Saunders, 1999, p 225, Figs. 19-20, 19-17, respectively.)*

Activation both pathways: ↓C4, factor B, C3

Fibrillar protein; interstitial tissue; pressure atrophy cells

Linear filament; β-pleated sheet

Eosinophilic staining H&E

Congo red +; apple green bfg when polarized

Ig: λ light chains > κ light chains

Urine light chains → BJ proteins

SAA is APR

APP gene chromosome 21

Transthyretin (carrier thyroxine, retinoic acid)

β₂-Microglobulin: component MHC

Prion proteins: maintain neuronal membranes

Majority have misfolded proteins

Large aggregates protein assemble in oligomers/ fibers

Dysfunctional proteasomes: cannot remove misfolded proteins

    d. Test results that indicate activation of both the classical and alternative systems include decreased C4, factor B, and C3.

VII. Amyloidosis

  A. Amyloid characteristics

    1. **Definition:** Amyloid is a fibrillar protein that is deposited in interstitial tissue, where it leads to organ dysfunction by pressure atrophy of adjacent cells.

    2. Composed of linear, nonbranching filaments (electron microscopy) in a β-pleated sheet (type of x-ray diffraction pattern) (Fig. 4-20 A; Link 4-32)

    3. Amyloid is eosinophilic staining with hematoxylin-eosin (H&E) stain (Fig. 4-20 B; Link 4-33).

    4. Congo red stain of tissue turns amyloid red, and polarizing microscopy shows an apple green (similar to a Granny Smith apple) birefringence (bfg; Fig. 4-20 C; Links 4-34 and 4-35). Polarization appearance is due to the β-pleated sheet conformation.

    5. Amyloid is derived from three major precursor proteins.

      a. Ig

        (1) Ig light chains, with λ light chains are more frequently involved than κ light chains

        (2) Light chains in urine are called Bence Jones (BJ) proteins.

      b. Serum amyloid A (SAA) protein: APR that is synthesized and released by the liver in inflammation (Link 4-36)

      c. Amyloid precursor protein (*APP*) gene is located on chromosome 21.

    6. Other important amyloid precursor proteins

      a. Transthyretin, which is a normal carrier protein for thyroxine and retinoic acid (vitamin A)

      b. β₂-Microglobulin, which is the light chain component of the MHC (see earlier)

      c. Prion proteins, which normally maintain neuronal membranes

  B. Pathogenesis of types of amyloidosis

    1. Majority of types of amyloidosis have misfolded proteins, which self-associate and accumulate in the interstitial tissue.

      a. **Definition:** A misfolded protein refers to an excessively large, incorrectly shaped aggregate of proteins that assembles in oligomers and fibers. Oligomers are a molecular complex that consists of a few monomer units, usually fewer than five.

      b. Misfolded proteins are normally removed by proteasomes, but in some types of amyloidosis, this system of removal is dysfunctional.

TABLE 4-11 Common Types of Amyloidosis and Associated Clinical Findings

TYPE OF AMYLOIDOSIS	DISEASE ASSOCIATIONS	FIBRIL PROTEIN DESIGNATION
SYSTEMIC AMYLOIDOSIS		
Immunocyte dyscrasias (primary amyloidosis)	• Plasma cell disorders (e.g., multiple myeloma, other monoclonal plasma cell dyscrasias [10% of all monoclonal gammopathies])	• **AL:** amyloid derived from immunoglobulin light chains, particularly λ light chains
Reactive systemic amyloidosis (secondary amyloidosis)	• Chronic inflammation: rheumatoid arthritis (MC), ankylosing spondylitis, inflammatory bowel disease (Crohn disease, ulcerative colitis), tuberculosis, leprosy, osteomyelitis, renal cell carcinoma, Hodgkin lymphoma, and heroin abusers ("skin popping")	• **AA:** amyloid derived from SAA protein
Hemodialysis-associated amyloidosis	• Chronic renal failure	• **Aβ₂m:** amyloid derived from β₂-microglobulin
HEREDITARY AMYLOIDOSIS		
Familial Mediterranean fever	• Autosomal recessive • Increased production of IL-1 • Fever, inflammation of serosal membranes (pleura, peritoneum, synovium)	• **AA:** amyloid derived from SAA protein
Familial amyloidotic neuropathies	• Autosomal dominant • Associated with peripheral and autonomic nerve disorders	• **ATTR:** amyloid derived from transthyretin (binding protein for thyroxine)
Systemic senile amyloidosis	• Amyloidosis of older patients (>70 yrs); autosomal dominant disease • Predominantly involves heart, producing restrictive cardiomyopathy associated with conduction defects	• **ATTR:** misfolded transthyretin (TTR) protein • Approximately 4% of blacks develop this type of amyloidosis
LOCALIZED AMYLOIDOSIS		
Senile cerebral amyloidosis	• Alzheimer disease (see Chapter 26)	• **Aβ:** amyloid derived from amyloid precursor protein (APP), coded for by chromosome 21
ENDOCRINE AMYLOID		
Medullary carcinoma of the thyroid	• Sporadic and familial (MEN IIa, IIb)	• **A Cal:** amyloid derived from the hormone calcitonin
Islets of Langerhans	• Type 2 diabetes mellitus	• **AIAPP:** amyloid derived from islet amyloid polypeptide

MC, Most common; *MEN,* multiple endocrine neoplasia; *SAA,* serum amyloid A.

    c. Other diseases associated with misfolded proteins include Alzheimer disease, bovine spongiform encephalopathy (BSE), Parkinson disease, and transthyretin amyloidosis.

  2. In amyloidosis due to SAA protein, enzyme defects in monocytes may be responsible for the accumulation of amyloid A protein (misfolded amyloid derived from SAA protein) in the interstitial tissue.

C. Classification of Amyloidosis (Table 4-11)

D. Clinical presentation of amyloidosis

  1. Common presenting signs in amyloidosis include fatigue, dyspnea, edema, paresthesias, and weight loss.

  2. Kidney involvement (see Fig. 4-20 B)

    a. Kidney is the most common organ involved in amyloidosis.

    b. Glomeruli, interstitial tissue, arteries, and arterioles are all involved.

    c. Proteinuria in the nephrotic range leads to generalized pitting edema and effusions due to loss of oncotic pressure from loss of albumin (see Chapters 4 and 20).

  3. Pulmonary involvement: findings include fatigue and dyspnea.

  4. Gastrointestinal involvement

    a. Macroglossia (enlarged tongue), which leads to problems with speech and swallowing

    b. Diarrhea, malabsorptive type, causing the loss of carbohydrates, proteins, and fat

  5. Cardiac involvement

    a. Restrictive cardiopathy is present because of infiltration of amyloid between myocardial fibers (see Chapter 11).

Margin notes:

Misfolded protein disorders: Alzheimer, BSE, Parkinson, transthyretin amyloidosis

SAA amyloidosis → enzyme defects monocytes → amyloid A misfolded proteins

Fatigue, dyspnea, edema, paresthesias, weight loss

Kidney MC site amyloidosis

All structures involved

Nephrotic syndrome → pitting edema/effusions; ↓oncotic pressure (↓albumin)

Pulmonary: fatigue, dyspnea

Macroglossia

Diarrhea (malabsorption type)

Restrictive cardiomyopathy

(1) Ejection fraction is frequently preserved (see Chapter 11).

(2) Produces a diastolic dysfunction type of left-sided heart failure (LHF; see Chapter 11)

b. Conduction defects are very common.

6. Nervous system involvement

a. Dementia (Alzheimer disease)

b. Peripheral neuropathies (paresthesias, muscle weakness)

c. Disabling autonomic neuropathies

7. Liver involvement

a. Hepatomegaly is a common finding in systemic amyloidosis.

b. Pressure atrophy of hepatocytes occurs; however, functional impairment is uncommon.

8. Spleen involvement

a. Splenic involvement (splenomegaly) is common in the systemic type of amyloidosis.

b. If the white pulp (splenic lymphoid follicles) is involved, the splenic surface looks like it is impregnated with grains of sand (called a sago spleen).

c. If the red pulp (venous sinuses with RBCs) is involved, the splenic surface has a waxy appearance (called a lardaceous spleen).

9. Hemodialysis-associated amyloidosis, musculoskeletal involvement is common. Clinical findings include carpal tunnel syndrome, destructive joint disease, bone cysts, and fractures.

10. Hemostasis abnormalities

a. Factor X deficiency may occur in the AL type (designation for amyloid derived from light chains) of systemic amyloidosis. Factor X binds to amyloid fibrils.

b. Skin hemorrhages are common around the orbit and in areas where the skin is pinched (called pinch purpura). Vascular instability is due to amyloid infiltration of small blood vessels.

E. **Techniques used to diagnose amyloidosis**

1. Serum immunoelectrophoresis (SIEP) and urine immunoelectrophoresis (UIEP) are useful in detecting monoclonal spikes in serum and light chains (BJ protein) in urine (see Chapter 14). Bone marrow aspiration and/or biopsy is useful to detect malignant plasma cell infiltrates (see Chapter 14).

2. Tissue biopsy is useful to detect amyloid.

a. Tissues commonly biopsied include the omental fat pad, rectum, and gingiva.

b. If these tissues do *not* reveal amyloidosis, then organ biopsy may be necessary (e.g., liver biopsy).

3. Two-dimensional Doppler echocardiography is useful in diagnosing ventricular filling problems (diastolic dysfunction) in cardiac involvement.

4. Nuclear imaging

a. Serum amyloid P component (SAP) scintigraphy has high sensitivity for detecting amyloid in multiple organ sites.

b. SAP has a high affinity for amyloid.

F. **Prognosis in amyloidosis**

1. In general, the prognosis is poor in systemic amyloidosis and more favorable with localized disease.

2. Better control of diseases that produce inflammation-associated types of amyloidosis has reduced the incidence of these types of systemic amyloidosis.

Diastolic dysfunction LHF

Conduction defects common

Dementia, peripheral/ autonomic neuropathy

Hepatomegaly

Functional impairment uncommon

Splenomegaly

White pulp (lymphoid follicles) → sago spleen

Red pulp (venous sinuses) → lardaceous (waxy) spleen

Hemodialysis-associated amyloidosis: musculoskeletal disorders

Factor X deficiency

Pinch purpura

Vascular instability → hemorrhage

SIEP/UIEP detect monoclonal spikes, BJ protein

Tissue Bx detects amyloid

Liver Bx

Doppler echocardiography

Nuclear imaging

SAP scintigraphy

SAP high affinity for amyloid

Prognosis poor if systemic, favorable if localized

Control diseases producing inflammation → reduced incidence systemic amyloidosis

CHAPTER 5

Water, Electrolyte, Acid-Base, and Hemodynamic Disorders

ABBREVIATIONS

Dx diagnosis
MC most common

MCC most common cause
Rx treatment

S/S signs/symptoms

I. Water and Electrolyte Disorders

A. Body fluid compartments

1. **Definition:** Total body water (TBW) accounts for 60% of the body weight in kilograms (kg) in men and 50% in women.

   ≈60% body weight kg

   a. TBW distribution (Fig. 5-1; Link 5-1)

   (1) Approximately two-thirds of TBW is in the intracellular fluid (ICF) compartment.

   ICF = 2/3 TBW

   (2) Approximately one-third of TBW is in the extracellular fluid (ECF) compartment.

   ECF = 1/3 TBW

   (3) The ECF compartment is subdivided into the interstitial fluid (ISF) compartment (three-fourths of the ECF compartment; fluid around the cells) and the intravascular fluid (IVF) compartment (one-fourth of the ECF compartment).

   ECF = ISF + IVF compartments

   (a) IVF compartment subdivisions include the blood (specifically the plasma component) within the heart, aorta, pulmonary artery, muscular arteries, arterioles, capillaries, venules, and veins.

   ICF > ECF; ISF > IVF

   (b) Because fat contains less water than lean muscle, water accounts for a lower percentage of total body weight in women, older adults, and obese individuals.

   Skin, kidneys, GI tract, respiratory tract

   (4) Water losses occur via the skin, kidneys, gastrointestinal (GI) tract, and respiratory tract.

   (a) Renal excretion of water is regulated via concentration (retain water) or dilution (lose water).

   Concentration (retain water) or dilution (lose water)

   (b) Insensible water loss refers to the total loss of water via the skin (predominantly) and the respiratory tract via evaporation (normal loss ranges from 500 to 1000 mL/day). Fever markedly increases insensible water loss and is often *not* considered in proper fluid replacement in a hospitalized person.

   Loss from skin/respiratory tract via evaporation

   Fever ↑insensible water loss

   Thirst corrects water deficits

   (c) Thirst is essential for preventing and correcting a water deficit. Increase in plasma osmolality (POsm) and hypovolemia stimulate thirst.

   ↑POsm, hypovolemia stimulate thirst

   b. Sodium (Na^+) is the major ECF cation (+ charge). Chloride (Cl^-) is the major ECF anion (− charge).

   Na^+ ECF cation, Cl^- ECF anion

   c. Potassium (K^+) is the major ICF cation. Phosphate (PO_4^{3-}) is the major ICF anion.

   K^+ ICF cation, PO_4^{3-} ICF anion

2. POsm

   a. **Definition:** The number of particles (osmoles) dissolved in plasma in mOsm/kg.

   POsm: number osmoles in plasma mOsm/kg

   b. Three different tonicity states may be present in a person.

   (1) Isotonic state = normal POsm

   Isotonic (normal POsm),

   (2) Hypotonic state = decreased POsm

   Hypotonic (↓POsm)

   (3) Hypertonic state = increased POsm

   Hypertonic (↑POsm)

   c. POsm = 2 (serum Na^+) + serum glucose/18 + serum blood urea nitrogen (BUN)/2.8 = 275–295 mOsm/kg

   POsm = 2 (serum Na^+) + serum glucose/18 + serum BUN/2.8 = 275–295 mOsm/kg

TOTAL BODY WATER

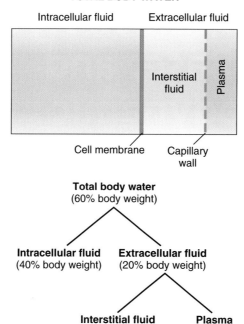

5-1: Body fluid compartments. The intracellular fluid compartment is the largest compartment, followed the extracellular fluid (ECF) compartment. The ECF compartment is subdivided into the interstitial fluid compartment and the vascular compartment, which includes the heart, arteries, arterioles, capillaries, venules, and veins. *(From Costanzo LS: Physiology, 5th ed, Saunders Elsevier, 2014, p 243, Fig. 6-4.)*

Normal fluid state POsm correlates with serum Na⁺

Na⁺ and glucose limited to ECF

Urea diffuses between ECF + ICF

Urea *not* involved in water movements

EOsm = 2 (serum Na⁺) + serum glucose/18

Glucose-6-phosphate traps glucose in the cell

Na⁺/glucose limited to ECF (effective osmoles)

Urea ineffective osmole

Osmotic gradient: ↓/↑ Na⁺ concentration; ↑glucose

Osmosis: Process H₂O moves between ECF/ICF

(1) In the normal fluid state, POsm correlates very closely with the serum Na⁺ concentration, which is actively pumped from the ICF to the ECF compartment by the Na⁺/K⁺-ATPase pump.

(2) Both Na⁺ and glucose are limited to the ECF compartment; however, urea diffuses freely between the ECF and the ICF compartment.

    (a) Because urea is present in both ECF and ICF compartments, it has *no effect* on controlling water movements between these two compartments by osmosis.

    (b) Because clinicians are concerned with water movements between the ECF and ICF compartments, they usually *exclude urea* from the POsm calculation and use the effective osmolality (EOsm) calculation.

    (c) Definition: EOsm = 2 (serum Na⁺) + serum glucose/18. EOsm best reflects osmoles that can alter water movements between the ECF and ICF compartments. Sodium and glucose are called *effective osmoles* (substances that do *not* cross cell membranes and remain in the ECF compartment). Recall that glucose is immediately metabolized when it enters the ICF compartment. The first reaction in glycolysis is phosphorylation of glucose to produce glucose-6-phosphate. This "traps" glucose in the cell so that it can be used to generate adenosine triphosphate (ATP).

      • Changes in the concentration of sodium and glucose in the ECF compartment can affect water movements between the ECF and ICF compartments.

      • Urea is an *ineffective osmole* and *cannot* alter water movements between the ECF and ICF compartments because it crosses cell membranes and distributes itself equally between the two compartments.

d. Changes in the concentration of sodium (low or high) and glucose (high only) alter the osmotic gradient between the ECF and ICF compartments, causing water to shift between the compartments in order to equalize the osmolality between the two compartments.

(1) Water shifts between the two compartments occur by osmosis.

      • **Definition:** Osmosis is the tendency for water to pass through a semipermeable cell membrane into a solution in which the solute concentration is higher, thus equalizing the concentrations of solutes on both sides of the membrane

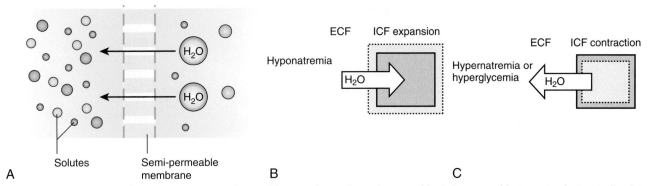

5-2: A, Osmotic movement of water across a membrane. The membrane is semi-permeable. It is permeable to water but *not* all solutes. In this schematic, water is moving from a point of low solute concentration (right side of the membrane) to high concentration (left side of the membrane). Eventually the solute concentration (osmolality) will be the same on both sides of the membrane. **B,** Osmotic shifts in hyponatremia. Note that water moves from the compartment with lowest solute concentration (extracellular fluid [ECF] compartment) to the compartment with highest solute concentration (intracellular fluid [ICF] compartment) by the law of osmosis; hence, there is expansion of the ICF compartment. **C,** In hypernatremia or hyperglycemia, water moves from the ICF compartment into the ECF compartment by osmosis; hence, the ICF compartment contracts. (*A from Naish J, Court DS: Medical Sciences, 2nd ed, Saunders Elsevier, 2015, p 8, Fig. 1.6.*)

(Fig. 5-2 A). If there is an osmotic gradient (difference in osmolality) between the two compartments, water moves from the compartment with the low osmolality to the compartment with the high osmolality.

> Osmosis: water from low to high solute concentration

    (2) Water shifts do *not* occur with an increase in urea concentration, because urea is a permeant solute and diffuses equally between the compartments *without* altering the osmotic gradient.

> *No* water shifts with increases in urea

  e. Hyponatremia (decreased serum sodium, decreased POsm) establishes an osmotic gradient, causing water to shift from the ECF compartment (low solute concentration) to the ICF compartment (high solute concentration). This causes the ICF compartment to expand (Fig. 5-2 B).

> Hyponatremia: ↓serum Na^+/POsm
>
> Osmotic gradient: H_2O moves from ECF to ICF (always expanded)

  f. Hypernatremia (increased serum sodium) and hyperglycemia produce an increased POsm, which causes water to shift from the ICF compartment (low solute concentration) into the ECF compartment (high solute concentration) causing the ICF compartment to contract (Fig. 5-2 C).

> H_2O moves from ICF (contracted) to ECF

B. Hypotonic, isotonic, and hypertonic disorders

  1. Serum Na^+ concentration (mEq/L) approximates the ratio of the total body Na^+ ($TBNa^+$) to the TBW.

> Serum Na^+ ≈ $TBNa^+$/TBW

    a. Serum Na^+ ≈ $TBNa^+$/TBW

      (1) $TBNa^+$ is the sum total of all ECF Na^+ (vascular compartment + interstitial compartment), unlike serum Na^+, which is the Na^+ concentration that is limited to the vascular compartment (i.e., 136–145 mEq/L).

> $TBNa^+$: all Na^+ in ECF + interstitial compartment

      (2) Whenever there is an increase in fluid, the ECF compartment always expands, and whenever there is a decrease in fluid, the ECF compartment contracts.

> Gain fluid → ECF always expands
>
> Loss fluid → ECF always contracts

    b. Hypotonic disorders: clinical findings that correlate with a decrease in $TBNa^+$

      (1) **Definition:** Hypotonic disorders are characterized by a decrease in POsm and serum Na^+ and expansion of the ICF compartment.

      (2) Decrease in $TBNa^+$ produces clinical signs (physical exam findings) of volume depletion (Link 5-2). Another term for volume depletion is *hypovolemia*.

> ↓$TBNa^+$ → signs volume depletion (hypovolemia)

        (a) Note: some authors incorrectly use the term *dehydration* interchangeably with *volume depletion*. **Definition:** Dehydration refers to a loss of only water, whereas volume depletion refers to the loss of both water and Na^+. Loss of pure water is present in diabetes insipidus and insensible water loss (see later under hypernatremia).

> Dehydration: loss pure water (diabetes insipidus, insensible water loss)
>
> Volume depletion: loss water + Na^+

        (b) Physical exam findings (signs) in patients with a decreased $TBNa^+$ include dry mucous membranes (Fig. 5-3 A) and decreased skin turgor (i.e., skin tenting when the skin is pinched; Fig. 5-3 B). Older adults commonly have decreased skin turgor as a result of a normal loss of subcutaneous connective tissue (*not* a decrease in $TBNa^+$).

> Signs ↓$TBNa^+$: dry mucous membranes; skin tenting (↓skin turgor)
>
> Older adults normally have ↓skin turgor

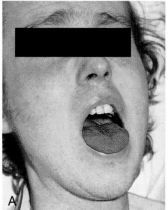 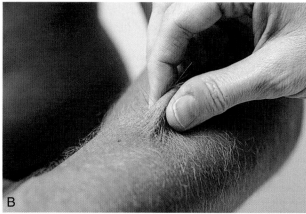 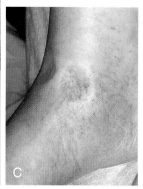

5-3: **A,** Patient with signs of volume depletion. The mucosal surface of the tongue is dry. Additional findings on examination of this patient would likely show hypotension, tachycardia, and decreased skin turgor. **B,** The patient has normal skin turgor with gentle pinching of the skin on the forearm. The skin should feel resilient, move easily when pinched, and return to place immediately when released. **C,** Dependent pitting edema showing depressions in the skin around the ankle after gentle pressure with the finger is applied and then released. Pitting edema is due to an increase in vascular hydrostatic pressure and/or a decrease in vascular oncotic pressure (hypoalbuminemia). *(A from Forbes C, Jackson W:* Color Atlas and Text of Clinical Medicine, *3rd ed, London, Mosby, 2004, p 318, Fig. 7-81; **B** from Seidel H, Ball J, Dains J, Benedict G:* Mosby's Guide to Physical Examination, *St. Louis, Mosby Elsevier, 6th ed, 2006, p 182, Fig. 8.9; **C** from Forbes C, Jackson W:* Color Atlas and Text of Clinical Medicine, *3rd ed, London, Mosby, 2004, p 200, Fig. 5-6.)*

Sitting/standing up from supine position → ↓BP (postural hypotension) + tachycardia

Positive tilt test

Weight loss

↓JVP

Soft sunken eyeball

Confusion, stupor, ↓urine output, lack of tears

↑Capillary filling time in children

↓TBNa⁺ children: capillary fill time >2 sec

Symptoms ↓TBNa⁺: thirst, dizziness (standing), weakness

Signs ↑TBNa⁺: cavity effusions, pulmonary edema; dependent pitting edema

Pitting edema: ↑Na⁺-containing fluid interstitial space (>2–3 liters)

Standing → ankles; supine → sacral area

Alteration Starling forces must be present

↑TBNa⁺: alteration of Starling forces (↑P$_H$ and/or ↓P$_O$); Starling forces: control fluid movements in ECF compartment

(c) Blood pressure (BP) decreases when standing (postural hypotension), and pulse increases (tachycardia) when sitting/standing up from a supine position (i.e., positive tilt test).

(d) Weight loss is due to a decrease in sodium-containing fluid.

(e) Jugular venous pressure (JVP) is decreased (decreased prominence of the internal jugular vein in the lateral neck; see Chapter 11).

(f) Gentle pressure with the index finger over the closed eye reveals a soft, sunken eyeball.

(g) Additional findings include confusion and stupor, decreased urine output, lack of tears, and increased capillary filling time.
   • Increased capillary filling time is the most reliable test to use in children to detect volume depletion. In children, the normal capillary fill time after pinching the fingertip is <2 seconds. In children with volume depletion, the capillary fill time after pinching the fingertip is >2 seconds.

(h) Symptoms (patient complaints) of a decrease in TBNa⁺ include thirst, dizziness on standing, and weakness.

(3) Increased TBNa⁺ produces clinical signs of body cavity effusions (e.g., ascites, pulmonary edema, pleural cavity effusions) and dependent pitting edema (Fig. 5-3 C), which is called hypervolemia (fluid overload).

(a) Dependent pitting edema is due to an excess of Na⁺-containing fluid in the interstitial space (>2–3 L). Because of the low protein content in edema fluid, the fluid obeys the law of gravity and moves to dependent portions of the body (e.g., ankles, if standing; sacral area, if supine). To test for pitting edema, apply gentle pressure with the middle three fingers and note a temporary depression in the skin.

(b) An alteration in Starling forces *must be* present to produce pitting edema and body cavity effusions (discussed later).

Fluid movement across a capillary/venule wall into the interstitial space is driven by Starling forces (*not* osmosis). The net direction of fluid movement depends on which Starling force is dominant. An increase in plasma hydrostatic pressure (P$_H$) and/or a decrease in plasma oncotic pressure (P$_O$; i.e., decrease in serum albumin) causes fluid to diffuse out of capillaries/venules into the interstitial space, resulting in dependent pitting edema and body cavity effusions. Starling forces are more fully discussed later in the chapter.

(c) Increase in TBNa$^+$ increases the plasma P$_H$. Increase in plasma volume (more Na$^+$-containing water is present) causes an increase in plasma P$_H$. Increase in plasma P$_H$ is responsible for pitting edema and body cavity effusions (e.g., ascites, pleural effusions). It may also produce pulmonary edema (fluid in the alveolar sacs and interstitium of the distal airways causing difficulty with breathing (called dyspnea).

$\uparrow$TBNa$^+$ → $\uparrow$plasma P$_H$ (more Na$^+$-containing water present)

$\uparrow$P$_H$ signs: pitting edema, cavity effusions, pulmonary edema

(d) Increase in TBNa$^+$ increases the body weight. Increase in TBNa$^+$ is the most common cause of weight gain in a hospitalized person; hence, it is important to weigh patients every morning. The most common causes of the increase in TBNa$^+$ in a hospitalized patient are heart failure (see Chapter 11) and/or infusion of a sodium-containing antibiotic.

$\uparrow$Patient weight hospital: MCC $\uparrow$TBNa$^+$

Heart failure and/or Na$^+$-containing antibiotic

(e) Increase in TBNa$^+$ increases the JVP, causing prominent distention of the internal jugular veins in the lateral neck.

$\uparrow$JVP

(4) Dyspnea (difficulty with breathing) is the most common symptom of an increase in TBNa$^+$. It is most often due to pulmonary edema and/or excess fluid in the interstitial spaces in the lungs.

Dyspnea MC symptom $\uparrow$TBNa$^+$

2. Isotonic fluid disorders (Table 5-1)

Understanding the fluid compartment boxes. The boxes are subdivided into the ECF compartment (one-third of TBW) and the ICF compartment (two-thirds of TBW). The height of the box is the POsm or serum sodium. If there is a loss of fluid, the ECF compartment is *always* contracted. If there is gain in fluid, the ECF compartment is *always* expanded. In hyponatremia, the height of the boxes is reduced, because the POsm is decreased. In hypernatremia or hyperglycemia, the height of the boxes is increased, because the POsm is increased. In all the hyponatremias, the ICF compartment is expanded, because water moves from the compartment with low solute concentration to the compartment with high concentration by osmosis. In all the hypernatremias and in hyperglycemia, the ICF compartment is contracted, because water moves from the compartment with low solute concentration (ICF) to the compartment with high solute concentration (ECF).

a. Isotonic loss of fluid (Table 5-1 A; Link 5-3)
(1) **Definition:** Isotonic loss of fluid refers to a loss of Na$^+$ and H$_2$O in equal proportions ($\leftrightarrow$ Serum Na = $\downarrow$TBNa$^+$/$\downarrow$TBW); therefore, the serum Na$^+$ concentration is normal. Number of arrows represents the magnitude of change in TBNa$^+$ and TBW (see Tables 5-1 and 5-2).
(2) Examples include a secretory type of diarrhea (e.g., cholera; see Chapter 18) and loss of whole blood (e.g., GI bleeding).
(3) POsm and serum Na$^+$ are normal (this is called hypovolemic normonatremia).
(4) There is *no* osmotic gradient; therefore, there are *no* fluid shifts between the ECF and ICF compartments. ECF volume contracts and the ICF volume remains unchanged (Link 5-3).
(5) Signs and symptoms of volume depletion are present (see earlier).
(6) Random urine Na$^+$ (UNa$^+$) should be <20 mEq/L. Diuretics falsely increase UNa$^+$.

$\leftrightarrow$ Serum Na$^+$ = $\downarrow$TBNa$^+$/$\downarrow$TBW

Secretory diarrhea (e.g., cholera), loss whole blood

POsm/serum Na$^+$ normal

No osmotic gradient; *no* fluid shifts; ECF contracted

S/S volume depletion

Random UNa$^+$ < 20 mEq/L

Diuretics falsely $\uparrow$UNa$^+$

Normal saline ≈ POsm

Normal saline $\uparrow$BP; equilibrates between vascular/interstitial space

Normal (isotonic) saline (0.9%) approximates plasma tonicity (POsm). It is infused in patients to maintain the BP when there is a significant loss of sodium-containing fluid (e.g., blood loss, diarrhea, sweat). As expected, some of the normal saline enters the interstitial compartment and some remains in the vascular compartment, the latter being responsible for raising the BP. Other solutions that are used include lactated Ringer and 5% albumin. Albumin, an impermeant solute, remains in the vascular compartment, so less is required to maintain the BP; however, it is more expensive.

b. Isotonic gain of fluid (Table 5-1 B; Link 5-4)
(1) **Definition:** Isotonic gain of fluid (hypervolemia) refers to an equal gain of Na$^+$ and H$_2$O ($\leftrightarrow$ serum Na$^+$ = $\uparrow$TBNa$^+$/$\uparrow$TBW); therefore, the serum Na$^+$ is normal. Example: excessive infusion of isotonic saline.
(2) POsm and serum Na$^+$ are normal (hypervolemic normonatremia).
(3) *No* osmotic gradient or fluid shift exists between the compartments. The ECF volume expands, while the ICF volume remains unchanged.
(4) Pitting edema and body cavity effusions may be present. Older adults and those with renal dysfunction are more likely to have pitting edema or effusions, because the kidneys are compromised in their ability to excrete excess sodium.
(5) Random UNa$^+$ will be >20 mEq/L. Diuretics falsely increase random\UNa$^+$.

Ringer's lactate, 5% albumin: maintain BP

$\leftrightarrow$ Serum Na$^+$ = $\uparrow$TBNa$^+$/$\uparrow$TBW

Excessive isotonic saline

POsm/serum Na$^+$ normal

No osmotic gradient; $\uparrow$ECF

Pitting edema, body cavity effusions

Random UNa$^+$ > 20 mEq/L

Diuretics falsely $\uparrow$ random UNa$^+$

TABLE 5-1   Isotonic and Hypotonic Disorders

COMPARTMENT ALTERATION	POSM/NA+	ECF VOLUME	ICF VOLUME	CONDITIONS
Normal ECF and ICF volume	Normal	Normal	Normal	Normal hydration
Isotonic net loss Na+ + H2O (**A**) Link 5-3 *Isotonic loss*	Normal ↓TBNa+/↓TBW	Contracted	Normal	**Hypovolemic normonatremia** • Adult diarrhea (secretory type; e.g., cholera) • Loss of whole blood
Isotonic net gain Na+ + H2O (**B**) Link 5-4 *Isotonic gain*	Normal ↑TBNa+/↑TBW	Expanded	Normal	**Hypervolemic normonatremia** • Infusion of excessive isotonic saline
Net loss Na+ in excess of H2O (**C**) *Hypertonic loss of Na+*	Decreased ↓↓TBNa+/↓TBW	Contracted	Expanded	**Hypovolemic hyponatremia** • Loop diuretics • Addison disease • 21-Hydroxylase deficiency
Net gain in water (no sodium) (**D**) Link 5-5 *Gain of water*	Decreased TBNa+/↑↑TBW	Expanded	Expanded	**Euvolemic hyponatremia** • SIADH • Compulsive water drinker
Net gain in H2O in excess of Na+ (**E**) *Hypotonic gain of Na+*	Decreased ↑TBNa+/↑↑TBW	Expanded Starling forces alteration	Expanded	**Hypervolemic hyponatremia** • Right-sided heart failure • Cirrhosis • Nephrotic syndrome

ECF, Extracellular fluid; *ICF,* intracellular fluid; *POsm,* plasma osmolality; *SIADH,* syndrome of inappropriate antidiuretic hormone; *TB,* total body; *TBW,* total body water.

Hyponatremia, ↓POsm

Osmotic gradient always present

H2O shifts ECF to ICF (low to high solute concentration)

ICF always expanded

Renal loss: random UNa+ > 20 mEq/L

3. Hypotonic fluid disorders (see Table 5-1)
   a. **Definition:** A hypotonic fluid disorder is characterized by hyponatremia and a decrease in POsm.
      (1) Osmotic gradient is always present.
      (2) Water shifts by osmosis from the ECF compartment into the ICF compartment (expands). ICF compartment is always expanded because of the movement of water into that compartment by osmosis.
      (3) If renal loss of Na+ is the cause of hyponatremia and the patient is *not* taking diuretics, the random UNa+ is >20 mEq/L.

(4) If hyponatremia is *not* due to a renal loss of Na^+ (e.g., GI loss of sodium), the random UNa^+ is <20 mEq/L.

Nonrenal loss: UNa^+ < 20 mEq/L

b. Hyponatremia caused by a hypertonic loss of Na^+ (Table 5-1 C)

(1) **Definition:** In a hypertonic loss of Na^+, hyponatremia occurs due to a net loss of Na^+ in excess of water ($\downarrow$serum $Na^+ = \downarrow\downarrow TBNa^+/\downarrow TBW$).

$\downarrow$Serum Na^+ = $\downarrow\downarrow TBNa^+/\downarrow TBW$

(2) POsm and serum Na^+ are *both* decreased (hypovolemic hyponatremia).

$\downarrow$POsm/serum Na^+

(3) Random urine sodium (UNa^+) is >20 mEq/L with renal loss of Na^+.

Random UNa^+ >20 mEq/L with renal loss Na^+

(4) ECF volume contracts while the ICF volume expands.

ECF contracts/ICF expands

(5) Signs of volume depletion are present.

Signs volume depletion

(6) Examples of a hypertonic loss in fluid include excessive use of loop diuretics/thiazides, Addison disease (loss of mineralocorticoids leads to sodium loss in the urine; see Chapter 23), 21-hydroxylase deficiency (loss of mineralocorticoids; see Chapter 23).

Loop diuretics/thiazides, Addison, $\downarrow$21-hydroxylase

In a patient with severe hyponatremia (Fig. 5-4 A, B), if there is a rapid intravenous fluid correction of the hyponatremia with saline, this may result in cerebral edema and an irreversible demyelinating disorder called central pontine myelinolysis (CPM; see Fig. 26-18). As a general rule of thumb, in the treatment of hyponatremia, all intravenous replacement of sodium-containing fluids should be given slowly over the first 24 hours regardless of the cause of the underlying serum sodium imbalance.

CPM due to rapid correction hyponatremia

c. Gain of pure water (Table 5-1 D)

(1) **Definition:** Gain of pure water hyponatremia refers to a net gain of water *without* sodium ($\downarrow$serum $Na^+ = TBNa^+/\uparrow\uparrow TBW$).

$\downarrow$Serum Na^+ = $TBNa^+/\uparrow\uparrow TBW$

(2) Decrease in POsm and serum Na^+ (euvolemic hyponatremia)

$\downarrow$POsm, $\downarrow$serum Na^+

(3) Expansion of ECF and ICF compartments

$\uparrow$ECF + ICF compartments

(4) *Normal* skin turgor, because the $TBNa^+$ is normal

Normal skin turgor ($TBNa^+$ normal)

(5) Examples of a gain in pure water include the syndrome of inappropriate secretion of antidiuretic hormone (SIADH; Link 5-5) and compulsive water drinking.

SIADH, compulsive water drinker

d. Hypotonic gain of Na^+ and water (Table 5-1 E)

(1) **Definition:** In a hypotonic gain of Na^+ and water, hyponatremia occurs due to a net gain of H_2O in excess of Na^+ ($\downarrow$serum $Na^+ = \uparrow TBNa^+/\uparrow\uparrow TBW$).

$\downarrow$Serum Na^+ = $\uparrow TBNa^+/\uparrow\uparrow TBW$

(2) Decrease in POsm and serum Na^+ (hypervolemic hyponatremia)

$\downarrow$POsm, $\downarrow$serum Na^+

(3) Expansion of *both* ECF and ICF compartments

$\uparrow$ECF/ICF compartments

(4) $TBNa^+$ is increased, causing pitting edema and body cavity effusions due to Starling force alterations. Examples:

(a) Right-sided heart failure (RHF) with an increase in venous P_H causing pitting edema in the lower legs

RHF ($\uparrow$venous P_H → pitting edema lower legs)

(b) Cirrhosis and nephrotic syndrome with a decrease in plasma oncotic pressure (P_O; the former from decreased synthesis of albumin and the latter from increased loss of albumin in the urine)

Cirrhosis, nephrotic syndrome → $\downarrow P_O$ → $\downarrow$cardiac output

In the previously discussed **pitting edema states,** the cardiac output is decreased, because fluid is trapped in the interstitial space and body cavities. A decrease in cardiac output causes the release of catecholamines, activation of the renin-angiotensin-aldosterone (RAA) system, stimulation of antidiuretic hormone (ADH) release, and increased renal retention of Na^+. The kidney reabsorbs a slightly hypotonic, Na^+-containing fluid ($\uparrow\uparrow TBNa^+/\uparrow\uparrow TBW$). Because these pitting edema states have alterations in Starling forces (increased P_H and/or decreased P_O), the Na^+-containing fluid reabsorbed by the kidneys is redirected into the interstitial space once it reaches the thin-walled capillaries and venules. This further exacerbates the pitting edema and body cavity effusions. In summary, despite compensatory mechanisms, the cardiac output will continue to be decreased until the cause of the decreased cardiac output is corrected.

e. Children with severe hyponatremia from any of the previously mentioned causes may have seizures *before* treatment is begun. This is less common in adults.

Child: seizures commonly occur

f. Pseudohyponatremia

(1) **Definition:** Pseudohyponatremia is a false decrease in serum Na^+ due to a marked increase in serum protein (e.g., multiple myeloma) or lipoproteins containing triglyceride (type IV and V hyperlipoproteinemia; see Chapter 10).

$\downarrow$Serum sodium, normal POsm → pseudohyponatremia

False $\downarrow$ in serum Na^+; $\uparrow$serum protein/triglycerides

(2) Sodium and other electrolytes are dissolved in the water fraction of plasma.

Sodium/electrolytes dissolved plasma water

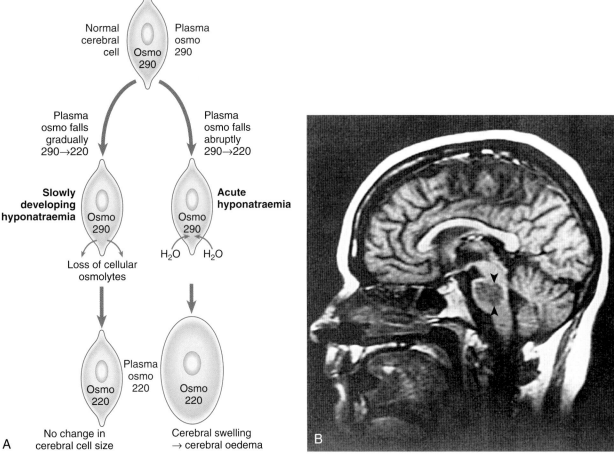

5-4: A, Numbers represent osmolality (osmo) in mmol/kg. Rapid correction of hyponatremia, especially when hyponatremia has developed over a long period of time (e.g., few weeks) is extremely dangerous. During this time, neurons have developed idiogenic osmoles (cellular osmolytes) that are lost from the neurons, so that there is no change in the size of the neurons *(left)*. If correction of the hyponatremia is too rapid, the abrupt increase in extracellular fluid osmolality can lead to water shifting into the neurons, causing cerebral edema. An additional serious effect is central pontine myelinolysis, where myelin detaches from the myelin sheaths. **B,** Central pontine myelinolysis. The black arrows show a central clear area of lucency in the pons. *(**A** from Walker BR, Colledge NR, Ralston SH, Penman ID: Davidson's Principles and Practice of Medicine, 22nd ed, Churchill Livingstone Elsevier, 2014, p 437, Fig. 16.6; **B** from Ashar BH, Miller RG, Sisson SD: The Johns Hopkins Internal Medicine Board Review, 4th ed, Elsevier, 2012, p 254, Fig. 32-3 A; taken from Goetz CG: Textbook of Clinical Neurology, ed 2, Philadelphia, Saunders, 2003.)*

↑Serum protein/lipoproteins
↓water fraction in plasma
→ false ↓serum Na⁺

POsm *not* altered by
↑proteins/triglyceride

Hypernatremia/
hyperglycemia

Osmotic gradient always
present

Water shifts from ICF
(contracted) to ECF
compartment

ECF expanded if TBNa⁺
increased

↑Serum Na⁺ =
↓TBNa⁺/↓↓TBW

↑POsm/serum Na⁺;
hypovolemic hypernatremia

ECF/ICF compartments
contracted

Signs volume depletion

(3) If serum proteins are markedly increased (e.g., multiple myeloma) or lipoproteins are increased (usually triglyceride and cholesterol to a lesser extent), this reduces the water fraction of plasma that sodium is dissolved in, leading to a false decrease in the serum sodium (pseudohyponatremia).

(4) If pseudohyponatremia is suspected, measuring the POsm is recommended, because it is *not* affected by an excess of protein or lipoproteins in plasma.

4. Hypertonic fluid disorders (Table 5-2)
   a. **Definition:** Hypertonic fluid disorders are characterized by hypernatremia or hyperglycemia and an increase in POsm and contraction of the ICF compartment.
   b. Increase in POsm is most often due to hypernatremia or hyperglycemia, the latter being more common due to the high incidence of diabetes mellitus.
      (1) Osmotic gradient is always present.
      (2) Water shifts from the ICF compartment (contracted) into the ECF compartment. ICF compartment is *always* contracted in hypertonic disorders.
      (3) ECF compartment is expanded *if* TBNa⁺ is increased.
   c. Hypotonic loss of Na⁺ (Table 5-2 A; Link 5-6)
      (1) **Definition:** In a hypotonic loss of Na⁺, hypernatremia occurs because the net loss of H_2O is greater than the loss of Na⁺ (↑serum Na⁺ = ↓TBNa⁺/↓↓TBW).
      (2) Both POsm and serum Na⁺ are increased (hypovolemic hypernatremia).
      (3) Both ECF and ICF compartments are contracted.
      (4) Signs of volume depletion are present.

TABLE 5-2   Hypertonic Disorders

COMPARTMENT ALTERATION	POSM/NA+	ECF VOLUME	ICF VOLUME	CONDITIONS
Net loss of H₂O in excess of Na⁺ (**A**) Link 5-6 Hypotonic loss of Na⁺	Increased ↓TBNa⁺/↓↓TBW	Contracted	Contracted	**Hypovolemic hypernatremia** • Osmotic diuresis: glucosuria, mannitol • Sweating • Diarrhea (osmotic type–laxatives, lactase deficiency) • Vomiting
Net loss of only water (**B**) Loss of water	Increased TBNa⁺/↓↓TBW	Contracted (mild)	Contracted	**Euvolemic hypernatremia** • Insensible water loss: fever • Diabetes insipidus: central and nephrogenic
Net gain Na⁺ in excess of H₂O (**C**) Link 5-7 Hypertonic gain of Na⁺	Increased ↑↑TBNa⁺/↑TBW	Expanded	Contracted	**Hypervolemic hypernatremia** • Infusion of a Na⁺- containing antibiotic • Excess infusion of sodium bicarbonate • Excessive ingestion of NaCl • Primary aldosteronism
Hyperglycemia (**D**) Hyperglycemia	↑Glucose ↓Na⁺ (dilutional effect from H₂O coming out of the ICF compartment into the ECF compartment)	Contracted	Contracted	• Diabetic ketoacidosis (type 1 diabetes mellitus) • Hyperglycemic hyperosmolar state (type 2 diabetes mellitus)

ECF, Extracellular fluid; *ICF,* intracellular fluid; *POsm,* plasma osmolality; *TB,* total body; *TBW,* total body water.

(5) Examples include sweating, osmotic diuresis (e.g., glucosuria, mannitol), diarrhea (osmotic type–laxatives; see Chapter 18), and vomiting.

d. Loss of pure water (Table 5-2 B)

  (1) **Definition:** Pure water loss hypernatremia occurs when there is a loss of water *without* the loss of sodium (↑serum Na⁺ = TBNa⁺/↓↓TBW).

  (2) Both POsm and serum Na⁺ are increased (euvolemic hypernatremia).

  (3) Both ECF and ICF compartments are contracted.

    (a) ECF contraction is mild, because there is no loss of Na⁺.

    (b) BP is normal, because the TBNa⁺ is normal.

  (4) Skin turgor is normal, because the TBNa⁺ is normal.

  (5) Examples of a pure water loss include diabetes insipidus (loss of ADH or refractoriness to ADH; discussed later) and insensible water loss (e.g., fever, where water evaporates from the warm skin surface).

e. Hypertonic gain of Na⁺ (Table 5-2 C, Link 5-7)

  (1) **Definition:** Hypertonic gain of Na⁺ hypernatremia occurs when the net gain in Na⁺ is greater than the gain in water (↑serum Na⁺ = ↑↑TBNa⁺/↑TBW).

  (2) Both POsm and serum Na⁺ are increased (hypervolemic hypernatremia).

  (3) ECF compartment expands, while the ICF compartment contracts.

  (4) Pitting edema and body cavity effusions may be present, because the TBNa⁺ is increased.

↑NaHCO₃, Na⁺-containing antibiotic

Glucose effective osmole; affects water movement ECF/ICF

DKA, HHS (enough insulin to prevent ketosis)

Both ECF/ICF contracted

Dilutional hyponatremia from excessive H₂O coming from ICF

↑POsm, ↓serum Na⁺ (dilutional hyponatremia)

Osmotic diuresis → hypovolemic shock

Reabsorb Na⁺, reclaims HCO₃⁻

↑Na⁺ reabsorption if ↓cardiac output

↓EABV → ↑FF → P₀ > Pₕ → ↑Na⁺ reabsorption

↓EABV: CHF, cirrhosis, hypovolemia

↑EABV → ↓FF → Pₕ > P₀ → ↓ Na⁺ reabsorption

↑EABV: 1° aldosteronism, isotonic gain fluid

1° site for reclamation HCO₃⁻

Not synthesizing HCO₃⁻

Reclaiming HCO₃⁻: retrieving filtered HCO₃⁻

H⁺ in PTCs exchanged for Na⁺ in urine

H⁺ combines with filtered HCO₃⁻ → H₂CO₃ in brush border

Function carbonic anhydrase: dissociates H₂CO₃ to H₂O and CO₂

H₂CO₃ reformed in PTCs

H₂CO₃ dissociates into H⁺ and HCO₃⁻.

HCO₃⁻ moves into blood → H₂CO₃

Normal renal threshold for reclaiming HCO₃⁻ is 24 mEq/L

Serum HCO₃⁻ always equals renal threshold for reclaiming HCO₃⁻

(5) Examples of a hypertonic gain in Na^+ include infusion of $NaHCO_3$ or Na^+-containing antibiotics or excessive ingestion of NaCl (uncommon).

f. Hypertonic state due to hyperglycemia (Table 5-2 D)

(1) **Definition:** Hyperglycemia produces a hypertonic state because, like sodium, it is an effective osmole that can influence water movements between the ECF and ICF compartments.

(2) Hypertonic state due to hyperglycemia primarily occurs in diabetic ketoacidosis (DKA), in which there is a complete lack of insulin (type 1 diabetes mellitus), and hyperglycemic hyperosmolar state (HHS), in which there is an insufficient amount of insulin to prevent hyperglycemia but enough to prevent ketoacidosis (type 2 diabetes mellitus; see Chapter 23).

(3) Hyperglycemia, both the ECF and ICF compartments are contracted (Table 5-2 D).

(a) With excessive amounts of water moving out of the ICF compartment into the ECF compartment by osmosis (much greater than with hypernatremia), there is a dilutional effect on the serum Na^+ in the ECF compartment causing *hypo*natremia.

(b) POsm is increased because of hyperglycemia, whereas serum sodium is decreased because of a dilutional hyponatremia from excess water entering the ECF compartment.

(c) However, the excess water does *not* remain in the ECF, because glucose in urine acts as an osmotic diuretic, causing a major urinary loss of both water and Na^+ (dilutional hyponatremia).

(4) Signs of volume depletion are invariably present. Glucosuria produces a hypotonic loss of water and Na^+ (osmotic diuresis), causing signs of volume depletion and a potential for developing hypovolemic shock. This is *not* uncommon in ketoacidosis associated with type 1 diabetes or HHS associated with type 2 diabetes mellitus.

C. **Volume control** (Box 5-1)

D. **Overview of functions of the major nephron segments**

1. Proximal renal tubule

a. Primary site for Na^+ reabsorption

(1) Na^+ reabsorption is increased when cardiac output is decreased (Box 5-1).

(a) ↓Effective arterial blood volume (EABV) → ↑filtration fraction (FF) → P_O (peritubular P_O) > P_H (peritubular P_H) → ↑Na^+ reabsorption (Box 5-1)

(b) Examples of conditions with a decreased EABV: congestive heart failure (CHF), cirrhosis, and hypovolemia

(2) Na^+ reabsorption is decreased when the cardiac output is increased.

(a) ↑EABV → ↓FF → P_H > P_O (Box 5-1)

(b) Examples of conditions with an increased EABV include mineralocorticoid excess (e.g., primary aldosteronism) and an isotonic gain in fluid.

b. Proximal tubule is the primary site for reclamation of bicarbonate (HCO_3^-; Fig. 5-5; Link 5-8; Link 5-9 **left schematic**).

(1) **Definition:** Reclamation is a mechanism for reclaiming filtered HCO_3^- back into the blood without having to synthesize HCO_3^-.

(a) Reclamation is *not* the same as regenerating (synthesizing) HCO_3^- (see later).

(b) In the proximal tubule, the filtered HCO_3^- is reclaimed ("retrieved" from the urine) and eventually delivered back into the bloodstream.

(2) Hydrogen ions (H^+) in proximal tubular cells (PTCs) are exchanged for Na^+ in the urine (Na^+/H^+ antiporter or exchanger).

(3) H^+ combines with filtered HCO_3^- to form carbonic acid (H_2CO_3) in the brush border of the proximal tubules.

(4) Carbonic anhydrase dissociates H_2CO_3 to H_2O and carbon dioxide (CO_2). CO_2 and H_2O are reabsorbed into PTCs.

(5) H_2CO_3 is reformed in the renal PTCs. H_2CO_3 dissociates into H^+ and HCO_3^-.

(6) HCO_3^- moves into the blood, where it forms H_2CO_3.

c. Clinical effect of lowering the renal threshold for reclaiming HCO_3^-

(1) Normal renal threshold for reclaiming HCO_3^- is 24 mEq/L, which means that the kidney can only reclaim (retrieve) HCO_3^- up to that threshold, and any excess of HCO_3^- is lost in the urine.

(a) Key point to remember is that the serum HCO_3^- concentration is equal to the renal threshold for reclaiming HCO_3^-.

BOX 5-1 Volume Control

Protection of the intravascular volume is paramount to normal survival. Maintenance of the extracellular fluid (ECF) volume involves the integration of factors that (1) control thirst (e.g., increased plasma osmolality [POsm] and angiotensin II); (2) activate the renin-angiotensin-aldosterone (RAA) system (e.g., reduced renal blood flow, sympathetic nervous system stimulation); (3) stimulate the baroreceptors in the arterial circulation (e.g., decreased effective arterial blood volume); (4) increase free water (fH_2O) reabsorption to concentrate the urine (e.g., antidiuretic hormone [ADH]); and (5) increase renal reabsorption of Na^+ and water (e.g., decreased effective arterial blood volume).

Effective Arterial Blood Volume

Effective arterial blood volume (EABV) is a conceptual term that refers to the portion of the ECF that is in the vascular space. In most instances, it correlates directly with the ECF volume and $TBNa^+$ status of the individual. For example, a $\downarrow$EABV (volume depletion) correlates with a $\downarrow$ECF and $\downarrow TBNa^+$ and an $\uparrow$EABV correlates with an $\uparrow$ECF and $\uparrow TBNa^+$. However, in edema states, where there is an alteration in Starling forces (e.g., right-sided heart failure [RHF], cirrhosis of the liver, nephrotic syndrome), the redistribution of fluid (a transudate) from the intravascular compartment into the interstitial fluid compartment increases the total ECF volume at the expense of reducing the venous return of blood to the right side of the heart, which in turn reduces the cardiac output and reduces the EABV ($\downarrow$EABV // $\uparrow$ECF/ $\uparrow TBNa^+$). Hence an increase in the total ECF volume and $TBNa^+$ does *not* always correlate with an increase in the EABV.

Baroreceptors and the Renin-Angiotensin-Aldosterone System

Control of the EABV is monitored by the pressure impacting on the high-pressure arterial baroreceptors located in the aortic arch and carotid sinus and the flow of blood to the renal arteries. When the baroreceptors are activated by a decreased EABV, signals are sent to the medulla to increase the sympathetic tone, leading to the release of catecholamines. The release of catecholamines causes vasoconstriction of peripheral resistance arterioles (increasing the diastolic blood pressure), venoconstriction (increasing venous return to the heart), an increase in heart rate (chronotropic effect), and an increase in cardiac contractility (inotropic effect). Signals are also sent to the supraoptic and paraventricular nuclei in the hypothalamus to synthesize and release ADH (vasopressin) from nerve endings located in the posterior pituitary. ADH enhances the reabsorption of fH_2O (water without electrolytes) from the collecting tubules in the kidneys and is also a potent vasoconstrictor of the peripheral resistance arterioles. Finally, the RAA system is activated owing to reduced blood flow to the juxtaglomerular (JG) apparatus located in the afferent arterioles and by direct sympathetic stimulation of the JG apparatus with subsequent release of the enzyme renin. Renin initiates the following reaction sequence: it cleaves renin substrate (angiotensinogen) into **angiotensin I** (ATI), which is converted by pulmonary **angiotensin-converting enzyme** (ACE) into **angiotensin II** (ATII). ATII has four important functions:

1. Vasoconstriction of peripheral resistance arterioles
2. Stimulation of aldosterone synthesis and release from the zona glomerulosa (aldosterone increases Na^+ reabsorption in exchange for potassium ions [K^+] and hydrogen ions [H^+])
3. Direct stimulation of the thirst center in the brain
4. Enhancement of the activity of the Na^+/H^+ antiporter in the proximal renal tubules to retrieve Na^+ from the urine
   All of these events are an attempt to increase the EABV *before* medical intervention.

   In contradistinction, when there is an **increase in EABV**, there are many counterregulatory mechanisms that act to eliminate the excess fluid *before* medical intervention. An increase in EABV is associated with a corresponding increase in cardiac output. This stretches the arterial baroreceptors, which triggers cessation of sympathetic outflow from the medulla. This, in turn, leads to inhibition of ADH synthesis and release, vasodilation of peripheral resistance arterioles, decreased cardiac contraction, inhibition of the RAA system, and decreased renal retention of Na^+ and water. Other counterregulatory factors include **atrial natriuretic peptide** (ANP), **prostaglandin E_2**, and **B-type natriuretic peptide** (BNP). ANP is released from the left and right atria in response to atrial distention (e.g., left-sided heart failure [LHF] and/or RHF). ANP has multiple functions, including (1) suppression of ADH release, (2) inhibition of the effect of ATII on stimulating thirst and aldosterone secretion, (3) vasodilation of the peripheral resistance arterioles, (4) direct inhibition of Na^+ reabsorption in the kidneys (diuretic/natriuretic effect), and (5) suppression of renin release from the JG apparatus. **Prostaglandin E_2** inhibits ADH, blocks Na^+ reabsorption in the kidneys, and is a potent intrarenal vasodilator (vasodilates the afferent arteriole) that offsets the vasoconstrictive effects of ATII (vasoconstrictor of the efferent arterioles in the kidney) and the catecholamines. BNP increases in the blood when the right and/or left ventricles are volume overloaded (e.g., LHF and/or RHF). It has a diuretic effect similar to ANP.

Renal Mechanisms in Volume Regulation

The response of the kidney to volume alterations is closely integrated with many of the events previously described. The reabsorption of solutes from the proximal tubules is dependent on the **filtration fraction** (FF) in the glomerulus in concert with Starling forces that operate in the peritubular capillaries. The FF is the fraction of the **renal plasma flow** (RPF) that is filtered across the glomerular capillaries into the tubular lumen. It is calculated by dividing the **glomerular filtration rate** (GFR) by the RPF (FF = GFR $\div$ RPF). Normally, the FF is $\approx 20\%$, with the remaining 80% of the RPF entering the efferent arterioles, which divide to form the intricate peritubular capillary microcirculation. Because prostaglandin E_2, a vasodilator, controls the afferent arteriolar blood flow into the glomerulus, and ATII, a vasoconstrictor, controls the efferent arteriolar blood flow leaving the glomerulus, the FF is significantly affected by alterations in the caliber of these arterioles. Starling forces in the peritubular capillaries determine how much of the fluid and solutes reabsorbed from urine by the proximal tubules is redirected back into the vascular component of the ECF compartment. For example, if the EABV is decreased (Box 5-1 B; e.g., ECF volume contraction, or hypovolemia), the peritubular capillary hydrostatic pressure (P_H) will be *decreased* and the peritubular oncotic pressure (P_O) will be *increased*. This enhances the reabsorption of solutes (e.g., sodium) from the tubular lumen into the tubular cell out into the lateral intercellular space and into the peritubular capillary (*thick dotted line*) and back into the vascular compartment. In addition, the FF is increased

Continued

BOX 5-1   Volume Control—cont'd

($\uparrow$FF = $\downarrow$GFR ÷ $\downarrow\downarrow$RPF), hence increasing the filtered load of Na$^+$ and other solutes so that it can be reabsorbed back into the blood. The previous mechanism is so effective that a random urine Na$^+$ (UNa$^+$) measurement is usually <20 mEq/L and is often 0 when hypovolemia is extreme. However, if the EABV is increased (e.g., ECF volume expansion or hypervolemia; Box 5-1 A), the peritubular capillary hydrostatic pressure (P$_H$) will be *increased* and the peritubular oncotic pressure (P$_O$) will be *decreased*. This enhances the loss of solutes in the urine and causes an increase in the UNa$^+$. In the presence of an increased EABV **(A)**, or hypervolemia, the FF is decreased ($\downarrow$FF = $\uparrow$GFR ÷ $\uparrow\uparrow$RPF) and the filtered load of Na$^+$ and other solutes is decreased, favoring loss of the filtered Na$^+$ plus other solutes (e.g., urea, uric acid) in the urine (random UNa$^+$ >20 mEq/L).

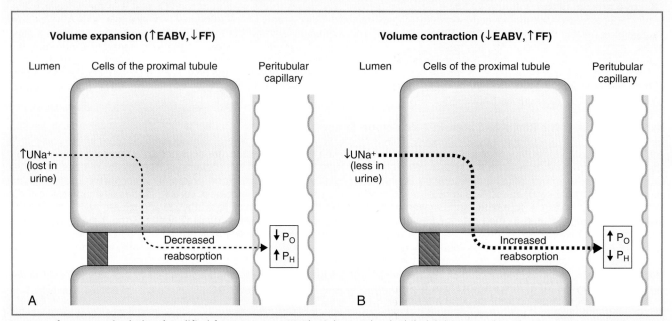

Lumen refers to renal tubules. *(Modified from Costanzo LS: Physiology, 5th ed, Philadelphia, Saunders Elsevier, 2014, p 276, Fig. 6-24.)*

5-5: Reclamation of bicarbonate (HCO$_3^-$) in the proximal tubule. The Na$^+$/H$^+$ antiporter (exchanger) is the primary site for Na$^+$ reabsorption in the kidneys and the reclamation (retrieving) of filtered HCO$_3^-$. The majority of filtered Na$^+$ is reabsorbed in the proximal tubule in exchange for H$^+$ ions. H$^+$ ions then bind to the filtered HCO$_3^-$ to form carbonic acid (H$_2$CO$_3$). Carbonic anhydrase *(c.a.)*, a brush border enzyme, then converts H$_2$CO$_3$ into CO$_2$ and H$_2$O, which diffuse back into the cell. Intracellular carbonic anhydrase then catalyzes a reaction to produce H$_2$CO$_3$, which immediately dissociates into HCO$_3^-$ and H$^+$. The HCO$_3^-$ is reclaimed and the H$^+$ ion exchanges with Na$^+$ (reabsorbed). *(From Goljan EF, Sloka KI: Rapid Review Laboratory Testing in Clinical Medicine, Philadelphia, Mosby Elsevier, 2007, p 32, Fig. 2-5.)*

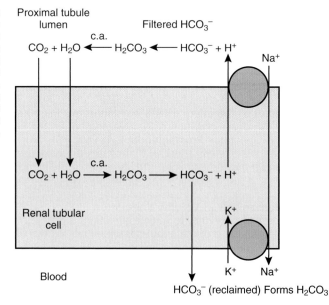

    (b) Normal serum HCO$_3^-$ is 24 mEq/L, which means that the renal threshold for reclaiming HCO$_3^-$ is set at 24 mEq/L.

(2) If the renal threshold is lowered from the normal of 24 mEq/L to 15 mEq/L, then the proximal tubule can only reclaim up to 15 mEq/L, causing the serum HCO$_3^-$ to drop to 15 mEq/L (metabolic acidosis), and the urine pH to become >5.5 from the loss of HCO$_3^-$ in the urine.

Renal threshold can be lowered

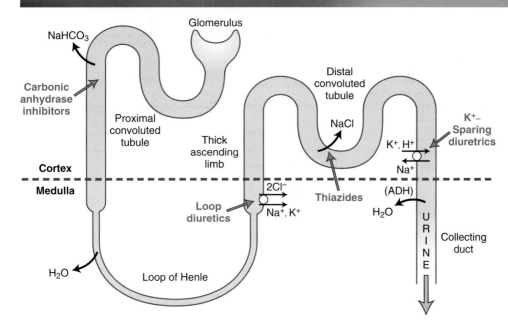

5-6: The nephron and sites of action of various diuretics. *(From O'Connell TX, Pedigo RA, Blair TE: Crush Step I: The Ultimate USMLE Step I Review, Saunders Elsevier, 2014, p 267, Fig. 8-40.)*

(a) Urine loss of HCO_3^- continues to occur until the serum HCO_3^- eventually matches the renal threshold.

(b) Mechanism for producing type II proximal renal tubular acidosis (RTA; discussed in section II: Acid-Base Disorders)

> Low renal threshold for reclaiming HCO_3^- occurs in type II proximal RTA
> CAI (acetazolamide): lowers renal threshold for reclaiming HCO_3^- → $NaHCO_3$ lost in urine → normal AG metabolic acidosis

Carbonic anhydrase inhibitors (CAIs; e.g., acetazolamide) lower the renal threshold for reclaiming HCO_3^-. HCO_3^- combines with Na^+ to form $NaHCO_3$, which is then excreted in the urine. Therefore, acetazolamide is acting as a proximal tubule diuretic in eliminating Na^+. Loss of HCO_3^- in the urine produces a normal anion gap (AG) metabolic acidosis (discussed later; Fig. 5-6 shows site of action of acetazolamide).

d. Clinical effect of raising the renal threshold for reclaiming HCO_3^-
   (1) Volume depletion due to excess vomiting is an example of raising the renal threshold for reclaiming (retrieving) HCO_3^-.
   (2) Raising the threshold means that proportionately more of the filtered HCO_3^- is reclaimed in the proximal tubule and the patient will develop and maintain metabolic alkalosis ($\uparrow HCO_3^-$ with an alkaline pH in the arterial blood). Raising the renal threshold for reclamation of HCO_3^- is the most important factor in maintaining the high serum HCO_3^- that occurs in metabolic alkalosis due to vomiting (see later).

> Renal threshold for reclaiming HCO_3^- can be increased
> Vomiting: renal threshold reclaiming HCO_3^- increased
> Raising threshold for reclaiming filtered HCO_3^- → reason for metabolic alkalosis
> Heavy metal poisoning (lead/mercury) → coagulation necrosis PTCs

In **heavy metal poisoning** with lead or mercury, the proximal tubule cells undergo coagulation necrosis, which produces a nephrotoxic acute tubular necrosis (see Chapter 20). All of the normal proximal renal tubule functions are destroyed, resulting in a loss of sodium (hyponatremia), glucose (hypoglycemia), uric acid (hypouricemia), phosphorus (hypophosphatemia), amino acids, HCO_3^- (type II RTA), and urea in the urine. This is called Fanconi syndrome.

2. Thick ascending limb (TAL; medullary segment; Fig. 5-6, Fig. 5-7)
   a. Primary function of the TAL is to generate free water (fH_2O) via the Na^+-K^+-$2Cl^-$ symporter.
      (1) By definition, fH_2O is water that is *not* attached to Na^+, K^+, or Cl^-.
      (2) Secondary function of the TAL is to reabsorb calcium (Ca^{2+}), in the absence of parathyroid hormone (PTH).
   b. Generation of fH_2O in the kidney primarily occurs in the active Na^+-K^+-$2Cl^-$ symporter (Fig. 5-7) in the TAL.
   c. All the water that is *proximal* to the Na^+-K^+-$2Cl^-$ symporter is obligated (o) water, which refers to water that is already bound to Na^+ (oNa^+), K^+ (oK^+), and Cl^- (oCl^-).
      (1) Obligated water *must* accompany every Na^+, K^+, or Cl^- that is excreted in the urine.
      (2) Obligated water in the kidney *cannot* be reabsorbed by ADH; only fH_2O can be reabsorbed by the renal tubules.

> Heavy metal poisoning: Fanconi syndrome
> Nephrotoxic ATN → hyponatremia, hypoglycemia, hypouricemia, hypophosphatemia, type II proximal RTA
> TAL: generates fH_2O via Na^+-K^+-$2Cl^-$ symporter
> fH_2O: water without electrolytes
> TAL: reabsorbs Ca^{2+} *without* PTH
> Proximal to TAL: all water obligated (oNa^+, oK^+, oCl^-)
> Excreted electrolytes in urine all obligated
> o Water cannot by reabsorbed by ADH; only fH_2O

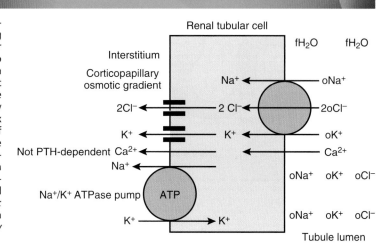

5-7: Na$^+$-K$^+$-2Cl$^-$ symporter in the medullary segment of the thick ascending limb. This is the primary symporter for generating free water *(fH$_2$O)* and is also is important in non-PTH reabsorption of calcium *(Ca^{2+})*. The electrolytes that are reabsorbed by this symporter are used to maintain the corticopapillary osmotic gradient, which in the cortex of the kidney has an osmolarity of ≈300 mOsm/L and at the tip of the papilla in the medulla has an osmolarity of 1200 mOsm/L. See the text for a full discussion. *ATP,* Adenosine triphosphate; *o,* obligated; *PTH,* parathyroid hormone. *(From Goljan EF, Sloka KI: Rapid Review Laboratory Testing in Clinical Medicine, Philadelphia, Mosby Elsevier, 2007, p 34, Fig. 2-6.)*

Na$^+$-K$^+$-2Cl$^-$ symporter: separate obligated water from Na$^+$, K$^+$, Cl$^-$ → becomes fH$_2$O

Reabsorption fH$_2$O in presence of ADH concentrates urine

Loss of fH$_2$O in absence of ADH concentrates urine

Cl$^-$ binding site Inhibited by loop diuretics

Rx of CHF (lose Na$^+$ and H$_2$O); Rx of hypercalcemia; loop diuretic electrolyte/acid-base problems: hyponatremia, hypokalemia, metabolic alkalosis

K$^+$ and 2Cl$^-$ move into interstium via channels

Na$^+$ entering interstitium requires ATP

Interstitium Na$^+$, K$^+$, Cl$^-$ maintains high osmolality in renal medulla

Renal cortex: corticopapillary osmolarity ≈300 mOsm/L

d. Primary function of the Na$^+$-K$^+$-2Cl$^-$ symporter is to separate the obligated H$_2$O that is attached to Na$^+$, K$^+$, and Cl$^-$, so that it becomes fH$_2$O, which is reabsorbed back into the blood in the presence of ADH or lost in the urine by the absence of ADH.
  (1) Remember that fH$_2$O is entirely free of electrolytes.
  (2) Reabsorption of fH$_2$O in the collecting tubules by ADH concentrates the urine (Link 5-10).
  (3) Loss of fH$_2$O in the collecting tubules in the absence of ADH dilutes urine (Link 5-10).
  (4) Loop diuretics block the Cl$^-$ binding site in the Na$^+$-K$^+$-2Cl$^-$ symporter (Figs. 5-6 and 5-7).

Loop diuretics (e.g., furosemide) are the mainstay for the treatment of CHF and hypercalcemia. They decrease TBNa$^+$ and TBW (see earlier) and also decrease reabsorption of Ca^{2+} by blocking the Cl$^-$ binding site in the Na$^+$-K$^+$-2Cl$^-$ symporter (Fig. 5-6). The drug attaches to the Cl$^-$ binding site of the symporter, which not only inhibits reabsorption of Na$^+$, K$^+$, and Cl$^-$ but also impairs the generation of fH$_2$O. Electrolytes are lost in the urine as obligated water and calcium are also lost. Because the normal dilution process is impaired (less fH$_2$O is generated), patients must be warned against consuming excess water. Loop diuretics also produce a hypertonic loss of Na$^+$ in the urine (see earlier), which, along with impaired dilution, may produce hyponatremia. Additional electrolyte abnormalities include hypokalemia and metabolic alkalosis (see later discussion).

Renal medulla: corticopapillary osmolarity 1200 mOsm/L

High interstitium osmotic gradient → normal concentration urine in presence of ADH

Early distal tubule; reabsorbs Na$^+$, Cl$^-$, Ca^{2+} (PTH-enhanced)

Na$^+$/Ca^{2+} share same site for reabsorption

Thiazides inhibit Cl$^-$ binding site in Na$^+$-Cl$^-$ symporter

Thiazide electrolyte abnormalities: hyponatremia, hypokalemia, ↑HCO$_3^-$ (metabolic alkalosis), hypercalcemia (if ↑PTH is present)

e. Fig. 5-7 shows reabsorbed K$^+$ *(asterisk)* and 2Cl$^-$ *(asterisk)* moving through channels into the interstitium *(not* into the bloodstream).
  (1) Na$^+$ entering the interstitium (left side) requires ATP. Na$^+$ exchanges with K$^+$, which moves into the cell.
  (2) Electrolytes in the interstitium (Na$^+$, K$^+$, Cl$^-$) are important in maintaining the extremely high osmolality in the corticopapillary osmotic gradient.
    (a) In the cortex of the kidney, the corticopapillary osmolarity is ≈300 mOsm/L.
    (b) At the tip of the papilla in the medulla, the corticopapillary osmolarity is 1200 mOsm/L.
    (c) Corticopapillary gradient is required for reabsorbing free H$_2$O from the urine in the late-distal and collecting ducts for concentration of urine in the presence of ADH.
3. Na$^+$-Cl$^-$ symporter in the early distal tubule (Fig. 5-8)
  a. Na$^+$-Cl$^-$ symporter primarily reabsorbs Na$^+$, Cl$^-$, and Ca^{2+}.
  b. Note that Na$^+$ and Ca^{2+} share the same site for reabsorption. Reabsorption of Ca^{2+} is enhanced by PTH.
  c. Thiazides inhibit the Cl$^-$ binding site in the Na$^+$-Cl$^-$ symporter (Figs. 5-6, 5-8).

Thiazides, in addition to being diuretics, are the mainstay for the treatment of hypertension in both black and older populations. In both groups, renal retention of Na$^+$ is the primary cause of the hypertension (see Chapter 10). Thiazides are also used in the treatment of hypercalciuria in people who develop Ca^{2+} renal stones (see Chapter 21). The drug attaches to the Cl$^-$ binding site and inhibits Na$^+$ and Cl$^-$ reabsorption. This leaves the Na$^+$ channel open for Ca^{2+} reabsorption, which is useful in treating hypercalciuria. Hyponatremia may occur because of a hypertonic loss of sodium (see previous discussion) in the urine, especially if the patient is indiscriminately drinking copious amounts of water. Additional electrolyte abnormalities include hypokalemia and metabolic alkalosis (mechanism discussed later), particularly if thiazides are taken in excess. Hypercalcemia may also be a complication; however, this is uncommon and is more likely to occur if the patient has an underlying primary hyperparathyroidism with an increase in PTH.

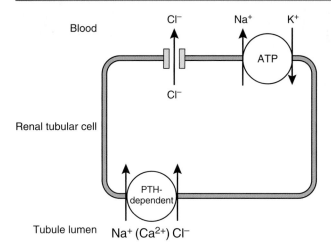

5-8: Na^+-Cl^- symporter in the early distal tubule. This symporter generates free water and also is the primary site for parathyroid hormone–dependent reabsorption of calcium (Ca^{2+}) using the Na^+ channel. See the text for the full discussion. *ATP,* Adenosine triphosphate; *PTH,* parathyroid hormone. *(From Goljan EF, Sloka KI: Rapid Review Laboratory Testing in Clinical Medicine, Philadelphia, Mosby Elsevier, 2007, p 35, Fig. 2-7.)*

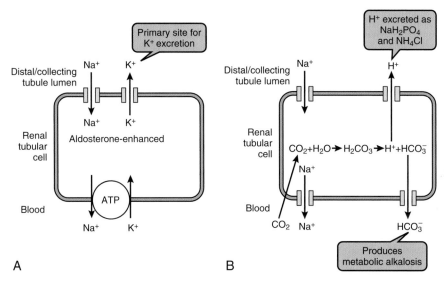

A   **B**

5-9: Na^+-K^+ epithelial channels **(A)** and Na^+-H^+ epithelial channels **(B)** in the late distal and collecting duct. The aldosterone-enhanced Na^+-K^+ epithelial channel **(A)** reabsorbs Na^+ in exchange for K^+. This is the primary channel for the excretion of K^+. If K^+ is depleted **(B;** hypokalemia), then Na^+ exchanges with H^+ ions. For every H^+ ion excreted in the urine, there is a corresponding gain of a bicarbonate (HCO_3^-) into the blood, which causes metabolic alkalosis. See the text for a full discussion. *ATP,* Adenosine triphosphate. *(From Goljan EF, Sloka KI: Rapid Review Laboratory Testing in Clinical Medicine, Philadelphia, Mosby Elsevier, 2007, p 36, Fig. 2-8.)*

4. Aldosterone-enhanced Na^+ and K^+ epithelial channels in the late distal tubule and collecting ducts
   a. Aldosterone-enhanced epithelial channels increase the reabsorption of Na^+ into the blood and the excretion of K^+ into urine (primary site for K^+ excretion; Fig. 5-9 A). Aldosterone-enhanced Na^+ and K^+ epithelial channels are the primary site for the excretion of excess K^+.
   b. Effect of K^+ depletion (hypokalemia) on these channels (Fig. 5-9 B)
      (1) If K^+ ions are depleted (e.g., hypokalemia), hydrogen (H^+) ions are excreted into the urine in exchange for Na^+.
      (2) Note in the schematic, that for every H^+ ion that is excreted in the urine, a corresponding HCO_3^- enters into the blood, which eventually produces metabolic alkalosis.
         (a) H^+ ions come from CO_2 diffusing into the renal tubular cell, combining with H_2O to form H_2CO_3, which then dissociates into H^+ ions and HCO_3^-.
         (b) Also note that the H^+ ions entering into the tubule lumen are excreted as titratable acid (NaH_2PO_4) and ammonium chloride (NH_4Cl).

> **Amiloride** and **triamterene** are diuretics with a K^+-sparing effect. By binding to Na^+ channels within the luminal membrane, they inhibit Na^+ reabsorption and K^+ excretion (see Fig. 5-6).

   c. Clinical effect of increased distal delivery of Na^+ from loop/thiazide diuretics acting proximal to these epithelial channels
      (1) Because more Na^+ is delivered to these channels than usual, there is an increase in Na^+ reabsorption and K^+ loss in the urine.

Na⁺/K⁺ epithelial channels late distal/collecting ducts aldosterone-enhanced

1° Site K⁺ excretion

Hypokalemia: ↑H⁺ excretion → ↑HCO₃⁻ in blood; metabolic alkalosis

H⁺ ions excreted as NaH₂PO₄ and NH₄Cl

Amiloride, triamterene: K⁺-sparing diuretics

5-10: H^+/K^+-ATPase pump in the collecting tubule. This is the primary pump for the excretion of excess H^+ ions, and it also reabsorbs K^+. It is an aldosterone-enhanced pump. Note that H^+ in the urine is excreted as titratable acid (NaH_2PO_4) or ammonium chloride (NH_4Cl). Note also that bicarbonate ($*HCO_3^-$) is regenerated (new synthesis) in this pump. This is the most important pump in regenerating bicarbonate. See the text for a full discussion. *ATP,* Adenosine triphosphate. *(From Goljan EF, Sloka KI:* Rapid Review Laboratory Testing in Clinical Medicine, *Philadelphia, Mosby Elsevier, 2007, p 37, Fig. 2-9.)*

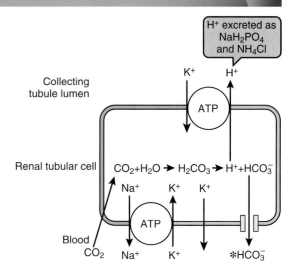

(2) This produces hypokalemia, particularly if K^+ supplements are *not* taken by the patient.

(3) Furthermore, when hypokalemia occurs, Na^+ exchanges with H^+ ions that are excreted as NaH_2PO_4 and NH_4Cl, while HCO_3^- enters into the bloodstream, producing metabolic alkalosis (see previous discussion and Fig. 5-9 B).

(4) This emphasizes the importance of potassium replacement in patients taking loop/thiazide diuretics.

5. Aldosterone-enhanced H^+/K^+-ATPase pump (Fig. 5-10)

a. Aldosterone-enhanced H^+/K^+-ATPase pump is located in the collecting tubules.

b. This is the primary pump for excretion of excess H^+ ions that must be eliminated on a daily basis.

(1) H^+ ions are excreted into the tubule lumen in exchange for K^+.

(2) H^+ combines with HPO_4^{3-} to produce NaH_2PO_4 (called titratable acidity).

(3) H^+ also combines with NH_3 and Cl^- to produce NH_4Cl. As important as NaH_2PO_4 is in eliminating excess H^+ ions, NH_4Cl is considered the *most effective* pump for removing excess H^+ ions.

(4) Both titratable acid and NH_4Cl acidify the urine.

c. Note also that HCO_3^- is synthesized de novo and is reabsorbed directly into the blood. Most important pump for regenerating (synthesizing) HCO_3^-. Recall that the proximal tubule reclaims HCO_3^-.

d. Link 5-9 (**right schematic**) shows the role of the proximal tubule in reclaiming HCO_3^- and the late distal and collecting ducts in regenerating HCO_3^-.

Spironolactone is a diuretic with a K^+-sparing effect (see Fig. 5-6). It inhibits aldosterone, which results in a loss of Na^+ in the urine and retention of K^+ in the blood (K^+-sparer). Hyperkalemia may occur in some cases. H^+ is retained, causing metabolic acidosis.

An **angiotensin-converting enzyme (ACE) inhibitor** is important in the treatment of CHF. Inhibition of the enzyme causes a decrease in angiotensin II (ATII) and aldosterone. ATII is normally a vasoconstrictor of peripheral resistance arterioles, which increases afterload (resistance the heart must contract against). Aldosterone normally causes the reabsorption of sodium, thus increasing preload (volume in the left ventricle). Therefore, an ACE inhibitor decreases both afterload and preload. The inhibition of aldosterone is short-lived and is frequently counterbalanced by the use of spironolactone or other K^+-sparing drugs.

6. Electrolyte changes in Addison disease (also see Chapter 23)

a. **Definition:** Addison disease is most often due to autoimmune destruction of the adrenal cortex.

b. Pathogenesis. Both aldosterone and other mineralocorticoids are deficient as well as cortisol (cortisol is *not* discussed in this chapter).

c. Clinical and laboratory findings

↑Distal delivery Na^+ (proximally acting diuretics): ↓K^+, metabolic alkalosis

K^+ replacement important!!!

Located in collecting tubules

1° pump for excretion excess H^+ ions

H^+ exchanges with K^+

Titratable acidity: excretion of NaH_2PO_4

NH_4Cl: most effective in removing H^+ not titratable acidity (NaH_2PO_4)

Both NH_4Cl and NaH_2PO_4 acidify the urine

Regenerates HCO_3^-

H^+-K^+-ATPase pump: excretes excess H^+; regenerates HCO_3^-

Spironolactone: aldosterone inhibitor; spares K^+; ACE inhibitor: ↓afterload (↓ATII), ↓preload (↓aldosterone)

Autoimmune destruction adrenal cortex

Aldosterone, other mineralocorticoids, cortisol are deficient

(1) Hyponatremia and hyperkalemia

    (a) Aldosterone-enhanced Na^+ and K^+ epithelial channels in the late distal tubule and collecting ducts are impaired (Fig. 5-9 A).

    (b) Hypertonic loss of Na^+ in the urine (more Na^+ in urine) causes hyponatremia, and decreased renal excretion of K^+ produces hyperkalemia.

    (c) Hypertonic loss of Na^+ produces signs of volume depletion (see Table 5-1 C; Fig. 5-9 B, C).

(2) Retention of H^+ ions produces acidosis.

    (a) Aldosterone-enhanced H^+/K^+-ATPase pump in the collecting ducts is impaired (Fig. 5-10).

    (b) This causes retention of H^+ ions (acidosis) and interferes with regeneration of HCO_3^-, causing a decrease in serum HCO_3^-, which, by definition, is metabolic acidosis.

    (c) Loss of K^+ does *not* significantly affect the serum K^+ level; therefore, hyperkalemia prevails in Addison disease.

7. Primary aldosteronism (see Chapter 23)

  a. **Definition:** Primary aldosteronism is an excess production of aldosterone by an adenoma or hyperplasia in the zona glomerulosa of the adrenal gland(s) leading to an increase in mineralocorticoids. This in turn can cause hypertension and electrolyte abnormalities (hypernatremia, hypokalemia) as well as acid-base abnormalities (metabolic alkalosis).

  b. Epidemiology

    (1) Most frequently caused by excessive production of aldosterone from a benign tumor called an adenoma (30%–50% of cases) arising in the zona glomerulosa of the adrenal cortex (normal site for mineralocorticoid synthesis).

    (2) Other causes: bilateral zona glomerulosa hyperplasia, malignant adrenal tumor producing aldosterone.

  c. Pathogenesis of electrolyte abnormalities: increased activity of the aldosterone-enhanced Na^+-K^+ epithelial channels in the late distal and collecting ducts as well as the H^+/K^+-ATPase pumps in the collecting ducts.

  d. Laboratory findings

    (1) Increased activity of the aldosterone-enhanced Na^+-K^+ epithelial channels (Fig. 5-9 A)

      (a) Increased Na^+ reabsorption causes *mild hypernatremia* (sometimes a high normal serum Na^+; Table 5-2 C), and increased K^+ excretion producing *hypokalemia*. Hypokalemia produces severe muscle weakness and polyuria (increased urination; hypokalemia is discussed later in the chapter).

      (b) When Na^+ begins to exchange with H^+ (Fig. 5-9 B), H^+ is lost in the urine in the form of NaH_2PO_4 and NH_4Cl. This is counterbalanced by a gain in HCO_3^-, causing *metabolic alkalosis* (Fig. 5-9 B).

    (2) Enhanced activity of the aldosterone-enhanced H^+/K^+-ATPase pump in the collecting ducts (Fig. 5-10)

      (a) H^+ is lost in the urine in the form of NaH_2PO_4 and NH_4Cl, and there is increased regeneration (synthesis) of HCO_3^-, which causes *metabolic alkalosis*.

      (b) Amount of K^+ reabsorbed by this pump does *not* override the amount of K^+ that is excreted by the Na^+-K^+ epithelial channels; hence, *hypokalemia* prevails as the primary K^+ abnormality in primary aldosteronism.

  e. Clinical findings relate to an increase in plasma volume (PV) from excess Na^+ in the ECF compartment (Table 5-2 C).

    (1) $\uparrow$PV $\rightarrow$ $\uparrow$stroke volume in the heart $\rightarrow$ $\uparrow$systolic blood pressure (SBP; see Chapter 10)

    (2) Excess Na^+ in the ECF compartment enters smooth muscle cells of the peripheral resistance arterioles (see Chapter 10). Excess Na^+ opens up Ca^{2+} channels in the smooth muscle, causing vasoconstriction and an increase in *diastolic blood pressure* (DBP; discussed further in Chapter 10).

    (3) $\uparrow$PV $\rightarrow$ $\uparrow$renal blood flow, which inhibits the RAA system $\rightarrow$ $\downarrow$plasma renin activity (PRA; see Chapter 10)

    (4) $\uparrow$PV $\rightarrow$ $\uparrow$glomerular filtration rate (GFR) $\rightarrow$ $\uparrow$peritubular capillary hydrostatic pressure (P_H) $\rightarrow$ $\downarrow$proximal tubule reabsorption of Na^+ (Box 5-1)

      (a) Excessive loss of Na^+ in the urine prevents pitting edema in primary aldosteronism and other mineralocorticoid excess states (i.e., the net gain in Na^+ is *not* enough to produce pitting edema).

Margin notes:

Hyponatremia/hyperkalemia

Hypertonic loss Na^+ in urine

Signs volume depletion

Retention H^+ ions $\rightarrow$ acidosis

$\downarrow$$HCO_3^-$: metabolic acidosis

Addison disease: hyponatremia, hyperkalemia, metabolic acidosis

Excess production of aldosterone

Adenoma or hyperplasia in zona glomerulosa

Hypernatremia, hypokalemia, metabolic acidosis

MCC benign adenoma

Hyperplasia, malignancy less common

$\uparrow$Activity Na^+-K^+ epithelial channels; H^+/K^+-ATPase pumps

Mild hypernatremia, hypokalemia

Hypokalemia $\rightarrow$ severe muscle weakness, polyuria

Metabolic alkalosis

H^+ lost as NaH_2PO_4 and NH_4Cl

$\uparrow$Regeneration of HCO_3^-

Metabolic alkalosis; hypokalemia

$\uparrow$SBP ($\uparrow$stroke volume)

$\uparrow$DBP

Low plasma renin type hypertension

Net gain in Na^+ *not* enough to produce pitting edema

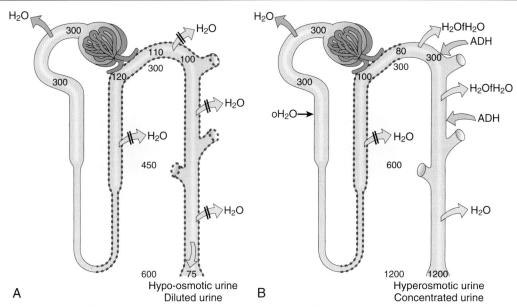

5-11: Production of hyperosmotic (concentrated urine) and hypo-osmotic urine (diluted urine) under the influence of antidiuretic hormone (ADH). **A,** Diuresis in the absence of ADH produces a diluted urine as free water is lost in the urine. The thicker, dotted line indicates impermeability to water. **B,** Diuresis in the presence of high serum ADH produces a concentrated urine (high specific gravity; increased urine osmolality) as free water is reabsorbed out of the urine in the late distal and collecting ducts. *(Further modified from my friend Ivan Damjanov, MD, PhD:* Pathophysiology, *Saunders Elsevier, 2009, p 415, Fig. 12-5; modified from Constanzo LS:* Physiology, *Philadelphia, Saunders, 1998, pp 258-259.)*

↑ANP, ↑BNP

- In addition, excess PV increases atrial dilation, causing the release of *atrial natriuretic peptide* (ANP), while ventricular dilation causes the release of *B-type natriuretic peptide* (BNP; see Box 5-1 discussion). Both of these peptides elicit sodium diuresis and play a major role in preventing pitting edema in primary aldosteronism.

No pitting edema

    (b) As stated previously, although Na^+-containing fluid is increased in the interstitial tissue, there is *not* enough (<2–3 liters) to produce pitting edema in primary aldosteronism.

Escape phenomenon ($P_H >$ P_O; lose Na^+ in urine)

    (c) In mineralocorticoid excess states, this paradox of *not* developing pitting edema is called the "escape phenomenon."

  E. Clinical conditions associated with dilution abnormalities (Fig. 5-11; Link 5-10)

    1. Overview of normal dilution of urine (Fig. 5-11 A)

Excretion excess fH_2O in urine

      a. **Definition:** Dilution is the process of excreting excess amounts of fH_2O in the urine.

      b. Dilution, the urine osmolality (UOsm) in the late distal tubule/collecting ducts is ≈150 mOsm/kg. Most of the water is fH_2O, and only a very small amount is oH_2O accompanying solute (e.g., oNa^+, oK^+) that has *not* been reabsorbed.

↓POsm → inhibits release of ADH → loss fH_2O → dilution

      c. Decrease in POsm inhibits the release of ADH from the posterior pituitary gland. Absence of ADH results in the loss of fH_2O in the urine, which defines dilution.

    2. Diabetes insipidus (see Chapter 23)

Diabetes insipidus: defect in dilution (loss fH_2O) in urine

      a. **Definition:** Diabetes insipidus refers to a defect in normal dilution due to absence of ADH or refractoriness of the collecting tubules to ADH, leading to a loss of fH_2O in the urine.

      b. Epidemiology

CDI: absence ADH; CNS tumors, trauma

        (1) In central diabetes insipidus (CDI), there is an absence of ADH. Common causes of CDI include central nervous system (CNS) trauma and tumors.

NDI: Collecting tubules refractory to ADH

Drugs, hypokalemia

        (2) In nephrogenic diabetes insipidus (NDI), the collecting tubules are refractory (do *not* respond) to ADH. Common causes of NDI include drugs (e.g., demeclocycline, lithium) and hypokalemia (discussed later).

Always diluting, never concentrating

      c. Pathogenesis of electrolyte abnormalities

        (1) Urine is always being diluted and never concentrated.

UOsm < POsm

        (2) As expected, UOsm is less than POsm because of excessive loss of fH_2O in the urine.

↑POsm → ↑thirst (polydipsia)

      d. Clinical and laboratory findings

        (1) Increase in POsm increases thirst (polydipsia).

Polyuria

        (2) Inability to reabsorb fH_2O causes polyuria (excess urination).

Hypernatremia (loss pure water)

        (3) Hypernatremia is due to loss of pure water ($TBNa^+$/↓↓TBW; see Table 5-2 B).

(4) POsm is >295 mOsm/kg (correlates with the high Na$^+$); UOsm is <500 mOsm/kg (correlates with the loss of water in the urine).

(5) Water deprivation studies distinguish CDI from NDI.

> **Water deprivation studies** help distinguish CDI from NDI. After water deprivation, UOsm is decreased in both CDI and NDI (<300 mOsm/kg). After injection of desmopressin acetate (ADH), UOsm is >800 mOsm/kg in CDI (indicating concentration), whereas in NDI, it is still <300 mOsm/kg, because the collecting tubules are refractory to the injected ADH.

F. **Clinical conditions associated with concentration abnormalities**
1. Overview of normal concentration of urine (Fig. 5-11 B; Link 5-10)
   a. **Definition:** Normal concentration refers to the reabsorption of water (fH$_2$O) from the collecting ducts of the kidneys due to the presence of ADH.
   b. Increase in POsm stimulates ADH synthesis and release into the blood.
   c. ADH reabsorbs fH$_2$O out of the collecting ducts and concentrates the urine. fH$_2$O is reabsorbed out of the urine and brings the increased POsm into the normal range.
   d. As expected, UOsm is greater than POsm in a concentrated urine.
   e. In chronic renal failure, both concentration and dilution are lost.
2. Syndrome of inappropriate antidiuretic hormone (SIADH)
   a. **Definition:** SIADH is most commonly due to ectopic production of ADH from a small cell carcinoma (SCC) of the lung leading to excessive reabsorption of water from the kidneys and severe hyponatremia.
   b. Epidemiology
      (1) SIADH accounts for ≈50% of hyponatremia in hospitalized patients.
      (2) Drugs that enhance the ADH effect that also may produce SIADH include chlorpropamide, cyclophosphamide, vincristine, vinblastine, amitriptyline, haloperidol, phenothiazines, and narcotics.
      (3) Other causes include hypothyroidism/hypocortisolism (thyroxine and cortisol normally inhibit ADH), pulmonary disorders (e.g., tuberculosis, aspergillosis, viral/bacterial pneumonia), intracranial pathology (e.g., trauma, infections, hemorrhage), postoperative period (e.g., surgical stress, ventilation with positive pressure, anesthetic agents), miscellaneous (e.g., acute intermittent porphyria).
   c. Pathophysiology of electrolyte abnormalities
      (1) Urine is always being concentrated, *never* diluted, because ADH is always present. As expected, UOsm is greater than POsm.
      (2) Hypotonic gain of water results in dilutional hyponatremia (TBNa$^+$/↑↑TBW) and an increase in PV (Table 5-1 D).
      (3) Increase in PV increases the peritubular capillary hydrostatic pressure (P$_H$). Because P$_H$ is greater than P$_O$, there is decreased PTC reabsorption of Na$^+$ (Box 5-1). Random UNa$^+$ > 40 mEq/L is characteristic of SIADH if the patient is *not* currently taking a diuretic.
   d. Clinical findings: mental status abnormalities, seizures, and coma may occur secondary to cerebral edema (H$_2$O movement into the ICF compartment).
   e. Laboratory findings: serum Na$^+$ < 120 mEq/L is diagnostic of SIADH; UOsm > 100 mOsm/kg of water (essential); and random UNa$^+$ > 20 mEq/L in a patient *not* taking diuretics (normal random UNa$^+$ is <20 mEq/L).

> **Pharmacology note:** Newer agents block the effect of ADH by inhibiting arginine vasopressin receptor 2 (AVPR2; e.g., conivaptan).

G. **Potassium (K$^+$) disorders**
1. Functions of potassium include regulation of the following:
   a. Neuromuscular excitability and muscle contraction
   b. Insulin secretion from β-islet cells in pancreas
      (1) Hypokalemia inhibits insulin secretion.
      (2) Hyperkalemia stimulates insulin secretion.
2. Potassium handling by the kidneys (Link 5-11)
3. Control of potassium

POsm >295 mOsm/kg; UOsm <500 mOsm/kg

CDI: desmopressin ↑UOsm (concentration); NDI: desmopressin no change in UOsm

Reabsorption fH$_2$O collecting ducts due to ADH

↑POsm stimulates ADH synthesis/release

ADH reabsorbs fH$_2$O out of collecting ducts

UOsm > POsm

Chronic renal failure: loss concentration/dilution

Ectopic ADH SCC lung → reabsorption excess water → severe hyponatremia

Common cause hyponatremia hospitalized patients

Drugs enhancing ADH effect (e.g., chlorpropamide)

Hypocortisolism/thyroidism

TB, aspergillosis, viral/bacterial pneumonia, intracranial pathology, postoperative, acute intermittent porphyria

Always concentrating never diluting

UOsm > POsm

Serum Na$^+$ < 120 mEq/L; TBNa$^+$/↑↑TBW

↑UOsm/random UNa$^+$

P$_H$ > P$_O$ → PTC cannot reabsorb Na$^+$

Random UNa$^+$ > 40 mEq/L diagnostic

Cerebral edema findings

Serum Na$^+$ < 120 mEq/L diagnostic SIADH

UOsm >100 mOsm/kg

Random UNa$^+$ > 20 mEq/L (not on diuretics)

Conivaptan inhibits AVPR2

Regulation neuromuscular excitability; muscle contraction

Regulation insulin secretion

Hypokalemia inhibits insulin secretion

Hyperkalemia stimulates insulin secretion, controls K$^+$

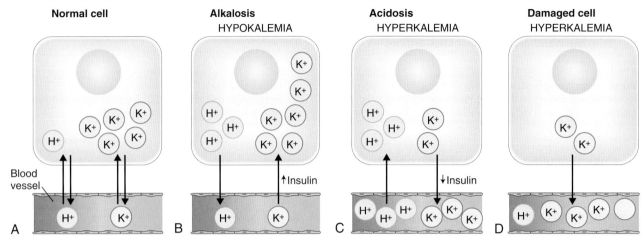

5-12: Potassium flux across the cell membrane. **A,** In the normal cell the intracellular potassium (K^+) concentration is several times higher than in the interstitial fluid. The gradient is maintained by the Na/K-ATPase in the cell membrane. **B,** In alkalosis the intracellular hydrogen ions (H^+) enter the interstitial fluid and the K^+ enters the cells, causing hypokalemia. Insulin also favors the entry of K^+ into the cells. **C,** In acidosis the H^+ enter the cells from the interstitial fluid, displacing K^+, which is translocated into the interstitial fluid and plasma, producing hyperkalemia. Lack of insulin in diabetes mellitus favors efflux of K^+ from cells. **D,** Cell injury leads to a leakage of K^+ from the cytoplasm into the interstitial fluid and plasma, causing hyperkalemia. *(Modified from my friend Ivan Damjanov, MD, PhD:* Pathophysiology, *Saunders Elsevier, 2009, p 13, Fig. 1-10.)*

TABLE 5-3   Causes of Hypokalemia

PATHOGENESIS	CAUSES
Decreased intake	• Older patients and those with eating disorders
Transcellular shift (intracellular)	• Alkalosis (intracellular shift of K^+; Fig. 5-12 B): vomiting, loop/thiazide diuretics, hyperventilation (respiratory alkalosis) • Drugs enhancing the Na^+/K^+-ATPase pump: insulin, β_2-agonists (e.g., albuterol)
Gastrointestinal loss	• Diarrhea ($\approx$30 mEq/L in stool) • Laxatives • Vomiting ($\approx$5 mEq/L in gastric juice)
Renal loss	• Loop and thiazide diuretics (most common cause): excessive exchange of Na^+ for K^+ in late distal and collecting tubules • Osmotic diuresis: glucosuria • Mineralocorticoid excess: primary aldosteronism, 11-hydroxylase deficiency, Cushing syndrome, glycyrrhizic acid (licorice, chewing tobacco), secondary aldosteronism (cirrhosis, congestive heart failure, nephrotic syndrome, conditions that result in a decrease in cardiac output, which decreases blood flow and activates the renin-angiotensin-aldosterone system)

Intracellular K^+ > interstitial tissue; maintained by Na/K-ATPase in cell membrane
Aldosterone 1° control of K^+
Aldosterone → ↑K^+ excretion in renal Na^+-K^+ epithelial channels
Aldosterone → ↑$K+$ reabsorption H^+/K^+-ATPase pump
Arterial pH effect on K^+
Alkalosis shifts K^+ into cells; hypokalemia
Acidosis shifts K^+ out of cells; hyperkalemia
Insulin, β_2-agonists enhance Na^+/K^+-ATPase pump: K^+ moves into cell; hypokalemia
Digitalis, β-blockers, succinylcholine inhibit $Na^+/$ K^+-ATPase pump: K^+ shifts out of cell; hyperkalemia
Serum K^+ < 3.5 mEq/L
Loop/thiazide diuretics: MCC hypokalemia
Muscle weakness/fatigue MC symptom; change K^+ membrane potential

a. Normal cell, the intracellular potassium (K^+) concentration is several times higher than in the ISF. Gradient is maintained by the Na/K-ATPase in the cell membrane (Fig. 5-12 A).
b. Aldosterone
   (1) Aldosterone increases K^+ excretion in renal Na^+-K^+ epithelial channels (Fig. 5-9 A).
   (2) Aldosterone increases K^+ reabsorption of K^+ in H^+/K^+-ATPase pump (Fig. 5-10).
c. Arterial pH effect on potassium
   (1) Alkalosis causes H^+ to shift out of cells and K^+ into cells (Fig. 5-12 B), creating potential for developing hypokalemia.
   (2) Acidosis causes H^+ to shift into cells (for buffering) and K^+ out of cells (Fig. 5-12 C), creating potential for developing hyperkalemia. ↓Insulin enhances hyperkalemia.
   (3) Insulin and β_2-agonists (e.g., albuterol) enhance the Na^+/K^+-ATPase pump → K^+ shifts into cells, creating potential for hypokalemia.
   (4) Digitalis, β-blockers, and succinylcholine inhibit the $Na+/K+$-ATPase pump → K^+ shifts out of cells, creating potential for hyperkalemia.
3. Hypokalemia
   a. **Definition:** Hypokalemia is a serum K^+ that is <3.5 mEq/L.
   b. Causes are discussed in Table 5-3.
   c. Clinical and laboratory findings
      (1) Muscle weakness and fatigue are the most common complaints. Muscle weakness is due to changes in intracellular/extracellular K^+ membrane potential.

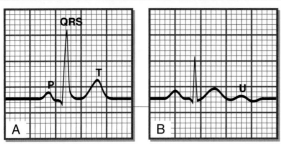

5-13: Electrocardiogram (ECG) changes associated with hypokalemia. **A,** Normal ECG in lead II. **B,** ECG with hypokalemia. A positive wave after the T wave is called a U wave, which is a sign of hypokalemia. *(From Gaw A, Murphy MJ, Srivastava R, Cowan RA, O'Reilly DSJ:* Clinical Biochemistry: An Illustrated Colour Text, *5th ed, Churchill Livingstone Elsevier, 2013, p 22, Fig. 11.2.)*

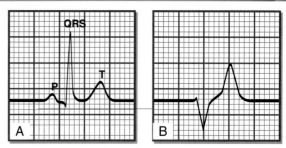

5-14: Electrocardiogram (ECG) changes associated with hyperkalemia. **A,** Normal ECG in lead II. **B,** ECG with hyperkalemia. Note the peaked T wave and widening of the QRS. *(From Gaw A, Murphy MJ, Srivastava R, Cowan RA, O'Reilly DSJ:* Clinical Biochemistry: An Illustrated Colour Text, *5th ed, Churchill Livingstone Elsevier, 2013, p 24, Fig. 12.1.)*

TABLE 5-4   Causes of Hyperkalemia

PATHOGENESIS	CAUSES
Tissue breakdown	• Pseudohyperkalemia (e.g., hemolysis of RBCs due to traumatic venipuncture, thrombocytosis, leukocytosis; Fig. 5-12 D) • Rhabdomyolysis (breakdown of skeletal muscle releases potassium)
Increased intake	• Increased intake of salt substitute (KCl) • Infusion old blood (leakage K^+ out of old RBCs) • K^+-containing antibiotics, e.g., TMP-SMX; urinary pH modifiers (e.g., potassium citrate)
Transcellular shift (extracellular)	• Acidosis (Fig. 5-12 C) • Drugs inhibiting the Na^+/K^+-ATPase pump: β-blocker (e.g., propranolol), digitalis toxicity, succinylcholine
Decreased renal excretion	• Renal disease: renal failure (MCC), interstitial nephritis (legionnaires disease, lead poisoning, sickle cell nephropathy, analgesic nephropathy, obstructive uropathy) • Mineralocorticoid deficiency: Addison disease, 21-hydroxylase deficiency, hyporeninemic hypoaldosteronism (destruction of juxtaglomerular apparatus; type IV RTA) • Drugs: spironolactone (inhibits aldosterone); triamterene, amiloride (inhibit Na^+ channels)

MCC, Most common cause; *RBCs,* red blood cells; *RTA,* renal tubular acidosis; *TMP-SMX,* trimethoprim-sulfamethoxazole.

(2) Electrocardiogram (ECG) shows U waves (Fig. 5-13).

(3) Polyuria (excessive urination). In severe hypokalemia, the collecting tubule cells become distended with fluid (vacuolar nephropathy), rendering them refractory to ADH (i.e., NDI).

(4) Rhabdomyolysis (breakdown of skeletal muscle tissue) may occur. Hypokalemia inhibits insulin → ↓muscle glycogenesis (less glucose available) → rhabdomyolysis due to a lack of ATP.

4. Hyperkalemia

a. **Definition:** Hyperkalemia is a serum K^+ that is > 5 mEq/L.

b. Causes are discussed in Table 5-4.

c. Clinical findings

(1) Ventricular arrhythmias. Severe hyperkalemia (e.g., 7–8 mEq/L) causes the heart to stop in diastole.

(2) Peaked T waves in an ECG (Fig. 5-14). Peaked T waves are due to accelerated repolarization of cardiac muscle.

(3) Muscle weakness and depressed/absent deep tendon reflexes. Hyperkalemia partially depolarizes the cell membrane, which interferes with membrane excitability.

II. Acid-Base Disorders

(margin notes)
U wave
Polyuria; vacuolar nephropathy (NDI) → refractory to ADH
NDI due to vacuolar nephropathy
Rhabdomyolysis (lack of ATP)
Serum K^+ > 5 mEq/L
Ventricular arrhythmias; heart stops in diastole
Peaked T waves; accelerated repolarization cardiac muscle
Muscle weakness, depressed/absent deep tendon reflexes; depolarizes cell membrane
Acidosis pH < 7.35, alkalosis pH > 7.45; No compensation: expected compensation remains in normal range; Partial compensation: expected compensation outside normal range; Full compensation: compensation brings pH into normal range (rarely occurs); pH defines the primary disorder

Definition: Compensation refers to respiratory and renal mechanisms that bring the arterial pH close to but *not* into the normal pH range (7.35–7.45). Acidosis refers to any pH that is <7.35, and alkalosis is any pH that is >7.45. In primary respiratory acidosis and alkalosis, compensation is metabolic alkalosis and metabolic acidosis, respectively. In primary metabolic acidosis and alkalosis, compensation is respiratory alkalosis and respiratory acidosis, respectively. When the expected compensation does *not* occur, the disorder is said to be *uncompensated*. If compensation occurs but does *not* bring pH into the normal range, a *partially compensated* disorder is present. When compensation brings the pH into the normal range, *full compensation* is present, which rarely occurs, with the exception of chronic respiratory alkalosis, particularly at high altitude. The pH defines the primary acid-base disorder. For example, if there is an acid pH (↓pH) associated with a metabolic acidosis (↓HCO_3^-) and a respiratory alkalosis (↓$PaCO_2$), the primary disorder is metabolic acidosis and the compensation is respiratory alkalosis.

Formulas are available that calculate the expected compensation for an arterial blood gas disorder. Calculation for the expected compensation of a blood gas disorder helps in identifying whether there is more than one primary acid-base disorder in a patient (called a mixed disorder; see section II.C.). The formulas and examples are located in the appendix.

Formulas help recognize single versus multiple acid-base disorders

Respiratory acidosis: $Paco_2$ > 45 mm Hg

A. Primary alterations in arterial Pco_2 (normal range of $Paco_2$ = 33–45 mm Hg)

1. Respiratory acidosis
   a. **Definition:** Respiratory acidosis is a $Paco_2$ that is >45 mm Hg.

Transport of carbon dioxide (CO_2) in the blood (Fig. 5-15; Link 5-12). CO_2 and H_2O are converted to H^+ and HCO_3^- inside red blood cells (RBCs). H^+ is buffered by hemoglobin (Hb-H; called carboxyhemoglobin) inside the RBCs. HCO_3^- exchanges for Cl^- (called the chloride shift) and is transported in plasma.
1. CO_2 diffuses from the tissue through the RBC membrane into the RBC.
2. Carbonic anhydrase in the RBC converts CO_2 + H_2O into H_2CO_3.
3. H_2CO_3 dissociates into H^+ + HCO_3^- in the RBC.
4. H^+ is buffered by deoxyhemoglobin (Hb-H).
5. HCO_3^- moves out of the RBC into the plasma, while Cl^- moves into the RBC (chloride shift).

Alveolar hypoventilation → retention CO_2

$Paco_2$ > 45 mm Hg; ↓pH ~ ↑HCO_3^-/↑↑Pco_2

Metabolic alkalosis: compensation

Serum HCO_3^- ≤ 30 mEq/L = acute respiratory acidosis

Serum HCO_3^- > 30 mEq/L = chronic respiratory acidosis

Chronic bronchitis: MCC respiratory acidosis

Somnolence, cerebral edema

Cyanosis, hypoxemia

Respiratory alkalosis

$Paco_2$ < 33 mm Hg; ↑pH ≈ ↑HCO_3^-/↓↓Pco_2

Anxiety (rapid breathing): MCC

   b. Causes (Table 5-5)
   c. Pathogenesis
      (1) Respiratory acidosis is due to alveolar hypoventilation with retention of CO_2.
      (2) $Paco_2$ is >45 mm Hg.
         (a) ↓pH ≈ ↑HCO_3^-/↑↑$Pco2$
         (b) Metabolic alkalosis (increased serum HCO_3^-) is the compensation for respiratory acidosis.
         (c) Serum HCO_3^- ≤ 30 mEq/L defines an acute respiratory acidosis.
         (d) Serum HCO_3^- > 30 mEq/L is characteristic of chronic respiratory acidosis (MCC; elevated HCO_3^- indicates that the kidneys have had time to compensate; i.e., metabolic compensation has occurred).
   d. Clinical findings
      (1) Somnolence (sleepiness); cerebral edema (due to vasodilation of cerebral vessels)
      (2) Cyanosis of the skin and mucous membranes (see Chapter 2); hypoxemia (↓Pao_2; see Chapter 2)
2. Respiratory alkalosis
   a. **Definition:** Respiratory alkalosis is a $Paco_2$ of <33 mm Hg.
      • ↑pH ~ ↑HCO_3^-/↓↓Pco_2
   b. Causes are discussed in Table 5-5.

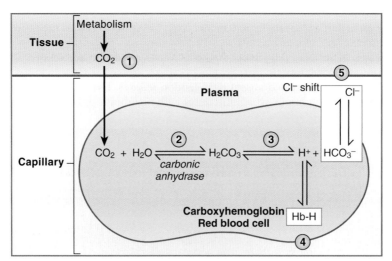

5-15: Transport of carbon dioxide (*CO₂*) in the blood. Refer to the text for discussion. (*Modified from Costanzo LS:* Physiology, *5th ed, Saunders Elsevier, 2014, p 219, Fig. 5-25.*)

TABLE 5-5   Causes of Respiratory Acidosis and Alkalosis

ANATOMIC SITE	RESPIRATORY ACIDOSIS	RESPIRATORY ALKALOSIS
CNS respiratory center	Depression of center: trauma, barbiturates, narcotics, brainstem disease	• Overstimulation: anxiety (MCC), high altitude, normal pregnancy (estrogen/progesterone effect), salicylate poisoning, endotoxic (septic) shock, cirrhosis
Upper airway	Obstruction: acute epiglottitis (*Haemophilus influenzae*), croup (parainfluenza virus), obstructive sleep apnea, obesity	
Chest wall disorders	• Severe kyphoscoliosis, flail chest, ankylosing spondylitis	• Rib fracture: hyperventilation from pain
Muscles of respiration	• Muscle weakness: ALS, phrenic nerve injury, Guillain-Barré syndrome, poliomyelitis, myasthenia gravis, hypokalemia, hypophosphatemia ($\downarrow$ATP), botulism, muscular dystrophy	
Lungs	• Obstructive disease: chronic bronchitis, cystic fibrosis • Other: pulmonary edema (severe), ARDS, RDS, severe asthma	• Restrictive disease: sarcoidosis, asbestosis • Others: pulmonary embolus, pulmonary edema (early), mild asthma (early phases before they become fatigued), early phase of ARDS, chronic illness in a hospital (chronic respiratory alkalosis; very common), pneumothorax (tension and spontaneous), mechanical ventilation

ALS, Amyotrophic lateral sclerosis; *ARDS,* acute respiratory distress syndrome; *ATP,* adenosine triphosphate; *CNS,* central nervous system; *MCC,* most common cause; *RDS,* respiratory distress syndrome.

c. Pathogenesis
   (1) Respiratory alkalosis is characterized by alveolar hyperventilation (breathing rapidly and/or more deeply) with elimination of CO_2.

   > Alveolar hyperventilation eliminating CO_2

   (2) $Paco_2$ is <33 mm Hg because of hyperventilation.
       (a) $\uparrow$pH ~ $\downarrow$HCO$_3^-$/$\downarrow\downarrow$Pco$_2$
       (b) Metabolic acidosis (decreased serum HCO$_3^-$) is the compensation for respiratory alkalosis.

   > Metabolic acidosis: compensation

       (c) Serum HCO$_3^-$ $\geq$ 18 mEq/L is characteristic of acute respiratory alkalosis.

   > Serum HCO$_3^-$ $\geq$ 18 mEq/L = acute respiratory alkalosis

       (d) Serum HCO$_3^-$ <18 mEq/L, but >12 mEq/L (indicates renal compensation) is characteristic of a chronic respiratory alkalosis.

   > Serum HCO$_3^-$ <18 mEq/L, but >12 mEq/L = chronic respiratory alkalosis

d. Clinical findings
   (1) Light-headedness and confusion

   > Light-headedness, confusion

   (2) Signs of tetany, which include thumb adduction into the palm (carpopedal spasm; see Fig. 23-13 A), perioral twitching when the facial nerve is tapped (Chvostek sign), and perioral numbness and tingling

   > Carpopedal spasm, perioral twitching when facial nerve is tapped (Chvostek sign)

Alkalosis increases the number of negative charges on albumin (more COO$^-$ groups on acidic amino acids). Therefore, calcium is displaced from the ionized calcium fraction and is bound to albumin, causing a decrease in ionized calcium levels and signs of tetany (see Fig. 23-13 A).

> Alkalosis: $\uparrow$COO$^-$ groups in acidic amino acids on albumin

B. **Primary alterations in HCO$_3^-$ (22–28 mEq/L)**
   1. Metabolic acidosis

   > Metabolic acidosis

      a. **Definition:** Metabolic acidosis is a serum HCO$_3^-$ that is <22 mEq/L.

   > Serum HCO$_3^-$ < 22 mEq/L

         (1) $\downarrow$pH ~ $\downarrow\downarrow$HCO$_3^-$/$\downarrow$Pco$_2$

   > $\downarrow$pH ~ $\downarrow\downarrow$HCO$_3^-$/$\downarrow$Pco$_2$

         (2) Respiratory alkalosis ($\downarrow$Pco$_2$) is the compensation for metabolic acidosis.

   > Respiratory alkalosis: compensation

      b. Pathogenesis
         (1) Addition of an acid to the ECF compartment produces an increased AG type of metabolic acidosis (discussed later).

   > Addition acid to ECF → $\uparrow$AG metabolic acidosis

         (2) Loss of HCO$_3^-$ or inability to synthesize or reclaim HCO$_3^-$ produces a normal AG type of metabolic acidosis (see later). Loss of HCO$_3^-$ is counterbalanced by a gain in Cl$^-$ anions (hyperchloremia).

   > Loss HCO$_3^-$/cannot reclaim/regenerate HCO$_3^-$ → normal AG metabolic acidosis

         (3) Figure 5-16 contrasts the two types of metabolic acidosis.

   > Loss HCO$_3^-$ counterbalanced by hyperchloremia

5-16: Comparison of increased anion gap (AG) metabolic acidosis and normal AG metabolic acidosis. Note that unmeasured anions *(UA)* are increased in the increased AG type of metabolic acidosis and are normal in the normal AG metabolic acidosis. Also note that the chloride *(Cl⁻)* is increased in normal AG metabolic acidosis and normal in increased AG metabolic acidosis. *(From Kliegman R: Nelson Textbook of Pediatrics, 19th ed, Philadelphia, Saunders Elsevier, 2011, p 234, Fig. 52.4.)*

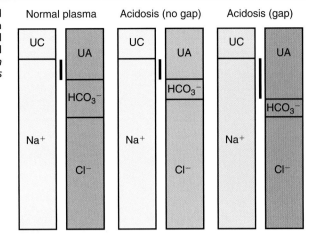

TABLE 5-6 Causes of Increased Anion Gap Metabolic Acidosis

CAUSES	PATHOGENESIS
Lactic acidosis	• Product of pyruvic acid metabolism; most common type ↑AG metabolic acidosis • Any cause of tissue hypoxia with concomitant anaerobic glycolysis: e.g., shock, CN poisoning, CO poisoning, severe hypoxemia (PaO₂ < 35 mm Hg), severe CHF, severe anemia (Hb < 6 g/dL), uncoupling of oxidative phosphorylation (e.g., dinitrophenol), respiratory failure, diabetic ketoacidosis and hyperglycemic hyperosmolar state (both produce shock from loss of Na⁺ fluid by osmotic diuresis) • Alcoholism: pyruvate is converted to lactate from the excess of NADH in alcohol metabolism. • Liver disease: the liver normally converts lactate to pyruvate, and pyruvate is used to synthesize glucose by gluconeogenesis (Cori cycle). Liver disease (e.g., hepatitis, cirrhosis) causes lactate to accumulate in the blood. • Renal failure • Drugs/chemicals: phenformin, salicylates, methanol and ethylene glycol metabolites
Ketoacidosis	• Diabetic ketoacidosis (type 1 diabetes mellitus): accumulation of AcAc and β-OHB • Alcoholism: acetyl CoA in alcohol metabolism is converted to ketoacids. Increase in NADH causes AcAc to convert to β-OHB, which is *not* detected with standard tests for ketone bodies. • Starvation, normal pregnancy, ketogenic diet
Renal failure	• Retention of acids: e.g., sulfuric acid, phosphoric acid, uric acid
Salicylate poisoning	• Salicylic acid is an acid and also a mitochondrial toxin that uncouples oxidative phosphorylation, leading to tissue hypoxia and lactic acidosis. In some cases, excess salicylate overstimulates the CNS respiratory center, producing a primary respiratory alkalosis.
Ethylene glycol poisoning	• Ethylene glycol is in antifreeze and is converted to glycolic and oxalic acid by alcohol dehydrogenase. Oxalate anions combine with calcium to produce calcium oxalate crystals that obstruct the renal tubules, causing renal failure. It increases the osmolar gap. IV infusion of ethanol decreases the metabolism of ethylene glycol, because alcohol dehydrogenase will preferentially metabolize alcohol. • Osmolal gap > 10 mOsm/kg
Methyl alcohol poisoning	• Methyl alcohol is present in windshield washer fluid, Sterno, and solvents for paints. It is converted into formic acid by alcohol dehydrogenase. Formic acid damages the optic nerve, causing optic neuritis and the potential for permanent blindness. IV infusion of ethanol decreases the metabolism of methyl alcohol, because alcohol dehydrogenase will preferentially metabolize alcohol. • Osmolal gap > 10 mOsm/kg

AcAc, Acetoacetate; *AG,* anion gap; *β-OHB,* β-hydroxybutyrate; *CHF,* congestive heart failure; *CN,* cyanide; *CNS,* central nervous system; *CO,* carbon monoxide; *Hb,* hemoglobin; *IV,* intravenous; *NADH,* reduced form of nicotinamide adenine dinucleotide.

Lactic acidosis MC metabolic acidosis

AG = serum Na⁺ − (serum Cl⁻ + serum HCO₃⁻) = 12 mEq/L ± 2

↑AG: anions present that should *not* be there

c. Increased AG type of metabolic acidosis
   (1) Causes of an increased AG metabolic acidosis are listed in Table 5-6.
   (2) The formula for calculating the AG follows.
      (a) **Definition:** AG = serum Na⁺ − (serum Cl⁻ + serum HCO₃⁻) = 12 mEq/L ± 2, in which 12 mEq/L represents the anions that are *not* accounted for in the formula (e.g., phosphate, albumin, sulfate); however, they are normally present in the serum.
      (b) Key point: if the AG is >12 mEq/L ± 2, there must be additional anions that are present that should *not be* there (e.g., lactate, salicylate, acetoacetate, β-hydroxybutyrate, oxalate, formate, sulfate, phosphate, or urate anions; Table 5-6).

(3) Excess H^+ ions of the acid (e.g., lactic acid) are buffered by HCO_3^-, which decreases the serum HCO_3^- ($H^+ + HCO_3^- \rightarrow H_2CO_3 \rightarrow H_2O + CO_2$).

$\downarrow HCO_3^-$ due to buffering excess H^+ from acid

(4) Loss of HCO_3^- (negative anions) related to the buffering of the excess H^+ ions is counterbalanced by an exact increase in the number of anions of the acid that has produced the metabolic acidosis (e.g., lactate anions). Example: for every HCO_3^- ion that is lost, there is a corresponding lactate anion to replace it.

Anions of acid replace buffered HCO_3^-

(5) Example of an AG calculation in lactic acidosis: serum Na^+ 130 mEq/L (135–147), serum Cl^- 88 mEq/L (95–105), serum HCO_3^- 10 mEq/L (22–28; mean 24)

   (a) AG = 130 − (88 + 10) = 32 mEq/L (normal 12 mEq/L ± 2)

   (b) The drop in HCO_3^- (i.e., from 24 mEq/L to 10 mEq/L; decrease of 14 mEq/L) was counterbalanced by an increase in 14 mEq/L of anions of the lactic acid.

Definition: Osmolal gap is the difference between the calculated POsm and the measured POsm. Calculation of the osmolal gap is useful in evaluating whether an increased AG metabolic acidosis is due to ethanol, methanol (windshield wiper fluid), ethylene glycol (antifreeze), isopropyl alcohol (rubbing alcohol), or acetone. All of these can be measured in the clinical laboratory using gas chromatography. The first step in calculating the osmolal gap is to calculate the POsm using the serum sodium, glucose, and blood urea nitrogen of the patient. The next step is to measure the POsm. If the difference between the calculated POsm and measured POsm (osmolal gap) is <10 mOsm/kg (set for high sensitivity), then ethanol, methanol, ethylene glycol, isopropyl alcohol, or acetone is *not* a cause of the increased AG metabolic acidosis. However, if the osmolal gap is >10 Osm/kg (set for high sensitivity), then ethanol, methanol, ethylene glycol, isopropyl alcohol, and acetone are potential causes of the increased AG metabolic acidosis. **Example:** serum sodium is 140 mEq/L, serum glucose 108 mg/dL, and serum blood urea nitrogen is 28 mg/dL. The calculated POsm is 140 × 2 + 108/18 + 28/2.8 = 296 mOsm/L. If the measured POsm = 300 mOsm/kg, the osmolal gap is <10 mOsm/kg indicating that the elevated POsm is *not* due to ethanol, methanol, ethylene glycol, isopropyl alcohol, or acetone. However, if the measured POsm is 340 mOsm/kg, the osmolal gap is 44 mOsm/kg (>10 mOsm/kg difference), then ethanol, methanol, ethylene glycol, isopropyl alcohol, and acetone are potential causes of the increased AG metabolic acidosis.

Osmolal gap: difference between calculated POsm and measured POsm

Useful in diagnosing ethanol, methanol, ethylene glycol, isopropyl alcohol, and acetone as causes of ↑AG metabolic acidosis

  c. Normal AG metabolic acidosis

    (1) **Definition:** Normal AG metabolic acidosis is a type of metabolic acidosis where the decrease in HCO_3^- anions is matched by an increase in chloride anions.

    (2) Causes are listed in Table 5-7.

    (3) Acidosis is due an inability to synthesize (regenerate) or reclaim (retrieve) HCO_3^- in the kidneys.

    (4) Cl^- anions increase to counterbalance the reduction in HCO_3^- anions—hence the term *hyperchloremic* normal AG metabolic acidosis.

      (a) AG = serum $Na^+ - (\uparrow\uparrow$ serum $Cl^- + \downarrow\downarrow$ serum HCO_3^-) = 12 mEq/L +/−

      (b) Note that a matching increase in anions of Cl^- are replacing the HCO_3^- anions that are lost; therefore, the AG calculation is "normal."

    (5) Example: serum Na^+ 136 mEq/L, serum Cl^- 110 mEq/L (normal Cl^- is 95–105 mEq/L), serum HCO_3^- 14 mEq/L

      (a) AG = 136 − (110 + 14) = 12 mEq/L

      (b) Note that the drop of 10 mEq/L of HCO_3^- from normal (24 − 14 = 10) is counterbalanced by a gain of 10 mEq/L of Cl^- ions (100 + 10 = 110); hence, the AG is normal.

  d. Clinical findings in both increased and normal AG metabolic acidosis

    (1) Hyperventilation (Kussmaul breathing). Produces respiratory alkalosis ($\downarrow Pco_2$), which is the compensation for metabolic acidosis.

    (2) Warm shock. Acidosis vasodilates the peripheral resistance arterioles.

    (3) Osteoporosis. Bone buffers excess H^+ ions causing loss of both organic and mineralized bone (see Chapter 24).

2. Metabolic alkalosis

  a. **Definition:** Metabolic alkalosis is a serum HCO_3^- that is >28 mEq/L.

  b. Pathogenesis

    (1) Metabolic alkalosis is due to a loss of H^+ ions or a gain in HCO_3^-.

    (2) Serum HCO_3^- is >28 mEq/L. $\uparrow$pH ≈ $\uparrow\uparrow HCO_3^-/\uparrow Pco_2$

    (3) Respiratory acidosis ($\uparrow Pco_2$) is the compensation for metabolic alkalosis.

  c. Causes are listed in Table 5-8. Vomiting is the most common cause of metabolic alkalosis.

  d. Types of metabolic alkalosis

    (1) Chloride-responsive

      (a) **Definition:** Chloride-responsive metabolic alkalosis is a type of metabolic alkalosis that can be corrected by the infusion of normal saline (Na<u>Cl</u>).

Normal AG metabolic acidosis: $\downarrow HCO_3^-/\uparrow Cl$

Diarrhea MCC adults/children

Inability to reclaim/regenerate HCO_3^-

AG = serum $Na^+ - (\uparrow\uparrow$ serum $Cl^- + \downarrow\downarrow$ serum HCO_3^-) = 12 mEq/L +/−

Cl^- anions replace HCO_3^-

Hyperventilation (Kussmaul breathing)

Warm shock; vasodilation peripheral resistance arterioles

Osteoporosis; bone buffers H^+ ions

Metabolic alkalosis

Serum HCO_3^- > 28 mEq/L

Lose H^+ or gain HCO_3^-

Serum HCO_3^- > 28 mEq/L; $\uparrow$pH ≈ $\uparrow\uparrow HCO_3^-/\uparrow Pco_2$

Respiratory acidosis compensation

Vomiting MCC metabolic alkalosis

Chloride-responsive

Corrected by infusion NaCl

TABLE 5-7 Causes of Normal Anion Gap Metabolic Acidosis

CAUSE	PATHOGENESIS
Diarrhea	• In adults and children, diarrhea is the most common cause of normal anion gap metabolic acidosis. There is a loss of HCO_3^- in diarrheal stool. • The source of HCO_3^- is from the pancreas, which alkalinizes the gastric meal so the pancreatic and small bowel enzymes are functional.
Cholestyramine	• Drug binds HCO_3^- as well as bile salts, vitamins, and some drugs.
Drainage of bile or pancreatic secretions	• Bile and pancreatic secretions contain large amounts of HCO_3^-.
Type I distal RTA	• Inability to regenerate HCO_3^- because of a dysfunctional H^+/K^+-ATPase pump in the collecting tubules (Fig. 5-10). Excess H^+ ions in the blood combine with Cl^- anions producing a normal anion gap metabolic acidosis. Hypokalemia is severe. • Inability to secrete H^+ ions decreases titratable acidity and the production of NH_4Cl causing the urine pH to be >5.5. Ammonia (NH_3), which normally diffuses into the urine from the medullary interstitium around the collecting ducts, cannot be excreted as NH_4Cl because H^+ ions are not being excreted into the urine by the dysfunctional H^+/K^+-ATPase pump. In addition, the lack of H^+ ions decreases the excretion of titratable acid (NaH_2PO_4). • Causes: amphotericin B, lithium, analgesics, light chains in multiple myeloma, autoimmune disease (e.g., SLE, RA, SS), sickle cell trait/disease
Type II proximal RTA	• Renal threshold for reclaiming HCO_3^- is lowered from a normal of ≈24 mEq/L to ≈18 mEq/L (Fig. 5-5). • Urine pH is initially >5.5 (alkaline), because of a loss of the filtered HCO_3^- in the urine. However, when the serum HCO_3^- eventually equals the renal threshold for reclaiming HCO_3^- (≈18 mEq/L), the proximal tubules can reclaim the filtered HCO_3^-, causing the urine pH to drop to <5.5 (acid). Therefore, early in the pathogenesis of proximal RTA, the urine is alkaline, but later in the disease, the urine is acidic. Hypokalemia may occur due to K^+ binding to HCO_3^- in the urine. • Causes: carbonic anhydrase inhibitors (most common cause), primary hyperparathyroidism (↑PTH, ↓proximal tubule HCO_3^- reclamation), proximal tubule nephrotoxic drugs (e.g., aminoglycosides, valproic acid, streptozotocin), proximal tubule nephrotoxic chemicals (e.g., lead, mercury), Wilson disease.
Type IV RTA	• Most common RTA in adults. It is also the only RTA with hyperkalemia. • Type IV RTA is due to aldosterone deficiency from destruction of the JG apparatus in the afferent arterioles. Two prominent causes of this destruction are hyaline arteriolosclerosis of afferent arterioles in DM (see Chapter 10) and acute or chronic tubulointerstitial inflammation (e.g., legionnaires disease). Destruction of JG apparatus produces a hyporeninemic hypoaldosteronism. Because aldosterone controls the Na^+-K^+ epithelial channels (Fig. 5-9), loss of aldosterone leads to loss of Na^+ in the urine and retention of K^+ in the blood, the latter producing hyperkalemia. Furthermore, aldosterone controls the H^+/K^+-ATPase pump in the collecting tubule (Fig. 5-10); therefore, there is less excretion of H^+ into the urine in type IV RTA. • The role of hyperkalemia is critical to understand the pathophysiology of type IV RTA, because it *inhibits* the synthesis of ammonia in the proximal tubules. Normally, glutamic dehydrogenase converts α-ketoglutarate to glutamine and NH_3. In the cell, NH_3 is converted to NH_4^+, which is excreted into the urine in exchange for Na^+. Some of the NH_4^+ remains in the urine to eventually become NH_4Cl, while the remainder is reabsorbed in the thick ascending limb and deposited in the medullary interstitial fluid around the collecting ducts. NH_3 in this latter site eventually diffuses into the urine and combines with H^+ that is excreted by the H^+/K^+-ATPase pump. With this as background, in type IV RTA, it is important to understand that hyperkalemia inhibits ammonia formation in the proximal tubule by altering the intracellular pH. K^+ enters the renal cells in exchange for H^+, which leaves the cell, causing an *intracellular alkalosis*. Intracellular alkalosis inhibits NH_3 synthesis from glutamine. Hence, type IV RTA is not only a problem with hypoaldosteronism and its effect on inhibiting the Na^+-K^+ epithelial channels and inhibiting the H^+/K^+-ATPase pumps, but it is also a problem in ammoniagenesis in the proximal tubule and excretion of NH_4Cl in the urine. In spite of this, the urine pH is usually acidic (pH < 5.5).

DM, Diabetes mellitus; *JG,* juxtaglomerular; *PTH,* parathyroid hormone; *RA,* rheumatoid arthritis; *RTA,* renal tubular acidosis; *SLE,* systemic lupus erythematosus; *SS,* Sjögren syndrome.

Vomiting, loop/thiazide diuretics

Volume depletion, ↓serum/urine Cl^-, ↑PRA, corrects with normal saline

Chloride-resistant metabolic alkalosis

No response to infusion normal saline

Mineralocorticoid excess (e.g., 1° aldosteronism)

Volume excess, ↑serum/urine Cl^-, ↓PRA; no correction with normal saline; ↑plasma aldosterone

(b) Causes of metabolic alkalosis that fall under this category include vomiting and loop/thiazide diuretics.

(c) Characteristic findings in this type of metabolic alkalosis include volume depletion, decreased serum/urine Cl^-, correction by infusion of normal saline (origin of the term *Cl⁻ responsive*), and increase in PRA due to activation of the RAA system by volume depletion.

(2) Chloride-resistant

  (a) **Definition:** Chloride-resistant metabolic alkalosis is a type of metabolic alkalosis that does *not* respond to infusion of normal saline.

  (b) Causes of chloride-resistant metabolic alkalosis that fall under this category are due to mineralocorticoid excess (e.g., primary aldosteronism).

  (c) Characteristic findings include volume excess, increased serum Cl^-, *no* correction of the metabolic alkalosis by infusion of normal saline (origin of the term *Cl⁻ resistant*), decrease in PRA, and increase in plasma aldosterone levels (see Chapter 23).

TABLE 5-8 Causes of Metabolic Alkalosis

CAUSE	PATHOGENESIS
Vomiting	• Vomiting is the most common cause of metabolic alkalosis. Loss of hydrochloric acid in vomiting results in volume depletion. For every H^+ ion lost in the vomitus, there is a corresponding HCO_3^- in the blood that eventually produces metabolic alkalosis. Because of volume depletion, the renal threshold for reclaiming HCO_3^- is increased. This occurs because in volume depletion, there is increased exchange of H^+ ions for Na^+ in the Na^+/H^+ antiporter (Fig. 5-5). An increase in H^+ ions in the urine allows for more of the filtered HCO_{3-} to be converted into H_2O and CO_2 in the brush border, which enters the proximal tubule and is reconverted to HCO_3^-, which, in turn, enters the blood. This increase in reclaiming of filtered HCO_3^- is what *maintains* the metabolic alkalosis in vomiting. However, if volume depletion is corrected (e.g., infusion of normal saline), the renal threshold for reclaiming HCO_3^- goes back to normal, and the excess HCO_3^- is lost in the urine. This defines a chloride-responsive type of metabolic alkalosis (i.e., infusion of normal saline corrects the metabolic alkalosis).
Mineralocorticoid excess	• Gain in HCO_3^- is due to enhanced function of the aldosterone-enhanced Na^+-H^+ epithelial channels in the late distal and collecting ducts leading to increased synthesis of HCO_3^- and metabolic alkalosis (Fig. 5-9 B). Infusion of normal saline does *not* correct the metabolic alkalosis (chloride-resistant). • Causes: primary aldosteronism, 11-hydroxylase deficiency, Cushing syndrome
Loop and thiazide diuretics	• Block in Na^+ reabsorption in the Na^+-K^+-$2Cl^-$ symporter (Fig. 5-7) by loop diuretics and the Na^+-Cl^- symporter by thiazides (Fig. 5-8) in the early distal tubule leads to augmented late distal and collecting tubule reabsorption of Na^+ and excretion of H^+ (Na^+-H^+ epithelial channels), leading to increased HCO_3^- entering the blood (Fig. 5-9 B). Volume depletion also increases the proximal tubule reclamation of HCO_3^- (Fig. 5-5), which maintains the metabolic alkalosis (chloride-responsive).
Other causes	• Nasogastric suction

    e. Both types of metabolic alkalosis carry an increased risk for developing ventricular arrhythmias. The reason is that alkalosis causes a leftward shift in the oxygen-dissociation curve (ODC), resulting in hypoxia (see Chapter 2).

C. **Mixed acid-base disorders**

    1. **Definition:** Mixed acid-base disorders are a blend of two or more primary acid-base disorders that are present at the same time.

    2. Clues that suggest a mixed acid-base disorder include a normal pH, an extreme acidemia, or an extreme alkalemia.

        a. Examples of a mixed acid-base disorder that has a *normal pH* due to a primary acidosis plus a primary alkalosis

           (1) Salicylate intoxication, particularly in adults

              (a) Salicylic acid produces a primary metabolic acidosis.

              (b) Salicylates can overstimulate the respiratory center, producing a primary respiratory alkalosis rather than a compensatory respiratory alkalosis.

              (c) If there is *no* respiratory center overstimulation, the pH is acidic, indicating a simple primary metabolic acidosis with compensatory respiratory alkalosis.

           (2) Patient with chronic bronchitis, who is taking a loop diuretic

              (a) Chronic bronchitis produces a primary respiratory acidosis.

              (b) Loop diuretics produce a primary metabolic alkalosis.

        b. Example of mixed acid-base disorder with *extreme acidemia* is cardiorespiratory arrest. In cardiorespiratory arrest, there is cardiogenic shock, causing metabolic acidosis due to lactic acidosis from hypoxia, and there is absence of breathing (hypoventilation), causing respiratory acidosis due to an increase in $PaCO_2$.

        c. Example of a mixed acid-base disorder with an *extreme alkalemia* is seen with vomiting (metabolic alkalosis) and hyperventilation (respiratory alkalosis). Severe vomiting produces metabolic alkalosis, while hyperventilation produces respiratory alkalosis.

D. **Schematic of acid-base disorders** (Fig. 5-17)

E. **Selected electrolyte profiles** (Table 5-9)

F. **Selected arterial blood gas profiles** (Table 5-10)

III. **Edema**

A. **Definition of edema**

    • Edema refers to the presence of increased fluid in the interstitial space of the ECF compartment.

B. **Types of edema** (Fig. 5-18 A)

    1. Transudate (see Chapter 3)

        a. **Definition:** Transudate is a protein-poor (<3 g/dL) and cell-poor fluid.

        b. Transudates are associated with dependent pitting edema (see Fig. 5-3 C) and body cavity effusions (see Fig. 19-7 E). Lack of significant amounts of protein and the complete

(margin notes)

↑Risk ventricular arrhythmias; leftward shift ODC

Two or more primary acid-base disorders

Normal pH, extreme acidemia/alkalemia

Normal pH: 1° metabolic acidosis + 1° respiratory alkalosis

Salicylate intoxication adults

Normal pH: chronic bronchitis + loop diuretic = 1° chronic respiratory acidosis + 1° metabolic alkalosis

Extreme acidemia: cardiorespiratory arrest (metabolic acidosis + respiratory acidosis)

Extreme alkalemia: vomiting (metabolic alkalosis) + hyperventilation (respiratory alkalosis)

Edema: excess fluid in interstitial space

Transudate

Protein-poor/cell-poor fluid

5-17: Acid-base graphs showing H⁺ (represented as pH on the y axis) and PCO₂ ranges (represented on the x axis) for various acute and chronic acid-base disorders. The hatched box represents the normal range or pH and arterial PCO₂. Note in chronic respiratory acidosis, that the compensation (metabolic alkalosis) has brought the pH closer to the normal range. *(From Gaw A, Murphy MJ, Srivastava R, Cowan RA, O'Reilly DSJ: Clinical Biochemistry: An Illustrated Colour Text, 5th ed, Churchill Livingstone Elsevier, 2013, p 45, Fig. 22.5.)*

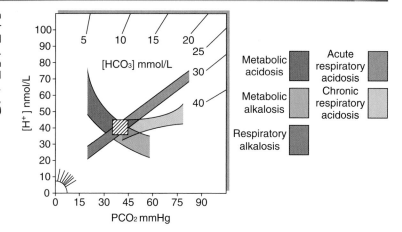

TABLE 5-9 Selected Electrolyte Profiles

SERUM NA⁺ (MEQ/L)	SERUM K⁺ (MEQ/L)	SERUM CL⁻ (MEQ/L)	SERUM HCO₃⁻ (MEQ/L)	DISCUSSION
136–145	3.5–5.0	95–105	22–28	Normal ranges
118	3.0	84	22	**SIADH:** excess water produces a dilutional effect on all electrolytes. In addition, excess sodium is lost in the urine due to volume overload.
128	5.9	110	14	**Addison disease:** lack of aldosterone causes Na⁺ loss in the urine (hyponatremia), retention of K⁺ (hyperkalemia), and decreased synthesis of HCO₃⁻ (normal AG metabolic acidosis; calculated AG is 14 mEq/L).
130	2.9	80	36	**Vomiting:** loss of Na⁺ and K⁺ in vomitus (hyponatremia, hypokalemia); volume depletion causes increased reclamation of HCO₃⁻ in the proximal tubule (metabolic alkalosis; Fig. 5-5).
				Loop and thiazide diuretics: hypertonic loss of Na⁺ in urine (hyponatremia); augmented exchange of Na⁺ for K⁺ in Na⁺-K⁺ epithelial channel (hypokalemia; Fig. 5-9 A) and increased loss of H⁺ and increased entry of HCO₃⁻ into the blood (metabolic alkalosis, Fig. 5-9 B)
146	2.8	110	33	**Mineralocorticoid excess:** primary aldosteronism; augmented exchange of Na⁺ for K⁺ (mild hypernatremia, severe hypokalemia; Fig. 5-9 A), and increased HCO₃⁻ enters the blood (metabolic alkalosis, Fig. 5-9B)
138	4.0	90	10	**Increased anion gap metabolic acidosis** (e.g., lactic acidosis); calculated anion gap is 38 mEq/L.
140	2.2	114	14	**Normal anion gap metabolic acidosis** (e.g., diarrhea); calculated anion gap is 12 mEq/L.

SIADH, Syndrome of inappropriate antidiuretic hormone.

Pitting edema, body cavity effusions

Alteration Starling forces

Exudate: protein-rich and cell-rich fluid

↑Viscosity (↑protein + cells); *no* pitting edema

Protein-rich lymphatic fluid; ISF/body cavities

No pitting edema

Myxedema

↑Hyaluronic acid

No pitting edema

Transudate: alteration in Starling forces

absence of cells allows a transudate to obey the law of gravity and to settle in dependent areas of the body (e.g., ankles when standing, sacral area when supine).
  c. Transudates are always associated with an alteration in Starling forces (see later).
2. Exudate (see Chapter 3)
  a. **Definition:** Exudate is a protein-rich (>3 g/dL) and cell-rich (e.g., neutrophils) fluid.
  b. Exudate produces swelling of tissue; however, because of increased viscosity due to increased protein and cells (neutrophils) there is *no* pitting edema.
3. Lymphedema (see Fig. 10-13 B, C)
  a. **Definition:** Lymphedema is a protein-rich lymphatic fluid that is present in the interstitial tissue and/or body cavities.
  b. Increased viscosity of the lymphedema fluid prevents pitting edema.
4. Myxedema
  a. **Definition:** Myxedema is a fluid that primarily consists of hyaluronic acid (a glycosaminoglycan; see Fig. 23-6 B; Fig. 23-7 C).
  b. Increased viscosity of the myxedema fluid prevents pitting edema.
C. Pathophysiology of edema
  1. Transudates are associated with an alteration in Starling forces.

TABLE 5-10   Selected Arterial Blood Gas Profiles

PH	PACO$_2$ (MM HG)	HCO$_3^-$ (MEQ/L)	DISCUSSION
7.35–7.45	33–45	22–28	Normal ranges
7.00	52	13	• Mixed disorder (extreme acidemia): primary metabolic acidosis (HCO$_3^-$ < 22 mEq/L), primary respiratory acidosis (PaCO$_2$ > 45 mm Hg) • *Example:* cardiorespiratory arrest
7.20	74	28	• Acute respiratory acidosis, uncompensated: PaCO$_2$ > 45 mm Hg, HCO$_3^-$ < 30 mEq/L • *Example:* CNS respiratory center depression (e.g., barbiturate poisoning)
7.33	60	31	• Chronic respiratory acidosis with partially compensated metabolic alkalosis: PaCO$_2$ > 45 mm Hg, HCO$_3^-$ > 30 mEq/L • *Examples:* chronic bronchitis, cystic fibrosis
7.28	28	12	• Metabolic acidosis with partially compensated respiratory alkalosis: HCO$_3^-$ < 22 mEq/L, PaCO$_2$ < 33 mm Hg • *Examples:* disorders associated with increased and normal anion gap metabolic acidosis
7.42	22	14	• Mixed disorder (normal pH): primary metabolic acidosis: HCO$_3^-$ < 22 mEq/L), primary respiratory alkalosis (PaCO$_2$ < 33 mm Hg) • *Examples:* salicylate poisoning, septic shock
7.50	47	35	• Metabolic alkalosis with partially compensated respiratory acidosis: HCO$_3^-$ > 28 mEq/L, PaCO$_2$ > 45 mm Hg) • *Causes:* loop/thiazide diuretics, vomiting, mineralocorticoid excess
7.56	24	21	• Acute respiratory alkalosis with partially compensated metabolic acidosis: PaCO$_2$ < 33 mm Hg, HCO$_3^-$ < 22 mEq/L) • *Causes:* anxiety, pulmonary embolus.

a. Two Starling forces that are present in the microcirculation (capillaries/venules) that affect the pathophysiology of edema are P_H and P_O (Fig. 5-18 A, B).

(1) P_H *favors* movement of fluid (transudate) out of the capillaries/venules.

(2) P_O equates with the serum albumin level and *opposes* movement of fluid out of the capillaries/venules.

(3) In normal circumstances, plasma P_O is greater than P_H ($P_O > P_H$) and fluid remains in the capillaries/venules.

b. Clinical examples of increased P_H producing edema

(1) Pulmonary edema in left-sided heart failure (LHF; Fig. 5-18 C)

(a) In LHF (see Chapter 11), blood builds up behind the failed heart (the lungs), causing increased P_H in the pulmonary vessels.

(b) Increased P_H in the pulmonary capillaries causes a transudate to enter the alveoli and interstitium of the lungs, producing pulmonary edema.

(2) Peripheral pitting edema in RHF (see Fig. 5-3 C)

(a) In RHF, blood builds up in the vena cava, causing a marked increase in P_H.

(b) Increase in P_H in the dependent vessels in the legs causes a transudate to enter the interstitial tissue around the ankles and lower leg causing pitting edema.

(3) Portal hypertension in cirrhosis, producing ascites (Fig. 5-18 D)

(a) Recall that the portal vein normally empties blood into the liver.

(b) In cirrhosis of the liver, the parenchyma is entirely replaced by fibrous tissue, causing the P_H within the portal vein to markedly increase (called portal vein hypertension).

(c) Increased portal vein pressure causes a fluid (a transudate) to enter the peritoneal cavity causing ascites.

c. Clinical examples of decreased P_O (hypoalbuminemia) producing peripheral pitting edema and ascites include malnutrition with decreased protein intake (see Fig. 5-18 A), cirrhosis with decreased synthesis of albumin, nephrotic syndrome with increased loss of protein in urine (>3.5 g/24 hr), and malabsorption with decreased absorption of protein.

d. Clinical examples of where both P_H and P_O are abnormal

(1) Ascites in cirrhosis (Fig. 5-18 A). Increase in P_H (portal vein hypertension) and decrease in P_O, due to decreased liver synthesis of albumin (hypoalbuminemia)

(2) Renal retention of sodium and water

(a) Retention of sodium and water in the vasculature increases the P_H (PV is increased) and decreases the P_O (dilutional effect of increased PV on albumin).

P_H: move transudate out of capillaries/venules

P_O (albumin): opposes movement fluid out of capillaries/venules

Normally $P_O > P_H$

↑P_H: pulmonary edema LHF

Blood backs up into lungs → pulmonary edema

↑P_H in pulmonary capillaries → pulmonary edema (transudate)

Peripheral pitting edema

↑P_H in vena cava due to RHF

↑P_H in vena cava → dependent pitting edema ankles/lower leg

Portal hypertension in cirrhosis → ascites

Portal vein normally empties into liver

Cirrhosis: ↑portal vein hypertension

↑Portal vein hypertension → ascites (transudate) in peritoneal cavity

↓P_O: nephrotic syndrome, malnutrition, cirrhosis, malabsorption

Both P_H and P_O abnormal

Ascites in cirrhosis: ↑P_H (portal vein hypertension), ↓P_O (hypoalbuminemia)

Renal retention sodium + water

↑P_H, ↓P_O (dilutional effect)

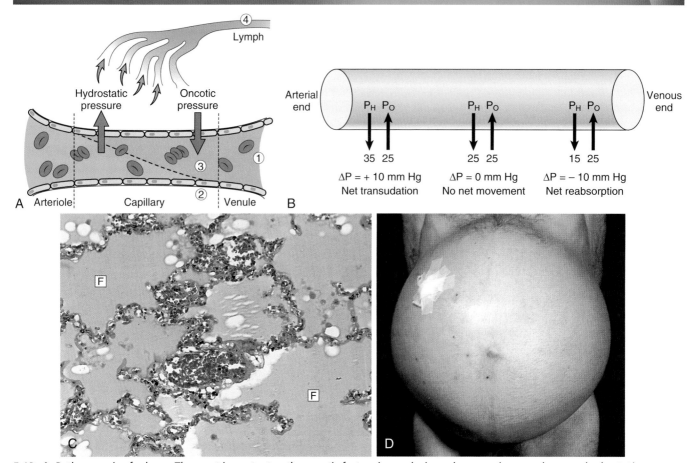

5-18: **A,** Pathogenesis of edema. The most important pathogenetic factors in producing edema are increased venous hydrostatic pressure *(1)*, increased permeability of the vessel wall from acute inflammation *(2)*, decreased oncotic pressure (P_O) of plasma resulting from a low albumin concentration *(3)*, and obstruction of lymphatics *(4)*. **B,** Starling forces in a capillary/venule. Hydrostatic pressure (P_H) pushes fluid out of capillaries/venules, while P_O keeps fluid in vessels. On the left of the schematic, P_H is greater than P_O, so fluid is leaving the vessel and entering the interstitial space (net transudation). In the middle of the schematic, both pressures are equal; therefore, there is no fluid movement into the interstitial space. On the right side of the schematic, P_O is greater than P_H; hence, there is net reabsorption of fluid. **C,** Pulmonary edema in a patient with left-sided heart failure (LHF). This histologic section shows lung alveoli filled with pink-stained edema fluid *(F)*, representing a transudate caused by increased P_H in the pulmonary capillaries from LHF. As will be discussed in Chapter 11 in greater detail, blood builds up behind the failed heart. Therefore, in LHF, blood builds up in the lungs. This increases the P_H in the pulmonary capillaries leading to fluid (a transudate) entering the alveoli in the lungs. **D,** Cirrhosis of the liver with ascites causing distention of the abdomen. In cirrhosis of the liver, the portal vein is unable to empty properly into the liver because of widespread replacement of the liver parenchyma by fibrous tissue. This increases the portal vein P_H leading to ascites. Ascitic fluid is a transudate. *(**A** from my friend Ivan Damjanov, MD, PhD: Pathology for the Health Professions, 4th ed, Saunders Elsevier, 2012, p 115, Fig. 6-2; **B** from Brown T: Rapid Review Physiology, 2nd ed, Philadelphia, Mosby Elsevier, 2012, p 133, Fig. 4.44; **C** from Stevens A, Lowe J, Scott I: Core Pathology, 3rd ed, Mosby Elsevier, 2009, 172, Fig. 10.33; **D** from Morse SA, Holmes KK, Ballard RC, Moreland AA: Atlas of Sexually Transmitted Diseases and AIDS, 4th ed, Saunders Elsevier, 2010, p 213, Fig. 12.16.)*

Periorbital edema

↑P_H, ↓P_O; acute/chronic renal failure, glomerulonephritis

↑Vascular permeability in venules

Acute inflammation; exudate (protein- + cell-rich fluid)

Tissue swelling after bee sting, cellulitis

Lymphatic obstruction

Lymphedema

(b) Periorbital edema is a common clinical finding with sodium and water retention due to the loose interstitial tissue in that area.

e. Examples of kidney diseases: acute and chronic renal failure, glomerulonephritis

2. Increased vascular permeability in venules (see Chapter 3)

a. Increased vascular permeability with production of an exudate occurs in acute inflammation. Unlike a transudate, an exudate is a protein- and cell-rich fluid (pus with neutrophils).

b. Examples of increased vascular permeability include tissue swelling after a bee sting and cellulitis.

3. Lymphatic obstruction

a. Lymphatic production produces lymphedema.

b. Examples

(1) Lymphedema after a modified radical mastectomy and radiation therapy (see Fig. 10-13 B)

(2) Lymphedema in filariasis, due to *Wuchereria bancrofti* (see Fig. 10-13 C)

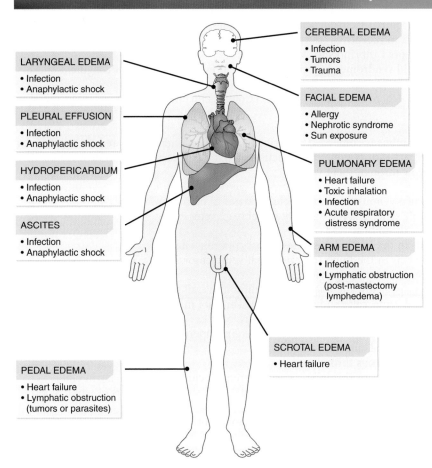

LARYNGEAL EDEMA
- Infection
- Anaphylactic shock

PLEURAL EFFUSION
- Infection
- Anaphylactic shock

HYDROPERICARDIUM
- Infection
- Anaphylactic shock

ASCITES
- Infection
- Anaphylactic shock

PEDAL EDEMA
- Heart failure
- Lymphatic obstruction
  (tumors or parasites)

CEREBRAL EDEMA
- Infection
- Tumors
- Trauma

FACIAL EDEMA
- Allergy
- Nephrotic syndrome
- Sun exposure

PULMONARY EDEMA
- Heart failure
- Toxic inhalation
- Infection
- Acute respiratory
  distress syndrome

ARM EDEMA
- Infection
- Lymphatic obstruction
  (post-mastectomy
  lymphedema)

SCROTAL EDEMA
- Heart failure

5-19: Clinically important forms of localized edema. *(From my friend Ivan Damjanov, MD, PhD:* Pathophysiology, *Saunders Elsevier, 2009, p 60, Fig. 2-25.)*

(3) Scrotal and vulvar lymphedema (see Fig. 22-1 C), due to lymphogranuloma venereum

(4) Breast lymphedema (inflammatory carcinoma), due to blockage of subcutaneous lymphatics by malignant cells (see Fig. 22-21 F)

4. Myxedema is produced when there is increased synthesis of extracellular matrix components (e.g., glycosaminoglycans).
  a. T-cell cytokines stimulate fibroblasts to synthesize excess amounts of hyaluronic acid leading to myxedema.
  b. Examples: pretibial myxedema and exophthalmos in Graves disease (see Fig. 23-7 C) and periorbital puffiness in Hashimoto thyroiditis (see Fig. 23-6 B)

D. Clinically important forms of localized edema (Fig. 5-19)

IV. Thrombosis

A. Definition: Thrombosis is the formation or presence of a blood clot (thrombus) in a blood vessel. A thrombus is composed of varying proportions of coagulation factors, RBCs, and platelets.

B. Pathogenesis (see Chapters 10 and 15)
  1. Endothelial cell injury
    a. Turbulent blood flow at arterial bifurcations
    b. Homocysteine
    c. Oxidized low-density lipoprotein (LDL)
    d. Cigarette smoke
    e. Cytokines
  2. Stasis of blood flow
    a. Prolonged bed rest or sitting (e.g., long airplane flight, immobilization in bed)
    b. Left atrial (LA) dilatation in mitral stenosis; LA dilatation also leads to atrial fibrillation (see Chapter 11)
  3. Hypercoagulability (see Chapter 15)
    a. Activation of the coagulation system. Example: disseminated intravascular coagulation.

Modified radical mastectomy/radiation; inflammatory carcinoma breast; filariasis

Increased synthesis extracellular glycosaminoglycans

T cells stimulate fibroblasts → ↑synthesis hyaluronic acid (myxedema)

Exophthalmos Graves disease; periorbital puffiness Hashimoto thyroiditis

Intravascular mass → attached to vessel wall → coagulation factors/RBCs/platelets

Endothelial cell injury

Bifurcations, homocysteine, oxidized LDL, cigarettes, cytokines

Stasis blood flow

Prolonged bed rest/sitting

LA dilatation in mitral stenosis

Hypercoagulability

Activation coagulation system: DIC

b. Hereditary or acquired factor deficiencies. Examples: hereditary antithrombin (ATIII) deficiency, oral contraceptives (estrogen decreases concentration of ATIII; increases the synthesis of factors I [fibrinogen], V, and VIII).

c. Antiphospholipid syndrome. Associated with the presence of lupus anticoagulant and/or anticardiolipin antibodies.

d. Thrombocytosis (increased platelet count). Etiologies include malignancy and essential thrombocytosis.

C. **Types**

1. **Definition:** A thrombus is composed of various blood components that are held together by fibrin leading to partial or complete obstruction of veins or arteries. This in turn results in reduced blood flow through these vessels.

2. Venous thrombus

   a. Pathogenesis of a venous thrombus includes stasis of blood flow (most common) and a hypercoagulable state, in a low-velocity vessel (e.g., vein).

   b. Sites of venous thrombosis

      (1) Deep veins in the lower extremities (most common site)

         (a) Deep veins in the thigh (e.g., popliteal vein, femoral vein). Thrombi extend (propagate) into the pelvic veins.

         (b) Deep veins below the knee (most common overall site; e.g., anterior, posterior, peroneal veins; calf venous sinusoids). Thrombi may extend into the popliteal and femoral veins and embolize to the heart.

      (2) Other sites of thrombosis include axillary vein, superior vena cava (SVC), hepatic vein, and the dural sinuses.

   c. Composition of a venous thrombus

      (1) **Definition:** A venous thrombus is an adherent, occlusive, dark red fibrin clot primarily composed of RBCs (red thrombus) with varying amounts of white blood cells (WBCs), and platelets.

      (2) Figure 5-20 A, B shows the sequence of venous clot formation in a vessel.

   d. Clinical findings

      (1) Thrombosis of a blood vessel within an extremity results in pain, swelling, and skin discoloration.

      (2) Lower extremity venous thrombus (LEVT) commonly embolizes ("chips off") to the pulmonary arteries, where it can produce sudden death and/or a pulmonary infarction (see Chapter 2).

      (3) Hepatic vein thrombosis (HVT) produces painful hepatomegaly (see Chapter 19).

      (4) Dural sinus thrombosis (DST) produces intracerebral hemorrhage (see Chapter 26).

      (5) SVC thrombosis produces jugular vein distention and stroke.

   e. Heparin/warfarin are anticoagulants that prevent venous thrombosis (see Chapter 15).

   f. Fibrinolytic system (plasmin) breaks down venous thrombi to restore blood flow.

3. Arterial thrombus

   a. **Definition:** An arterial thrombus is primarily composed of platelets held together by fibrin.

   b. Pathogenesis

      (1) Most commonly caused by endothelial cell injury related to turbulent blood flow at bifurcations and/or over disrupted atherosclerotic plaques in high-velocity vessels (see Chapter 10)

      (2) Hypercoagulability and stasis of blood flow are *uncommon* causes of an arterial thrombus.

   c. Sites

      (1) Most arterial thrombi develop in high-velocity vessels (e.g., elastic and muscular arteries).

         (a) Most arterial thrombi overlie disrupted atherosclerotic plaques. In descending order of frequency, these sites include coronary (Fig. 5-21), cerebral, and femoral arteries. Carotid artery is a less common site.

         (b) Arterial thrombi are adherent, usually occlusive (in muscular arteries), gray-white fibrin clots that are primarily composed of platelets (see Chapter 15). Inhibitors of platelet aggregation prevent their formation (e.g., aspirin, P2Y12 receptor antagonists). P2Y12 receptors normally initiate ADP-induced platelet aggregation.

         (c) Examples of outcomes of arterial thrombosis include infarction (e.g., myocardial infarction, small bowel infarction, renal infarction) and stroke (e.g., thrombosis of the middle cerebral artery or branch of the carotid artery).

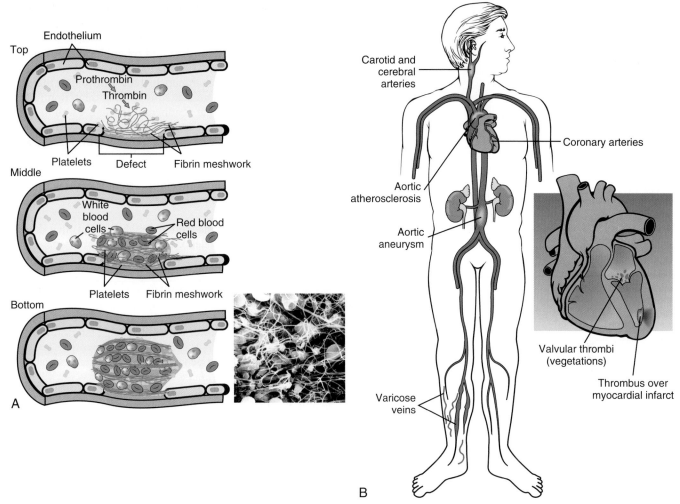

5-20: A, Formation of a venous clot in the lower extremity. **Top,** Disruption of the endothelium with platelet adhesion and early formation of fibrin strands from activation of the coagulation system. **Middle,** Fibrin from activation of the coagulation system is forming a meshwork that anchors the clot to the wall of the vessel and traps red blood cells (predominant component), white blood cells, and platelets. **Bottom,** Clot is fully formed and consists of layers of fibrin with entrapped blood cells. **Inset,** Fibrin clot appearance with a scanning electron microscope. Fibrin strands are trapping predominantly red blood cells and a few platelets (small white structures). **B,** Common sites of thrombus formation. *(A from my friend Ivan Damjanov, MD, PhD: Pathology for the Health-Related Professions, 2nd ed, Philadelphia, Saunders, 2000, p 129, Fig. 6-6; **Inset** from my friend Ivan Damjanov, MD, PhD, Linder J: Anderson's Pathology, 10th ed, St. Louis, Mosby, 1996, p 479, Fig. 22.4 C; **B** from my friend Ivan Damjanov, MD, PhD: Pathology for the Health Professions, 4th ed, Saunders Elsevier, 2012, p 121, Fig. 6-7.)*

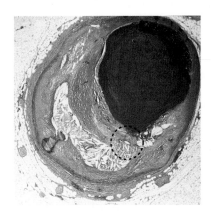

5-21: Coronary artery thrombosis. In this specially stained cross-section of a coronary artery, collagen is blue and the thrombus is red. The red thrombus in the vessel lumen is composed of platelets held together by fibrin. Directly beneath the thrombus is a fibrous plaque (fibrous cap), which stains blue. Beneath the plaque is necrotic atheromatous debris. The circle shows disruption of the fibrous plaque with cholesterol crystals extending through the wall to the lumen. *(From my friend Ivan Damjanov, MD, PhD, Linder J: Pathology: A Color Atlas, St. Louis, Mosby, 2000, p 21, Fig. 1-44.)*

(2) Thrombus composition in the heart chambers and aorta

    (a) Thrombi are laminated with alternating pale and red areas (lines of Zahn; Link 5-13). Mixed type of thrombus. Pale areas are composed of platelets held together by fibrin. Red areas are composed of RBCs and other blood cells held together by fibrin.

    (b) Examples of thrombi that develop in heart chambers include a thrombus that is adherent to the left ventricular (LV) wall in an acute myocardial infarction (AMI; called a mural thrombus) and a thrombus that is adherent to the LA wall in mitral stenosis.

    (c) Thrombi in the aorta usually develop in aneurysms (outpouching of the vessel; see Chapter 10). Example: abdominal aortic aneurysm (AAA; see Fig. 10-8 A, B)

    (d) Embolization to distant sites is the most common clinical complication with these types of thrombi.

4. Postmortem clot

    a. **Definition:** Postmortem clot is a fibrin clot of plasma (resembles chicken fat) that does *not* contain entrapped cells (e.g., RBCs, WBCs, platelets).

    b. A postmortem clot is *not* attached to the vessel wall.

V. Embolism

  A. Definition: Detached mass (e.g., clot, fat, gas) that is carried through the blood to a distant site

  B. Pulmonary thromboembolism (see Chapter 17)

    1. Sites of origin of an embolus

      a. Most emboli originate from the deep veins of the lower extremities (e.g., femoral vein) and pelvis.

      b. Less commons sites of origin for emboli include the pelvic veins and the venae cavae.

    2. Clinical findings

      a. Sudden death

        (1) Usually caused by a saddle embolus that occludes the major pulmonary artery branches on both sides (see Fig. 17-9 A)

        (2) Cause of death is acute right-sided heart strain (acute cor pulmonale).

      b. Pulmonary infarction

        (1) Small thromboemboli occlude medium-sized or small pulmonary arteries, which in some cases produces a hemorrhagic infarction (see Fig. 2-16 C).

        (2) Less than 10% of thromboemboli to the lungs produce infarction; this is due to the dual blood supply of the lungs, mainly the pulmonary arteries and the bronchial arteries (see Chapters 2 and 17).

        (3) Clinical findings in pulmonary infarction include sudden onset of dyspnea (difficulty breathing) and tachypnea (rapid breathing), with or without pleuritic chest pain (pain on inspiration caused by distention of inflamed pleura) and hemoptysis (coughing up blood).

  C. Paradoxical embolism

    • **Definition:** Venous embolus that passes through an atrial septal defect (ASD) or a ventricular septal defect (VSD) thereby gaining access to the systemic (arterial) circulation

  D. Systemic embolism

    1. **Definition:** Embolus that is traveling in the arterial rather than the venous vascular system

    2. Causes

      a. Most systemic emboli originate from the left side of the heart (80% of cases).

        (1) Mural thrombus in the left ventricle

        (2) Thrombus in the left atrium in patient with mitral stenosis. Atrial fibrillation (an irregular fluttering of the left atrium) predisposes to atrial clot formation and embolization.

        (3) Atrial myxoma (benign tumor of the left atrium; see Fig. 11-25)

        (4) Sterile/infected vegetations (e.g., colonies of *Staphylococcus aureus* entrapped in fibrin) involving the aortic and/or mitral valve (see Fig. 11-20 A)

      b. Another cause of systemic embolization is a mixed-type of thrombus developing in an AAA (see Fig. 10-8 A). Embolization material includes particles of ulcerated atherosclerotic plaque material composed of calcium and cholesterol. Another common location for atherosclerotic embolization is the middle cerebral artery (MCA), where embolic material produces a cerebrovascular stroke (see Chapter 26).

    3. Target sites for systemic embolization

      a. Lower extremities (most common site; 75% of cases; Fig. 5-22 A)

      b. Brain (via the MCA; Fig. 5-22 B)

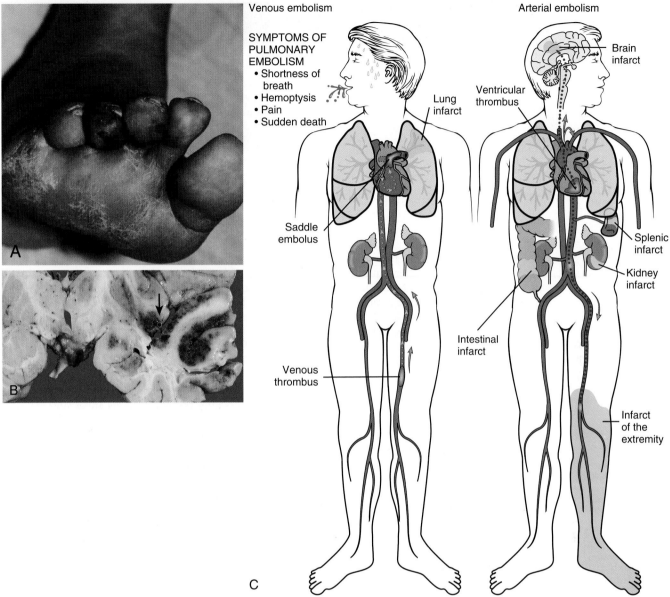

5-22: A, Atheromatous emboli with infarction of digit 4. Note the red and black areas representing infarction (dry gangrene). Digits 2 to 5 have a dusky appearance and there is a blue discoloration (cyanosis) over the dorsum of the foot. **B,** Hemorrhagic embolic infarction. Note the recent hemorrhagic infarct involving the superior part of the temporal lobe, the insula, and inferior part of the frontal lobe resulting from an embolus, which is visible in the middle cerebral artery *(arrow)*. **C,** Venous and arterial emboli. *Left,* Venous emboli can lodge in the lung, causing a variety of symptoms and conditions. *Right,* Arterial emboli may occlude arteries in many organs. *(A from Marx J: Rosen's Emergency Medicine Concepts and Clinical Practice, 7th ed, Philadelphia, Mosby Elsevier, 2010, p 1110, Fig. 85.2; courtesy Gary R. Seabrook, MD; B from Ellison D, Love S, et al: Neuropathology: A Reference Text of CNS Pathology, 3rd ed, Mosby Elsevier, 2013, p 210, Fig. 9.33c; C from my friend Ivan Damjanov, MD, PhD: Pathology for the Health Professions, 4th ed, Saunders Elsevier, 2012, p 123, Fig. 6-10.)*

      c. Small bowel (via the superior mesenteric artery [SMA])

      d. Spleen, kidneys, or upper extremities (via the aorta)

   4. Complications of systemic embolization include (see Chapter 2; Fig. 5-22 C) pale infarctions of the digits, spleen, and/or kidneys and hemorrhagic infarctions in the brain and/or small bowel.

E. Fat embolism

   1. **Definition:** Composed of microglobules of fat most commonly the result of a traumatic fracture

   2. Epidemiology

      a. Clinical diagnosis in most cases

      b. Most often due to a traumatic fracture of long bones (e.g., femur) or pelvis. Less common causes include trauma to fat-laden tissues (liposuction), fatty liver, and decompression sickness.

Small bowel via SMA

Spleen, kidney, upper extremity via aorta

Pale or hemorrhagic infarctions

Fat embolism

Microglobules fat post traumatic fracture

Clinical diagnosis

Traumatic fracture long bones (femur) or pelvis

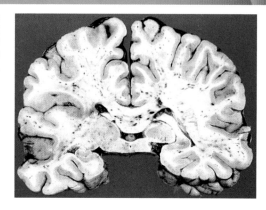

5-23: Fat embolism in the brain. Note the hemorrhages in the white matter, which correspond to small vessel occlusion and injury by microglobules of fat. *(From my friend Ivan Damjanov, MD, PhD, Linder J: Anderson's Pathology, 10th ed, St. Louis, Mosby, 1996, p 98, Fig. 5-24 A.)*

Marrow fat enters ruptured marrow sinusoids/venules

Pulmonary capillaries

Arteriovenous shunts to disperse to distant sites

Obstruct microvasculature

Fatty acids damage vessel endothelium → platelets/WBCs adhere to areas of injury

S/S fat embolism 1–3 days

Delirium/coma

Dyspnea, tachypnea, hypoxemia (perfusion defect)

Petechiae chest/upper extremities (↓platelets)

Platelets consumed in platelet thrombi

Mortality rate low

Hypoxemia; ↑A-a gradient

Lipiduria; fat in BAL

Thrombocytopenia

Amniotic fluid embolism

Tears placental membranes; rupture uterine veins postpartum

During labor or immediately postpartum; mortality 80%

Pathogenesis: tears in placental membrane, rupture uterine veins

Cardiorespiratory collapse + DIC

   c. Pathogenesis
     • At the fracture site, microglobules of marrow fat with or without hematopoietic tissue enter ruptured marrow sinusoids and venules.
       Microglobules initially deposit in pulmonary capillaries. Microglobules of fat enter arteriovenous shunts in the lungs, from which they embolize to distant sites (e.g., brain, spleen, kidneys). In these sites, they obstruct the microvasculature particularly in the lungs and brain (Fig. 5-23), where they produce ischemia and inflammation. Fatty acids, derived from the breakdown of fat in the microglobules, ↓damage vessel endothelium, causing platelet/WBC adherence to areas of injury.
 3. Clinical findings
     a. Symptoms and signs (S/S) begin 24 to 72 hours after trauma. Patients are symptomatic in less than 10% of cases.
     b. Delirium and coma are common neurologic findings.
     c. Pulmonary findings include dyspnea and tachypnea. Fat microglobules blocking pulmonary capillaries cause hypoxemia, due to a perfusion defect (see Chapter 2).
     d. Petechiae (pinpoint areas of hemorrhage) commonly develop over the chest and upper extremities. Petechiae are due to thrombocytopenia (decreased number of platelets) from platelet adhesion to microglobules and to damaged endothelial tissue, which then develop platelet thrombi over the areas of injury. Platelets are also consumed in formation of the platelet thrombi causing thrombocytopenia (reduced number of platelets).
     e. Mortality rate, though low, is more likely to occur in older patients or those with underlying medical problems.
 4. Laboratory findings
     a. Hypoxemia (↓Pao_2) occurs with an increase in the alveolar-arterial (A-a) gradient related to the perfusion defect (see Chapter 2).
     b. Fat globules may be present in the urine (lipiduria), pulmonary capillary blood, and bronchoalveolar lavage (BAL) material.
     c. Thrombocytopenia (decreased platelets) is commonly present.
 F. **Amniotic fluid embolism**
 1. **Definition:** Result of tears in placental membranes or rupture of uterine veins during labor or immediately postpartum
 2. Epidemiology
     a. Maternal mortality approaches 80%.
     b. Pathogenesis
       (1) Tears in the placental membranes and/or rupture of the uterine veins
       (2) Amniotic fluid enters the maternal circulation. Amniotic fluid in the systemic circulation precipitates cardiorespiratory collapse (possibly an anaphylactic reaction to fetal antigens) and disseminated intravascular coagulation (DIC), because procoagulants present in amniotic fluid stimulate clot formation. This precipitates cardiorespiratory collapse (possibly an anaphylactic reaction to fetal antigens) and DIC, because procoagulants that stimulate clot formation are present in amniotic fluid.
 3. Clinical findings

a. Abrupt onset of dyspnea, cyanosis, hypotension, and bleeding
  (1) Dyspnea is due to pulmonary edema and/or the acute respiratory distress syndrome (ARDS; see Chapter 17).
  (2) Bleeding is due to DIC (see Chapter 15).
  (3) Over 50% of patients die within an hour of the previously mentioned symptoms and signs.
b. Diagnosis is confirmed at autopsy. Fetal squamous cells, lanugo hair, fat from vernix caseosa are present in the maternal pulmonary vessels.
c. Women who survive usually have permanent neurologic impairment (85% of cases).
4. Laboratory findings
  a. Respiratory acidosis occurs with associated hypoxemia.
  b. Prothrombin time (PT) is usually prolonged (see Chapter 15) due to the consumption of coagulation factors that are used up in the formation of thrombi in DIC.

G. Decompression sickness
1. **Definition:** Type of gas embolism that is most often caused by scuba diving and deep sea diving
2. Epidemiology; pathogenesis
  a. Atmospheric pressure increases with depth.
  b. Nitrogen (N) gas is forced out of the alveoli and dissolves in the blood and tissues.
  c. Rapid ascent causes nitrogen to come out of solution to form gas bubbles in the tissue and in vessel lumens.
3. Clinical findings
  a. Severe pain develops in joints, skeletal muscles, and bones ("the bends").
  b. Gas bubbles block pulmonary vessels, causing edema, hemorrhage, and atelectasis (collapse of small airways).
  c. Vertebral back pain and symptoms occur that mimic spinal cord trauma (e.g., loss of anal sphincter tone).
  d. Other complications
    (1) Pneumothorax (see Chapter 17)
      (a) Most often associated with a sudden rise to the surface
      (b) Changes in pressure cause the rupture of preexisting subpleural or intrapleural blebs in the lungs.
      (c) Results in a collapsed lung and sudden onset of dyspnea and pleuritic chest pain (sharp pain on inspiration)
    (2) Pulmonary thromboembolism
      (a) Increased external venous pressure at increased depth produces stasis and thrombus formation in the lower extremities.
      (b) Pulmonary thromboembolism occurs, causing dyspnea and pleuritic chest pain (pain on inspiration).
  e. Chronic changes (called caisson disease)
    (1) Caused by a persistence of gas emboli in the bones
    (2) Produces aseptic necrosis (bone infarctions; see Chapter 24) in the femur, tibia, and humerus
4. Recompression in a high-pressure chamber forces nitrogen gas back into solution. This is followed by slow decompression.

VI. Shock
  A. Definition: Reduced perfusion of tissue, which results in impaired oxygenation of tissue
  B. Types of shock
    1. Hypovolemic shock. **Definition:** Type of shock that is due to an excessive loss of sodium-containing fluid (e.g., blood, sweat), causing hypotension and multiorgan failure (MOF).
      a. Epidemiology
        (1) Massive blood loss is the most common cause of hypovolemic shock.
        (2) Loss of > 20% of the blood volume (≈1000 mL) results in hypovolemic shock.
        (3) Common causes of external blood loss include penetrating trauma and GI bleeding.
        (4) Common causes of internal blood loss are trauma to a solid organ (e.g., spleen, liver) and a ruptured AAA (abdominal aortic aneurysm).
        (5) *No* initial drop in hemoglobin (Hb) and hematocrit (Hct) concentration, because there is an equal loss of RBCs and plasma.
          (a) Plasma is replaced first with fluid from the interstitial space. Uncovers the RBC deficit within hours to days.

Normal saline immediately uncovers RBC deficit

Reticulocyte response begins 5–7 days

↓Volume blood → ↓cardiac output

↓LVEDP: loss blood volume in left ventricle

↑PVR: arteriole vasoconstriction (catecholamines, ADH, ATII)

↓MVO$_2$

Best indicator of tissue hypoxia

Degree extraction O$_2$ from blood to tissue

↓CO, ↓LVEDP, ↑PVR, ↓MVO$_2$

Cold, clammy skin

Hypotension; rapid, weak pulse

↓Urine output; ↓GFR

↑AG metabolic acidosis (lactic acidosis)

MCC AMI

Myocarditis, infective endocarditis, cardiomyopathy

↓Contraction damaged LV muscle → ↓cardiac output

↓Cardiac output → blood accumulates in left ventricle → ↑LVEDP

Arteriole vasoconstriction (catecholamines, ADH, ATII)

↓MVO$_2$

↓CO, ↑LVEDP, ↑PVR, ↓MVO$_2$

↑CK-MB, ↑troponin I/T

Septic shock

Bloodstream infection: septicemia

Microbes invade bloodstream

Lungs MC site for septicemia

MCC death in ICU

MC G+ organisms (coagulase-negative *Staphylococci*; *S. aureus*)

E. coli MC G−

Candida species MC fungal cause

Lipoteichoic acid in G+ pathogens

Endotoxins G− pathogens

(b) Infusion of 0.9% normal saline immediately uncovers the RBC deficit. Normal saline "acts like" plasma *except* it lacks the proteins that are present in plasma (especially albumin).

(c) Increase in peripheral blood reticulocytes (indicators of effective marrow erythropoiesis) begins in 5 to 7 days (see Chapter 12).

(6) Pathophysiology

(a) Cardiac output is decreased, due to a decreased volume of blood.

(b) Left ventricular end-diastolic pressure (LVEDP) is decreased. Loss of blood volume in the left ventricle lowers the LVEDP.

(c) Peripheral vascular resistance (PVR) is increased. Due to vasoconstriction of peripheral resistance arterioles by catecholamines, ADH (vasopressin), and ATII, which are released in response to the decreased cardiac output.

(d) Mixed venous oxygen content (MVO$_2$) is decreased. *Best indicator* of tissue hypoxia. Measured in the right side of the heart by a Swan-Ganz catheter. Indicates the degree of extraction of O$_2$ from blood delivered to tissue. In hypovolemic shock, decreased blood flow through the microcirculation leads to increased extraction of O$_2$ from the blood resulting in a decreased MVO$_2$.

b. Clinical findings

(1) Exam reveals cold, clammy skin due to vasoconstriction of the superficial skin vessels.

(2) Hypotension is present along with a rapid, weak pulse (a compensatory response to a decreased cardiac output).

(3) Urine output is decreased because of a decreased renal blood flow and glomerular filtration rate (GFR).

c. Laboratory findings

• Increased AG type of metabolic acidosis due to lactic acidosis, the end-product of anaerobic glycolysis (see previous discussion)

2. Cardiogenic shock

a. **Definition:** Type of shock that is most commonly caused by an AMI. Other causes of cardiogenic shock include myocarditis (inflammation of the heart), acute valvular dysfunction (e.g., infective endocarditis), and cardiomyopathy.

b. Pathophysiology

(1) Cardiac output is decreased due to decreased force of contraction by the damaged LV myocardial tissue.

(2) LVEDP is increased; because cardiac output is decreased, blood accumulates in the left ventricle, causing an increase in pressure and volume.

(3) PVR is increased because of vasoconstriction of arterioles by catecholamines, ADH (vasopressin), and ATII, which are released in response to the decreased cardiac output.

(4) MVO$_2$ is decreased; decreased blood flow through the microcirculation leads to increased extraction of O$_2$ from the blood and a decreased MVO$_2$.

c. Clinical findings (see Chapter 11). Chest pain is followed by signs similar to those seen in hypovolemic shock (i.e., cold, clammy skin; hypotension; decreased urine output).

d. Laboratory findings. Increased creatine kinase MB fraction and troponin I and T (the gold standard; see Chapter 11).

3. Septic shock

a. **Definition:** Type of shock associated with bloodstream infection by microbial pathogens (bacterial and/or fungal)

b. Epidemiology

(1) Microbes invade the bloodstream (called septicemia).

(2) Most common sites for infection leading to sepsis in descending order are the lungs, blood, abdomen, urinary tract, and skin.

(3) Most common cause of death in intensive care units (ICU). Mortality rate in septic shock is 20% to 30%.

(4) Microbial pathogens involved in septic shock.

(a) Gram-positive organisms (65% of cases): coagulase-negative *Staphylococci* and *Staphylococcus aureus* are the most common pathogens.

(b) Gram-negative organisms (25% of cases): most commonly *Escherichia coli*

(c) Systemic fungi (9% of cases): *Candida* species is the most common pathogen.

(5) Pathogenesis

(a) Lipoteichoic acid in gram-positive pathogens causes the release of tumor necrosis factor (TNF) and interleukin-1 (IL-1; see Chapter 3).

(b) Endotoxins (lipopolysaccharide) are released by gram-negative bacteria.

TABLE 5-11   Summary of Pathophysiologic Findings in Hypovolemic, Cardiogenic, and Septic Shock

TYPE OF SHOCK	CO	PVR	LVEDP	MVO$_2$
Hypovolemic	↓	↑	↓	↓
Cardiogenic	↓	↑	↑	↓
Endotoxic (septic)	↑	↓	↓	↑

CO, Cardiac output; *LVEDP,* left ventricular end-diastolic pressure; *MVO$_2$,* mixed venous oxygen content; *PVR,* peripheral vascular resistance.

Endotoxins activate macrophages, causing the release of IL-1 and TNF. IL-1 produces fever (see Chapter 3). TNF damages endothelial cells, causing them to release vasodilators like nitric oxide (NO) and prostaglandin I$_2$ (PGI$_2$). Endotoxins activate the alternative complement pathway producing anaphylatoxins (C3a and C5a), which stimulate mast cell release of histamine (vasodilator). Endotoxins damage tissue, causing the release of tissue thromboplastin, which activates the coagulation cascade resulting in DIC (see Chapter 15). Endotoxins activate neutrophil adhesion molecules causing adherence of circulation neutrophils to the vascular lumen, resulting in neutropenia (↓neutrophil count; see Chapter 3).

(6) Pathophysiology
    (a) Cardiac output is initially increased (bounding pulses) due to rapid blood flow through dilated PVR arterioles (NO and PGI$_2$ are vasodilators), causing increased venous return of blood to the right heart (analogous to opening up the flood gates in a dam).
    (b) LVEDP is decreased due to decreased compliance (filling) in the left ventricle ("stiff ventricle").
    (c) PVR is decreased due to vasodilation of the PVR arterioles.
    (d) MVO$_2$ is decreased. Tissues are unable to extract O$_2$ because of the increased blood flow through the microcirculation related to the dilated PVR arterioles. Good analogy is opening up the flood gates in a dam and releasing water. The dam represents the peripheral resistance arterioles.
    (e) Table 5-11 shows a summary of the pathophysiologic findings in shock.
c. Clinical and laboratory findings
    (1) Skin is warm, due to vasodilation of the superficial blood vessels.
    (2) Hypotension is due to vasodilation of arterioles and increased vascular permeability, related to damage of the endothelial cells. Fluid leaks into the interstitial space.
    (3) Peripheral pulses are strong as the cardiac output increases in a compensatory response to the hypotension.
    (4) Activation of the coagulation system leads to DIC (see Chapter 15).
    (5) There is an increased risk for developing acute respiratory distress syndrome (see Chapter 17).
    (6) Hematologic findings include anemia (from bleeding and venipuncture), thrombocytopenia (platelets are trapped and consumed in thrombi), and neutropenia (margination of neutrophils from adhesion molecule activation; see Chapter 3).
    (7) Complications
        (a) Ischemic acute tubular necrosis (see Chapter 20). Coagulation necrosis occurs in the proximal tubule cells and the tubular cells in the thick ascending limb (TAL). This produces renal tubular cell (RTC) casts (detached RTCs held together by proteinaceous material) that occlude tubular lumens producing oliguria (decreased urine flow) and renal failure. This is called ischemic acute tubular necrosis (ATN).
        (b) Multiple organ dysfunction syndrome (MODS) is the most common cause of death in septic shock. Associated with widespread endothelial cell and parenchymal cell injury.
            • Multifactorial pathophysiology. Widespread tissue hypoxia results in a lack of ATP.
            • Endotoxins and various cytokines have direct cytotoxic effects.
            • Damage to tissue serves as a stimulus for apoptosis (see Chapter 2).
            • DIC produces fibrin thrombi in the microvasculature of most organs, leading to tissue damage.
            • Myocardial depressants (e.g., endotoxins, TNF) produce myocardial dysfunction.

Margin notes:

IL-1: fever, activate neutrophil adhesion molecules (neutropenia): TNF: damages endothelial cells (releases vasodilators; NO, PGI$_2$); Endotoxins: activate macrophages, complement system, tissue thromboplastin (DIC)

Cardiac output initially increased

↓LVEDP; stiff left ventricle

↓PVR: vasodilation of PVR arterioles

↓MVO$_2$

↑CO, ↓LVEDP, ↓PVR, ↑MVO$_2$

Warm skin: vasodilation blood vessels

Hypotension: vasodilation arterioles, ↑vascular permeability

Strong peripheral pulses (↑cardiac output), hypotension

DIC

↑Risk ARDS

Anemia, thrombocytopenia, neutropenia

Ischemic ATN with RTC casts

MODS: MCC death in shock

Endothelial/parenchymal cell injury

Tissue hypoxia (lack of ATP)

Endotoxins/cytokines direct cytotoxic effects

Tissue damage stimulates apoptosis

DIC → fibrin thrombi in microvasculature → tissue damage

Myocardial depressants → myocardial dysfunction

ABBREVIATIONS

MC most common   MCC most common cause

Permanent change in DNA

I. Mutations
   A. Definition: Permanent change in the nucleotide sequence or arrangement of DNA (Link 6-1)
   1. Mutations involving germ cells (e.g., ovum) can be transmitted to offspring.
   2. Mutations involving somatic cells are *not* transmitted to offspring.

Change in single nucleotide base within a gene

Silent: Altered DNA codes for same amino acid; no phenotypic effect

Missense: Altered DNA codes for different amino acid; change phenotypic effect
Sickle cell disease/trait

   B. Point mutations
   1. **Definition:** Change in a *single* nucleotide base in a nucleotide sequence
   2. Silent mutation (Fig. 6-1 A). **Definition:** DNA codes are altered for the *same* amino acid *without* changing the phenotypic effect.
   3. Missense mutation (Fig. 6-1 B; Link 6-2 A). **Definition:** Point mutation in which a single nucleotide change results in a codon that codes for a different amino acid (e.g., sickle cell trait/disease); accounts for 50% of disease-causing mutations

In both **sickle cell trait** and **sickle cell disease,** a missense mutation occurs when adenine replaces thymidine, causing valine to replace glutamic acid in the sixth position of the β-globin chain. As a result, red blood cells spontaneously sickle in the peripheral blood if the amount of sickle hemoglobin is greater than 60%.

Nonsense: Stop codon; premature termination protein synthesis

Nonsense mutation; no synthesis β-globin chain

   4. Nonsense mutation (Fig. 6-1 C; Link 6-2 B). **Definition:** Altered DNA codes for a stop codon that causes premature termination of protein synthesis; accounts for 10% of disease-producing mutations

In **β-thalassemia major,** a nonsense mutation produces a stop codon that causes premature termination of DNA transcription of the β-globin chain. Consequently, there is no synthesis of hemoglobin A ($\alpha_2\beta_2$). There is a corresponding increase in hemoglobin A_2 ($\alpha_2\delta_2$) and hemoglobin F ($\alpha_2\gamma_2$).

Insertion/deletion one or more nucleotides shifts reading frame DNA strand

Frame mutation; 4-base insertion; ↓synthesis hexosaminidase A

 # Base pairs deleted/added multiple 3; *not* frame mutation;

Translated protein gained/ lost amino acids

   C. Frameshift mutation
   1. **Definition:** Insertion or deletion of one or more nucleotide bases shifts the reading frame of the DNA strand.
   2. If the number of bases that is added or deleted is *not* a multiple of three, a frameshift results in premature termination of protein synthesis downstream from the mutation. This type of mutation accounts for 25% of disease-causing mutations. Example of a frameshift mutation: in Tay-Sachs disease, a four-base insertion results in an altered DNA code leading to decreased synthesis of hexosaminidase (stop codon; Fig. 6-2; Link 6-3).
   3. If the number of base pairs that is either deleted or inserted is a multiple of three, it is *not* a frameshift mutation. Translated protein has either gained or lost amino acids.

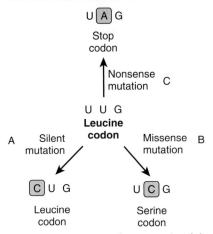

6-1: Point mutations: silent mutation (A), missense mutation (B), nonsense mutation (C). In a silent mutation, the altered DNA codes for the same amino acid and thus does not change the phenotypic effect. In a missense mutation, the altered DNA codes for a different amino acid, which changes the phenotypic effect. In a nonsense mutation, the altered DNA codes for a stop codon that causes premature termination of protein synthesis. (From Pelley JW, Goljan E: Rapid Review Biochemistry, 2nd ed, Philadelphia, Mosby Elsevier, 2007, p 190, Fig. 10-11.)

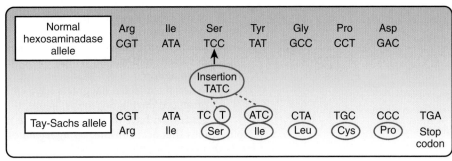

6-2: Frameshift mutation in Tay-Sachs disease. In a frameshift mutation, insertion or deletion of one or more nucleotides shifts the reading frame of the DNA strand. In Tay-Sachs disease, a four-base insertion (TATC) alters the reading frame for the synthesis of hexosaminidase, leading to formation of a stop codon that reduces the synthesis of the enzyme.

- Example: in cystic fibrosis, a three-nucleotide deletion that normally codes for phenylalanine produces a protein (i.e., cystic fibrosis transmembrane regulator [CFTR]) that is missing phenylalanine (see Chapter 17). The defective CFTR is degraded in the Golgi apparatus.

D. **Trinucleotide repeat disorder**

1. A trinucleotide repeat disorder is an example of a DNA replication error. It is an *uncommon* cause of a disease-causing mutation.
2. **Definition:** There is amplification of a sequence of three nucleotides, which prevents the normal expression of the gene.
   a. Most trinucleotide repeats (TRs) contain guanine (G) and/or cytosine (C).
   b. Examples of TR disorders and their triplet repeats include fragile X syndrome (FXS) with a CGG repeat; myotonic dystrophy (MD) with a CTG repeat; Friedrich ataxia (FA) with a GAA repeat; and Huntington disease (HD) with a CAG repeat.
3. Tendency for expanding (amplifying) TRs is highly dependent on the sex of the parent transmitting the disease. For example, expansion of TRs in FXS primarily occurs in oogenesis, whereas in Huntington disease, it occurs in spermatogenesis.
4. Number of TRs determines the severity of the disease. For example, in FXS, unaffected individuals have 5 to 54 CGG repeats, individuals with premutations have 55 to 200 CGG repeats (normal to mild disease), and those with full mutations have more than 200 repeats (more severe disease).
5. Amplification that occurs in *noncoding areas* of the gene (intron) produce a loss-of-function type of mutation manifested as a decrease in protein synthesis.
   a. Examples of diseases that fit under this category include FXS, myotonic dystrophy, and Friedrich ataxia. Because protein synthesis is decreased in the these disorders, multiple organ systems are adversely affected.
   b. Another characteristic is the progression from premutations to full mutations in germ cells in future generations, due to increased amplification of triplet repeats in gametogenesis.
      (1) Disease activity that increases in severity with each generation is called anticipation.
      (2) Example of anticipation: FXS, a sex-linked disease
         (a) Carrier males with a premutation are phenotypically normal or mildly affected (mild mental impairment).

Cystic fibrosis: 3-nucleotide deletion; phenylalanine lost from CFTR

Defective CFTR degraded in Golgi

DNA replication error

Amplified sequence 3 nucleotides; prevent normal gene expression

Most TRs contain G and/or C

FXS (CGG), MD (CTG), FA (GAA), HD (CAG)

TR amplification sex dependent

Amplification in oogenesis (FXS), spermatogenesis (HD)

TRs determines disease severity

Amplification in intron → loss-of-function mutation

FXS, MD, FA; multisystem diseases

Premutation → full mutation

↑Disease severity each generation → anticipation

(b) Because FXS is an X-linked recessive disease, all female children of carrier males are carriers with a premutation (phenotypically normal or mild mental impairment), but all the male children are normal.

(c) When a carrier female with a premutation has children, 50% of the males will have a full mutation, because in oogenesis, there is amplification of the CGG repeats and a premutation is converted into a full mutation (>200 repeats).

(d) Furthermore, 50% of a carrier female's daughters have the potential for full mutations and will be symptomatic (more severe mental impairment than a premutation).

(e) When the affected daughters have children, even more triplet repeats are produced during oogenesis; hence, the affected males and females in this generation have more severe disease than those in the previous generation.

6. Amplifications that occur in the *coding region* of the gene (exon) all have CAG triplet repeats that code for glutamine residues.

a. Expansion of CAG repeats that encode for glutamine residues produces neurodegenerative types of disorders (polyglutamine disorders); examples include Huntington disease (HD) and various subtypes of spinocerebellar ataxia.

b. Proteins that are produced with an excess of glutamine residues are *misfolded* and produce aggregates that suppress transcription of other genes, interfere with mitochondrial function, and trigger apoptosis of neurons.

c. Aggregates also produce intranuclear inclusions, which are a key feature of the previously mentioned neurodegenerative diseases.

II. Mendelian Disorders

A. Overview of Mendelian disorders (Table 6-1)

1. **Definition:** Single-gene mutations that produce large effects
2. The majority of mendelian disorders are familial (80%–85% of cases); however, the remainder are new mutations.
3. Patterns of single-gene mutations chiefly depend on whether a dominant or recessive phenotype is present in a chromosome pair.
   a. Dominant phenotype is expressed when only one chromosome of a pair carries the mutant allele (gene).
   b. Recessive phenotype is expressed only when both chromosomes of a pair carry mutant alleles.
4. Chromosomal location of the gene locus of the mutation may be on an autosome (chromosomes 1 to 22) or on a sex chromosome (chromosomes X and Y). The vast majority of sex chromosome disorders are X-linked.
5. The four basic single-gene mutation disorders are autosomal recessive (most common [MC] type), autosomal dominant, X-linked recessive (XR), and X-linked dominant (XD).

B. Autosomal recessive disorders

1. Inheritance pattern characteristics of autosomal recessive disorders (Fig. 6-3 A; Link 6-4 A, B)
   a. **Definition:** Individuals with autosomal recessive disorders must be homozygous (aa) for the mutant recessive gene (a) to express the disorder.
   b. Homozygotes (aa) are symptomatic early in life.
   c. Heterozygous individuals (Aa) are usually asymptomatic carriers. Dominant gene (A) overrides the mutant recessive gene (a).

↑Amplification of repeats in gametogenesis

Amplification in exon → CAG repeats code glutamine residues

CAG repeats → neurodegenerative disease

HD, spinocerebellar ataxia subtypes

Misfolded proteins

Suppress transcription other genes

Disrupt mitochondrial function

Trigger neuron apoptosis

Aggregates produce intranuclear inclusions

Mendelian disorders

Single-gene mutations produce large effects

Majority familial; remainder new mutations

Patterns single-gene mutations: dominant or recessive

Dominant: expressed when only 1 chromosome carries mutant allele

Recessive: expressed when both chromosomes carry mutant alleles

Autosomes (1 to 22), sex chromosomes (X and Y)

Autosomal recessive (MC), autosomal dominant, XR, XD

MC Mendelian disorder

Homozygotes (aa) symptomatic early

Heterozygotes (Aa) asymptomatic carrier

Dominant gene (A) overrides mutant recessive gene (a)

TABLE 6-1   Protein Defects Associated With Selected Mendelian Disorders

PROTEIN TYPE	SPECIFIC PROTEIN	DISORDER	INHERITANCE PATTERN
Enzyme	C1 esterase inhibitor deficiency	Hereditary angioedema	Autosomal dominant
Structural	Sickle hemoglobin	Sickle cell disease	Autosomal recessive
Transport	Cystic fibrosis transmembrane regulator	Cystic fibrosis	Autosomal recessive
Receptor	Low-density lipoprotein receptor	Familial hyper-cholesterolemia	Autosomal dominant
Growth regulating	Neurofibromin	Neurofibromatosis	Autosomal dominant
Hemostasis	Factor VIII	Hemophilia A	X-linked recessive

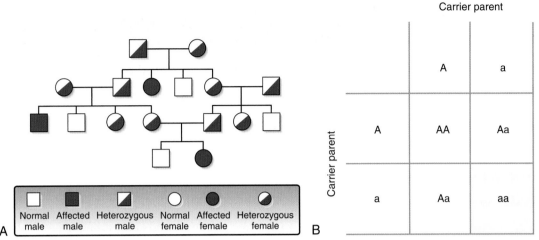

6-3: A, Pedigree of an autosomal recessive disorder. Both parents must have the mutant gene (a) to transmit the disorder to their children. Approximately 25% of the children of heterozygous parents are normal (AA), 50% are asymptomatic heterozygous carriers (Aa), and 25% express the disorder (aa). **B,** The Punnett square illustrates the mating of two heterozygous carriers of an autosomal recessive gene (Aa). Note that 25% of the offspring are affected (shaded area aa), 50% are asymptomatic carriers (Aa), and 25% are normal (AA). **(B** *from Jorde LB, Carey JC, Bamshad MJ: Medical Genetics, 4th ed, Philadelphia, Mosby Elsevier, 2010, p 61, Fig. 4-5.)*

d. Both parents must be heterozygous (Aa) to transmit the disorder to their children (Link 6-4 A, B; Fig. 6-3 B). Example of an autosomal recessive disorder: Aa × Aa → AA, Aa, Aa, aa (25% without disorder [AA]; 50% asymptomatic carriers [Aa]; 25% with disorder [**aa**])

e. New mutations are uncommon.

f. Complete penetrance is common (i.e., homozygotes express the disease). *Penetrance* refers to the proportion of individuals with the mutation who exhibit clinical symptoms.

Both parents heterozygous

Aa × Aa: 25% AA (normal), 25% (homozygous; aa), 50% heterozygous (Aa)

New mutations uncommon

Complete penetrance common (aa)

Penetrance: proportion individuals who express disease

Most autosomal recessive disorders involve enzyme deficiencies

Cystic fibrosis is an autosomal recessive disorder with a carrier rate of 1 in 25. To calculate the prevalence of cystic fibrosis in the population, the number of couples at risk of having a child with cystic fibrosis (1/25 × 1/25, or 1/625) is multiplied by the chance of having a child with cystic fibrosis (1/4). Prevalence of cystic fibrosis = 1/625 × 1/4, or 1/2500. Note how it is possible to calculate the carrier rate if given the prevalence of the disease by dividing 1/2500 by 4 to get the number of couples at risk, and then taking the square root of 1/625 to get the carrier rate of 1 in 25.

2. Autosomal recessive protein defects are listed in Table 6-1.

3. Selected inborn errors of metabolism are discussed in Table 6-2 and shown in Figs. 6-4 through 6-8.

a. Most metabolic disorders are due to an enzyme deficiency.

b. Substrate and intermediates proximal to the enzyme block increase.

c. Intermediates and the end-product distal to the enzyme block decrease (Link 6-5). Example: In phenylketonuria, where there is a phenylalanine hydroxylase deficiency, phenylalanine increases and tyrosine decreases (Link 6-6).

d. Lysosomal storage diseases (Table 6-3; Fig. 6-9 A–E)

• Enzyme deficiencies lead to accumulation of undigested substrates (e.g., glycosaminoglycans [GAGs], sphingolipids, glycogen) in lysosomes.

Most metabolic disorders due to enzyme deficiency

↑Substrate proximal to enzyme block; ↓substrate distal to block

↓Phenylalanine hydroxylase ↑phenylalanine, ↓tyrosine

Lysosomal storage diseases

Undigested substrates (GAGS, sphingolipids, glycogen) accumulate in lysosomes

Overview of the glycogenoses (Table 6-2; Fig. 6-10). In the glycogenoses, there may be an increase in glycogen synthesis (e.g., von Gierke disease) or inhibition of glycogenolysis (glycogen breakdown; e.g., debranching enzyme deficiency). There may be an increase in normal glycogen in tissue (e.g., von Gierke disease) or structurally abnormal glycogen in tissue (e.g., debranching enzyme deficiencies). Glycogen deposition in tissue produces organ dysfunction (e.g., restrictive heart disease in Pompe disease and hepatorenomegaly in von Gierke disease). In some glycogenoses, there is fasting hypoglycemia due to a decrease in gluconeogenesis (e.g., glucose-6-phosphatase deficiency in von Gierke disease) or a decrease in liver glycogenolysis (e.g., liver phosphorylase deficiency).

TABLE 6-2 Selected Inborn Errors of Metabolism

ERROR	DEFICIENT ENZYME	ACCUMULATED SUBSTRATE(S)	COMMENTS
Alkaptonuria (Figs. 6-4, 6-5)	**Homogentisate oxidase** ↑Homogentisate ⇏ ↓Maleylacetoacetate	Homogentisate (black pigment); binds to collagen (connective tissue, tendons, cartilage)	• Black urine undergoes oxidation when exposed to light); black pigmentation nose, ears, cheeks; black cartilage in joints and intervertebral disc producing degenerative arthritis
Galactosemia (Fig. 6-6 A, B)	**GALT** ↑Galactose 1-P ⇏ ↓Glucose 1-P → ↓Glucose 6-P → ↓Glucose (fasting state)	Galactose 1-phosphate (toxic to liver, CNS) Galactose (in urine) Galactitol (alcohol sugar; increase produces osmotic damage in lens)	• Mental impairment, cirrhosis, fasting hyperglycemia (decrease in gluconeogenic substrates distal to the block), cataracts (osmotic damage) • Avoid dairy products (galactose derives from lactose).
Hereditary fructose intolerance (Fig. 6-7)	**Aldolase B** ↑Fructose 1-P ⇏ ↓G3P + ↓DHAP → ↓Glucose (fasting state)	Fructose 1-phosphate (toxic substrate)	• Cirrhosis, hypoglycemia (decrease in gluconeogenic substrates), hypophosphatemia (used up in phosphorylating fructose) • Avoid fructose (e.g., honey) and sucrose (glucose + fructose).
Homocystinuria (Fig. 6-8)	**Cystathionine synthase** ↑Homocysteine ⇏ ↓Cystathionine	Homocysteine and methionine	• Mental impairment, vessel thrombosis (homocysteine is thrombogenic); lens dislocation, arachnodactyly (similar to Marfan syndrome; called genetic heterogeneity)
Maple syrup urine disease	**Branched chain α-keto-acid dehydrogenase** ↑Isoleucine ⇏ ↓AcCoA + ↓Succinyl CoA ↑Leucine ⇏ ↓AcCoA + ↓AcAc ↑Valine ⇏ ↓Succinyl CoA	Leucine, valine, isoleucine, and their ketoacids	• Mental impairment, seizures, feeding problems, sweet-smelling urine
Phenylketonuria (see Fig. 6-4; Link 6-6)	**Phenylalanine hydroxylase** ↑Phenylalanine ⇏ ↓Tyrosine	Phenylalanine Neurotoxic by-products	• Mental impairment, microcephaly, mousy odor (phenylalanine converted into phenyl-acids), ↓pigmentation (melanin derives from tyrosine) • Must be exposed to phenyllanine (milk) *before* phenylalanine is increased • Restrict phenylalanine; avoid sweeteners containing phenylalanine (e.g., NutraSweet). • Add tyrosine to diet. • Pregnant women with PKU must be on a phenylalanine-free diet or newborns will have mental impairment at birth.
"Malignant" phenylketonuria (Fig. 6-4)	**Dihydropterin reductase**	Phenylalanine Neurotoxic by-products	• Similar to PKU • Inability to metabolize tryptophan (not shown in figure) or tyrosine, which both require BH₄. This ↓synthesis of neurotransmitters (serotonin and dopamine, respectively). • Neurologic problems occur despite adequate dietary therapy. • Restrict phenylalanine in the diet. • Administer L-dopa and 5-hydroxytryptophan to replace neurotransmitters. • Administer BH₄.
McArdle disease	**Muscle phosphorylase** ↑Glycogen ⇏ ↓Glucose	Glycogen	• Glycogenosis with muscle fatigue and a propensity for rhabdomyolysis with myoglobinuria • There is *no* lactic acid increase with exercise due to lack of glucose in muscle and a corresponding lack in anaerobic glycolysis (lactic acid is the end-product).
Pompe disease	**α-1,4-Glucosidase** (lysosomal enzyme)	Glycogen	• Glycogenosis, cardiomegaly with early death from heart failure (restrictive cardiomyopathy)
Von Gierke disease	**Glucose 6-phosphatase** (gluconeogenic enzyme) ↑G6P ⇏ ↓Glucose	Glucose 6-phosphate	• Glycogenosis, enlarged liver and kidneys (both contain gluconeogenic enzymes), fasting hypoglycemia (no response to glucagon or other gluconeogenesis stimulators)

AcAc, Acetoacetate; *AcCoA,* acetyl CoA; *DHAP,* dihydroxyacetone phosphate; *GALT,* galactose-1-phosphate uridyltransferase; *G3P,* glyceraldehyde 3-phosphate; *G6P,* glucose 6-phosphate; *PKU,* phenylketonuria.
*Site of enzyme activity.

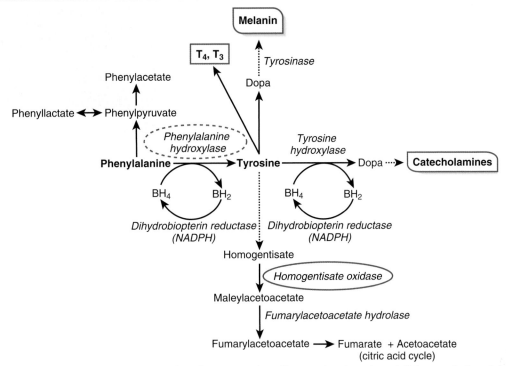

6-4: Phenylketonuria and alkaptonuria biochemical pathways. In phenylketonuria, there is a deficiency of phenylalanine hydroxylase *(interrupted ellipse)* with a buildup of products proximal to the enzyme block (e.g., phenylalanine, phenyllactate, phenylacetate) and a decrease in substrates distal to the block (e.g., tyrosine, which is a precursor of melanin). In alkaptonuria, there is a deficiency of homogentisate (homogentisic acid) oxidase (solid ellipse) with proximal accumulation of homogentisic acid, which turns black in urine on oxidation. It also deposits in cartilage (e.g., intervertebral disks and joints), producing degenerative arthritis. *NADPH,* Reduced nicotinamide adenine dinucleotide phosphate. *(From Pelley JW, Goljan E:* Rapid Review Biochemistry, *2nd ed, Philadelphia, Mosby Elsevier, 2007, p 139, Fig. 8-4.)*

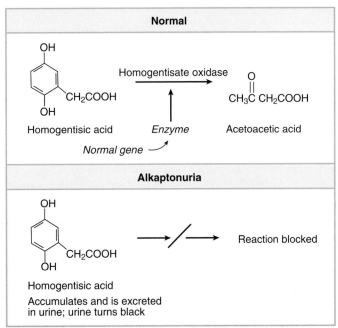

6-5: Alkaptonuria. Lack of the enzyme homogentisate oxidase leads to an increase in homogentisic acid. On exposure to air, homogentisic acid gradually darkens to a black color. *(From Adkison LR:* Elsevier's Integrated Review Genetics, *2 ed, Philadelphia, 2012, Saunders, p. 51, Fig. 4-1.)*

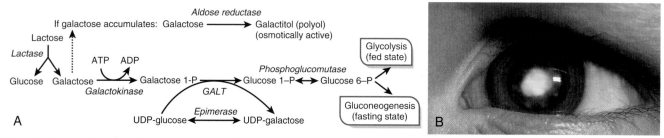

6-6: A, Galactosemia. There is an increase in galactose and galactitol (alcohol sugar) proximal to the block and a decrease in glucose 1-phosphate (G1P) distal to the block (hypoglycemia in fasting state). **B,** Galactosemia cataract. The accumulation of galactose in the lens leads to the production of galactitol. This sugar alcohol exerts increased osmotic pressure within the lens because it diffuses very slowly. The induced swelling is not solely responsible for subsequent cataract formation; however, evidence supports its role in cataract formation rather than G1P because a galactokinase deficiency in which G1P is absent will still yield cataracts. *ADP,* Adenosine diphosphate; *ATP,* adenosine triphosphate; *GALT,* galactose-1-phosphate uridyltransferase; *P,* phosphate; *UDP,* uridine diphosphate. *(A from Pelley JW, Goljan E: Rapid Review Biochemistry, 2nd ed, Philadelphia, Mosby Elsevier, 2007, p 104, Fig. 6-10; B from Kanski J: Clinical Ophthalmology: A Systemic Approach, 4th ed, London, Butterworth Heinemann, 1999, p 177.)*

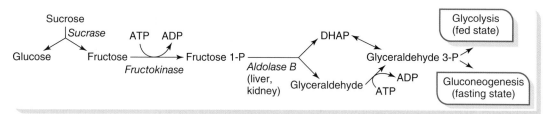

6-7: Hereditary fructose intolerance. Hereditary fructose intolerance is caused by a deficiency of aldolase B. This causes an increase in fructose 1-phosphate (toxic substance) and fructose (proximal) and a decrease in DHAP and glyceraldehyde (distal), which, in normal circumstances, is converted to glyceraldehyde 3-phosphate, a three-carbon intermediate in glycolysis and gluconeogenesis. In hereditary fructose intolerance, hypoglycemia occurs in the fasting state. *ADP,* Adenosine diphosphate; *ATP,* adenosine triphosphate; *DHAP,* dihydroxyacetone phosphate; *P,* phosphate. *(From Pelley JW, Goljan EF: Rapid Review Biochemistry, 2nd ed, Philadelphia, Mosby Elsevier, 2007, p 104, Fig. 6-11.)*

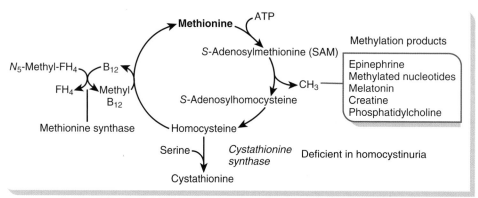

6-8: Homocystinuria. In this inborn error of metabolism, cystathionine synthase is deficient, causing an increase in homocysteine and methionine. An increase in homocysteine produces vessel thrombosis. *CH₃,* Methyl group. *(From Pelley JW, Goljan EF: Rapid Review Biochemistry, 2nd ed, Philadelphia, Mosby Elsevier, 2007, p 143, Fig. 8-5.)*

Hemochromatosis MC autosomal recessive disorder

Heterozygotes (Aa) express the disorder

Homozygotes (AA) spontaneously aborted

Heterozygotes (Aa) living

Aa × aa → Aa, Aa, aa, aa; 50% have disorder (Aa); 50% normal (aa)

4. Other autosomal recessive disorders include hemochromatosis (MC), 21-hydroxylase deficiency, Wilson disease, and thalassemia.

C. **Autosomal dominant disorders**
   1. Inheritance pattern characteristics (Fig. 6-11 A).
      a. **Definition:** One dominant mutant gene (A) is required to express the disorder (Fig. 6-11 A, **left schematic**).
         (1) Heterozygotes (Aa) express the disorder.
         (2) Most homozygotes (AA) are spontaneously aborted. Most of the living individuals with autosomal dominant disorders are heterozygotes (Aa).
         (3) Example of an autosomal dominant disorder: Aa × aa → Aa, Aa, aa, aa (50% have the disorder [Aa]; 50% do *not* have the disorder [aa]) (Fig. 6-11 B)

TABLE 6-3   Selected Lysosomal Storage Disorders

DISORDER	DEFICIENT ENZYME	ACCUMULATED SUBSTRATE	CLINICAL FINDINGS
Gaucher disease (adult type) (Fig. 14-15 A)	Glucocerebrosidase	Glucocerebroside	• Most common lysosomal storage disease • Seen in Eastern European (Ashkenazic) Jews (1/14 carrier rate) • In type I disease, there is hepatosplenomegaly; fibrillar-appearing macrophages are found in the liver, spleen, and bone marrow. Pancytopenia results from marrow involvement and hypersplenism from an enlarged spleen. There is *no* CNS involvement. • Replacement therapy with recombinant enzyme is effective.
Hurler syndrome (Fig. 6-9 C)	α-1-Iduronidase	Dermatan and heparan sulfate (mucopolysaccharides or glycosaminoglycans) accumulate in mononuclear phagocytic cells, lymphocytes, endothelial cells, intimal smooth muscle cells, and fibroblasts.	• Normal at birth but patients develop severe mental impairment and hepatosplenomegaly by 6–24 months. • Characteristics include coarse facial features, short neck, corneal clouding, coronary artery disease, and vacuoles in circulating lymphocytes. • The XR form (Hunter syndrome) is milder.
Niemann-Pick disease (Fig. 14-15 B)	Sphingomyelinase	Sphingomyelin	• Seen in Eastern European (Ashkenazic) Jews (1/90 carrier rate) • Signs and symptoms begin at birth. • Type A is very severe and involves CNS (psychomotor dysfunction, short lifespan). • Type B does *not* have CNS involvement and patients survive into adulthood. Phagocytic cells are involved in the liver (hepatomegaly), spleen (massive splenomegaly), lymph nodes, and bone marrow. Phagocytes have a foamy appearance (zebra bodies on EM). A cherry red macula is present in 30%–50% of cases.
Tay-Sachs disease (Figs. 6-9 D, E)	Hexosaminidase	GM₂ ganglioside	• Seen in Eastern European (Ashkenazic) Jews (1/30 carrier rate) • Normal at birth but manifest signs and symptoms by 6 months of age • Motor (muscle weakness) and mental deterioration, whorled configurations in neurons, cherry red macula (pale ganglion cells with excess gangliosides accentuate the normal red color of the macular choroid)

CNS, Central nervous system; *EM*, electron microscopy; *XR*, X-linked recessive.

   b. Some disorders arise by new mutations. Most new mutations occur in germ cells of older males (paternally inherited).

   c. Delayed manifestations of disease. **Definition:** Symptoms and signs may *not* occur early in life.
      • Some examples include adult polycystic kidney disease (cysts are *not* present at birth) and familial polyposis (polyps are *not* present at birth).

   d. Penetrance. **Definition:** Proportion of individuals with the mutation who exhibit clinical symptoms
     (1) Complete penetrance (Fig. 6-11 A; Link 6-7 A)
      • **Definition:** All individuals with the mutant gene express the disorder (e.g., familial polyposis).
     (2) Incomplete penetrance (Fig. 6-11 B; Link 6-7 B)
      • **Definition:** Individuals with the mutant gene are phenotypically normal. However, they can transmit the disorder to their offspring (e.g., Marfan syndrome).

   e. Variable expressivity
     (1) **Definition:** All individuals with the mutant gene express the disorder but at *different levels* of severity.
     (2) Example: In neurofibromatosis, some patients may have a few café au lait spots (coffee-colored flat lesions) or numerous neurofibromas (pedunculated, pigmented lesions; see Fig. 26-5 A).

New mutations: paternally inherited

Delayed manifestations

Symptoms/signs occur later in life

Proportion individuals with mutation exhibit clinical symptoms

Complete penetrance

All individuals with mutation express disease

Phenotypically normal

Can transmit disease to offspring

Variable expressivity

Express disease but severity varies

Neurofibromatosis

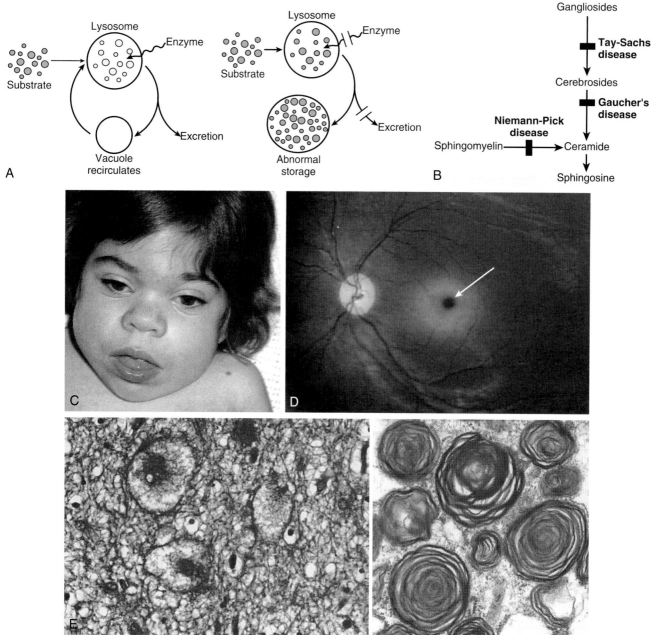

6-9: **A,** Pathogenesis of lysosomal storage disease. *Left,* Normal lysosomes digest the material included within the lytic bodies. *Right,* Lack of degradation enzymes leads to the accumulation of metabolic residues inside the lysosomes. **B,** Sphingolipid metabolism. See Table 6-3 for discussion of selected sphingolipidoses. **C,** Hurler syndrome. Note the coarse facial features and short neck. **D,** Cherry red spot *(arrow)* in Tay-Sachs disease is due to glycolipid deposits in the retinal ganglion cells, giving a whitish appearance to the retina. Because the parafoveal area has many ganglion cells and the fovea has none, the fovea has its normal orange-red color, whereas the retina peripheral to the fovea is white. This produces a "cherry red spot" in the macula. Recall that the fovea is a tiny pit located in the macula of the retina that provides the clearest vision. **E,** Tay-Sachs disease. *Left,* On light microscopy the neural system cells appear to be swollen and vacuolated because their cytoplasm contains an increased number of lipid-rich lysosomes. *Right,* On electron microscopy the cells are seen to contain myelin figures composed of concentric membranes. *(A, E from my friend Ivan Damjanov, MD, PhD: Pathology for the Health Professions, 4th ed, Saunders Elsevier, 2012, pp 104, 105, Figs. 5-18, 5-19; B from Pelley JW, Goljan EF: Rapid Review Biochemistry, 2nd ed, Philadelphia, Mosby Elsevier, 2007, p 104, Fig. 6-11; C from Seidel HM, Ball JW, Danis JE, Benedict GW: Mosby's Guide to Physical Examination, 6th ed, St. Louis, Mosby Elsevier, 2006, p 273, Fig. 10-26; D from Digre K, Corbett JJ: Practical Viewing of the Optic Disc, Philadelphia, Butterworth Heinemann, 2003, p 518.)*

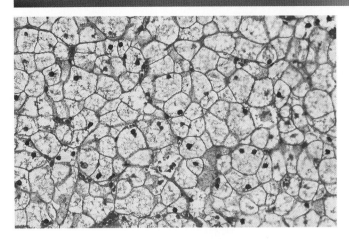

6-10: Glycogenosis. Liver cells are swollen and have pyknotic centrally or eccentrically located nuclei. The cytoplasm is rarefied. This micrograph could be confused with fatty change, but in fatty change the nucleus is pushed to the side. (From Burt AD, Portmann BC, Ferrell LD: MacSween's Pathology of the Liver, 6th ed, Churchill Livingstone Elsevier, 2013, p 164, Fig. 4.6.)

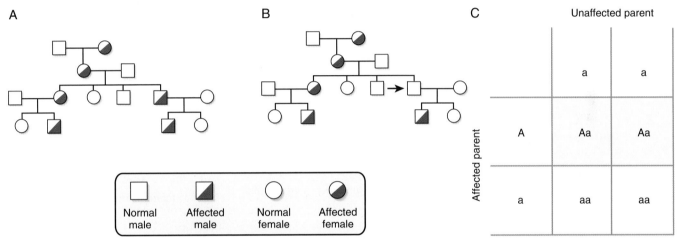

6-11: A, Pedigree showing complete penetrance in an autosomal dominant disorder. Complete penetrance means that all individuals with the mutant gene express the disease. B, Reduced (incomplete) penetrance means that an individual has the mutant gene but does not express the disorder. The unaffected father with the mutant gene (arrow) has transmitted the disorder to his son. C, The Punnett square illustrates the mating of an unaffected parent (aa) with an individual who is heterozygous for an autosomal dominant disease gene (Aa). Note than 50% of the offspring are affected (shaded areas). (C from Jorde LB, Carey JC, Bamshad MJ: Medical Genetics, 4th ed. Philadelphia, Mosby Elsevier, 2010, p 60, Fig. 4-2.)

     f.　A male-to-male transmission essentially confirms an autosomal dominant inheritance.

  2.　Autosomal dominant protein defects (see Table 6-1). Enzyme deficiencies are relatively uncommon in autosomal dominant disorders.

  3.　Other autosomal dominant disorders include von Willebrand disease (vWD; MC autosomal dominant disorder), Huntington disease, osteogenesis imperfecta, achondroplasia, tuberous sclerosis, hereditary spherocytosis, myotonic dystrophy, and familial hypercholesterolemia.

D. X-linked recessive (XR) disorders

  1.　Inheritance pattern characteristics of XR disorders

    a.　**Definition:** Males must have the mutant recessive gene on the X chromosome to express the disorder.

      (1)　Y chromosome disorders are more likely to involve defects in spermatogenesis.

      (2)　X chromosome in a male is active, whereas in females, random inactivation of one of their two X chromosomes leaves ≈50% of their X chromosomes active while the other X chromosome is an inactive Barr body located on the cell's nuclear membrane (Fig. 6-12 A, Link 6-8).

    b.　Affected males (XY) transmit the mutant gene to *all* of their daughters (Fig. 6-12 B, C; Links 6-9 and 6-10).

      (1)　Males are hemizygous for the X-linked mutant gene. Y chromosome is *not* homologous to the X chromosome; hence the term *hemizygous*.

      (2)　Example of an X-linked disorder is shown in Figure 6-12.

Male-to-male transmission confirms autosomal dominant disease

Autosomal dominant disorders: enzyme deficiencies uncommon

vWD MC autosomal dominant disorder

XR disorders

Males with XR disorder; mutant gene on male X chromosome

Y chromosome disorders: defects in spermatogenesis

Male X chromosomes active; 50% female X chromosomes active

Males hemizygous for X-linked mutant gene

XY × XX → XX, XX, XY, XY

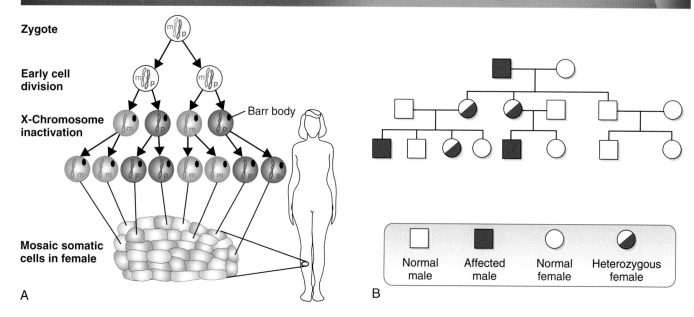

6-12: **A,** The X chromosome inactivation. Both maternal *(m)* and paternal *(p)* X chromosomes are active in the zygote and in early embryonic cells. X inactivation then takes place, resulting in cells having either an active paternal X or an active maternal X chromosome. Females are thus X chromosome mosaics, as shown in the tissue sample at the bottom of the figure. **B,** Pedigree of an X-linked recessive (XR) disorder. The affected male transmits the mutant gene on the X chromosome to *both* of his daughters and *none* of his sons. Both daughters are asymptomatic heterozygous carriers of the mutant gene. The daughter with four children has transmitted the mutant gene to 50% of her sons. **C,** Inheritance possibilities in XR inheritance (Punnett squares). *X, carrier gene. (**A** from Jorde LB, Carey JC, Bamshad MJ: Medical Genetics, 4th ed, Philadelphia, Mosby Elsevier, 2010, p 77, Fig. 5-1; **B** from; **C** from Stevens A, Lowe J, Scott I: Core Pathology, 3rd ed, Mosby Elsevier, 2009, p 68, Fig. 5-25.)

XX heterozygous carriers asymptomatic; paired normal allele (X)

50% sons symptomatic; 50% daughters asymptomatic carriers

Female carriers rarely symptomatic

(3) Daughters (XX) are usually asymptomatic carriers. Heterozygous females (XX) usually are asymptomatic because of the paired normal allele, unlike affected males (XY), who do *not* have a paired homologous allele.

   c. Asymptomatic female carriers (X mutant gene) transmit the disorder to 50% of their male offspring and 50% of their female offspring, who are asymptomatic carriers (see Fig. 6-12 A).

   d. In rare cases, female carriers are symptomatic.

     (1) Female carriers can be symptomatic if maternally derived X chromosomes *without* the mutant gene are preferentially inactivated. Therefore, only paternally derived X chromosomes *with* the mutant gene remain.

     (2) Offspring of a symptomatic male and asymptomatic female carrier can have a symptomatic female child (<u>XX</u>).

       (a) Example: <u>XX</u> × <u>XY</u> → <u>XX</u>, <u>XX</u>, <u>XY</u>, <u>XY</u>

       (b) However, because of random inactivation of one of the X chromosomes, the disease is usually *not* as severe as in a male.

Usually involve enzyme deficiencies

XR TR disorder with CGG

2. Sex-linked recessive protein defects (see Table 6-1). Enzymes are the most common type of proteins affected in sex-linked recessive disorders.

3. Fragile X syndrome (FXS)

   a. **Definition:** FXS is an X-linked triple repeat disorder (CGG). See previous discussion.

   b. Epidemiology

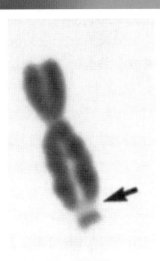

6-13: Fragile site *(arrow)* at Xq27.3 in fragile X syndrome. *(From Nussbaum R, McInnes R, Willard H:* Thompson & Thompson Genetics in Medicine, *7th ed, Philadelphia, Saunders Elsevier, 2007, p 142, Fig. 7-30.)*

(1) Carrier rate for affected males is 1/1550 (some authors say 1/2500–4000) and 1/8000 for affected females.

(2) Most common Mendelian disorder causing mental impairment

(3) Pathogenesis

    (a) Genetic defect is at the distal end of the long arm of the X chromosome (band Xq27.3).

        • At this site, CGG amplification produces a constriction that gives the appearance of a fragile portion of the X chromosome; hence the term *fragile X* (Fig. 6-13 A).

        • Familial mental impairment-1 *(FMR1)* gene is located at this site.

        • Loss of function of this gene, which is most abundantly expressed in the brain and testis, is responsible for mental impairment in FXS as well as other findings listed later.

    (b) Males with a premutation (60–200 repeats) are usually asymptomatic or mildly affected and can transmit the premutation to their daughters.

    (c) Males with the full mutation (>200 CGG repeats, see earlier discussion) have manifestations of FXS. Mothers of nearly all males with FXS have premutation (60–200 repeats) or FXS (>200 repeats).

    (d) Females with a premutation (60–200 repeats) are usually asymptomatic, or they have a mild degree of mental impairment and/or premature ovarian failure (25% of cases). However, during oogenesis, the number of CGG multiples is amplified and exceeds 200 CGG repeats; hence, a male child will have the full mutation and develop FXS, whereas the female child will have a 50% chance of having FXS (see later for explanation).

    (e) Half of the females with the full mutation on a single X chromosome are asymptomatic because of random inactivation of more than half of the affected X chromosomes. The other 50% of females have FXS, although the degree of mental impairment is much less than in males with FXS.

c. Clinical findings

    (1) Affected males have mental impairment with an IQ range of 20 to 70.

    (2) Females with FXS and less affected males have IQs that approach 80.

    (3) Facial changes include long face, large mandible, everted ears, and high-arched palate.

    (4) Macro-orchidism (enlarged testes) at puberty is almost universal. Normal testicular volume at puberty is 17 mL, whereas in individuals with FXS, the volume is >25 mL.

    (5) Other findings include mitral valve prolapse (MVP), pectus excavatum, scoliosis, and hyperextensible joints.

d. Diagnosis

    (1) DNA analysis (polymerase chain reaction) to identify TRs is the best test.

    (2) Fragile X chromosome study (false negative rate of 20%)

MC Mendelian disorder causing mental impairment

Genetic defect distal end long arm of X chromosome (band Xq27.3)

FMR1 gene located at fragile X site

Females full mutation: normal/mild ↓IQ with/without premature ovarian failure

Mental impairment (IQ 20–70)

Long face, large mandible, everted ears, high-arched palate

Macro-orchidism at puberty

MVP, pectus excavatum, scoliosis, hyperextensible joints

DNA analysis for TRs is best

Fragile X chromosome study

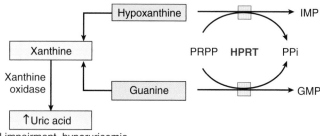

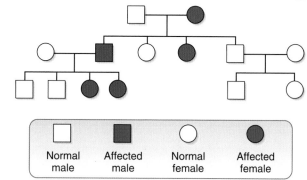

6-14: Hypoxanthine and guanine pathway. A deficiency in hypoxanthine-guanine phosphoribosyltransferase *(HPRT)* leads to the overproduction of uric acid and the symptoms associated with Lesch-Nyhan syndrome. *GMP,* Guanosine 5′-monophosphate; *IMP,* inosine 5′-monophosphate; *PPi,* inorganic pyrophosphate; *PRPP,* 5-phospho-α-D-ribosyl-1-pyrophosphate. *(Modified from Adkison LR:* Elsevier's Integrated Review Genetics, *2nd ed, Saunders Elsevier, 2012, p 136, Fig. 8-5.)*

6-15: Pedigree of an X-linked dominant disorder. In these rare disorders, female carriers and males with the mutant dominant gene express the disorder. The distribution is similar to that of X-linked recessive disorders, *except* that carrier females are symptomatic. It is distinguished from an autosomal dominant disorder because there is no male-to-male transmission, as noted in the pedigree.

XR disorder, ↓HGPRT

HGPRT involved in salvaging purines

Mental impairment, hyperuricemia, self-mutilation

AIS, CGD, BAG, G6PD deficiency

XD disorders

Dominant mutant gene → disease males/females

No male-to-male transmission

Defect renal/gastrointestinal reabsorption phosphate → hypophosphatemia

Defective bone mineralization (osteomalacia)

46 chromosomes (diploid)

Autosomes 22 pairs

1 pair sex chromosomes

Products of meiosis → haploid (23 chromosomes)

Lyon hypothesis

1 of 2 X chromosomes randomly inactivated

Inactivated X chromosome Barr body

Attached to nuclear membrane

Normal female 1 Barr body, none in males

≈50% X chromosomes paternal, ≈50% are maternal

Barr bodies = number of X chromosomes − 1

Chromosome alterations

Numeric/structural abnormalities → autosomes or sex chromosomes

Nondisjunction: unequal separation chromosomes in meiosis

22 or 24 chromosomes egg or sperm

4. Lesch-Nyhan syndrome (Fig. 6-14). **Definition:** XR disorder with a deficiency of hypoxanthine-guanine phosphoribosyltransferase (HGPRT). HGPRT is normally involved in salvaging the purines hypoxanthine and guanine.
   • Clinical findings include mental impairment, hyperuricemia, and self-mutilation.
5. Other XR disorders include androgen insensitivity syndrome (AIS), chronic granulomatous disease (CGD), Bruton agammaglobulinemia (BAG), and glucose-6-phosphate dehydrogenase (G6PD) deficiency.

E. **X-linked dominant (XD) disorders**
   1. Inheritance pattern characteristics
      a. **Definition:** An XD disorder is the same as an XR disorder *except* the dominant mutant gene causes disease in males and females (Fig. 6-15; Link 6-11). Female carriers are symptomatic.
      b. Distinguished from autosomal dominant disorders by the fact that there is *no* male-to-male transmission. Impossible in X-linked inheritance, because males transmit the Y chromosome to their sons.
   2. Vitamin D–resistant rickets
      a. **Definition:** Defect in renal and gastrointestinal reabsorption of phosphate (hypophosphatemia)
      b. Defective bone mineralization (i.e., osteomalacia), because phosphate is required to drive calcium into bone

III. **Chromosomal Disorders**
   A. **General considerations in chromosomal disorders**
      1. Overview of mitosis (Link 6-12) and meiosis (Link 6-13)
      2. Most human cells are diploid (46 chromosomes).
         a. Autosomes: 22 pairs
         b. Sex chromosomes (XX in females and XY in males): 1 pair
      3. Gametes, the products of meiosis, are haploid (23 chromosomes).
      4. Lyon hypothesis
         a. In females, one of the two X chromosomes (X paternal, X maternal) is randomly inactivated (Fig. 6-12 A, Link 6-8). Inactivation occurs on day 16 of embryonic development.
         b. Inactivated X chromosome is called a Barr body. It is attached to the nuclear membrane of cells and can be counted in squamous cells obtained by scraping the buccal mucosa.
         c. Normal females have one Barr body per cell, and normal males have none.
         d. Inactivation accounts for parental derivation of the X chromosomes in females.
            (1) ≈50% of X chromosomes are paternal and ≈50% are maternal.
            (2) Number of Barr bodies = number of X chromosomes − 1
   B. **Chromosomal alterations**
      1. **Definition:** Numeric or structural abnormalities of autosomes or sex chromosomes
      2. Nondisjunction (Fig. 6-16)
         a. **Definition:** Unequal separation of chromosomes in *meiosis*
         b. Results in 22 or 24 chromosomes in the egg or sperm

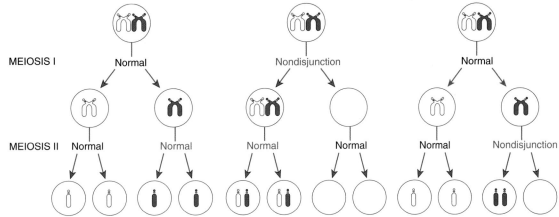

6-16: The different consequences of nondisjunction at meiosis I *(center)* and meiosis II *(right)*, compared with normal meiosis *(left)*, using chromosome 21 as an example. If the error occurs in meiosis I, the gametes either contain a representative of both members of the chromosome 21 pair (maternal and paternal members of the pair) or lack a chromosome 21 altogether. If nondisjunction occurs in meiosis II, the abnormal gametes contain two copies of one parental chromosome 21 (maternal or paternal) or lack a chromosome 21. *(From Nussbaum R, McInnes R, Willard H:* Thompson & Thompson Genetics in Medicine, *7th ed, Philadelphia, Saunders, 2008, p 68, Fig. 5-7.)*

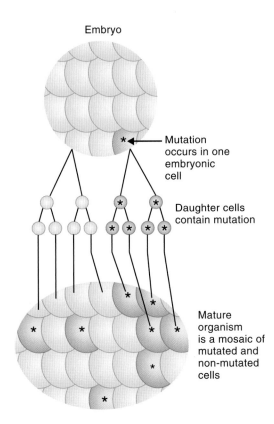

Embryo

Mutation occurs in one embryonic cell

Daughter cells contain mutation

Mature organism is a mosaic of mutated and non-mutated cells

6-17: Mosaicism: a mutation occurs in one cell of the developing embryo. All descendants of that cell have the same mutation, resulting in mosaicism. If the first mutated cell is part of the germline, mosaicism results. *(From Jorde LB, Carey JC, Bamshad MJ:* Medical Genetics, *4th ed, Philadelphia, Mosby Elsevier, 2010, p 64, Fig. 4-9.)*

c. Examples: Turner syndrome (22 + 23 = 45 chromosomes); Down syndrome (24 + 23 = 47 chromosomes; trisomy)

3. Mosaicism
   a. **Definition:** Nondisjunction of chromosomes during *mitosis* in the early embryonic period (Fig. 6-17)
   b. Two chromosomally different cell lines are derived from a single fertilized egg.
   c. Mosaicism most often involves sex chromosomes (e.g., Turner syndrome).

4. Translocation
   a. **Definition:** Transfer of chromosome parts between nonhomologous chromosomes
   b. In a **balanced translocation** the translocated fragment is *functional.*
      A **robertsonian** translocation is a balanced translocation between two acrocentric chromosomes (centromere is near the end of the chromosome; e.g., chromosomes 14 and 21).

Turner syndrome (45 chromosomes); Down syndrome (47 chromosomes)

Mosaicism: nondisjunction in mitosis

Two chromosomally different cell lines from one fertilized egg

Most often involves sex chromosomes

Transfer chromosome parts between nonhomologous chromosomes

Balanced: translocated fraction functional

Robertsonian: balanced translocation between acrocentric chromosomes; 14;21

6-18: Robertsonian translocation. This is a type of translocation between two acrocentric chromosomes, in this case chromosomes 14 and 21. The mother of an affected child has 45 (*not* 46) chromosomes because of a robertsonian translocation between the long arms of chromosomes 21 and 14. This produces one long chromosome (14;21) and one very short chromosome. The short chromosome is lost in subsequent divisions. The mother also has one chromosome 14 and one chromosome 21. The father has the normal 46 chromosomes. The affected child has 46 chromosomes with three functional 21 chromosomes. This includes chromosome (14;21) and chromosome 21 from the mother and chromosome 14 and chromosome 21 from the father.

Mother
45 chromosomes

Father
46 chromosomes

Lost chromosome

Down syndrome
46 chromosomes

Down syndrome balanced translocation (Fig. 6-18) is a type of translocation (robertsonian translocation; 4% of cases of Down syndrome) between two acrocentric chromosomes, in this case chromosomes 14 and 21. The mother of an affected child with Down syndrome has 45 (*not* 46) chromosomes because of a robertsonian translocation between the long arms of chromosomes 21 and 14. The **mother** has one chromosome 14, one chromosome 21, one long chromosome 14;21, and one very short chromosome that is lost in subsequent divisions for a total of 45 chromosomes. The **father** has the normal 46 chromosomes (2) 14 chromosomes and (2) 21 chromosomes. The **affected child** has 46 chromosomes with three functional 21 chromosomes, including chromosome 14;21 and chromosome 21 from the mother and chromosome 14 and chromosome 21 from the father.

Balanced translocation in Down syndrome: mother affected child 45 chromosomes, father 46 chromosomes

Deletion: loss of portion of chromosome

Cri du chat: short arm chromosome 5 deleted;

Mental impairment, cat-like cry, VSD

Down syndrome: facial features, mental impairment

Most cases due to nondisjunction

Robertsonian translocation

Mosaicism

↑Maternal age major risk factor

Meiotic disjunction chromosome 21 oogenesis in meiosis I

1/25 live births women >45 yrs old

Majority conceptions die embryonic/fetal life

Female with Down syndrome: 50% risk children with Down

Mental impairment

MC chromosomal abnormality with mental impairment

Mild (usually mosaics) to severe impairment

5. Deletion. **Definition:** Loss of a portion of a chromosome
   - Cri du chat syndrome. **Definition:** Loss of the short arm of chromosome 5. Clinical findings include mental impairment, cat-like cry, and ventricular septal defect (VSD).

C. **Disorders involving autosomes**
   1. Down syndrome
      a. **Definition:** Chromosomal disorder characterized by distinct facial features, multiple malformations, and moderate to severe mental impairment
      b. Epidemiology
         (1) Causes
            (a) Nondisjunction (95% of cases, trisomy 21; Fig. 6-19 A karyotype)
            (b) Robertsonian translocation (4% of cases; 46 chromosomes; Fig. 6-18)
            (c) Mosaicism (1% of cases)
         (2) Risk factors
            (a) Increased maternal age is the major risk factor.
               - Meiotic nondisjunction of chromosome 21 occurs in oogenesis, usually in meiosis I.
               - It occurs in 1 in 25 live births in women over 45 years of age.
               - Approximately 75% of conceptions with trisomy 21 die in embryonic or fetal life.
            (b) A female with Down syndrome has a 50% risk of having children with Down syndrome.
         (3) Median age at death: 47 years
      c. Clinical findings (Fig. 6-19 B–G)
         (1) Mental impairment
            (a) Down syndrome is the most common *chromosomal abnormality* associated with mental impairment.
            (b) Patients may have mild impairment (IQ 50–75; usually mosaics) or severe impairment (IQ 20–35).

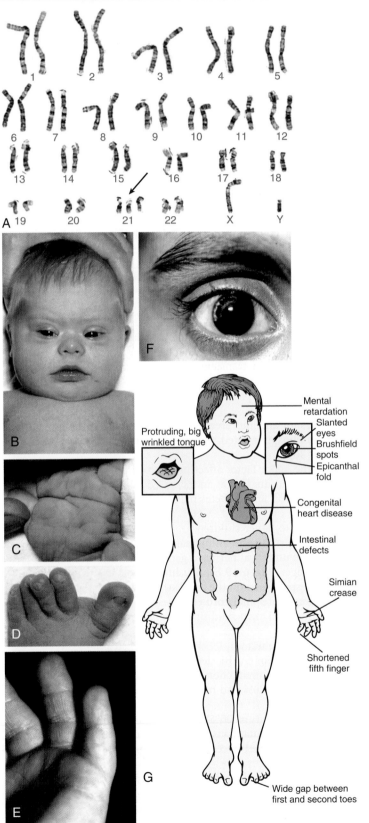

6-19: Down syndrome. A, Karyotype of male with trisomy 21 as seen in Down syndrome. This karyotype reveals 47 chromosomes instead of 46, with an extra chromosome in pair 21 *(arrow)*. **B,** The face shows a mongoloid slant of the palpebral fissures (separation between the upper and lower lids), prominent upward slanting of the epicanthal folds (skin folds of the upper eyelids), a flat nasal root (portion between the eyes) and small nose, low-set ears, and a small mouth. The tongue is not completely visible, but it was large (macroglossia). Not shown is the short stature of the child. **C,** The hand shows a palmar (simian) crease *(arrow)*. **D,** Wide space between first and second toes. **E,** Short fifth finger. **F,** Brushfield spots. Brushfield spots are white or yellow spots seen on the anterior surface of the iris. The spots may be arranged concentrically to the pupils or, as seen here, along the pupillary periphery. They are present in 85% of blue- or hazel-eyed patients with trisomy 21. **G,** Typical features of Down syndrome. *(A, F, From Adkison LR:* Elsevier's Integrated Review Genetics, *2 ed, Philadelphia, 2012, Saunders, p 18-19, Figs. 2-6A, 2-7; B, C, D, E, From Zitelli B, McIntire S. Nowalk A:* Zitelli's and Davis' Atlas of Pediatric Physical Diagnosis, *6th ed, Philadelphia, 2012, Saunders, p 11, Fig. 1.22D; G, From my friend Ivan Damjanov MD, PhD:* Pathology for the Health Professions, *4th ed, Philadelphia, 2012, Saunders, p 98, Fig. 5-7.)*

Mental retardation

Protruding, big wrinkled tongue

Slanted eyes

Brushfield spots

Epicanthal fold

Congenital heart disease

Intestinal defects

Simian crease

Shortened fifth finger

Wide gap between first and second toes

(2) General appearance

(a) Muscle hypotonia is present at birth. Down syndrome is the most common cause of the "floppy baby" syndrome.

(b) Upslanting of the palpebral fissures, epicanthic folds, a flat facial profile, and macroglossia with a protuberant tongue (Fig. 6-19 B)

(c) Simian crease (Fig. 6-19 C)

(3) Congenital heart defects

(a) Heart defects are present in 40% to 60% of patients.

(b) Heart defects are the major factor affecting survival in early childhood.

(c) Heart defects include endocardial cushion defect (ECD, atrioventricular defect; 43%), VSD (32%), atrial septal defect (10%), tetralogy of Fallot (6%), and isolated patent ductus arteriosus (PDA; 4%).

(4) Gastrointestinal tract abnormalities

(a) Tracheoesophageal (TE) fistula. Proximal esophagus ends blindly and the distal esophagus arises from the trachea (see Fig. 18-10).

(b) Duodenal atresia. Atresia (incomplete formation of a lumen) of the small bowel distal to where the common bile duct empties into the duodenum; vomiting of bile-stained fluid at birth (see Fig. 18-22 C)

(c) Hirschsprung disease. An aganglionic segment in the large bowel, which causes problems with stooling at birth (see Fig. 18-22 D, F)

(5) Hematologic abnormalities

(a) Increased risk for developing leukemia

(b) Acute lymphoblastic leukemia (ALL) and acute megakaryocytic leukemia are the most common types of leukemia (see Chapter 13).

(c) Leukemia is usually preceded by transient myeloproliferative diseases (MPDs).

(6) Central nervous system (CNS) abnormalities

(a) Most patients develop the neuropathologic signs of Alzheimer disease by 35 to 40 years of age.

(b) Chromosome 21 codes for amyloid precursor protein, which is the progenitor for Aβ protein. When phosphorylated, this protein induces apoptosis of neurons (see Chapter 26).

(c) Alzheimer disease is the major factor affecting survival in older individuals.

(7) Immune abnormalities. Patients are also at an increased risk of developing hypothyroidism, lung infections, and diabetes mellitus (DM).

(8) Fertility abnormalities

(a) Males are usually unable to father children.

(b) Females have decreased fertility and an increased incidence of miscarriages.

(9) Other abnormalities include umbilical hernia, a gap between first and second toes (Fig. 6-19 D), short fifth finger (Fig. 6-19 E), Brushfield spots in the eyes (Fig. 6-19 F; white or yellow-colored spots seen on the anterior surface of the iris), and atlantoaxial instability (danger of spinal cord compression).

(10) Overview of clinical findings in Down syndrome (Fig. 6-19 G)

d. Diagnosis

(1) Maternal screening with the triple test

(a) Decrease in serum α-fetoprotein (AFP), decrease in urine unconjugated estriol (uE3), and increase in serum human chorionic gonadotropin (hCG)

(b) Triple test has a sensitivity of ≈70% and must be followed by invasive diagnostic tests.

(2) Invasive diagnostic testing (sensitivity ≈100%) includes amniocentesis with chorionic villous sampling and percutaneous umbilical blood sampling.

(3) Cytogenetic and DNA studies are used to confirm the diagnosis.

2. Trisomy 18: Edwards syndrome

a. **Definition:** Chromosomal disorder caused by the presence of all, or part of, an extra 18th chromosome

b. Second most common trisomy syndrome (incidence 1/8000 births)

c. Clinical findings

(1) Mental impairment; clenched fist with overlapping fingers (Fig. 6-20 **A**)

(2) Rocker-bottom feet (Fig. 6-20 B), VSD, early death

3. Patau syndrome

a. **Definition:** Trisomy 13 chromosome disorder

b. Epidemiology: incidence of 1 in 15,000 births

c. Clinical findings

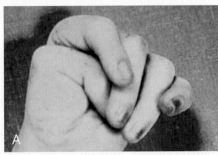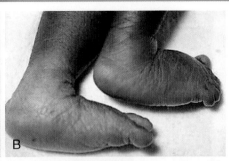

6-20: **A,** Trisomy 18. Note the clenched fist and overlapping fingers. **B,** Trisomy 18 with rocker-bottom foot. Trisomy 16 also has rocker-bottom feet. *(From Kliegman RM:* Nelson Textbook of Pediatrics, *20th ed, Philadelphia, 2016, Elsevier, p. 14, Figs 1-24 B, C.)*

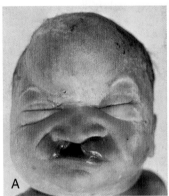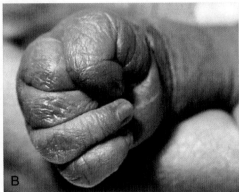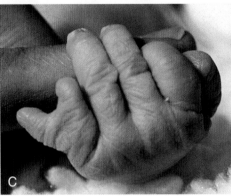

6-21: Several physical manifestations of trisomy 13. **A,** Facies showing midline defect. **B,** Clenched hand with overlapping fingers. **C,** Postaxial polydactyly. *(**A** courtesy T. Kelly, MD, University of Virginia Medical Center, Charlottesville; **B, C** courtesy Kenneth Garver, MD, Pittsburgh, PA; **A–C** from Zitelli B, McIntire S, Nowalk A:* Zitelli and Davis' Atlas of Pediatric Physical Diagnosis, *6th ed, Saunders Elsevier, 2012, p 13, Fig. 1-23 A, B, C.)*

(1) Mental impairment, midline defects (cleft lip and palate; (Fig. 6-21 A), clenched hand with overlapping fingers (Fig. 6-21 B), polydactyly (Fig. 6-21 C)

(2) VSD, cystic kidneys, early death

D. Disorders involving sex chromosomes

1. Turner syndrome

   a. **Definition:** Chromosomal condition in females in which the complete or partial absence of a second normal X chromosome results in short stature, primary ovarian failure, and other phenotypic defects

   b. Epidemiology

      (1) Most common sex chromosome abnormality in females (1/3000 female births)

      (2) Fifteen percent (15%) of spontaneous abortions are due to Turner syndrome.

      (3) Normal intelligence

      (4) Karyotype abnormalities

         (a) 45,X karyotype (most conceptuses are nonviable). Majority are due to paternal nondisjunction. *No* Barr bodies are present in the XO types of Turner syndrome.

         (b) Structural abnormalities (e.g., isochromosomes [chromosome produced by transverse splitting of the centromere so that both arms are from the same side of the centromere, are of equal length, and possess identical genes], deletion)

         (c) Mosaicism (most common cause of Turner syndrome; see later)

            - 45,X/46,XX karyotype (most common type).

            - 45,X/46,XY (risk for developing gonadoblastoma of the ovary; see Chapter 22)

            - Using sensitive DNA techniques, mosaicism accounts for up to 75% of all cases of Turner syndrome, because most 45,XO conceptuses are nonviable.

   c. Clinical and laboratory findings (Fig. 6-22 A–D)

      (1) General abnormalities on physical exam

         (a) Short stature is a cardinal finding in Turner syndrome (>95% of cases).

            - Growth hormone (GH) and insulin-like growth factor-1 (IGF-1) are normal.

Mental impairment, cleft lip/palate

Clenched hand overlapping fingers

VSD, cystic kidneys, early death

Turner syndrome

Complete/partial absence 2nd normal X chromosome

MC female sex chromosome abnormality

15% of spontaneous abortions

Normal intelligence

45X karyotype: paternal nondisjunction

No Barr bodies

Isochromosomes, deletion

Mosaicism: 45,X/46,XX karyotype (MC type)

45,X/46,XY; ↑risk gonadoblastoma of ovary

Sensitive DNA techniques: mosaicism 75% of all cases

Short stature

GH/IGF-1 normal

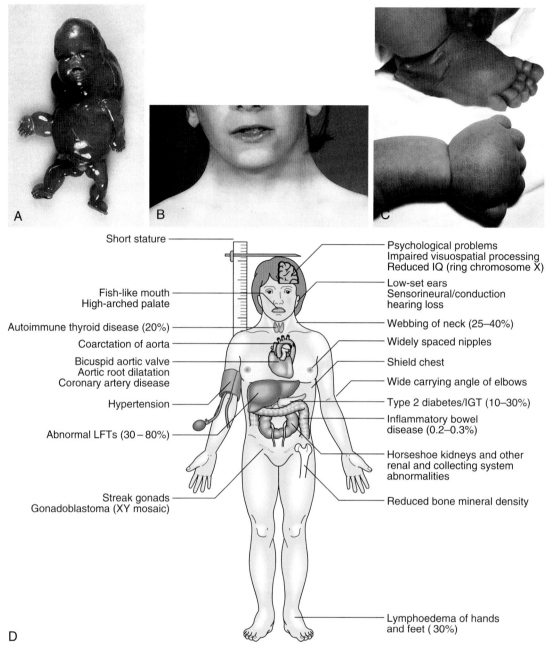

6-22: **A,** Aborted Turner syndrome fetus with a 45,X karyotype showing lymphedema of the hands, feet, and neck. Most 45,X karyotypes are aborted. **B,** Turner syndrome is characterized by a webbed neck. Other findings include short stature, primary amenorrhea, and delayed secondary sex characteristics (e.g., underdeveloped breasts). **C,** Clinical photographs in a newborn showing prominent lymphedema of the hands and feet. **D,** Summary of clinical features of Turner syndrome. IGT, impaired glucose tolerance; LFTs, liver function tests. *(A from my friend Ivan Damjanov, MD, PhD, Linder J: Anderson's Pathology, 10th ed, St. Louis, Mosby, 1996, p 338, Fig. 16.21; B from Bouloux P-M: Self-Assessment Picture Tests: Medicine, Vol 1, London, Mosby-Wolfe, 1996, p 45, Fig. 90; C from Zitelli B, McIntire S, Nowalk A: Zitelli and Davis' Atlas of Pediatric Physical Diagnosis, 6th ed, Saunders Elsevier, 2012, p 15, Fig. 1-25 D, E; D from Walker BR, Colledge NR, Ralston SH, Penman ID: Davidson's Principles and Practice of Medicine, 22nd ed, Churchill Livingstone Elsevier, 2014, p 765, Fig. 20.15.)*

Deletion 2nd *SHOX* gene on X chromosome

SHOX gene critical for growth regulation

Cubitus valgus

Knuckle-knuckle-dimple sign

Shield chest, underdeveloped breasts

Pubic hair development normal

- Short stature is due to deletion of a second *SHOX* gene located on the X chromosome.
- *SHOX* gene is critical for regulation of growth and, unlike most genes, remains active on both X chromosomes; hence, a deletion of one of the two *SHOX* genes causes the short stature.

(b) Carrying angle of the arms is increased (cubitus valgus).

(c) Short fourth metacarpal or metatarsal bone produces the knuckle (index finger)-knuckle-dimple (short fourth metacarpal/metatarsal bone)-knuckle sign.

(d) Shield chest has widely spaced nipples and underdeveloped breasts.

(e) Pubic hair development is normal.

(2) Lymphedema may occur in the hands, feet, and neck in infancy (Fig. 6-22 A–C). Webbed neck in Turner syndrome is caused by dilated lymphatic channels (cystic hygroma) and persists into adult life.

(3) Cardiovascular abnormalities

    (a) Congenital heart disease (CHD) occurs in 20% to 50% of cases.

    (b) A hypoplastic left heart is the major cause of mortality in early infancy.

    (c) Preductal coarctation commonly occurs and often presents with left-sided heart failure.

    (d) Bicuspid aortic valves are another common cardiac abnormality.

(4) Genitourinary abnormalities

    (a) Both ovaries are replaced by fibrous stroma (called streak gonads). Increased risk for developing ovarian dysgerminoma.

    (b) Ovaries are devoid of oocytes by 2 years of age. Some women with mosaicism are fertile.

    (c) Primary amenorrhea occurs with delayed sexual maturation.

- Turner syndrome is the most common genetic cause of primary amenorrhea.
- Estradiol and progesterone are decreased.
- Follicle-stimulating hormone (FSH) and luteinizing hormone (LH) are increased.

    (d) Incidence of horseshoe kidneys is increased.

(5) Hypothyroidism, due to Hashimoto thyroiditis, occurs in 10% to 30% of cases.

(6) Figure 6-22 D summarizes the clinical findings in Turner syndrome.

2. Klinefelter syndrome

  a. **Definition:** Male-dominant disease characterized by the presence of a 47,XXY chromosome pattern

  b. Epidemiology

    (1) Most common genetic cause of male hypogonadism and occurs in 1 in 500 to 1 in 1000 live male births.

    (2) Causes

      (a) Nondisjunction is the most common cause of the syndrome (90% of cases) and produces 47 chromosomes with an XXY karyotype. Maternal and paternal nondisjunction in meiosis I occurs in roughly equal proportions. One Barr body forms through random inactivation of one of the two X chromosomes.

      (b) Mosaicism is the remaining cause of the syndrome, with the most common karyotype being 46,XY/47,XXY.

    (3) Testicular abnormalities and female secondary sex characteristics do *not* develop until puberty.

  c. Pathophysiology

    (1) Testicular volume at puberty is decreased (<17 mL) and is due to atrophy.

      (a) Histologic exam reveals fibrosis of seminiferous tubules with absence of spermatogenesis (azoospermia; infertility), loss of Sertoli cells, and presence of Leydig cells.

      (b) Loss of Sertoli cells leads to a decrease in inhibin and a corresponding increase in FSH (loss of negative feedback with inhibin). Increase in FSH increases the synthesis of aromatase in the Leydig cells.

      (c) Leydig cells are prominent because of atrophy of other portions of the testis. Increased synthesis of aromatase very likely converts a little of the testosterone synthesized by the Leydig cells into estradiol; however, this does *not* fully explain why patients with Klinefelter syndrome have hypogonadism and feminization.

    (2) Primary reason for hypogonadism and feminization is that testosterone does *not* have a normal interaction with androgen receptors.

      (a) X chromosome carries genes that encode for androgen receptors, testis function, brain development, and growth.

      (b) Testosterone mediates its function through the androgen receptors.

      (c) Gene on the X chromosome that is responsible for androgen receptor synthesis contains CAG TRs.

      (d) Functional response of testosterone is dependent on the number of CAG repeats in the androgen receptor.

- Testosterone interacts better with androgen receptors that have the *smallest* number of CAG repeats.

Margin notes:

Lymphedema hands, feet, neck (webbed neck)

CHD common

Hypoplastic left heart major cause infant mortality

Preductal coarctation

Bicuspid aortic valves common

Streak gonads → ↑risk dysgerminoma

Ovaries devoid of oocytes (2 yrs age)

MC genetic cause 1° amenorrhea

↓Estradiol/progesterone; ↑FSH/LH

Horseshoe kidneys

Hashimoto thyroiditis

No Barr bodies in buccal smear

Klinefelter syndrome: male dominant

47,XXY chromosome pattern

MC genetic cause male hypogonadism

Maternal or paternal nondisjunction MCC; 47 chromosomes, XXY

1 Barr body

Random inactivity of one of two X chromosomes

Mosaicism 46,XY/47,XXY

Testicular abnormalities; female characteristics delayed until puberty

↓Testicular volume at puberty

Fibrosis of seminiferous tubules, azoospermia, loss Sertoli cells, Leydig cells present

↓Inhibin (loss Sertoli cells) → ↑FSH → ↑aromatase synthesis (Leydig cells)

Leydig cells prominent (synthesize aromatase, testosterone)

Aromatase converts testosterone to estradiol (partial role in feminization)

Testosterone *cannot* interact with androgen receptors → hypogonadism/feminization

X genes: androgen receptors, testis function, brain development, growth

Testosterone requires androgen receptors

X chromosome gene for androgen receptor synthesis contains CAG TRs

Testosterone reacts best with androgen receptors containing least # CAG repeats

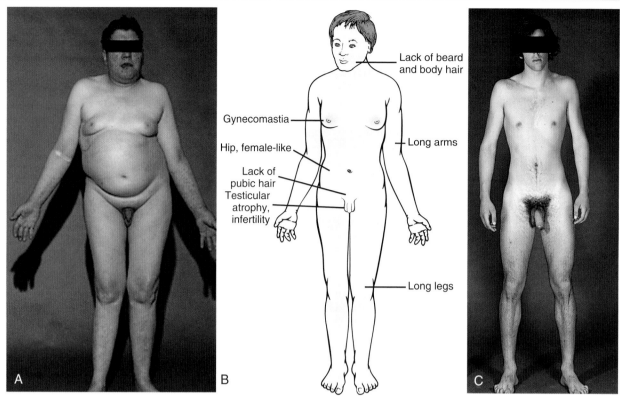

6-23: **A,** Klinefelter syndrome is characterized by female secondary sex characteristics, including gynecomastia (male breast development) and a female distribution of pubic hair (note that the hair does not extend from the mons pubis to the umbilicus). The penis is small (micropenis). The legs are disproportionately long, giving the patient a eunuchoid appearance. **B,** Clinical features of Klinefelter syndrome. **C,** XYY syndrome. Individuals with this syndrome are tall and extremely aggressive. **(A** from *Bouloux P-M:* Self-Assessment Picture Tests: Medicine, *Vol 1, London, Mosby-Wolfe, 1996, p 82, Fig. 163;* **B** from my friend Ivan Damjanov, MD, PhD: Pathology for the Health Professions, *4th ed, Saunders Elsevier, 2012, p 99, Fig. 5-10;* **C** from *Bouloux P-M:* Self-Assessment Picture Tests: Medicine, *Vol 4, London, Mosby-Wolfe, 1997, p 99, Fig. 196.)*

X chromosome with least # CAG repeats preferentially inactivated

Testosterone cannot interact with androgen receptors containing longest CAG repeats → hypogonadism

Signs male hypogonadism/feminization begin at puberty

Persistent gynecomastia in late puberty

Facial/body/pubic hair diminished

Pubic hair distribution resembles female

Micropenis (↓testosterone in utero)

↓Testicular volume (atrophy)

Eunuchoid body habitus: disproportionately long legs

Mean IQ lower than normal

Developmental/learning disabilities

Variants >2 X chromosomes greater mental impairment

MVP common

Type 2 DM, metabolic syndrome

- In Klinefelter syndrome, the X chromosome with the smallest number of CAG repeats is preferentially inactivated, leaving behind androgen receptors that have the longest CAG repeats.
- Testosterone does *not* interact with androgen receptors with the longest CAG repeats, which, along with increased conversion into estradiol by aromatase, causes hypogonadism and leaves estradiol unopposed by any androgen effects resulting in feminization.

d. Clinical and laboratory findings (Fig. 6-23 A, B)

(1) Signs of male hypogonadism/feminization begin at puberty.

(a) Persistent gynecomastia (breast development in a male) is a characteristic feature in late puberty.

(b) Facial, body, and pubic hair are diminished.

(c) Hair distribution in the pubic region resembles that of a female (lack of extension of hair from the genitalia to the umbilicus).

(d) Penis is small (micropenis) because of decreased fetal production of testosterone in utero.

(e) Testicular volume is decreased from testicular atrophy.

(2) Eunuchoid body habitus with disproportionately long legs.

(3) Intelligence in Klinefelter syndrome

- Mean IQ is lower than normal.
- Minor developmental and learning disabilities are present in most cases.
- Variants with more than two X chromosomes (e.g., XXXY, XXXXY) have even lower IQ.

(4) Cardiovascular abnormalities in Klinefelter syndrome. Mitral valve penetrance (MVP; sometimes severe) is present in 50% of adults.

(5) Endocrine abnormalities in Klinefelter syndrome. Increased incidence of type 2 DM and metabolic syndrome (insulin resistance; see Chapter 23).

(6) Findings
    (a) Decreased serum testosterone and increased serum LH
    (b) Increased serum FSH and estradiol
    (c) Decreased serum inhibin; azoospermia (no sperm)
(7) Increased risk for developing autoimmune disease (e.g., systemic lupus erythematosus [SLE], rheumatoid arthritis, Sjögren syndrome), breast cancer, and osteoporosis.

3. XYY syndrome (Fig. 6-23 C)
  a. **Definition:** Sex chromosome aneuploidy where males tend to be taller than average and have a 10- to 15-point lower IQ
  b. Epidemiology
    (1) Caused by a *paternal* nondisjunction
    (2) Occurs in 1 in 2000 live births
    (3) Associated with aggressive (sometimes criminal) behavior. In the prison population, its incidence in the male population may be as high as 1 in 30 compared with 1 in 1000 in the general male population.
    (4) Normal gonadal function

IV. Other Patterns of Inheritance
  A. **Multifactorial (complex) inheritance**
    1. **Definition:** Result of complex interactions between a number of genetic and environmental factors
    2. Epidemiology
      a. Incidence of multifactorial inheritance is ≈50 in 1000 live births.
      b. Examples
        (1) Open neural tube (ONT) defects. Associated with decreased maternal folic acid levels.
        (2) Type 2 DM. Associated with obesity, which down-regulates insulin receptor synthesis.
        (3) Other examples of multifactorial inheritance include gout, cleft lip/palate, congenital heart defects, pyloric stenosis, and coronary artery disease.
  B. **Mitochondrial DNA (mtDNA) disorders**
    1. **Definition:** A group of disorders caused by mutations in mtDNA that display characteristic modes of inheritance that have a large degree of phenotypic variability
    2. Epidemiology
      a. Mitochondrial DNA codes for enzymes that are involved in mitochondrial oxidative phosphorylation (OP) reactions.
      b. Inheritance pattern
        (1) Affected *females* transmit the mutant gene to *all* their children (Fig. 6-24; Link 6-14). Ova contain mitochondria with the mutant gene.
        (2) Affected males do *not* transmit the mutant gene to any of their children. Sperm lose their mitochondria during fertilization.
        (3) Examples: Leber hereditary optic neuropathy and myoclonic epilepsy
  C. **Genomic imprinting**
    1. **Definition:** Allelic expression is parent-of-origin specific for some alleles.
    2. Inheritance pattern
      a. Examples include Prader-Willi (PW) syndrome and Angelman syndrome.
      b. Epidemiology; pathogenesis (Fig. 6-25 A)

Margin notes

↓Testosterone → ↑LH

↑FSH, ↑estradiol

↓Serum inhibin; azoospermia

↑Risk autoimmune disease (SLE, rheumatoid arthritis, Sjögren syndrome), breast cancer, osteoporosis

XYY syndrome

Sex chromosome aneuploidy; males tall, low IQ

Paternal nondisjunction

Aggressive criminal behavior

Normal gonadal function

Multifactorial inheritance

Interaction genetic + environmental factors

ONT defects (↓maternal folic acid)

Type 2 DM

Gout, cleft lip/palate, congenital heart defects, pyloric stenosis, coronary artery disease

Mutation mtDNA; large degree phenotypic variability

mtDNA: codes for OP enzymes

Affected females transmit mutant gene to all children

Ova mitochondria contain mutant gene

Affected males do *not* transmit mutant gene

Sperm lose mitochondria during fertilization

Leber hereditary optic neuropathy, myoclonic epilepsy

Genomic imprinting

Allelic expression is parent-of-origin specific for some alleles

PW, Angelman syndromes

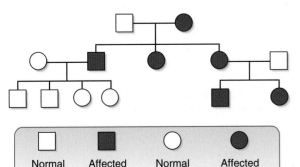

6-24: Pedigree showing transmission of mitochondrial DNA. Affected females transmit the disorder to *all* their children, whereas affected males do not (spermatozoa lack the mutant gene).

| Normal male | Affected male | Normal female | Affected female |

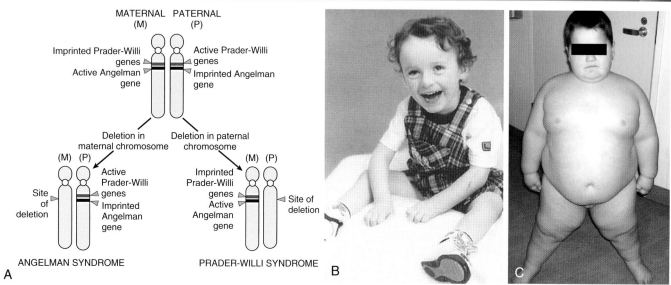

MATERNAL PATERNAL
(M) (P)

Imprinted Prader-Willi genes
Active Angelman gene

Active Prader-Willi genes
Imprinted Angelman gene

Deletion in maternal chromosome

Deletion in paternal chromosome

(M) (P)

Site of deletion

Active Prader-Willi genes
Imprinted Angelman gene

(M) (P)

Imprinted Prader-Willi genes
Active Angelman gene

Site of deletion

ANGELMAN SYNDROME

PRADER-WILLI SYNDROME

A

B

C

6-25: **A,** Genetics of Angelman and Prader-Willi (PW) syndromes. Normal changes in the maternal chromosome 15 during gametogenesis *(top)* is inactivation of the PW genes expression by methylation (imprinted) and activation (not methylated) of the Angelman gene. Normal changes in the paternal chromosome 15 during gametogenesis *(top)* are inactivation of the Angelman gene expression by methylation (imprinted) and activation (not methylated) of the PW genes. In the PW syndrome *(right)*, there is a microdeletion of the entire gene site on paternal chromosome 15, resulting in a complete loss of the PW genes expression. In Angelman syndrome *(left),* there is a microdeletion of the entire gene site on maternal chromosome 15, resulting in a complete loss of Angelman gene expression. **B,** Angelman syndrome. Note the happy face. When walking, the child had a wide-based gait; hence the term "happy puppet" for this syndrome. The child also had intellectual disability. **C,** Prader-Willi syndrome. Note the marked obesity in this child and small penis. (*A from Kumar V, Abbas AK, Fausto N, Mitchell RN: Robbins Basic Pathology, 8th ed, Philadelphia, Saunders Elsevier, 2007, p 251, Fig. 7-18; **B,** From Kliegman RM: Nelson Textbook of Pediatrics, 20th ed, Philadelphia, 2016, Elsevier, p 620, Fig. 81-16C. From Hyme HE, Greydanus D, editors: Genetic Disorders in Adolescents: State of the Art Reviews. Adolescent Medicine, Philadelphia, 2002, Hanley and Belfus, pp: 305-313; **C,** From Sahoo T, del Gaudio D, German JR, et al: Prader-Willi phenotype caused by paternal deficiency for the HBII-85 C/D box small nucleolar RNA cluster, Nat Genet 40:719–721, 2008.*)*

Normal changes maternal chromosome 15 during gametogenesis

PW gene imprinted (inactivated by methylation)

Angelman gene activated (*not* methylated)

Normal changes paternal chromosome 15 during gametogenesis

PW genes active

Angelman gene imprinted by methylation

PW: microdeletion entire gene site *paternal* chromosome

Complete loss expression PW genes

Maternal chromosome PW genes imprinted, Angelman gene active

Angelman: microdeletion entire gene site *maternal* chromosome 15

Complete loss Angelman gene expression

Paternal chromosome 15: Angelman gene imprinted, PW genes active

Mental impairment

"Marionette"

"Happy puppet"

Neonatal hypotonia, genital hypoplasia

Short stature (↓GH)

Hyperphagia (obesity)

Satiety defect (↑gherlin)

Y chromosome

(1) Normal changes in the maternal chromosome 15 occur during gametogenesis.
   (a) Expression of PW genes (series of genes) is imprinted. Imprinted means that the gene has been inactivated by methylation.
   (b) Angelman gene *(UBE3A)* is active. Active means that the gene has *not* been methylated.
(2) Normal changes in the paternal chromosome 15 occur during gametogenesis.
   (a) PW genes are active.
   (b) Angelman gene expression is imprinted (inactivated) by methylation.
(3) Microdeletion of the entire gene site on *paternal* chromosome 15 (C15) causes PW syndrome.
   (a) Complete loss of expression of the PW genes
   (b) On the maternal chromosome, the PW genes are imprinted and the Angelman gene is active.
(4) Microdeletion of the entire gene site on *maternal* chromosome 15 causes Angelman syndrome.
   (a) Complete loss of Angelman gene expression
   (b) On the paternal chromosome 15, the Angelman gene is imprinted and the PW genes are active.
3. Clinical findings in Angelman syndrome include (Fig. 6-25 B) mental impairment, jerky, wide-based gait with hand flapping (resembles a marionette), and outbursts of inappropriate laughter ("happy puppet" syndrome).
4. Clinical findings in PW syndrome include (Fig. 6-25 C) neonatal hypotonia and genital hypoplasia at birth, short stature (due to GH deficiency), and hyperphagia (insatiable appetite) leading to obesity.
  • Satiety defect is due to increased levels of gherlin, a polypeptide hormone produced by the stomach and arcuate nucleus in the hypothalamus that increases food intake (see Chapter 8).

V. Disorders of Sex Differentiation
  A. Normal sex differentiation
    1. Normal karyotype is demonstrated in Link 6-15.
    2. Y chromosome

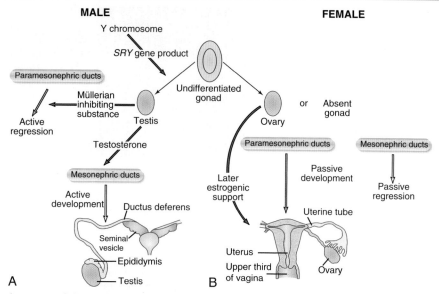

MALE   FEMALE

6-26: A, Progressive development of the male genitalia. The *SRY* gene on the Y chromosome encodes testis-determining factor, which causes the undifferentiated gonad to develop into a testis. The Sertoli cells produce müllerian inhibitory substance, which causes parame-sonephric structure to regress. Testosterone induces development of the epididymis, seminal vesicle, and ductus deferens from mesonephric duct structures. Dihydrotestosterone (not shown) causes development of the external genitalia (penis, scrotum, and prostate gland). **B,** Development of the female genitalia. In the absence of the Y chromosome, the undifferentiated gonad develops into an ovary. Mesonephric ducts undergo regression, and the paramesonephric ducts are developed into fallopian (uterine) tubes, uterus, and the upper one-third of the vagina. The lower two-thirds of the vagina develops from the urogenital sinus (not shown). *(From Moore A, Roy W:* Rapid Review Gross and Developmental Anatomy, *3rd ed, Philadelphia, Mosby Elsevier, 2010, p 130, Fig. 4.32.)*

a. Compared to other chromosomes, Y is relatively gene poor (contains ≈50 genes).

b. *SRY* gene is the sex-determining gene on the Y chromosome.

c. Presence of a single Y gene determines the male sex.

3. Presence of the Y chromosome (Fig. 6-26 A)

a. *SRY* gene encodes a testis-determining factor that causes the undifferentiated gonad to develop into a testis.

b. Müllerian inhibitory substance (MIS), synthesized in the Sertoli cells of the testes, causes the paramesonephric ducts to undergo apoptosis.

c. Function of fetal testosterone. Develops the mesonephric duct structures (MDSs), which include the epididymis, seminal vesicles, and vas (ductus) deferens.

d. 5α-Reductase, in peripheral tissue, converts testosterone to dihydrotestosterone (DHT).

e. Functions of fetal DHT

(1) In the male embryo, the genitalia are phenotypically female *before* DHT is produced.

(2) In the presence of DHT, what phenotypically appears to be labia fuses to become the scrotum.

(3) In the presence of DHT, what phenotypically appears to be a clitoris becomes elongated into a penis.

(4) Fetal DHT also develops the prostate gland.

4. Absence of the Y chromosome (Fig. 6-26 B).

a. Absence of the Y chromosome causes gonadal tissue to differentiate into an ovary beginning as early as the eighth week of gestation and continuing for several weeks.

b. Fallopian tubes, uterus, and upper vagina develop from the paramesonephric ducts (müllerian ducts), while mesonephric duct structures undergo apoptosis.

c. Contact of the uterovaginal primordium (sinus tubercle) with the urogenital sinus induces the formation of sinovaginal bulbs that fuse to form a vaginal plate, which canalizes to form the lumen of the vagina.

B. True hermaphrodite

1. **Definition:** Fetus has a testis on one side and an ovary on the other side or a fusion of ovarian and testicular tissue (ovotestes).

2. Karyotype is 46,XX in 50% of cases, whereas the remaining 50% are mosaics with a 46,XX/46,XY karyotype.

Relatively gene poor

SRY gene: sex-determining gene on Y chromosome

Single Y gene determines male sex

Testis-determining factor → undifferentiated gonad becomes testis

Sertoli cells synthesize MIS

MIS causes apoptosis paramesonephric ducts

Fetal testosterone: develop MDSs → epididymis, seminal vesicles, vas deferens

5α-Reductase converts testosterone to DHT

Genitalia female until DHT produced

"Labia" fuses → scrotum

"Clitoris" → penis

DHT develops prostate gland

Absence Y chromosome

Undifferentiated gonads develop into ovaries

Paramesonephric ducts: fallopian tubes, uterus, upper vagina

Sinus tubercle fuses with urogenital sinus → sinovaginal bulbs → vaginal plate → vagina

Testis 1 side, ovary other side; or ovotestes

46, XX 50%; other 50% mosaics 46,XX/46,XY karyotype

6-27: A, Androgen insensitivity syndrome. The patient is genotypically male but phenotypically female. The vagina ends as a blind pouch. **B,** Ambiguous genitalia in a child with an XY karyotype and partial androgen insensitivity. *(A from Bouloux, P-M: Self-Assessment Picture Tests: Medicine, Vol 3, London, Mosby-Wolfe, 1997, p 24, Fig. 48; B from McKay M: Vulvar manifestations of skin disorders. In Black M, McKay M, Braude P, et al, eds: Obstetric and Gynecologic Dermatology, 2nd ed, Edinburgh, Mosby, 2003, p 121.)*

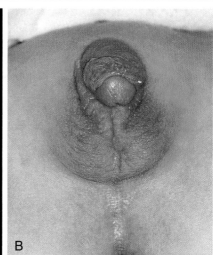
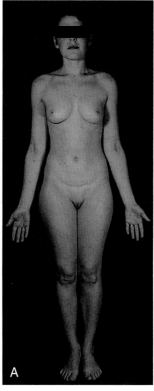

Phenotype (external appearance) and genotype (true genetic sex) do *not* match

Male pseudohermaphroditism

Genotype XY; phenotype ambiguous or completely female

AIS, ↓5α-reductase

Female pseudohermaphroditism

Genotypically female; phenotypically ambiguous or virilized

Normal ovaries/internal genitalia

Adrenogenital syndrome: MCC female pseudohermaphroditism

AIS (testicular feminization)

Male pseudohermaphroditism; loss-of-function mutation androgen receptor gene

XR disorder

AIS MCC male pseudohermaphroditism

Loss-of-function mutation androgen receptor gene on X chromosome

Prenatal undervirilization external genitalia

Loss pubertal changes: voice changes, male hair distribution hair, acne

Complete loss androgen receptor or alteration testosterone binding affinity for receptor

Birth: testicles inguinal canal/abdominal cavity

PMD structures absent: fallopian tubes, uterus, cervix, upper vagina; MIS functional

C. Pseudohermaphrodite
   1. **Definition:** Phenotype (external appearance) and genotype (true genetic sex) do *not* match.
   2. Male pseudohermaphroditism
      a. **Definition:** Male pseudohermaphrodite is genotypically a male (XY with testes); however, phenotypically, the external genitalia is ambiguous (male and female looking) or completely female.
      b. Examples include AIS (see section V.D.) and deficiency of 5α-reductase.
   3. Female pseudohermaphroditism
      a. **Definition:** Female pseudohermaphrodite is genotypically a female (XX with ovaries), but phenotypically she has ambiguous genitalia or the genitalia is virilized.
      b. Ovaries and internal genitalia are normal.
      c. Most common cause of female pseudohermaphoditism is adrenogenital syndrome due to 21- or 11-hydroxylase deficiency (see Chapter 23).
D. Androgen insensitivity syndrome (AIS; testicular feminization) (Fig. 6-27)
   1. **Definition:** Type of male pseudohermaphroditism due to a loss-of-function mutation in the androgen receptor gene
   2. Epidemiology
      a. XR disorder
      b. Most common cause of male pseudohermaphroditism
      c. Pathogenesis
         (1) Loss-of-function mutation in the androgen receptor gene on the long arm of the X chromosome (Xq11-13). Loss of receptor function means that even though male hormone synthesis is normal, the effects of the hormone in tissue do *not* occur, resulting in prenatal undervirilization of external genitalia and loss of pubertal changes one would expect in a male (e.g., voice changes, male distribution of hair, acne).
         (2) Complete loss of the androgen receptor or an alteration in the substrate (testosterone) binding affinity to the receptor
   3. Clinical and laboratory findings
      a. At birth, testicles are in inguinal canal or abdominal cavity.
      b. Paramesonephric duct (PMD) structures are *absent* (fallopian tubes, uterus, cervix, upper vagina), because MIS is present and initiates apoptosis of those structures in utero.

c. Male accessory structures (epididymis, seminal vesicles, vas deferens, prostate gland) are *absent*.

d. External genitalia remain female in appearance.
  (1) *No* DHT effect on the external genitalia
  (2) Vagina ends as a blind pouch. Lower two-thirds of the vagina is *not* of paramesonephric duct origin (see previous discussion); therefore, it is present and the vagina ends as a blind pouch.

e. If *not* identified in the newborn period, patients present with primary amenorrhea (lack of menses) in their teenage years.

f. Gynecomastia (swelling of breast tissue) is usually present as a postpubertal finding.

g. If testes *not* surgically removed, there is an increased risk for developing a gonadoblastoma (see Chapter 22).

h. Laboratory test findings
  (1) Karyotype is essential in order to differentiate an undermasculinized male from a virilized female.
  (2) Serum testosterone/DHT levels are those of a normal male.
  (3) Slight increase in serum LH
  (4) Slight increase in serum estradiol
    (a) Since estrogen activity is unopposed and estrogen receptors are present, the patient has female phenotypic findings.
    (b) Term *unopposed* means that testosterone function is neutralized by the absence or nonfunctionality of the androgen receptors.
  (5) Mutation analysis of the androgen receptor gene detects up to 95% of the mutations.

4. Majority are reared as a female.

VI. Congenital Anomalies
A. Definition: Defects that are recognized only at birth ("born with").
B. Epidemiology (Link 6-16)
1. Occur in 3% to 5% of all newborns
2. Most common cause of death in children <1 year of age.
3. Major causes
  a. Genetic abnormalities. Examples: chromosome abnormalities (most common; 10%–15% of cases) and single-gene mutations (2%–10% of cases)
  b. Maternal abnormalities (6%–8% of cases)
    (1) DM
      (a) Increased risk of neural tube defects (NTDs) and CHD
      (b) Hyperglycemia causes fetal macrosomia, because hyperinsulinemia in the fetus increases muscle mass and stores of fat in the adipose (see Chapter 23). Hyperinsulinemia is present in the fetus, because increased glucose from the mother enters the fetus and the fetal pancreas responds by increasing insulin synthesis.
    (2) SLE. Newborn may develop congenital heart block if the mother has anti-Ro antibodies that cross the placenta (see Chapter 4).
    (3) Hypothyroidism (see Chapter 23)
      (a) Newborn may develop cretinism with severe mental impairment.
      (b) Thyroid hormone is necessary for normal development of the brain.
  c. Maternal intake of drugs and chemicals (1% of cases; Table 6-4; Fig. 6-28 A, B; Fig. 6-29)
  d. Congenital infections (2%–3% of cases; Table 6-5; Fig. 6-30)
    (1) TORCH syndrome = <u>t</u>oxoplasmosis, <u>o</u>ther agents, <u>r</u>ubella, <u>c</u>ytomegalovirus (CMV), <u>h</u>erpes simplex virus
    (2) Newborns with a congenital infection have an increase in cord blood immunoglobulin M (IgM).
      (a) IgM normally is *not* synthesized in the fetus *unless* there is a congenital infection.
      (b) Normally, IgM synthesis begins *after* birth.
      (c) CMV is the most common congenital infection.
    (3) Vertical transmission (mother to baby during the period immediately before and after birth)
      Routes of vertical transmission
      (a) Transplacental (most common route)
      (b) Birth canal
      (c) Breastfeeding

Absence of epididymis, seminal vesicles, vas deferens, prostate gland

External genitalia remain female

No DHT effect external genitalia

Vagina ends as blind pouch; lower two-thirds *not* paramesonephric duct origin

Present with primary amenorrhea as teenager

Gynecomastia postpubertal finding

Testes at risk for gonadoblastoma

Karyotype (male or female)

Normal serum testosterone/DHT for male

↑Serum LH

↑Serum estradiol

Female phenotypic findings; estrogen activity unopposed; estrogen receptors present

Testosterone function neutralized due to absent/nonfunctioning receptors

Mutation analysis androgen receptor gene detects mutations

Majority reared female

Defect recognized only at birth

MCC death children <1 year old

Genetic abnormalities

Chromosome aberrations MC; single-gene mutations

Maternal abnormalities

Maternal DM

NTDs/CHD

Fetal macrosomia (↑fetal insulin)

Hyperinsulinemia ↑muscle mass/fat

Maternal SLE

Congenital heart block (anti-Ro antibodies)

Maternal hypothyroidism

Cretinism/mental impairment

Thyroid hormone required for brain development

Alcohol: MC teratogen (fetal alcohol syndrome)

Congenital infections

TORCH: toxoplasmosis, other agents, rubella, CMV, herpes simplex virus

Newborns: ↑cord blood IgM

Newborns should *not* have IgM

CMV MC congenital infection

Vertical transmission (mother to baby)

Transplacental MC

Birth canal, breast-feeding

TABLE 6-4 **Teratogens Acting on Pregnant Women That May Adversely Affect Structure and Function of the Fetus and Newborn**

TERATOGEN	DEFECTS
ACE inhibitor and angiotensin receptor antagonists	• IUGR, renal failure, Potter-like syndrome, pulmonary hypoplasia, increased risk of orofacial clefts and cardiovascular defects (especially cardiac septal defects) • Mechanism: inhibiting fetal urine production (oligohydramnios) leads to renal dysplasia and renal failure, hypoplastic calvaria (skullcap covering the cranial cavity containing the brain is not fully developed), and IUGR
Alcohol (Fig. 6-28 A, B)	• Mental impairment (leading cause in the Western Hemisphere), microcephaly, congenital heart defects (VSD, ASD), attention deficit, diagnostic facial features (upper lip thinning, epicanthal folds, flat nasal bridge, short nose, hirsute forehead, and short palpebral fissures) • Mechanism: acetaldehyde (breakdown product of alcohol metabolism) disrupts cellular differentiation and growth (disrupts retinoic acid and hedgehog signaling pathways), disrupts DNA and protein synthesis, and inhibits cell migration
Amphetamine	• Congenital heart defects, IUGR, behavioral deficiencies, learning disabilities, cranial abnormalities, oral cleft and limb defects, and abnormal brain development closely resembling those in ill, asphyxiated infants • Mechanism: neurotoxicity on mature neurons due to the production of reactive oxygen species and nitric oxide, and p53 activation resulting in apoptosis, and mitochondrial dysfunction
Aspirin (acetylsalicylic acid)	• Increased risk of orofacial clefts and cardiovascular defects, especially cardiac septal defects • Mechanism: acetylsalicylic acid (aspirin) is the only NSAID that irreversibly inhibits cyclooxygenase by acetylation. Cyclooxygenases produce prostaglandins that play a significant role in keeping the ductus arteriosus open and increasing blood flow in the placenta.
Carbon monoxide	• Cerebral atrophy, microcephaly, seizures • Mechanism: activation of an inflammatory cascade resulting in oxidative damage and brain lipid peroxidation (free radical damage)
Cocaine	• Microcephaly, low birth weight, renal agenesis, intestinal atresia, congenital heart disease, urinary tract abnormalities (urethral obstruction, hydronephrosis, hypospadias [urethra opens on undersurface of penis]) • Mechanism: disruption of normal growth and development as a result of vascular insufficiency
DES	• Vaginal and/or cervical clear cell carcinoma (develops from remnants of paramesonephric ducts; see Fig. 22-3 B) paramesonephric duct defects (uterine abnormalities, cervical incompetence) • Mechanism: DES inhibits normal differentiation of paramesonephric structures.
Phenytoin	• Nail and distal phalanx hypoplasia, cleft lip and/or palate, neuroblastoma, bleeding (vitamin K deficiency) • Mechanism: embryonic hypoxia during susceptible periods. Oxidative stress (free radical damage).
Progesterone	• Virilization of female fetus • Mechanism: progesterone structurally related to testosterone and can virilize female fetuses (enlarged clitoris)
Retinoic acid	• Craniofacial dysmorphisms, cleft palate, thymic aplasia, and neural tube defects • Mechanism: disrupts *Hox* gene function (important in determining the different structures that develop in the anterior-posterior axis)
Statin drugs	• IUGR, limb deficiencies, VACTERAL (vertebral, anal, cardiac, TE fistula, renal, arterial, limb) • Mechanism: interference with Hedgehog proteins, which are key regulators of embryonic growth, patterning and morphogenesis of many structures; therefore, downregulation of the synthesis of these proteins may lead to birth defects.
Thalidomide (Fig. 6-29)	• Amelia (absent limbs), phocomelia (seal-like limbs), deafness • Mechanism: oxidative stress and anti-angiogenesis; drug binds to thalidomide-binding protein, cereblon (CRBN), and inhibiting its ubiquitin ligase activity
Tobacco (nicotine)	• IUGR, low birth weight, prone to sudden infant death syndrome; does not produce congenital malformations • Mechanism: oxidative stresses (free radicals)
Valproate	• Neural tube defects (valproate is a folate antagonist), autism • Spina bifida, facial and cardiac anomalies, limb defects, impaired neurologic function, autism spectrum disorder • Mechanism: folic acid antagonist (neural tube defects) • Oxidative stress
Warfarin	• Nasal hypoplasia, agenesis corpus callosum, fetal bleeding, death • Mechanism: hemorrhages into developing organs
Methotrexate	• Craniofacial and limb abnormalities • Mechanism: folic acid antagonist
Tetracycline	• Teeth pigmentation, hypoplasia of enamel, retarded skeletal growth, cataract, limb malformations • Mechanism: crosses the placental membrane and deposits in bones and teeth in the embryo
Lithium	• Ebstein tricuspid valve abnormalities • Mechanism: targets glycogen synthase kinase-3, which is a negative regulator of the Wnt signaling pathway, which regulates embryonic patterning and organogenesis
Streptomycin	• Ototoxicity • Mechanism: enters hair cells where it induces cell death via free radicals, disruption of mitochondrial protein synthesis, and activation of caspases and nucleases leading to apoptosis

ACE, Angiotensin-converting enzyme; *ASD,* atrial septal defect; *DES,* diethylstilbestrol; *IUGR,* intrauterine growth impairment; *TE,* tracheoesophageal; *VSD,* ventricular septal defect.

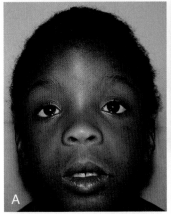
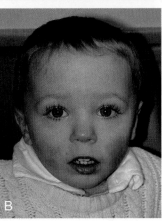

6-28: Fetal alcohol syndrome. **A,** Note the wide-spread eyes (hyper-telorism), inner epicanthal folds, short nose, hirsute forehead, and thin upper lip. **B,** Note the low nasal root, short palpebral fissures, smooth philtrum, and thin upper lip. *(A from Zitelli B: Atlas of Pediatric Physical Diagnosis, 3rd ed, London, Mosby, 1997; B from Jorde LB, Carey JC, Bamshad MJ: Medical Genetics, 4th ed, Philadelphia, Mosby Elsevier, 2010, p 307, Clinical Commentary 15-5: Fetal Alcohol Syndrome.)*

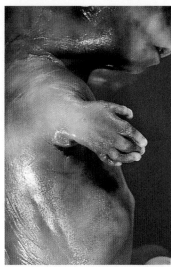

6-29: Phocomelia. This fetus shows incomplete development of the arm. This congenital malformation may occur spontaneously but is particularly associated with the chemical teratogen thalidomide. *(From Stevens A, Lowe J, Scott I: Core Pathology, 3rd ed, Mosby Elsevier, 2009, p 56, Fig. 5.3.)*

TABLE 6-5 Congenital Infections Associated With Congenital Defects

INFECTION	TRANSMISSION	CLINICAL FINDINGS
Cytomegalovirus (Fig. 6-30 A, B)	Transplacental	• Deafness, IUGR, CNS calcification (periventricular in 40% of cases), petechiae (50% of cases), hepatomegaly with jaundice (40% of cases), thrombocytopenia • Culture urine (best fluid to culture); urine cytology findings: large cells with eosinophilic intranuclear inclusions
Herpes simplex type 2	Birth canal	• IUGR, vesicular lesions or scarring, keratoconjunctivitis, microcephaly
Rubella (Fig. 6-30 C, D, E)	Transplacental	• Deafness (sensorineural), PDA, cataract, thrombocytopenia ("blueberry muffin" rash), hepatomegaly
Syphilis (Fig. 6-30 F, G; Fig. 18-3 H)	Transplacental	• Occurs after 20 weeks gestation • Hepatitis, saddle nose, blindness, notched/peg teeth
Toxoplasmosis (Fig. 26-16 D, E)	Transplacental	• Blindness (chorioretinitis), deafness (sensorineural), CNS calcification (basal ganglia), IUGR, hydrocephalus, hepatosplenomegaly • Pregnant women should avoid cat litter, raw meat
Varicella	Transplacental	• Limb defects, mental impairment, blindness (chorioretinitis), cataracts, skin scars
HIV	Transplacental, birth canal, breast-feeding	• Oral thrush, recurrent bacterial infections, intracranial calcification, failure to thrive

CNS, Central nervous system; *HIV,* human immunodeficiency virus; *IUGR,* intrauterine growth impairment; *PDA,* patent ductus arteriosus.

   e. Ionizing radiation (1% of cases). Produces malformations (see later) in the embryonic period (see later) causing microcephaly, skull defects, blindness, and ONT defects (NTDs; e.g., spina bifida).
   f. Multifactorial inheritance (20%–25% of cases), including ONT defects (see Fig. 26-4 A–D), CHD, and cleft lip/palate (Fig. 6-31)
4. Types of errors in morphogenesis
   a. Malformation
      (1) **Definition:** Disturbance in the morphogenesis (development) of an organ
      (2) Malformations mainly occur during embryogenesis (first 9 weeks of pregnancy; Fig. 6-32).
         (a) Most malformations occur between the third and ninth weeks of embryogenesis.
         (b) Most susceptible embryonic period for developing a malformation is during the *fourth* and *fifth weeks*, when organs are being formed from the germ cell layers (ectoderm, endoderm, and mesoderm).

Ionizing radiation

Microcephaly, skull defects, blindness, open NTDs

Overall MCC congenital anomalies

ONT defects, CHD, cleft lip/palate

Malformation

Disturbance organ morphogenesis embryonic period

Embryogenesis first 9 wks pregnancy

Most occur between 3rd–9th weeks

4th–5th week most susceptible embryonic period

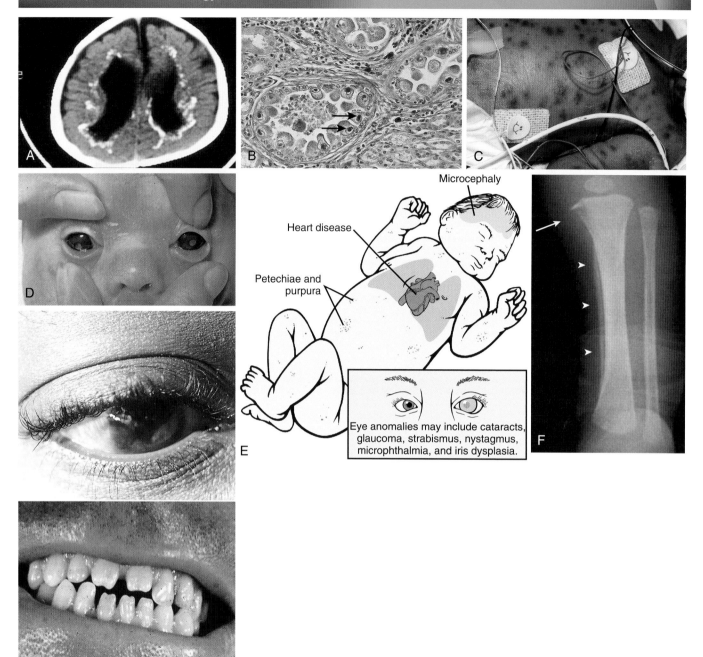

6-30: **A,** Computerized tomography of an infant with congenital cytomegalovirus (CMV) infection with periventricular calcification, a classic finding in congenital CMV. **B,** Congenital CMV infection. Note the characteristic **enlarged** renal tubular cells with basophilic (**usually eosinophilic**) nuclear inclusions *(arrows).* **C,** Congenital rubella with blueberry muffin lesions. Multiple violaceous, infiltrative papules and nodules in this newborn with congenital rubella. **D,** Bilateral cataracts and blindness in a newborn with congenital rubella. Note the opaque lenses in both eyes. Congenital rubella syndrome is marked by a triad that includes microcephaly, microphthalmia, and congenital heart disease. **E, G,** Hutchinson triad of late congenital syphilis: Top slide shows interstitial keratitis (white patches over pupil), which may lead to blindness. Bottom slide shows Hutchinson notched incisors. **F,** Radiograph of an infant with congenital syphilis showing a periosteal reaction along the shaft of the left tibia *(arrowheads;* saber shin) and a characteristic lucency of the medial proximal tibial metaphysis *(long white arrow)* called the Wimberger sign, which represents bony destruction. *(A from Shakoor A, Sy A, Acharya N: Ocular manifestations of intrauterine infections. In Pediatric Ophthalmology and Strabismus, ed 4, Philadelphia, Elsevier, 2013, p 81; B from my friend Ivan Damjanov, MD, PhD, Linder J: Anderson's Pathology, 10th ed, St. Louis, Mosby, 1996, p 349, Fig. 16.28 A; C from Paller AS, Mancini AJ: Hurwitz Clinical Pediatric Dermatology, 4th ed, Saunders, 2011, p 29, Fig. 2.39; D from Forbes CD, Jackson WF: Color Atlas and Text of Clinical Medicine, 3rd ed, Mosby, 2003 p 13, Fig. 1.43; E from my friend Ivan Damjanov, MD, PhD: Pathology for the Health Professions, 4th ed, Saunders Elsevier, 2012, p 96, Fig. 5-4; F from Donnelly LF: Pediatric Imaging: The Fundamentals, Philadelphia, 2009, Saunders, p 171; G courtesy of CDC Still Pictures Archives; from Morse SA, Holmes KK, Ballard RC, Moreland AA: Atlas of Sexually Transmitted Diseases and AIDS, 4th ed, Saunders Elsevier, 2010, p 292, Figs. 16.24 and 16.25.)*

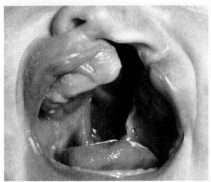

6-31: Cleft palate. Note the absence of the palate. *(Courtesy Christine L. Williams, MD; from Zitelli B, McIntire S, Nowalk A:* Zitelli and Davis' Atlas of Pediatric Physical Diagnosis, *6th ed, Saunders Elsevier, 2012, p 9, Fig. 1.20 B.)*

b. Deformation
  (1) **Definition:** Congenital anomaly caused by extrinsic factors that physically impinge on fetal development in utero
  (2) Occurs between the ninth week and term *after* fetal organs have developed
  (3) Most often associated with restricted movement of the fetus in the uterine cavity (called uterine restraint)
    (a) Maternal factors such as a malformed uterus or large leiomyomas (smooth muscle tumors) in the uterine wall that bulge into the uterine cavity
    (b) Placental factors such as oligohydramnios (reduced amount of amniotic fluid; see later) or twin pregnancies

> **Amniotic fluid** is predominantly composed of fetal urine. **Oligohydramnios** (decreased amniotic fluid) occurs from decreased production of fetal urine (e.g., renal agenesis, cystic disease of the kidneys). Oligohydramnios restricts fetal movement in the uterine cavity. As a result, newborns have flat facial features (Potter facies), compression of the skull vault, dysplastic/displaced ears, underdevelopment of the chest wall, and club feet (talipes equinovarus; Fig. 6-33 A, B; Links 6-17 and 6-18).

c. Disruption
  (1) **Definition:** Type of deformation that results from destruction of irreplaceable normal fetal tissue
  (2) Deformation may be due to vascular insufficiency (e.g., thrombosis of vessels in the placenta), trauma, or teratogens.
  (3) Disruption may be due to amniotic bands (Link 6-19). Rupture of the amnion (lines the fetal sac) is associated with the formation of fibrous bands that encircle parts of the fetus leading to partial amputation of a limb or constriction rings around digits (Fig. 6-34 A, B).
d. Agenesis
  (1) **Definition:** Complete absence of an organ due to absence of the anlage (primordial tissue)
  Example: renal agenesis
e. Aplasia
  (1) **Definition:** Defective development or congenital absence of an organ or tissue. The anlage (primordial tissue) is present but it *never develops* into an organ.
  (2) Example: In lung aplasia, the tissue only contains rudimentary ducts and connective tissue.
f. Hypoplasia
  (1) **Definition:** Primordial tissue develops incompletely, but the tissue is histologically normal.
  (2) Examples: microcephaly (small brain), hypoplastic left heart
g. Atresia
  (1) **Definition:** Incomplete formation of a lumen
  (2) Example: small bowel atresia (Fig. 6-35; Fig. 18-22 C)
C. **Pathogenesis of congenital anomalies**
  1. Timing of the teratogenic insult (see Fig. 6-32)
    a. Malformations occur during the embryonic period (from 3 to 9 weeks).
    b. Deformations occur during the fetal period (ninth week to term).

Deformation

Extrinsic disturbance *after* fetal organs developed

9th week to term

Uterine restraint

Maternal factors: malformed uterus, uterine leiomyomas

Placental factors: oligohydramnios, twin pregnancies

Amniotic fluid: fetal urine. Deformation: oligohydramnios causing Potter facies, club feet

Disruption

Destruction irreplaceable normal fetal tissue

Vascular insufficiency, trauma, teratogens

Rupture amnion → fibrous bands constrict fetal parts (e.g., digits)

Agenesis

Complete absence organ; absence primordial tissue

Renal agenesis

Aplasia

Defective development/ congenital absence of organ or tissue

Lung aplasia

Hypoplasia

Incomplete development primordial tissue; tissue normal

Atresia

Incomplete lumen formation

Timing teratogenic insult

Malformation: embryonic period (3rd–9th week)

Deformation: fetal period (9th week to term)

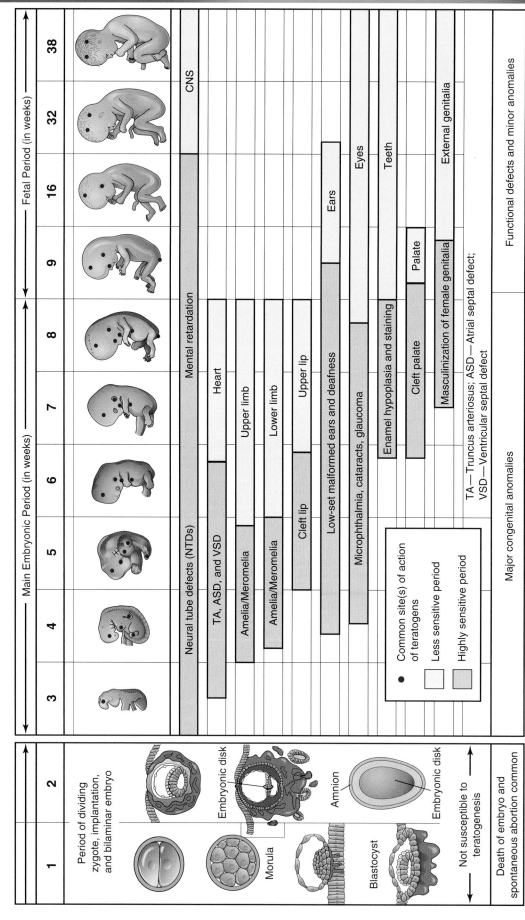

6-32: Sensitive or critical periods in embryonic development. Congenital anomalies that occur in the embryonic period (first 9 weeks of pregnancy) produce malformations. Anomalies after that period produce deformations. (*From Seidel H, Ball J, Dains J, Benedict G: Mosby's Guide to Physical Examination, 6th ed, St. Louis, Mosby Elsevier, 2006, p 111, Fig. 5.5.*)

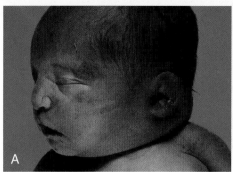
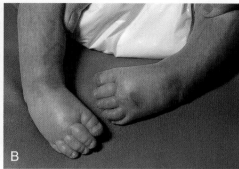

6-33: A, Potter facies. Note the flattened nose and facial features, micrognathia (small lower jaw), dysplastic/displaced ears, and the compression of the skull vault. These changes occurred because of oligohydramnios (decreased amniotic fluid), which restricted fetal movement in the uterine cavity. **B,** Club feet (talipes equinovarus). (*A from Zitelli B, McIntire S. Nowalk A: Zitelli's and Davis' Atlas of Pediatric Physical Diagnosis, 6th ed, Philadelphia, Saunders, 2012, p 551, Fig. 13-38; B from Swartz M: Textbook of Physical Diagnosis: History and Examination, 5th ed, Philadelphia, Saunders Elsevier, 2006, p 784, Fig. 24.22.)*

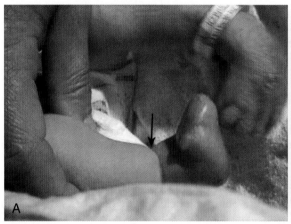
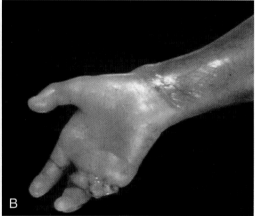

6-34: A, Amniotic band syndrome. Note the constriction ring at the ankle and amputation of the toes, a sequela to the amniotic bands. **B,** The amniotic band sequence includes fetal hand deformities. Note the missing fingers. (*A from Zitelli B, McIntire S, Nowalk A: Zitelli and Davis' Atlas of Pediatric Physical Diagnosis, 6th ed, Saunders Elsevier, 2012, p 10, Fig. 1-21; B from Crum CP, Nucci MR, Lee KR, et al: Diagnostic Gynecologic and Obstetric Pathology, 2nd ed, Saunders Elsevier, 2011, p 1013, Fig. 32.26 A.)*

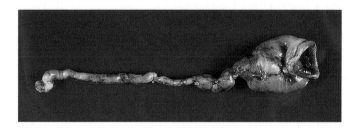

6-35: Congenital small bowel atresia. Note the long atretic segment of the small bowel. Normal small bowel is at the end of the atretic segment. (*From Rosai J: Rosai and Ackerman's Surgical Pathology, 10th ed, Mosby Elsevier, 2011, p 674, Fig. 11.78.)*

2. Alterations occur during key steps in morphogenesis.
   a. Mutations may occur in genes normally involved in morphogenesis. Example: Mutations of the *Hox* genes alter the development of craniofacial structures.
   b. Alterations in cell proliferation, migration, and apoptosis may occur.

> Alterations key steps in morphogenesis
>
> *HOX* genes involved in morphogenesis craniofacial structures
>
> Alterations cell proliferation, migration; ↑apoptosis

Pregnant women should *not* be treated for acne with retinoic acid. Retinoic acid disrupts the function of the *Hox* genes, which are important in producing proteins that are involved in the patterning of craniofacial structures, vertebrae, and limbs. Dysfunction of these genes results in craniofacial, CNS, and cardiovascular defects.

VII. Perinatal and Infant Disorders
A. Stillbirth
1. **Definition:** The birth of a dead child
2. Epidemiology

> *Hox* genes involved in patterning craniofacial structures, vertebrae, limbs; retinoic acid disrupts *Hox* genes
>
> Stillbirth
>
> Birth of dead child

a. Most frequently caused by an abruptio placentae. In placental abruption, there is premature separation of the placenta because of a retroplacental blood clot (see Fig. 22-15 E).

b. Other causes include maternal DM, infection, and Rh hemolytic disease (RHD) of newborn.

B. **Spontaneous abortion (miscarriage)**

1. **Definition:** Any pregnancy that is not viable or in which the fetus is born before the 20th week of pregnancy

2. Epidemiology

a. Most common complication in early pregnancy

(1) Overall spontaneous abortion rate is 15% to 20%.

(2) Majority occur in the first trimester of pregnancy.

b. Most often (≈50% of cases) caused by a fetal karyotypic abnormality (e.g., trisomy 16).

c. Predisposing factors include advanced maternal age, infections (e.g., *Streptococcus agalactiae*, *Listeria monocytogenes*), and tobacco and alcohol use.

C. **Sudden infant death syndrome (SIDS)**

1. **Definition:** Sudden and unexpected death of an apparently healthy infant under 1 year of age, which remains unexplained after a thorough case investigation and autopsy

2. Epidemiology

a. In the United States, SIDS is the most common cause of death of an infant between age 1 month and 1 year.

b. Most SIDS deaths occur between 2 and 4 months of age. Approximately 90% of SIDS cases occur in infants <6 months of age.

c. Death usually occurs during sleep.

d. Pathogenesis

(1) No single cause of SIDS (multifactorial condition)

(2) Maternal risk factors include smoking, young age, frequent childbirths, and inadequate prenatal care.

(3) Infant risk factors include prematurity, prior sibling with SIDS, prior history of a mild respiratory infection, sleeping prone or on the side (should be supine), neural developmental delay, and a brainstem defect, which increases the risk for not being able to be aroused from slow wave sleep.

3. Autopsy findings

a. Petechiae on the visceral and parietal pleura, epicardium, and thymus are the most common findings (≈80% of cases).

b. Nonspecific signs of tissue hypoxia are present (e.g., extramedullary hematopoiesis [hematopoiesis outside the bone marrow]; see Chapter 12).

c. Thickened pulmonary arteries (sign of pulmonary hypertension) are present with pulmonary vascular engorgement and edema.

d. Brainstem shows microscopic changes from hypoxia (e.g., hypoplasia of the arcuate nucleus).

e. Astrogliosis (hypertrophy and hyperplasia of astrocytes) is present in the cerebellum and brainstem.

D. **Prematurity and intrauterine growth impairment**

1. Newborn classification is based on weight and gestational age.

a. Appropriate for gestational age (AGA)

b. Small for gestational age (SGA); has the highest mortality rate

c. Large for gestational age (LGA); most often associated with maternal DM

2. Prematurity

a. **Definition:** Gestational age of the newborn that is <37 weeks. Premature newborns usually weigh <2500 g.

b. Epidemiology

(1) Prematurity is the most common cause of neonatal death and morbidity.

(2) Risk factors for prematurity

(a) Premature rupture of the membranes (PROM; most common cause)

(b) Intrauterine infections

• Chorioamnionitis: inflammation of the placental membranes

• Funisitis: inflammation of the umbilical cord

• Pathogens that have been implicated in intrauterine infections include *Streptococcus agalactiae* (MCC), *Ureaplasma urealyticum*, *Mycoplasma hominis*, *Gardnerella vaginalis*, *Trichomonas vaginalis*, *Neisseria gonorrhoeae*, and *Chlamydia trachomatis*.

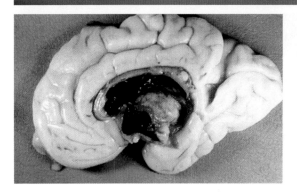

6-36: Intraventricular hemorrhage in an infant with prematurity. *(From my friend Ivan Damjanov, MD, PhD: Pathology for the Health-Related Professions, 2nd ed, Philadelphia, Saunders, 2000, p 120, Fig. 5-29.)*

      (c) Placental abnormalities: placenta previa, abruptio placentae (see Chapter 22)

      (d) Twin pregnancies (see Chapter 22)

      (e) Maternal factors: poor nutrition, low socioeconomic status, and smoking

    (3) Complications

      (a) Respiratory distress syndrome (decreased surfactant; see Chapter 17)

      (b) Necrotizing enterocolitis (intestinal ischemia; see Chapter 18)

      (c) Intraventricular hemorrhage (Fig. 6-36; Link 6-20)

  3. Intrauterine growth retardation (IUGR)

    a. **Definition:** Newborn that is <10% of the predicted fetal weight for the gestational age

    b. Epidemiology

      (1) IUGR usually occurs in SGA infants.

      (2) Majority of cases of IUGR in SGA infants are of maternal origin and are associated with preeclampsia (see Chapter 22), poor nutrition, drug addiction, alcoholism, and smoking.

      (3) Fetal causes of IUGR include chromosomal disorders, congenital malformations, and congenital infections. *Symmetric* growth impairment is found in all organ systems.

      (4) Placental causes of IUGR include abruptio placentae (premature separation of the placenta from the implantation site), placental infarction due to vessel thrombosis, and a single umbilical artery (umbilical cord should contain one umbilical vein and two umbilical arteries).

        • Unlike fetal causes of intrauterine growth retardation, which show symmetric growth retardation, in placental causes of IGUR there is an asymmetric growth impairment. Example: The brain is spared relative to visceral organs such as the liver.

      (5) About 85% of infants with IUGR have oligohydramnios (decreased amount of amniotic fluid) caused by diversion of blood flow from peripheral organs (kidneys) to the brain and reduced renal perfusion and urinary flow rates (amniotic fluid is predominantly fetal urine).

    c. Ultrasonography is a common initial step in the workup of IUGR.

 E. **Neonatal period**

  1. **Definition:** The first 4 weeks of life

  2. Epidemiology

    a. Majority of deaths in childhood occur during this period.

    b. Common causes of death include respiratory distress syndrome and congenital anomalies.

    c. Selected neonatal period extracranial hemorrhages are associated with delivery (Fig. 6-37).

VIII. Diagnosis of Genetic and Developmental Disorders

 A. **Invasive testing**

  1. Amniocentesis (Link 6-21)

    a. Amniocentesis (needle removal of fluid from the amniotic sac) is used to identify prenatal genetic defects.

    b. Risk of complications is increased if amniocentesis is performed early in the pregnancy (e.g., 10th to 14th weeks).

    c. Amniotic fluid, primarily composed of fetal urine, contains fetal cells that can be cultured for fetal tests.

Marginal notes:

Placental abnormalities: placenta previa, abruption placentae

Twin pregnancies

Maternal factors: poor nutrition, smoking

Respiratory distress syndrome

Necrotizing enterocolitis

Intraventricular hemorrhage

IUGR

Newborn <10% predicted fetal weight for gestational age

MC in SGA infants

Majority SGAs maternal origin: preeclampsia, drugs, smoking, alcohol

Fetal causes: chromosome disorders, malformations, infections

Fetal: symmetric growth impairment

Placental causes: abruption, infarction, single umbilical artery

Placental asymmetric growth impairment

Brain spared relative to visceral organs

85% IUGR have oligohydramnios

Ultrasonography: common initial step in workup of IUGR

Neonatal period: first 4 weeks of life

Majority of deaths in childhood

Respiratory distress syndrome/congenital anomalies

Amniocentesis: removal fluid from amniotic sac

Identifies prenatal genetic defects

↑Complications if amniocentesis early in pregnancy

Amniotic fluid: primarily fetal urine; contains fetal cells (fetal tests)

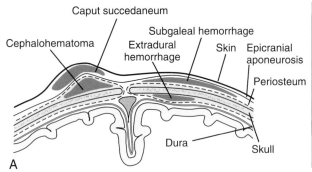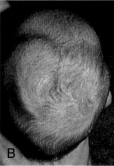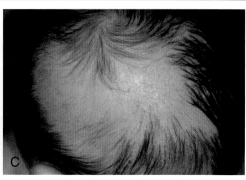

6-37: A, Sites of extracranial (and extradural) hemorrhages in the newborn. Schematic diagram of the important tissue planes from skin to dura. **B,** Cephalohematoma. A cephalohematoma is a subperiosteal hematoma overlying the calvarium. These lesions are more common following prolonged labor, instrument-assisted deliveries, and abnormal presentations. They usually develop over the first hours of life and present as subcutaneous swellings in the scalp. They do not cross the midline, as they are limited to one cranial bone, which helps distinguish them from caput succedaneum. Note the sharp demarcation at the midline. **C,** Caput succedaneum is a localized edema of the newborn scalp related to the mechanical forces involved in parturition. It is probably related to venous congestion and edema secondary to cervical and uterine pressure and, as such, is more common with prolonged parturition and seen most often in primigravidas. Caput presents as a boggy scalp mass and may result in varying degrees of bruising and necrosis in addition to the edema, at times with tissue loss. In distinction to cephalohematoma, caput succedaneum lesions often cross the midline. These lesions tend to resolve spontaneously over 48 hours, and treatment is generally unnecessary. This 4-month-old boy shows generalized thinning of scalp hair, reflecting telogen effluvium. He also had suction, leading to caput succedaneum and "halo alopecia." **(A** from Pape KE, Wigglesworth JS: Haemorrhage, Ischaemia and the Perinatal Brain, *Philadelphia, JB Lippincott, 1979; as modified in Zitelli B, McIntire S, Nowalk A:* Zitelli and Davis' Atlas of Pediatric Physical Diagnosis, *6th ed, Saunders Elsevier, 2012, p 55, Fig. 2-32;* **B, C** from Paller AS, Mancini AJ: Hurwitz Clinical Pediatric Dermatology, *4th ed, Saunders, 2011, pp 12, 131, Figs. 2-3, 7-2, respectively.)*

AFP measured in amniotic fluid	d. α-Fetoprotein (AFP) is commonly measured in amniotic fluid.
Fetal glycoprotein synthesized fetal liver; enters maternal blood	(1) Fetal glycoprotein is produced mainly in the fetal liver, secreted into the circulation, and excreted by the kidneys.
AFP measured in amniotic fluid/maternal serum	(2) Fetal glycoprotein enters the maternal bloodstream via the placenta, amniotic membranes, and maternal-fetal circulation, which explains why AFP is measured in amniotic fluid and maternal serum.
Chorionic villus sampling	2. Chorionic villus sampling
Transcervical or transabdominal	a. Test is performed transcervically or transabdominally between the 10th and 12th weeks of pregnancy.
Detects fetal abnormalities earlier than amniocentesis	b. Results of possible fetal abnormalities are available earlier in the pregnancy than with amniocentesis.

B. Noninvasive testing

Ultrasonography	1. Ultrasonography
Fetal age/sex/viability, multiple pregnancies, morphologic abnormalities	a. Ultrasonography is important in the assessment of fetal age, fetal sex, multiple pregnancies, fetal viability, and for detection of possible fetal morphologic abnormalities.
ONT defects, Turner syndrome, osteogenesis imperfecta	b. Examples of fetal abnormalities that are detected include ONT defects (e.g., anencephaly, meningomyelocele), cystic hygroma (Turner syndrome), chromosomal aneuploidy syndromes (e.g., trisomy syndromes, Turner syndrome), and certain types of single-gene disorders (e.g., osteogenesis imperfecta).
AFP	2. Maternal triple marker screening
↑AFP ONT defects; ↓AFP Down syndrome	a. AFP
ONT defects: due to folic acid deficiency *before* conception	(1) Increased in ONT defects and decreased in Down syndrome
	(2) ONT defects are causally related to folic acid deficiency *before* conception. Emphasizes the importance of providing folic acid as a vitamin supplement.
Serum hCG	b. Serum human chorionic gonadotropin (hCG)
↑hCG with gestational age	(1) Levels of hCG increase with gestational age.
↑hCG in Down syndrome	(2) In Down syndrome, serum hCG is increased.
uE3	c. Unconjugated estriol (uE3)
uE3 excellent marker fetal/ placental/maternal dysfunction	(1) Estriol is an excellent marker of fetal, placental, and maternal dysfunction (see Chapter 22). It is a form of estrogen that is produced during pregnancy.
↓uE3 in Down syndrome	(2) In Down syndrome, there is a decrease in uE3.
Karyotyping; ID numeric/ structural abnormalities	**C. Genetic analysis**
	1. Chromosome karyotyping: karyotyping identifies numeric and structural abnormalities.
DNA molecular assays: PCR, FISH	2. DNA molecular assays (e.g., polymerase chain reaction [PCR], fluorescence in situ hybridization [FISH]). Highly sensitive and specific tests that are useful in diagnosing
Dx mutations	a spectrum of mutations.

IX. Aging

A. Theories of aging

1. Stochastic (random error) theories

   a. Somatic mutation theory
      - **Definition:** Proposes that genetic damage from ionizing radiation produces mutations in DNA leading to failure in critical bodily functions

   b. DNA repair theory
      - **Definition:** States that the inability to repair DNA damage is responsible for age-related and dependent detrimental effects

   c. Cross-linking theory
      (1) **Definition:** Suggests that increased cross-linking of proteins in the extracellular matrix (e.g., collagen, elastin, crystallin) impairs the diffusion of essential nutrients to tissue
      (2) Nonenzymatic glycosylation (NEG; a type of cross-linking involving glucose attachment to proteins) is also thought to impair diffusion of essential nutrients to tissue. Example: Glycosylation of collagen and the eye lens protein crystallin is associated with cataracts in older people.

   d. Free radical theory (see Chapter 2)
      (1) **Definition:** Suggests that most aging changes are due to free radical damage of cell membranes and nuclear proteins
      (2) High levels of free radical metabolizing enzymes (e.g., superoxide dismutase) have been found in longer-lived species.

2. Programmed cell death theory

   a. **Definition:** Proposes that the process of aging is part of a genetically programmed continuum of development and maturation

   b. Supported by the similarity of attained age in identical versus nonidentical twins, increased longevity in certain families, and the presence of genetic defects in people with premature aging (e.g., Down syndrome; progeria)

B. Age-dependent changes
- **Definition:** Changes are inevitable with age (Table 6-6).

C. Age-related changes
- **Definition:** Changes of greater incidence with age but *not* inevitable with age (Table 6-7)

D. Changes with aging and clinical consequences (Figs. 6-38, 6-39, and 6-40)

Margin notes:
Stochastic theories
Somatic mutation theory
Genetic damage from ionizing radiation
DNA repair theory
Inability to repair DNA damage
Cross-linking theory
↑Cross-linking proteins impairs diffusion nutrients to tissue
NEG impairs diffusion nutrients to tissues
NEG collagen and crystalline in lens → cataracts in aging
Free radical theory of aging
Free radical injury cell membranes/nuclear proteins
↑Superoxide dismutase found in long-lived species
Programmed cell death theory
Genetically programmed continuum development/maturation
Age-dependent: changes inevitable with age (e.g., ↓glomerular filtration rate [GFR])
Age-related: changes common but *not* inevitable; e.g., Alzheimer disease

TABLE 6-6   Age-Dependent Changes (Figs. 6-38, 6-39)

SYSTEM	DESCRIPTION
Auditory	• Presbycusis: sensorineural hearing loss, particularly at high frequency • Otosclerosis: fusion of ear ossicles producing conductive hearing loss
Body composition	• Total body fat increases while total body water and lean body mass decrease. Water-soluble medications (e.g., cimetidine, digoxin, ethanol) have decreased volume of distribution causing higher levels in the plasma. Fat-soluble drugs (e.g., chlordiazepoxide) have a larger volume of distribution causing a decreased plasma concentration. Excretion from the body is at a slower rate, which increases half-life and extends pharmacologic effects. • Energy balance in old age. Body composition is altered (muscle mass is decreased and percentage of body fat is increased). With the fall in lean body mass, the basal metabolic rate is decreased and energy requirements are reduced (see Chapter 8). • Weight often decreases after age 70 years. Reflects decreased appetite (sense of smell and taste is reduced) and decreased interest in food, particularly if there is a recent loss of a partner or close friend. • Body mass index is less reliable as height is lost due to kyphosis (anterior curvature of the spine), osteoporosis (collapse of the vertebra), and loss of intervertebral space, which results from degeneration of the intervertebral disks. • Although energy requirements decrease, the need for micronutrients does not decrease. A vitamin-rich diet is important. Vitamin D levels are frequently decreased (e.g., poor diet, lack of sun exposure, liver disease, renal disease, gastrointestinal disease). Vitamin D deficiency leads to bone loss and increased risk for fractures. Vitamin B_{12} deficiency may lead to dementia and demyelination syndromes in the spinal cord (subacute combined degeneration; see Chapter 12) and macrocytic anemia with pancytopenia (see Chapter 12). Lack of adequate amounts of folic acid may also lead to macrocytic anemia (see Chapter 12).

Continued

TABLE 6-6   Age-Dependent Changes (Figs. 6-38, 6-39)—cont'd

SYSTEM	DESCRIPTION
Cardiovascular	• Blunted maximal cardiovascular responses to exercise
Central nervous	• Cerebral atrophy with mild forgetfulness (see Fig. 2-15 A) • Impaired sleep patterns such as insomnia, early wakening • Decreased dopaminergic synthesis: parkinsonian-like gait • Decrease in cerebral blood flow and increase in blood-brain barrier permeability: increases sensitivity to medications that affect CNS • Increased sensitivity to drug effects • Drug adherence may be poor because of cognitive impairment, difficulty in swallowing (dry mouth), and complex polypharmacy regimes.
Female reproductive	• Breast and vulvar atrophy (see Fig. 22-2 A) • Decreased estrogen and progesterone: ↑FSH and LH, respectively
Gastrointestinal	• Decreased gastric acidity: predisposes to *Helicobacter pylori* infection • Decreased colonic motility: constipation predisposing to diverticulosis
General	• Increased body fat: decreased number of insulin receptors (glucose intolerance) • Genetic disease may present for the first time (e.g., Huntington disease). • Thermoregulatory problems are more common. Impairments in vasomotor function, skeletal muscle response, and sweating mean that older people will react more slowly to changes in temperature. Problems with thermoregulation are more likely in the presence of atherosclerosis and hypothyroidism as well as with medications such as sedatives and hypnotics. Hypothermia commonly complicates other acute illnesses such as pneumonia, stroke, and fractures. Financial pressures and old or nonfunctional heating systems may result in inadequate heating during cold weather.
Hepatobiliary	• Liver mass decreases 25%–35% with increasing age: liver blood flow decreases 35%–45%; hence, medications have a longer duration of effect.
Immune	• Decreased skin response to antigens (called anergy). • T-cell response declines with reduced delayed hypersensitivity responses. • Antibody function decreases for many exogenous antigens. Autoantibodies are more common; however, autoimmune diseases are less common. Up to 30% of healthy older people do not develop protective immunity after influenza vaccination. • Allergic reactions and transplant rejections are less common. • Susceptibility to infections increases (e.g., community acquired pneumonia). Latent infections such as tuberculosis and herpes zoster may be reactivated.
Male reproductive	• Prostate hyperplasia: predisposes to urinary retention (see Fig. 21-4 A) • Prostate cancer: most common cancer in men (see Fig. 21-4 C)
Musculoskeletal	• Osteoarthritis in weight-bearing joints: wearing down of articular cartilage in the femoral head (see Fig. 24-7 B)
Renal	• Kidney loses 20%–25% of renal mass as people age from 30 to 80 years. • Decreased GFR (↓10% per decade from the age of 30 years): increased risk of drug toxicity from slow clearance of drugs
Respiratory	• FEV_1/FVC ratio decreases with age due to decreased elastic recoil in the small airways with age. Smoking accelerates the decline. Symptoms occur when the FEV_1 drops below 50% of the predicted value. • Increased $\bar{V}/\dot{Q}$ mismatch due to a decrease in elastic recoil in the lung, particularly in dependent areas of the lung, thus reducing ventilation • Mild obstructive pattern in pulmonary function tests: e.g., ↑TLC, ↓vital capacity • Mild hypoxemia and increased A-a gradient
Skin	• Decreased skin elasticity due to increased cross-bridge formation between collagen fibers • Senile purpura over the dorsum of the hands (see Fig. 15-7) and lower legs
Visual	• Cataracts: visual impairment, increased risk for falls (see Fig. 26-26 N) • Presbyopia: inability to focus on near objects

A-a, Alveolar-arterial; *FEV₁*, forced expiratory volume in 1 sec; *FSH*, follicle-stimulating hormone; *FVC*, forced vital capacity; *GFR*, glomerular filtration rate; *LH*, luteinizing hormone; *TLC*, total lung capacity; $\bar{V}/\dot{Q}$, ventilation/perfusion.

TABLE 6-7   Age-Related Changes (See Figs. 6-38 and 6-39)

SYSTEM	DESCRIPTION
Cardiovascular	• Atherosclerosis: increased risk for coronary artery disease, heart failure, peripheral vascular disease, strokes (see Fig. 10-5 C) • Aortic stenosis: most common valvular abnormality in older adults (see Fig. 11-18 A); common cause of syncope, angina, and heart failure (see Chapter 11) • Hypertension: Almost 50% of individuals older than 60 years have hypertension. This includes systolic hypertension, which commonly occurs due to loss of aortic elasticity. Treatment of the hypertension is essential to prevent myocardial infarction, heart failure, and stroke. • Increased risk for giant cell (temporal) arteritis: large vessel vasculitis involving aortic arch vessels (see Fig. 10-17 B) • Increased risk for congestive heart failure (CHF): CHF affects 5%–10% of individuals in their 80s. Causes of CHF include hypertension, atherosclerotic coronary artery disease, and calcific aortic valve stenosis. Diastolic dysfunction types of CHF (see Chapter 11) are more common, particularly in individuals with a history of poorly controlled hypertension. • Atrial fibrillation increases with age: This arrhythmia is present in 9% of individuals older than 80 years. Frequently complicated by diastolic heart failure. Common causes of atrial fibrillation should be excluded (e.g., hyperthyroidism). Atrial fibrillation increases the risk for developing embolic strokes, due to stasis of blood in the left atrium leading to thrombus formation (see Chapters 11 and 26). Anticoagulation to prevent thrombosis imposes additional risks; hence, the target International Normalized Ration (INR) needs to be lower because of increased risk for intracranial hemorrhage from embolic strokes. Direct thrombin inhibitors and factor Xa inhibitors are often used rather than warfarin. • Coronary artery atherosclerotic disease (see Fig. 10-5 B) causing angina increases with age: Women and men are almost equally at risk in the older population. Coexisting diseases such as anemia and thyroid disease exacerbate angina. Calcific aortic stenosis is also a common cause of angina and must be excluded. • Acute myocardial infarction (AMI; see Fig. 11-6) may have an atypical presentation in older adults. Lack of appetite (anorexia), generalized weakness or fatigue rather than bouts of chest pain may be the presentation rather than chest pain with radiation into the left arm. Hospital mortality often exceeds 25% in those individuals over 75 years old who have an AMI. Hazards of various treatments for an AMI also increase in older adults. • Infective endocarditis: Signs and symptoms are often *not* as dramatic as they are in younger individuals. Confusion, weight loss, malaise, and weakness may be the only clinical findings. Common causative agents for endocarditis are enterococci from the urinary tract (particularly if the patient has a urinary catheter) and *Streptococcus bovis* from the gastrointestinal tract (see Chapter 11). As expected, morbidity and mortality are much higher in the older than in the younger population. • Deep vein thrombosis of lower extremities (see Fig. 10-12 A): increased risk for patients who are bed-ridden at home, in nursing homes, or in hospitals
Central nervous system	• Alzheimer disease: most common cause of dementia in people older than 65 years (see Fig. 26-19 A, B) • Parkinson disease (see Fig. 26-20 A) • Subdural hematomas: due to falls (see Fig. 26-7 D, E) • Delirium: transient, reversible cognitive dysfunction. Occurs in 30% of older hospital patients either at admission or during their hospital stay. Precipitating factors include intercurrent illness (cardiac problems), surgery (hip replacement), change of environment, medications, sensory deprivation (no visitors), volume depletion (loss of insensible water from fever), pain, hypoxia, fever, acute urinary retention (more likely in older males), or alcohol withdrawal.
Endocrine	• Increase in type 2 DM (10% in older adults) • Renal threshold for glucose increases in older adults; hence, glucosuria may *not* develop until the blood glucose is markedly elevated. This may delay suspecting the presence of DM. • Pancreatic carcinoma in old age often presents with DM (loss of endocrine function) along with weight loss and diminished appetite (cachectins). • Increased risk for hyperthyroidism due to one or more nodules in multinodular goiter increasing the synthesis of thyroid hormone • Increased risk for euthyroid sick syndrome (see Chapter 23) • Nonspecific findings such as apathy, slowness, and constipation may be interpreted as part of aging and a diagnosis of hypothyroidism is missed. • Myxedema coma (severe hypothyroidism) is more common in older adults. • Rigorous treatment of hypothyroidism may exacerbate underlying disorders involving the heart. • Glucocorticoid therapy may be hazardous in older patients who have osteoporosis, DM, and hypertension. • Spontaneous hypoglycemia in older adults presents with focal neurologic abnormalities that can be confused with a stroke; hence, it is important to order a blood glucose test. • Pituitary tumors causing visual disturbances, amenorrhea, or sexual disturbances may be missed because these findings are often expected to be present in younger adults. • Diabetic foot ulcers are commonly associated with osteomyelitis.
Female reproductive	• Increased incidence of cancers of the breast, endometrium, ovary • Increased incidence of postmenopausal osteoporosis due to a lack in estrogen in women and testosterone in men (see Fig. 24-3 B) • Hirsutism and balding may occur in women due to an increase in androgens.

Continued

TABLE 6-7 Age-Related Changes (See Figs. 6-38 and 6-39)—cont'd

SYSTEM	DESCRIPTION
Gastrointestinal	• Increased incidence of colorectal cancer (see Fig. 18-28 F) • Diarrhea: Incidence is *not* increased but potential complications are more common (e.g., volume depletion, hypokalemia, metabolic acidosis). Pseudomembranous colitis from *Clostridium difficile* is more common, especially in hospitalized patients or those in nursing homes, owing to the loss of protective bacteria (e.g., patient is on antibiotics; Links 18-78 and 18-79). • Abdominal pain: Severity of pain and location are often blunted with age; hence, the presentation of pain may be atypical in appendicitis, diverticulitis, and cholecystitis. Older patients are more likely to have confusion, anorexia, or lack of pain to palpation. Cancer is more likely to be a cause of pain in older compared with younger people. • Gastroesophageal reflux (see Fig. 18-13 A) is increased; hence, esophagitis, strictures, and bleeding are more common. • Malabsorption due to small bowel bacterial overgrowth (jejunal diverticulosis, adverse effects of previous gastric surgery) and celiac disease is increased and often undiagnosed. • Constipation: Causes include lack of fiber intake, immobility, drugs that reduce colon transit time (antidepressants, antacids containing aluminum or calcium, antihistamines, diuretics, and anti-Parkinsonism drugs), and depression. • Common liver diseases in older adults include primary biliary cirrhosis, alcoholic liver disease (hepatitis, fatty change, cirrhosis), liver abscesses (majority from direct extension, biliary tract, portal vein, in decreasing order of occurrence), and hepatocellular carcinoma (arising out of a preexisting cirrhosis). • Gallbladder disease: Gallstones are present in ≈30% in women and ≈20% in men over 70 years of age (see Fig. 19-9 B). Complications related to acute cholecystitis are more likely to occur in older adults (i.e., perforation, empyema (gallbladder lumen is filled with pus).
Immune/Hematology	• Increased risk for MGUS: most common cause of monoclonal gammopathy (see Fig. 14-13) • Although the hemoglobin concentration normally declines in older adults, it is still within the normal reference interval. As expected, reduced volume of blood has its greatest effect on the central nervous system (dizziness, apathy) and the cardiovascular system (dyspnea, edema). Iron deficiency is more likely due to blood loss from the gastrointestinal system (serum ferritin is the best screening test). Anemia of chronic disease is likely to accompany chronic lung disease, rheumatologic disease, and malignancy. Macrocytic anemias are more likely to be due to vitamin B_{12} (pernicious anemia from chronic gastritis) and/or folic acid deficiency (related to poor diet). Chronic lymphocytic leukemia is commonly seen in older adults.
Musculoskeletal	• Osteoporosis: vertebral column in females and femoral head in males (see Fig. 24-3 A–C); age-related defect switch in which bone marrow stromal cells differentiate into adipocytes rather than osteoblasts. • Polymyalgia rheumatica: muscle and joint pain associated with an increased erythrocyte sedimentation rate • Secondary gout (see Fig. 24-9 A-D): Hyperuricemia causing gout in older adults is most often associated with thiazides and chronic kidney disease. Painful tophi and chronic symptoms are more common than acute gouty arthritis. Joints in the upper extremity are most commonly involved. • Peripheral vascular disease most likely affects the joints in the feet. • Prosthetic devices, hips and knees: Group D enterococci (*Streptococcus bovis*) are the organisms most commonly isolated (33% of cases).
Renal/lower urinary tract	• Renovascular hypertension secondary to atherosclerosis of the renal artery is more likely to occur (see Fig. 10-18 A). • Urinary incontinence (involuntary loss of urine) occurs in 15% of older women and 10% of older men. See Chapter 21 for a full discussion. • Nephrons decline in number with age; hence, the glomerular filtration rate progressively declines. The creatinine clearance decreases (normal 140 mL/min/1.73 m² at age 30 years to about 97 mL/min/1.73 m² at age 80 years). Renal tubular function declines with old age, leading to a decline in urinary concentration ability. Serum creatinine levels are also misleading in old age because of functional limitation of the kidneys. Use of drugs like diuretics, ACE inhibitors, and NSAIDS may increase the risk for developing acute kidney injury, especially if the dose of the drug or drugs is *not* age-adjusted. • Concurrent diseases increase the risk for acute kidney injury. Examples include prostate hyperplasia with urinary tract obstruction, renovascular hypertension due to atherosclerosis of the renal arteries, heart failure with a reduced cardiac output leading to decreased renal artery blood flow. • Asymptomatic bacteriuria increases with age. Up to 30% of older individuals will develop symptoms within a year. • Urinary catheters increase the risk for gram-negative bacteremia fivefold.
Respiratory	• Older people are less tachypneic (breathing rate less than expected) with a decrease in PaO_2 or increase in $PaCO_2$ (respiratory acidosis). • Impaired defenses against bacteria due to reduced numbers of glandular epithelial cells, which leads to a reduction of mucus production (normally has a protective effect against bacteria) • Maximum uptake of oxygen is decreased due to a combination of impairments in muscle and the cardiorespiratory system. • Loss of chest compliance (ability of the lungs to expand) is due to a combination of kyphosis (anterior curvature of the spine), reduced respiratory muscle strength, and endurance. This is usually *not* a major problem in older adults unless there is underlying respiratory disease. • Pneumonia: usually *Streptococcus pneumoniae* (see Fig. 17-5 A–D). Recurrent pneumonia is often due to aspiration of gastric contents and gastroesophageal reflux disease. • Primary lung cancer: particularly in smokers (see Fig. 17-17 A–D)

TABLE 6-7   Age-Related Changes (See Figs. 6-38 and 6-39)—cont'd

SYSTEM	DESCRIPTION
Skin	• Skin begins to show signs of aging between ages 30 and 35. Aged skin is thin (atrophic), fragile, and inelastic. Signs of atrophy include a thin epidermis and a gradual loss in blood vessels, dermal collagen, fat, and the number of elastic fibers (normally give skin elasticity and resilience [skin turgor when pinched]). Hair follicles, sweat ducts, and sebaceous glands are reduced, resulting in a decrease in perspiration and sebum production. Loss of elastic tissue causes shallow wrinkling of the skin that disappears when it is stretched. Sun-damaged skin is characterized by coarsening and yellowish discoloration, irregular pigmentation, roughness or dryness, telangiectasia (dilated capillaries), atrophy, and deep wrinkling. • UVB-induced cancers: e.g., basal cell carcinoma (most common; see Fig. 25-11 B, C) • Actinic (solar) keratosis: precursor for squamous cell carcinoma (see Fig. 25-11 A) • Pressure sores (Fig. 6-40): Pressure on capillaries is the most important risk factor.
Visual	• Macular degeneration: most common cause of blindness in older adults (see Fig. 26-26 L)
Miscellaneous	• Falls: Approximately 30%–40% of people over 60 years of age fall each year. Falls account for 90% of hip fractures in older adults. Acute illness may be an underlying cause (e.g., infection, stroke, heart failure, medications). • Dizziness: Occurs in approximately 30% of people over 65 years of age. Causes include hypotension, arrhythmia, myocardial infarction, posterior fossa stroke, vestibular disorder. • Adverse drug reactions: Account for 20% of hospital admissions in older adults. Polypharmacy (use of four or more drugs) is a common cause. Common drug offenders include opiates, NSAIDs, warfarin, diuretics, β-blockers, antidepressants, ACE inhibitors, benzodiazepines, and anticholinergics. • Antimicrobial therapy: Antibiotics may predispose to *Clostridium difficile* infection (see Chapter 18); nephrotoxicity (e.g., aminoglycosides); hypersensitivity reactions; renal impairment even though the serum creatinine is normal; increased penicillin reabsorption due to reduced gastric acid production causing a higher pH; hepatotoxicity (e.g., isoniazid; due to reduced hepatic metabolism); confusion and seizures (e.g., quinolones). • Fever: core body temperature >38.0° C. Oral temperatures are unreliable (eardrum reflectance should be utilized). Confusion is common especially in patients with dementia or cerebrovascular disease. Common noninfectious causes include polymyalgia rheumatica, tuberculosis, cancer, urinary tract infection, intra-abdominal abscess (e.g., ruptured appendix, diverticulitis perforation), tumors (e.g., renal cell carcinoma), and infective endocarditis. • Hyponatremia/hypernatremia: Older people are more disposed to these electrolyte disturbances. Factors that are responsible include increased free water intake (hyponatremia), thiazides/loop diuretics (hyponatremia), increased ADH release (patient in heart failure, small cell carcinoma of lung; severe hyponatremia), excess sweating (hypernatremia), reduced intake of water (blunted thirst; physical restriction; hypernatremia), drugs containing sodium (ceftriaxone sodium, sodium bicarbonate for ulcers; hypernatremia). • Cancer: Approximately 50% of cancers occur in the 15% of the population older than 65 years. Rate of progression is slow due to a decrease in angiogenesis with age, which increases the time frame for metastasis to occur. • Polypharmacy: Common in older adults especially in those residing in nursing homes. Currently, close to 50% of men and women older than age 65 take five or more medications per week. Approximately 10% of both men and women take 10 or more medications per week. Medications include both prescription and over-the-counter (OTC) preparations, such as vitamin/mineral supplements and herbal products. Acetaminophen, ibuprofen, and aspirin are the most common OTC preparations. The most common group of drugs causing adverse reactions include diuretics, anticoagulants, cardiovascular agents, antibiotics, hypoglycemic agents (e.g., insulin), steroids, NSAIDs, opioids, anticholinergics, and benzodiazepines. Common herbal supplements that are used by older people include St. John's wort, gingko biloba, garlic, ginseng, aloe vera, chamomile, spearmint, and ginger. Clinicians should be aware of what herbal supplements are being used by their patients, because of important adverse interactions that may affect the medications that have been prescribed.

ACE, Angiotensin-converting enzyme; *ADH*, antidiuretic hormone; *DM*, diabetes mellitus; *MGUS*, monoclonal gammopathy of undetermined significance; *NSAIDs*, nonsteroidal anti-inflammatory drugs; *UVB*, ultraviolet light B.

E. **Progeria** (Fig. 6-41)
   1. **Definition:** Rare autosomal dominant disease (less commonly autosomal recessive) that produces premature aging
   2. Epidemiology
       a. Progeria is due to a mutation that results in the formation of progerin, a component of the nuclear laminin.
       b. Progerin is defective and cannot insert into the nuclear lamina, which leads to progressive deformities in the nuclei. Nuclear lamina is a fibrillar network found inside the nucleus of most cells. Composed of intermediate filaments and membrane-associated proteins. It provides mechanical support and also regulates cellular events such as DNA replication and cell division.
   3. Clinical findings
       a. Reduced birth weight and growth retardation

Progeria

Rare autosomal dominant disease with premature aging

Mutation forms progerin (component nuclear laminin)

Progerin defective: cannot insert into nuclear lamina → nuclear deformities

Nuclear lamina: composed intermediate filaments/ membrane-associated proteins

Provides mechanical support, regulated DNA replication/cell division

Reduced birth weight, growth retardation

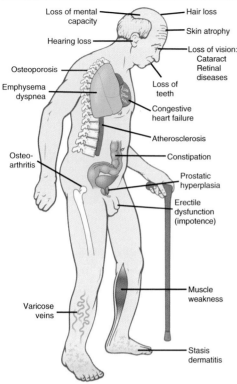

6-38: Common pathologic changes in older people. *(From my friend Ivan Damjanov, MD, PhD: Pathology for the Health Professions, 4th ed, Saunders Elsevier, 2012, p 16, Fig. 1-20.)*

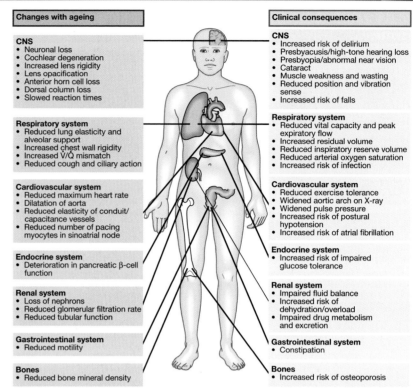

6-39: Changes with aging and clinical consequences. *CNS,* Central nervous system; $\dot{V}/\dot{Q}$, ventilation/perfusion. *(From Walker BR, Colledge NR, Ralston SH, Penman ID: Davidson's Principles and Practice of Medicine, 22nd ed, Churchill Livingstone Elsevier, 2014, p 169, Fig. 7.2.)*

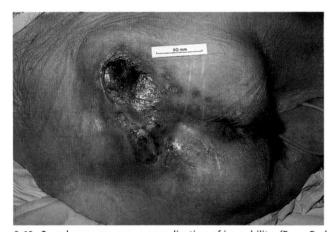

6-40: Sacral pressure sore, a complication of immobility. *(From Forbes CD, Jackson WF: Color Atlas and Text of Clinical Medicine, 3rd ed, Mosby, 2003, p 275, Fig. 11.69.)*

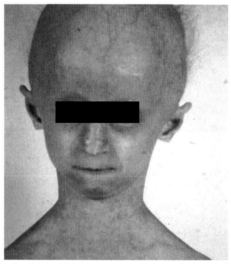

6-41: Progeria. Alopecia, subcutaneous atrophy, prominent scalp veins, and bird-like facies. *(Courtesy Schachner LA, Hansen RC, eds: Pediatric Dermatology, 3rd ed, New York, Elsevier, 2003.)*

Manifests at 6–18 months of age; skin changes

Osteopenia → fractures

Micrognathia

Generalized muscle atrophy, beaked nose (bird-like)

Normal intelligence

b. First manifests at 6 to 18 months of age with skin changes including abnormal pigmentation and scleroderma-like changes, loss of hair
c. Additional findings
  (1) Osteopenia with fractures; micrognathia
  (2) Generalized atrophy of muscle and subcutaneous tissue with a beaked nose and a bird-like appearance
  (3) Normal intelligence

CHAPTER 7

Environmental Pathology

ABBREVIATIONS

MC most common	MCC most common cause	COD cause of death

I. Chemical Injury

A. Tobacco use

1. Epidemiology
   a. Leading cause of premature death in developed countries
   b. Most preventable cause of death worldwide
   c. Rate of cigarette smoking: increasing in females and decreasing in males
   d. Chemical components of tobacco
      (1) Nicotine
         (a) Rapidly absorbed; addictive chemical in tobacco smoke
         (b) Cotinine is the most important metabolite of nicotine. Cotinine screening test for blood or urine is used to detect whether a person is a smoker.
      (2) Noxious chemicals in cigarette smoke
         (a) Polycyclic hydrocarbons are carcinogens that damage DNA.
         (b) Tar is a resinous compound that contains most of the carcinogenic agents in cigarette smoke. Tar is the tacky, brown material left behind in a cigarette filter that gives the teeth and fingers holding the cigarette a brownish yellow film.
         (c) Phenol is carcinogenic and irritates mucosa.
         (d) Nitrosamine is a carcinogen that damages DNA.
         (e) Nitrogen oxides damage cilia and irritate mucosa. Also a major component of smog.
         (f) Carbon monoxide attaches to heme groups (decreases arterial oxygen saturation), shifts the oxygen dissociation curve (ODC) to the left, and inhibits cytochrome oxidase in the electron transport chain (refer to Chapter 2).
         (g) Formaldehyde damages cilia and irritates the mucosa.
   e. Smokeless tobacco (e.g., chewing tobacco)
      (1) Can cause nicotine addiction
      (2) Increases the risk for developing squamous cell cancer of the buccal mucosa and gums
   f. Passive (secondhand) smoke inhalation
      (1) Secondhand smoke has its most serious impact on children. It increases the risk for developing respiratory and middle ear infections, and it exacerbates asthma.
      (2) Passive smoke inhalation also increases one's risk for lung cancer and coronary artery disease (CAD).
2. Systemic effects (Table 7-1)
3. Beneficial effects of smoking cessation
   a. Nonsmokers live longer, regardless of age, than individuals who continue to smoke. If cessation is *before* age 50 years, the reduction in risk of dying in the next 15 years is cut in half compared with those who continue to smoke.
   b. Lower risk for developing cardiovascular (CV) disease. Risk approaches that of a nonsmoker after 15 years.

Leading cause of premature death in developed countries

Most preventable COD worldwide

Nicotine

Addictive component

Cotinine metabolite nicotine; screening test

Polycyclic hydrocarbons carcinogens; damage DNA

Tar contains carcinogenic agents

Brownish yellow film on teeth/fingers

Phenol carcinogenic

Nitrosamine carcinogenic

Nitrogen oxides irritants; smog

Formaldehyde

Smokeless tobacco

Nicotine addiction

Risk for oral squamous cancer

Secondhand smoke

Respiratory/middle ear infections in children

Exacerbates asthma

Passive inhalation: risk lung cancer; CAD

Live longer

↓Risk CV disease

TABLE 7-1 Systemic Effects Associated With Tobacco Use

SYSTEM	EFFECTS
Cardiovascular	• Acute myocardial infarction: increases atherosclerosis in coronary arteries • Sudden cardiac death • Peripheral vascular disease: increases atherosclerosis of the femoral and popliteal arteries • Hypertension
Central nervous	• Strokes: intracerebral bleeding, subarachnoid hemorrhage
Gastrointestinal	• Increased risk for oropharyngeal cancer: squamous cell carcinoma • Increased risk for upper and midesophageal cancer: squamous cell carcinoma • Increased risk for stomach cancer: adenocarcinoma • Gastroesophageal reflux disease: decreases tone of lower esophageal sphincter • Increased risk for peptic ulcers and delayed healing of peptic ulcers • Increased risk for pancreatic cancer: adenocarcinoma
General	• Low birth weight in newborns, intrauterine growth retardation • Neutrophilic leukocytosis: decreased activation of neutrophil adhesion molecules • Decreased concentration of ascorbic acid (used up in neutralizing hydroxyl free radicals) and β-carotenes
Genitourinary	• Increased risk for cervical cancer: squamous cell carcinoma • Decreased free testosterone in males ($\uparrow$SHBG; $\uparrow$binding of free testosterone) • Decreased estrogen in females (early menopause) • Increased risk for kidney cancer: renal cell carcinoma • Increased risk for urinary bladder cancer: urothelial cell carcinoma
Hematopoietic	• Increased risk for acute myeloblastic leukemia
Integument	• Increased facial wrinkling
Musculoskeletal	• Osteoporosis: due to decreased estrogen in females and decreased free testosterone in males
Respiratory	• Increased risk for laryngeal cancer: squamous cell carcinoma • Chronic obstructive pulmonary disease: chronic bronchitis, emphysema • Increased risk for lung cancer: squamous cell carcinoma, small cell carcinoma, some types of adenocarcinoma
Special senses	• Decreased sense of smell and taste • Blindness: macular degeneration • Cataracts

SHBG, Sex hormone–binding globulin.

↓Risk lung cancer

↓Risk stroke

↓Risk cancers mouth, larynx, esophagus, pancreas, kidney, urinary bladder

Improved pulmonary function

↓Risk pneumonia, flu, bronchitis

Alcohol MC recreational drug

Amount/duration

Female sex, Asian descent

Legal limit 80 mg/dL

Absorbed stomach (most)/small intestine

Metabolized liver (most), stomach

Alcohol → acetaldehyde; enzyme alcohol dehydrogenase

c. Lower risk for developing lung cancer. Risk approaches that of a nonsmoker after 15 years.
d. Lower risk for developing a stroke. Risk approaches that of a nonsmoker after 5 to 15 years.
e. Other benefits of smoking cessation
(1) Reduced risk for cancers of the mouth, larynx, esophagus, pancreas, kidney, and urinary bladder
(2) Improved pulmonary function regardless of severity of the disease
(3) Reduced risk for pneumonia, influenza, and bronchitis
B. **Alcohol use disorder**
1. **Definition:** Pattern of drinking that results in harm to an individual's health, interpersonal relationships, or ability to work
2. Epidemiology
a. Alcohol is the most common recreational drug taken in the United States.
b. Alcohol is the third leading cause of preventable death in the United States.
c. Risk factors for alcohol-related disease include amount and duration of alcohol intake and female sex or Asian descent (see later).
d. Legal blood alcohol limit for driving in the United States is 80 mg/dL (0.08%).
3. Alcohol absorption and metabolism
a. Alcohol is absorbed in the stomach (most) and small intestine predominantly through diffusion.
b. Metabolism of alcohol occurs primarily in the liver. Gastric metabolism occurs to a smaller degree.
(1) Alcohol is metabolized into acetaldehyde by the enzyme alcohol dehydrogenase. Because levels of this enzyme are lower in the gastric mucosa of women, their degree of gastric metabolism is decreased compared with that of men.

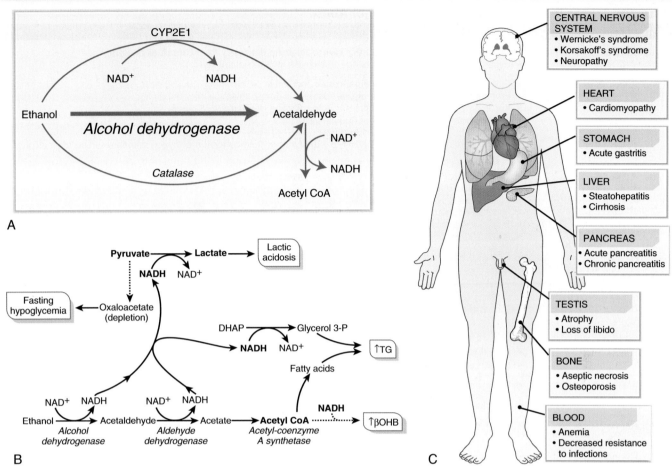

7-1: A, Three enzymes play a key function in the metabolism of alcohol in liver cells: alcohol dehydrogenase, CYP2E (cytochrome P450 enzyme in the smooth endoplasmic reticulum of the microsomal fraction), and catalase in peroxisomes. Alcohol dehydrogenase is the most important liver enzyme involved in oxidation of alcohol, transforming it into acetaldehyde, which is then oxidized to acetyl coenzyme A (CoA). Nicotine adenine dinucleotide (NAD$^+$) is reduced to NADH in this process, as well as during the action of CYP2E, a toxic metabolite, which is in turn oxidized to acetyl CoA by aldehyde dehydrogenase. **B,** Laboratory findings that occur in the metabolism of alcohol. Note that there is an increase in NADH in ethanol metabolism. An increase in NADH increases the conversion of pyruvate to lactate causing lactic acidosis (increased anion gap metabolic acidosis). The decrease in pyruvate leads to less oxaloacetate, a substrate for gluconeogenesis. This produces a fasting hypoglycemia. There is an increased conversion of DHAP to glycerol 3-phosphate. Finally, excess acetyl CoA is used to synthesize fatty acids, which, together with the increase in glycerol 3-phosphate, increases triglyceride synthesis (hypertriglyceridemia). **C,** The most common clinical consequences of chronic alcohol abuse. *β-OHB,* β-hydroxybutyrate; *DHAP,* dihydroxyacetone phosphate; *NADH,* reduced nicotinamide adenine dinucleotide; *steatohepatitis,* fatty change; *TG,* triglyceride. (**A, C** from my friend Ivan Damjanov, MD, PhD: Pathophysiology, *Saunders Elsevier, 2009, pp 75, 77, Figs. 3-9, 3-11, respectively;* **B** from Pelley JW, Goljan EF: Rapid Review Biochemistry, *2nd ed, Philadelphia, Mosby, 2007, p 172,* Fig. 9-6.)

(2) Unmetabolized alcohol diffuses into the blood, causing higher levels of alcohol than in individuals with normal amounts of alcohol dehydrogenase. Furthermore, women have a lower total body fluid volume than men of the same weight (more fat, less muscle); therefore the same amount of alcohol intake leads to a higher serum concentration of alcohol in women than in men.
- These reasons explain why there is enhanced vulnerability of women to acute and chronic complications of alcohol.

(3) Three enzyme systems in the liver are involved in the biotransformation of alcohol to acetaldehyde.
  (a) Cytosol of the liver: alcohol dehydrogenase (rate-limiting enzyme of alcohol metabolism) is key enzyme
  (b) Microsomal ethanol-oxidizing system (MEOS): CYP2E1 isoenzyme is key enzyme (Fig. 7-1 A; see Chapter 2)
  (c) Peroxisomes: catalase is key enzyme

(4) Conversion of acetaldehyde by acetaldehyde dehydrogenase to acetic acid occurs in the mitochondria. Acetic acid (acetate) is then converted into acetyl coenzyme A (CoA) by acetyl CoA synthetase.

Margin notes:

Unmetabolized alcohol diffuses into blood

↑Women risk acute/chronic alcohol complications; ↓alcohol dehydrogenase gastric mucosa

Alcohol dehydrogenase: rate-limiting enzyme

MEOS (CYP2E1 isoenzyme)

Peroxisome catalase

mt site conversion acetaldehyde to acetic acid

Acetic acid → acetyl CoA

TABLE 7-2 Systemic Effects Associated With Alcohol Abuse

SYSTEM	EFFECTS
Cardiovascular	• Dilated (congestive) cardiomyopathy: due to thiamine deficiency from chronic alcoholism • Hypertension: vasopressor effects due to increase in catecholamines
Central nervous system	• CNS depressant: particularly cerebral cortex and limbic system • Wernicke syndrome: confusion, ataxia, nystagmus due to thiamine deficiency • Korsakoff psychosis: memory deficits due to thiamine deficiency • Cerebellar atrophy: due to loss of Purkinje cells • Cerebral atrophy: due to loss of neurons • Central pontine myelinolysis: due to rapid intravenous fluid correction of hyponatremia resulting from alcohol abuse
Gastrointestinal	• Oropharyngeal and upper to midesophageal cancer: squamous cell carcinoma • Acute hemorrhagic gastritis • Mallory-Weiss syndrome: tear of distal esophagus caused by retching • Boerhaave syndrome: rupture of the distal esophagus caused by retching • Esophageal varices: caused by portal vein hypertension in alcoholic cirrhosis • Acute and chronic pancreatitis
General	• Fetal alcohol syndrome: mental retardation, microcephaly, atrial septal and ventricular septal defects
Genitourinary	• Testicular atrophy: decreased testosterone, decreased spermatogenesis • Increased risk for spontaneous abortion
Hematopoietic	• Folic acid deficiency: decreased absorption of folic acid in the jejunum; macrocytic anemia • Acquired sideroblastic anemia: microcytic anemia due to a defect in heme synthesis • Anemia chronic disease: most common anemia comorbid with alcoholic abuse.
Hepatobiliary	• Fatty liver, alcoholic hepatitis, cirrhosis • Hepatocellular carcinoma: preexisting cirrhosis
Integument	• Porphyria cutanea tarda: photosensitive bullous skin lesions
Musculoskeletal	• Rhabdomyolysis: direct alcohol effect on muscle
Peripheral nervous system	• Peripheral neuropathy: due to thiamine deficiency

↑NADH key to lab abnormalities

Synthesis lactic/β-OHB acids; ↑liver triglyceride synthesis

Acetyl CoA used to synthesize fatty acids/ketoacids

Fasting hypoglycemia

Pyruvate → lactate → ↓pyruvate → fasting hypoglycemia

↑AG lactic acidosis

↑AG β-OHB ketoacidosis

β-OHB *not* detected with urine dipstick

Hyperuricemia

Hypertriglyceridemia

AST > ALT in liver disease

Alcohol mt toxin: causes mitochondria to release AST

c. Important products of alcohol metabolism (Fig. 7-1 B)
  (1) Increase in reduced nicotinamide adenine dinucleotide (NADH) causes conversion of the following:
    (a) Pyruvate to lactate, leading to lactic acidosis
    (b) Acetoacetate to β-hydroxybutyrate (β-OHB), producing β-OHB ketoacidosis
    (c) Dihydroxyacetone phosphate to glycerol 3-phosphate, which increases liver synthesis of triglyceride (see Chapter 2)
  (2) Acetyl CoA is used to synthesize fatty acids for triglyceride synthesis and is also used to synthesize ketoacids.
4. Systemic effects (Table 7-2; Fig. 7-1 C)
5. Laboratory findings (see Chapter 19)
  a. Increased risk for developing fasting hypoglycemia. Excess NADH in alcohol metabolism causes pyruvate (substrate for gluconeogenesis) to be converted to lactate (see Fig. 7-1).
  b. Increased risk for developing an increased anion gap (AG) metabolic acidosis (see Chapter 5) due to:
    (1) Lactic acidosis (as just mentioned, when pyruvate is converted to lactate)
    (2) β-OHB ketoacidosis. Excess acetyl CoA is converted to β-OHB acid in the liver. β-OHB acid is *not* detected with a urine dipstick or by the blood test for ketone bodies.
  c. Other findings
    (1) Hyperuricemia (potential for developing gout). Lactic acid/β-OHB acid excretion into urine increases uric acid reabsorption in the proximal tubules resulting in hyperuricemia.
    (2) Hypertriglyceridemia. Hypertriglyceridemia is due to increased production of glycerol 3-phosphate, the key substrate for triglyceride synthesis in the liver (see Chapters 2 and 10).
    (3) Increased serum aminotransferases
      (a) Serum aspartate aminotransferase (AST) is greater than serum alanine aminotransferase (ALT) in liver disease (90% sensitivity, 75% specificity).
      (b) Alcohol is a mitochondrial (mt) toxin that causes release of AST, which is located in the mitochondria (see Chapter 2).

TABLE 7-3   Selected Drugs of Abuse and Their Effects

DRUG	DESCRIPTION	TOXIC EFFECTS
Cocaine	Stimulant	• Mydriasis, tachycardia, hypertension • Associated risk of AMI, CNS infarction, perforation of nasal septum (intranasal use)
Heroin (Link 7-1)	Opiate	• Miotic pupils, noncardiogenic pulmonary edema (frothing from the nose and mouth), focal segmental glomerulosclerosis (nephrotic syndrome) • Granulomatous reactions in skin and lungs from material used to "cut" (dilute) drug
Marijuana *(Cannabis)**	THC-containing psychoactive stimulant	• Red conjunctivae, euphoria, delayed reaction time
MPTP	By-product of synthesis of meperidine	• Irreversible Parkinson disease: MPTP is cytotoxic to neurons in nigrostriatal dopaminergic pathways

*Used medically to decrease nausea and vomiting associated with chemotherapy, decrease intraocular pressure in glaucoma, and treat epilepsy and seizures.
AMI, Acute myocardial infarction; *CNS,* central nervous system; *MPTP,* 1-methyl-4-phenyl-1,2,3,6-tetrahydropyridine; *THC,* Δ9-tetrahydrocannabinol.

(4) Increased serum γ-glutamyltransferase (GGT; 75% sensitivity, 90% specificity). Alcohol induces smooth endoplasmic reticulum (SER) hyperplasia, causing increased synthesis of GGT (an enzyme located in the SER, see Chapter 2).

> Alcohol ↑serum GGT (SER hyperplasia)

(5) Increased urine ethyl glucuronide (excellent indicator of recent alcohol ingestion; better than blood alcohol levels)

> ↑Urine ethyl glucuronide; better than blood alcohol

C. Other drugs of abuse
1. Sedatives, stimulants, and hallucinogens are summarized in Table 7-3 (Link 7-1).
2. Central nervous system (CNS) effects of long-term drug abuse include damage to neurotransmitter receptor sites and increased risk for developing cerebral atrophy (e.g., alcohol abuse).

> Damage neurotransmitter sites; danger cerebral atrophy

3. Complications of intravenous drug use (IVDU)

> Complications IVDU

   a. Hepatitis C (HCV). Recently, HCV surpassed hepatitis B (HCB) as the most common hepatitis due to IVDU (see Chapter 19).

> IVDU: HCV > HBV

   b. Human immunodeficiency virus infection (HIV; see Chapter 4); *Staphylococcus aureus* from contaminated needles

> ↑HIV, *S. aureus*

   c. Tetanus. May result as a complication of "skin popping" using a dirty needle (see Chapter 24).

> Tetanus: skin popping

D. Adverse effects of therapeutic drug use (Table 7-4; Fig. 7-2)
1. Acetaminophen is converted into free radicals in the liver causing possible damage to the liver (e.g., mild to fulminant hepatitis; see Fig. 19-4 B) and the kidneys (e.g., renal papillary necrosis; see Fig. 20-6 E).

> Acetaminophen: chemical hepatitis; renal papillary necrosis

2. Aspirin (acetylsalicylic acid) overdose

> Aspirin overdose

   a. General symptoms of aspirin overdose include tinnitus (ringing in the ears), vertigo (loss of balance), change in mental status (confusion, seizures), and tachypnea (rapid breathing).

> Tinnitus, vertigo, confusion, tachypnea

   b. Acid-base disorders associated with aspirin overdose
      (1) Respiratory alkalosis may occur as the initial disorder (within 12–24 hours; see Chapter 5).

> Initial respiratory alkalosis

         (a) Respiratory alkalosis (hyperventilation) is due to direct stimulation of the respiratory center. Increased loss of carbon dioxide in the breath (↓$Paco_2$; see Chapter 5).

> Hyperventilation

         (b) Respiratory acidosis (hypoventilation) may occur as a late finding.

> Respiratory acidosis (hypoventilation) late finding

      (2) After respiratory alkalosis, there is a shift to an increased AG metabolic acidosis (see Chapter 5), particularly in children.

> Shift to developing ↑AG metabolic acidosis (children)

      (3) Mixed primary respiratory alkalosis and metabolic acidosis is more likely to occur in adults than in children (see Chapter 5).

> Mixed 1° respiratory alkalosis + 1° metabolic acidosis (adults)

   c. Hyperthermia with aspirin overdose (see Chapter 2)
      (1) Salicylates damage the inner mitochondrial membrane.

> Salicylates damage inner mt membrane

      (2) Oxidative energy is released as heat, *not* as adenosine triphosphate.

> Danger hyperthermia (oxidative energy released as heat)

   d. Other potential complications of aspirin include hemorrhagic gastritis (see Link 18-57) and fulminant hepatitis (see Links 19-35, 19-36).

> Acetaminophen/aspirin toxicity → fulminant hepatitis

3. Disorders associated with exogenous estrogen *without* progestin (unopposed estrogen)
   a. Increased risk for cancer (adenocarcinoma) of the endometrium and breast (see Chapter 22)

> Adenocarcinoma endometrium/breast

TABLE 7-4 Adverse Reactions Associated With Therapeutic Drug Use

REACTION	DRUG(S)
Blood Dyscrasias	
Aplastic anemia	• Chloramphenicol, alkylating agents
Hemolytic anemia	• Penicillin, methyldopa, quinidine
Macrocytic anemia	• Methotrexate (most common), phenytoin, oral contraceptives, 5-fluorouracil
Platelet dysfunction	• Aspirin, other NSAIDs
Thrombocytopenia	• Heparin (most common cause in hospital), quinidine
Cardiac	
Dilated cardiomyopathy	• Doxorubicin, daunorubicin
Central Nervous System	
Tinnitus (ringing in the ears), vertigo (room spinning around)	• Salicylates
Cutaneous	
Angioedema	• ACE inhibitors (↑bradykinin)
Maculopapular rash	• Penicillin
Photosensitive rash	• Tetracycline
Urticaria	• Penicillin
Gastrointestinal	
Hemorrhagic gastritis	• Iron, salicylates
Hepatic	
Cholestasis	• Oral contraceptives, estrogen, anabolic steroids
Fatty change	• Amiodarone, tetracycline, methotrexate
Hepatic adenoma	• Oral contraceptives, anabolic steroids
Liver necrosis	• Acetaminophen (most common), isoniazid, salicylates, halothane, iron
Pulmonary	
Asthma	• Aspirin, other NSAIDs
Interstitial fibrosis	• Bleomycin, busulfan, nitrofurantoin, methotrexate
Systemic	
Drug-induced lupus	• Procainamide, hydralazine

ACE, Angiotensin-converting enzyme; *NSAIDs,* nonsteroidal antiinflammatory drugs.

AT normally neutralizes active coagulation factors

Estrogen ↑synthesis factors I, V, VIII

Estrogen ↓antithrombin → ↑venous thromboembolism

Estrogen ↑risk for intrahepatic cholestasis/jaundice

Estrogen ↑risk AMI/stroke

OCP: estrogen + progestins

OCP: risk adenocarcinoma breast, SCC cervix

OCP: risk venous thromboembolism

OCP: folic acid deficiency (macrocytic anemia)

OCPs ↓jejunal absorption folic acid

OCP: risk for HTN

OCP: ↑ATG → ↑ATII (vasoconstrictor)

OCP MCC HTN young women

Hepatic adenoma → rupture → intraperitoneal hemorrhage

b. Decrease in the synthesis of antithrombin (see Chapter 15)
   (1) Antithrombin normally neutralizes activated coagulation factors.
   (2) Estrogen increases the synthesis of clotting factors I (fibrinogen), V, and VIII, causing a hypercoagulable state.
   (3) Venous thromboembolism in the lower extremity may result in a pulmonary embolus with subsequent infarction (see Chapter 17).
c. Increased risk for developing intrahepatic cholestasis with jaundice (see Chapter 19)
d. Increased risk for developing an acute myocardial infarction (AMI; see Chapter 11) and stroke (see Chapter 26)
4. Disorders associated with oral contraceptive pills (OCPs; estrogen + progestin) include an increased risk for developing:
   a. Adenocarcinoma of the breast and squamous cell carcinoma (SCC) of the cervix (see Chapter 22)
   b. Venous thromboembolism. Pathogenesis is similar to the previous discussion of estrogen without progestin.
   c. Folic acid deficiency (macrocytic anemia). OCPs decrease jejunal absorption of folic acid.
   d. Hypertension (HTN)
      (1) HTN is due to increased synthesis of angiotensinogen (ATG), which is converted into angiotensin II (ATII), a vasoconstrictor.
      (2) OCPs are the most common cause of HTN in young women.
   e. Hepatic adenoma (see Link 19-67)
      • **Definition:** Benign liver tumor with increased risk for rupture and associated intraperitoneal hemorrhage

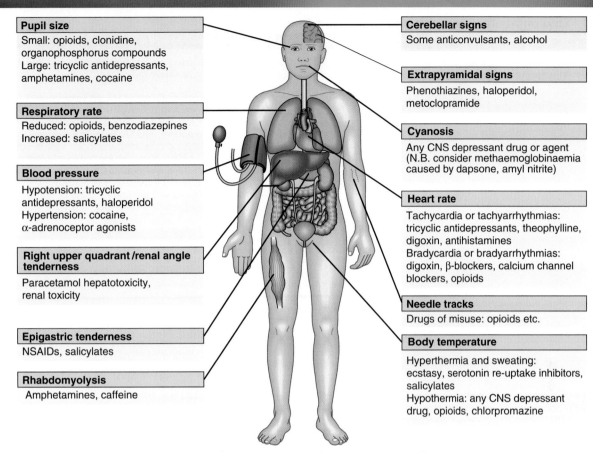

Pupil size
Small: opioids, clonidine, organophosphorus compounds
Large: tricyclic antidepressants, amphetamines, cocaine

Respiratory rate
Reduced: opioids, benzodiazepines
Increased: salicylates

Blood pressure
Hypotension: tricyclic antidepressants, haloperidol
Hypertension: cocaine, α-adrenoceptor agonists

Right upper quadrant/renal angle tenderness
Paracetamol hepatotoxicity, renal toxicity

Epigastric tenderness
NSAIDs, salicylates

Rhabdomyolysis
Amphetamines, caffeine

Cerebellar signs
Some anticonvulsants, alcohol

Extrapyramidal signs
Phenothiazines, haloperidol, metoclopramide

Cyanosis
Any CNS depressant drug or agent (N.B. consider methaemoglobinaemia caused by dapsone, amyl nitrite)

Heart rate
Tachycardia or tachyarrhythmias: tricyclic antidepressants, theophylline, digoxin, antihistamines
Bradycardia or bradyarrhythmias: digoxin, β-blockers, calcium channel blockers, opioids

Needle tracks
Drugs of misuse: opioids etc.

Body temperature
Hyperthermia and sweating: ecstasy, serotonin re-uptake inhibitors, salicylates
Hypothermia: any CNS depressant drug, opioids, chlorpromazine

7-2: Schematic showing clinical signs of poisoning from pharmaceutical agents. *CNS,* Central nervous system; *NSAIDs,* nonsteroidal anti-inflammatory drugs. *(From Walker BR, Colledge NR, Ralston SH, Penman ID:* Davidson's Principles and Practice of Medicine, *22nd ed, Churchill Livingstone Elsevier, 2014, p 207.)*

    f. Intrahepatic cholestasis (obstruction of bile flow; see Fig. 19-6 A) with jaundice

    g. Cholesterol gallstones (yellow color; see Fig. 19-9 B). Estrogen increases cholesterol excretion in the bile.

  E. Injuries caused by environmental chemicals (Table 7-5; Link 7-2, Link 7-3)

  F. Injuries caused by arthropods and reptiles (Table 7-6; Fig. 7-3; Link 7-4, Link 7-5)

II. Physical Injury

  A. Mechanical injury

    1. Types of skin wounds (Fig. 7-4)

      a. Contusion (bruise): due to blunt force injury to blood vessels with subsequent escape of blood into tissue

      b. Abrasion: due to superficial excoriation of the epidermis

      c. Laceration: due to jagged tear of skin with intact bridging blood vessels, nerves, and connective tissue; usually caused by the force of a blunt object (e.g., baseball bat)

      d. Incision: skin wound produced by a sharp object (e.g., knife, razor); sharp margins and severed bridging blood vessels

    2. Gunshot wounds

      a. Contact wounds

        (1) **Definition:** Stellate-shaped wounds

        (2) Contain soot and gunpowder (called fouling)

      b. Intermediate-range wounds

        • **Definition:** Powder tattooing (stippling) of the skin present around the entrance site (Fig. 7-5)

      c. Long-range wounds

        • **Definition:** Absence of powder tattooing

      d. Exit wounds

        • **Definition:** Larger and more irregularly shaped than entrance wounds

    3. Motor vehicle accidents (MVAs)

Intrahepatic cholestasis → jaundice

→ Cholesterol gallstones
Bee/wasp/hornet sting: MCC death due to venomous bite

Contusion: blunt force injury
Abrasion: superficial excoriation epidermis
Laceration: jagged tear/ intact bridging vessels
Incision: produced by sharp object
Wound with sharp margins
Severed blood vessels
Gunshot wounds
Contact wound; stellate-shaped
Fouling (soot + gunpowder)
Intermediate-range wound
Powder tattooing
Long-range wound
No powder tattooing
Exit wounds
Larger than entrance wound

TABLE 7-5   Environmental Chemicals and Associated Toxic Effects

CHEMICAL	SOURCE	TOXIC EFFECTS
Air pollution chemicals	Smog	• Sulfur dioxide: produces a burning sensation in the nose and throat, dyspnea, asthma attacks in susceptible individuals • Carbon monoxide • Ozone: produced by interaction of O_2 with UV light to produce O_3. The ozone layer 10–30 miles above earth's surface is beneficial (absorbs dangerous solar emission). Ground-level ozone is produced by interaction of nitrogen oxides, organic compounds, and UV light. The chemicals just mentioned are present in industrial emissions and motor vehicle exhaust. This type of ozone produces free radicals that damage respiratory epithelial cells, inflame the upper respiratory tract, and exacerbate asthma. • Nitrogen dioxide: damages cilia and irritates airway mucosa • Particulate matter (soot): particles <10 μm enter the alveoli and are phagocytosed by macrophages, causing the release of inflammatory mediators. • Lead: can accumulate over time and cause damage (see Link 7-3)
Arsenic	Pesticides, contaminated ground water, vineyard workers	• Arsenic inhibits enzymes that require lipoic acid as a cofactor (e.g., pyruvate dehydrogenase), causing increased conversion of pyruvate to lactate (lactic acidosis) • Severe headaches, abdominal pain, diarrhea, delirium, convulsions, transverse bands in nails (Mees lines), death • Squamous cell carcinoma of the skin, liver angiosarcoma, lung cancer
Asbestos (see Chapter 17)	Insulation, roofing material, shipyard worker	• Primary lung cancer, mesothelioma
Benzene	Solvent, chemical industry workers	• Acute leukemia, aplastic anemia
Carbon monoxide (see Chapter 2)	Automobile exhaust, house fires, generators	• Headache (first sign), cherry red skin, coma • $\downarrow O_2$ saturation, normal PaO_2; lactic acidosis (due to hypoxia)
Cyanide (see Chapter 2)	House fires	• Odor of bitter almonds; coma, seizures, heart dysfunction, metabolic acidosis (serum lactate >10 mmol/L), due to inhibition of cytochrome oxidase in ETC and subsequent shift to anaerobic glycolysis as only ATP source
Ethylene glycol (Link 7-2)	Antifreeze: end-product oxalic acid	• Increased anion gap metabolic acidosis • Acute renal failure
Isopropyl alcohol	Rubbing alcohol: end-product acetone	• Fruity odor to breath (acetone); can progress into deep coma • Does *not* produce increased anion gap like ethanol, methanol, and ethylene glycol, but does increase the osmolal gap (see Chapter 5)
Lead (see Chapter 12); Link 7-3	Lead-based paint, batteries, metal casting	• Microcytic anemia with coarse basophilic stippling, nephrotoxicity in proximal tubule
Mercury	Fish most important source	• Diarrhea, constricted visual fields, nephrotoxicity in proximal tubule, tachycardia, hyperhidrosis (↑sweating), peripheral neuropathy, hypertension
Methanol (see Chapter 5)	Windshield washer fluid: end-product formic acid	• Increased anion gap metabolic acidosis • Blindness due to optic atrophy
Organophosphates	Pesticides	• Salivation, lacrimation, urinary/fecal incontinence, diaphoresis, blurred vision, hypotension, bradycardia, muscle fasciculations • Decreased serum and RBC cholinesterase levels
Polyvinyl chloride	Plastics industry	• Liver angiosarcoma

ATP, Adenosine triphosphate; *ETC,* electron transport chain; *FRs,* free radicals; *PaO2,* partial pressure of oxygen; *RBC,* red blood cell; *UV,* ultraviolet.

TABLE 7-6   Injuries Caused by Arthropods and Reptiles

AGENT	VENOM	TOXIC EFFECTS
Coral snake (elapid)	Neurotoxin: binds to presynaptic nerve terminals and acetylcholine	• "Red on yellow" bands ("red and yellow kill a fellow"); "red on black" is a harmless scarlet king snake ("red and black, friend of Jack") • Toxic effects: paralysis (diplopia, respiratory muscles), fixed and contracted pupils, death by respiratory failure
Rattlesnake, copperhead, water moccasin (crotalids) (Fig. 7-3 A; Link 7-4)	Venom is cytohemoneurotoxic	• Toxic effects: local edema/pain with progressive development of ecchymoses and bleeding into tissue, shock, DIC

TABLE 7-6   Injuries Caused by Arthropods and Reptiles—cont'd

AGENT	VENOM	TOXIC EFFECTS
Latrodectus spp. (black widow spiders) (Fig. 7-3 B)	Latrotoxin (acts through Ca^{2+}-mediated channels to cause release of acetylcholine and norepinephrine from nerve terminals)	• Painful bite followed by increasing local pain; small erythematous macule develops within an hour, which then becomes a "target" lesion with a pale center surrounded by erythema; severe muscle cramps/spasms develop in trunk, thighs, and abdomen, the latter simulating an acute abdomen; possible hypertension
Loxosceles (brown recluse spider) (Fig. 7-3 C, D)	Necrotoxins	• Initially painless bite; painful reddish blister forms in several hours, which develops a bluish discoloration in 24 hours; extensive skin necrosis occurs over next 3–4 days, with eschar formation by the end of the first week; may become infected; surgical débridement may be necessary
Scorpion (Fig. 7-3 E)	Neurotoxin	• Poisonous species in southwestern U.S. deserts (*Centruroides* spp.) • Toxic effects: initial painful sting followed by numbness, hypertension, ascending motor paralysis leading to death; may cause acute pancreatitis
Bees, wasps, hornets (Link 7-5)	Histamine and other components	• As a group, the most common cause of death due to a venomous bite in the United States • Range of reactions from localized erythema and swelling to an anaphylactic reaction (dyspnea, wheezing, inspiratory stridor [laryngeal swelling], shock, death)
Fire ants (Link 7-5)	Insoluble alkaloid	• Swarm when provoked and attack in great numbers; painful bites with papules becoming sterile pustules in several hours; necrosis, scarring, secondary infection can occur; death possible in some cases

DIC, Disseminated intravascular coagulation.

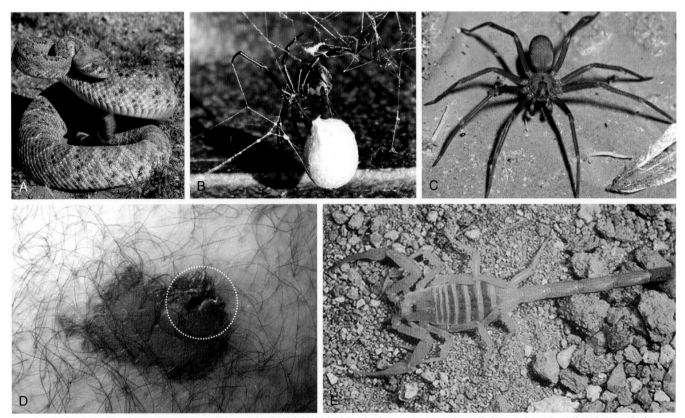

7-3: A, Diamondback rattlesnake. Note the triangular head and black and white stripes on the tail that ends with a vibrating rattle (reason for the blurry picture). **B,** Black widow spider with egg case. Note the glossy black color and the characteristic red hourglass marking on the ventral abdomen. **C,** Brown recluse spider (*Loxosceles* spp.). Note the long legs and the violin-shaped dark brown mark on the dorsum of the cephalothorax of the spider. **D,** Brown recluse spider bite showing a severe, local necrotic reaction with ulceration (*interrupted white circle*). **E,** Scorpion. *Centruroides* species are the most poisonous scorpions in the United States. (*A from Townsend C:* Sabiston Textbook of Surgery, *18th ed, Philadelphia, Saunders Elsevier, 2008, p 587, Fig. 23-1; B courtesy Vania Revell DO; C from Kliegman RM:* Nelson Textbook of Pediatrics, *20th ed, Elsevier, 2016, p 3457, Fig. 725-4; courtesy Michael Cardwell/Extreme Wildlife Photography; D from Marks JG, Miller JJ:* Lookingbill and Marks' Principles of Dermatology, *5th ed, Saunders Elsevier, 2013, p 144, Fig. 11.3; E courtesy Dr. JC Cockendolpher, from Peters W:* A Colour Atlas of Arthropods in Clinical Medicine, *London, Wolfe, 1992.*)

MARKS from INSTRUMENTS

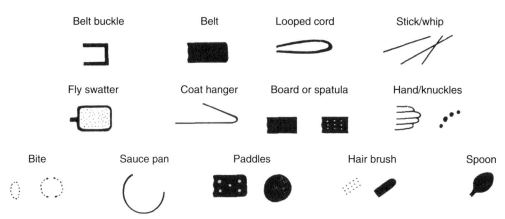

7-4: Marks from instruments. *(From Kliegman RM: Nelson Textbook of Pediatrics, 20th ed, Elsevier, 2016, p 238, Fig. 40-3.)*

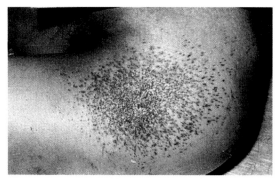

7-5: Intermediate-range gunshot wound showing powder tattooing (tippling). *(From my friend Ivan Damjanov, MD, PhD, Linder J: Anderson's Pathology, 10th ed, St. Louis, Mosby, 1996, p 90, Fig. 5.12 B.)*

MVAs MC COD ages 1–44 yrs

Frequently alcohol-related

Shaken baby syndrome

Injury from violent shaking

>50% deaths in child abuse

Majority infants (<1 yr old)

Retinal hemorrhages key sign

Multiple fractures long bones

Subdural hematoma

Exposure to excessive heat/ flame

Fire MCC burns

Upper extremities MC site

Protein denaturation

Irreversible coagulation necrosis

a. Most common cause of death in people ages 1 to 44 years
b. Account for 26% of all injury-related deaths and are frequently alcohol-related (≈20% of cases)
4. Shaken baby syndrome
   a. **Definition:** Injury to a baby caused by repeated violent shaking
   b. Epidemiology
      (1) Greater than 50% of deaths in child abuse are due to shaken baby syndrome.
      (2) Majority are infants (those <1 year old).
   c. Characteristic signs
      (1) Retinal hemorrhages (key sign). May be the only sign of the shaken baby syndrome and should be confirmed by an ophthalmologist.
      (2) Multiple fractures of long bones (Link 7-6)
      (3) Subdural hematomas (see Chapter 26)
B. **Thermal injury**
   1. Burns
      a. **Definition:** Injury caused by exposure to excessive heat or flame
      b. Epidemiology
         (1) Causes of burns in descending order include fire/flame, scalds, contact with hot objects, electricity, and chemicals.
         (2) Most common sites for burns in descending order include upper extremities, lower extremities, and head and neck.
      c. Pathophysiology
         (1) Common denominator in all burns is protein denaturation.
         (2) Burn injury is divided into three concentric zones.
            (a) Center of the burn exhibits irreversible injury with coagulation necrosis (see Chapter 2).

TABLE 7-7   Burn Classification

TYPE OF BURN	APPEARANCE	SURFACE	SENSATION	HEALING TIME
First degree	Red	Dry	Painful	Few days
Second degree Superficial	Red, clear blisters; blanches with pressure	Moist	Painful	2–3 weeks
Deep	White with some red areas, hemorrhagic blisters, less blanching with pressure	Less moist than superficial	Painful	Weeks; danger of progressing to third-degree burn
Third degree	White, brown	Dry, leathery	Painless in area of burn	Requires excision and graft
Fourth degree	Brown, charred, visibly thrombosed vessels	Dry	Painless in area of burn	Requires excision and graft

Modified from Marx J: *Rosen's Emergency Medicine,* 7th ed, Philadelphia, Mosby Elsevier, 2010, p 759, Table 60-1.

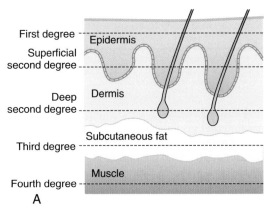
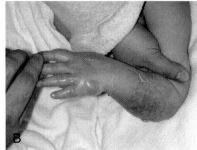
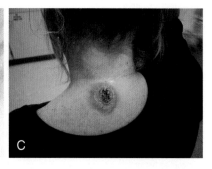

7-6: A, Depths of a burn. First-degree burns are confined to the epidermis. Second-degree burns extend into the dermis (dermal burns). Third-degree burns are full thickness through the epidermis and dermis. Fourth-degree burns involve injury to underlying tissue structures such as muscle, tendons, and bone. **B,** Superficial second-degree burn. Note the redness of the skin and clear vesicles. **C,** Third-degree burn. Note the central area of coagulation necrosis and the surrounding area of erythema. *(A from Townsend CM, Beauchamp RD, Evers BM, Mattox KL: Sabiston Textbook of Surgery: The Biological Basis of Modern Surgical Practice, 19th ed, Saunders Elsevier, 2012, p 523, Fig. 21-2; B, C from Marx J: Rosen's Emergency Medicine, 7th ed, Philadelphia, Mosby Elsevier, 2010, p 760, Fig. 60-1, 60-3, respectively.)*

(b) Zone of ischemia around the center yields reduction in the dermal microcirculation, putting this area at risk for irreversible damage.

> Reduction in dermal microcirculation

(c) Zone of hyperemia around the area of ischemia is characterized by redness of the skin due to an immediate and transient increase in perfusion.

> Immediate/transient increase in perfusion

(3) Ability of the skin to regenerate depends on the depth of the burn.

> Regeneration depends on depth of burn

(4) Regeneration of the damaged epidermis derives from two primary sources.

> Regeneration damaged epidermis two sources

(a) In small burns, proliferation of the basal layer of cells from the uninjured adjacent epidermis can reepithelialize the burn.

> Small burns: basal layer cells uninjured epidermis

(b) In large burns, the major source of regenerative epithelial cells comes from the dermal skin appendages (hair follicles and sebaceous glands).

> Large burns: dermal skin appendages

d. Classification of burns (see Table 7-7; Fig. 7-6 A)

(1) First-degree burns

> 1st-degree burns: limited to epidermis

(a) **Definition:** Burns limited to the epidermis (e.g., sunburn)

(b) Heal in a few days without scarring

> Heal *without* scarring

(2) Second-degree burns are subdivided into superficial and deep.

> 2nd-degree burns: superficial and deep

(a) **Definition:** Superficial second-degree burns extend into the superficial, papillary dermis (partial-thickness burn; Fig. 7-6 B).

> Superficial 2nd-degree: extend into superficial, papillary dermis (partial-thickness burn)

(b) **Definition:** Deep second-degree burns extend into the deep, reticular dermis (partial-thickness burn).

> Deep 2nd-degree: extends into reticular dermis; partial-thickness burn

(3) Third-degree burns

> 3rd-degree burns

(a) **Definition:** Burns that extend through both the epidermis and dermis (full-thickness burn; Fig. 7-6 C)

> Extends through epidermis/dermis; full-thickness

(b) Destruction of adnexa and nerves (painless)

> Destruction adnexa/nerves (painless)

(c) Scarring is inevitable. Keloids commonly occur (see Chapter 3). Potential for developing SCC in the scar (see Chapter 9).

> Scarring; keloids
>
> SCC risk in keloids

4th-degree burns

Extends thru skin, sc fat, muscle/bone

Hypovolemic shock: loss of plasma

P. aeruginosa MCC infection of burn wound

S. aureus, Candida

Curling ulcers proximal duodenum

Hypermetabolic syndrome

Heat loss from damaged skin surface → ↑BMR

Smoke inhalation: carbon monoxide/cyanide poisoning

Heat edema

Mild swelling feet, ankles, hands

Cutaneous vasodilation with gravitational pooling

Older adults tropical climates

Healthy traveler coming from cold to hot area

Self-limited

Heat cramps

Painful, spasmodic muscle contractions after exercise

Begins in calves

Deficiency Na⁺, Cl⁻, and fluids in muscle

Electrolytes: hyponatremia/hypochloremia

Heat exhaustion

Volume depletion under conditions of heat stress

Hypotension, nausea, vomiting

Core temp <40° C (104° F)

Profuse sweating

Mental status normal

↑Hb/Hct from ↓PV

(4) Fourth-degree burns
  - **Definition:** Burns that extend through the skin and subcutaneous (sc) fat into the underlying muscle and bone
e. "Rule of nines" in determining the extent of burns (Link 7-7)
f. Various marks of burns (Link 7-8)
g. Complications of severe burns
  (1) Hypovolemic shock may occur due to loss of plasma from the burn surface (see Chapter 5). Loss of protein from the plasma loss may result in generalized pitting edema.
  (2) Infection of the wound site and sepsis may occur.
    (a) Sepsis due to *Pseudomonas aeruginosa* is the most common cause of infection in burn patients.
    (b) Other pathogens include methicillin-resistant *Staphylococcus aureus* and *Candida* species.
  (3) Ulcers may occur in the proximal duodenum (known as Curling ulcer; see Chapter 18).
  (4) Hypermetabolic syndrome may occur if >40% of the body surface is burned.
    - Excess heat loss from the damaged skin surface leads to an increase in the resting (basal) metabolic rate (BMR).
  (5) Smoke inhalation may result in carbon monoxide and cyanide poisoning (see Chapter 2).
2. Minor heat syndromes
  a. Heat edema
    (1) **Definition:** Mild swelling of the feet, ankles, and hands
    (2) Due to cutaneous vasodilation with gravitational pooling of the blood into the extremities
    (3) Commonly occurs in nonacclimatized older adults, who encounter climactic stresses when visiting tropical and semitropical areas
    (4) May also occur in healthy travelers moving from a cold to a hot environment
    (5) Self-limited and does *not* require treatment
  b. Heat cramps (Table 7-8)
    (1) **Definition:** Painful, involuntary spasmodic contractions of muscle that occur after exercise
    (2) Muscle cramps begin to occur when the person has stopped exercising and is relaxing.
    (3) Pain usually starts in the calves but may progress to other muscle groups.
    (4) Cramps are due to deficiency of sodium (Na⁺), chloride (Cl⁻), and fluids in muscle fibers. Serum electrolytes frequently show hyponatremia and hypochloremia.
  c. Heat exhaustion (see Table 7-8)
    (1) **Definition:** Significant volume depletion (salt and water depletion) under conditions of heat stress
    (2) Clinical findings
      (a) Malaise, orthostatic hypotension (from volume depletion), dizziness, headache, nausea, and vomiting are common findings.
      (b) Core temperature is variable and ranges from normal to <40° C (104° F).
      (c) Profuse sweating may occur.
      (d) Mental status examination is normal.
    (3) Laboratory findings
      (a) Hemoconcentration of blood (e.g., ↑hemoglobin [Hb]/hematocrit [Hct]) occurs because of a decrease in plasma volume.

TABLE 7-8 Heat Injuries*

TYPE OF INJURY	BODY TEMPERATURE	SKIN	MENTAL STATUS
Heat cramps	37°C (98.6°F)	Moist and cool	Normal
Heat exhaustion	<40°C (<104°F)	Profuse sweating	Normal
Heat stroke	>40°C (>104°F)	Hot and dry (anhidrosis)	Impaired consciousness CNS dysfunction

*Heat injury is exacerbated by high humidity.
CNS, Central nervous system.

(b) Serum Na⁺ is variable depending on the previous intake of fluid.

- Hypernatremia (indicates no intake of fluid), normonatremia, or hyponatremia (patient drank too much water *without* electrolytes)

3. Major heat syndrome: classic heatstroke (CHS; see Table 7-8)
   a. **Definition:** CHS usually occurs in periods of sustained, high ambient temperatures and humidity during the summer months.
   b. Epidemiology; predisposing factors
      (1) Victims are often older adults as well as the poor who live in underventilated apartments/homes without air conditioning.
      (2) Infants, children, older adults are at risk.
      (3) Majority of victims have chronic disorders (e.g., psychiatric disorders, alcoholism) that require medication (e.g., diuretics, neuroleptics).
   c. Clinical presentation is similar to heat exhaustion, *except* for the following:
      (1) Core body temperature is >40° C (104° F).
      (2) Skin is hot and dry (anhidrosis), mental status exam is abnormal (e.g., do not know time, date), and CNS dysfunction is present (e.g., coma, seizures, delirium).
   d. Laboratory findings in CHS include mild respiratory alkalosis and a slight increase in serum creatine kinase (CK).

4. Major heat syndrome: exertional heatstroke (EHS)
   a. **Definition:** EHS usually occurs in athletes and military recruits, whose cooling mechanisms are overridden by endogenous heat production from heavy exercising.
   b. Epidemiology; predisposing factors: Victims are young and healthy as opposed to those with CHS, who are usually older with predisposing factors and medications.
   c. Clinical presentation is much more severe in EHS than in CHS.
      (1) Core body temperature is >40° C (104° F).
      (2) Profuse sweating is present in 50% of cases. CNS dysfunction is present (e.g., coma, seizures, delirium, convulsions [75% of cases]).
   d. Laboratory findings
      (1) Marked lactic acidosis is present.
      (2) Marked increase in serum CK may occur, with myoglobinuria secondary to rhabdomyolysis (breakdown of muscle).
      (3) Acute renal failure (ARF) with oliguria may occur, causing an increase in blood urea nitrogen and creatinine (see Chapter 20).
      (4) Coagulation abnormalities are common, the worst of which is disseminated intravascular coagulation (DIC; see Chapter 15).
      (5) Hepatic damage is common, causing an increase in serum transaminases.
      (6) Hypocalcemia occurs because of calcium binding to damaged muscle.

5. Frostbite and related cold injuries
   a. **Definition:** Direct damage to tissue caused by ice crystallization in cells
   b. Epidemiology
      (1) Most common freezing injury to tissue
      (2) Trench foot and immersion foot are *nonfreezing injuries* related to exposure to wet cold.
      (3) Chilblain (pernio) is a *nonfreezing injury* due to exposure to dry cold.
      (4) Pathogenesis
         (a) Frostbite occurs when tissue is exposed to temperatures less than 0° C.
         (b) Direct damage to tissue is caused by ice crystallization in cells.
         (c) Stasis of blood flow, due to vasodilation, leads to thrombosis and ischemia of tissue.
   c. Clinical findings
      (1) Prefreeze phase: Anesthesia of the affected tissue occurs. Physiologic changes include endothelial cell leakage of plasma, constriction of the microvasculature, and increased plasma viscosity.
      (2) Freeze-thaw phase: Ice crystallization occurs in the extracellular tissue, causing water to exit the cell. This results in intracellular volume depletion and cell death.
      (3) Immediately after thawing, there is microvascular collapse, sludging, stasis, and cessation of blood flow in the capillaries, venules, and arterioles. Tissues are deprived of nutrients and oxygen, and necrosis occurs (Fig. 7-7 A).
      (4) Frozen tissue is yellow-white, waxy, mottled, or violaceous-white in color. Numbness and edema occur as well (Fig. 7-7 B).
      (5) Clear to hemorrhagic blisters may occur.
      (6) Favorable signs after thawing are normal sensation, warm skin, and normal skin color.

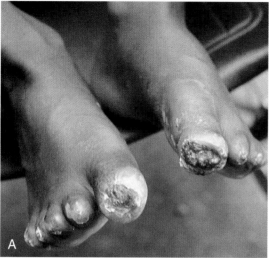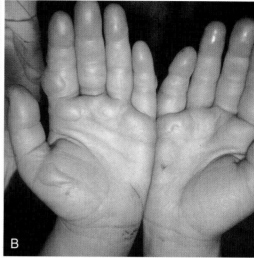

7-7: **A,** Frostbite of toes. Localized cold injury has caused necrosis of toes exposed to extreme cold on a climbing expedition in the Himalayas. **B,** Hands with frostbite showing clear vesiculations, waxy appearance of the skin, and edema. *(**A** from Stevens A, Lowe J, Scott I:* Core Pathology, *3rd ed, London, Elsevier, 2009; **B** courtesy Bill Mills, MD; from Marx J:* Rosen's Emergency Medicine Concepts and Clinical Practice, *7th ed, Philadelphia, Mosby Elsevier, 2010, p 1865, Fig. 137-1.)*

Electrical injury

Children/work-related

5th leading cause fatal occupational injuries

Current (amperes) main determinant tissue injury

AC: changing direction current flow

DC: unchanging direction current flow

Frequency: #transitions form + to − in AC

Resistance: tendency for material to resist electrical current

Voltage: difference in electrical potential between two points

Determined by electrical source

Current (I) = voltage (V)/resistance (R)

U.S. household wiring 120 volts AC

Current main determinant tissue damage

↑R or ↓V = ↓I through tissue

↓R or ↑V = ↑I

AC more dangerous than DC at same voltage

AC induces tetanic contractions (hold on)

DC induces single muscle spasm (throws patient away)

Wet skin ↓R causing ↑I

Dry skin ↑R causing ↓I

↑Tissue damage with ↑voltage + duration of exposure

Current from left arm to right leg most dangerous

Cardiorespiratory arrest MCC death due to electrical injury

C. Electrical injury
1. Epidemiology
   a. Most injuries occur in children or in adults at work.
   b. Fifth leading cause of fatal occupational injuries
   c. Electricity terms
      (1) **Definition:** Current is the measure of the amount of energy that flows through an object. It is expressed in amperes and is the main determinant of tissue injury.
      (2) **Definition:** Alternating current (AC) is the electrical source with changing direction of current flow.
      (3) **Definition:** Direct current (DC) is the electrical source with unchanging direction of current flow.
      (4) **Definition:** Frequency is the number of transitions from positive to negative per second in alternating current.
      (5) **Definition:** Resistance is the tendency of a material to resist the flow of electrical current.
      (6) **Definition:** Voltage is a measure of the difference in electrical potential between two points, and it is determined by the electrical source.
      (7) **Definition:** Ohm's law is current (I) = voltage (V)/resistance (R). An equivalent expression of the law is V = I × R.
      (8) In the United States, household wiring has 120 volts of alternating current.
      (9) Voltage in high-tension transmission lines exceeds 100,000 volts, whereas voltage in distribution lines is 7000 to 8000 volts. This voltage is further stepped down *before* delivery to homes.
2. Pathophysiology
   a. Current is the main determinant of tissue damage.
      (1) According to Ohm's law (I = V/R), increasing resistance or decreasing voltage decreases current through tissue.
      (2) Decreasing resistance or increasing voltage increases current through tissue.
   b. AC exposure at the same voltage is three times more dangerous than DC.
      (1) AC induces tetanic (continuous) muscle contractions; therefore, it is more difficult for the victim to separate themselves from the source.
      (2) DC produces a single muscle spasm, often throwing the victim from the source.
   c. Wet skin decreases resistance, which increases current.
   d. Dry skin increases resistance, which decreases current.
   e. Tissue damage increases with increased voltage and duration of exposure (Link 7-9). High-voltage injuries (>1000 volts) are more dangerous than low voltage injuries (<1000 volts).
   f. Current moving from the left arm to the right leg is the most dangerous route because it affects the heart and may cause cardiorespiratory arrest, the most common cause of death due to electrical injury.

3. Lightning injury
   a. **Definition:** Lightning is a discharge of electricity.
   b. Lightning accounts for 100 to 200 deaths/year.
   c. Case fatality rate is 25% to 35%, with ≈70% of victims having permanent damage (e.g., chronic pain syndromes, sympathetic nervous system injury, neurocognitive injury).
   d. Current surge can affect all major organ systems.
   e. Most common cause of death from lightning is cardiorespiratory arrest.

D. **Drowning**
   1. **Definition:** Death by suffocation from immersion in a liquid
   2. Epidemiology
      a. Fourth most common cause of accidental death in the United States
      b. Second most common cause of accidental death in the United States in children 1 to 4 and 10 to 14 years old
      c. Risk factors for drowning
         (1) Acute ethanol intoxication is a contributing factor to drowning among adults and teenagers in 30% to 50% of cases.
         (2) Other factors include seizures, trauma, child abuse/neglect, suicide, and cardiovascular disease.
      d. Terminology and pathophysiology
         (1) **Definition: Near drowning** is survival following asphyxia secondary to submersion.
         (2) **Definition: Wet drowning** is aspiration of water during the event.
            (a) Approximately 80% to 90% of drownings are classified as wet drowning.
            (b) Initial laryngospasm on contact with water is followed by relaxation and aspiration of water.
            (c) Amount of water that is aspirated is variable; possible complications include pulmonary edema, atelectasis due to loss of surfactant, and risk for pulmonary infections.
         (3) **Definition: Immersion syndrome** is sudden death after submersion in very cold water that is most likely due to a vagally mediated asystolic cardiac arrest.
         (4) **Definition: Dry drowning** is asphyxia caused by intense laryngospasm *without* aspiration.
         (5) **Definition:** A **diving reflex** occurs in water that is colder than 20° C (70° F). Characteristics include bradycardia, peripheral vasoconstriction (shunts blood to more vital areas), blood shifting (shift of blood to the thoracic cavity to prevent atelectasis of the lungs), and prolonged survival without O_2 in both conscious and unconscious people.
   3. Cause of death in drowning
      a. Most commonly due to asphyxia caused by laryngospasm and closure of the glottis, followed by hypoxemia and combined respiratory and metabolic acidosis.
      b. Tonicity of the water (fresh water vs. salt water) does *not* appear to play a significant role as a cause of death in drowning, because not all drowning victims have water in their lungs.

E. **High-altitude injury**
   1. Overview of changes in high altitude (see Chapter 2)
      a. O_2 concentration is 21%; however, the barometric pressure is decreased.
      b. Hypoxemia stimulates the peripheral chemoreceptors, which increases the respiratory rate and causes respiratory alkalosis. A decrease in alveolar P_{CO_2} causes a corresponding increase in alveolar P_{O_2}, which slightly increases the arterial P_{O_2} (see Chapter 2).
      c. Respiratory alkalosis increases glycolysis by activating phosphofructokinase (PFK), the rate-limiting reaction of glycolysis. This results in an increased synthesis of 2,3-bisphosphoglycerate (2,3-BPG), which rightward shifts the ODC, causing increased delivery of oxygen to tissue.
   2. Acute mountain sickness
      a. **Definition:** Usually occurs at elevations >8000 feet (>2440 m)
         (1) At this altitude, the arterial saturation of O_2 (Sa_{O_2}) is <90%.
         (2) Moderate altitude is between 8000 and 10,000 feet (2438–3048 m), high altitude is between 10,000 and 18,000 feet (3048–5486 m), and extreme altitude is >18,000 feet (>5486 m).
      b. Risk factors include rate of ascent, extreme altitude, previous symptoms of acute mountain sickness, and duration of stay at high altitude.

Headache (MC), fatigue, insomnia

HAPE

Elevation >14,500 feet

Noncardiogenic PE

Immediate descent

HACE

HACE: > 12,000 feet; ataxia, stupor, coma

Ionizing radiation injury

Atom becomes charged/ ionized

X-rays, γ-rays

Injury: type, dose, surface area exposed

Radon/thoron

Direct/indirect DNA damage by hydroxyl FRs

Production thymidine dimers

Lymphoid tissue most sensitive

Hematopoietic cells

Mucosa GI, germinal tissue

Bone least sensitive

Lymphopenia first hematologic sign

Thrombosis/fibrosis; ischemia

Skin effects

Acute: erythema, edema, blisters

Chronic: radiodermatitis; danger SCC

Diarrhea (acute)

Bowel adhesions (chronic)

   c. Clinical findings include headache (most common), fatigue, dizziness, anorexia, nausea, and insomnia.

  3. High-altitude pulmonary edema (HAPE)
- More common above 14,500 feet (4420 m); noncardiogenic pulmonary edema (PE) with increased protein (exudate); immediate descent required

  4. Acute cerebral edema, or high-altitude cerebral edema (HACE)
    a. More common above 12,000 feet (3658 m)
    b. Clinical findings include ataxia, stupor, and coma.

III. Radiation Injury

  A. Ionizing radiation injury

    1. **Definition** (WHO definition): **Ionizing radiation** is radiation with enough energy so that during an interaction with an atom, it can remove tightly bound electrons from the orbit of an atom, causing the atom to become charged or ionized.

    2. Epidemiology
      a. Examples include x-rays and γ-rays.
      b. Pathophysiology
        (1) Injury correlates with the type of radiation, cumulative dose, and amount of surface area exposed.
        (2) Radon and thoron (background) account for 37% of radiation exposure (Link 7-10).
        (3) Direct or indirect DNA injury occurs via formation of hydroxyl free radicals (see Chapter 2). Causes production of thymidine dimers (Link 7-11).
      c. Tissue susceptibility (Fig. 7-8)
        (1) Most radiosensitive tissues (highest mitotic activity)
          (a) Lymphoid tissue (most sensitive tissue)
          (b) Hematopoietic cells in the bone marrow
          (c) Mucosa of the gastrointestinal tract and germinal tissue (e.g., ovaries, testes)
        (2) Least radiosensitive tissues: bone (least sensitive), brain, muscle, and skin
      d. Radiation effects in different tissues (Table 7-9)
        (1) Hematopoietic system effects include lymphopenia (initial change), thrombocytopenia, and bone marrow hypoplasia.
        (2) Vascular system effects include thrombosis (early), fibrinoid necrosis (Link 7-12), and fibrosis (late finding) leading to ischemic damage.
        (3) Integumentary system effects
          (a) Acute changes (e.g., erythema, edema, and blister formation)
          (b) Chronic changes (e.g., radiodermatitis); potential for developing SCC
        (4) Gastrointestinal system effects include diarrhea (acute effect) and development of adhesions with a potential for bowel obstruction (chronic effect; see Chapter 18).
        (5) Responses to total body radiation (see Fig. 7-8)

TABLE 7-9 Summary of Effects of Radiation on Various Tissues*

TISSUE	ACUTE EFFECT	CHRONIC EFFECT
Skin	Erythema, edema, blistering	Radiodermatitis Cancer
Bone		Bone necrosis Closure of epiphyses in children Osteosarcoma
Bone marrow	Lymphopenia (first change), thrombocytopenia, bone marrow hypoplasia	Acute leukemia
Ovary/testis	Destruction of germ cells	Atrophy and fibrosis
Lungs	Acute radiation pneumonitis	Chronic interstitial fibrosis
Gastrointestinal	Diarrhea, mucosal necrosis	Fibrosis and strictures in the bowel
Vascular	Thrombosis (early) and fibrinoid necrosis, ischemic damage (Link 7-12)	Fibrosis
Kidney	Acute radiation nephritis, acute renal failure	Gradual loss of renal parenchyma with eventual chronic renal failure
Brain	Transient somnolence	Developmental delay in young children
Eye		Cataracts
Ear		Deafness
Thyroid		Hypothyroidism, papillary carcinoma

*See Link 7-12.
Modified from Stevens A, Lowe J, Scott I: *Core Pathology*, 3rd ed, Mosby Elsevier, 2009, p 143, Fig. 9.5.

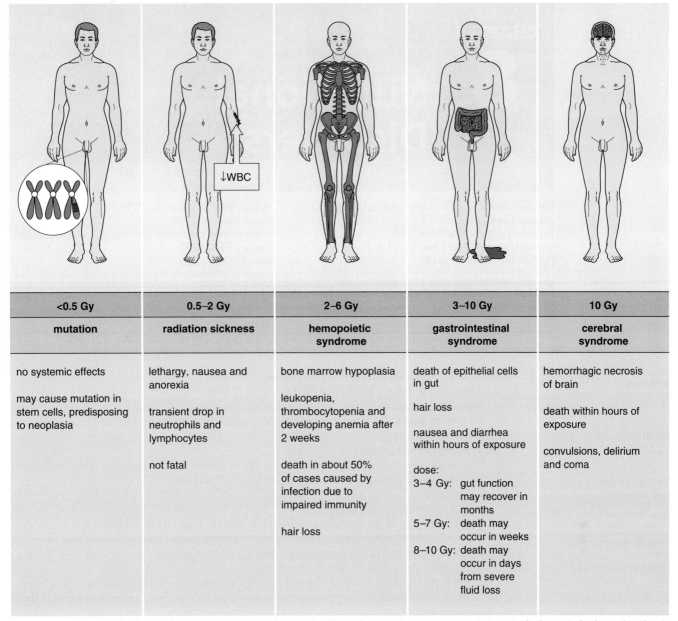

<0.5 Gy	0.5–2 Gy	2–6 Gy	3–10 Gy	10 Gy
mutation	**radiation sickness**	**hemopoietic syndrome**	**gastrointestinal syndrome**	**cerebral syndrome**
no systemic effects may cause mutation in stem cells, predisposing to neoplasia	lethargy, nausea and anorexia transient drop in neutrophils and lymphocytes not fatal	bone marrow hypoplasia leukopenia, thrombocytopenia and developing anemia after 2 weeks death in about 50% of cases caused by infection due to impaired immunity hair loss	death of epithelial cells in gut hair loss nausea and diarrhea within hours of exposure dose: 3–4 Gy: gut function may recover in months 5–7 Gy: death may occur in weeks 8–10 Gy: death may occur in days from severe fluid loss	hemorrhagic necrosis of brain death within hours of exposure convulsions, delirium and coma

7-8: Responses to total body irradiation. *WBC,* White blood cells. *(From Stevens A, Lowe J, Scott I:* Core Pathology, *3rd ed, Mosby Elsevier, 2009, p 142, Fig. 9.3.)*

    e. Cancers caused by radiation include acute leukemia (most common overall cancer; see Chapter 13), papillary carcinoma of the thyroid (see Chapter 23), and osteosarcoma (see Chapter 24).

B. Nonionizing radiation injury

    1. **Definition:** Skin or cornea exposure to ultraviolet (UV) light

    2. Epidemiology

      a. Ultraviolet light B (UVB) is most damaging to the skin.

      b. Pathogenesis of injury (see Chapter 9)

        (1) Pyrimidine (thymine) dimers distort the DNA helix (see Fig. 9-13), *p53* suppressor gene is inactivated, and the *RAS* proto-oncogene is activated.

        (2) General effects include sunburn; actinic (solar) keratosis, a precursor of SCC (2%–5% of cases; see Fig. 25-11 A); and corneal burns from skiing.

      c. Cancer associations include basal cell carcinoma (BCC; most common; see Fig. 25-11 B), SCC (see Fig. 25-11 D), and malignant melanoma (see Fig. 25-9 H).

    3. Laser radiation may cause third-degree burns.

Acute leukemia MC

Papillary thyroid cancer

Osteosarcoma

Non-ionizing radiation injury

Skin/cornea exposure UV light

UVB most damaging

Pyrimidine dimers distort DNA

p53 suppressor gene inactivated

RAS proto-oncogene activated

Sunburn; actinic keratosis

SCC, corneal burns (skiing)

BCC MC

SCC, melanoma

Laser radiation: 3rd-degree burns

ABBREVIATIONS

COD cause of death
MC most common

MCC most common cause

Rx treatment

Nutrient/energy requirements

RDA

Optimal dietary intake nutrients good health

Daily energy expenditure

BMR most important

Energy to support *involuntary* activities that sustain life

Circulation, respiration, ion pumps

Thyroid hormones control BMR

BMR ≈ 60% daily energy expenditure

Body mass

Lean body tissue most metabolically active

Men > women

Hypothyroidism: ↓BMR

Hyperthyroidism: ↑BMR

Thermic effect of food

Energy expended eating

Degree physical activity

Dietary fuels

Carbohydrates

Glucose

Stored as glycogen in liver/muscle

I. Nutrient and Energy Requirements in Humans

A. Recommended dietary allowance (RDA)

- **Definition:** Optimal dietary intake of nutrients that, under ordinary conditions, will keep the general population in good health; varies with sex, age, body weight, diet, and physiologic status

B. Daily energy expenditure

1. Factors influencing the daily energy expenditure include basal metabolic rate (BMR; most important) and thermic effect of food and physical activity.
   a. **Definition:** Rate at which the body uses energy to support all the *involuntary* activities that are necessary to sustain life
      (1) Examples of involuntary activities: circulation, respiration, temperature maintenance, hormone secretion, nerve activity, new tissue synthesis, and maintenance of ion pumps (e.g., Na^+/K^+-ATPase pump)
      (2) BMR controlled by thyroid hormones
   b. BMR accounts for ≈60% of the daily energy expenditure. For example, a person who needs 2000 calories a day may spend as many as 1000 to 1600 calories to support basal metabolism.
   c. Key factors affecting the BMR
      (1) Body mass
         (a) The greater the amount of lean body tissue, the higher the BMR will be.
         (b) Lean body tissue is more metabolically active than fat; therefore, the way to increase the BMR to the maximal rate is to make endurance and strength-building activities a daily habit.
      (2) Gender. Lean body mass is greater in men than women.
      (3) Hypothyroidism. BMR is decreased (hypometabolic).
      (4) Hyperthyroidism. BMR is increased (hypermetabolic).
2. Thermic effect of food
   a. **Definition:** Energy expended in response to having eaten a meal; sometimes called diet-induced thermogenesis
   b. Thermic effect of food uses about 5% to 10% of a meal's energy value.
3. Degree of physical activity affects the daily energy expenditure. As expected, less physical activity has little effect on the daily energy expenditure, whereas increased physical activity increases the daily energy expenditure.

II. Dietary Fuels

A. Carbohydrates

1. Glucose
   a. Glucose is stored primarily as glycogen in the liver and muscle.

(1) Muscle uses glycogen to support its own energy needs.

(2) Liver uses glycogen to supply glucose to other tissues during the fasting state.

   b. Mature red blood cells (RBCs) use only glucose for energy. They lack mitochondria and use anaerobic glycolysis for generating adenosine triphosphate (ATP).

   c. Complete oxidation of glucose produces 4 kcal/g.

2. Enzymatic digestion of carbohydrates

   a. Begins in the mouth.

     (1) Amylase from the salivary glands breaks down polysaccharides (e.g., starch) into disaccharides (lactose, maltose, sucrose).

     (2) In Sjögren syndrome (see Chapter 24), there is immune destruction of the salivary glands and amylase is *not* available to digest polysaccharides. In addition, patients have a dry mouth and poor dentition.

   b. Pancreatic amylase. In chronic pancreatitis, carbohydrates are absorbed, because predigestion by salivary amylase occurs in the mouth, *not* in the small bowel.

   c. Brush border intestinal enzymes are called disaccharidases; examples include lactase, maltase, and sucrase.

     (1) Lactase hydrolyzes lactose to produce galactose and glucose, maltase hydrolyzes maltose to produce two glucoses, and sucrase hydrolyzes sucrose to form fructose and glucose.

     (2) Disaccharidases produce glucose, galactose, and fructose.

       (a) In certain types of diarrhea (e.g., *Rotavirus*), the brush border is temporarily destroyed and disaccharidases *cannot* hydrolyze disaccharides.

       (b) People with lactase deficiency *cannot* hydrolyze lactose in dairy products.

         • Lactase deficiency produces an osmotic type of diarrhea if dairy products are consumed (see Chapter 18).

B. Proteins

1. Amino acids (AAs) are substrates for gluconeogenesis.

   a. Transaminases remove amine groups to form a corresponding α-ketoacid.

   b. Examples of transaminases: alanine aminotransferase (ALT) removes the amine group from alanine to form pyruvate, whereas aspartate aminotransferase (AST) removes an amine group from aspartate to produce oxaloacetate (OAA). Pyruvate and OAA are substrates for gluconeogenesis in the fasting state.

2. Digestion of protein

   a. Begins in the stomach (pepsin and acid)

     (1) Hydrochloric acid (HCl) synthesized in parietal cells cleaves pepsinogen into pepsin.

     (2) If acid is absent (e.g., chronic atrophic gastritis involving the body and fundus), protein *cannot* be digested.

     (3) Pepsin cleaves proteins into smaller polypeptides.

   b. Pancreatic proteases (e.g., trypsin) and peptidases secreted by intestinal epithelial cells hydrolyze polypeptides to release AAs. In chronic pancreatitis, pancreatic proteases are deficient and polypeptides *cannot* be hydrolyzed to AAs.

   c. AAs are absorbed by villi in the small intestine. In celiac disease, there is autoimmune destruction of the villi; therefore, absorption of AAs is compromised.

3. Complete oxidation of protein produces 4 kcal/g.

C. Fats

1. Triglyceride (TG)

   a. TG is the major dietary lipid and is transported by very-low-density lipoprotein (VLDL) and in chylomicrons.

   b. Long-chain free fatty acids (FAs) are the major source of energy for all cells *except* RBCs and brain tissue.

   c. Plants contain unsaturated fats and saturated fats.

     (1) Monounsaturated fats are present in olive oil and canola oil.

     (2) Polyunsaturated fats are present in soybean oil and corn oil.

     (3) Saturated fats are present in coconut oil and palm oil.

   d. Animal fats contain unsaturated and saturated fats.

     (1) Animal fats from the adipose contain saturated fats.

     (2) Animal fats from muscle and organ tissues contain polyunsaturated and monounsaturated fats.

2. Essential FAs

   a. Dietary fats also contain polyunsaturated essential FAs (linolenic acid, linoleic acid).

   b. Functions of linolenic acid (ω-3) and linoleic acid (ω-6)

(1) Important in the synthesis of eicosanoids (see arachidonic acid metabolism in Chapter 3), which are important in muscle contraction and relaxation, blood vessel constriction and relaxation, blood clot formation, blood lipid regulation, and immune response to injury and infection (including fever, inflammation, and pain)

(2) Important as structural and functional components in cell membranes

(3) Contribute lipids to the brain and nerves

(4) Important in normal growth and vision

(5) Assist in gene regulation and genetic activities affecting metabolism

(6) Help maintain the outer structures of the skin, which protects against water loss

(7) Support immune functions

   c. Clinical findings associated with deficiency of essential FAs include scaly dermatitis, hair loss, and poor wound healing.

3. Digestion of dietary TG

   a. Digestion of TG occurs in the small intestine.

(1) Dietary TG is hydrolyzed by pancreatic lipase.

(a) Hydrolysis products of dietary TG are monoglycerides (MGs) and FAs.

(b) In chronic pancreatitis, pancreatic lipase is deficient and fats are undigested, which produces a fatty stool (called steatorrhea).

(2) Bile salts/acid produce micelles to enhance reabsorption of fats by villi in the small intestine.

(a) Micelles contain MGs, FAs, fat-soluble vitamins, and cholesterol esters. Note that all the fat-soluble vitamins (vitamins A, D, E, and K) are packaged in micelles along with the products of fat digestion; hence, any disease producing maldigestion of fats will result in a deficiency of fat-soluble vitamins.

(b) In bile acid deficiency, micelles are not formed, resulting in a fatty stool.

(3) Once absorbed, intestinal cells resynthesize TGs and package them into chylomicrons. Chylomicrons are absorbed into the lymphatics for transport to the bloodstream.

(a) Formation and secretion of chylomicrons requires apolipoprotein B48 (apoB-48). Absence of apoB-48 in abetalipoproteinemia compromises both the formation and the secretion of chylomicrons into the blood (see Chapter 10).

(b) Loss of the villus surface in celiac disease results in fatty stools and deficiencies of fat-soluble vitamins.

   b. Complete oxidation of fat produces 9 kcal/g.

III. Protein-Energy Malnutrition (PEM)

   A. Overview of PEM

1. **Definition:** Inadequate dietary protein

2. PEM is best determined by using the body mass index (BMI), which correlates extremely well with body fatness.

3. BMI = weight in kilograms/height in meters squared. Normal range for the BMI is 18.5 to 24.9 kg/m². PEM is defined as a BMI < 16 kg/m².

4. Measurement of body fat stores

   a. Measuring thickness of skinfolds in various parts of the body with standardized calipers; density measurements (e.g., underwater weighing)

   b. Measurement of conductivity of tissue using bioelectrical impedance; dual energy x-ray absorptiometry (DEXA), which measures total body fatness, fat distribution, and bone density

5. Somatic protein stores in skeletal muscle are evaluated by measuring the circumference of the mid-arm.

6. Visceral protein stores in organs (most is in the liver) are evaluated by measuring serum albumin and transferrin levels.

   B. Kwashiorkor

1. **Definition:** Total caloric intake is normal, but a majority of the calories are from carbohydrates. Dietary protein is notably decreased.

2. Protein findings associated with kwashiorkor

   a. Visceral protein is decreased, whereas somatic protein is relatively unchanged.

   b. Somatic protein is relatively unchanged, because carbohydrates are protein sparing.

(1) Breakdown of liver glycogen (glycogenolysis) into glucose provides the main source of energy.

(2) Proteins in muscle do *not* need to be degraded into AAs and converted into glucose by gluconeogenesis.

c. Visceral protein is decreased, because the liver is unable to synthesize proteins (e.g., albumin and other proteins).

(1) Related to oxidative (free radical [FR]) damage to cellular protein synthesis brought on by infections (e.g., parasitic, fungal, bacterial) superimposed on malnutrition

(2) Pathophysiology explains why antioxidants, antibiotics, and normal protein diets are imperative in the treatment of kwashiorkor.

3. Clinical findings (Fig. 8-1 A, left; B, C; Links 8-1, 8-2, and 8-3)

a. Pitting edema and ascites. Due to a loss of plasma oncotic pressure from hypoalbuminemia (see Chapter 5).

b. Massive hepatomegaly secondary to a fatty liver, the pathogenesis of which is due to:

(1) Decreased synthesis of apolipoproteins. ApoB-100 is required for assembly and secretion of VLDLs in the liver.

(2) Increased synthesis of VLDL from glycerol 3-phosphate (G3P), a three-carbon intermediate substrate of glycolysis

c. Diarrhea

(1) Diarrhea is due to mucosal atrophy in the small intestine with loss of the villi and concurrent loss of the brush border disaccharidases.

Margin notes:

Liver glycogen → glucose for energy

Somatic protein not degraded

↓Visceral protein

FR damage cellular protein synthesis; infections

Pitting edema/ascites; ↓oncotic pressure

Massive hepatomegaly: fatty liver

↓ApoB synthesis; assembly/secretion VLDL in liver

↑VLDL synthesis from G3P

Diarrhea

Mucosal atrophy small intestine

Loss of villi/disaccharidases

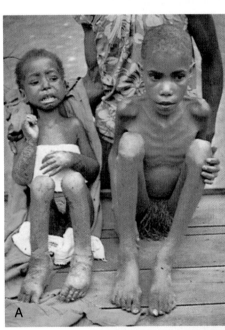
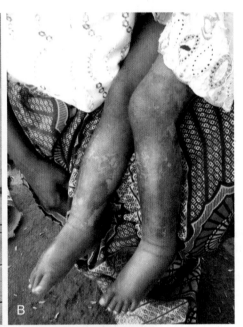
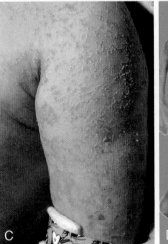
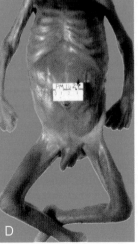

8-1: **A,** Kwashiorkor and marasmus. *Left,* Child with kwashiorkor, showing dependent pitting edema involving the lower legs. Also, there are multiple areas of desquamation on the legs and arms, giving a "flaky paint" appearance. Alternating dark and light areas are noted in the hair. *Right,* Child with marasmus, showing "broomstick" extremities with loss of muscle mass and subcutaneous tissue. **B,** Pitting edema of the legs in a child with kwashiorkor. **C,** Kwashiorkor: "flaky paint" dermatitis. **D,** Marasmus. This emaciated infant died as a result of marasmus, complicated by gastroenteritis. *(A from Forbes C, Jackson W: Color Atlas and Text of Clinical Medicine, 2nd ed, London, Mosby, 2002, p 343, Fig. 7-138; B from Goldman L, Schafer A: Goldman's Cecil Medicine, 25th ed, Saunders Elsevier, 2016, p 1435, Fig. 215-2; C from Katz KA, Mahlberg MH, Honig PJ, et al: Rice nightmare: kwashiorkor in 2 Philadelphia-area infants fed Rice Dream beverage, J Am Acad Dermatol 52(5 Suppl 1):S69-S72, 2005; D from Stevens A, Lowe J, Scott I: Core Pathology, 3rd ed, Mosby Elsevier, 2009, p 148, Fig. 9-7.)*

(2) In addition, problems with cell-mediated immunity (CMI) predispose patients to parasitic infections in the bowel.

(3) Loss of lactase, a disaccharidase, causes problems in using milk-based products as a food supplement.

d. Anemia

(1) RBC precursors in bone are decreased (hypoplasia), leading to anemia.

(2) Multiple vitamin deficiencies are usually present, which also predispose to anemia.

(a) Folic acid and vitamin B$_{12}$ are commonly deficient and may produce a macrocytic anemia (see Chapter 12).

(b) Iron deficiency, due to decreased intake of iron and loss of blood from parasitic infections in the small intestine, produces a microcytic anemia (see Chapter 12).

e. Cutaneous changes

(1) Alternating zones of hyperpigmentation and hypopigmentation in areas of desquamation give the skin a "flaky paint" appearance (Fig. 8-1 A, C).

(2) Hair changes with loss of color, leading to alternating bands of dark hair and light hair ("flag sign"; Fig. 8-1 A)

f. Increased risk for infections. CMI (T cells) is compromised, predisposing patients to parasitic infections.

g. Growth retardation. Due to the lack of essential nutrients in the diet.

h. Psychological disturbances

• Patients are usually apathetic, listless, and anorexic, which contributes to the poor prognosis in kwashiorkor.

C. **Marasmus**

1. **Definition:** Total calorie deprivation with a dietary deficiency of both protein and carbohydrates

2. Epidemiology

• Marasmus results in a decrease in somatic protein (muscle protein).

3. Clinical findings (Fig. 8-1 B, right; D; Link 8-4)

a. Extreme muscle wasting ("broomstick extremities")

(1) Due to the breakdown of muscle protein for energy. AAs from muscle breakdown are used as substrates for gluconeogenesis.

(2) Loss of subcutaneous fat is due to a decrease in leptin stores in the adipose, which stimulates the hypothalamic-pituitary axis to release cortisol, a lipolytic agent (see section IV.D.).

b. Growth retardation, anemia, defects in CMI similar to kwashiorkor

4. Table 8-1 compares findings in kwashiorkor and marasmus.

D. **Secondary PEM**

1. **Definition:** PEM due to inadequate intake of food related to illness, age, alcohol excess, medications, or other causes

2. Epidemiology

a. Secondary PEM is common in older adults (living alone or in hospitals or nursing homes), chronic alcoholics, the homeless population, and bedridden patients.

b. Occurs in 30% to 50% of older individuals in hospitals or nursing homes

(1) Older patients commonly consume less than two-thirds of the RDA.

(2) Accumulated illnesses, medications, and social circumstances deplete body caloric reserves.

(3) Factors responsible for reduced intake

(a) Diminished sense of taste and smell, rendering food less palatable

(b) Suppressed appetite and/or absorption of nutrients in the gastrointestinal tract from accumulated illnesses and medications

(c) Social factors such as reduced income, social isolation, and depression

(d) Advanced age

3. Clinical findings

a. Depletion of subcutaneous fat and skeletal muscle, similar to marasmus

b. Ankle or sacral edema, similar to kwashiorkor

c. Increased risk for infection, impaired wound healing from nutrient deficiencies, and increased risk for death after surgery, particularly hip replacement

IV. **Eating Disorders and Obesity**

A. **Anorexia nervosa**

1. **Definition:** Self-induced starvation leading to secondary PEM (Fig. 8-2); intense fear of gaining weight or becoming fat even while underweight

TABLE 8-1   Clinical Findings in Kwashiorkor and Marasmus

CLINICAL FINDINGS	KWASHIORKOR	MARASMUS
Total caloric intake	Normal	Decreased
Protein intake	Decreased	Decreased
Carbohydrate intake	Increased	Decreased
Pitting edema and ascites	Present	Not present
Growth retardation	Present	Present
Muscle wasting	Not present	Present
Loss subcutaneous fat	Not present	Present
Somatic protein loss	Not present	Present
Visceral protein loss	Present	Not present
Decreased serum albumin/transferrin	Present	Slightly present
Anemia	Present	Present
Mucosal atrophy small bowel villi	Present	Not present
Hepatomegaly	Present	Not present
Defect in cellular immunity	Present	Present
Multiple vitamin deficiencies	Present	Present
"Flaky paint" dermatitis	Present	Not present
"Flag sign" in hair	Present	Not present
Apathy, listlessness, poor appetite	Present	Not present
Prognosis	Poor	Excellent

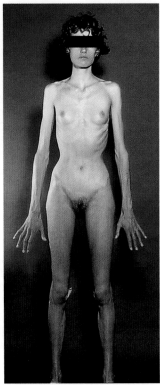

8-2 Anorexia nervosa. Note the loss of muscle and subcutaneous tissue consistent with total calorie deprivation. *(From Forbes C, Jackson W: Color Atlas and Text of Clinical Medicine, 2nd ed, London, Mosby, 2002, p 344, Fig. 7-147.)*

2. Epidemiology
   a. Anorexics view themselves as "fat" even when they are emaciated.
   b. Cause is unknown; however, it is probably multifactorial (sociocultural, psychological, familial, genetic factors, possibly altered serotonin metabolism).
   c. Anorexia has the highest death rate of all the psychiatric disorders.
   d. Laxative abuse is common and often results in a laxative bowel and hypokalemia, the latter precipitating cardiac arrhythmias and possible death.
   e. The disease most commonly occurs in teenage girls and young women. Female/male ratio is 9:1.
   f. Anorexia is common among participants of activities that promote thinness (e.g., athletics, modeling, ballet).
   g. History of sexual abuse is found in 50% of cases.
3. Clinical findings
   a. Secondary amenorrhea (see Chapter 22)
      (1) Excessive loss of body fat and weight results in decreased secretion of gonadotropin-releasing hormone (GnRH) from the hypothalamus.
      (2) Decrease in GnRH causes a decrease in serum gonadotropins (i.e., follicle-stimulating hormone [FSH] and luteinizing hormone [LH]), leading to decreased levels of serum estradiol.
   b. Osteoporosis (loss of both organic bone matrix [osteoid] and mineralized bone)
      (1) In women, this is caused by hypoestrinism (see Chapter 24). In men, it is caused by a decrease in testosterone.
      (2) Estrogen normally enhances osteoblastic activity and inhibits osteoclastic activity. Lack of estrogen leads to decreased osteoblastic activity and increased osteoclastic activity.
   c. Cutaneous findings
      (1) Lanugo hair (fine, downy hair) is present on the face.
      (2) Skin is dry and may also be yellow because of increased carotene levels.

Distorted body image

Multifactorial etiology

Highest death rate all psychiatric disorders

Danger laxative bowel/hypokalemia

Teenage girls/young women; female/male ratio 9:1

Athletics, modeling, ballet

History sexual abuse in 50%

2° Amenorrhea

↓GnRH; excessive ↓body fat/weight

↓FSH, LH, estradiol

Osteoporosis: loss organic/mineralized bone

Osteoporosis → hypoestrinism; males ↓testosterone

Estrogen: normally ↑osteoblastic/↓osteoclastic activity

↓Estrogen → ↓osteoblastic/↑osteoclastic activity → osteoporosis

Lanugo hair (fine, downy hair) on face

Skin dry; ↑carotene (yellow skin)

↓Metabolism carotenes (euthyroid sick syndrome)

Brittle nails, scalp hair sparse

Axillary/pubic hair preserved.

Euthyroid sick syndrome: ↓thyroid hormone

Bradycardia, hypotension, cold intolerance

Peripheral edema

Cardiac arrhythmias, sudden death

↓Serum GnRH, estradiol, FSH, LH

Anovulation; *no* LH surge

↑Serum growth hormone, cortisol (stress hormones)

MC COD ventricular arrhythmia (↓K⁺ laxative abuse)

Bulimia nervosa

Bingeing, self-induced vomiting

More common than anorexia

Teenage girls/young women

Sociocultural, psychological, familial

Western society

Associated with anorexia

(3) Decreased metabolism of carotenes in the diet is caused by the euthyroid sick syndrome (see Chapter 23).

(4) Nails are brittle and scalp hair is sparse. Axillary and pubic hair is preserved.

d. Euthyroid sick syndrome (see Chapter 23); decreased thyroid hormone associated with bradycardia, hypotension, cold intolerance, and the changes in the skin, nails, and hair just listed

e. Mild peripheral edema; increased risk for cardiac arrhythmias and sudden death

4. Laboratory findings

a. Decreased serum GnRH, estradiol, FSH, and LH. Ovulation does *not* occur (anovulation) because there is an absence of the menstrual cycle surge in LH (see Chapter 22).

b. Increased serum growth hormone and cortisol (stress hormones)

5. Most common cause of death: ventricular arrhythmia usually related to hypokalemia from laxative abuse

B. **Some other important causes of weight loss** (Fig. 8-3 A)

C. **Bulimia nervosa**

1. **Definition:** Characterized by bingeing (overeating/drinking) followed by self-induced vomiting

2. Epidemiology

a. More common than anorexia nervosa

b. Predominantly seen in teenage girls and young women; female/male ratio is 10 : 1

c. Etiology is unknown; probably multifactorial (sociocultural, psychological, and familial)

d. More common in Western society, where there is a strong cultural pressure to be slender

e. Commonly associated with anorexia nervosa

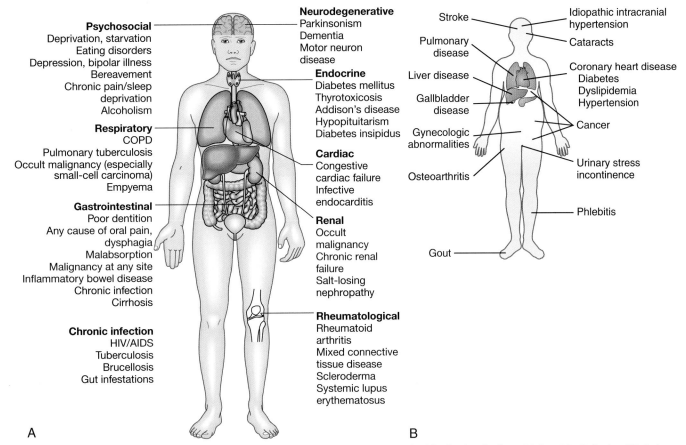

Psychosocial
Deprivation, starvation
Eating disorders
Depression, bipolar illness
Bereavement
Chronic pain/sleep deprivation
Alcoholism

Respiratory
COPD
Pulmonary tuberculosis
Occult malignancy (especially small-cell carcinoma)
Empyema

Gastrointestinal
Poor dentition
Any cause of oral pain, dysphagia
Malabsorption
Malignancy at any site
Inflammatory bowel disease
Chronic infection
Cirrhosis

Chronic infection
HIV/AIDS
Tuberculosis
Brucellosis
Gut infestations

Neurodegenerative
Parkinsonism
Dementia
Motor neuron disease

Endocrine
Diabetes mellitus
Thyrotoxicosis
Addison's disease
Hypopituitarism
Diabetes insipidus

Cardiac
Congestive cardiac failure
Infective endocarditis

Renal
Occult malignancy
Chronic renal failure
Salt-losing nephropathy

Rheumatological
Rheumatoid arthritis
Mixed connective tissue disease
Scleroderma
Systemic lupus erythematosus

Stroke
Pulmonary disease
Liver disease
Gallbladder disease
Gynecologic abnormalities
Osteoarthritis
Gout

Idiopathic intracranial hypertension
Cataracts
Coronary heart disease
Diabetes
Dyslipidemia
Hypertension
Cancer
Urinary stress incontinence
Phlebitis

A

B

8-3: **A,** Some important causes of weight loss. **B,** Medical complications associated with obesity. (**A** *from Walker BR, Colledge NR, Ralston SH, Penman ID:* Davidson's Principles and Practice of Medicine, *22nd ed, Churchill Livingstone Elsevier, 2014, p 859, Fig. 22.23;* **B** *from Melmed S, Polonsky KS, Larsen PR, Kronenberg HM:* Williams Textbook of Endocrinology, *12th ed, Saunders Elsevier, 2011, p 1614, Fig. 36-4.)*

3. Clinical findings
   a. Complications related to vomiting
      (1) Eroded enamel due to acid injury
      (2) Hypokalemia and metabolic alkalosis (see Chapter 5)
      (3) Parotid and salivary gland swelling
      (4) Hematemesis (vomiting blood) from tears/rupture of the distal esophagus (see Chapter 18)
   b. Unlike anorexia nervosa, emaciation and amenorrhea are *not* present unless the patient also has anorexia nervosa.
4. Laboratory findings
   a. Electrolyte abnormalities from vomiting: hyponatremia, hypokalemia, metabolic alkalosis (increased serum bicarbonate; see Chapter 5)
   b. Diarrhea from laxative abuse: hyponatremia, hypokalemia, hypomagnesemia (magnesium is required for the synthesis and release of parathyroid hormone), hypocalcemia, and a normal anion gap (NAG) metabolic acidosis (see Chapter 5)
   c. Because both metabolic alkalosis and metabolic acidosis may be present, the pH may be normal (see mixed arterial blood gas disorders in Chapter 5).
   d. Most common cause of death is a ventricular arrhythmia, usually related to hypokalemia from laxative abuse and vomiting.

D. Obesity
1. **Definition:** BMI that is greater than 30 kg/m^2
   Epidemiology
   a. Morbid obesity is a BMI that is ≥ 40 kg/m^2.
   b. Worldwide epidemic; prevalence increases with advancing age and levels off after the sixth decade, when weight begins to decline.
   c. Obesity is an independent risk factor for ischemic heart disease (IHD).
   d. Obesity in adolescence is significantly associated with an increased risk of severe obesity in adulthood.
   e. Major preventable cause of death and disability in the United States
   f. Evidence suggests that weight loss can reverse or arrest the harmful effects of obesity.
   g. Risk factors for increased morbidity/mortality in obesity are associated with the type of fat distribution.
      (1) Excess fat in the waist and flanks is a more important risk factor than excess fat in the thighs and buttocks.
      (2) Excess visceral fat in the abdominal cavity has greater significance than excess subcutaneous fat. Magnetic resonance imaging (MRI) is used to access the amount of visceral fat.
2. Pathogenesis
   a. Energy balance dysfunction
      (1) Energy balance involves complex neuron circuits in the arcuate nucleus and the paraventricular nuclei of the hypothalamus of the brain, which control food intake and energy expenditure.
      (2) It involves signals from the adipose (leptin) and stomach (ghrelin) that affect the arcuate nucleus and paraventricular nuclei to control food intake and energy expenditure.
      (3) Leptin, a hormone secreted by the adipose tissue, *stimulates* the anorexigenic neurons (suppresses appetite) in the paraventricular nuclei and *inhibits* the orexigenic neurons (normally stimulate appetite) in the lateral hypothalamus.
         (a) Net effect of leptin is suppression of appetite.
         (b) Leptin also *increases* energy expenditure by *stimulating* the sympathetic nervous system, which increases the BMR and stimulates the release of cortisol (breaks down fat stores) and thyroxine (increases the BMR).
      (4) Ghrelin, a gut hormone secreted from the stomach, *stimulates* the orexigenic neurons in the hypothalamus (stimulates appetite) and *inhibits* the anorexigenic neurons (normally suppresses appetite).
         (a) Net effect of ghrelin is to stimulate appetite.
         (b) Ghrelin also *decreases* energy expenditure by *inhibiting* the anorexigenic center (normally activates the sympathetic nervous system and increases the release of cortisol and thyroxine).
      (5) Decrease/dysfunction of leptin produces energy balance dysfunction by leaving ghrelin activity unopposed (↑appetite, ↓energy expenditure), which increases the risk for developing obesity.

Vomiting related

Eroded enamel; acid injury

↓K^+, metabolic alkalosis

Parotid/salivary gland swelling

Hematemesis (tear/rupture distal esophagus)

Absence emaciation/amenorrhea

Vomiting: ↓Na^+/↓K^+/met alkalosis

Diarrhea (laxative abuse)

Diarrhea: ↓Na^+/↓K^+/↓Mg^{2+}, ↓Ca^{2+}, NAG metabolic acidosis

Mixed acid-base disorder; normal pH

MC COD ventricular arrhythmia (↓K^+)

Obesity

Obesity = BMI > 30 kg/m^2

Morbid: BMI $\geq$ 40 kg/m^2

↑With age; ↓after 6th decade

Risk factor IHD

Obesity adolescence → severe obesity adult

Major preventable COD/disability in United States

Weight loss can reverse harmful effects

Risk factors associated with fat distribution

Waist/flanks worse than thighs/buttocks

Abdominal visceral fat > significance than subcutaneous fat

Energy balance dysfunction

Arcuate nucleus, paraventricular nuclei

Leptin hormone from adipose

Net effect leptin: suppression appetite

↑Leptin → ↓food intake, ↑energy expenditure (↑BMR, ↑cortisol, ↑thyroxine)

Ghrelin: hormone secreted by stomach

Net effect: stimulate appetite

↑Ghrelin → ↑food intake, ↓energy expenditure

↓/Dysfunction leptin; ↑ghrelin (↑appetite, ↓energy expenditure)

TABLE 8-2 Clinical Findings Associated With Obesity

CLINICAL FINDING	COMMENTS
Cancer	Increased incidence of estrogen-related cancers (e.g., endometrial, breast) occurs because of increased aromatase stores in adipose and conversion of androgens to estrogens.
Cholelithiasis	Increased incidence of cholecystitis and cholesterol stones occurs, because bile is supersaturated with cholesterol.
Diabetes mellitus, type 2	Increased adipose downregulates insulin receptor synthesis. Hyperinsulinemia increases adipose stores. Weight reduction upregulates insulin receptor synthesis.
Hepatomegaly	Fatty change is accompanied by liver cell injury and repair by fibrosis.
Hypertension	Hyperinsulinemia increases sodium retention (mineralocorticoid function), leading to an increase in plasma volume which increases the blood pressure. Left ventricular hypertrophy and stroke complicate hypertension.
Hypertriglyceridemia	Hypertriglyceridemia decreases serum high-density lipoprotein levels, which increases the risk of developing coronary artery disease.
Increased low-density lipoprotein levels	Low-density lipoprotein predisposes to coronary artery disease. It is the main vehicle for carrying cholesterol. If oxidized, it damages endothelial cells leading to atherosclerosis.
Obstructive sleep apnea	Weight of adipose tissue compresses the upper airways, causing respiratory acidosis (retention of CO_2) and hypoxemia ($\downarrow$arterial PO_2). Hypoxemia and respiratory acidosis cause smooth muscle cells in the pulmonary vessels to vasoconstrict, which leads to pulmonary hypertension. Once pulmonary hypertension develops, the right ventricle becomes hypertrophied. The combination of pulmonary hypertension and right ventricular hypertrophy is called cor pulmonale.
Osteoarthritis	Degenerative arthritis occurs in weight-bearing joints (e.g., femoral heads).

CO_2, Carbon dioxide; PO_2, oxygen partial pressure.

Genetic factors 5%–10%

Chronic ingestion excess calories, hypothalamic lesions

Insulin role

Insulin inhibits lipolysis TG in adipose to FAs

Type 2 diabetes mellitus: $\uparrow$insulin → $\uparrow$TG adipose stores

b. Genetic factors account for 5% to 10% of obesity. Metabolic syndrome (obesity, hypertension, diabetes) is one example.

c. Acquired causes of obesity include chronic ingestion of excess calories and hypothalamic lesions.

d. Insulin has a role in obesity.

(1) Insulin normally inhibits lipolysis or the breakdown of TG in the adipose to FAs.

(2) In type 2 diabetes mellitus, there is an increase in insulin due to fewer insulin receptors and post-receptor defects (see Chapter 23). Hyperinsulinemia increases TG storage in the adipose.

3. Clinical findings (Table 8-2; Fig. 8-3 B)

V. Fat-Soluble Vitamins

A. Overview of fat- and water-soluble vitamins

1. Figure 8-4 summarizes the primary functions of the fat-soluble and water-soluble vitamins.

2. Absorption of fat-soluble vitamins depends on normal fat absorption in the small bowel.

Absorption fat-soluble vitamins → micelles

Malabsorption fat → fat-soluble vitamin deficiencies

Vitamin toxicities: fat-soluble > water-soluble

Water-soluble vitamins: cofactors enzyme reactions (*except* folic acid)

Microflora large intestine: synthesize water-soluble vitamins/vitamin K

Retinol

Dietary β-carotenes/retinol esters sources retinol

Dietary β-carotenes → retinol

$\uparrow$Dietary β-carotenes → yellow skin

a. Recall from the previous discussion of fat digestion, that MGs, FAs, fat-soluble vitamins (A, D, E, K), and cholesterol esters are packaged in micelles, which are then reabsorbed by the villi.

b. Therefore, factors that interfere with fat reabsorption (e.g., chronic pancreatitis, bile salt deficiency, loss of villi) also lead to deficiencies of fat-soluble vitamins.

3. Vitamin toxicities are more common with fat-soluble vitamins than water-soluble vitamins; excesses of the latter are lost in the urine.

4. All the water-soluble vitamins are cofactors for enzyme reactions, with the *exception* of folic acid.

5. In addition to food intake, microflora in the large intestine can synthesize water-soluble vitamins (e.g., thiamine, folic acid, biotin, riboflavin, vitamin $B_{12,}$ and vitamin K).

B. Vitamin A

1. Retinol

a. Retinol (Fig. 8-5)

(1) **Definition:** Dietary β-carotenes and retinol esters are sources of retinol.

(2) After absorption in the small intestine, β-carotenes are converted into retinol.

(a) Increased β-carotenes in the diet cause the skin to turn yellow (hypercarotenemia).

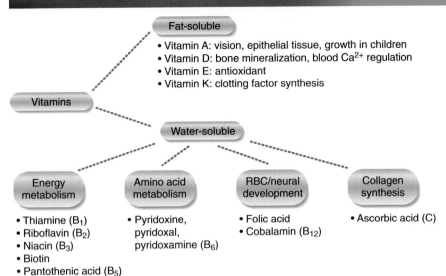

8-4: Classification and functions of the vitamins. Water-soluble vitamins are usually cofactors in key biochemical reactions, whereas fat-soluble vitamins are involved in growth and development of tissue (vitamin A), neutralization of free radicals (vitamin E), bone mineralization and maintenance of serum calcium (vitamin D), and hemostasis (vitamin K). *Ca²⁺*, Calcium ion; *RBC*, red blood cell. *(From Pelley J, Goljan E:* Rapid Review Biochemistry, *3rd ed, Philadelphia, Mosby Elsevier, 2011, p 40, Fig. 4-2.)*

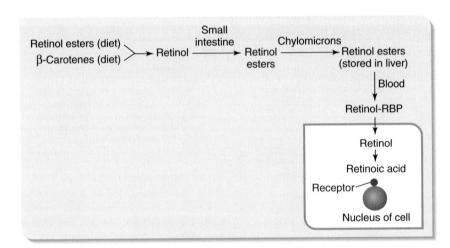

8-5: Vitamin A absorption and transport. Ingested retinol esters and β-carotenes are converted to retinol, the key absorption and transport form of vitamin A. In the small intestine, retinol is converted to retinol esters, the key storage form of vitamin A. When needed, retinol is released from the liver into the bloodstream, where it complexes with retinol-binding protein *(RBP)*. Within cells, retinol is irreversibly oxidized to retinoic acid, which binds to nuclear receptors and activates gene transcription. *(From Pelley J, Goljan E:* Rapid Review Biochemistry, *3rd ed, Philadelphia, Mosby Elsevier, 2011, p 45, Fig. 4-4.)*

    (b) Sclera remains white, whereas in jaundice the sclera is yellow (a distinguishing factor between the two conditions).

    (c) Vitamin toxicity does *not* occur with an increase in serum carotene.

  (3) Retinol is taken up by apoE receptors in the liver and stored in Ito cells as retinyl esters, the storage form of vitamin A.

  (4) When retinyl esters are mobilized, retinol is bound to retinol-binding protein (RBP) and transported to tissue where there are receptors for RBP.

  (5) In tissue, RBP is released and enters the blood, whereas retinol is oxidized to retinoic acid. Retinoic acid binds to nuclear receptors, which activates gene transcription.

  (6) Retinoic acid is important in the differentiation of epithelial tissue and in growth and reproduction.

2. Retinal
  a. **Definition:** Product of the oxidation of retinol
  b. Eye (important in reduced light)
3. Sources
  a. Preformed vitamin A is present in liver, egg yolk, butter, and milk.
  b. β-Carotenes are present in dark-green and yellow vegetables.
  c. Absorption of vitamin A occurs in the small intestine along with TG breakdown products of pancreatic lipase (MGs and FAs), which are packaged in micelles formed by bile salts and acids.
4. Functions
  a. Important in normal vision in reduced light (night vision)
  b. Maintains mucus-secreting epithelium, stimulates immune system, and stimulates growth and reproduction

Yellow skin, white sclera

↑Serum carotene: *no* vitamin toxicity

Retinol, stored in liver Ito cells as retinyl esters

Retinol released from liver binds to RBP in blood

Cells: retinol oxidized to retinoic acid → binds to nuclear receptors → gene transcription

Retinoic acid: differentiation epithelial tissue; growth/reproduction

Retinal

Oxidation product of retinol

Synthesize rhodopsin in rods → important in reduced light

Packaged in micelles

Night vision

Maintains mucus-secreting epithelium

Stimulates immune system, growth/reproduction

Deficiency: diet lacking yellow/green vegetables; fat malabsorption

Toxicity

Eating liver from polar bears, whales, sharks, tuna

Megadoses vitamin A

Rx acne with isotretinoin

Acne (isotretinoin)

APL

Measles

Vitamin A deficiency malnourished children

Post-measles blindness

5. Causes of vitamin A deficiency include a diet lacking sufficient yellow and green vegetables and fat malabsorption (e.g., celiac disease; see **II.C.3.**)
6. Causes of toxicity
   a. Consumption of the liver of polar bears, whales, sharks, and tuna. Toxicity is a common finding in Eskimos, who hunt and eat polar bear and whale livers.
   b. Taking megadoses of vitamin A; treatment of acne with isotretinoin
7. Clinical findings in deficiency and toxicity (Table 8-3)
8. Clinical uses include the treatment of:
   a. Acne (e.g., isotretinoin)
   b. Acute promyelocytic leukemia (APL; see Chapter 13), where it causes leukemic cells to differentiate into neutrophils, which subsequently undergo apoptosis and die
   c. Measles
      (1) Vitamin A deficiency is almost universally present in malnourished children in underdeveloped countries. When these children develop measles, post-measles blindness is a common complication of the infection because of underlying vitamin A deficiency.

TABLE 8-3   Fat-Soluble Vitamins: Clinical Findings in Deficiency and Toxicity

VITAMIN	SIGNS OF DEFICIENCY	SIGNS OF TOXICITY
Vitamin A	• Impaired night vision is an early finding. Blindness may occur due to squamous metaplasia of the corneal epithelium, which is normally nonkeratinizing squamous epithelium (produces keratomalacia; Fig. 8-7 A, B). Conjunctival epithelium (normally pseudostratified columnar epithelium with goblet cells) undergoes squamous metaplasia, producing localized keratin debris (called Bitot spot) or more extensive areas of keratinization (called xerophthalmia). • Vitamin A deficiency is a major cause of blindness worldwide. • Follicular hyperkeratosis may occur from loss of sebaceous gland function related to plugging of the ducts by excess keratin (Fig. 8-7 C). • Vitamin A deficiency is a major cause of growth retardation in children worldwide. • Other findings in vitamin A deficiency include pneumonia (squamous metaplasia of the ciliated columnar epithelium of the bronchi) and renal calculi.	Signs of hypervitaminosis A include papilledema with blurred vision, seizures (due to an increase in intracranial pressure), hepatitis, bone pain (due to periosteal proliferation), and bone resorption and fractures (retinoic acid stimulates osteoclast production and activation).
Vitamin D	• Signs of vitamin D deficiency in both adults and children include pathologic fractures due to an excess of unmineralized osteoid, tibial bowing due to soft bones (Fig. 8-7 D), and continuous muscle contraction (tetany) due to low serum ionized calcium levels (see Chapter 23). • Signs of vitamin D deficiency (rickets) exclusively seen in *children* include craniotabes (soft skull bones with delayed suture and fontanel closing), rachitic rosary (defective mineralization and overgrowth of unmineralized epiphyseal cartilage in the costochondral junctions), frontal bone thickening and bossing of the forehead, short stature (often in the 3rd percentile), and pectus carinatum ("pigeon breast," anterior protrusion of the sternum). • Adults who develop vitamin D deficiency do *not* have craniotabes or rachitic rosaries, because the bone or cartilage in these areas has already been mineralized. Bone remodeling is defective, because newly formed osteoid is excessive and left unmineralized, causing the bone to be soft, hence the term *osteomalacia* (soft bone; Link 8-5).	Signs of hypervitaminosis D include hypercalcemia with metastatic calcification of soft tissue, renal calculi, and bone pain.
Vitamin E	• Hemolytic anemia may result from free radical damage to the lipid in the RBC membrane. • Peripheral neuropathy and degeneration of the posterior column (poor joint sensation) and spinocerebellar tracts (ataxia) may result from free radical damage. • In the neonate, vitamin E deficiency presents with hemolytic anemia, peripheral edema, and thrombocytosis.	• Excessive intake of vitamin E has a synergistic effect with warfarin anticoagulation. It causes over-anticoagulation manifested by bleeding and a markedly prolonged prothrombin time and calculated INR. • Giving vitamin K reverses the over-anticoagulation.
Vitamin K	• Newborns with vitamin K deficiency develop hemorrhagic disease (CNS bleeding, ecchymoses) due to deficiency of the vitamin K–dependent coagulation factors (II, VII, IX, and X). • Adults with vitamin K deficiency develop gastrointestinal bleeding and ecchymoses (bleeding) in the skin. • Prothrombin time and partial thromboplastin time are prolonged (see Chapter 15).	If a pregnant woman is taking excessive amounts of vitamin K, the newborn child may develop a hemolytic anemia, jaundice, and kernicterus (see Chapter 16).

CNS, Central nervous system; *INR,* International normalized ratio; *RBC,* red blood cell.

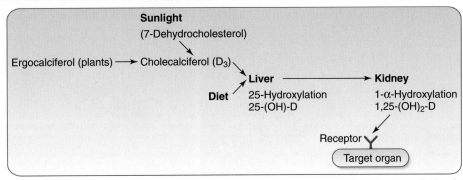

8-6: Vitamin D metabolism. Most vitamin D comes from photoconversion of 7-dehydrocholesterol to cholecalciferol (vitamin D₃).

(2) Treatment with vitamin A decreases the risk for developing blindness by increasing corneal stromal repair.

d. Hairy leukoplakia, due to Epstein-Barr virus (used topically); retinitis pigmentosum

C. Vitamin D

1. Sources of vitamin D include fish oil, egg yolk, liver, grains, and fortified milk, which contribute 10% of the daily required vitamin D.

2. Metabolism (Fig. 8-6; see Chapter 23)

   a. Preformed vitamin D in plants called ergocalciferol is converted to cholecalciferol (vitamin D₃).

   b. Endogenous synthesis of vitamin D in the skin occurs by photoconversion of 7-dehydrocholesterol via sunlight into cholecalciferol (vitamin D₃).

      (1) Accounts for ≈90% of endogenously derived vitamin D

      (2) Cholecalciferol (vitamin D₃) is an over-the-counter (OTC) vitamin supplement and is frequently measured to determine a person's vitamin D status.

   c. Absorption occurs in the small intestine in association with fat absorption (see vitamin A discussion).

   d. Liver hydroxylation of vitamin D to 25-hydroxyvitamin D (25-[OH]D, calcidiol) occurs in the cytochrome P450 (CYP450) system. 25-Hydroxylases are CYP27A1 and other cytochrome P isoenzymes.

   e. Kidney hydroxylation by 1-α-hydroxylase in the proximal tubule produces 1,25-(OH)₂D (active form of vitamin D, calcitriol).

      (1) Parathyroid hormone (PTH) synthesizes 1-α-hydroxylase in the proximal tubules.

      (2) In sarcoidosis, macrophages in granulomas synthesize 1-α-hydroxylase and synthesize vitamin D, producing hypervitaminosis D (see Chapter 17).

   f. Calcitriol attaches to nuclear receptors in target tissues (e.g., osteoblasts).

   g. Feedback control of calcitriol synthesis is calcium mediated.

      (1) Hypocalcemia stimulates the release of PTH, which increases the synthesis of 1-α-hydroxylase (1-α-OHase), which in turn increases the synthesis of calcitriol.

      (2) Hypercalcemia inhibits the release of PTH. Decreased levels of PTH decrease the synthesis of 1-α-hydroxylase, which decreases the synthesis of calcitriol.

3. Functions of calcitriol

   a. Functions as a hormone

   b. Important in the maintenance of serum calcium and phosphorus. Increases calcium and phosphorus absorption from the small bowel and reabsorption in the kidneys

   c. Required for mineralization of epiphyseal cartilage and osteoid matrix in bone formation

      (1) Vitamin D receptors are located on osteoblasts and mature chondrocytes.

      (2) Attachment to the receptor stimulates the release of alkaline phosphatase (AP). AP dephosphorylates pyrophosphate (PP), which normally inhibits bone mineralization.

      (3) Calcitriol also stimulates osteoblasts to synthesize osteocalcin, a calcium-binding protein that is involved in the deposition of calcium in bone.

   d. Calcitriol stimulates conversion of macrophage stem cells into osteoclasts in the bone marrow.

   e. Calcitriol stimulates the maturation of cells, including those in the immune system.

Rx vitamin A: ↓risk blindness from measles

Hairy leukoplakia (Epstein-Barr virus)

Retinitis pigmentosum

Fish oil, egg yolk, liver, fortified milk

Ergocalciferol (plants) → cholecalciferol (vitamin D₃)

Photoconversion 7-dehydrocholesterol → cholecalciferol

Vitamin D₃ (OTC drug)

Determine patient vitamin D status

Absorption small intestine

25-Hydroxylation liver CYP450 system

Kidney hydroxylation: 1,25-(OH)₂D active form

PTH synthesizes 1-α-hydroxylase in proximal tubules

Sarcoidosis: macrophages synthesize 1-α-hydroxylase → hypervitaminosis D

Calcitriol attaches to nuclear receptors (osteoblasts)

Feedback control calcitriol synthesis calcium mediated

↓Serum Ca²⁺ → ↑PTH → ↑1-α-OHase → ↑calcitriol

↑Serum Ca²⁺ → ↓PTH → ↓1-α-OHase → ↓calcitriol

Functions as a hormone

Maintain serum Ca²⁺/PO₄³⁻

↑Calcium/phosphorus reabsorption small bowel/kidneys

Bone mineralization

Vitamin D receptors osteoblasts/chondrocytes

Attachment releases AP

AP dephosphorylates PP (inhibitor bone mineralization)

Calcium-binding protein; bone mineralization

Macrophage stem cells → osteoclasts

Maturation of cells; immune system

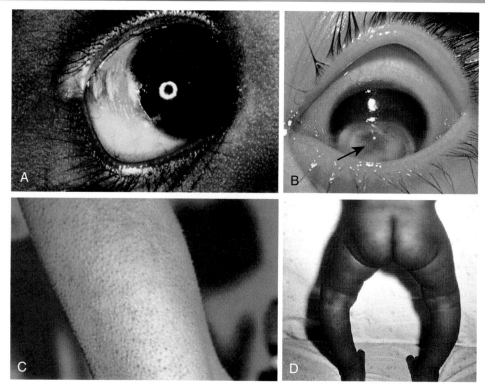

8-7: **A**, Squamous metaplasia of conjunctiva (Bitot spot; *arrow*) in vitamin A deficiency. Note the raised white area on the conjunctiva *(arrow)* encroaching on the cornea. **B**, Keratomalacia. Liquefactive necrosis *(black arrow)* is affecting most of the cornea. **C**, Follicular hyperkeratosis in vitamin A deficiency. Note the "goose-bump" appearance of the raised, hyperkeratotic lesions. **D**, Child with rickets. Note the bow legs. (**A** *reprinted with permission from Oomen HAPC: Vitamin A deficiency, xerophthalmia and blindness.* Nutr Rev *1974:32:161-166, Wiley-Blackwell; **B** from Walker BR, Colledge NR, Ralston SH, Penman ID:* Davidson's Principles and Practice of Medicine, *22nd ed, Churchill Livingstone Elsevier, 2014, p 126, Fig. 5.18 A; **C** from Morgan SL, Weinsier RL:* Fundamentals of Clinical Nutrition, *2nd ed, St. Louis, Mosby, 1998; **D** from Kumar V, Fausto N, Abbas A:* Robbins and Cotran's Pathologic Basis of Disease, *8th ed, Philadelphia, Saunders, 2007, p 455, Fig. 8-21.)*

Vitamin D deficiency

Renal failure

Renal failure MCC vitamin D deficiency

↓1-α-Hydroxylation vitamin D in proximal tubule cells

↓Sun exposure → ↓skin photoconversion to vitamin D₃

Fat malabsorption → ↓micelle formation → ↓vitamin D/fat reabsorption

Chronic liver disease → ↓25-(OH)D

Induction CYP450 system → ↑conversion 25-(OH)D → inactive metabolite

Exclusive breast-feeding

Megadoses, sarcoidosis

Vitamin E

Nuts, green vegetables, wheat germ

Antioxidant: protect cell membranes FR damage

↓Oxidization LDL (FR form causes atherosclerosis)

Prevent lung FR damage by superoxide (Rx with high concentration O₂; RDS)

4. Causes of vitamin D deficiency
   a. Renal failure
      (1) Most common cause of vitamin D deficiency
      (2) Renal failure causes a decrease in 1-α-hydroxylation of vitamin D, due to the loss of proximal tubule cells that synthesize 1-α-hydroxylase.
   b. Inadequate exposure to sunlight (e.g., clothes, black skin, sunscreen) decreases photoconversion of 7-dehydrocholesterol to cholecalciferol.
   c. Fat malabsorption. Decreased micelle formation with concomitant decrease in vitamin D and fat reabsorption.
   d. Chronic liver disease. Due to decreased synthesis of 25-(OH)D in the CYP450 system.
   e. Induction of the liver CYP450 enzyme system (e.g., alcohol) increases the metabolism of 25-(OH)D into an inactive metabolite.
   f. Infants who breast-feed exclusively *without* vitamin D supplementation because human breast milk has low levels of vitamin D
5. Causes of vitamin D toxicity include megadoses of vitamin D and increased synthesis of vitamin D in granulomas (e.g., sarcoidosis (see Chapter 17).
6. Clinical findings in vitamin D deficiency and toxicity (see Table 8-3; Fig. 8-7 D)

D. Vitamin E
1. Sources of vitamin E include nuts (almonds, seeds), green leafy vegetables, olives, vegetable oil, and wheat germ.
2. Functions
   a. Antioxidant that protects cell membranes from lipid peroxidation by FRs (see Chapter 2)
   b. Prevents the oxidation of low-density lipoprotein (LDL) to a FR form (oxidized LDL), which is more atherogenic than non-oxidized LDL
   c. Protects cell membranes in the lungs from FR damage by superoxide when high concentrations of O₂ are used (e.g., treatment of respiratory distress syndrome [RDS] in neonates)

3. Causes of deficiency
   a. Fat malabsorption in children with cystic fibrosis
      - Chronic pancreatitis is universal in cystic fibrosis; therefore, pancreatic lipase is deficient and unable to hydrolyze dietary fat into MGs and FAs.
   b. Abetalipoproteinemia, due to chylomicrons accumulating in villi and preventing micelle absorption into the small intestine (see Chapter 10)
4. Megadoses of vitamin E may be toxic.
5. Clinical findings in vitamin E deficiency and toxicity (see Table 8-3)

E. Vitamin K
   1. Sources of vitamin K include bacteria within the colon, which synthesize vitamin K (most common source), and dark green vegetables.
   2. Endogenously synthesized vitamin K is activated by the liver microsomal enzyme epoxide reductase. Anticoagulant effect of coumarin derivatives is due to inhibition of epoxide reductase.
   3. Function (see Chapter 15)
      a. γ-Carboxylates glutamate residues in vitamin K–dependent procoagulants and anticoagulants (proteins C and S, which degrade activated factors V and VIII)
         (1) Procoagulants include factors II (prothrombin), VII, IX, and X.
         (2) Procoagulants that are synthesized by the liver are nonfunctional.
      b. γ-Carboxylation allows vitamin K–dependent procoagulants to actively bind to calcium in fibrin clot formation. Calcium is important in the normal coagulation pathway because it binds to the vitamin K–dependent coagulation factors that are involved in the formation of a fibrin clot.
   4. Causes of deficiency
      a. Use of broad-spectrum antibiotics
         (1) Antibiotics destroy bacteria in the colon that synthesize vitamin K.
         (2) Antibiotics are the most common cause of vitamin K deficiency in hospitalized patients.
      b. Newborns
         (1) Bacterial colonization of the bowel does *not* occur until newborns are 5 to 6 days old.
         (2) Newborns must receive an intramuscular (IM) injection of vitamin K at birth, because they are essentially anticoagulated from birth until approximately 1 week of life. In this time period, vitamin K–dependent factors are nonfunctional because they are *not* γ-carboxylated.
         (3) Vitamin K injection prevents vitamin K deficiency bleeding (previously known as hemorrhagic disease of the newborn (see Chapter 15).
            - Breast milk is deficient in vitamin K.
      c. Coumarin derivatives/cirrhosis
         (1) Both decrease epoxide reductase activation of vitamin K
         (2) Rat poison is warfarin; hence, children/adults who inadvertently or purposely ingest rat poisoning may develop life-threatening bleeding that can be reversed only by infusion of fresh frozen plasma.
         (3) Recall that the liver synthesizes the microsomal enzyme epoxide reductase. This is compromised when the liver is cirrhotic (replaced by fibrosis).

Warfarin is an anticoagulant that inhibits epoxide reductase, which prevents any further γ-carboxylation of the vitamin K–dependent coagulation factors. However, full anticoagulation does *not* immediately occur, because previously γ-carboxylated factors are still present. Prothrombin has the longest half-life; therefore, full anticoagulation requires at least 3 to 4 days *before* all the functional prothrombin has disappeared. This explains why patients are initially placed on both heparin and warfarin, because heparin provides immediate anticoagulation in the patient by enhancing antithrombin activity.

      d. Fat malabsorption. Because vitamin K is normally absorbed with fat in micelles, fat malabsorption (e.g., celiac disease) causes decreased intestinal absorption of the vitamin, as well as all the other fat-soluble vitamins (i.e., A, D, E).
   5. Toxicity caused by excessive intake of vitamin K is uncommon.
   6. Clinical findings in vitamin K deficiency and toxicity are discussed in Table 8-3.

VI. Water-Soluble Vitamins
   A. Thiamine (vitamin B₁)
      1. Sources of thiamine include liver, eggs, whole grain cereal, rice, and wheat. Removal of the outer layer of grain in the refining process (white rice, white bread) significantly

---

Chronic pancreatitis child with cystic fibrosis → ↓lipase → fat malabsorption

Abetalipoproteinemia → prevent micelle absorption

Megadoses are toxic

Vitamin K

Majority synthesized by colonic bacteria

Liver epoxide reductase activates vitamin K

Coumarin derivatives inhibit epoxide reductase

γ-Carboxylates II, VII, IX, X; protein C/S

Can bind to calcium in fibrin clot formation

Calcium binds to vitamin K–dependent coagulation factors

Broad-spectrum antibiotics destroy bacteria that synthesize vitamin K

Antibiotics MC hospital cause vitamin K deficiency

Lack bacterial colonization bowel until 5–6 days old

Newborns must receive IM injection vitamin K

Prevent hemorrhagic disease of newborn

Breast milk lacks vitamin K

Coumarin/liver disease ↓epoxide reductase

Rat poison is warfarin

↓Intestinal absorption fat-soluble vitamins (celiac disease)

Toxicity uncommon

Outer layer grain has thiamine; refined rice deficient in thiamine

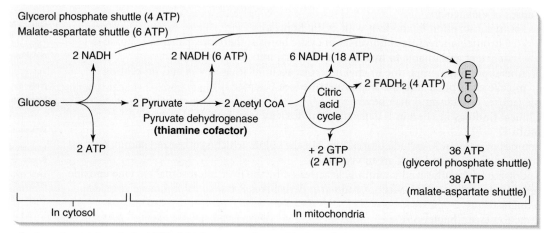

8-8: Overview of adenosine triphosphate *(ATP)* yield from complete oxidation of glucose. Substrate-level phosphorylation generates two ATP per glucose molecule in the cytosol; however, the bulk of the energy output is derived from electron flow through the electron transport chain *(ETC)* and coupled oxidative phosphorylation. Electrons from cytosolic reduced nicotinamide adenine dinucleotide *(NADH)* move into mitochondria by the malate-aspartate shuttle to produce 38 ATP, or by the glycerol phosphate shuttle, which results in a slightly lower ATP yield (i.e., 36 ATP). Note that thiamine is a cofactor for pyruvate dehydrogenase conversion to acetyl coenzyme A *(CoA)*, which is used to synthesize citrate for the citric acid cycle (acetyl CoA + oxaloacetic acid → citrate), which is the main source of ATP. Therefore, a deficiency of thiamine plays a key role in the overall synthesis of ATP. *FADH₂*, Flavin adenine dinucleotide (reduced form). *(From Pelley J, Goljan E: Rapid Review Biochemistry, 3rd ed, Philadelphia, Mosby Elsevier, 2011, p 66, Fig. 6-2.)*

lowers thiamine content. Eating refined rice is the most common cause of thiamine deficiency worldwide.

2. Functions

   a. Cofactor in biochemical reactions that produce ATP. For example, thiamine is a cofactor in the conversion of pyruvate to acetyl CoA by pyruvate dehydrogenase.
   b. This reaction produces 2 NADH, which produces a total of 6 ATP in oxidative phosphorylation (Fig. 8-8).

   c. Thiamine is a cofactor in transketolase reactions in the pentose phosphate pathway.
      (1) Transketolase is involved in two-carbon transfer reactions that provide fructose 6-phosphate and glyceraldehyde 3-phosphate intermediates for glycolysis in the fed state and gluconeogenesis in the fasting state.

      (2) Thiamine levels are evaluated by measuring RBC transketolase activity.
3. Causes of deficiency

   a. Chronic alcoholism is the most common cause of thiamine deficiency in the United States.
   b. Diet of unenriched rice (rice with the outer layer removed) is the most common cause of deficiency in developing countries.
4. Clinical findings in deficiency are summarized in Table 8-4.

B. Riboflavin (vitamin B₂)

1. Sources of riboflavin include liver, dairy products, nuts, green leafy vegetables, and soybeans.

2. Active forms of riboflavin include flavin adenine dinucleotide (FAD) and flavin mononucleotide (FMN).
   a. FAD is a cofactor associated with succinate dehydrogenase conversion of succinate to fumarate in the citric acid cycle.

   b. FMN is in complex I and FAD in complex II of the electron transport chain (ETC; primary site for ATP synthesis). Both accept two electrons in these locations to produce their reduced forms, FMNH₂ and FADH₂, respectively.
3. Deficiency is uncommon but is most often caused by severe malnourishment.
4. Clinical findings in deficiency are summarized in Table 8-4.

C. Niacin (vitamin B₃, nicotinic acid; Fig. 8-9 A)

1. Sources include most animal products, fruits and vegetables, and seeds.
2. Functions
   a. Active forms

      (1) Oxidized nicotinamide adenine dinucleotide (NAD⁺)
      (2) Oxidized nicotinamide adenine dinucleotide phosphate (NADP⁺)

TABLE 8-4 Water-Soluble Vitamins: Clinical Findings in Deficiency

VITAMIN	SIGNS OF DEFICIENCY
Thiamine (vitamin B$_1$)	• Dry beriberi: peripheral neuropathy (due to demyelination) • Wernicke syndrome: ataxia, confusion, nystagmus, ophthalmoplegia; hemorrhages present in the mammillary bodies (see Chapter 26, see Fig. 26-21 B) • Korsakoff syndrome: antegrade and retrograde amnesia; demyelination in the limbic system (see Chapter 26) • Wet beriberi: dilated cardiomyopathy with biventricular heart failure and dependent pitting edema; cardiac muscle lacks ATP; intravenous thiamine reverses cardiomyopathy in some cases (see Chapter 11)
Riboflavin (vitamin B$_2$)	Corneal neovascularization, glossitis (magenta tongue), cheilosis (cracked lips), angular stomatitis (fissuring at the angles of the mouth)
Niacin (vitamin B$_3$)	Pellagra: diarrhea, dermatitis (hyperpigmentation in sun-exposed areas; see Fig. 8-10 A), dementia (3 Ds)
Pyridoxine (vitamin B$_6$)	Sideroblastic anemia (microcytic anemia with ringed sideroblasts; see Fig. 12-13), convulsions, peripheral neuropathy
Cobalamin (vitamin B$_{12}$)	• Megaloblastic anemia with hypersegmented neutrophils (see Fig. 12-18 D), pancytopenia, neurologic disease (posterior column and lateral corticospinal tract demyelination [see Fig. 12-18 C], peripheral neuropathy, dementia), glossitis (see Chapter 12) • Vitamin B$_{12}$ deficiency in infants seen exclusively in breast-fed infants of vitamin B$_{12}$–deficient mothers
Folic acid	• Megaloblastic anemia with hypersegmented neutrophils (more than five lobes), pancytopenia (RBCs, WBCs, platelets all decreased), and glossitis (inflamed tongue); no neurologic abnormalities (see Chapter 12) • Open neural tube defects: several gene defects affecting enzymes and proteins involved in transport and metabolism of folic acid implicated in the pathogenesis of open neural tube defects (see Fig. 26-4 A–E; see Chapter 26)
Biotin	• Dermatitis, alopecia, and lactic acidosis possible • Biotin is cofactor in the pyruvate carboxylase reaction where pyruvate is converted to oxaloacetate; with biotin deficiency, conversion to oxaloacetate blocked; pyruvate level increases and is converted by pyruvate dehydrogenase to lactic acid (increased anion gap metabolic acidosis)
Ascorbic acid (vitamin C)	• In vitamin C deficiency (scurvy), collagen weakened from insufficient cross-bridge formation between tropocollagen molecules; resulting decrease in tensile strength of collagen in the walls of capillaries and venules causing them to rupture, producing skin hemorrhages, perifollicular hemorrhages (ring of hemorrhage around hair follicles; see Fig. 8-10 B), hemarthrosis (bleeding into joints), and bleeding gums with loose teeth (see Fig. 8-10 C) • Additional findings in scurvy: anemia (combined iron and folic acid deficiency), glossitis, poor wound healing, bone fragility and joint pains, calcium oxalate stones in the urine, corkscrew hairs (see Fig. 8-10 D, E)

ATP, Adenosine triphosphate; *RBCs,* red blood cells; *WBCs,* white blood cells.

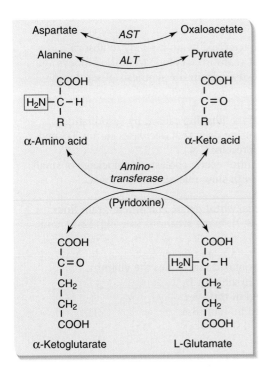

8-9: Transamination. In transamination reactions, amino acids can be synthesized from α-ketoacids, or ketoacids can be synthesized from amino acids. Pyridoxine is the cofactor for aminotransferase for these reaction. Note that if the amine group *(H$_2$N–; square)* is removed from alanine by alanine aminotransferase *(ALT),* pyruvate is formed and is used as a substrate for gluconeogenesis. Similarly, if the amine group *(H$_2$N–; square)* is removed from aspartate by aspartate aminotransferase *(AST),* oxaloacetate is formed and is used as a substrate for gluconeogenesis. *(Modified from Pelley J, Goljan E: Rapid Review Biochemistry, 3rd ed, Philadelphia, Mosby Elsevier, 2011, p 99, Fig. 8-1.)*

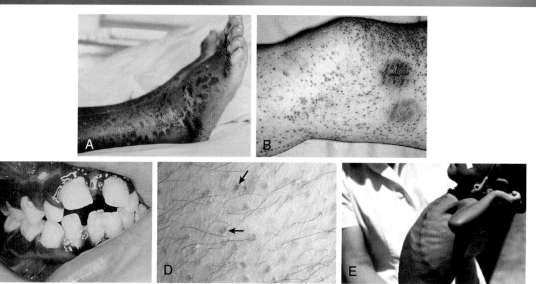

8-10: **A,** Pellagra. Note the areas of irregular hyperpigmented skin. **B,** Perifollicular hemorrhage in vitamin C deficiency. The areas of hemorrhage surround hair follicles. **C,** Gums showing the effects of scurvy. The swelling, inflammation, and bleeding of the gingival papillae are prominent. **D,** Corkscrew hairs in vitamin C deficiency. Note the coiled hairs lying within plugged follicles. **E,** Scorbutic rosary in vitamin C deficiency (excess osteoid). *(A, C from Morgan SL, Weinsier RL: Fundamentals of Clinical Nutrition, 2nd ed, St. Louis, Mosby, 1998; B from Callen JP, Palier AS, Creer KE, Swinyer LJ: Color Atlas of Dermatology, 2nd ed, Philadelphia, Saunders, 2000; D from Savin JA, Hunter JAA, Hepburn NC: Diagnosis in Color: Skin Signs in Clinical Medicine, London, Mosby-Wolfe, 1997, p 85, Fig. 3-8; E courtesy of Dr. JD Maclean, McGill Centre for Tropical Diseases, Montreal; from Kliegman RM: Nelson Textbook of Pediatrics, 20th ed, Elsevier, 2016, p 329, Fig. 50-1.)*

Cofactors oxidation-reduction reactions

NAD⁺ reactions catabolic

NADP⁺ reactions anabolic

Pellagra: deficiency niacin

Corn-based diets deficient tryptophan/niacin

Tryptophan used to synthesize niacin

Corn-based diet

Hartnup disease

Carcinoid syndrome

Tryptophan used to synthesize serotonin

Three Ds of pellagra: dermatitis, diarrhea, dementia

Excessive intake: flushing caused by vasodilation

Adverse effect nicotinic acid (lipid-lowering agent)

Intrahepatic cholestasis

Pyridoxine

Heme synthesis, transamination reactions, neurotransmitters

INH inactivates pyridoxine

Goat mild deficient in pyridoxine

Chronic alcoholism pyridoxine degraded in liver

Biotin

Most foods

    b. NAD^+ and $NADP^+$ are cofactors in oxidation-reduction reactions.
      (1) In general, NAD^+ oxidation-reduction reactions are catabolic (e.g., glycolysis).
      (2) In general, $NADP^+$ oxidation-reduction reactions are anabolic (e.g., FA and cholesterol synthesis).
  3. Causes of deficiency (pellagra; Fig. 8-10 A)
    a. Corn-based diets are the major cause of niacin deficiency, because corn is deficient in tryptophan and niacin.
    b. Deficiency of tryptophan
      (1) Used to synthesize niacin
      (2) Causes of tryptophan deficiency
        (a) Corn-based diet
        (b) Hartnup disease
          • Inborn error of metabolism characterized by an inability to absorb tryptophan in the small bowel or reabsorb tryptophan in the kidneys
        (c) Carcinoid syndrome. Tryptophan is used up in the synthesis of serotonin (see Chapter 18).
  4. Clinical findings in deficiency are summarized in Table 8-4.
  5. Excessive intake of niacin (nicotinic acid) leads to flushing caused by vasodilation.
    a. Adverse effect of nicotinic acid, a lipid-lowering drug that decreases serum TG and cholesterol and increases high-density lipoproteins
    b. Another adverse effect of nicotinic acid is intrahepatic cholestasis (blockage of small bile ducts), leading to jaundice (less likely with slow-release preparations).

D. Pyridoxine (vitamin B_6)
  1. Sources of pyridoxine include meats, fish, seeds, wheat germ, and whole-grain flour.
  2. Functions: Required for transamination (Fig. 8-9), heme synthesis (see Fig. 12-8), and neurotransmitter synthesis
  3. Causes of deficiency
    a. Isoniazid (used in treating tuberculosis). Isoniazid inactivates the vitamin.
    b. Drinking goat milk. Goat milk is deficient in vitamin B_6.
    c. Chronic alcoholism. Pyridoxine is degraded in the liver.
  4. Clinical findings in deficiency are summarized in Table 8-4.

E. Vitamin B_{12} (cobalamin) (see Chapter 12)

F. Folic acid (see Chapter 12)

G. Biotin
  1. Present in most foods
  2. Function of biotin

a. Cofactor in carboxylase reactions
b. Examples of carboxylase reactions
   (1) Conversion of pyruvate to OAA by pyruvate carboxylase in gluconeogenesis
   (2) Conversion of propionyl CoA to methylmalonyl CoA by propionyl CoA carboxylase in odd-chain FA metabolism, the end-product of which is succinyl CoA
3. Causes of deficiency
   a. Eating raw eggs (avidin in eggs binds biotin). One would have to consistently consume more than 20 raw eggs a day to become biotin deficient.
   b. Taking antibiotics (destroys colonic microflora that synthesize the vitamin)
4. Clinical findings in deficiency are summarized in Table 8-4.

H. **Ascorbic acid (vitamin C;** see Fig. 8-10 B–E)
1. Sources of ascorbic acid include fruits, vegetables, liver, fish, and milk.
2. Functions
   a. Important in collagen synthesis
      (1) Vitamin C hydroxylates lysine and proline residues in the rough endoplasmic reticulum (RER) of fibroblasts.
      (2) Lysyl oxidase, a copper-containing enzyme, oxidizes the lysine side chain to reactive aldehydes that spontaneously form cross-links between tropocollagen molecules.
      (3) Cross-linking of collagen molecules is responsible for the tensile strength of collagen (see Chapter 3).
         (a) In vitamin C deficiency (scurvy), tropocollagen molecules have defective cross-linking, causing them to have decreased tensile strength. Abnormal tropocollagen molecules with defective cross-linking are poorly secreted from the fibroblast and are also subject to enzymatic degradation; hence the amount of collagen that is synthesized is not only decreased but also structurally abnormal.
         (b) Because osteoid in bone is composed of collagen, there is inadequate synthesis of structurally weak osteoid in vitamin C deficiency (called scurvy). This causes bone fragility and joint pain.
         (c) Structurally abnormal collagen in small blood vessels (venules, capillaries) results in a bleeding diathesis (e.g., bleeding gums, bleeding into the skin [perifollicular hemorrhage], hemarthrosis) and poor wound healing.
   b. Antioxidant activity
      (1) Regenerates vitamin E (also an antioxidant)
      (2) Neutralizes hydroxyl FR (see Chapter 2)
   c. Reduces nonheme iron (oxidized; Fe^{3+}) in plants to heme iron (reduced; Fe^{2+}), which allows iron to be absorbed in the duodenum. In vitamin C deficiency, there is decreased absorption of heme iron in the duodenum, which could lead to iron deficiency anemia (microcytic anemia; see Chapter 12).
   d. Keeps tetrahydrofolate (FH_4) in folic acid metabolism in its reduced form (see Fig. 12-16)
      (1) FH_4 in its reduced form is important in single-carbon transfer reactions (methyl group CH_3; e.g., DNA synthesis, synthesis of methionine; see Chapter 12 for full discussion).
      (2) Vitamin C deficiency is a cause of folic acid deficiency (macrocytic anemia).
   e. Cofactor for the conversion of dopamine to norepinephrine (NOR) in catecholamine synthesis (see Fig. 23-19 A)
3. Causes of deficiency
   a. Diets lacking fruits and vegetables
   b. Cigarette smoking. Vitamin C is depleted, neutralizing FRs in cigarette smoke.
4. Clinical findings in deficiency are summarized in Table 8-4.

VII. **Trace Elements**
A. **Definition**: Micronutrients that are required in the normal diet
B. **Zinc**
1. Functions
   a. Cofactor for metalloenzymes (e.g., collagenase in wound remodeling; see Chapter 3)
   b. Important in growth and spermatogenesis in children
2. Causes of deficiency
   a. Alcoholism, diabetes mellitus, and chronic diarrhea
   b. Acrodermatitis enteropathica (ADE)
      (1) **Definition:** Autosomal recessive disease associated with zinc deficiency
      (2) Clinical findings in ADE include dermatitis, growth retardation, decreased spermatogenesis, and poor wound healing.
3. Clinical findings in deficiency (Table 8-5)

TABLE 8-5   Trace Metals: Clinical Findings in Deficiency

TRACE METAL	EFFECTS OF DEFICIENCY
Chromium	Metabolic: impaired glucose tolerance, peripheral neuropathy
Copper	Blood: microcytic anemia (cofactor in ferroxidase) Vessels: aortic dissection (weak elastic tissue) Metabolic: poor wound healing (cofactor in lysyl oxidase)
Fluoride	Teeth: dental caries
Iodide	Thyroid: thyroid enlargement (goiter; see Fig. 23-8 A), hypothyroidism
Selenium	Muscle: muscle pain and weakness, dilated cardiomyopathy
Zinc	Metabolic: poor wound healing (cofactor in collagenase) Mouth: dysgeusia (*cannot* taste), anosmia (*cannot* smell), perioral rash (see Fig. 8-11) Children: hypogonadism, growth retardation

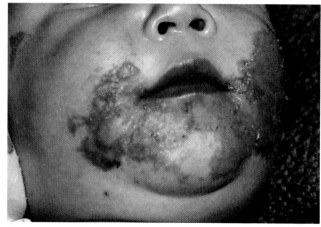

8-11: Zinc deficiency is a child. Note the perioral rash. *(From Marks JG, Miller JJ: Lookingbill and Marks' Principles of Dermatology, 5th ed, Saunders Elsevier, 2013, p 105, Fig. 8-22.)*

Copper

Cofactor ferroxidase, lysyl oxidase, tyrosinase

Deficiency: TPN

Wilson disease: ↑copper

Iodine

Used to synthesize thyroid hormone

↓Intake iodized table salt

Chromium

Insulin cofactor: facilitates binding of glucose to muscle/adipose

Supplement in diabetes mellitus

Deficiency: TPN

Selenium

Component glutathione peroxidase

Deficiency: TPN

Fluoride

Part of calcium hydroxyapatite bone/teeth; prevent dental caries

C. Copper
1. Functions of copper. Cofactor for ferroxidase (binds iron to transferrin), lysyl oxidase (cross-linking of collagen and elastic tissue), and tyrosinase (melanin synthesis)
2. Copper deficiency: most often due to total parenteral nutrition (TPN)
3. Clinical findings in deficiency (see Table 8-5)
4. Copper excess: seen in Wilson disease (see Chapter 19)

D. Iodine
1. Iodine is used to synthesize thyroid hormone (see Chapter 23).
2. Deficiency is most often due to inadequate intake of iodized table salt. Some countries do *not* use iodized table salt.
3. Clinical findings in deficiency (Table 8-4)

E. Chromium
1. Functions
   a. Cofactor for insulin that facilitates the binding of glucose to adipose and muscle glucose transport units
   b. Useful supplement in patients with diabetes mellitus
2. Deficiency most often due to TPN
3. Clinical findings in deficiency (see Table 8-5)

F. Selenium
1. Functions. Component of glutathione peroxidase, which produces reduced glutathione, an antioxidant that converts hydrogen peroxide to water.
2. Deficiency is most often due to TPN.
3. Clinical findings in deficiency (Table 8-5)

G. Fluoride
1. Function. Component of calcium hydroxyapatite in bone and teeth, which prevents the formation of dental caries.

TABLE 8-6   Mineral and Electrolyte Deficiency and Excess

	SIGNS AND SYMPTOMS OF DEFICIENCY	SIGNS AND SYMPTOMS OF EXCESS
Calcium	• Tetany (hypocalcemia lowers muscle and nerve threshold potential). • Signs of tetany: carpopedal spasm (thumb adducts into palm; see Fig. 23-12 A), Chvostek sign (facial twitch after tapping VII nerve), muscle twitching. • Osteoporosis (decreased bone mass).	• Kidney stones (calcium oxalate and phosphate). • Metastatic calcification (calcification of normal tissues; e.g., deposition in the kidneys is called nephrocalcinosis). • Polyuria (increased urination due to calcification of the renal tubule basement membranes and lack of response to antidiuretic hormone; nephrogenic diabetes insipidus).
Phosphorus	• Muscle weakness: rhabdomyolysis with myoglobinuria (due to decreased ATP). • Hemolytic anemia (due to decreased ATP).	• Hypocalcemia (increased phosphorus drives calcium into bone and soft tissue (metastatic calcification). • Hypovitaminosis D (hyperphosphatemia inhibits the activity of 1-α-hydroxylase).
Sodium	• Mental status abnormalities (cerebral edema, water shifts into the cells by osmosis), convulsions (see Chapter 5).	• Mental status abnormalities (intracellular shrinkage of neuroglial cells and neurons), convulsions, pitting edema (increases plasma hydrostatic pressure) (see Chapter 5)
Potassium	• Muscle weakness (cannot repolarize muscle) • Polyuria (renders the collecting tubules resistant to antidiuretic hormone; nephrogenic diabetes insipidus) (see Chapter 5)	• Heart stops in diastole (must protect the heart with an injection of calcium gluconate) (see Chapter 5)
Magnesium	• Hypocalcemia with tetany (acquired hypoparathyroidism due to impaired PTH secretion and resistance to PTH in target tissues) • Tachycardia	• Neuromuscular depression (depressed deep tendon reflexes, muscle weakness) • Bradycardia

PTH, Parathyroid hormone.

2. Deficiency is due to inadequate intake of fluoridated water.
3. Clinical findings in deficiency (Table 8-5)
4. Clinical findings of excess include chalky deposits on the teeth, calcification of ligaments, and increased risk for bone fractures.

VIII. Mineral and Electrolyte Deficiency and Excess (Table 8-6)
IX. Dietary Fiber
  A. Types of dietary fiber
    1. Insoluble fiber
      a. Nonfermentable. Examples: wheat bran, wheat germ, fruits, and vegetables.
      b. Absorbs water, which increases the bulk of stool
      c. Softens the stool and causes more frequent elimination
    2. Soluble fiber
      a. Fermentable. Examples: oat bran, psyllium seeds, fruits.
      b. Softens stool
      c. Increases fecal bacterial mass
  B. Benefits of increased dietary fiber
    1. Binds potential carcinogens and excretes them in stool
      a. Lithocholic acid (LCA) and deoxycholic acid (DOC) are secondary bile acids.
        (1) In the presence of a high dietary intake of fat, LCA and DOC increase the production of reactive oxygen/nitrogen species that damage DNA, increase resistance to apoptosis, and increase the risk for mutation and genomic instability in colonic epithelium, leading to colorectal cancer. They have also been implicated as causal agents of other gastrointestinal tract cancers, including cancers of the esophagus, stomach, small intestine, liver, pancreas, and biliary tract.
        (2) Insoluble fiber eliminates secondary bile acids.
      b. Estrogen
        (1) Some estrogen in the stool is reabsorbed back into the blood. Insoluble fiber eliminates the estrogen that is normally absorbed.
        (2) Increased estrogen increases the risk for endometrial and breast cancer.
    2. Decreases the risk for developing diverticulosis by preventing constipation
    3. Decreases the risk for developing heart disease. Soluble fiber increases the loss of cholesterol in stool. Cholesterol is important in the formation of atheromatous plaques.

Deficiency: inadequate intake fluoridated water

Excess: chalky tooth deposits, calcification ligaments, ↑risk bone fractures

Fiber types: insoluble, soluble

Nonfermentable
Absorbs water → ↑bulk of stool
Softens stool

Fermentable
Softens stool
↑Fecal bacterial mass

Binds potential carcinogens

LCA/DOC ↑risk GI cancers
Insoluble fiber eliminates secondary bile acids
Estrogen
Insoluble fiber eliminates excess estrogen
↑Estrogen ↑risk endometrial, breast cancer
↓Risk for sigmoid diverticulosis by preventing constipation
Soluble fiber lowers serum cholesterol; ↓heart disease

X. Special Diets
   A. Sodium-restricted diets; nonpharmacologic treatment for:
   - Primary hypertension (HTN; see Chapter 10), congestive heart failure (CHF; see Chapter 11), chronic renal failure (CRF; see Chapter 20), and cirrhosis (see Chapter 19)
   B. Protein-restricted diets
   1. Reduces the formation of urea and ammonia (see Chapter 19)
   2. Used in the treatment of:
      a. CRF (see Chapter 20)
         (1) Kidney is the primary site for the removal of urea produced by the urea cycle in the liver.
         (2) In CRF, the urea *cannot* be excreted and its accumulation in the blood (blood urea nitrogen [BUN]) produces toxic changes in multiple organ systems.
      b. Cirrhosis of the liver (see Chapter 19)
         (1) In cirrhosis, the urea cycle is impaired; hence the normal conversion of ammonia to urea in the urea cycle *cannot* occur, leading to an increase in serum ammonia and a decrease in serum BUN. Protein restriction is essential to reduce ammonia levels.
         (2) Increased serum ammonia produces hepatic encephalopathy (drowsiness, mental status abnormalities, coma).

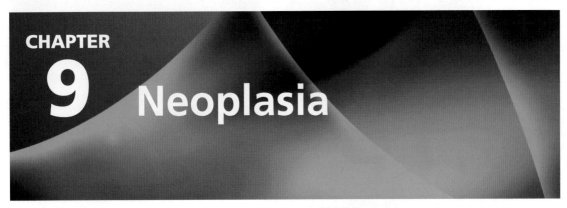

ABBREVIATIONS

MC most common
MCC most common cause

1° primary

Rx treatment

I. Nomenclature

A. Benign tumors

1. **Definition:** Characterized by an unregulated proliferation of cells of epithelial or connective tissue origin that do not invade or spread to other sites

2. Suffix *-oma* generally indicates a benign tumor.
   - *Exceptions* to the rule are seminoma (testicular cancer), lymphoma (malignancy of lymph nodes), glioma (malignancy of glial cells in the brain), mesothelioma (malignancy of pleural/peritoneal serosa), and neuroblastoma (malignancy of neuroblasts).

3. Derivation of benign tumors of epithelial origin
   a. Epithelial tumors arise from ectoderm (e.g., squamous and transitional epithelium) or endoderm (e.g., glandular epithelium).
   b. An example of a benign tumor is a tubular adenoma (adenomatous polyp) that derives from glands in the colon (Fig. 9-1 A; Link 9-1).

4. Benign tumors of connective tissue origin
   a. Arise from the mesoderm
   b. Examples
      (1) Lipomas derive from adipose tissue (Fig. 9-1 B; Link 9-2).
      (2) Leiomyomas of the uterus derived from smooth muscle (Link 9-3).

5. Unusual tumors that are *usually* benign
   a. Mixed tumors
      (1) **Definition:** Composed of neoplastic cells that have two different morphologic patterns, but derive from the *same* germ cell layer
         - *Not* the same as a teratoma (see later)
      (2) Example: pleomorphic adenoma of the parotid gland
   b. Teratomas
      (1) **Definition:** Derive from *more than one* germ layer—ectoderm, endoderm, and/or mesoderm (Fig. 9-1 C; Link 9-4); may be benign or malignant
      (2) Sites: ovaries (most common site), testes, anterior mediastinum, and pineal gland; tend to have a midline location (pineal gland, anterior mediastinum) or close to the midline (ovaries and testes)

B. Malignant tumors (cancer)

1. **Definition:** Characterized by an unregulated proliferation of cells that invade tissue and are capable of spreading to other sites that are remote from the primary site of origin

2. Carcinomas
   a. **Definition:** Derive from epithelial tissue—squamous, glandular, or transitional epithelium
   b. Primary sites for squamous cell carcinoma (SCC) include oropharynx, larynx, upper/ middle esophagus, lung, cervix, penis, and skin (Figs. 9-1 D, E). Squamous cell cancers commonly have keratin pearls that stain bright red with a hematoxylin-eosin (H&E stain; Fig. 9-1 E).

Margin notes:
Unregulated benign proliferation epithelial/connective tissue

Exceptions: seminoma, lymphoma

Benign: epithelial origin

Epithelial tumors: squamous/transitional/glandular epithelium

Tubular adenoma in colon

Benign: connective tissue origin

Mesoderm origin

Lipoma, leiomyoma

Mixed tumors

Two patterns; *same* germ cell layer; e.g., parotid gland tumors

Not same as teratoma

Pleomorphic adenoma parotid

Teratomas

Derive from ecto-, endo-, mesoderm

At/close to midline; ovary MC site

Malignant tumors

Unregulated proliferation; invasion; possible spread

Carcinomas

Derives from epithelial tissue

Squamous, glandular, transitional

1° sites SCC: mouth, larynx, cervix

Keratin pearls (bright red)

9-1: A, Tubular adenoma (adenomatous polyp) of the colon. Note the fibrovascular stalk *(arrow)* lined by normal colonic mucosa and a branching head surfaced by dysplastic (blue-staining) epithelial glands. The epithelium is glandular; therefore it derives from the endoderm. **B,** Lipoma showing a well-circumscribed yellow tumor. Adipose tissue is connective tissue; therefore it derives from the mesoderm. **C,** Cystic teratoma of the ovary, showing the cystic nature of the tumor. Hair is present, and a tooth is visible *(arrow).* Teratomas can arise from ectoderm (this photograph), endoderm, and mesoderm. **D,** Schematic shows keratin pearls (concentric layers of eosin-staining keratin similar to the layers of a pearl). **E,** Squamous cell carcinoma. The many well-differentiated foci of eosinophilic-staining neoplastic cells produce keratin in layers (keratin pearls). Note how squamous epithelium takes up the red eosin stain. **F,** Schematic shows glands lined by neoplastic glandular cells with hyperchromatic and irregular nuclei, and a gland lumen with material in the lumen. **G,** Adenocarcinoma. Irregular glands infiltrate the stroma. The nuclei lining the gland lumens are cuboidal and contain nuclei with hyperchromatic nuclear chromatin. Glandular cells appear to pile up on each other. Many of the gland lumens contain secretory material *(arrow).* **H,** Osteogenic sarcoma of the distal femur. The light-colored mass of tumor in the metaphysis abuts the epiphyseal plate *(arrow)* and has spread laterally out through the cortex and into the surrounding tissue. *(**A** from Kumar V, Fausto N, Abbas A:* Robbins and Cotran's Pathologic Basis of Disease, *7th ed, Philadelphia, Saunders, 2004, p 860, Fig. 17-57 A;* **B–D** *and* **F** *from my friend Ivan Damjanov, MD, PhD:* Pathology for the Health-Related Professions, *2nd ed, Philadelphia, Saunders, 2000, pp 77, 79, 78, 78, Figs. 4-7, 4-11, 4-10 A, 4-10 B, respectively;* **E** *from Klatt F:* Robbins and Cotran's Atlas of Pathology, *Philadelphia, Saunders, 2006, p 302, Fig. 13-35;* **G, H** *from my friend Ivan Damjanov, MD, PhD, Linder J:* Pathology: A Color Atlas, *St. Louis, Mosby, 2000, pp 139, 369, Figs. 7-59, 17-35 B, respectively.)*

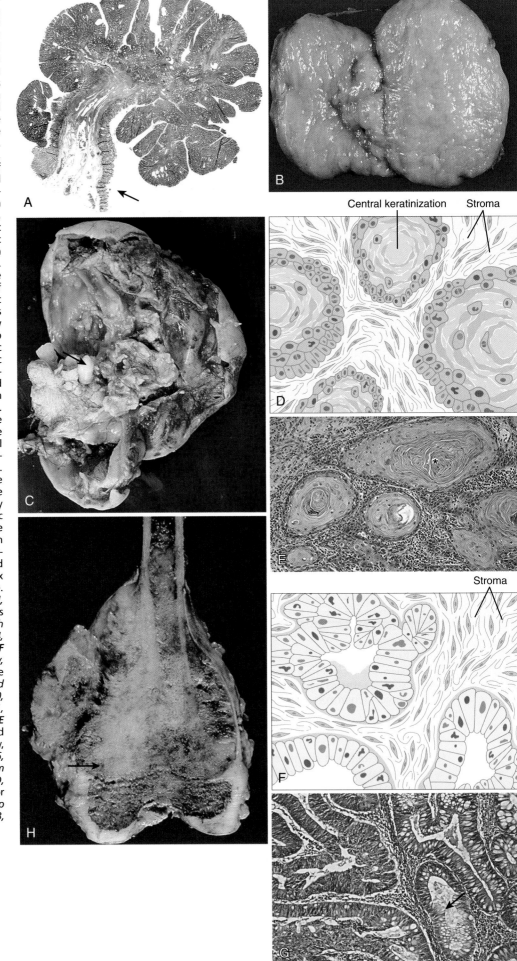

    c. Primary sites for adenocarcinoma (glandular epithelium) include lung, distal esophagus to rectum, pancreas, liver, breast, endometrium, ovaries, kidneys, and prostate (Fig. 9-1 F, G). Adenocarcinomas commonly have glands with secretions in the lumen (Fig. 9-1 G).

    d. Primary sites for transitional cell carcinoma (TCC) include urinary bladder, ureter, and renal pelvis.

  3. Sarcomas

    a. **Definition:** Derive from connective tissue (mesoderm origin)

    b. Approximately 40% of sarcomas are located in the lower extremity.

    c. Examples include those that arise from bone (osteosarcoma; Fig. 9-1 H) and skeletal muscle (rhabdomyosarcoma; Link 9-5; see also Link 24-23 A, B).

C. Tumor-like conditions

  1. Hamartoma

    a. **Definition:** Nonneoplastic overgrowth of disorganized tissue that is indigenous to a particular site

    b. Examples: bronchial hamartoma (contains cartilage; Link 9-6), Peutz-Jeghers (PJ) polyp (contains glandular tissue)

  2. Choristoma (heterotopic rest)

    a. **Definition:** Mass of nonneoplastic tissue that is located in a foreign place

    b. Examples: pancreatic tissue in wall of the stomach (Link 9-7), brain tissue in the nasal cavity, functioning thyroid tissue in the liver (Link 9-8)

II. Properties of Benign and Malignant Tumors

A. Components of benign and malignant tumors

  1. Parenchyma

    • **Definition:** Neoplastic component of a tumor that determines its biological behavior

  2. Stroma

    a. **Definition:** Nonneoplastic supportive tissue of a tumor

    b. Most infiltrating carcinomas induce production of a dense, fibrous stroma (called desmoplasia) that surrounds the invading cancer.

B. Differentiation in benign and malignant tumors

  1. Benign tumors

    • **Definition:** Usually well differentiated (resembles the parent tissue) and does *not* have the capacity to spread to distant sites

  2. Malignant tumors

    a. Well-differentiated or low-grade cancer

      (1) **Definition:** Cancer cells histologically resemble the parent tissue

      (2) Examples: parenchyma showing keratin pearls (characteristic of squamous tissue; Fig. 9-1 D; Link 9-9) or glandular lumens with secretions (characteristic of normal gland lumens with secretions; see Fig. 9-1 F, G; Link 9-10)

    b. Poorly differentiated, high-grade, or anaplastic cancer

      • **Definition:** Do *not* resemble the parent tissue histologically (e.g., *no* glands, keratin)

    c. Moderately well-differentiated (intermediate-grade) cancer

      • **Definition:** Exhibit histologic features that are between those of low- and high-grade cancer (i.e., occasional gland-like structures are seen, or areas that look like keratin are present, whereas the rest of the tumor has no characteristics of the tissue of origin)

C. Cell organelles in malignant versus normal cells

  1. Organelles in the cytoplasm when compared to a normal cell (Fig. 9-2)

    a. Less mitochondria

    b. Rough endoplasmic reticulum (RER) is less prominent.

    c. Loss of cell-to-cell adhesion molecules (cadherins). Cadherins are a group of calcium-dependent transmembrane proteins that play an important role in cell-to-cell adhesion. Loss of adhesion allows malignant cells to extend into surrounding tissue.

  2. Nuclear features when compared to a normal cell

    a. Nucleus is larger, has irregular borders, and has more chromatin (hyperchromatic).

    b. Nucleolus is larger and has irregular borders.

    c. Mitoses have normal and *atypical* mitotic spindles (Fig. 9-3; Link 9-11).

D. Biochemical changes in malignant cells

  1. Rely on anaerobic glycolysis for energy. Explains why there is more lactic acid produced under hypoxic conditions than one would see in a normal cell.

Margin notes:

1° sites adeno: distal esophagus to rectum; pancreas, breast, kidneys

TCC: bladder, ureter, renal pelvis

Sarcomas

Connective tissue origin (mesoderm)

Lower extremity common site

Osteogenic sarcoma (bone)

Rhabdomyosarcoma (skeletal muscle)

Tumor-like conditions

Hamartoma

Nonneoplastic overgrowth

Bronchial hamartoma; PJ polyp

Choristoma

Normal tissue in foreign location

Pancreatic tissue in stomach wall, thyroid tissue in liver

Parenchyma

Neoplastic component

Stroma

Nonneoplastic (supportive)

Infiltrating cancer: desmoplasia

Benign tumors

Well-differentiated; *no* metastasis

Malignant tumors

Well-differentiated (low-grade)

Cancer cells resemble parent tissue

Low-grade: keratin pearls, glands with lumens

Poorly differentiated (high-grade)

No differentiating features

Moderately well-differentiated (intermediate)

Cell organelles

Less mitochondria

Less prominent RER

Loss cadherins

Loss cell-to-cell adhesion

Nuclear features

Larger, irregular, hyperchromatic

Nucleolus larger/irregular borders

Normal/abnormal mitotic spindles; hyperchromatic nuclei

Anaerobic glycolysis

↑Lactic acid in neoplastic cells

9-2: Schematic showing normal organelles in a normal cell on the left **(A)** and a malignant cell **(B)** on the right. Note that when compared to a normal cell, a malignant cell has fewer mitochondria, less prominence of the rough endoplasmic reticulum with an increase in free ribosomes, loss of cell adhesion molecules between cells (cadherins and occludens), and a larger nucleus with irregular borders, excess chromatin, and a larger, irregular nucleolus. Tumor antigens are sometimes expressed on the surface of malignant cells *(CEA)*. **C,** Comparison of normal glands with carcinoma. Normal glands have smooth contours and uniform nuclei. Adenocarcinoma is composed of irregular glands. Anaplastic or undifferentiated carcinoma forms cell groups that show little resemblance to glands *(far right)*. CEA, Carcinoembryonic antigen. *(A–C from my friend Ivan Damjanov, MD, PhD: Pathology for the Health-Related Professions, 2nd ed, Philadelphia, Saunders, 2000, p 80, 70, Figs. 4-12, 4-2, respectively.)*

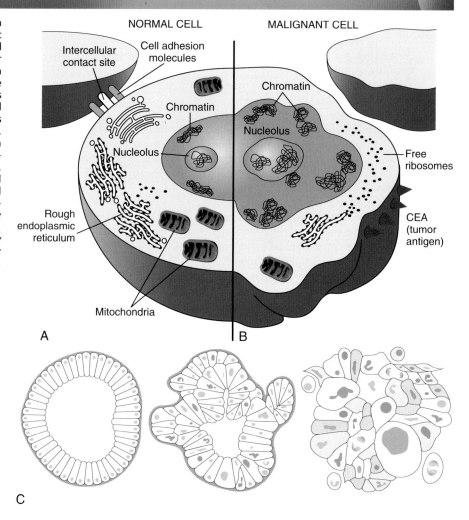

↑Uptake of glucose analog

PET scan

Diagnosis, staging, monitoring therapy

Store glycogen in cytosol

β-oxidation fatty acids or anaerobic glycolysis for energy

Benign: usually low growth rate

Malignant: variable growth rate

Correlates with degree of differentiation

High-grade cancer: ↑growth rate

Clinically detectable: 30 population doublings to produce 10^9 cells (1 g tissue)

↑Growth rate: use cell cycle–specific chemo

MTX inhibits S phase; vincristine inhibits M phase

Malignant cells killed: other cells enter cycle

Nonneoplastic tumors polyclonal

Benign/malignant cells: from single precursor cell

2. Increased uptake of a glucose analog
   a. A special test has been developed in which cancer cells take up a glucose analog with positron emission tomography (PET).
   b. PET scan is widely used in the diagnosis, staging, and monitoring of therapy of various kinds of cancer.
3. Cancer cells do *not* process glucose as well as normal cells, and store glucose in the form of glycogen within the cytosol.
4. Some cancers (e.g., prostate cancer) derive energy from β-oxidation of fatty acids rather than anaerobic glycolysis.

E. **Growth rate in benign and malignant tumors**
   1. Benign tumors usually have a slow growth rate.
   2. Malignant tumors have a variable growth rate.
      a. Growth rate correlates with degree of differentiation of the malignant tumor.
      b. Example: Anaplastic (high-grade) cancers have an increased growth rate, whereas low-grade cancers tend to grow more slowly.
   3. Clinically detectable tumor mass must have 30 population doublings to produce 10^9 cells, which equals 1 g of tissue.
   4. Malignant cells with an increased growth rate (e.g., acute myelogenous leukemia) are treated with cell cycle–specific chemotherapy agents.
      a. Methotrexate (MTX) inhibits the synthesis (S) phase of the cell cycle (duplication of DNA), whereas vincristine inhibits the mitotic (M) phase of the cell cycle.
      b. When malignant cells are killed, other malignant cells quickly enter the cycle, and the cycle repeats itself so that the size of the tumor begins to shrink.

F. **Monoclonality in benign and malignant tumors**
   1. Nonneoplastic tumors derive from multiple cells (polyclonal).
   2. Benign and *most* malignant tumors derive from a single precursor cell.

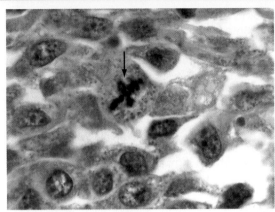

9-3: Abnormal mitotic figure H&E. This micrograph of a malignant tumor of the skin contains an abnormal mitotic figure *(arrow)*. The cell is in metaphase, but rather than a metaphase plate with two sets of chromatids and two spindles, the cell has produced four sets of chromatids and four spindles, a quadripolar mitosis. Such abnormalities are frequently seen in malignant tumors and are virtually never found in normal tissues and benign tumors. *(From Young B, O'Dowd G, Woodford P:* Wheater's Functional Histology: A Colour Text and Atlas, *6th ed, Churchill Livingstone Elsevier, 2014, p 44, Fig. 2.9.)*

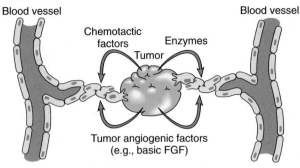

9-4: The schematic shows tumor-induced angiogenesis, which refers to the sprouting of new capillaries from preexisting vessels. For a tumor to survive, it must have an adequate blood supply to provide oxygen and nutrients. Refer to the text for a full discussion. *FGF,* Fibroblast growth factor. *(Modified from my friend Ivan Damjanov, MD, PhD:* Pathology for the Health-Related Professions, *2nd ed, Philadelphia, Saunders, 2000, p 76, Fig. 4-6.)*

The **monoclonal origin** of neoplasms has been shown by studying glucose-6-phosphate dehydrogenase (G6PD) isoenzymes A and B in selected neoplasms (e.g., leiomyoma of the uterus). All the neoplastic smooth muscle cells in uterine leiomyomas have either the A or the B G6PD isoenzyme. Nonneoplastic smooth muscle proliferations in the uterus (e.g., pregnant uterus) have some cells with the A isoenzyme and others with the B isoenzyme, indicating their polyclonal origin.

G. **Telomerase activity in benign and malignant tumors**
   1. Telomere complexes (Link 9-12)
      a. **Definition:** Repetitive sequences of nontranscribed DNA located at the ends of chromosomes
      b. Prevent end-to-end fusion of chromosomes during normal mitosis and, along with other factors, are important in determining the longevity of a cell
      c. Shorten with each round of replication and eventually, when only a few nucleotide bases remain, genome becomes unstable, which produces a signal for apoptosis
   2. Benign tumors have normal telomerase activity.
   3. Malignant cells have upregulation of telomerase activity, which *prevents* the naturally programmed shortening of telomere complexes with cell replication; hence the cell no longer undergoes apoptosis.
H. **Upregulation of decay accelerating factor (DAF) by malignant cells**
   1. DAF normally degrades C3 convertase and C5 convertase in the classical and alternative complement pathways (see Fig. 4-18).
   2. Upregulation of DAF ensures that degradation of the convertases just mentioned prevents formation of the membrane attack complex (MAC; C5b-9); therefore cancer cells *cannot* be killed by the MAC.
I. **Local invasion and metastasis**
   1. Benign tumors do *not* invade. Exception is a dermatofibroma, which invades tissue but does *not* metastasize (see Link 25-150). Benign tumors are usually enclosed by a fibrous tissue capsule. Exception is a uterine leiomyoma (benign tumor of smooth muscle), which does *not have* a fibrous tissue capsule.
   2. Malignant tumors
      a. Invade tissue. Invasion is an important criterion for malignancy.
      b. Some tissues resist invasion. Examples include mature cartilage and the elastic tissue of arteries.
      c. All malignant tumors require oxygen and nutrients to survive and do so by stimulating angiogenesis within the tumor and its metastatic sites (Fig. 9-4).
         (1) Angiogenesis, or new blood vessel formation, occurs by forming capillary sprouts from preexisting capillaries (parent capillaries) and/or by stimulating the synthesis of endothelial precursor cells (EPCs) from the bone marrow that migrate to the tumor site.

Neoplastic cells monoclonal; nonneoplastic cells polyclonal

Telomere complexes

Repetitive sequences nontranscribed DNA ends chromosomes

Prevent end-to-end chromosome fusion during mitosis

Shorten with each cell division → signal apoptosis

Benign tumors: normal telomerase activity

Malignant tumors: upregulation telomerase activity; prevents apoptosis

DAF: normally degrades C3/C5 convertase

Upregulation DAF prevents MAC formation

Benign tumors: do *not* invade

Exception: dermatofibroma

Enclosed by fibrous tissue capsule

Exception: uterine leiomyoma

Malignant tumors

Invade tissue: important criterion for malignancy

Resist invasion: cartilage, elastic tissue artery

Stimulate angiogenesis

New blood vessel formation

New capillary sprouts parent capillaries; EPC synthesis

(2) Vascular endothelial growth factor (VEGF) and other growth factors produced by the tumor (see Chapter 3) directly act on endothelial cells in the parent capillaries to develop new capillary sprouts. Tumor necrosis factor (TNF) released by macrophages is important in stimulating tumor cells to produce these angiogenesis factors.

(3) Chemotactic factors produced by the tumor cells and inflammatory cells (particularly macrophages) assist in attracting endothelial cells from the parent capillaries to form the new capillary sprouts.

(4) Enzymes (e.g., proteases) regulate the balance between angiogenesis and the many factors that can inhibit angiogenesis (e.g., angiostatin, endostatin).

(5) Enzymes also degrade basement membranes in parent vessels to allow endothelial cells to migrate and form new capillary sprouts.

(6) EPCs from the bone marrow are also used in new vessel formation.

(7) Monoclonal antibodies have been developed to inhibit tumor angiogenesis. For example, bevacizumab is a recombinant humanized antibody that inhibits the binding of VEGF to endothelial cells in new capillary sprouts. Monoclonal antibodies are indicated for the treatment of metastatic colon cancer and non–small cell carcinoma of the lung.

d. Sequence of hematogenous (capillary) invasion by malignant tumors is illustrated in Figure 9-5.

(1) Same sequence of invasion also applies to invasion of a lymphatic vessel or a venule.

(2) Schematic (Fig. 9-5) shows the primary tumor resting on top of the basement membrane of a capillary. Note the importance of angiogenesis in maintaining the viability of the primary tumor as well as the metastatic foci.

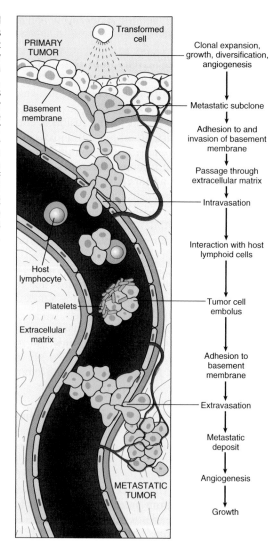

9-5: Sequential steps involved in the hematogenous spread of cancer from a primary to a distant site. Initially there is clonal proliferation of a subset of primary tumor cells that have the capacity to metastasize. To invade from the primary site, the cancer cells must lose their cell-to-cell adhesion molecules, obtain the capacity to move through tissue, adhere to and degrade the basement membrane, pass through the extracellular matrix, and penetrate the vascular wall of a capillary (intravasation). In the bloodstream, the cancer cells encounter host defense cells (e.g., cytotoxic T cells, killer cells) and some are destroyed (type IV hypersensitivity reaction; see Chapter 4). Those that survive form tumor cell emboli that attach to the capillary endothelium of a distant organ (e.g., lung) and repeat the process of invasion of the capillary wall into the tissue of the distal organ, where it sets up a metastatic focus of tumor that will grow and continue to spread. *(From Kumar V, Fausto N, Abbas A, Aster J: Robbins and Cotran Pathologic Basis of Disease, 8th ed, Philadelphia, Saunders Elsevier, 2010, p 298, Fig. 7-36.)*

(3) Within the primary tumor, there is *clonal proliferation of cells* that develops the capacity to invade and metastasize. All other primary tumor cells *cannot* invade and metastasize.

(4) *First key step* in invasion is for malignant cells to lose their cell-to-cell adhesion molecules (cadherins).

(5) *Second key step* is for cell receptors to attach to laminin (a glycoprotein) in the basement membrane and to release metalloproteinases (e.g., collagenases, stromelysins, gelatinases) to degrade the basement membrane and other enzymes to degrade the interstitial connective tissue. Tissue inhibitors of metalloproteinases neutralize these tumor-produced enzymes and limit the degree of invasion.

(6) *Third key step* is for cell receptors to attach to fibronectin and other proteins in the extracellular matrix (ECM) and to break it down.

(7) *Fourth key step* is for malignant cells to produce cytokines that stimulate locomotion, so that they can move through basement membranes and the intracellular and extracellular matrices.

(8) When malignant cells encounter capillaries, they must penetrate the blood vessels (called intravasation) in order to enter the microcirculation.

(9) While in the circulation, some malignant cells encounter host defense cells (e.g., cytotoxic T cells, killer cells; see Chapter 4) and are destroyed, whereas other cells escape destruction. In cancer surgery, malignant cells that enter the circulation from manipulation of tissue may produce metastasis.

(10) Tumor cells that escape destruction form tumor cell emboli that are coated by platelets and fibrin.

(11) Tumor emboli enter capillaries of a target organ, attach to the blood vessel wall, and repeat the four-step process of invasion (called extravasation) to set up a metastatic focus that will grow and continue to spread throughout the target organ.

(12) Where these tumor emboli eventually settle depends on several factors.
    (a) Sometimes the metastatic site is the first capillary bed it encounters.
    (b) Sometimes it travels through the Batson paravertebral plexus and ends up in the vertebral column (discussed later).
    (c) Sometimes the primary cancer releases chemokines that go specifically to sites that have chemokine receptors similar to those in the primary tumor.
    (d) Sometimes target organs release chemoattractants that signal tumor cells to deposit at that site.

J. **Types of metastasis**
  1. Benign tumors do *not* metastasize.
  2. Malignant tumors metastasize (exception: basal cell carcinoma [BCC] of skin).
    a. Metastasis is the most important criterion for malignancy.
    b. Invasion of tissue is the second most important criterion for malignancy.
  3. Pathways of dissemination (overview Figs. 9-6 and 9-7)
    a. Lymphatic spread
      (1) Lymphatic spread to regional lymph nodes is the first step for dissemination in carcinomas. Lymph nodes are the first line of defense against the spread of carcinomas.
      (2) Using the model of invasion and metastasis discussed in Figure 9-5, in carcinomas, the vessel that is invaded is an afferent lymphatic vessel. The tumor emboli enter the sinuses of the regional lymph nodes and invade the parenchymal tissue of the lymph node.
      (3) Tumor cells that invade efferent lymphatics send tumor emboli into the thoracic duct, and from there they enter the systemic circulation, where they disperse to capillaries in target organs to form metastatic foci. This is the *hematogenous phase* of cancer dissemination in carcinomas.
    b. Hematogenous spread
      (1) Sarcomas initially invade capillaries and/or venules and directly spread to distant sites *without* involving the lymph nodes.
      (2) Malignant cells entering the portal vein metastasize to the liver (Fig. 9-7 A), whereas those that enter the vena cava metastasize to the lungs.
      (3) Both carcinomas and sarcomas have hematogenous dissemination; however, carcinomas usually invade regional lymph nodes *before* entering the systemic circulation.

Marginal notes:

Clonal proliferation cells can invade/metastasize

1st step: lose cell-to-cell adhesion molecules (cadherins)

2nd step: attach to basement membrane; degrade it

3rd step: attach to ECM; degrade it

4th step: stimulate cell motility

Invade capillaries; enter circulation (intravasation)

Evade/destroyed by host defense cells

Tumor emboli coated by fibrin/platelets

Attach to capillaries target organ; repeat steps of invasion

Batson paravertebral plexus → invade vertebra

Directed metastasis with chemokines

Chemoattractants

Benign tumors: do *not* metastasize

Malignant tumors metastasize

Exception BCC skin

Metastasis most important criterion malignancy

Invasion 2nd most important criterion

Pathways dissemination

Lymphatic spread

Lymphatic spread → regional nodes; 1st line defense

Invade efferent lymphatics → systemic circulation

Sarcomas invade capillaries without involving nodes

Portal vein → liver; vena cava → lungs

Carcinomas/sarcomas have hematogenous spread

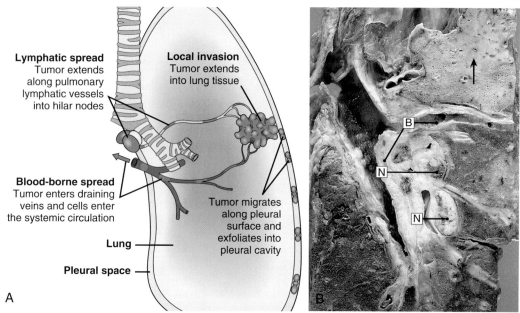

9-6: Main routes of tumor spread. The spread of a malignant tumor is shown diagrammatically **(A)** and in a real specimen **(B)** for a carcinoma of the lung. The four main routes—local, lymphatic, blood-borne, and transcoelomic—are shown. **B,** The malignant neoplasm originated in a bronchus *(B)* and spread locally into adjacent lung *(arrow)*. Tumor has also spread via lymphatics and is evident as white deposits in hilar lymph nodes *(N)*, which also contain black carbon pigment. *(From Stevens A, Lowe J, Scott I: Core Pathology, 3rd ed, Mosby Elsevier, 2009, p 75, Fig. 6-7.)*

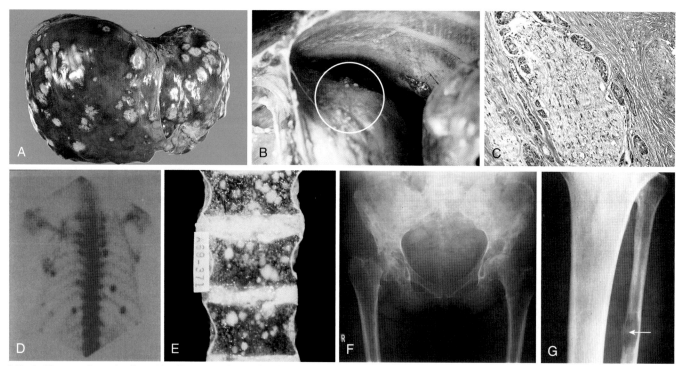

9-7: A, Metastasis to the liver. The liver contains multiple nodules that have a depressed central area ("umbilicated") and stellate-shaped borders. **B,** Seeding of the peritoneum *(white circle* showing numerous white nodules) from a primary ovarian cancer. **C,** Perineural invasion by cancer (adenoid cystic carcinoma of salivary gland). Note the nests of tumor completely surrounding the nerve sheath. **D,** Radionuclide scan. Radionuclide uptake is increased throughout the skeleton, with a very heavy uptake in the vertebral column. The patient had a primary breast cancer, which is the most common cancer metastatic to bone. **E,** Prostate cancer metastatic to the vertebral column. Multiple white foci of metastatic prostate cancer produce an osteoblastic response in the bone. **F,** Multiple osteolytic metastases and a pathologic fracture of the right femoral neck in a woman with breast cancer. Lytic lesions are scattered throughout the pelvis and in the proximal femoral bones. **G,** Radiograph showing osteolytic lesions. Note the radiolucent areas in the midshaft of the fibula *(arrow)* in metastatic breast cancer. *(A from my friend Ivan Damjanov, MD, PhD: Pathology for the Health-Related Professions, 2nd ed, Philadelphia, Saunders, 2000, p 303, Fig. 11-18; B, C from Rosai J: Rosai and Ackerman's Surgical Pathology, 10th ed, Mosby Elsevier, 2011, pp 1579, 835, Figs. 19.272, 12.31, respectively; D from Bouloux P: Self-Assessment Picture Tests: Medicine, Vol. 1, London, Mosby-Wolfe, 1997, p 70, Fig. 140; E from Kumar V, Fausto N, Abbas A: Robbins and Cotran's Pathologic Basis of Disease, 7th ed, Philadelphia, Saunders, 2004, p 1052, Fig. 21-35; F from Forbes C, Jackson W: Color Atlas and Text of Clinical Medicine, 3rd ed, London, Mosby, 2004, p 145, Fig. 3.156; G from Rosai J, Ackerman LV: Surgical Pathology, 9th ed, St. Louis, Mosby, 2004, p 2187, Fig. 24-92.)*

Renal cell carcinomas (RCCs) commonly invade the renal vein, where the tumor has the potential for extending into the vena cava to as far as the right side of the heart. RCCs also have lymphatic spread to regional lymph nodes. Hepatocellular carcinomas (HCCs) invade the portal and hepatic veins. Tumor obstruction of either vein produces portal hypertension, splenomegaly, and ascites. HCCs also spread to regional lymph nodes. Follicular carcinomas of the thyroid invade blood vessels and have hematogenous spread. Lymph nodes are usually spared.

c. Seeding (transcoelomic) spread (Fig. 9-7 B)
  (1) **Definition:** Malignant cells exfoliate from a serosal surface and implant and invade tissue in a body cavity (pleural, pericardial, or peritoneal).
    (a) This process is analogous to a farmer spreading seeds in a field, which develop roots and grow.
    (b) Some authors use the term *transcoelomic* for seeding.
  (2) Primary surface-derived ovarian cancers (e.g., serous cystadenocarcinoma) commonly seed the omentum and produce malignant effusions in the peritoneal cavity.
  (3) Peripherally located lung cancers (usually adenocarcinomas) commonly seed the parietal and visceral pleurae, causing malignant pleural effusions. A variant of seeding is a medulloblastoma, a high-grade cancer arising in the brain that commonly exfoliates malignant cells into the cerebrospinal fluid and seeds the brainstem and spinal cord.
d. Perineural invasion by malignant cells (Fig. 9-7 C). Usually produces pain.
4. Bone metastasis
  a. Vertebral column
    (1) Most common metastatic site in bone (Fig. 9-7 D, E)
      (a) Breast cancer is the most common cancer metastatic to bone.
      (b) Prostate cancer is the second most common cancer metastatic to bone.
    (2) Batson paravertebral venous plexus is responsible for the predilection of bone metastases to the vertebrae.
      (a) Connections with the vena cava and the vertebral bodies
      (b) Using breast cancer as an example, a tumor embolus in the intercostal vein enters the vena cava and from there enters the paravertebral venous plexus, which has tributaries that enter the vertebral bodies.
  b. Osteoblastic metastasis
    (1) Malignant cells in metastatic sites secrete cytokines that specifically activate osteoblasts, which initiate reactive bone formation (Fig. 9-7 E).
      (a) Prostate cancer is the most common cancer producing osteoblastic metastases. The second most common cancer producing osteoblastic metastases is breast cancer.
      (b) Serum alkaline phosphatase (ALP) is elevated, because osteoblasts use this enzyme in bone formation.
    (2) Bone formation in metastatic sites produces radiodensities that are identified in radiographs (e.g., prostate cancer).
  c. Osteolytic metastases
    (1) Osteolytic metastases produce radiolucencies in bone that are identified in radiographs (Figs. 9-7 F, G).
    (2) Pathogenesis
      (a) Malignant cells in metastatic sites produce chemicals (e.g., prostaglandin E_2 [PGE_2], interleukin [IL]-1) that locally activate osteoclasts.
      (b) Cancers that commonly produce lytic metastases include lung cancer, RCCs, and breast cancer.
    (3) Clinical findings include pathologic fractures and/or hypercalcemia, if osteolytic lesions are extensive.
  d. Bone pain from metastasis requires localized radiation.
5. Metastasis is more common than a primary cancer in the following sites:
  a. Lymph nodes (e.g., metastatic breast/lung cancer most common). Lymph nodes are the most common overall site for metastasis.
  b. Lungs (e.g., metastatic breast cancer most common cause)
  c. Liver (e.g., metastatic colorectal cancer most common cause; Fig. 9-7 A)
  d. Bone (e.g., metastatic breast cancer most common cause; Figs. 9-7 F, G)
  e. Brain (e.g., metastatic lung cancer most common cause)
K. **Comparison between benign and malignant tumors (Fig. 9-8 A, B)**

RCC commonly invades veins; spares lymph nodes. HCC invades hepatic/portal veins. Follicular cancer thyroid hematogenous spread, spares nodes.

Seeding, transcoelomic spread

Exfoliation serosal surface; invade tissue body cavity

Malignant surface-derived ovarian cancers; omental implants

Peripheral lung adenocarcinomas seed pleural cavity

Medulloblastoma uses spinal fluid to seed distant sites (brainstem, spinal cord)

Perineural invasion; produces pain

Bone metastasis

Vertebrae MC bone site

Breast cancer MC cancer metastatic to bone

Prostate cancer 2nd MC cancer metastatic to bone

Batson paravertebral venous plexus

Connections with vena cava and vertebral bodies

Osteoblastic metastasis

Cytokines activate local osteoblasts

Prostate cancer MC cancer osteoblastic

Breast cancer 2nd MC cancer osteoblastic

↑Serum ALP

Radiodensities in radiographs

Osteolytic metastases

Radiolucencies in bone

PGE_2, IL-1 produced by tumor locally activate osteoclasts

Osteolytic metastasis: lung, kidney, breast

Pathologic fractures

Hypercalcemia

Bone pain: localized radiation

Lymph nodes: breast/lung cancer

Lymph nodes: MC overall site for metastasis

Lungs: breast cancer

Liver: colorectal MCC

Bone: breast cancer MCC

Brain: lung cancer MCC

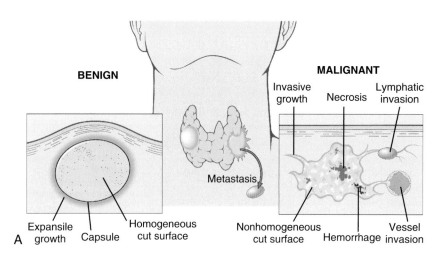

9-8: Comparison of a benign and a malignant tumor using thyroid neoplasms as an example. (*From my friend Ivan Damjanov, MD, PhD: Pathology for the Health Professions, 4th ed, Saunders Elsevier, 2012, pp 69, 71, Fig. 4-1, Table 4-1, respectively.*)

Comparison of benign and malignant tumors

Feature	Benign	Malignant
Growth	Slow Expansive	Fast Invasive
Metastases	No	Yes
Gross appearance		
External surface	Smooth	Irregular
Capsule	Yes	No
Necrosis	No	Yes
Hemorrhage	No	Yes
Microscopic appearance		
Architecture	Resembles that of tissues of origin	Does not resemble that of tissues of origin
Cells	Well differentiated	Poorly differentiated
Nuclei	Normal size and shape	Pleomorphic
Mitoses	Few	Many irregular

III. Cancer Epidemiology

A. General epidemiology of cancer

1. Second most common cause of death in the United States
2. Causes
   a. External factors: Tobacco (#1), alcohol, chemicals, radiation, microbial pathogens
   b. Internal factors: Hormones, immune conditions, inherited mutations
   c. Geographic and ethnic factors
3. Age is an important risk factor for cancer.
   a. Incidence increases with age; the majority are in persons 55 years or older.
   b. Colorectal, lung, and prostate cancer progressively increase in incidence with age, whereas others reach a peak and begin to decline (e.g., malignant melanoma).
4. Racial and ethnic differences affect cancer incidence.
   a. Blacks have a greater risk for developing prostate cancer than white Americans.
   b. Japanese men have a low incidence of prostate cancer.
   c. Skin cancer is more common in fair-skinned people than dark-skinned people because of the protective effect of melanin against ultraviolet (UV) light.
   d. Breast cancer has a low incidence in Japanese and Asian women, whereas the incidence is high in North American and European women.

B. Cancer incidence by age and sex

1. Cancers in children
   a. Malignant neoplasms are the leading cause of disease-related (noninjury) mortality among children 1 to 14 years of age.
   b. Top three cancers in children, in decreasing order, are leukemia (acute lymphoblastic leukemia is the most common leukemia), central nervous system (CNS; cerebellar tumors are the most common), and neuroblastoma (malignant tumor arising from postganglionic sympathetic neurons).
   c. Other common cancers in children that are *not* common in adults include embryonal rhabdomyosarcoma (malignancy of skeletal muscle), Wilms tumor (malignant tumor of the kidney that is derived from the metanephric blastema), retinoblastoma (malignant tumor in the eye), osteosarcoma (malignancy of osteoid in bone), and Ewing sarcoma (neuroectodermal malignancy of bone).

Margin notes:

2nd MCC death in U.S.

Tobacco MC external cause cancer

Increasing age important risk factor for cancer

Majority >55 yrs old

Colorectal/lung/prostate cancers increase with age

Racial/ethnic differences

Prostate cancer blacks > whites

Japanese men: low incidence prostate cancer

Skin cancer: ↓blacks

North American/European women: ↑incidence breast cancer

Cancer MCC disease-related (noninjury) mortality 1–14 years of age

Children: leukemia (#1), CNS, neuroblastoma

Children: embryonal rhabdomyosarcoma, Wilms, retinoblastoma, Ewing sarcoma

d. Epithelial tumors of organs, such as lung, colon, and breast, are common in adults but uncommon in children.

2. Top three noncutaneous cancer sites in men, in decreasing order, are prostate, lung/bronchus, and colorectal.

3. Top three noncutaneous cancer sites in women, in decreasing order, are breast, lung/bronchus, and colorectal.

4. Top three sites for gynecologic cancers, in decreasing order, are ovary, uterine corpus (endometrium), and cervix.

C. **Sites for cancer-related deaths**

1. Top three sites for cancer-related deaths in men, in decreasing order, are lung/bronchus, prostate, and colorectal.

2. Top three sites for cancer-related deaths in women, in decreasing order, are lung/bronchus, breast, and colorectal.

3. Top three gynecologic sites for cancer-related deaths in women, in decreasing order, are ovary, uterine corpus (endometrium), and cervix.

D. **Cancer and heredity**

1. Inherited predisposition to cancer accounts for 5% of all cancers.

2. Categories of inherited cancers include autosomal dominant cancer syndromes, autosomal recessive disorders involving DNA repair, and familial cancers (Table 9-1; Figs. 9-9 and 9-10).

E. **Cancer and geography**

1. Worldwide. Malignant melanoma is the most rapidly increasing cancer in the world.

2. China

Margin notes:

Common sites in adults: lung, colon, breast

Men: prostate, lung, colorectal

Women: breast, lung/bronchus, colorectal

Ovary, uterine corpus, cervix

Cancer-related death men: lung/bronchus, prostate, colorectal

Sites cancer-related death women: lung/bronchus, breast, colorectal

Gynecologic cancers: ovary, uterus, cervix

Heredity 5% all cancers

Autosomal dominant, autosomal recessive, familial cancers

Malignant melanoma: most rapidly increasing worldwide

China

TABLE 9-1 Selected Inherited Cancer Syndromes

CATEGORY	CANCER
Autosomal dominant cancer syndromes (Figs. 9-9 A–C)	• **Retinoblastoma:** malignancy of the eye, nearly always occurring before age 5. Of all cases of retinoblastoma, 60% are nonhereditary and are usually unilateral, 15% are autosomal dominant and have unilateral retinoblastomas, and 25% are autosomal dominant and have bilateral retinoblastomas. In the autosomal dominant type, one of the *RB1* genes on chromosome 13 is mutated in germ cells. A second mutation of the *RB1* gene on the remaining chromosome 13 (deletion or recombination mutation) must occur after birth ("two hits") to produce a unilateral retinoblastoma or a bilateral retinoblastoma. In the sporadic type of retinoblastoma, the two somatic mutations of the *RB1* suppressor gene on chromosome 13 occur in early childhood and produce unilateral retinoblastomas. In the autosomal dominant type of retinoblastoma, there is an additional risk for developing second malignancies, which include osteosarcoma (malignancy of bone; most common), a soft tissue sarcoma (malignancy of connective tissue), or a malignant melanoma (malignancy of melanocytes). • **Familial adenomatous polyposis:** colorectal cancer from malignant transformation of polyps develops by age 50 years. There is inactivation of the <u>a</u>denomatous <u>p</u>olyposis <u>c</u>oli *(APC)* suppressor gene and an increased incidence of desmoid tumors (fibromatosis of the anterior abdominal wall). • **Li-Fraumeni syndrome:** increased risk for developing brain tumors, sarcomas, leukemias (malignant transformation marrow stem cells), carcinomas (e.g., breast, brain) before age 50. There is a heterozygous loss-of-function mutation (see Chapter 6) in the suppressor gene encoding p53. • **Hereditary nonpolyposis colon cancer (Lynch syndrome):** increased risk for developing colorectal cancers (especially in the proximal colon) without having previous polyps. It is caused by a germ line mutation that inactivates DNA mismatch repair genes, which causes a microsatellite repeat replication error (called microsatellite instability). Microsatellites are repeated sequences that predispose to replication errors if there are mutations in DNA repair enzymes (e.g., mismatch repair genes). The microsatellites become unstable (become longer or shorter) and produce frameshift mutations (see Chapter 6) that inactivate or alter tumor suppressor gene function leading to cancer. Microsatellite instability is found in the majority of patients with hereditary nonpolyposis colon cancer. • *BRCA1* and *BRCA2* **genes:** Inactivation of these genes increases the risk for developing breast cancer (sometimes bilateral) and ovarian cancer. Because of the very high risk for these cancers, many women with these mutations elect to have prophylactic bilateral mastectomy and oophorectomy in the absence of a detectable tumor in these sites.
Autosomal recessive syndromes with defects in DNA repair	• **Xeroderma pigmentosum (Fig. 9-10):** increased risk at an early age for developing skin cancers (basal cell carcinoma, squamous cell carcinoma, and malignant melanoma) due to inability to repair pyridine dimers produced by exposure to ultraviolet light. • **Chromosome instability syndromes:** Chromosomes are susceptible to damage by ionizing radiation and drugs. In **ataxia telangiectasia,** there is an increased risk for developing malignant lymphomas. In **Bloom syndrome,** there is an increased risk for developing gastrointestinal tumors and malignant lymphoma. In **Fanconi syndrome,** there is an increased risk for developing malignant lymphomas, squamous cell carcinoma, and hepatocellular carcinomas.
Familial cancer syndromes	• No clearly defined pattern of inheritance; however, certain cancers (e.g., breast, ovary, colon) develop with increased frequency in families. This syndrome sometimes involves inactivation of the *BRCA1* and *BRCA2* suppressor genes.

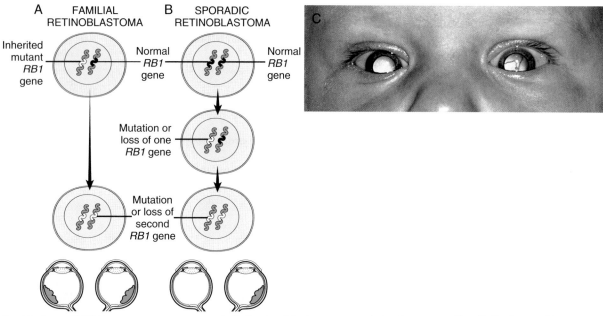

9-9: Retinoblastoma *(RB1)* tumor suppressor gene. **A,** Patients with the autosomal dominant type (familial) of retinoblastoma are born with only one normal *RB1* gene; the other one is deleted in germ cells (first "hit"). After birth, the normal *RB1* gene is mutated in retinoblasts as a result of a spontaneous somatic mutation (second "hit"), which allows oncogenes in those cells to express themselves and produce a retinoblastoma either in one or both eyes. **B,** Patients with the sporadic type of retinoblastoma have normal *RB1* genes at birth, and both of the normal *RB1* genes must undergo a spontaneous somatic mutation in the same retinoblast ("two hits"), causing a retinoblastoma to develop in one eye. Retinoblastomas usually develop before 5 years of age, hence the importance of genetic counseling of the parents. **C,** Leukocoria in a child with retinoblastoma. The normal red reflex to light, which may be red, orange, or yellow, is replaced by a white reflex in 60% of patients with retinoblastoma. *(A, B modified from my friend Ivan Damjanov, MD, PhD: Pathology for the Health-Related Professions, 2nd ed, Philadelphia, Saunders, 2000, p 89, Fig. 4-21; C from Adkison LR: Elsevier's Integrated Review Genetics, 2nd ed, Saunders Elsevier, 2012, p 77, Fig.5-11; taken from Augsburger JJ, Bornfeld N, Giblin ME: Retinoblastoma. In Yanoff M, Duker JS, eds: Ophthalmology, 2nd ed, St. Louis, Mosby, 2004.)*

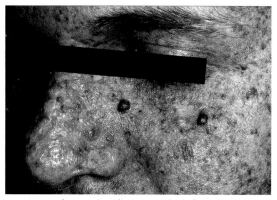

9-10: Xeroderma pigmentosum. This is an autosomal recessive disease with defects in DNA repair. Note the numerous hyperpigmented lesions and nodular and scaly growths on the face. Many of these lesions are precancerous or ultraviolet light–related cancers. *(Courtesy RA Marsden, MD, St. George's Hospital, London.)*

Nasopharyngeal carcinoma (EBV)

Esophageal SCC (smoking/alcohol)

Japan

Stomach adenocarcinoma (smoked foods)

Southeast Asia

HCC (HBV, HCV cirrhosis; aflatoxins)

Sub-Saharan Africa

Burkitt lymphoma (EBV); KS (HHV-8)

    a. Nasopharyngeal carcinoma is causally associated with the Epstein-Barr virus (EBV).
    b. SCC of the esophagus is causally associated with alcohol abuse, smoking, and other unknown factors.
  3. Japan. Adenocarcinoma of the stomach is causally associated with smoked foods.
  4. Southeast Asia. HCC is causally associated with chronic liver disease such as that caused by hepatitis B virus (HBV) or hepatitis C virus (HCV). Other associations include cirrhosis of any etiology as well as aflatoxin, a toxin derived from *Aspergillus* that contaminates improperly stored food crops.
  5. Sub-Saharan Africa. Burkitt lymphoma is causally associated with EBV. Kaposi sarcoma (KS) is causally associated with human herpesvirus 8 (HHV-8).
  F. Acquired preneoplastic disorders (Table 9-2)
  G. Prevention modalities in cancer

TABLE 9-2   Acquired Preneoplastic Disorders*

PRECURSOR LESION	CANCER
Actinic (solar) keratosis (see Fig. 25-11 A)	Squamous cell carcinoma
Atypical hyperplasia of ductal epithelium of the breast	Adenocarcinoma
Chronic irritation at sinus orifices, third-degree burn scars	Squamous cell carcinoma
Chronic ulcerative colitis (see Fig. 18-26 A)	Adenocarcinoma
Complete hydatidiform mole (see Fig. 22-17 A)	Choriocarcinoma
Dysplastic nevus (see Fig. 25-9 G)	Malignant melanoma
Endometrial hyperplasia (see Fig. 22-11 D)	Adenocarcinoma
Glandular metaplasia of esophagus (Barrett esophagus; see Fig. 18-13 B)	Adenocarcinoma
Glandular metaplasia of stomach (*Helicobacter pylori*)	Adenocarcinoma
Myelodysplastic syndrome	Acute leukemia
Regenerative nodules in cirrhosis (see Fig. 19-7 C)	Adenocarcinoma
Scar tissue in lung (see Fig. 17-17 E)	Adenocarcinoma
Squamous dysplasia of oropharynx, larynx, bronchus, cervix (see Fig. 2-15 H)	Squamous cell carcinoma
Tubular adenoma of colon (see Fig. 9-1 A)	Adenocarcinoma
Vaginal adenosis (diethylstilbestrol exposure; Link 22-50)	Adenocarcinoma
Villous adenoma of rectum (see Fig. 18-28 D)	Adenocarcinoma

*Metaplastic and hyperplastic cells become dysplastic *before* progressing to cancer.

1. Modify lifestyle
    a. Cessation of smoking cigarettes
        • Most important lifestyle modification to prevent cancer (see Chapter 7 for the list of cancers)
    b. Increasing dietary fiber and decreasing dietary saturated animal fat
        • Previously mentioned modifications decrease the risk for developing colorectal cancer.
    c. Reducing alcohol intake (see Chapter 7 for the list of cancers)
    d. Reducing weight
        (1) More adipose tissue increases aromatase conversion of androgens to estrogen.
        (2) Increased levels of estrogen increase the risk for developing endometrial and breast cancer.
    e. Sunscreen protection. Decreases the risk for developing BCC, SCC, and malignant melanoma of skin (see Chapter 25)
2. Immunization
    a. HBV immunization. Decreases the risk for developing HCC, due to HBV-induced cirrhosis
    b. Human papillomavirus (HPV) immunization. Immunization against HPV decreases the risk for developing SCC of the cervix and penis
3. Screening procedures to detect cancer
    a. Cervical Papanicolaou (Pap) smears
        (1) Pap smears decrease the risk for cervical cancer due to HPV. HPV subtypes 16 and 18 are the most common. Explains why cervical cancer is the *least* common gynecologic cancer and the *least* common gynecologic cancer causing death.
        (2) Pap smears detect dysplasia of the cervical mucosa, the precursor to invasive cervical cancer (Link 9-13). Cervical dysplasia is treated by cervical conization and other interventions (see Chapter 22).
    b. Colonoscopy. Detects and removes precancerous polyps.
    c. Mammography. Detects nonpalpable breast masses.
    d. Prostate-specific antigen (PSA). Prostate-specific antigen is more sensitive than specific for diagnosing prostate cancer. Specificity is decreased, because other conditions such as benign prostatic hyperplasia and prostatitis can cause elevated PSA as well.

Cessation smoking: most important

↑Fiber, ↓animal saturated fat: ↓risk colorectal cancer

↓Alcohol intake: ↓risk for alcohol-related cancers

Reduce weight

↓Risk estrogen-related endometrial/breast cancer

Sunscreen protection

↓Risk BCC, SCC, melanoma

Immunization

HBV immunization

↓HCC risk from HBV-cirrhosis

HPV immunization

↓Risk cervical/penile SCC

↓Risk HPV 16/18 induced cervical cancer

Cervical cancer least common gynecologic cancer

Cervical cancer least common gynecologic cancer causing death

Pap smears: detect dysplasia, precursor cervical cancer

Colonoscopy: detects/removes precancerous polyps

Mammography: detects nonpalpable breast masses

PSA

More sensitive than specific for Dx prostate cancer

4. Treatment of conditions that predispose to cancer decreases the risk for cancer.
   a. Treatment of *Helicobacter pylori* infections (peptic ulcer disease, gastritis)
      (1) Treatment decreases the risk for developing malignant lymphoma (lymphoid hyperplasia → malignant lymphoma).
      (2) Treatment does *not* decrease the risk for developing adenocarcinoma of the stomach.
   b. Treatment of gastroesophageal reflux disease (GERD). Treatment of GERD decreases the risk for developing distal adenocarcinoma arising from a Barrett esophagus (glandular metaplasia → adenocarcinoma; see Chapters 2 and 18).

IV. **Carcinogenesis**
   A. **Overview of carcinogenesis**
      • Cancer is a multistep process involving gene mutations, telomerase activation, angiogenesis, invasion, and metastasis (Link 9-14).
   B. **Types of gene mutations producing cancer**
      1. Point mutations (most common mutation; see Fig. 6-1)
      2. Balanced translocations (Fig. 9-11)
      3. Insertion of a viral genome (insertional mutagenesis). Disrupts normal chromosome structure and increases genetic dysregulation.
      4. Other mutations, such as deletion, gene amplification (multiple copies of a gene), and overexpression (increased gene transcription resulting in the production of too much protein product)
   C. **Genes involved in cancer**
      1. Mutations involving proto-oncogenes
         a. Proto-oncogenes are involved in normal growth and repair.
         b. Functions of proto-oncogene protein products include synthesis of growth factors, growth factor receptors, signal transducers, and nuclear transcribers.
         c. Mutations of proto-oncogenes cause *sustained activity* of the genes (Table 9-3; Fig. 9-9; Link 9-15).
      2. Mutations involving suppressor genes (antioncogenes)
         a. Suppressor genes protect against unregulated cell growth.
         b. Main sites of suppressor gene control in the cell cycle are the G₁ to S phase and nuclear transcription (see Chapter 3).
         c. Mutations of suppressor genes cause *unregulated cell proliferation* (Table 9-4).
      3. Mutations involving antiapoptosis genes; *BCL2* family of genes (see Chapter 3)
         a. *BCL2* gene family that is located on chromosome 18 produces gene products that prevent mitochondrial (mt) leakage of cytochrome *c* (an antiapoptosis gene).
         b. Cytochrome *c* in the cytosol activates caspases initiating apoptosis.
         c. Translocation t(14;18) in B cells causes an overexpression type of mutation of the *BCL2* protein product. Prevents apoptosis of B lymphocytes (cytochrome *c* cannot enter the cytosol), which produces a B-cell follicular lymphoma (see Chapter 14).

TABLE 9-3 Some Proto-oncogenes and Their Functions, Mutations, and Associated Cancers

PROTO-ONCOGENE	NORMAL FUNCTION	MUTATION	CANCER ASSOCIATIONS
ABL (Fig. 9-11)	Nonreceptor tyrosine kinase activity	Translocation t(9;22); forms a fusion gene (*BCR-ABL*)	• Chronic myelogenous leukemia: chromosome 22 with the translocation is called the Philadelphia chromosome.
ERBB2 (also called *Her-2/Neu*)	Receptor synthesis	Amplification or overexpression	• In breast carcinoma, *ERBB2* is a marker of aggressiveness (poor prognosis). It is amplified or overexpressed in 25% of breast cancers.
C-MYC (Fig. 9-12)	Nuclear transcription	Translocation t(8;14)	• Burkitt lymphoma
N-MYC	Nuclear transcription	Amplification	• Neuroblastoma, small cell carcinoma of the lung
RAS	Guanosine. triphosphate signal transduction	Point mutation	• Accounts for 15%–20% of all cancers: pancreatic carcinomas (90%); ≈50% of endometrial, colon, and thyroid cancers; 30% of lung adenocarcinomas and myeloid leukemias; and urinary bladder cancer
RET	Receptor synthesis	Point mutation	• Multiple endocrine neoplasia IIa/IIb syndromes; leukemia
SIS (*PBGFB*)	Growth factor synthesis	Overexpression	• Osteosarcoma, astrocytoma

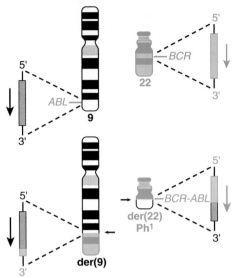

9-11: The Philadelphia chromosome translocation, t(9;22). The Philadelphia chromosome (Ph[1]) is the derivative of chromosome 22, which has exchanged part of its long arm for a segment of material from chromosome 9q that contains the *ABL* oncogene (nonreceptor tyrosine kinase). Formation of the *BCR-ABL* fusion gene on the Ph[1] chromosome is the critical genetic event in the development of chronic myelogenous leukemia. *(From Nussbaum R, McInnes R, Willard H: Thompson & Thompson Genetics in Medicine, 7th ed, Philadelphia, Saunders Elsevier, 2007, p 466, Fig. 16-4.)*

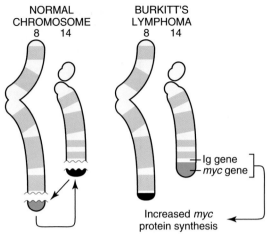

9-12: Translocation of the *MYC* oncogene from chromosome 8 to chromosome 14 activates the *MYC* oncogene and produces Burkitt lymphoma. The immunoglobulin *(Ig)* gene juxtaposed to the *MYC* gene on chromosome 14 acts as a promoter. *(Adapted from Kumar V, Abbas AK, Fausto N, Aster JC: Robbins and Cotran Pathologic Basis of Disease, 9th ed, Philadelphia, Saunders, 2015, p 287, Fig. 7-26.)*

TABLE 9-4 Some Tumor Suppressor Genes, Their Functions, and Associated Cancers

GENE	NORMAL FUNCTION	ASSOCIATED CANCERS
APC	Prevents nuclear transcription (degrades catenin, an activator of nuclear transcription)	• Inherited mutation (AD): familial polyposis (colorectal carcinoma) • Somatic mutations: colon and stomach cancer
BRCA1/BRCA2	Regulates DNA repair	• Inherited mutation: female breast, ovary carcinomas; carcinoma of the male breast
NF1	Inhibits RAS signal transduction; cell cycle inhibitor	• Inherited mutation (AD): neurofibromatosis type 1: pheochromocytoma, Wilms tumor, neurofibrosarcomas • Somatic mutation: neuroblastoma
NF2	Cytoskeletal stability	• Inherited mutation (AD): neurofibromatosis type 2: bilateral acoustic neuromas (schwannoma), meningioma • Somatic mutation: schwannoma, meningioma
p53	Inhibits G1 to S phase Repairs DNA, inhibits the *BCL2* antiapoptosis gene (initiates apoptosis)	• Inherited mutation (AD): Li-Fraumeni syndrome: breast carcinoma, brain tumors, leukemia, sarcomas • Somatic mutation: most human cancers (*p53* gene is the most common gene producing cancer)
RB1	Inhibits G1 to S phase	• Inherited mutation (AD): retinoblastoma, osteosarcoma • Somatic mutation: retinoblastoma, osteosarcoma, carcinomas of breast, lung, colon
TGF-β	Inhibits G1 to S phase	• Inherited mutation: familial stomach cancer • Somatic mutation: pancreatic and colorectal carcinomas
VHL	Regulates nuclear transcription	• Inherited mutation (AD): von Hippel–Lindau syndrome: cerebellar hemangioblastoma, retinal angioma, renal cell carcinoma (bilateral), pheochromocytoma (bilateral)
WT1	Regulates nuclear transcription	• Inherited mutation (AD): Wilms tumor • Sporadic mutation: Wilms tumor

AD, Autosomal dominant; *APC,* adenomatous polyposis coli; *BRCA,* breast cancer; *RB,* retinoblastoma; *TGF-β,* transforming growth factor β; *VHL,* von Hippel–Lindau; *WT,* Wilms tumor.

1 A DNA molecule is distorted by ultraviolet light-induced pyrimidine dimer

2 A specific endonuclease breaks one chain near the dimer

3 An exonuclease excises a small region containing the pyrimidine dimer

4 5′–3′ synthesis of a new strand takes place, the correct bases inserted by pairing with bases on the intact strand

5 Polynucleotide ligase effects the joining of the strands, completing the repaired molecule

9-13: Excision-repair mechanism of a pyrimidine dimer. *(Modified from McKee PH, Calonje E, Granter SR: Pathology of the Skin with Clinical Correlations, 3rd ed, St. Louis, Mosby Elsevier, 2005, p 1228, Fig. 22.193.)*

Mismatch repair genes: correct errors nucleotide pairing

Lynch syndrome

DNA repair enzymes (in order): endonuclease, exonuclease, polymerase, ligase

Allow cells with nonlethal damage to proliferate (↑risk cancer)

PAHs in tobacco smoke MC carcinogen

React with electron-rich atoms in DNA (e.g., alkylating agents)

Carcinogens require metabolic conversion (e.g., PAHs)

Initiation → promotion → progression

Initiation: irreversible mutation

IR, UVB light, nitrosamines, asbestos, PHCs, HPV

Stimulate mutated cells to enter cell cycle

Cannot induce cancer on their own

Estrogen a promoter

Development tumor heterogeneity

Clonal production cells that invade/metastasize

HBV, HPV, HCV, EBV

H. pylori gastric adenocarcinoma/lymphoma

S. haematobium: SCC bladder

4. Mutations involving DNA repair genes (see Table 9-1 and Table 9-4)
   a. Examples of DNA repair
      (1) Mismatch repair genes produce proteins that correct errors in nucleotide pairing. Mutations in mismatch repair genes are associated with hereditary nonpolyposis colon cancer syndrome (Lynch syndrome; see Table 9-1).
      (2) Nucleotide excision repair pathway removes pyrimidine dimers in UV-damaged skin (Fig. 9-13). DNA repair enzymes in order are endonuclease, exonuclease, polymerase, ligase.
   b. Effect of mutations involving the DNA repair genes. Mutations in repair genes allow cells with nonlethal damage to proliferate, increasing the risk for cancer.

V. **Carcinogenic Agents**
   A. **Chemical carcinogens (Table 9-5; see Chapter 7)**
      1. Polycyclic aromatic hydrocarbons (PAHs) in tobacco smoke. Most common group of carcinogens in the United States.
      2. Mechanism of action of chemical carcinogens
         a. Direct-acting carcinogens. Contain electron-deficient atoms that react with electron-rich atoms in DNA (e.g., alkylating agents, nickel).
         b. Indirect-acting carcinogens
            (1) Require metabolic conversion to a carcinogen *before* they become active
            (2) For example, PAHs from cigarette smoke, smoked meats, or meats cooked at a high temperature over an open flame are metabolized in the liver cytochrome P450 system and converted into DNA-binding epoxides that are carcinogenic.
      3. Sequence of chemical carcinogenesis
         a. Initiation
            (1) Initiation produces an irreversible mutation.
            (2) Examples of initiators include ionizing radiation (IR), UVB light, nitrosamines, asbestos, polycyclic hydrocarbons (PHCs), and HPV.
         b. Promotion
            (1) Promoters stimulate mutated cells to enter the cell cycle.
            (2) Promoters *cannot* induce cancer on their own.
            (3) An example of a promoter is estrogen.
         c. Progression
            (1) Progression is involved in the development of tumor heterogeneity.
            (2) Example of progression is the clonal production of cells that invade or metastasize (Fig. 9-5).
   B. **Carcinogenic microbial agents**
      1. Oncogenic viruses (Table 9-6): HBV, HCV, EBV, HTLV-1, HHV-8, HPV types 16, 18
      2. Oncogenic bacteria
         a. *Helicobacter pylori,* which produces adenocarcinoma and low-grade malignant lymphoma of the stomach
         b. *Fusobacterium nucleatum* in the early stages of colorectal cancer development
      3. Oncogenic parasites
         a. *Schistosoma haematobium.* Causes SCC of the urinary bladder (see Chapter 21).

TABLE 9-5 Chemical Carcinogens

CARCINOGEN	MEANS OF EXPOSURE/SOURCES	ASSOCIATED CANCERS
Aflatoxin (from *Aspergillus*)	Ingestion of maize and peanuts grown in hot/humid climates	• Hepatocellular carcinoma in association with HBV
Alkylating agents	Oncology chemotherapy	• Malignant lymphoma
Arsenic	Herbicides (common in vineyard workers), fungicides, animal dips; metal smelting; intentional/accidental poisoning	• Squamous cell carcinoma of skin, lung cancer, liver angiosarcoma (malignancy of blood vessels)
Asbestos	Roofing material (roofers with over 20 years of experience have had contact with asbestos); insulation for pipes in ships in shipyards (no longer used for insulation), old homes; old cars with brake liners	• Bronchogenic carcinoma (most common), pleural mesothelioma
Azo dyes	Used in paints, printing inks, varnishes, leather products, carpets, food products	• Hepatocellular carcinoma
Benzene	Component of light oil; used in printing industry, dry cleaning, paint, adhesives and coatings	• Acute leukemia, Hodgkin lymphoma
Beryllium	Used in the space industry (missile fuel and space vehicles; metal alloys in aerospace appliances and nuclear reactors)	• Bronchogenic carcinoma
Cadmium	Used in industries where ore is being smelted; electroplating; welders who have welded on cadmium-containing alloys or worked with silver solders; found in some batteries	• Prostate and lung cancer
Cyclophosphamide	Chemotherapy agent	• Transitional cell carcinoma of urinary bladder
Diethylstilbestrol (DES)	Once used to treat women with threatened abortions	• Daughters exposed to mothers who took DES may develop clear cell carcinoma of vagina/cervix
β-Naphthylamine (aniline dyes) and aromatic amines	Workers in the rubber, chemical, leather, textile, metal, and printing industries	• Transitional cell carcinoma of urinary bladder
Nickel	Nickel plating, by-product of stainless steel welding, ceramics, batteries, spark plugs	• Bronchogenic carcinoma, nasal cavity cancer
Oral contraceptives	Birth control pill	• Breast and cervical cancer; hepatic adenoma (tendency to rupture)
Polycyclic hydrocarbons	Formed when coal, soot (chimney sweeper), wood, gasoline, oil, tobacco, or other organic materials are burned; also formed in food when fish or meats are charbroiled on an open flame	• Squamous cell carcinoma: skin (scrotum with soot in chimney sweeper), oral cavity, mid-esophagus, larynx, lung • Adenocarcinoma: distal esophagus, pancreas, kidney • Transitional cell carcinoma: urinary bladder, renal pelvis
Polyvinyl chloride	Found in plastic piping material, adhesive plastics, refrigerant	• Liver angiosarcoma
Radon and decay products	By-product of decay of uranium, hazard in quarries and underground mines	• Bronchogenic carcinoma
Silica	Chemical of silicon dioxide, rock quarries, sandblasting	• Bronchogenic carcinoma

      b. *Clonorchis sinensis* and *Opisthorchis viverrini*. Cause cholangiocarcinoma of bile ducts (see Chapter 19).
    4. Order of importance of microbial agents causing cancer: viruses > bacteria > parasites
  C. Radiation
    1. Ionizing radiation–induced cancers
      a. Mechanism of ionizing radiation: induces hydroxyl free radical injury of DNA in exposed tissue
      b. Examples of ionizing radiation–induced cancers
        (1) Acute myeloblastic leukemia (AML) and chronic myelogenous leukemia (CML)
          (a) Leukemia is the most common overall cancer due to ionizing radiation.
          (b) Radiologists and individuals exposed to radiation in nuclear reactors are at increased risk of developing leukemia.
        (2) Papillary thyroid carcinoma

Clonorchis sinensis, Opisthorchis viverrini: cholangiocarcinoma bile ducts

Viruses > bacteria > parasites

Hydroxyl FRs damage DNA

AML, CML

MC overall cancer due to ionizing radiation

Papillary cancer thyroid

TABLE 9-6 Oncogenic RNA and DNA Viruses

VIRUS	MECHANISM	ASSOCIATED CANCER(S)
RNA		
HCV	Produces cirrhosis	• Hepatocellular carcinoma
HTLV-1	Activates *TAX* gene, stimulates polyclonal T-cell proliferation, inhibits *p53* suppressor gene	• T-cell leukemia and lymphoma
DNA		
EBV	Promotes polyclonal B-cell proliferation, which increases the risk for a t(8;14) translocation	• Burkitt lymphoma, CNS lymphoma in AIDS, mixed cellularity Hodgkin lymphoma, nasopharyngeal carcinoma
HBV	Activates proto-oncogenes, inactivates *p53* suppressor gene	• Hepatocellular carcinoma
HHV-8	Acts via cytokines released from HIV and HSV	• Kaposi sarcoma
HPV types 16 and 18	• Type 16 (≈50% of cancers): E6 gene product inhibits the *p53* suppressor gene • Type 18 (≈10% of cancers): E7 gene product inhibits the *RB1* suppressor gene	• Squamous cell carcinoma of vulva, vagina, cervix, anus (associated with anal intercourse), larynx, oropharynx

AIDS, Acquired immunodeficiency syndrome; *CNS,* central nervous system; *EBV,* Epstein-Barr virus; *HBV,* hepatitis B virus; *HCV,* hepatitis C virus; *HHV,* human herpesvirus; *HPV,* human papillomavirus; *HSV,* herpes simplex virus; *HTLV,* human T-cell lymphotropic virus.

Lung, breast, bone cancers	(3) Lung, breast, and bone cancers
	(4) Liver angiosarcoma. Due to radioactive thorium dioxide that is used to visualize the arterial tree. Yttrium oxide (or sometimes zirconium oxide) is used increasingly as a replacement for thorium dioxide.
	2. UVB light–induced cancers
Pyrimidine dimers that distort DNA	a. UVB light produces pyrimidine dimers that distort DNA structure (Fig. 9-13).
BCC MC cancer; SCC, melanoma	b. Examples of UVB light–induced cancers are BCC (see Fig. 25-11 B), SCC (see Fig. 25-11 D), and malignant melanoma (see Fig. 25-9 H).
	D. Physical injury
SCC 3rd-degree burns	1. SCC may develop in third-degree burn scars.
SCC orifice draining sinus	2. SCC may develop at the orifices of chronically draining sinuses (e.g., chronic osteomyelitis).
	VI. Clinical Oncology
	A. Host defenses against cancer (see Chapter 4)
Humoral immunity: antibodies, complement	1. Humoral immunity. Humoral immunity involves antibodies and complement.
	2. Type IV cell-mediated immunity (CMI)
CMI most effective	a. CMI is the most efficient mechanism for killing cancer cells.
Cytotoxic CD8 T cells most effective defense	b. Cytotoxic CD8 T cells. Recognize altered class I antigens on neoplastic cells and destroy them.
NK cells kill cell directly (type IV HSR)/indirectly via type II HSR	3. Natural killer (NK) cells. Directly kill malignant cells (type IV hypersensitivity) or use indirect killing of cells via type II hypersensitivity reactions.
Macrophages kill cancer cells	4. Macrophages kill cancer cells; however, they are *not* as effective as cytotoxic T cells and NK cells.
	B. Grading and staging of cancer
	1. Grading criteria for cancer
Degree differentiation	a. Degree of differentiation (e.g., low, intermediate, or high grade [anaplastic])
Nuclear features, invasiveness	b. Nuclear features, invasiveness
Stage more important than grade cancer	2. Staging criteria (Fig. 9-14)
	a. Most important prognostic factor for survival
	b. TNM system for staging cancer
Least to most important	(1) TNM progresses from the least to the most important prognostic factor.
T tumor size	(2) *T* refers to tumor size. Malignant tumor that is ≥2 cm is inherently capable of metastasizing.
Malignant tumor ≥2 cm: inherent ability to metastasize	
N nodes	(3) *N* refers to whether lymph nodes are involved.
M extranodal metastasis	(4) *M* refers to extranodal metastases (e.g., liver, lung).
	(a) For a carcinoma to reach M, it already has passed through N (lymph nodes) and spread to other organ sites via the bloodstream.
M > N > T	(b) If there are *no* extranodal metastases, then N (lymph nodes) is the most important prognostic factor for survival.
	C. Cancer effects on the host
	1. Cachexia (wasting disease) (Fig. 9-15)
Generalized catabolic reaction	a. **Definition:** Generalized catabolic reaction that is associated with anorexia, muscle wasting, loss of subcutaneous fat, and fatigue

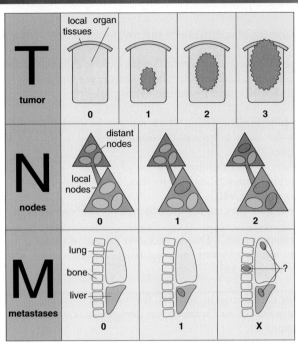

9-14: Staging of carcinoma by TNM system. The general principles of TNM staging are as follows: **T** refers to primary tumor. The accompanying number denotes the size of tumor and its local extent. The number varies according to site. **N** refers to lymph node involvement, and a high number denotes increasing extent of involvement. **M** refers to the extent of distant metastases. *(From Stevens A, Lowe J, Scott I: Core Pathology, 3rd ed, Mosby Elsevier, 2009, p 80, Fig. 6-13.)*

SIGNS AND SYMPTOMS OF MALIGNANT TUMORS

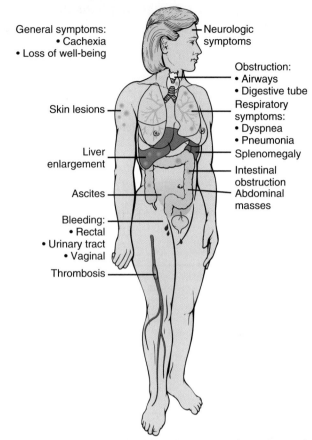

9-15: Signs (e.g., splenomegaly) and symptoms (e.g., dyspnea) of malignant tumors. *(From my friend Ivan Damjanov, MD, PhD: Pathology for the Health Professions, 4th ed, Saunders Elsevier, 2012, p 87, Fig. 4-24.)*

  b. Epidemiology
    (1) Very common complication of disseminated cancer (weight loss syndrome)
    (2) Includes anorexia, muscle wasting, body fat loss
    (3) Accounts for ≈30% of deaths due to cancer
  c. Pathogenesis
    (1) Cancer cells release cachectic agents.
      (a) Proteolysis-inducing factor (PIF)
      (b) Lipolysis-mobilizing factor (LMF)
    (2) PIF uses NF-κB (nuclear factor kappa-light-chain-enhancer of activated B cells) to activate the ubiquitin-proteasome pathway (see Chapter 2). Activation of this pathway causes degradation of myosin heavy chains in skeletal muscle.
    (3) LMF has multiple functions.
      (a) Activates hormone-sensitive lipase (HSL) in adipose cells, which reduces body fat and increases free fatty acids
      (b) Increases release of TNF from macrophages and monocytes. TNF suppresses the appetite center in the hypothalamus, which leads to weight loss. TNF stimulates apoptosis (see Chapter 2).
  2. Anemia in cancer (see Chapter 12)
    a. Anemia of chronic disease (ACD) is the most common anemia in malignancy.
    b. Iron deficiency is most often due to gastrointestinal blood loss (e.g., colorectal cancer).
    c. Macrocytic anemia is most often due to folic acid deficiency from rapid tumor growth and the use of folic acid for DNA synthesis.
    d. Cold autoimmune hemolytic anemia (AIHA) due to immunoglobulin M (IgM) cold agglutinins is associated with chronic lymphocytic leukemia (CLL) and certain types of malignant lymphoma.

Complication disseminated cancer

Anorexia, muscle wasting, body fat loss

Cachectic agents PIF, LMF

PIF uses NF-κB to activate ubiquitin-proteasome pathway

Degradation skeletal muscle

LMF activates HSL → ↓body fat, ↑fatty acids

LMF ↑ release TNF from macrophages/monocytes

TNF suppresses appetite; stimulates apoptosis

ACD MC anemia

Iron deficiency usually colorectal cancer

Macrocytic anemia: folic acid deficiency; tumor uses folic acid for DNA synthesis

Cold AIHA: IgM cold agglutinins (CLL), malignant lymphoma

Myelophthisic anemia

Marrow replacement by cancer and/or fibrous tissue

Leukoerythroblastic smear

NRBCs, metamyelocytes

Teardrop RBCs: marker myelofibrosis due to metastasis

Hemostasis abnormalities

Vessel thrombosis

Thrombocytosis, ↑synthesis coagulation factors

Procoagulants released from cancer cells

DIC from cancer releasing tissue thromboplastin

Fever

Infection MCC

Gram-negative sepsis: common COD in cancer

Paraneoplastic syndromes

Distant effects unrelated to metastasis

Predate metastasis

Mimic metastatic disease

Ectopic secretion hormones

e. Myelophthisic anemia
   (1) **Definition:** Due to the replacement of normal bone marrow by malignant cells and/or fibrosis
   (2) In the peripheral blood, there are immature, normal hematopoietic cells mixed in with normal hematopoietic cells (i.e., leukoerythroblastic smear; see Fig. 13-2).
      (a) Nucleated red blood cells (NRBCs) and immature neutrophils (e.g., metamyelocytes)
      (b) Presence of teardrop red blood cells (RBCs), which are a good marker for the presence of myelofibrosis due to metastasis in the bone marrow
3. Hemostasis abnormalities (see Chapter 15)
   a. Increased risk for blood vessel thrombosis in malignancy
      (1) Due to thrombocytosis (increased platelets) and/or increased synthesis of coagulation factors (e.g., fibrinogen, factors V and VIII)
      (2) In addition, cancer cells may release procoagulants, which is notably common in pancreatic carcinoma.
   b. Disseminated intravascular coagulation (DIC). Due to excessive release of tissue thromboplastin from cancer cells, which activates the coagulation system to form fibrin clots in the microcirculation (see Chapter 15).
4. Fever in malignancy
   a. Most often due to infection rather than pyrogens secreted from cancer cells
   b. Gram-negative sepsis from *Escherichia coli* or *Pseudomonas aeruginosa* is a common cause of death in cancer (see Chapter 5).
5. Paraneoplastic syndromes
   a. **Definition:** Distant effects of a tumor that are unrelated to metastasis
   b. Epidemiology of paraneoplastic syndromes
      (1) Predate the onset of metastasis
      (2) Occur in 10% to 15% of cancer patients
      (3) Involve multiple organ systems and mimic metastatic disease (Table 9-7; Fig. 9-12)
      (4) Some cancers may ectopically secrete hormones (Table 9-8).

TABLE 9-7 Paraneoplastic Syndromes

SYNDROME	ASSOCIATED CANCER(S)	COMMENTS
Acanthosis nigricans (see Fig. 25-10 B)	Stomach carcinoma	Black, verrucous lesion
Eaton-Lambert syndrome	Small cell carcinoma of lung	Myasthenia gravis–like symptoms (e.g., muscle weakness); antibody directed against calcium channel
Hypertrophic osteoarthropathy (Fig. 9-16 A)	Bronchogenic carcinoma	Periosteal reaction of distal phalanx (often associated with clubbing of nail)
Nonbacterial thrombotic endocarditis	Mucus-secreting pancreatic and colorectal carcinomas	Sterile vegetations on mitral valve
Seborrheic keratosis (see Fig. 25-10 A)	Stomach carcinoma	Sudden appearance of numerous pigmented seborrheic keratoses (Leser-Trélat sign)
Superficial migratory thrombophlebitis	Pancreatic carcinoma	Release of procoagulants (Trousseau sign)
Nephrotic syndrome	Lung, breast, stomach carcinomas	Diffuse membranous glomerulopathy

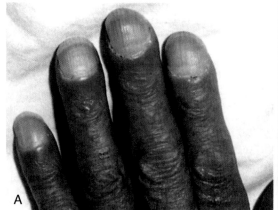
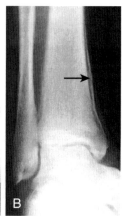

9-16: **A,** Hypertrophic osteoarthropathy with finger clubbing. Note the bulbous swelling of the connective tissue in the terminal phalanxes. **B,** Hypertrophic osteoarthropathy of the tibia showing periosteal elevation of the tibia (black arrow). (**A** from Grieg JD: Color Atlas of Surgical Diagnosis, London, Mosby-Wolfe, 1996, p 57, Fig. 8.33; **B** from Goldman L, Schafer A: Goldman's Cecil Medicine, 25th ed, Saunders Elsevier, 2016, p 1221, Fig. 179-1; courtesy of Dr. Lynne S. Steinbach.)

TABLE 9-8   Paraneoplastic Syndrome Endocrinopathies

DISORDER	ASSOCIATED CANCER(S)	ECTOPIC HORMONE(S)
Cushing syndrome	Small cell carcinoma of lung, medullary carcinoma of thyroid, pancreatic cancer	ACTH
Gynecomastia	Choriocarcinoma (testis), seminoma	hCG
Hypercalcemia	• Renal cell carcinoma, primary squamous cell carcinoma of lung, breast carcinoma, adult T-cell leukemia/lymphoma • Malignant lymphomas (contain 1α-hydroxylase)	• PTH-related protein • Calcitriol (vitamin D)
Hypocalcemia	Medullary carcinoma of the thyroid	Calcitonin
Hypoglycemia	Hepatocellular carcinoma, ovarian carcinoma, fibrosarcoma	Insulin-like factor
Hyponatremia	Small cell carcinoma of lung	Antidiuretic hormone
Secondary polycythemia	Renal cell carcinoma, hepatocellular carcinoma, cerebellar hemangioma	Erythropoietin

ACTH, Adrenocorticotropic hormone; *hCG,* human chorionic gonadotropin; *PTH,* parathyroid hormone.

TABLE 9-9   Tumor Markers and Associated Cancers

TUMOR MARKER	ASSOCIATED CANCER(S)
AFP	Hepatocellular carcinoma, yolk sac tumor (endodermal sinus tumor) of ovary or testis
Bence Jones protein (light chains)	Multiple myeloma, Waldenström macroglobulinemia (represent light chains in urine)
CA 15-3	Breast cancer
CA19-9	Pancreatic, colorectal carcinomas
CA125	Surface-derived ovarian cancer (e.g., serous cystadenocarcinoma; helpful in distinguishing benign from malignant tumors)
CEA	Colorectal and pancreatic carcinomas (monitor for recurrences); cancers of lung, stomach, heart
LDH	Malignant lymphoma (prognostic factor for response to standard therapy)
Neuron specific enolase	Small cell carcinoma of lung
PSA	Prostate carcinoma (also increased in prostate hyperplasia)

AFP, α-Fetoprotein; *CEA,* carcinoembryonic antigen; *LDH,* lactate dehydrogenase; *PSA,* prostate-specific antigen.

D. Tumor markers (biomarkers) in cancer
  1. Biological markers of cancer include hormones, enzymes, oncofetal antigens, immunoglobulins, and glycoproteins (Table 9-9).
  2. Pathologists use special stains and techniques that help define the origin of different types of cancer.
     a. Cytokeratin stain positive: epithelial tissue origin
     b. Vimentin stain positive: connective tissue origin
     c. CD45 positive: malignant lymphoma
  3. Tumor markers are used to diagnose cancer, estimate tumor burden, detect recurrences, and predict the tumor response to treatment.

Tumor markers

Hormones, enzymes, oncofetal antigens, immunoglobulins, glycoproteins

Cytokeratin +: epithelial tissue origin

Vimentin +: connective tissue origin

CD45 +: malignant lymphoma

Dx cancer, estimate tumor burden, detect recurrences, predict tumor response to Rx

ABBREVIATIONS

MC most common   MCC most common cause

I. Lipoprotein Disorders
A. Lipoproteins
1. **Definition:** Lipoproteins are structures composed of varying proportions of protein, triglyceride (TG), cholesterol (CH), and phospholipids.
2. **Structure:** All lipoprotein fractions must be coated by protein so they can be carried in the water phase of plasma (Fig. 10-1; Link 10-1).
3. Overview
   a. Five lipoprotein fractions that have varying proportions of protein, TG, CH, and phospholipid (Link 10-2). They include chylomicrons, very-low-density lipoprotein (VLDL), intermediate-density lipoproteins (IDL), low-density lipoprotein (LDL), and high-density lipoprotein (HDL).
   b. The *exogenous cycle* of lipoprotein metabolism involves the metabolism of chylomicrons (Fig. 10-2 A). Chylomicrons derived from the small bowel are hydrolyzed by capillary lipoprotein lipase (CLL) into chylomicron remnants, which are then taken up by the liver.
   c. In the *endogenous cycle* of lipoprotein metabolism (Fig. 10-2 B), VLDL is synthesized by the liver (nascent VLDL) and then enters the circulation. In the circulation, CLL hydrolyzes VLDL into IDL, which is further hydrolyzed into LDL. Some of the LDL is taken up by extrahepatic cells, some by scavenger cells, and some by the liver. CH released from scavenger cells is bound to HDL, which delivers the CH to the liver.
4. Chylomicron formation (exogenous cycle)
   a. **Definition:** Chylomicrons are lipoproteins that transport *diet-derived* TGs in the blood and are *absent* during fasting.
   b. The composition of chylomicrons is protein (2%), TG (87%), CH (3%), and phospholipid (8%).
   c. Formation of chylomicrons in the small intestine
      (1) Enterocytes lining the villi absorb monoglycerides and fatty acids, which are then converted into TG in the cytosol (see Chapters 8 and 10).
      (2) TG is then packaged into a chylomicron, which requires apolipoprotein B48 (apoB-48) for assembly and secretion.
      (3) Nascent (newly made) chylomicrons enter intestinal lymphatics that drain into the thoracic duct, which empties into the bloodstream.
   d. Chylomicrons in the circulation (Fig. 10-2 A; Links 10-2 and 10-3)
      (1) Nascent chylomicrons obtain apoCII and apoE from HDL and become mature chylomicrons.
      (2) TG in chylomicrons is hydrolyzed by CLL into fatty acids and glycerol. Fatty acids and glycerol are taken up by the liver, where they are used to synthesize TGs (see later) and adipose tissue, the latter being a storage site for fat.

Margin notes (left column):

Coated by protein → water phase of plasma

Chylomicrons
VLDL
IDL, LDL, HDL

Chylomicrons → chylomicron remnants → liver

VLDL→IDL→LDL→ liver, extrahepatic cells, scavenger cells→ liver

Chylomicrons

Diet-derived TGs; absent during fasting

Least dense (protein 2%) all lipoproteins

Enterocytes absorb monoglycerides + fatty acids → TG

Requires apoB-48 assembly/secretion

Enterocytes → lymphatics → thoracic duct → blood

Obtain apoCII/apoE from HDL

CLL hydrolyze TG → fatty acids, glycerol

Fatty acids + glycerol in liver → synthesize TG

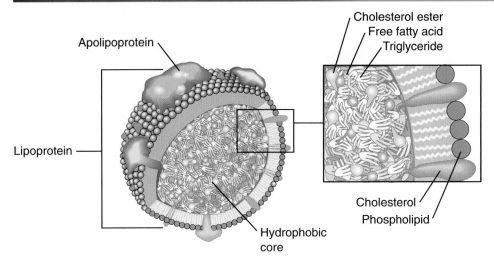

10-1: Lipoprotein structure. Lipoproteins are spherical particles with a hydrophobic core and an amphiphilic surface. The surface consists of a single layer of phospholipids. This surface layer also contains proteins (makes it soluble in the water phase of plasma) and free cholesterol. The hydrophobic core mainly contains triglycerides and cholesterol esters. (*From McPherson, R, Pincus, M: Henry's Clinical Diagnosis and Management by Laboratory Methods, 21st ed, Philadelphia, Saunders, 2007, p 227, Fig. 17-1.*)

   (3) Hydrolysis of chylomicrons in capillaries by CLL leaves *chylomicron remnants,* which contain much less TG than mature chylomicrons.

      (a) In the fed state, insulin is responsible for the synthesis of CLL. CLL is located in capillaries in the adipose tissue, muscle, and myocardium.

      (b) In the fed state, apoCII is responsible for activating CLL.

   (4) Chylomicron remnants are removed from the circulation by apoE receptors in the liver.

  5. VLDL (Fig. 10-2 B; Link 10-3)

    a. TG in the liver is synthesized by adding three fatty acids to glycerol 3-phosphate (G3P) (see Chapter 2). G3P is a three-carbon intermediate of glucose metabolism.

    b. With the aid of apoB-100, TG is packaged into VLDL and secreted into the blood as nascent VLDL.

    c. Composition of VLDL is as follows: protein (9%), TG (55%), CH (17%), and phospholipid (19%).

    d. VLDL is a source of fatty acids and glycerol.

      (1) TG in VLDL is hydrolyzed by CLL into fatty acids and glycerol. Fatty acids and glycerol are used to synthesize TG in the liver (see later) and adipose tissue.

      (2) Hydrolysis of nascent VLDL by CLL first produces IDL. Further hydrolysis of IDL then results in the production of LDL.

      (3) Some of the IDL is removed from the blood by apoE receptors in the liver.

    e. Cholesterol ester transport protein (CETP)

      (1) CETP transfers CH from HDL to VLDL and TG from VLDL to HDL. CETP interferes with HDL's main function of transferring CH from peripheral tissue to the liver for excretion in bile or for the synthesis of bile salts/acids.

      (2) Increase in VLDL always causes a decrease in HDL, which explains why an increase in VLDL is a risk factor for developing coronary artery disease (CAD).

    f. VLDL concentration is directly measured or calculated with the following formula: VLDL = TG ÷ 5.

    g. There are four clinically important serum TG levels. They are: optimal level: <150 mg/dL; borderline high level: 150–199 mg/dL; high level: 200–499 mg/dL; and very high level: >500 mg/dL

  6. Causes of increased plasma turbidity (Fig. 10-3)

    a. Increased turbidity, or a milky appearance of plasma, is due to very high levels of TGs in the serum (usually >1000 mg/dL). An increase in CH does *not* produce turbidity.

    b. An increase in serum TG is due to an increase in chylomicrons and/or VLDL.

    c. Standing chylomicron test distinguishes which lipoprotein component is increased.

      (1) Test tube is left upright in a refrigerator overnight to give the TG a chance to settle, based on the density of the lipoprotein (percent protein) that is present.

      (2) In the morning, if milky material is floating on the surface of the plasma (supranate), chylomicrons are increased. This indicates that the person did *not* fast before the lipid study (most common cause) or that the person has a type I hyperlipoproteinemia (discussed later).

Margin notes:

Chylomicrons capillaries hydrolyzed → CHLYO remnants (↓↓TG)

Insulin (fed state) responsible for synthesis of CLL

CLL in adipose, muscle, myocardium

Fed state: apoCII activates CLL

Chylomicron remnants removed by apoE receptors in liver

VLDL: liver-derived TG

G3P + 3 fatty acids → TG → VLDL

ApoB-100 important in synthesis/secretion VLDL

VLDL: source fatty acids + glycerol

CLL hydrolyzes TG

TG synthesis liver, TG stores in adipose

CLL: VLDL → IDL → LDL

CETP

Transfers CH from HDL to VLDL

CETP transfers TG from VLDL → HDL

HDL transfers CH → VLDL

↑VLDL/↓HDL; ↑VLDL risk factor CAD

VLDL = TG ÷ 5

↑Plasma turbidity: ↑TG

↑TG from ↑chylomicrons/VLDL

↑Turbidity → ↑↑TG

Turbid supranate → ↑chylomicrons (type I)

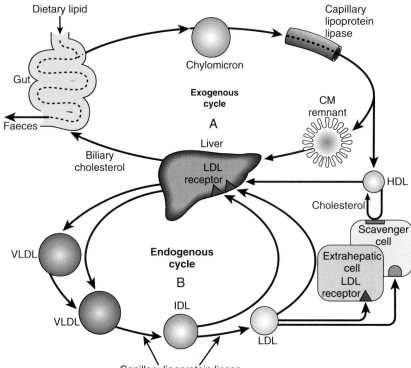

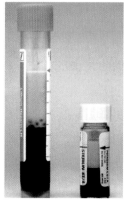

10-3: Turbidity in plasma. The turbidity could be due to an increase in chylomicrons and/or very-low-density lipoprotein. *(From Kliegman R: Nelson Textbook of Pediatrics, 19th ed, Philadelphia, Saunders Elsevier, 2011, p 476, Fig. 80-13; courtesy Durrington P: Dyslipidmia, Lancet 2003;362:717-731.)*

10-2: Schematic of lipid metabolism. The **exogenous cycle** on the top shows chylomicron *(CM)* synthesis from enterocytes in the small bowel. Chylomicrons that are synthesized in the small intestine enter the circulation. Capillary lipoprotein lipase hydrolyzes triglyceride in the chylomicron releasing fatty acids and glycerol (not shown) and produces a chylomicron remnant that is removed by the liver. The **endogenous cycle** on the bottom shows the liver synthesizing very-low-density lipoprotein *(VLDL)*. VLDL enters the circulation, where capillary lipoprotein lipase hydrolyzes the triglyceride into fatty acids and glycerol (not shown) eventually producing intermediate-density lipoprotein *(IDL)*, a remnant of VLDL. IDL is taken up by the liver, or it continues to be hydrolyzed until it becomes low-density lipoprotein *(LDL)*. LDL is the primary carrier of cholesterol (CH). Most extrahepatic cells have receptors for LDL because they all need CH for cell membrane synthesis or, in some cases, for hormone synthesis (e.g., vitamin D and adrenal cortex hormones). Some of the CH returns to the liver and some goes to scavenger cells. CH released from scavenger cells is bound to high-density lipoprotein *(HDL)* to produce HDL-CH. HDL transports the CH to the liver, where it is used to synthesize bile salts and acids. *(Modified from Gaw A, Murphy MJ, Srivastava R, et al: Clinical Biochemistry: An Illustrated Colour Text, 5th ed, Churchill Livingstone Elsevier, 2013, p 133, Fig. 66.2.)*

Turbid infranate: ↑VLDL (type IV)	(3) If the milky material is dispersed throughout the plasma (infranate), then only VLDL is increased. This occurs because VLDL has more protein in it than chylomicrons; hence, it sinks in the upright test tube. This is a type IV hyperlipoproteinemia (discussed later).
Supranate/infranate: type V	(4) If both a supranate and an infranate are present, then chylomicrons and VLDL are increased. This is a type V hyperlipoproteinemia (discussed later).
LDL	7. LDL
LDL transports CH	a. Primary vehicle for transporting CH in the blood
IDL → LDL	b. Derives from continued hydrolysis of IDL by CLL (Fig. 10-2 B, Link 10-3)
Removed by LDL receptors peripheral tissue	c. Removed from the blood by LDL receptors in the peripheral tissue
Small, dense LDL particles	d. Small, dense LDL particles
↑Risk atherosclerosis, CAD	(1) Increased levels of small LDL are associated with an increased risk of atherosclerosis and CAD. Small particle size allows them to penetrate the endothelium of arteries, making it easier to form atherosclerotic plaques.
↑Diets high in carbohydrates	(2) Levels of small LDL are increased in diets that are high in carbohydrates.
LDL mainly CH	e. Composed of protein (22%), TG (10%), CH (47%), and phospholipid (21%)
Calculated LDL = CH − HDL − TG ÷ 5 (VLDL)	f. Calculated using the formula CH − HDL − TG ÷ 5 (represents the VLDL)
Chylomicrons falsely ↓calculated LDL	(1) Chylomicrons falsely lower the calculated LDL by increasing diet-derived TG; therefore, fasting is required for an accurate calculated LDL.
Chylomicrons falsely ↑calculated VLDL	(2) Chylomicrons falsely increase the calculated VLDL (TG ÷ 5).
CH functions	g. Functions of CH

(1) Major component of the cell membrane

(2) Important in the synthesis of vitamin D, adrenal cortex hormones (e.g., cortisol), and bile salts and acids in the liver

h. Clinically important serum LDL levels

(1) Optimal level: <100 mg/dL (risk for coronary artery disease [CAD] is markedly reduced); near optimal level: 100–129 mg/dL; borderline high level: 130–159 mg/d; high level: 160–189 mg/dL; and very high level: >190 mg/dL increased serum LDL level—greatest risk factor for CAD)

i. Fasting is *not* required for measuring serum CH accurately. CH content in chylomicrons is <3%; therefore, fasting does *not* have a medically significant effect on the serum CH level. However, because other lipid components are measured or calculated, it is best to have a fasting level for all lipid studies.

Intensity of **treatment to lower cholesterol (CH)** is directly related to the degree of risk for coronary artery disease (CAD). Risk groups include high risk, moderately high risk, moderate risk, and low risk. The risk factors include age (male >45 years, female ≥55 years); family history of premature CAD (e.g., family member with myocardial infarction *before* 55 years of age); LDL > 160 mg/dL; current cigarette smoking; blood pressure ≥140/90 mm Hg (or on antihypertensive medicine); and HDL < 40 mg/dL (if ≥60 mg/dL, subtract 1 from the total).

---

8. High-density lipoprotein (HDL) (Fig. 10-2 B)

a. Often called the "good cholesterol" because it delivers CH to the liver and removes CH from atherosclerotic plaques

b. Composed of protein (50%), TG (3%; unless VLDL is increased), CH (20%), and phospholipid (27%)

c. Synthesized in the liver and small intestine

d. Functions of HDL

(1) Source of apoE and apoCII to attach to other lipoprotein fractions

(2) Removal of CH from fatty streaks and atherosclerotic plaques

(a) HDL delivers CH from peripheral tissue to the liver.

(b) In the liver, CH is either excreted into bile or converted into bile acids/salts.

e. Reverse CH transport and HDL metabolism

(1) Unesterified cholesterol (UCH) in peripheral cells can be transferred to HDL and esterified by lecithin-cholesterol acyltransferase (LCAT).

(2) Cholesterol ester in HDL is transferred to the liver directly through a scavenger receptor.

(3) Alternatively, cholesterol ester can be transferred to apoB-100–containing lipoproteins in exchange for TGs through the action of CETP.

f. Factors that increase HDL: nicotinic acid and exercise

(1) Nicotinic acid is the best lipid-lowering agent for increasing HDL.

(2) Dietary alterations are *not* effective for increasing HDL.

g. Laboratory measurement of HDL

(1) Reported as HDL-CH

(2) Increased HDL-CH is associated with a decreased risk for CAD.

(3) HDL-CH is decreased if VLDL is increased.

(4) Ranges of HDL-CH and their significance

(a) High level (optimal; >60 g/dL)

(b) Low level (suboptimal; <40 mg/dL)

B. **Lipoprotein disorders** (Table 10-1; Fig. 10-3; Links 10-4, 10-5, 10-6, and 10-7)

II. **Arteriosclerosis**

A. **Definition:** Thickening and loss of elasticity of arterial walls

B. **Medial calcification**

1. **Definition**: Dystrophic calcification in the wall of muscular arteries

• Visible in plain radiographs. Examples: calcification in uterine arteries and radial arteries

2. *No* clinical significance unless it is associated with atherosclerosis

C. **Atherosclerosis**

1. **Definition:** Result of endothelial injury to muscular and elastic arteries (sometimes veins) leading to the development of raised, yellow plaques that contain leukocytes, foam cells, smooth muscle cells, and necrotic debris

2. Epidemiology

Margin notes:

CH in cell membranes

CH synthesis vitamin D, cortisol, bile salts/acids

↑LDL greatest CAD risk factor

Fasting *not* required

HDL-CH "good CH"

HDL mainly protein

Synthesized liver/small intestine

Functions

Source apoE, apoCII

Remove CH from plaques

Delivers CH from peripheral tissue to liver

Liver: CH excreted in bile or converted bile salts/acids

Reverse CH transport/HDL metabolism

UCH transferred to HDL, esterified by LCAT

HDL-CH ester liver

↑HDL: nicotinic acid/exercise

Nicotinic acid best lipid-lowering agent to ↑HDL

Diet alterations not effective

Reported as HDL-CH

↑HDL-CH, ↓risk CAD

↓HDL-CH if ↑VLDL

Arteriosclerosis

Thickening arterial wall; loss elasticity

Medial calcification

Dystrophic calcification muscular arteries

Calcification uterine/radial arteries

No clinical significance *except* atherosclerosis

Endothelial injury: muscular/elastic arteries

Raised yellow plaques

TABLE 10-1   Lipoprotein Disorders

TYPE	COMMENTS
Type I	• **Familial chylomicronemia**: AR inheritance, childhood disease • **Pathogenesis:** deficiency of CLL or apoCII (normally activates CLL). Chylomicrons are primarily increased in early childhood. VLDL also increases later in life. • **Clinical findings:** presents with acute pancreatitis (chylomicrons block the circulation and cause rupture of pancreatic vessels) • **Laboratory findings in children:** increase in serum TG (>1,000 mg/dL; primarily chylomicrons); turbid supranate (chylomicrons) and a clear infranate with refrigeration (no VLDL). Serum CH levels are typically normal.

Type II	• **Type IIa hypercholesterolemia:** increase in serum CH (>260 mg/dL) and LDL (>190 mg/dL); serum TG < 300 mg/dL
	• **Type IIb hypercholesterolemia:** increase in serum CH (>260 mg/dL) and LDL (>190 mg/dL); serum TG > 300 mg/dL. Note that the increased TG distinguishes type IIb from type IIa hyperlipoproteinemia.
	• **Acquired causes**
	  • *Primary hypothyroidism:* decreased synthesis of LDL receptors
	  • *Blockage of bile flow:* bile contains CH
	  • *Nephrotic syndrome:* increased liver synthesis of CH
	• **Genetic causes**
	  • *Polygenic hypercholesterolemia* (type IIa): most common type (85% of cases); multifactorial (polygenic) inheritance; alteration in the regulation of LDL levels with a primary increase in serum LDL and serum TG < 300 mg/dL
	  • *Familial combined hypercholesterolemia* (type IIb): AD inheritance; CH and TG begin to increase around puberty; associated with metabolic syndrome (see Chapter 23); increase in CH and TG that is >300 mg/dL; decrease in HDL
	  • *Familial hypercholesterolemia* (type IIa): AD inheritance associated with a deficiency of LDL receptors
	• Achilles tendon xanthoma (diagnostic; Fig. 10-4 A; Link 10-4), xanthelasma (yellow plaques on the eyelid; Fig. 10-4 B; Link 10-5), and tuberous xanthomas (Link 10-6)
	• Increased incidence of premature CAD and atherosclerotic types of stroke; increased serum CH and LDL; serum TG < 300 mg/dL; decreased HDL

Type III	• **Familial dysbetalipoproteinemia "remnant disease"**: AR inheritance • **Pathogenesis:** deficiency of apolipoprotein E (apoE), resulting in decreased liver uptake of IDL and chylomicron remnants • **Clinical findings:** palmar xanthomas in flexor creases (Fig. 10-4 C); increased risk for CAD and peripheral vascular disease • **Laboratory findings:** serum CH and TG > 300 mg/dL; LDL < 190 mg/dL. Diagnosis is confirmed with ultracentrifugation to identify the remnants. Lipoprotein electrophoresis identifies the *apoE* gene defect.

Type IV	• **Familial hypertriglyceridemia:** AD inheritance (**most common hyperlipoproteinemia**)
	• **Pathogenesis:** Increased production (most common) or decreased clearance of VLDL
	• **Clinical findings:** increased risk for CAD and peripheral vascular disease; eruptive xanthomas (yellow, papular lesions; Fig. 10-4 D; Link 10-7)
	• **Laboratory findings:** increase in serum TG (>300 mg/dL). Serum CH normal to moderately increased (250–500 mg/dL); serum LDL < 190 mg/dL; decreased HDL (inverse relationship with the increase in VLDL); results in a turbid infranate after refrigeration overnight
	• **Acquired causes of type IV hyperlipoproteinemia:** more common than genetic causes
	  • *Excess alcohol intake:* most common acquired cause of type IV hyperlipoproteinemia; increased production of VLDL and decreased activity of CLL
	  • *Oral contraceptives:* estrogen increases synthesis of VLDL
	  • *Diabetes mellitus:* decreased adipose and muscle CLL, which decreases the clearance of VLDL. The decrease in insulin is responsible for the decreased synthesis of CLL. Serum LDL is increased. Serum HDL is decreased.
	  • *Chronic renal failure:* increased synthesis and decreased clearance of VLDL
	  • *Thiazide diuretics, β-blockers:* inhibit CLL, which decreases the VLDL clearance

Type V	• Most commonly due to familial hypertriglyceridemia plus an exacerbating disorder (e.g., diabetic ketoacidosis, alcoholism) • **Pathogenesis:** increase in chylomicrons and VLDL due to decreased activation and release of CLL • **Clinical findings:** hyperchylomicronemia syndrome, characterized by eruptive xanthomas (same as those in type IV), acute pancreatitis, and lipemia retinalis (the retinal vessels look like milk with associated blurry vision (Fig. 10-4 E). Dyspnea and hypoxemia (impaired gas exchange in the pulmonary capillaries) and hepatosplenomegaly are also noted. • **Laboratory findings:** increased serum TG (usually >1000 mg/dL); normal serum CH and LDL; turbid supranate (chylomicrons) and infranate (TG) after refrigeration

AD, Autosomal dominant; *AR,* autosomal recessive; *CH,* cholesterol; *CHD,* coronary heart disease; *CLL,* capillary lipoprotein lipase; *HDL,* high-density lipoprotein; *IDL,* intermediate-density lipoprotein; *LDL,* low-density lipoprotein; *TG,* triglyceride; *VLDL,* very-low-density lipoprotein.

↑Age; men/women equal

Blacks > whites

HTN: endothelial dysfunction

DM: hyperlipidemia, HTN

DM: coagulation/platelets; ↑oxidative stress, endothelial dysfunction

Smoking, hyperlipoproteinemia, *C. pneumoniae*

a. Prevalence increases with age and is equal in men and women. Blacks are at greater risk than whites.

b. Risk factors
   (1) Hypertension (HTN). Accelerates atherosclerosis by producing endothelial cell dysfunction.
   (2) Diabetes mellitus (DM). It is associated with hyperlipidemias and hypertension, which are risk factors for atherosclerosis. It is also associated with a variety of abnormalities involving coagulation, platelet adhesion and aggregation, oxidative stress, and endothelial dysfunction.
   (3) Additional risk factors include cigarette smoking, hyperlipoproteinemia, previous *Chlamydophila pneumoniae* infections (see Chapter 17).

3. Pathogenesis
   a. Atherosclerosis is the result of endothelial cell damage of muscular and elastic arteries. Veins under increased pressure (e.g., pulmonary venous HTN, saphenous veins used in coronary artery bypass [CAB]) may also undergo atherosclerosis.
   b. Causes of endothelial cell injury include stress areas in the vasculature (e.g., vessel bifurcations), HTN, smoking tobacco, homocysteine, oxidized LDL (free radical), small dense LDL (see previous text).
   c. Cell response to endothelial injury ("reaction to injury" theory) (Links 10-8 and 10-9)
      (1) Macrophages infiltrate the intima, and platelets adhere to damaged endothelium in muscular and elastic arteries.
         (a) Platelet products induce inflammatory responses in both leukocytes and endothelial cells (see Chapter 15).
         (b) Platelet-mediated inflammatory responses occur even with the widespread use of platelet-inhibiting drugs.
      (2) Inflammatory cells release cytokines and growth factors (e.g., platelet-derived growth factor [PDGF]), the latter causing hyperplasia of smooth muscle cells (SMCs).
      (3) SMCs migrate to the tunica intima. CH enters the smooth muscles and macrophages, producing foam cells. Grossly, these early lesions have the appearance of fatty streaks.
      (4) SMCs and macrophages release cytokines that produce extracellular matrix. Matrix components include collagen, proteoglycans, and elastin.
   d. Development of a fibrous plaque (cap) (Fig. 10-5 A)
      (1) Pathognomonic lesion of atherosclerosis
      (2) Components of an atherosclerotic plaque include fibrous plaque, SMCs, foam cells, inflammatory cells, calcium salts, and extracellular matrix.
      (3) Fibrous plaque overlies a necrotic center. Necrotic center consists of cellular debris, CH crystals (slit-like spaces), and foam cells (CH in SMCs and macrophages).
      (4) Disrupted (inflammatory) plaques may expose underlying necrotic material, which serves as a nidus for thrombus formation. The thrombus is composed predominantly of platelets held together by fibrin (Fig. 10-5 B; Link 10-10).

Endothelial cell damage muscular/elastic arteries

Veins under pressure: pulmonary venous HTN, saphenous veins CAB

Endothelial cell injury: HTN, smoking, homocysteine, oxidized/small dense LDL

"Reaction to injury"

Macrophages infiltrate, platelets adhere

Platelet products affect leukocytes/endothelial cells

PDGF hyperplasia SMCs

Foam cells: macrophages, SMCs with CH

Fatty streaks

SMCs/macrophages → cytokines → ↑extracellular matrix collagen/proteoglycans/elastin

Fibrous plaque (cap)

Pathognomonic lesion atherosclerosis

Fibrous plaque, SMCs, foam cells, inflammatory cells, calcium, extracellular matrix

Fibrous plaque overlies necrotic center

Cell debris, CH crystals, foam cells, macrophages

Disrupted inflammatory plaque nidus for platelet thrombus (platelets and fibrin)

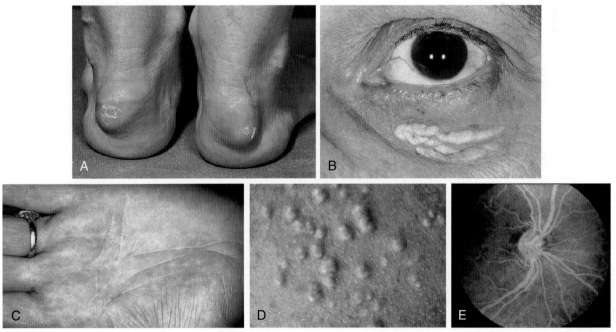

10-4: **A,** Achilles tendon xanthoma. Note the slightly yellow nodular lesions at the distal end of the Achilles tendon. **B,** Xanthelasma. Note the yellow, raised lesions on the lower left eyelid. **C,** Palmar xanthomas. Note the yellow macules on the palm that are accentuated in the creases. **D,** Eruptive xanthomas. Note the numerous small yellow papular lesions distributed over on the skin. **E,** Lipemia retinalis. Note the milk-like retinal vessels. (*A courtesy AF Lant, MD, and J Dequeker, MD, London; B from Yanoff M, Duker J:* Ophthalmology, *3rd ed, St. Louis, Mosby, 2009, Fig. 12-9-18; C courtesy RA Marsden, MD, St. George's Hospital, London; D, E from Melmed S, Polonsky KS, Larsen PR, Kronenberg HM:* Williams Textbook of Endocrinology, *12th ed, Saunders Elsevier, 2011, p 1651, Fig. 37-17 G, B, respectively.*)

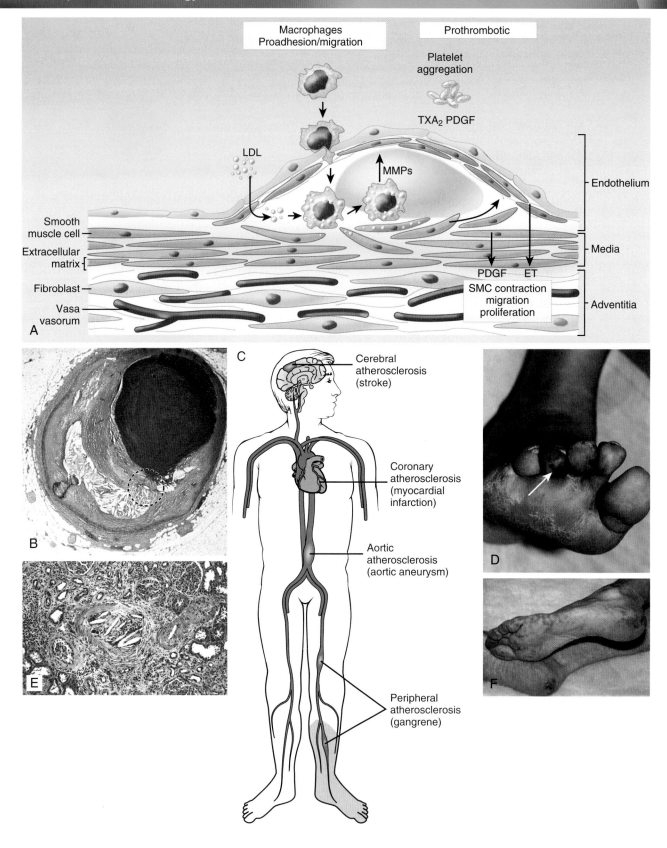

Serum C-reactive protein (CRP) is increased in patients with disrupted inflammatory plaques (see Chapter 3). Plaques may rupture and produce vessel thrombosis, which leads to an acute myocardial infarction. CRP may be a stronger predictor of cardiovascular events than LDL.

(5) Fibrous plaques frequently become dystrophically calcified (see Chapter 2) and ulcerated (complicated plaque).

4. Sites of atherosclerosis include (descending order of common locations) (Fig. 10-5 C)

   a. Abdominal aorta. Below L2 (level of renal arteries), the abdominal aorta lacks vasa vasorum and requires diffusion of nutrients from blood for its energy needs (Links 10-11 and 10-12).

   b. Coronary artery, popliteal artery, internal carotid artery

5. Complications of atherosclerosis

   a. Vessel weakness (e.g., vessel aneurysms; discussed later)

   b. Vessel thrombosis (platelet thrombus overlying disrupted atheromatous plaques; see Chapter 5)

     (1) Acute myocardial infarction (AMI; coronary artery) (see Chapter 11)

     (2) Stroke (internal carotid artery, middle cerebral artery) (see Chapter 26)

     (3) Small bowel infarction (superior mesenteric artery [SMA]) (see Chapter 18)

   c. HTN

     • Decreased renal blood flow secondary to atherosclerosis of the renal artery results in activation of the renin-angiotensin-aldosterone (RAA) system (discussed later), producing HTN (discussed later).

   d. Cerebral atrophy. Reduction of cerebral blood flood flow secondary to atherosclerosis can cause cerebral atrophy (see Chapter 26). Atherosclerosis may involve circle of Willis vessels and/or the internal carotid artery (see Chapter 26).

   e. Atherosclerotic embolization (Fig. 10-5 D–F).

   f. Peripheral vascular disease (PVD) (Link 10-13)

     (1) Risk factors: smoking, DM, HTN, hypercholesterolemia, increase in serum homocysteine (damages endothelial tissue), and increased alcohol

     (2) Clinical findings associated with PVD due to atherosclerosis

       (a) Claudication

         • **Definition**: Unilateral, gradual, and consistent cramping pain in the buttock, thigh, and calf that may be associated with weakness and numbness. It is due to decreased arterial blood flow to the affected leg. Pain is relieved by resting.

       (b) Ulcers in the lower leg/foot (Link 10-14) that heal slowly; danger for developing gangrene (dry and wet; see Fig. 2-16 D, F)

       (c) Dependent rubor (redness) of the foot

       (d) Cool skin temperature

       (e) Diminished hair and nail growth on the dorsum of the toes

Margin notes:

Serum CRP marker disrupted inflammatory plaques

Dystrophic calcification/ ulceration → complicated plaque

Abdominal aorta: MC site atherosclerosis; lacks vasa vasorum

↓Order: abdominal aorta; coronary, popliteal, internal carotid

Vessel weakness

Vessel thrombosis

AMI: coronary artery

Stroke: internal carotid artery, middle cerebral artery

Small bowel infarction: SMA

HTN (renal artery atherosclerosis): activation RAA system

Cerebral atrophy

Circle of Willis, internal carotid artery

Atherosclerotic embolization

Peripheral vascular disease

Smoking, DM, HTN, ↑CH, ↑homocysteine, ↑alcohol

Clinical findings PVD

Claudication: key sign PVD

Pain buttocks/thighs, calf; weakness/numbness; relieved by resting

Ulcers lower leg/foot; danger gangrene

Dependent rubor

Cool skin

↓Hair/nail growth distal toes

10-5: A, Early stages of formation of a fibrous plaque. Macrophages are entering the areas of endothelial disruption and are phagocytosing yellow lipid drops carried by low-density lipoprotein *(LDL)* to form foam cells. They release numerous cytokines including matrix metalloproteinases *(MMPs)*. Platelets release thromboxane A_2 *(TXA$_2$)* and platelet-derived growth factor *(PDGF)* as well as inflammatory cytokines that attract macrophages and produce endothelial cell dysfunction that are *not* shown in the schematic. Smooth muscle cells *(SMCs)* and macrophages endocytose LDL and form foam cells. SMCs also contract (endothelin *[ET]*), proliferate (undergo hyperplasia), and migrate beneath endothelial cells. The yellow material beneath the endothelium represents necrotic debris. In later stages, matrix components produce collagen, proteoglycans, and elastin forming the mature fibrous plaque, the primary lesion of atherosclerosis. **B,** Coronary artery thrombosis. In this specially stained cross-section of a coronary artery, collagen is blue and the thrombus is red. The red thrombus in the vessel lumen is composed of platelets held together by fibrin. Directly beneath the thrombus is a fibrous plaque (fibrous cap), which stains blue. Beneath the plaque is necrotic atheromatous debris. The circle shows disruption of the fibrous plaque with cholesterol crystals extending through the wall to the lumen. This is the area of injury that leads to the formation of a platelet thrombus. **C,** Major forms of atherosclerosis. **D,** Clinical presentation of atheromatous emboli, or blue toe syndrome *(arrow)*. **E,** Atheroemboli lodge in arterioles and smaller arteries of the kidneys (most common site for atheroemboli). Note the multiple cleft-shaped spaces, reflecting the empty space left after dissolution of the cholesterol by standard processing. **F,** Livedo reticularis on the lateral portion of the left foot and both heels. The second and fourth toes are cyanotic. These findings are typical of atheromatous embolization, and the fact that both feet are involved indicates a source above the aortic bifurcation. Also note the reticular (fishnet, lacy appearance) red lesion on the left foot. *(A modified from Goldman L, Ausiello D: Cecil's Medicine, 23rd ed, Philadelphia, Saunders Elsevier, 2008, p 473, Fig. 69-1 B; **B** from my friend Ivan Damjanov, MD, PhD, Linder J: Pathology: A Color Atlas, St. Louis, Mosby, 2000; **C** from my friend Ivan Damjanov, MD, PhD: Pathology for the Health Professions, 4th ed, Saunders Elsevier, 2012; **D** from Marx JA, Hockberger RS, Walls RM: Rosen's Emergency Medicine Concepts and Clinical Practice, 8th ed, Saunders Elsevier, 2014, p 1144, Fig. 87-2; courtesy Gary R. Seabrook, MD; **E** from Fogo AB, Kashgarian M: Diagnostic Atlas of Renal Pathology, 2nd ed, Elsevier, 2012, p 370, Fig. 2.100; **F** from Bartholomew JR, Olin JW: Atheromatous embolization. In Young JR, Olin JW, Bartholomew JR, eds: Peripheral Vascular Diseases, 2nd ed, St. Louis, Mosby, 1996.)*

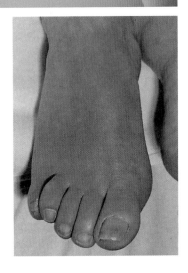

10-6: Patient with previous intermittent claudication from atheromatous peripheral arterial occlusive disease now has a history of sudden onset of pain in the foot along with coldness and loss of sensation due to acute peripheral artery occlusion. The foot is cyanotic. Note the absence of hair on the dorsum of the toes. The toenails are thick (dystrophic nails). *(From Forbes CD, Jackson WF: Color Atlas and Text of Clinical Medicine, 3rd ed, Mosby, 2003, p 240, Fig. 5.151.)*

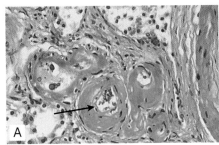 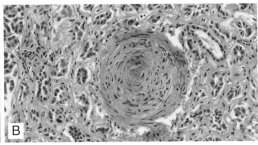

10-7: **A,** Hyaline arteriolosclerosis. The arrow depicts eosinophilic material representing protein that has leaked through the basement membrane and deposited in the wall of an arteriole. Other neighboring arterioles demonstrate similar changes. Diabetes mellitus and hypertension are the most common causes. **B,** Hyperplastic arteriolosclerosis. Hyperplastic arteriolosclerosis of an arteriole in the kidney in malignant hypertension due to systemic sclerosis. *(A from my friend Ivan Damjanov, MD, PhD, Linder J: Pathology: A Color Atlas. St. Louis, Mosby, 2000, p 32, Fig. 2-1 A; B from Ellison D, Love S, et al: Neuropathology: A Reference Text of CNS Pathology, 3rd ed, Mosby Elsevier, 2013, p 250, Fig. 10.33 d.)*

↓Pedal pulses, bruits femoral/popliteal arteries

Pain

Pallor

Paresthesias

Paralysis

Pulselessness

Collapsed superficial veins/ cold skin

Resting ABI ratio, angiography, duplex US

Arteriolosclerosis: arteriole occlusion

Hyaline/hyperplastic types

Hyaline arteriolosclerosis

Arteriole occlusion by protein in vessel wall

    (f) Diminished pedal pulses, bruits over the femoral and/or popliteal arteries (harsh sound heard with the microscope due to blood flowing through a narrow opening)

    (g) Acute peripheral artery vessel occlusion: the five *P*s
- Pain: shooting pain that is followed by numbness and weakness
- Pallor: pale color that progresses to a mottled cyanosis (Fig. 10-6)
- Paresthesias (tingling numbness): portends serious consequences if it progresses rapidly
- Paralysis: weakness of dorsiflexion of the foot or toe in the peroneal nerve distribution (anterolateral aspect of the leg and dorsum of the foot)
- Pulselessness: absent pulse below the area of occlusion
- Also, collapsed superficial veins and cold skin

(3) Diagnostic techniques for detecting peripheral arterial disease due to atherosclerosis
    (a) Measurement of the resting ankle-brachial index (ABI ratio <0.9 is consistent with PVD)
    (b) Angiography, duplex ultrasonography (US)

D. Arteriolosclerosis
1. **Definition:** Pathologic processes that result in arteriole occlusion
- Two types: hyaline arteriolosclerosis and hyperplastic arteriolosclerosis
2. Hyaline arteriolosclerosis
    a. **Definition:** Arteriole occlusion that is caused by increased protein deposition within the vessel wall
    b. Pathogenesis
        (1) Increased protein is deposited in the vessel wall and occludes the arteriole lumen (Fig. 10-7 A; Link 10-15).
        (2) Causes of hyaline arteriolosclerosis
            (a) In poorly controlled diabetes mellitus, glucose combines with proteins in the basement membrane of arterioles, a process called nonenzymatic glycosylation

(NEG) (see Chapter 23). NEG causes the basement membrane to leak proteins from the plasma into the vessel wall (pink-staining material on H&E stain).

  (b) HTN. Increased luminal pressure in arterioles pushes plasma proteins into the vessel wall.

 (3) Hyaline arteriolosclerosis causes increased rigidity, which limits the capacity for expansion and constriction of the vessel and also reduces the luminal size and blood flow through the vessel, leading to tissue ischemia. Ischemia leads to atrophy of tissue.

3. Hyperplastic arteriolosclerosis
 a. **Definition:** Arteriole occlusion due to basement membrane duplication and SMC hyperplasia as a reaction to a rapid increase in blood pressure (BP).
 b. Commonly seen in the afferent and efferent arterioles of the kidneys in patients with severe HTN (malignant HTN; e.g., systemic sclerosis). Malignant HTN is accompanied by renal failure and cerebral edema.
 c. Renal arterioles have an "onion skin" appearance (Fig. 10-7 B).

III. Vessel Aneurysms
 A. Definition: Dilation of a vessel wall due to increased wall stress; "vessel weakening plus outpouching" (Link 10-16)
  1. True aneurysm involves all layers from intima to the adventitia.
  2. In an aortic dissection, blood enters the media of the vessel and "splits" the aortic wall under pressure and dilates the aorta only in the area where the dissection is present. This is a *false aneurysm*.
 B. Abdominal aortic aneurysm (AAA)
  1. **Definition:** Result of weakening of the wall of the abdominal aorta, leading to localized dilation of the aorta from increased wall stress
  2. Epidemiology
   a. Most common vessel aneurysm
   b. Usually occurs in men >60 years old (4:1 male/female ratio)
   c. Tenth leading cause of death in men >65 years old
   d. Usually located *below* the renal artery orifices (*no* vasa vasorum in abdominal aorta; see following)
  3. Pathogenesis
   a. Atherosclerosis of the aorta weakens the vessel wall.
    (1) Vessel wall stress increases with increase in vessel diameter (law of Laplace).
    (2) Vessel lumen fills with atheromatous debris and blood clots (Fig. 10-8 A).
   b. Other factors that contribute to an increased risk of developing an AAA include family history (e.g., connective tissue defects) and the absence of vasa vasorum in the abdominal aorta (vessel that supplies the blood vessel). *No* vasa vasorum is present in the aorta *below* the orifices of the renal arteries. This renders the aorta susceptible to endothelial injury and atherosclerosis with eventual weakening of the vessel.
  4. Clinical findings
   a. Usually asymptomatic
   b. Physical exam findings
    (1) Pulsatile epigastric mass (may or may not be tender). There is a risk of rupture if palpated, so it is much safer to perform an ultrasound if an AAA is suspected. In very thin individuals, the abdominal wall will frequently show visible pulsations, giving a false impression of an AAA.
    (2) A bruit (harsh sound) may be auscultated if renal artery stenosis and/or arterial stenosis involving the orifices of the mesenteric arteries are present along with the AAA.
   c. Portions of the atherosclerotic plaques may break off the aneurysm and embolize to the distal extremities (Fig. 10-5 D, E). This may produce the "blue toe syndrome" from decreased blood flow and cyanosis of the overlying tissue.
   d. Rupture is the most common complication of an AAA.
    (1) *Rupture triad* is the sudden onset of severe left flank pain (bleed is initially retroperitoneal), followed by hypotension from blood loss into the retroperitoneum and the presence of a pulsatile mass on physical examination.
    (2) Greatest predictor of rupture is the diameter of the aneurysm. Surgeons have criteria for when to treat AAAs that are *not* symptomatic. Endovascular repair is the usual treatment rather than surgical removal of the aneurysm.
  5. Diagnosis

Hyaline arteriolosclerosis: DM

NEG: glucose + proteins in basement membrane arterioles

Leaky basement membranes permeable to plasma protein

HTN: Hyaline arteriolosclerosis

HTN: ↑intraluminal pressure

Hyaline arteriolosclerosis causes: DM, HTN

Hyaline arteriolosclerosis: vessel rigidity, ↓luminal size → ↓blood flow → tissue atrophy

Hyperplastic arteriolosclerosis: Rapid ↑BP → basement membrane duplication → SMC hyperplasia

Hyperplastic arteriolosclerosis: involves afferent/efferent arterioles; malignant HTN

Malignant HTN: renal failure, cerebral edema

Malignant HTN: "onion skinning" renal arterioles

Vessel aneurysms

↑Wall stress → "weakening + outpouching" → aneurysm

True all layers: intima to adventia

Aortic dissection: blood enters media; false aneurysm

AAA: weakening wall → localized dilation from ↑wall stress

AAA MC vessel aneurysm

Men >60 yrs; male dominant

Below renal artery orifices: *no* vasa vasorum in abdominal aorta

Atherosclerosis weakens wall → ↑wall stress with ↑vessel diameter

Lumen: atheromatous debris/blood clots

Risk for AAA: *no* vasa vasorum below orifices of renal arteries

Usually asymptomatic

Pulsatile epigastric mass (below xiphoid bone)

Bruit: renal artery and/or mesenteric artery stenosis

Blue toe syndrome from embolization

Rupture MC complication

Rupture triad: left flank pain, hypotension, pulsatile mass

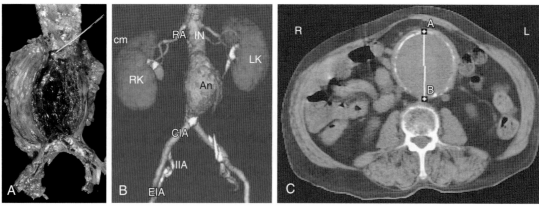

10-8: **A,** Abdominal aortic aneurysm (AAA). The aneurysmal dilation of the aorta is just above the bifurcation of the aorta. The probe is located at the rupture site. The lumen is filled with atherosclerotic debris and clot material. Ulcerated atheromatous plaques are proximal and distal to the aneurysm. The common iliac arteries have extensive atherosclerosis as well. It is likely that this patient had signs and symptoms of peripheral vascular disease. **B,** AAA (three-dimensional computed tomography [CT] image). Note the aneurysm *(An)* below the renal artery *(RA)*. **C,** CT showing an AAA. *A* and *B* show the size of the aneurysm. *CIA,* Common iliac artery; *EIA,* external iliac artery; *IIA,* internal iliac artery; *IN,* intrarenal neck; *LK,* left kidney; *RK,* right kidney. (**A** *from Kumar V, Fausto N, Abbas A:* Robbins and Cotran Pathologic Basis of Disease, *7th ed, Philadelphia, Saunders, 2004, p 531, Fig. 11-19 B;* **B** *from Ferri FF:* 2016 Ferri's Clinical Advisor, *Elsevier, 2016, p 5, Fig. A1-3; from* Sabiston Textbook of Surgery, *ed 17, Philadelphia, 2004, Saunders;* **C** *from Forbes CD, Jackson WF:* Color Atlas and Text of Clinical Medicine, *3rd ed, Mosby, 2003 p 246, Fig. 5.173.)*

Ultrasound best initial screen	a. Ultrasound is 100% accurate (excellent initial screen).
	b. Computed tomography (CT) scan is used preoperatively to localize extent into renal vessels and evaluate the integrity of the vessel wall to exclude rupture (Fig. 10-8 B, C). Angiography gives detailed arterial anatomy.
CT, angiography	**C. Popliteal artery aneurysm**
Popliteal artery aneurysm	1. Predominantly in males (>95% of cases)
Male dominant	2. Most common peripheral artery aneurysm; presents as a pulsatile mass behind the knee
MC peripheral artery aneurysm	**D. Mycotic aneurysm**
Pulsatile mass behind knee	1. **Definition:** Aneurysm that is secondary to weakening of the vessel wall due to an infection (fungal or bacterial)
Mycotic aneurysm	2. Epidemiology
Aneurysm fungal/bacterial; weakening vessel wall	a. Fungi that commonly invade vessels and weaken them include *Aspergillus, Candida,* and *Mucor.*
Aspergillus, Candida, Mucor	b. Bacteria that invade vessels and weaken them include *Bacteroides fragilis, Pseudomonas aeruginosa,* and *Salmonella* species.
B. fragilis, P. aeruginosa, Salmonella spp.	3. Clinical findings include thrombosis with or without infarction, rupture.
Thrombosis, rupture	**E. Berry (saccular) aneurysm of cerebral arteries** (see Chapter 26)
Berry aneurysm cerebral arteries	1. **Definition:** Saccular dilatation of a cerebral artery that is typically located at the base of the brain around the circle of Willis
Saccular dilatation; base brain around circle of Willis	2. Epidemiology
Circle of Willis, base brain	a. Risk factors
Normal stress	(1) Normal hemodynamic stress
HTN	(2) Presence of HTN of any cause
	(3) Coarctation of the aorta
Coarctation aorta; constriction Ao below arch vessels	• **Definition:** Constriction of the aorta (Ao) that is usually located *below* the arch vessels, which increases the arterial pressure proximal to the constriction, including the arch vessels, the aortic valve, and the left ventricle (see Chapter 11)
Atherosclerosis	(4) Atherosclerosis
MC site berry aneurysm: junction communicating branch with anterior cerebral artery	b. Most common site of a berry aneurysm is at the junction of the communicating branches with the anterior cerebral artery (see Fig. 26-12 A).
	3. Pathogenesis
Lack internal elastic lamina/ smooth muscle	a. At the junction of the communicating branches with the main cerebral vessels, the vessel normally lacks an internal elastic lamina and smooth muscle.
Blood subarachnoid space/ brain	b. Rupture of the aneurysm releases blood into the subarachnoid space and/or into the brain parenchyma (see Fig. 26-12 B).
	4. Clinical findings of a ruptured berry aneurysm
"Worst headache I've ever had"	a. Sudden onset of severe occipital headache that is described as the "worst headache I've ever had"
Severe nuchal pain	b. Severe nuchal (neck) rigidity from irritation of the meninges

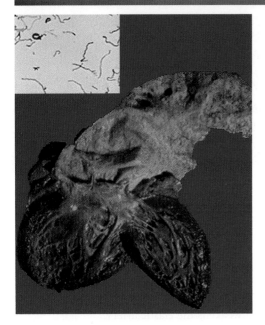

10-9: Syphilitic aortitis. Note the dilated aortic valve root and the irregular intimal wrinkling ("tree barking") due to scarring in the wall of the aorta from inflammation and repair of the vasa vasorum. The inset shows a silver stain with spirochetes. *(From Klatt F:* Robbins and Cotran Atlas of Pathology, *Philadelphia, Saunders, 2006, p 9, Figs. 1-22 [gross picture], 1-24 [inset].)*

    5. Complications of a ruptured berry aneurysm
      a. Death may occur shortly after the bleed.
      b. Rebleeding. This may produce hydrocephalus from blockage of foramina in the ventricles by blood.
      c. Severe neurologic deficits
    6. Diagnosis is made using a CT scan and angiography (definitive test).
F. Syphilitic aneurysm
    1. **Definition:** Complication of tertiary syphilis due to the spirochete *Treponema pallidum*
    2. Epidemiology
      a. Men 40 to 55 years of age
      b. Pathogenesis
        (1) *Treponema pallidum* infects the vasa vasorum of the ascending and transverse portions of aortic arch (Fig. 10-9).
        (2) Vasculitis is called endarteritis obliterans.
        (3) Histologic sections of the aneurysm shows a plasma cell infiltrate in the vessel wall. Plasma cell infiltrates are characteristic in all three stages of syphilis (primary, secondary, and tertiary).
        (4) Inflammation is intense and often occludes the lumen of the vessel, causing reduced blood flow to the aorta.
      c. Vessel ischemia of the medial tissue leads to weakness and subsequent dilation of the aorta and aortic valve (AV) ring.
      d. Involved areas of the aorta show irregular intimal wrinkling ("tree barking") due to scarring in the wall of the aorta from inflammation and repair of the vasa vasorum.
    3. Clinical findings
      a. AV regurgitation (see shaded area).

Aortic valve regurgitation is a problem in closing the aortic valve. Because the aortic valve closes in diastole, the murmur occurs in early diastole as blood leaks back into the ventricle. The increase in left ventricular end-diastolic volume results in an increase in stroke volume (increased systolic pressure). Blood rapidly draining back into the left ventricle decreases the diastolic pressure and also produces an early diastolic heart murmur right after the second heart sound (discussed in Chapter 11). An increase in the systolic pressure along with a decrease in the diastolic blood pressure produces a wide pulse pressure (difference between the systolic and diastolic pressure). This is clinically manifested by a hyperdynamic circulation (e.g., pulsating uvula, bounding pulses, visible pulsations beneath the finger nail beds). Excessive blood flowing back onto the anterior mitral valve leaflet produces another diastolic murmur called the Austin Flint murmur (discussed in Chapter 11). The presence of an Austin Flint murmur indicates the need for an aortic valve replacement.

---

      b. Brassy cough. Left recurrent laryngeal nerve is stretched by the aneurysm.
    4. Linear calcifications (dystrophic calcification) are usually seen in the aortic wall on a plain radiograph. The definitive diagnosis of a syphilitic aneurysm is made by aortography.

Margin notes:

Death

Rebleeding, hydrocephalus

Severe neurologic deficits

CT, angiography

Syphilitic aneurysm

Complication tertiary syphilis; *Treponema pallidum* (spirochete)

Male dominant

Infects vasa vasorum ascending/transverse aortic arch

Vasculitis called endarteritis obliterans

Plasma cell vasculitis

Plasma cell key inflammatory cell all stages syphilis

Inflammation occludes vasa vasorum

Weakness aortic wall → dilation aorta → dilation AV ring

"Tree barking" appearance; scarring of aorta

AV regurgitation; dilation aorta/valve ring

AV regurgitation: early diastolic murmur; wide pulse pressure; bounding pulses;

Austin Flint murmur

Brassy cough; stretching left recurrent laryngeal nerve

Linear calcifications aortic wall; aortography

Aortic dissection

Intimal tear with dissection blood in media of aorta

Male dominant; history HTN

MCC death Marfan syndrome/EDS

G. Aortic dissection

1. **Definition:** Blood under pressure enters an intimal tear and dissects proximally and/or distally through the elastic tissue in the media of the aorta
2. Epidemiology
   a. Most often occurs in men (3:1 male/female ratio) with a mean age of 40 to 60 years and a history of antecedent HTN
   b. May also occur in young people with an underlying connective tissue disorder (e.g., Marfan syndrome or Ehlers-Danlos syndrome (EDS) (see Chapter 3)

Marfan syndrome (Links 10-17, 10-18, 10-19, and 10-20) is an autosomal dominant disorder resulting in the production of weak elastic tissue due to a defect in fibrillin synthesis (missense mutation). Cardiovascular abnormalities dominate. Dilation of the ascending aorta may progress to aortic dissection and/or AV regurgitation. Mitral valve prolapse (discussed later) is the most common valvular defect and is often associated with conduction defects causing sudden death. Skeletal defects include hypermobile joints, eunuchoid proportions (lower body length > upper body length, arm span > height), and arachnodactyly (spider hands; Fig. 10-10 A). Dislocation of the lens is another finding, because the suspensory ligament holding the lens is composed of elastic tissue.

Aortic dissection, missense mutation in fibrillin synthesis; arachnodactyly, dislocated lens, mitral valve prolapse, AV regurgitation, eunuchoid

Cystic medial degeneration

Elastic tissue fragmentation; weakens media elastic artery

Degraded matrix material

↑Wall stress; HTN, pregnancy, coarctation

Defects connective tissue: Marfan (elastic tissue), EDS (collagen)

Intimal tear in aorta

Tear: HTN, structural weakness

Tear 10 cm from AV

Blood dissects under pressure

Blood dissects proximal and/or distal

Pain radiates into back; absent pulse

AMI pain radiates down inner arms

AV ring dilation → AV regurgitation

Radiograph/echocardiogram widening AV root

Axial CT shows false/true lumen

Loss upper extremity pulse: compression subclavian artery

Cardiac tamponade MCC death

Venous system

Saphenous vein system

Superficial saphenous veins → perforators → deep veins

Perforator branch valves prevent reversal blood

Deep veins → back to right heart

Varicose veins

Abnormally distended veins

Superficial saphenous veins MC site

Distal esophagus: portal HTN

3. Pathogenesis
   a. Cystic medial degeneration
      (1) Elastic tissue fragmentation in the media weakens the elastic artery.
      (2) Degraded matrix material collects in areas of fragmentation in the media.
   b. Risk factors for cystic medial degeneration
      (1) Increased wall stress: causes include HTN, pregnancy (increased plasma volume), and coarctation of the aorta.
      (2) Defects in connective tissue; diseases include Marfan syndrome (defect in elastic tissue) and EDS (defect in collagen).
   c. Intimal tear in the aorta
      (1) Tear is due to HTN or underlying structural weakness in the media.
      (2) Usually occurs within 10 cm of the AV (Fig. 10-10 B)
      (3) Blood dissects under arterial pressure through the areas of weakness in the media of the aorta.
      (4) Blood dissects proximally and/or distally (Fig. 10-10 C, D).
4. Clinical findings of cystic medial degeneration
   a. Acute onset of severe retrosternal chest pain radiating to the back
      (1) Dissections peak between 0800 and 1100 and decline from 1100 to 1800.
      (2) AMI, pain usually radiates down the inner arms (see Chapter 11).
   b. AV regurgitation
      (1) Due to AV ring dilation
      (2) Radiograph or echocardiogram shows widening of the aortic valve root (Fig. 10-10 E).
   c. Axial CT shows true and false lumen of dissection (Fig. 10-10 F).
   d. Loss of the upper extremity pulse is due to compression of subclavian artery by blood in the false lumen.
   e. Rupture sites include the pericardial sac (most common site; cardiac tamponade), thoracic cavity, and internal rupture (within the wall of the aorta), with blood tracking back into the lumen by rupturing through the inner media and intima to produce a double-channeled aorta (rare complication).

IV. Venous System Disorders
A. Saphenous venous system
1. Superficial saphenous veins drain blood into the deep veins via the perforating branches.
2. Valves in the perforator branches prevent the reversal of blood flow into the superficial system.
3. Deep veins direct blood back to the heart.
B. Varicose veins
1. **Definition:** Abnormally distended (>3 mm) and often tortuous veins that arise underneath the skin or mucosal surface
2. Epidemiology
   a. Locations
      (1) Superficial saphenous veins (most common site)
      (2) Distal esophagus (due to portal HTN) (see Chapter 18)

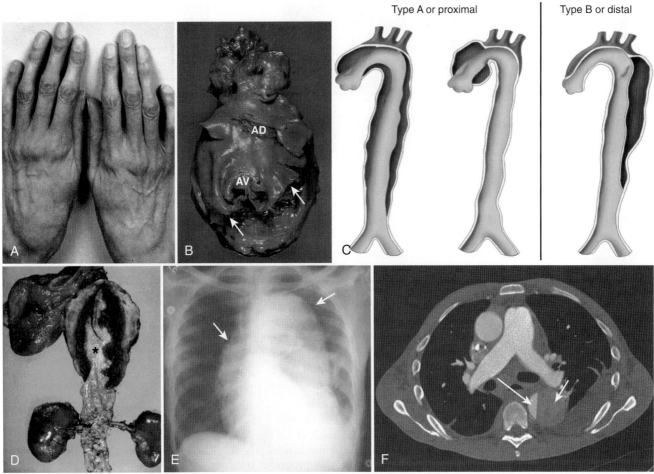

Type A or proximal

Type B or distal

10-10: **A,** Marfan syndrome. Note the arachnodactyly ("spider" fingers) in both hands. **B,** Aortic dissection. The aortic valve (AV) is depicted. A large, irregular tear in the intima (AD) of the aorta shows clot material in the false lumen beneath the surface. The white arrows show blood in the false lumen that is proximal to the tear, indicating that it probably emptied into the pericardial sac, producing cardiac tamponade as the cause of death. **C,** Type A (proximal) and type B (distal) aortic dissection. Note that the proximal type can be limited to the arch or involve the arch and distal aorta, whereas type B (distal) spares the proximal aorta and primarily involves the distal aorta. **D,** Aortic dissection showing blood in the false lumen of the aorta distal to the heart. The true lumen of the aorta is marked with a black asterisk. **E,** Radiograph of an aortic dissection. The white arrows show widening of the aortic valve root. **F,** Axial computed tomography angiography of an aortic dissection. The long arrow indicates the location of the true lumen, and the short arrow indicates the false lumen. (*A from Doherty M, George E: Self-Assessment Picture Tests in Medicine: Rheumatology, London, Mosby-Wolfe, 1995, p 40, Fig. 60 B; B from Grieg JD, Garden JO: Color Atlas of Surgical Diagnosis, London, Mosby-Wolfe, 1996, p 102, Fig. 75-4; C from Braunwald E, Zipes DP, Libby P, Bonow RO, eds: Braunwald's Heart Disease: A Textbook of Cardiovascular Medicine, 7th ed, Philadelphia, Saunders, 2004, p 1416; D from my friend Ivan Damjanov, MD, PhD, Linder J: Anderson's Pathology, 10th ed, St. Louis, Mosby, 1996, p 1411, Fig. 47-12; E from Herring W: Learning Radiology: Recognizing the Basics, St. Louis, Mosby Elsevier, 2007, Fig. 13-11; F from Pretorius ES, Solomon JA: Radiology Secrets Plus, 3rd ed, Philadelphia, Mosby Elsevier, 2011, p 66, Fig. 10.3 A.)*

(3) Anorectal region (e.g., internal hemorrhoids) (see Chapter 18)

(4) Left scrotal sac (e.g., varicocele) (see Chapter 21)

b. Superficial varicosities in the lower extremities

(1) Most common clinical manifestation of chronic venous insufficiency

(2) Risk factors: female gender, family history of varicose veins, multiple pregnancies, jobs with prolonged standing, obesity, and advanced age

(3) Pathogenesis

(a) Varicose veins occur secondary to valve incompetence of the perforator branches. This allows retrograde blood flow from the high-pressure deep venous system into the superficial system (Fig. 10-11 A, B; Link 10-21).

(b) Varicose veins may be secondary to deep venous thrombosis (DVT) (Fig. 10-11 C). Increased pressure in the deep veins causes retrograde blood flow through the perforating branches into the superficial system. Increased pressure in the superficial venous systems produces dilation of the vessels and superficial varicosities.

Anorectal: internal hemorrhoids

Left scrotal sac: varicocele

Superficial varices lower extremity

MC clinical manifestation of chronic venous insufficiency

Female, family history

↑Standing, obesity, older adults

Defective perforator branches

Varicose veins 2nd to DVT

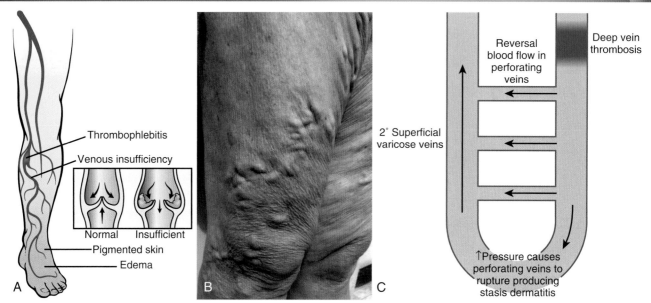

10-11: A, Varicose veins of the calf. The inset shows venous valvular insufficiency, which accounts for the reflux of blood and the serpiginous dilation of the veins. Complications are also depicted, including thrombophlebitis (inflammation of the vein), pigmented skin from rupture of perforating branches around the malleolus (called stasis dermatitis), and edema due to increased hydrostatic pressure in the venous system. **B,** Note the marked bilateral superficial varicosities on the lower extremity. The veins in the thighs are distended and tortuous. **C,** Secondary superficial varicose veins from a deep vein thrombosis. Increased pressure behind the thrombus reverses blood flow through the perforating branches (damages the valves) and increases pressure in the superficial vessels, causing dilation. Increased pressure around the medial malleolus of the ankles ruptures the vessels and causes stasis dermatitis. (*A from my friend Ivan Damjanov, MD, PhD: Pathology for the Health Professions, 4th ed, Saunders Elsevier, 2012, p 158, Fig. 7-32; B from Swartz MH: Textbook of Physical Diagnosis: History and Examination, 7th ed, Saunders Elsevier, 2014, p 397, Fig. 12-7.)*

Venous thromboses

Thrombus: fibrin entrapped RBCs, WBCs, platelets

MCC stasis blood flow; hypercoagulability

Locations

MC deep veins lower extremity

Veins in calf, popliteal/femoral veins

Less common: portal vein, hepatic vein, dural sinuses

DVT calf

Acute signs

Swelling

Pain (dorsiflexion/compression)

Pitting edema distal to thrombus (↑HP)

Chronic signs DVT

Stasis dermatitis

Hemorrhage/orange; ulcers; medial malleolus

Causes: DVT MCC, trauma, pregnancy

CDVI → rupture malleolus perforators

CDVI → reversal venous blood flow → rupture perforating branches

Secondary varicosities

C. Venous thromboses (see Chapter 5)
   1. **Definition:** Contains entrapped red blood cells (RBCs; primary component), white blood cells (WBCs), and platelets held together by fibrin
   2. Causes include stasis blood flow (MCC; e.g., prolonged immobilization [≥3 days], postoperative state) and hypercoagulability (e.g., antithrombin deficiency, oral contraceptives; pancreatic cancer, factor V deficiency, protein C and S deficiencies; see Chapter 15).
   3. Locations
      a. Most often occur in the deep veins of the lower extremity (e.g., veins in the calf [anterior, posterior, peroneal veins; calf venous sinusoids]; popliteal vein; and the femoral vein)
      b. Less common sites include the portal vein, hepatic vein, and dural sinuses in the brain.
   4. DVT in the calf (see Chapter 5)
      a. Acute signs of DVT
         (1) Swelling of the affected leg relative to the other leg (>3 cm in circumference; Fig. 10-12 A)
         (2) Pain on dorsiflexion of the foot (Homans sign) and compression of the calf.
         (3) Pitting edema distal to the thrombosis due to increased hydrostatic pressure (HP).
      b. Chronic signs of DVT in the lower leg include stasis dermatitis and secondary varicose veins.
         (1) Stasis dermatitis (Fig. 10-12 B; Link 10-22)
            (a) **Definition:** Hemorrhagic or orange discoloration of the skin associated with ischemic ulcers (poor oxygen perfusion). It is located around the medial malleolus of the ankle. The orange discoloration is due to hemosiderin deposited in the skin from ruptured blood vessels.
            (b) Causes of stasis dermatitis include DVT (most common), trauma, or pregnancy (increased venous pressure in the legs).
            (c) Pathogenesis. Chronic deep vein insufficiency (CDVI) produces reversal of the venous blood flow in the leg and increased venous pressure that ruptures the perforating branches around the malleolus. Blood in the tissue degrades into hemosiderin and ischemia produces ulceration of the skin (Fig. 10-12 C).
         (2) Secondary varicosities may also develop in the superficial venous system (see Fig. 10-11 C).

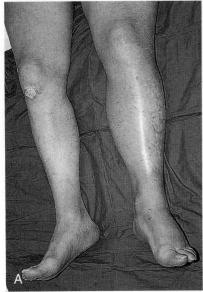
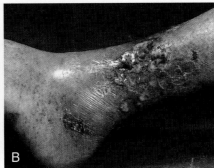
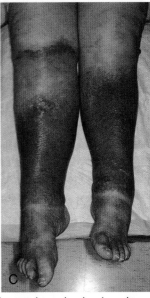

10-12: A, Deep vein thrombosis presenting as an acutely swollen left leg. The leg was hot to the touch, and palpation along the line of the left popliteal and femoral veins caused pain. Note the coincidental psoriatic lesion below the patient's right knee. **B,** Stasis dermatitis. Note the red discoloration of the skin and punctate areas of hemorrhage from ruptured perforator branches around the malleolus. There is an extensive area of ulceration above the malleolus with a yellow exudate covering the surface. Over time, the areas of hemorrhage will turn orange-brown as hemosiderin accumulates in the subcutaneous tissue. **C,** Chronic venous insufficiency. Note the marked discoloration of the skin from stagnation of venous blood and swelling (pitting edema) in the lower extremities due to increased hydrostatic pressure in the venous system. *(**A** from Goldman L, Schafer A:* Goldman's Cecil Medicine, *Saunders Elsevier, 2012, p 505, Fig. 81-6; from Forbes CD, Jackson WF:* Color Atlas and Text of Clinical Medicine, *3rd ed, London, Mosby, 2003;* **B** *from Bouloux P:* Self-Assessment Picture Tests Medicine, *Vol 1, London, Mosby-Wolfe, 1997, p 9, Fig. 195;* **C** *from Swartz MH:* Textbook of Physical Diagnosis: History and Examination, *7th ed, Saunders Elsevier, 2014, p 396, Fig. 12-5.)*

   c. Diagnosis (Dx) of DVT is confirmed by using venous duplex US (95% sensitivity/specificity) plus a serum D-dimer assay (88%–97% sensitivity; see Chapter 15). D-Dimers are a sign that the fibrinolytic system is active in breaking down fibrin in the clot.

   d. Serum D-dimer assays are also useful in predicting the recurrence of a DVT after withdrawal of anticoagulation (<250 mg/mL, low risk for recurrence; >250 mg/dL, high risk for recurrence).

D. Superficial thrombophlebitis

  1. **Definition:** Acute inflammation of a superficial vein

  2. Epidemiology

    a. 10% to 20% are associated with an occult DVT.

    b. Pathogenesis

      (1) Intravenous cannulation of a vein most commonly associated with plastic catheters that are inserted into veins in the lower extremities

      (2) Infection (*Staphylococcus aureus* in 65%–78% of cases)

      (3) Carcinoma of the head of the pancreas. Pancreatic cancers produce superficial migratory thrombophlebitis (Trousseau sign), due to the release of procoagulants by the cancer.

      (4) Hypercoagulable state (see Chapter 15)

  3. Clinical findings

    a. Pain and tenderness to palpation along the course of the inflamed superficial vein

    b. Erythema and edema of the overlying skin and subcutaneous tissue

E. Superior vena cava (SVC) syndrome

  1. **Definition:** Clinical findings that are associated with external compression of the SVC

  2. Pathogenesis. Most often caused by external compression of the SVC by a primary lung cancer (90% of cases); most common type is small cell carcinoma (SCC).

  3. Clinical findings

    a. "Puffiness" and blue to purple discoloration of the face, arms, and shoulders (see Fig. 17-19 B)

    b. Retinal hemorrhage, stroke

Dx DVT: duplex US + D-dimer assay

D-Dimers sign fibrinolytic activity

D-Dimers: useful in predicting recurrence DVT

Superficial thrombophlebitis

Acute inflammation superficial vein

Occult DVT may be present

IV catheters lower extremities MCC

Infection: *S. aureus* MCC

Ca head pancreas

Hypercoagulable state

Pain, tenderness

Erythema/edema of overlying skin/subcutaneous tissue

SVC syndrome

External compression SVC

MCC compression 1° lung cancer; usually SCC

Discoloration/puffiness face, arms, shoulders

Retinal hemorrhages; stroke

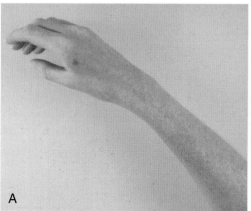 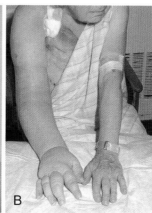 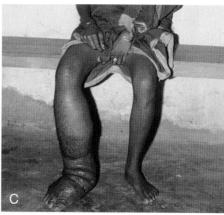

10-13: **A,** At the base of the index finger is an ulceration from the bite of a brown recluse spider (see Chapter 7). Redness of the skin extends around the bite and down the lymphatics on the medial side of the wrist and forearm. **B,** Lymphedema. Note the swelling of the entire right arm. The patient had a modified radical mastectomy followed by radiation. **C,** Elephantiasis (lymphedema) of the right leg due to filariasis *(Wuchereria bancrofti). (A courtesy Edward Goljan, MD; B from Swartz M:* Textbook of Physical Diagnosis History and Examination, *5th ed, Philadelphia, Saunders Elsevier, 2006, p 444, Fig. 15-3; C from Cohen J, Powderly W, Opal S:* Infectious Diseases, *3rd ed, Philadelphia, Elsevier, 2010, Fig. 115.1 a.)*

Thoracic outlet syndrome

Compression neurovascular compartment in neck

Cervical rib, tight scalene muscles, positional changes neck/arms

Arm "falls asleep" while sleeping

Numbness/paresthesias

+ Adson test

Lymphatic disorders

Incomplete basement membranes → infection, tumor invasion

Acute lymphangitis

Cellulitis with inflammation lymphatic vessels

MCC *Streptococcus pyogenes*

Tender "red streaks"

Sporotrichosis: nodular lymphangitis

Lymphedema

Lymph fluid interstitial space

Post–radical mastectomy radiation

Congenital, Turner syndrome, filariasis (MCC in world)

Pitting edema early; nonpitting advanced cases

Painless, progressive

Chylous effusions

Contains chylomicrons

Malignant lymphoma, surgery

F. **Thoracic outlet syndrome (TOS)**
1. **Definition:** Compression of the neurovascular compartment in the neck
2. Causes include cervical rib, spastic anterior scalene muscles, or positional changes in the neck and arms, particularly in muscular individuals.
3. Clinical findings
   a. Vascular signs (e.g., arm "falls asleep" while the person is sleeping)
   b. Nerve root signs (e.g., numbness, paresthesias [numbness and tingling])
   c. Positive Adson test. Diminished to absent pulse when the arm is outstretched and person looks to the side of the outstretched arm.

V. **Lymphatic Disorders**
   A. **Structure of lymphatic vessels**
   • Lymphatic vessels are predisposed to infection and tumor invasion because they have incomplete basement membranes.
   B. **Acute lymphangitis**
   1. **Definition:** Acute lymphangitis is inflammation of lymphatic vessels usually associated with a cellulitis (Fig. 10-13 A).
   2. Cellulitis is most often due to *Streptococcus pyogenes.*
   3. Lymphatic vessels in the area of the cellulitis appear as tender "red streaks" beneath the skin.
   C. **Nodular lymphangitis**
   • Nodular lymphangitis (chain of subcutaneous tender nodules) is most often caused by sporotrichosis (see Chapter 25; Fig. 25-7 K).
   D. **Lymphedema** (see Chapter 5)
   1. **Definition:** Collection of lymphatic fluid in the interstitial tissue or body cavities
   2. Epidemiology and causes
      a. In the United States, lymphedema is most often associated with post–radical mastectomy followed by irradiation of the axilla (Fig. 10-13 B).
      b. Other causes include filariasis (most common cause of lymphedema in the world; Fig. 10-13 C), congenital origin (birth, teenager, >30 years old), and Turner syndrome (see Fig. 6-22 C).
   3. Clinical findings
      a. Early in interstitial fluid lymphedema, there is pitting with compression; however, in advanced cases it is nonpitting, due to increased fibrosis.
      b. Lymphedema is usually painless and progressive.
   4. Chylous effusions (e.g., pleural cavity)
      a. **Definition:** Effusions that contain chylomicrons with TG (milky appearance; Fig. 10-3)
      b. Causes in the thoracic cavity include damage to the thoracic duct by malignant lymphoma or trauma (usually surgery).

VI. **Vascular Tumors and Tumor-like Conditions** (Table 10-2; Fig. 10-14; Links 10-23, 10-24, 10-25, 10-26, 10-27, 10-28, 10-29, 10-30, 10-31, 10-32, 10-33, and 10-34)
   • Most tumors derive from small vessels or arteriovenous anastomoses in glomus bodies.

TABLE 10-2 Vascular Tumors and Tumor-Like Conditions

TUMOR/CONDITION	CLINICAL FINDINGS

Angiomyolipoma	• **Definition:** Nonneoplastic tumor composed of blood vessels, smooth muscle, and mature adipose tissue
	• Associated with tuberous sclerosis (see Chapter 26), an AD disorder associated with various clinical manifestations
	  • Mental retardation and seizures (infantile spasms) that begin in infancy
	  • Angiofibromas (adenoma sebaceum, benign tumors with fibrous tissue containing vascular channels) occurring on the face (see Fig. 26-5 D)
	  • Hypopigmented skin lesions called shagreen patches (ash leaf spots) on the skin (see Fig. 26-5 E)

Angiosarcoma	• **Definition:** Malignancy of blood vessels. Liver angiosarcomas are associated with exposure to polyvinyl chloride, arsenic, or thorium dioxide.
Bacillary angiomatosis (Fig. 10-14 A; Link 10-23)	• **Definition:** Benign capillary proliferation involving the skin and visceral organs in AIDS patients • Caused by *Bartonella henselae*, a gram-negative bacillus (also causes cat-scratch disease) • Gross appearance on the skin simulates Kaposi sarcoma in AIDS.
Capillary hemangioma (Fig. 10-14 B; Links 10-24, 10-25, 10-26)	• **Definition:** Benign tumor derived from capillaries; commonly seen on the face of newborns. Advise parents that these normally regress with age.
Cavernous hemangioma (Link 10-27)	• **Definition:** Benign vascular tumor; most common benign tumor of liver and spleen • May rupture if large and produce a hemoperitoneum (blood in the peritoneal cavity)
Cystic hygroma (see Fig. 6-22 A, B)	• **Definition:** Lymphatic cyst in the neck that is commonly associated with Turner syndrome (responsible for the webbed neck)
Glomus tumor Link 10-28	• **Definition:** Benign tumors arising from arteriovenous shunts in glomus bodies • Present as a painful, red subungual nodule in a digit or as multiple nodules on other sites in the body
Hereditary telangiectasia (AD) (Fig. 10-14 D; Links 10-29, 10-30)	• **Definition:** Dilated blood vessels on the skin and mucous membranes in the mouth and throughout the GI tract • Chronic iron deficiency anemia may occur because of bleeding from telangiectasias (vessel dilation) in the GI tract.
Kaposi sarcoma (Fig. 4-16 B–D)	• **Definition:** Malignant tumor arising from endothelial cells or primitive mesenchymal cells, associated with human herpesvirus type 8 • AIDS-defining lesion and the most common cancer in AIDS • Presents as a raised, red-purple discoloration that progresses from a flat lesion to a plaque to a nodule that ulcerates • Common sites: skin (most common site), mouth (2nd most common site), and GI tract
Lymphangiosarcoma	• **Definition:** Malignancy of lymphatic vessels that arises out of long-standing chronic lymphedema (e.g., after a modified radical mastectomy; filariasis)

Pyogenic granuloma (Fig. 10-14 E; Link 10-31)	• **Definition:** Nonneoplastic vascular, red pedunculated mass that ulcerates and bleeds easily
	• Commonly occurs following trauma or in association with pregnancy
	  • Caused by increased estrogen
	  • Usually regresses postpartum without a scar

Spider telangiectasia (see Fig. 19-7 F)	• **Definition:** Arteriovenous fistula that disappears when the central body is compressed • Associated with hyperestrinism (e.g., cirrhosis, normal pregnancy)
Sturge-Weber syndrome (Fig. 10-14 F; Links 10-32, 10-33)	• **Definition:** Syndrome characterized by a nevus flammeus ("birthmark," "port-wine stain") on the face in the distribution of the ophthalmic branch and/or maxillary branch of cranial nerve V (trigeminal) • Some cases have an ipsilateral malformation of the pia mater vessels overlying the occipital and parietal lobes. Vessels can bleed and produce a subarachnoid hemorrhage.
von Hippel–Lindau syndrome (AD)	• **Definition:** AD disease characterized by the presence of cavernous hemangiomas in the cerebellum and the retina • Increased incidence of bilateral pheochromocytoma (benign tumor secreting catecholamines) and bilateral renal cell carcinomas
Salmon patch (Link 10-34)	• **Definition:** Blanchable vascular patch usually on the face of a newborn that becomes more prominent with crying or increased body temperature; most common vascular lesion in childhood

AD, Autosomal dominant; *AIDS,* acquired immunodeficiency syndrome; *GI,* gastrointestinal.

VII. Vasculitic Disorders
A. Definition of vasculitis
- Vasculitis refers to inflammation involving the vessel wall; may include small vessels (arterioles, venules, capillaries), medium-sized vessels (muscular arteries), large vessels (elastic arteries), or combinations of these vessel types (Figs. 10-15 and 10-16 A; Link 10-35).

Vasculitis: inflammation any caliber of vessel

10-14: **A,** Bacillary angiomatosis. Note the nodular red mass and satellite lesions at the periphery. **B,** Capillary hemangioma. Note the raised, red lesion above the right eyelid in this child. **C,** Cystic hygroma in the neck of a newborn that did not have Turner syndrome. **D,** Hereditary telangiectasia. Note the telangiectasias scattered over the dorsal surface of the tongue. **E,** Pyogenic granuloma. Note the nodular, bleeding, red mass erupting from the skin surface. **F,** Sturge-Weber syndrome. There is a nevus flammeus ("birthmark") on the face in the distribution of the ophthalmic and maxillary branch of cranial nerve V (trigeminal). *(A courtesy Richard Johnson, MD, Beth Israel Deaconess Medical Center, Boston; B from Habif T: Clinical Dermatology, 4th ed, St. Louis, Mosby, 2004; C from Townsend C: Sabiston Textbook of Surgery, 18th ed, Philadelphia, Saunders Elsevier, 2008, p 2052, Fig. 71.3; D, F from Swartz MH: Textbook of Physical Diagnosis, 5th ed, Philadelphia, Saunders Elsevier, 2006, pp 333, 770, Figs. 12-11, 24-8, respectively; E from Fitzpatrick JE, Morelli JG: Dermatology Secrets Plus, 4th ed, Philadelphia, Mosby Elsevier, 2011, p 303, Fig. 42.7.)*

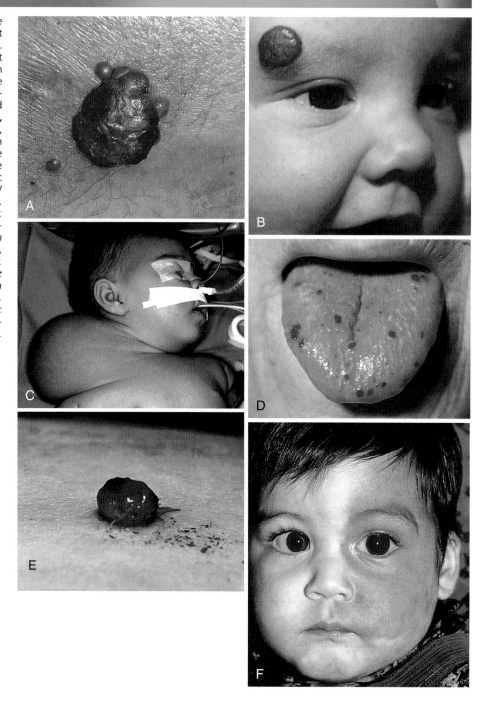

Type III HSRs with immunocomplexes; e.g., HSP

Type II HSRs with antibodies; GPS

ANCA antibodies against cytoplasmic components neutrophils

Abs activate neutrophils: release enzymes, FRs

c-ANCA: Abs against proteinase 3

Granulomatosis with polyangiitis

p-ANCA: antibodies against MPO

Microscopic polyangiitis, CSS

Direct microbial invasion

B. Pathogenesis
1. Type III hypersensitivity reactions (HSRs; immunocomplexes; see Chapter 4). Example: Henoch-Schönlein purpura (HSP).
2. Type II hypersensitivity reactions (antigen-antibody). Example: Goodpasture syndrome (GPS; anti–basement membrane antibodies; see Chapter 4)
3. Antineutrophil cytoplasmic antibodies (ANCA) (Fig. 10-16 B)
   a. Antibodies activate neutrophils, causing release of their enzymes and free radicals (FRs) resulting in vessel damage.
   b. In c-ANCA type of vasculitides, antibodies are directed against proteinase 3 in neutrophil cytoplasmic granules. Example: granulomatosis with polyangiitis (formerly known as Wegener granulomatosis).
   c. In p-ANCA type of vasculitides, antibodies are directed against myeloperoxidase (MPO) in neutrophils. Examples: microscopic polyangiitis, Churg-Strauss syndrome (CSS).
4. Direct invasion by all classes of microbial pathogens

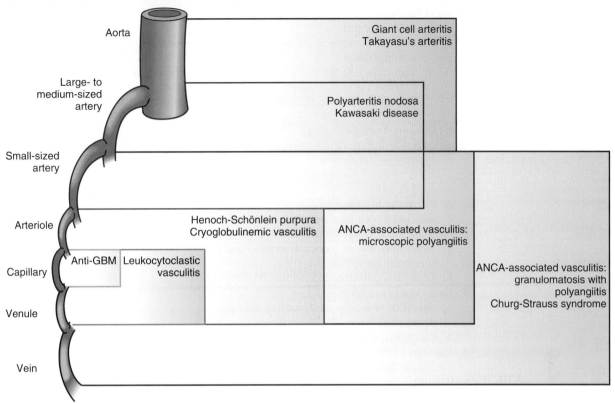

10-15: Classification of vasculitis by blood vessel size. Granulomatosis with polyangiitis (formerly known as Wegener's granulomatosis). *ANCA,* Antineutrophil cytoplasmic antibody; *GBM,* glomerular basement membrane. *(From Firestein GS, Budd RC, Gabriel SE, et al: Kelley's Textbook of Rheumatology, 9th ed, Saunders Elsevier, 2013, p 1455, Fig. 87-1.)*

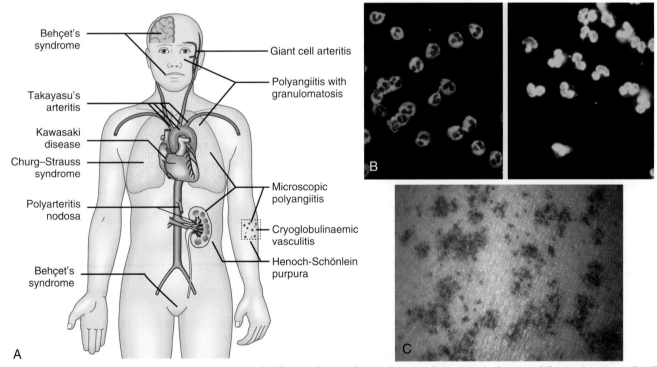

10-16: A, Types of vasculitis. The anatomic targets of different forms of vasculitis are shown. **B,** Antineutrophil cytoplasmic antibodies *(ANCA)* demonstrated by fluorescent microscopy following the application of the patient's serum to test smears. Left schematic shows cytoplasmic antibodies (c-ANCA); right schematic shows perinuclear antibodies (p-ANCA). **C,** The red lesions on the skin were palpable (tumor of acute inflammation); hence, the term *palpable purpura.* This patient has leukocytoclastic vasculitis. *(A from Walker BR, Colledge NR, Ralston SH, Penman ID: Davidson's Principles and Practice of Medicine, 22nd ed, Churchill Livingstone Elsevier, 2014, p 1116, Fig. 25.47; B from Corrin B, Nicholson AG, Burke M, Rice A: Pathology of the Lungs, 3rd ed, Churchill Livingstone Elsevier, 2011, p 432, Fig. 8.3.1; courtesy Dr. G. Valesini, Rome, Italy; C from Firestein GS, Budd RC, Gabriel SE, et al: Kelley's Textbook of Rheumatology, 9th ed, Saunders Elsevier, 2013, p 609, Fig. 43-13.)*

C. Clinical findings
1. Small vessel vasculitis
   a. Known as leukocytoclastic or hypersensitivity vasculitis
   b. Gross appearance
      (1) Skin overlying the vasculitis is hemorrhagic, raised, and painful to palpation. Called palpable purpura ("tumor" of acute inflammation) (see Chapter 15; Fig. 10-16 C).
      (2) Examples: Henoch-Schönlein purpura (HSP) and microscopic polyangiitis

Purpura due to thrombocytopenia or vessel instability (e.g., scurvy) is *not* palpable, because acute inflammation is *not* involved (see Chapter 15).

   c. Microscopic appearance. Vessel is disrupted and contains a neutrophilic infiltrate associated with nuclear debris and fibrinoid necrosis (see Chapter 2).
2. Medium-sized vessel vasculitis
   a. Vasculitis involves muscular arteries and may present with thrombosis, infarction, or aneurysm formation.
   b. Examples: polyarteritis nodosa (PAN) and Kawasaki disease (KD)
3. Large vessel vasculitis
   a. Vasculitis of a large elastic artery may present with decreased to absent pulse and/or stroke.
   b. Examples: Takayasu arteritis (TA) and giant cell (temporal arteritis)
4. Summary table of vasculitides (Table 10-3; Fig. 10-17; Links 10-35, 10-36, 10-37, 10-38, 10-39, 10-40, 10-41, 10-42, 10-43, 10-44, 10-45, 10-46, and 10-47)

VIII. Hypertension
   A. Definition
   1. Normal blood pressure: <120 mm Hg systolic, <80 mm Hg diastolic
   2. Prehypertension: 120–139 mm Hg systolic, 80–90 mm Hg diastolic
   3. Stage 1 HTN: 140–159 mm Hg systolic, 91–99 mm Hg diastolic
   4. Stage 2 HTN: ≥160 mm Hg systolic, ≥100 mm Hg diastolic
   B. Epidemiology
   1. Primary (formerly "essential") HTN accounts for 85% of cases. Remaining 15% represent secondary HTN.
   2. In the United States, 25% to 30% of the adult population has HTN.
   C. Pathophysiology
   1. Systolic blood pressure (SBP)
      a. **Definition:** Correlates with the stroke volume and the compliance of the aorta
      b. Primary determinants of the stroke volume
         (1) Preload, or the volume of blood in the left ventricle (LV)
         (2) Afterload, or the resistance the left ventricle contracts against to eject blood from the heart. The usual resistance is in the peripheral vascular arterioles. Examples of afterload: aortic stenosis is an afterload that is present at the level of the aortic valve; vasoconstriction of peripheral vascular resistance (PVR) vessels
         (3) Contractility of the heart
      c. Vessel elasticity determines the compliance of the aorta, or the ability of the aorta to expand with blood during systole.
         (1) Compliance decreases with age because of reduced elasticity in the aorta.
         (2) Decreased compliance is the mechanism for systolic HTN in people >60 years of age.
      d. Increase in SBP is caused by an increase in preload, an increase in contractility, or a decrease in the compliance of the aorta.
      e. Decrease in SBP is caused by a decrease in preload, a decrease in contractility, or an increase in afterload (e.g., severe aortic stenosis).
   2. Diastolic blood pressure (DBP)
      a. Correlates with the volume of blood in the aorta during diastole
      b. Primarily depends on the state of contraction (tonicity) of the SMCs in the PVR arterioles, the viscosity of blood, and the heart rate (HR)
      c. Causes of increased diastolic blood pressure
         (1) Vasoconstriction of the PVR arterioles. A greater volume of blood is present in the artery while the heart is filling up in diastole.
         (2) Increase in blood viscosity (hyperviscosity; e.g., polycythemia)

Small vessel vasculitis

Leukocytoclastic vasculitis/hypersensitivity vasculitis

Palpable purpura; painful; acute inflammation

HSP, microscopic polyangiitis

Purpura thrombocytopenia/vessel instability *not* acute inflammation

Disrupted, neutrophils, fibrinoid necrosis

Medium-sized vessel vasculitis: muscular arteries

Muscular artery vasculitis: thrombosis, infarction, aneurysm

PAN, KD

Large vessel vasculitis

Absent pulse, stroke

TA, temporal arteritis

Hypertension

Normal: <120 mm Hg systolic, <80 mm Hg diastolic

Primary HTN: 85% all HTN cases

SBP

Correlates with stroke volume, aorta compliance

Determinants stroke volume

Preload (blood in LV)

Afterload (resistance LV contracts against)

Aortic stenosis; vasoconstriction PVR vessels

Contractility of heart

Vessel elasticity determines aortic compliance

Aortic compliance ↓with age

Systolic HTN: >60 yrs old; loss aortic compliance

↑SBP: ↑preload, ↑contractility, ↓aortic compliance

↓SBP: ↓preload, ↓contractility, ↑afterload (aortic stenosis)

DBP

Correlates with blood volume in aorta while heart fills in diastole

DBP: tonicity SMCs PVR arterioles, blood viscosity, HR

↑DBP causes: Vasoconstriction of PVR arterioles, ↑blood hyperviscosity (polycythemia)

TABLE 10-3   Vasculitic Disorders: Elastic Artery, Muscular Artery, and Small Vessel

DISORDER	VASCULITIS	EPIDEMIOLOGY/ETIOLOGY	CLINICAL/LABORATORY FINDINGS
Takayasu arteritis ("pulseless disease") (Fig. 10-17 A)	Granulomatous large vessel vasculitis involving aortic arch vessels	Seen in young Asian women and children	• Absent upper extremity pulse • Discrepancy in blood pressure between the arms that is >10 mm Hg • Visual defects and stroke possible
Giant cell (temporal) arteritis (Fig. 10-17 B; Links 10-36 and 10-37)	Granulomatous large vessel vasculitis with multinucleated giant cells and a lymphoid infiltrate involving the superficial temporal and ophthalmic arteries	Occurs in adults >50 years of age	• Temporal headache, due to inflamed temporal artery and jaw claudication (pain when chewing due to ischemia); ipsilateral blindness possible due to involvement of the ophthalmic artery • Polymyalgia rheumatica (muscle and joint pain; normal serum creatine kinase) present in most cases • Increased ESR and CRP (useful screening tests; see Chapter 3)
Polyarteritis nodosa (Fig. 10-17 C, Link 10-38)	Necrotizing medium-sized vessel vasculitis that may involve the renal, coronary, and mesenteric arteries Does *not* involve pulmonary arteries Only affects part of the vessel, which, when weakened, produces an aneurysm ("nodosa")	• Affects middle-aged men • Association with HBsAg (30% of cases) • Hepatitis B–associated polyarteritis nodosa is an immunocomplex disease (type III hypersensitivity); otherwise, cause for polyarteritis nodosa is unknown	• Vessels at *all stages* of acute and chronic inflammation • Fever commonly present, often as fever of unknown origin • Focal vasculitis produces aneurysms (detected with angiography) • Organ infarction possible in kidneys (renal failure, hematuria), heart (AMI), bowels (bloody diarrhea), skin (ischemic ulcer), testicle (testicular pain) • Angiography shows aneurysms; lesion biopsy confirms diagnosis
Kawasaki disease (Fig. 10-17 E, F, Links 10-39, 10-40, 10-41)	Necrotizing medium-sized vessel vasculitis involving coronary arteries (e.g., thrombosis, aneurysms)	• Occurs in children <5 years of age; more common in boys than girls • Children of Asian descent have highest incidence, with the highest incidence in Japan • Surpassed acute rheumatic heart disease as the most common acquired heart disease in children • Leading cause of acquired heart disease in children in developed countries • Likely has infectious etiology that precipitates immune reaction in genetically susceptible individuals	• Fever, erythema and edema of hands and feet • Conjunctivitis, painful cervical adenopathy, oral erythema and cracking of the lips, strawberry-appearing tongue from glossitis • Abnormal ECG possible; possible AMI • Most common cause of AMI in children
Thromboangiitis obliterans (Buerger disease) (Link 10-42)	Medium-sized vessel vasculitis with digital vessel thrombosis and damage to the neurovascular compartment	• Typically occurs in men aged 25–50 who smoke cigarettes; may occur in women (10% of cases) • Most commonly occurs in Jews of Ashkenazi ancestry living in Israel • High morbidity in India, Korea, and Japan • Genetic mechanism proposed	• Lower extremity involved in 100% of cases • Resting pain on the forefoot is characteristic finding • Ischemic ulcers or gangrene of the foot/toes possible • Upper extremity involved in 40%–50% of cases • Upper limb ischemia with ulceration and gangrene (amputation is common) • Raynaud phenomenon possible
Raynaud disease	• Medium-sized vessel vasculitis that involves digital vessels in fingers and toes • May also affect tip of nose and ears	• Most commonly occurs in young women • Thought to be an exaggerated vasomotor response to cold or stress	• Paroxysmal digital color changes in the fingers and toes with a white to blue to red sequence • Ulceration and gangrene possible in chronic cases
Raynaud phenomenon (Fig. 10-17 G, Link 10-43)	Medium-sized vessel vasculitis that involves digital vessels in fingers, toes, tip of the nose, ears	• Most often occurs in adult men and women • May be associated with collagen vascular diseases (see Chapter 4), including systemic sclerosis, CREST syndrome, and systemic lupus erythematosus	• Systemic sclerosis and CREST syndrome (see Chapter 4): digital vasculitis with vessel fibrosis, dystrophic calcification, ulceration, gangrene, Raynaud phenomenon, sclerodactyly, telangiectasia (dilated vessels on the face)

Continued

TABLE 10-3 Vasculitic Disorders: Elastic Artery, Muscular Artery, and Small Vessel—cont'd

DISORDER	VASCULITIS	EPIDEMIOLOGY/ETIOLOGY	CLINICAL/LABORATORY FINDINGS
Granulomatosis with polyangiitis (formerly known as Wegener's granulomatosis) (Fig. 10-17 H; Links 10-44, 10-45, 10-46, 10-47)	Necrotizing medium and small-sized vessel vasculitis that involves vessels in lung (infarctions) and kidneys (infarctions and glomerulonephritis)	• Mean age 41 years • Incidence equal in men and women • Symptoms involving upper and/or lower airways (≈90% of patients)	• Necrotizing granulomas in skin, upper respiratory tract (nasopharynx–saddle nose deformity, chronic sinusitis, collapse of the trachea), and lower respiratory tract (cavitating nodular lesions in the lungs) • Necrotizing vasculitis in lungs produces infarctions and hemoptysis (coughing up blood); lung is most reliable site for biopsy to secure diagnosis • In kidneys, crescentic type of glomerulonephritis, with c-ANCA antibodies present in >90% of cases
Microscopic polyangiitis	Small vessel vasculitis that involves skin, lung, brain, GI tract, and kidneys (postcapillary venules and glomerular capillaries)	• Occurs in children and adults • Precipitated by drugs (e.g., penicillin), infections (e.g., streptococci), and immune disorders (e.g., system lupus erythematosus)	• Vessels are at *same* stage of inflammation • Palpable purpura and crescentic glomerulonephritis associated with p-ANCA antibodies (>80% of cases; see Chapter 20)
Churg-Strauss syndrome	Small vessel vasculitis that involves skin, lung, and heart vessels	• Occurs at a mean of 51 years of age • May be an autoimmune disease	• Allergic rhinitis and asthma common • p-ANCA antibodies (70% of cases), eosinophilia
Henoch-Schönlein purpura (Fig. 10-17 I)	Small vessel vasculitis that involves skin, GI tract, kidney, and joints	• Most common vasculitis in children; usually seen in children 1–15 years old • Some cases occur in young adults • Occurs in males more often than females • More common in whites and Asians than in blacks • Peak incidence in the spring and rarely the summer • IgA–anti-IgA immunocomplex (type III hypersensitivity disease)	• Often follows viral upper respiratory infection, group A streptococcal pharyngeal infection • Pathogens may act as an antigen trigger that causes antibody formation and eventually immunocomplexes (type III hypersensitivity). • Palpable purpura on buttocks and lower extremities is characteristic (95%–100% of cases) • Polyarthritis (80%), glomerulonephritis (80%), abdominal pain and vomiting (85%), and GI bleeding possible • Recurrence in one-third of cases • Most patients have spontaneous recovery in 4 months without therapy.
Cryoglobulinemia	• Small vessel vasculitis involving skin, GI tract, and renal vessels • Different types of cryoglobulinemia (mixed, monoclonal, polyclonal)	• Primarily occurs in adults • More common in females than males (3 : 1 ratio) • Association with hepatitis C (>50% of cases), type 1 MPGN, multiple myeloma (monoclonal type), lymphoproliferative disorders, and connective tissue disorders	• Cryoglobulins: proteins in plasma that gel at cold temperatures, particularly in areas exposed to cold temperature (nose, fingers, ears) • Palpable purpura (small vessel vasculitis), acral cyanosis (nose and ears), and Raynaud phenomenon in cold temperatures (reverses when in a warm room) • Crescentic type of glomerulonephritis with rapid renal failure (see Chapter 20)
Infectious vasculitis Figs. 10-17 J, K	Small vessel vasculitis involving skin vessels	• Occurs in children and adults • Involves all microbial pathogens • Rocky Mountain spotted fever: most prevalent in the Southeast, followed by south central states	• **Rocky Mountain spotted fever:** transmitted by dog tick (*Dermacentor variabilis*) or wood tick (*Dermacentor andersoni*); *Rickettsia rickettsii* present in tick's salivary glands; organisms invade endothelial cells, producing vasculitis; fever in 100% of cases. Petechiae (vasculitis) begin on palms and spread to trunk; appear in first days in 50% of cases and by 5th day in 80% of cases; no petechiae in 10% of cases • **Disseminated meningococcemia:** Due to *Neisseria meningitidis* • Capillary thromboses develop, usually in the setting of disseminated intravascular coagulation (see Chapter 15). Initially, there are hemorrhages into the skin (petechiae) that eventually become confluent ecchymoses as the disease progresses. Hemorrhagic infarctions of both adrenal glands commonly occurs, producing acute hypocortisolism and death (called Waterhouse-Friderichsen syndrome).

AMI, Acute myocardial infarction; *c-ANCA*, cytoplasmic antineutrophil cytoplasmic antibodies; *CRP*, C-reactive protein; *ECG*, electrocardiogram; *ESR*, erythrocyte sedimentation rate; *GI*, gastrointestinal; *MPGN*, membranoproliferative glomerulonephritis; *p-ANCA*, perinuclear antineutrophil cytoplasmic antibodies.

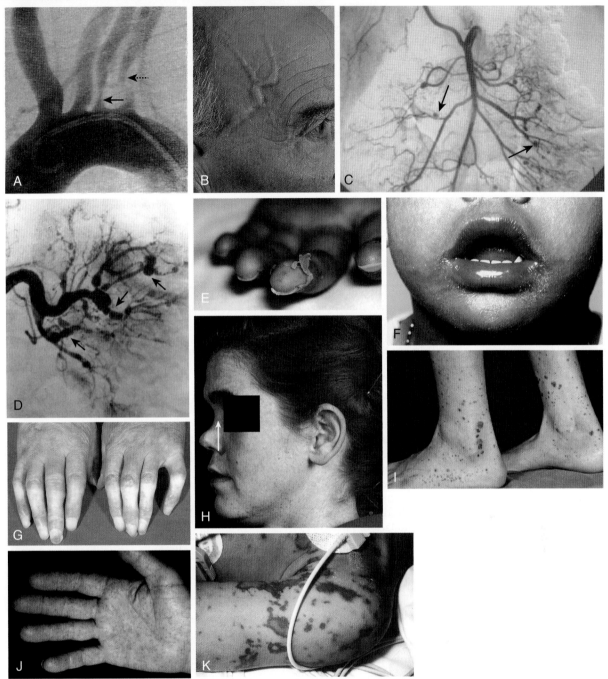

10-17: **A:** Digital subtraction angiogram in Takayasu arteritis involving some of the aortic branches. From left to right, the vessels are innominate, left common carotid, an anomalous origin of the left vertebral artery, and the left subclavian artery. The left vertebral artery *(solid arrow)* and the left subclavian artery *(interrupted arrow)* have significant stenoses near their origin. **B,** Older man with right temporal arteritis. Note the bulging vessels. The vessels were tender to palpation. **C,** Mesenteric angiogram in polyarteritis nodosa. Note the numerous small aneurysms *(arrows)* in the medium-sized vessels. **D,** Renal angiogram showing vascular aneurysms *(arrows)* in a patient with hepatitis B–associated polyarteritis nodosa. **E,** Kawasaki disease. Note the desquamation of the skin of the finger, which is a characteristic skin finding in this disease. **F,** Kawasaki disease. Note the swollen, erythematous lips and the erythema in the angles of the lips (angular cheilosis). The child also had glossitis. The tongue had an erythematous appearance resembling the surface of a strawberry ("strawberry" tongue). **G,** Raynaud phenomenon. Note the extreme pallor of the digits in both hands in this patient with systemic lupus erythematosus. **H,** Saddle nose deformity in granulomatosis with polyangiitis. Note the concavity *(arrow)* below the bridge of the nose having the appearance of a saddle. **I,** Henoch-Schönlein purpura. Multiple erythematous, raised, palpable lesions around the ankles show areas of hemorrhage into the skin overlying areas of immunocomplex vasculitis involving small vessels. The lesions extended up to the buttocks. **J,** Rocky Mountain spotted fever. The palm shows a few petechial lesions in this patient with a history of a tick bite. **K,** Disseminated meningococcemia showing confluent ecchymoses. *(A from Forbes CD, Jackson WF: Color Atlas and Text of Clinical Medicine, 3rd ed, Mosby, 2003 p 248, Fig. 5.182; B from Forbes CD, Jackson WF: Color Atlas and Text of Clinical Medicine, 3rd ed, Mosby, 2003 p 129, Fig. 3.98; C from Goldman L, Ausiello D: Cecil's Textbook of Medicine, 2nd ed, Philadelphia, Saunders Elsevier, 2008, p 2054, Fig. 291-2 A; D from McNally PR: GI/Liver Secrets Plus, 5th ed, Mosby Elsevier, 2015, p 170, Fig. 22-1; E from Gwin: Immune disorders. In Pediatric Nursing: An Introductory Text, 2012, pp 355–373; F from McKee PH, Calonje E, Granter RS: Pathology of the Skin with Clinical Correlations, 3rd ed, St. Louis, Mosby Elsevier, 2005, p 736, Fig. 15.63; G from Savin JA, Hunter JAA, Hepburn NC: Diagnosis in Color: Skin Signs in Clinical Medicine, London, Mosby-Wolfe, 1997, p 205, Fig. 8.43; H, I, K from Bouloux P-M: Self-Assessment Picture Tests: Medicine, Vol 3, London, Mosby-Wolfe, 1996, pp 41, 66, 96, Figs. 92, 75, 191, respectively; J from Habif TB: Clinical Dermatology: A Color Guide to Diagnosis and Therapy, ed 6, Elsevier, 2016, p 609, Fig. 15-42.)*

↑Heart rate → ↓filling coronary arteries → ↑volume blood in aorta in diastole

↓DBP causes

Vasodilation PVR arterioles

↓Blood viscosity (anemia)

↓Heart rate

(3) Increase in heart rate (HR). Increasing heart rate decreases filling of the coronary arteries, leaving a greater volume of blood in the aorta during diastole.
d. Causes of decreased diastolic blood pressure
(1) Vasodilation of the PVR arterioles
(2) Severe anemia, which decreases the viscosity of blood
(3) Decreasing the heart rate (HR). Decreasing heart rate increases filling of the coronary arteries, leaving less blood in the aorta during diastole.

Factors that contract arteriole smooth muscle cells causing vasoconstriction include α-adrenergic stimuli, catecholamines, angiotensin II, vasopressin, endothelin, and increased total body sodium.

Sodium in HTN

↑Sodium retention: ↑plasma volume → ↑stroke volume → ↑SBP

↑Sodium retention: ↑vasoconstriction PVR arterioles → ↑DBP

Primary HTN

No known secondary cause

BP: force blood directed against arterial walls as heart contracts

MC in non-Hispanic black adults

Linked to increasing age

↑Risk AMI, CHF, stroke, renal disease

Pathogenesis

Genetic factors reduce renal sodium excretion

↓Na⁺ excretion → ↑plasma volume → ↑stroke volume ↑SBP

↓Na⁺ excretion → ↑PVR (vasoconstriction) → ↑DBP

Obesity, stress, smoking, ↑dietary salt, lack exercise

3. Role of sodium in HTN
a. Excess sodium increases plasma volume. Excess plasma volume increases stroke volume, which in turn increases the SBP.
b. Excess sodium produces vasoconstriction of the PVR arterioles. Increase of sodium in smooth muscle increases calcium-mediated contraction of the muscle, causing an increase in the diastolic blood pressure.
D. Primary HTN
1. **Definition:** High blood pressure that has no known secondary cause (e.g., primary aldosteronism). Blood pressure (BP) is the force of blood directed against the arterial walls as the heart pumps blood throughout the body.
2. Epidemiology (old term essential HTN)
a. Primary HTN is most common in non-Hispanic black adults.
b. Approximately 50% of people 60 to 69 years have HTN. Greater than 75% of people over 70 years of age have HTN.
c. HTN increases the risk for AMI, congestive heart failure (CHF), stroke, and renal disease.
d. Pathogenesis
(1) Genetic factors reduce renal sodium excretion (85% cases).
(a) Decreased sodium excretion increases plasma volume, which increases stroke volume, which increases SBP.
(b) Decreased sodium excretion increases vasoconstriction of PVR arterioles, which increases the DBP.
(2) Additional important factors include obesity, stress, smoking, increased salt intake, and lack of physical exercise.

Reduced renal sodium excretion is the primary mechanism of primary HTN in the black population and older adults. Increased plasma volume suppresses renin release from the juxtaglomerular apparatus, producing a low-renin type of HTN.

↓Renal sodium excretion: mechanism blacks/older adults. Primary HTN blacks/older adults: ↑plasma volume suppresses renin release JG apparatus (low renin HTN).

Secondary HTN

Renovascular HTN and drugs leading causes

• Descending order complications: acute MI, stroke, renal failure

• Control HTN greatest benefit in reducing incidence of strokes; however, it also significantly reduces risk for developing chronic heart disease and renal disease.

• Control of HTN has greatest benefit in reducing incidence of strokes.

E. Secondary hypertension
1. Accounts for 15% of cases of HTN
2. Causes (Table 10-4; Fig. 10-16)
F. Complications of HTN (Table 10-5; Box 10-1; see margin note)

TABLE 10-4 Causes of Secondary Hypertension

SYSTEM OR SOURCE	DESCRIPTION
Adrenal	• **Cushing syndrome:** increased mineralocorticoids (see Chapter 23) • **Pheochromocytoma:** increased catecholamines (see Chapter 23) • **Neuroblastoma:** increased catecholamines (see Chapter 23) • **11-Hydroxylase deficiency:** increased mineralocorticoids (i.e., deoxycorticosterone; see Chapter 23) • **Primary aldosteronism** (Conn syndrome): increased aldosterone (see Chapter 5)
Aorta	• **Postductal coarctation:** causes activation of the RAA system due to decreased blood flow to the renal arteries (see Chapter 11) • **Older adults:** systolic hypertension due to decreased elasticity of the aorta (see Chapter 6)
CNS	• **Intracranial hypertension:** increased release of catecholamines
Drugs	• **Oral contraceptives:** estrogen increases synthesis of angiotensinogen; most common cause of hypertension in young women; resolves with discontinuing contraceptives (see Chapter 22) • **Cocaine:** increased sympathetic activity (see Chapter 7)

TABLE 10-4   Causes of Secondary Hypertension—cont'd

SYSTEM OR SOURCE	DESCRIPTION
Parathyroid	• **Primary hyperparathyroidism:** calcium increases PVR arteriole smooth muscle cell contraction (see Chapter 23)
Pregnancy	• **Preeclampsia:** increased production of angiotensin II (see Chapter 22)
Renal	• **Renovascular disease:** atherosclerosis (older men; Fig. 10-18 A), fibromuscular hyperplasia (women; Fig. 10-18B). In both conditions, there is an epigastric bruit due to blood being forced through a narrow lumen. In both conditions, there is activation of the RAA system (high renin hypertension). Angiotensin II causes vasoconstriction of PVR arterioles and increases sodium absorption in the kidneys (increases plasma volume → stroke volume; increases calcium-mediated vasoconstriction of PVR arterioles). Increased aldosterone increases renal absorption of sodium. The increased plasma volume from sodium retention increases renal blood flow in the *unaffected* renal artery, causing suppression of plasma renin activity. • **Renal parenchymal disease:** e.g., diabetic nephropathy, adult polycystic kidney disease, glomerulonephritis; retention of sodium produces hypertension
Thyroid	• **Graves disease:** systolic hypertension from increased cardiac contraction (see Chapter 23) • **Hypothyroidism:** diastolic hypertension due to retention of sodium (see Chapter 23)

CNS, Central nervous system; *PVR,* peripheral vascular resistance; *RAA,* renin-angiotensin-aldosterone.

TABLE 10-5   Complications of Hypertension

SYSTEM	COMPLICATIONS
Cardiovascular	• **Left ventricular hypertrophy:** most common overall complication • **Acute myocardial infarction:** most common cause of death associated with hypertension • **Atherosclerosis:** hypertension is risk factor for atherosclerosis (see previous discussion)
Central nervous system	• **Intracerebral hematoma:** rupture of Charcot-Bouchard aneurysms (see Chapter 26) • **Berry aneurysm:** rupture produces a subarachnoid hemorrhage (see previous discussion; see Chapter 26) • **Lacunar infarcts:** small infarcts due to hyaline arteriolosclerosis (see previous discussion; see Chapter 26)
Renal	• **Benign nephrosclerosis:** kidney disease of hypertension; due to hyaline arteriolosclerosis; causes atrophy of the tubules and sclerosis of the glomeruli; progresses to renal failure (see Chapter 20) • **Malignant hypertension:** associated with a rapid increase in blood pressure accompanied by renal failure and cerebral edema (see Chapter 20); hyperplastic arteriolosclerosis of renal vessels (see previous discussion)
Eyes (Links 10-48, 10-49, 10-50)	• **Hypertensive retinopathy:** arteriovenous nicking, hemorrhage of retinal vessels, exudates (increased vessel permeability, retinal infarction), and papilledema (swelling of the optic nerve) (see Box 10-1)

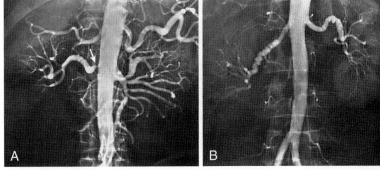

10-18: A, Angiogram showing right renal artery stenosis with poststenotic dilatation *(arrow).* **B,** Angiogram showing bilateral renal artery fibromuscular hyperplasia. Note the beading effect in both vessels. **(A** *from Katz D, Math K, Groskin S: Radiology Secrets, Philadelphia, Hanley & Belfus, 1998, p 184, Fig. 7;* **B** *from Katz D, Math K, Groskin S: Radiology Secrets, Philadelphia, Hanley & Belfus, 1998, p 180, Fig. 27.)*

BOX 10-1 Hypertensive Retinopathy

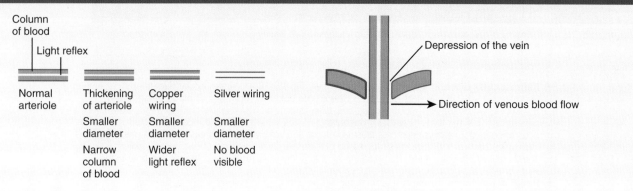

The sequence of events in hypertensive retinopathy involves focal spasm of the arterioles followed by progressive sclerosis and narrowing of the arterioles, leading eventually to flame hemorrhages from rupture of the vessels, formation of exudates (soft and hard), and papilledema (swelling of the optic disk). Normal arteriole walls are transparent; hence the column of blood is visible and the light reflex is narrow. Sclerotic changes in the vessels are first described as "copper wiring," because blood is still visible through the vessel wall. The light reflex becomes wider. When the vessel wall is thickened enough to prevent visualization of the blood, the light reflects back from the vessel wall to produce a "silver wiring" effect. In some cases, no blood is visible in portions of the vessel. Because arterioles cross over the veins (normal ratio of arteriole/venous diameters is 3:4), as arterioles thicken, they create a depression in the wall of the venule, which is called an arteriovenous nicking defect. The distal vein becomes slightly distended owing to the backup of blood. More advanced nicking literally cuts off the blood flow, and the veins appear to end abruptly. Hemorrhages in the retina are usually the result of rupture of microaneurysms that develop from increased pressure on the arterioles. Grayish white exudates that are soft, like cotton wool, are due to microinfarctions, whereas exudates that have clear margins (hard exudates) are due to leakage of protein from increased vessel permeability. A brief summary of the Keith-Wagener-Barker classification of hypertensive retinopathy follows (other classification schema are also available):

Grade I: focal narrowing of the arterioles, mild arteriovenous nicking
Grade II: arteriole narrowing, copper wiring present, arteriovenous nicking more accentuated
Grade III: arteriole narrowing, silver wiring present, hemorrhages, soft and hard exudates, disappearance of the vein under the arteriole, disk normal
Grade IV: arterioles are fine fibrous cords; same as grade III except papilledema is present

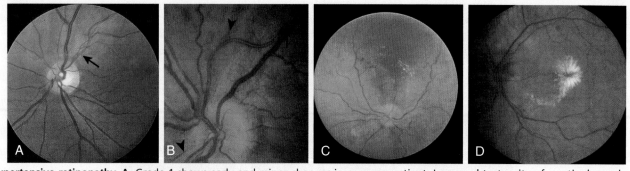

Hypertensive retinopathy. A, Grade 1 shows early and minor changes in a young patient. Increased tortuosity of a retinal vessel and increased reflectiveness (silver wiring) of a retinal artery are seen at 1 o'clock in this view. Otherwise, the fundus is completely normal. **B,** Grade 2 also shows increased tortuosity and silver wiring *(arrowheads)*. In addition, there is "nipping" of the venules at arteriovenous crossings *(arrow)*. **C,** Grade 3 shows the same changes as grade 2 plus flame-shaped retinal hemorrhages and soft "cotton-wool" exudates. **D,** In grade 4, there is swelling of the optic disk (papilledema [left]), retinal edema is present, and hard exudates may collect around the fovea, producing a typical "macular star." *(From Forbes CD, Jackson WF: Color Atlas and Text of Clinical Medicine, 3rd ed, Mosby, 2003, p 238, Figs. 5.142–5.145.)*

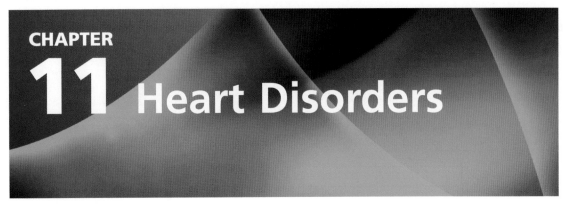

ABBREVIATIONS

MC   most common
MCC most common cause

COD cause of death
Hx   history

Dx   diagnosis
R/O rule out

I. **Cardiac Physical Diagnosis** (Box 11-1)
  A. **Overview of Normal Anatomy** (Link 11-1 to Link 11-8)
II. **Ventricular Hypertrophy**
  A. **Definition of ventricular hypertrophy**
   • Ventricular hypertrophy is a compensatory change related to alterations in pressure and/or volume imposed on the wall of the ventricle.

  | Compensatory change pressure/volume changes

  B. **Pathogenesis of left ventricular hypertrophy (LVH) and right ventricular hypertrophy (RVH)**
   1. Sustained pressure in the ventricles increases wall stress.

   ↑Pressure ↑wall stress

   2. Changes in wall stress alter gene expression in the muscle.

   Wall stress ↑sarcomere duplication

   3. Changes in gene expression lead to duplication of sarcomeres. **Definition:** Sarcomeres are the contractile elements of muscle.

   Contractile element muscle

   4. Changes occur in wall stress when there is an increase in afterload.
     a. **Definition:** Afterload is the resistance the ventricle contracts against to eject blood in systole.

   ↑Wall stress ↑ventricle afterload

     b. Increased afterload produces concentric hypertrophy of the ventricular wall (Fig. 11-1 A). Sarcomeres duplicate parallel to the long axis of the cells, causing the individual muscle fibers to be thicker.

   ↑Afterload, concentric hypertrophy ventricle

   Sarcomeres duplicate parallel to long axis

     c. Causes of concentric LVH due to increased afterload include primary hypertension (HTN; most common), aortic valve (AV) stenosis, and hypertrophic cardiomyopathy (HCM).

   1°HTN (MC), AV stenosis, HCM

     d. Causes of concentric RVH due to increased afterload include pulmonary HTN (PH; see Link 17-66) and pulmonary valve (PV) stenosis.

   PH, PV stenosis

   5. Changes occur in wall stress when there is an increase in preload.
     a. **Definition:** Preload refers to the volume of blood in the ventricle that must be expelled during systole.

   Volume blood ventricle must expel in systole

     b. Preload correlates with left and right ventricle end-diastolic volumes (LVEDV, RVEDV).

   Preload = LVEDV, RVEDV

     c. Increased preload increases stroke volume (SV; volume of blood ejected) via the Frank-Starling pressure relationship.

   ↑Preload ↑SV

     d. Increased preload causes dilation and hypertrophy (eccentric hypertrophy) of the ventricular wall (Fig. 11-1 B). Sarcomeres duplicate in series (on top of each other), causing the individual muscle fibers to increase in length and width.

   ↑Preload→eccentric hypertrophy

   Sarcomeres duplicate in series

     e. Causes of eccentric hypertrophy of the left ventricle (LV) due to increased preload include:
      (1) mitral valve (MV) or AV regurgitation.

   Eccentric LVH: MV/AV regurgitation

      (2) left-to-right shunting of blood (e.g., ventricular septal defect [VSD]). In left-to-right shunting, more blood returns to the left side of the heart because the right side of the heart is receiving more blood than usual.

   Left-to-right shunt

BOX 11-1   Cardiac Physical Diagnosis

Valve Locations for Auscultation

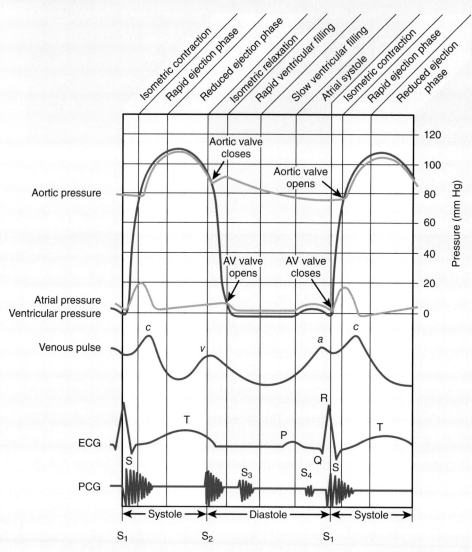

(From Seidel H, Ball J, Dains J, Benedict G: Mosby's Guide to Physical Examination, 6th ed, St. Louis, Mosby Elsevier, 2006, p 419, Fig. 14.7.)

Locations where heart sounds are best heard do *not* always correlate with their anatomic location. The mitral valve (MV) is best heard at the apex; the tricuspid valve (TV), at the left parasternal border; the pulmonary valve (PV), at the left second and third intercostal spaces; and the aortic valve (AV), at the left sternal border for regurgitation murmurs and right second intercostal space for ejection murmurs.

Cardiac Cycle Relationships With Heart Sounds

The P wave represents atrial depolarization; the PR interval, atrioventricular conduction time; the QRS, ventricular depolarization; and, the T wave, ventricular repolarization, or recovery. The S_1 heart sound co-occurs with the QRS complex and marks the beginning of systole, and the S_2 heart sound occurs after the T wave and marks the beginning of diastole.

Heart Sounds

The **S_1 heart sound** corresponds with closure of the MV and TV during systole. This causes moving columns of blood to abruptly decelerate, which sets up vibrations of the chordae tendineae, ventricles, and blood as a unit. The MV closes *before* the TV. It is best heard at the apex and corresponds with the carotid or radial pulse. The **S_2 heart sound** is caused by closure of the AV and PV (doors make noise when they close) and marks the beginning of diastole. It is best heard at the left second or third intercostal space. The aortic component (A_2) normally precedes the pulmonary component (P_2) of the S_2 heart sound. Unlike the S_1 heart sound, the S_2 heart sound splits on inspiration. As the diaphragm descends, it causes a further decrease in intrathoracic pressure, which increases the flow of blood out of the vena cava into the right side of the heart. This causes flattening of the jugular neck veins. The excess amount of blood in the right side of the heart delays closure of the PV, causing P_2 to separate more from A_2 (see

BOX 11-1   Cardiac Physical Diagnosis—cont'd

schematic; called wide physiologic splitting of the second heart sound). This physiologic split is best heard over the PV area. A_2 and P_2 become a single sound on expiration as intrathoracic pressure becomes less negative. An **accentuated A_2** is heard in primary hypertension (increased pressure causes it to snap shut), and an **accentuated P_2** is heard in pulmonary hypertension (increased pressure causes it to snap shut).

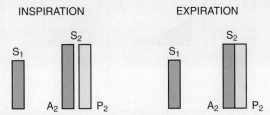

An **S_3 heart sound** (see schematic) is the most clinically significant extra heart sound. It may be a normal finding in children and young adults, in whom it reflects a more energetic expansion and filling of the left ventricle; however, it is considered a pathologic finding after 40 years of age. It is thought to be caused by a sudden rush of blood entering a volume-overloaded left or right ventricle (stiff ventricle). This is analogous to a river emptying into a large volume of water. Turbulence occurs where the two bodies of water interact. The S_3 heart sound is best heard at the apex with the patient in the left lateral decubitus position. It commonly occurs with regurgitant types of murmurs involving any of the valves. It is the first cardiac sign of congestive heart failure, in which increased ventricular volume stretches the MV or TV ring, causing volume overload from mitral or tricuspid regurgitation. An S_3 heart sound produces a ventricular gallop. An **S_4 heart sound** (see schematic) coincides with atrial contraction in late diastole and the a wave in the jugular venous pulse (JVP; see later). The finding of the S_4 heart sound has less diagnostic value than the S3 because disorders causing stiff ventricles are so diverse and because the S_4 does not predict the patient's hemodynamic findings (ejection fraction, left heart filling pressures, or postoperative complications). It is never a normal finding and is caused by increased resistance to filling (decreased compliance) in the left or the right heart after a vigorous atrial contraction. It is heard best at the apex. Causes of decreased ventricular compliance include concentric ventricular hypertrophy (left/right) and a volume overloaded ventricle (no more room to expand). In a volume-overloaded left or right ventricle, it is commonly present along with an S_3 heart sound. An S_4 heart sound and the a wave of a JVP are absent in atrial fibrillation. The presence of an S_4 heart sound produces an atrial gallop. The presence of an S_3 and S_4 heart sound is called a summation gallop (see schematic) and sounds like a galloping horse.

Heart Murmurs

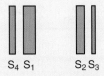

Heart murmurs may occur in systole and diastole. They may be caused by structural valve disease (e.g., damage caused by rheumatic fever) or stretching of the valve ring (e.g., volume overload in left- or right-sided heart failure). Murmurs caused by stretching of valve rings are often called functional murmurs. Murmurs often radiate. For example, AV stenosis radiates into the neck, and MV regurgitation radiates into the axilla. They are graded 1 to 6 in terms of their intensity. Grade 1 and 2 murmurs are very hard to hear, but grade 3 murmurs are easy to hear. Grade 4 to 6 murmurs are often accompanied by a palpable precordial thrill. Grade 6 murmurs are audible without a stethoscope. Murmurs and abnormal heart sounds (e.g., S_3 and S_4 heart sounds) change their intensity with respirations. Right-sided murmurs and abnormal heart sounds have increased intensity when the patient takes a deep inspiration and holds the breath for 3 to 5 seconds. This occurs as the intrathoracic pressure becomes increasingly negative, essentially drawing blood out of the venous system into the right side of the heart, hence accentuating the murmur and abnormal heart sound on that side. In contradistinction, left-sided heart murmurs and abnormal heart sounds do *not* change their intensity with deep held inspiration. **Continuous murmurs** occur through systole and diastole. The most common cause of a continuous murmur in children is a cervical venous hum. A patent ductus arteriosus also produces a continuous murmur. **Innocent murmurs** occur in children from 3 to 7 years old. They are usually grade 2 systolic murmurs that are caused by increased blood flow through the PV. They are best heard in the PV area, and as expected, their intensity increases with deep held inspiration. **Stenosis murmurs** occur when there is a problem in opening the valves. Because the AV and PV normally open in systole, the murmurs of AV and PV stenosis occur in systole. They produce an ejection type of murmur (schematic A), which has a diamond-shaped (crescendo-decrescendo) configuration. The MV and TV normally open in diastole; therefore, the murmurs of MV and TV stenosis are heard in diastole. MV stenosis is accompanied by an opening snap (schematic B), which occurs when the thickened valve is forced open by a strong atrial contraction. An opening snap is usually absent in TV stenosis. **Regurgitation (insufficiency) murmurs** occur when there is defective valve closure. Because the MV and TV normally close in systole, these murmurs occur in systole. They are even-intensity pansystolic murmurs (schematic C) that often obliterate the S_1 and S_2 heart sounds. AV and PV regurgitation murmurs occur in diastole immediately after the S_2 heart sound (schematic D).

Continued

BOX 11-1 Cardiac Physical Diagnosis—cont'd

Jugular Venous Pulses

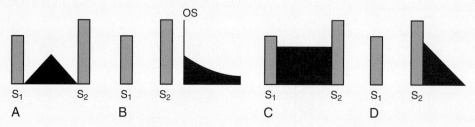

Normal JVPs (see schematic) have three positive waves (*a, c,* and *v*) and two negative waves (*x* and *y*). The **a wave** is a positive wave caused by atrial contraction in late diastole. It occurs after the P wave in an electrocardiogram. It disappears in atrial fibrillation. A **giant a wave** occurs when there is restricted filling of the right side of the heart (e.g., TV stenosis, pulmonary hypertension, right ventricular hypertrophy). The **c wave** is a positive wave caused by right ventricular contraction in systole causing bulging of the TV into the right atrium, producing increased pressure in the atrium and jugular vein. It correlates with the S_1 heart sound and the upstroke of the carotid pulse. The **x wave** is a large negative wave occupying most of systole. It is caused by downward displacement of the TV when blood is ejected out of the right ventricle into the pulmonary artery. The **v wave** is a positive wave that correlates with right atrial filling in systole when the TV is closed. The peak of the v wave marks the end of systole and beginning of diastole. A **giant c-v wave** occurs in TV regurgitation as blood refluxes back into the right atrium during systole. The **y wave** is a negative wave occupying most of diastole. It is due to opening of the TV with rapid flow of blood into the right ventricle in diastole.

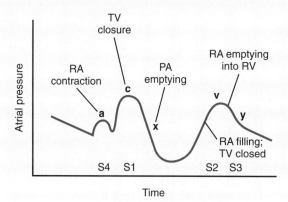

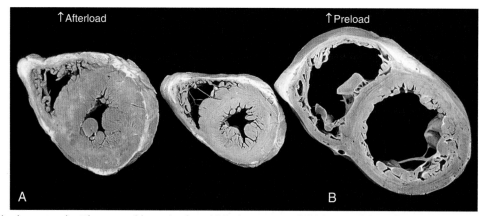

11-1: Left ventricular hypertrophy. The normal heart in the middle has a normal thickness of the left ventricle (LV). The heart on the left **(A)** has concentric hypertrophy of the left ventricle that is related to an increase in afterload, and the heart on the right **(B)** has eccentric hypertrophy of the left ventricle that is related to an increase in preload. *(Reproduced with permission from Allen HD, Driscoll DJ, Shaddy RE, Feltes TF [eds]: Moss and Adams Heart Disease in Infants, Children, and Adolescents: Including the Fetus and Young Adults, 7th ed, Philadelphia, Williams & Wilkins, 2008, Fig. 1.12B.)*

f. Causes of eccentric hypertrophy of the right ventricle (RV) due to increased preload include tricuspid valve (TV) and PV regurgitation.

C. **Consequences of ventricular hypertrophy**
   1. Left- and right-sided heart failure (LHF, RHF discussed later)
      a. Excess work is imposed on the ventricles (LVH and/or RVH).
      b. Excess work is caused by either an increase in afterload or an increase in preload.
   2. Angina pectoris (AP; chest pain) with exercise (only a complication of LVH; discussed later)
      a. In the normal LV, the subendocardium receives the least amount of blood from the coronary arteries (CAs).
      b. Therefore, if the muscle is concentrically thickened, angina may occur with exercise because the muscle wall is so thick that the subendocardium tissue receives dangerously low levels of O_2, causing chest pain. Recall that with exercise, the heart rate (HR) increases, which decreases the time for diastole and the filling of the CAs. Therefore, there is even less blood flow to the subendocardium.
   3. Pathologic S_4 heart sound is commonly present in either LVH and/or RVH.
      a. Abnormal heart sound that correlates with atrial contraction in late diastole. S_4 heart sound produces an atrial gallop (see Box 11-1).
      b. Caused by blood entering a noncompliant ventricle (problem in filling the ventricle)
         (1) Noncompliant ventricle is present in concentric hypertrophy involving the LV and/or RV.
         (2) Noncompliant ventricle is also present in left- and/or right-sided eccentric hypertrophy because the ventricles are volume overloaded and resist receiving more blood in late diastole.
      c. Examples of a noncompliant ventricle producing an S_4 heart sound include:
         (1) concentric LVH in primary HTN or AV stenosis ($\uparrow$afterload).
         (2) concentric RVH in pulmonary hypertension (PH) or PV stenosis ($\uparrow$afterload).
         (3) eccentric hypertrophy from volume overload in MV or TV regurgitation ($\uparrow$preload).
         (4) eccentric hypertrophy from volume overload in AV or PV regurgitation ($\uparrow$preload).
   4. Pathologic S_3 heart sound is commonly present in either left- or right-sided eccentric hypertrophy.
      a. S_3 heart sound is caused by blood entering a volume overloaded chamber in early diastole (see Box 11-1). An analogy is the Mississippi River emptying into the Gulf of Mexico. The water is very turbulent where the two bodies of water meet.
      b. Examples of volume overloaded ventricles producing an S_3 heart sound include:
         (1) volume overload in MV or TV regurgitation.
         (2) volume overload in AV or PV regurgitation.

III. **Congestive Heart Failure (CHF)**
   A. **Definition:** CHF is a heart that fails when it is unable to eject blood delivered to it by the venous system. The inferior vena cava (IVC) empties blood into the right atrium (RA), and the pulmonary vein empties blood into the left atrium (LA).
   B. **Epidemiology**
      1. CHF is the most common hospital admission diagnosis for those >65 years of age.
      2. Types of CHF include:
         a. LHF (most common type).
         b. RHF.
         c. biventricular heart failure (LHF and RHF).
         d. high-output heart failure (HOF; least common heart failure).
      3. Blood builds up behind the failed ventricle.
         a. In LHF, blood backs up into the lungs (pulmonary congestion).
         b. In RHF, blood builds up in the systemic venous system (vena cava and its tributaries).
   C. **LHF**
      1. **Definition:** In LHF, the LV cannot efficiently eject blood into the aorta (Ao), causing blood to backup into the lungs ("blood builds up behind the failed heart").
         a. Causes an increase in the LVEDV and left ventricular end-diastolic pressure (LVEDP; hydrostatic pressure)
         b. Backup of blood into the lungs produces pulmonary edema (see Chapter 5).
      2. Pathogenesis of LHF.
         a. Decrease in LV contraction
            (1) Decreased LV contraction defines systolic heart failure (SHF).
               (a) SHF is the most common type of LHF.
               (b) Some clinicians use the term *systolic dysfunction* rather than SHF.

Marginal notes:

Eccentric RVH: TV/PV regurgitation

LHF and RHF
Excess work LV/RV
$\uparrow$Afterload and/or $\uparrow$preload
AP with exercise
Subendocardium least amount blood flow

Thick muscle less blood to subendocardium
$\uparrow$HR, $\downarrow$diastole, $\downarrow$filling CAs, $\downarrow$blood to subendocardium

S_4: LVH and/or RVH

S_4 abnormal sound late diastole

S_4 blood entering noncompliant ventricle

Noncompliant ventricle: concentric hypertrophy LV/RV

Noncompliant ventricle: eccentric hypertrophy LV/RV

S_4: concentric LVH: PH, AV stenosis

S_4: concentric RVH: PH, PV stenosis

S_4: eccentric MV/TV regurgitation

S_4: eccentric AV/PV regurgitation

Pathologic S_3

S_3: blood entering volume overloaded ventricle(s)

MV/TV regurgitation

MV/PV regurgitation

Congestive heart failure

Heart fails if unable to eject blood from venous system

MCC hospital admission persons >65 years old

LHF MC
RHF
LHF + RHF
HOF least common
Blood builds up behind failed ventricle
LHF: blood backs up into lungs
RHF: blood backs up into venous system
LHF: blood backs up into lungs
$\uparrow$LVEDV, $\uparrow$LVEDP
LHF $\rightarrow$ pulmonary edema

$\downarrow$LV contraction $\rightarrow$ SHF
SHF MC type LHF
SHF, systolic dysfunction same

Ischemia MCC SHF
SHF: post-MI, myocarditis, dilated cardiomyopathy
Stiff ventricle with impaired relaxation → DHF
↑LVEDP
DHF, diastolic dysfunction same
Causes DHF
Concentric hypertrophy from 1° HTN MCC DHF
AV stenosis, HCM, restrictive cardiomyopathy

(2) Causes of SHF include:
   (a) ischemia caused by atherosclerosis of the CAs (most common cause of SHF).
   (b) post–myocardial infarction (MI), myocarditis, and dilated cardiomyopathy.
  b. Noncompliant LV (stiff ventricle) with impaired relaxation
   (1) Noncompliant LV with impaired relaxation defines diastolic heart failure (DHF).
    (a) Increased LVEDP (*not* volume)
    (b) Some clinicians use the term *diastolic dysfunction* rather than DHF.
   (2) Causes of DHF include:
    (a) concentric LVH due to primary HTN is the most common cause of DHF.
    (b) other causes include AV stenosis, HCM, and restrictive cardiomyopathy (amyloidosis or glycogenosis).

Systolic heart failure (SHF) is characterized by a low ejection fraction (EF <40%; some clinicians use <50%). The EF equals the SV divided by LVEDV. The normal value ranges from 55% to 80%. **Diastolic heart failure (DHF)** is characterized by a normal EF (>60%) at *rest*. In addition, there is usually an S_4 atrial gallop because of increased resistance to filling in late diastole. There is an increase in left atrial and LVEDP. Pulmonary congestion commonly occurs when the heart cannot meet the metabolic demands of peripheral tissue (e.g., when the patient exercises) at which point the EF is decreased.

EF = SV/LVEDV; SHF: ↓EF; DHF: normal EF at rest

Lungs heavy, congested

Alveoli filled with transudate/ "heart failure" cells

3. Gross and microscopic findings in LHF
  a. Lungs are heavy and congested and exude a frothy pink transudate (edema) on the cut surface or in the airways.
  b. Alveoli are filled with a pink-staining fluid (Fig. 11-2 A; Links 11-9 and 11-10) and alveolar macrophages (MPs) often contain hemosiderin ("HF," heart failure cells).
   (1) Presence of hemosiderin implies that the pulmonary capillaries ruptured under pressure and red blood cells (RBCs) entering the alveoli were phagocytosed by alveolar MPs.

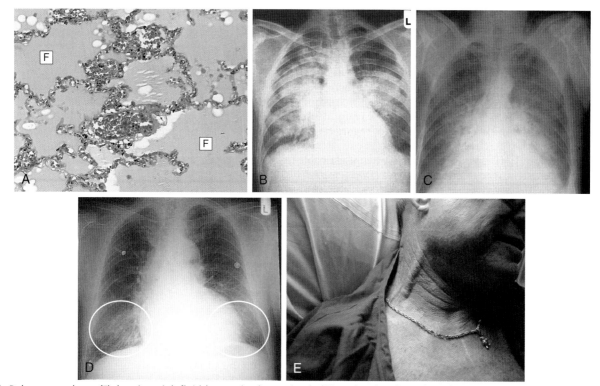

11-2: A, Pulmonary edema *(F)* showing pink fluid (transudate) completely filling the alveoli. **B,** Chest frontal radiograph showing pulmonary edema. Note the fluffy alveolar infiltrates ("bat-wing" or "angel wing" configuration) throughout both lung fields. Careful observation in the opaque fluffy infiltrates shows air bronchograms (lucent areas around opaque regions). **C,** Pulmonary edema with "ground-glass" appearance of alveolar edema. **D,** Kerley B lines (septal edema; circles) in both lower lobes in a patient with pulmonary edema. **E,** Distention of the internal jugular vein. The patient has right-sided heart failure. *(A from Stevens A, Lowe J, Scott I: Core Pathology, 3rd ed, Mosby Elsevier, 2009, p 172, Fig. 10.33; B from Walker BR, Colledge NR, Ralston SH, Penman ID: Davidson's Principles and Practice of Medicine, 22nd ed, St. Louis, Churchill Livingstone Elsevier, 2014, p 482, Fig. 17.11; C from Ashar BH, Miller RG, Sisso SD: The Johns Hopkins Internal Medicine Board Review, 4th ed, St. Louis, Elsevier, 2012, p 53, Fig. 6-3A. Taken from Haslett C, Chilvers ER: Davidson's Principles and Practice of Medicine, 19th ed, Philadelphia, Churchill Livingstone, 2003, Fig. 12.22A; D from Forbes CD, Jackson WF: Color Atlas and Text of Clinical Medicine, 3rd ed, St. Louis, Mosby, 2003 p 223, Fig. 5.97; E from http://courses.cvcc.vccs.edu/WisemcmDIjugular.)*

(2) Excess iron in the macrophage binds to ferritin, which degrades into hemosiderin (rust-colored granules with hematoxylin and eosin stain or blue with Prussian blue stain), producing a rust-colored sputum (Link 11-11).

4. Clinical and laboratory findings in LHF include:
   a. difficulty with breathing (dyspnea).
      (1) **Definition:** In dyspnea, the patient has difficulty with breathing because she or he *cannot* take a full inspiration.
      (2) Interstitial fluid stimulates the juxtacapillary (J) receptors that are innervated by the vagus nerve, the latter inhibiting the patient from taking a full inspiration.
   b. pulmonary edema.
      (1) An increase in LVEDV and pressure leads to a backup of blood into the pulmonary veins and pulmonary capillaries.
         (a) When pulmonary capillary hydrostatic pressure is greater than the oncotic pressure (OP), fluid (a transudate) enters the interstitial space and then the alveoli, producing pulmonary edema (see Chapter 5; see Fig. 11-2 A; Link 11-9, left schematic).
         (b) Peribronchiolar edema narrows the small airways and produces expiratory wheezing (called cardiac asthma).
      (2) Bibasilar (base of the lungs) inspiratory crackles (rales) are present.
         (a) Inspiratory crackles are caused by air expanding alveoli filled with fluid.
         (b) Rust-colored sputum (Links 11-10 and 11-11). Hemorrhage into the alveoli from increased hydrostatic pressure in the pulmonary capillaries results in the phagocytosis of the extravasated RBCs by alveolar MPs. The MPs break hemoglobin down into hemosiderin (called heart failure cells).
      (3) Chest radiograph findings in LHF include:
         (a) congestion in the upper lobes (early finding).
         (b) perihilar congestion ("bat-wing configuration" or "angel-wing configuration"; Fig. 11-2 B).
         (c) fluffy ("ground glass") alveolar infiltrates (Fig. 11-2 C).
         (d) Kerley B lines (septal edema; Fig. 11-2 D).
         (e) air bronchograms (air is visible in the small airways because fluid surrounds the airways).
   c. left-sided S_3 (first cardiac sign of LHF) and S_4 heart sounds (see Box 11-1). Excess fluid in the LV produces the S_3 heart sound, and the increased left-ventricular end-diastolic pressure produces the S_4 heart sound.
   d. functional MV regurgitation. Stretching of the MV ring by the increased LVEDV causes a regurgitant murmur. This is why it is called functional MV regurgitation. When the LVEDV is normalized with treatment, the murmur disappears.
   e. paroxysmal nocturnal dyspnea (PND).
      (1) **Definition:** PND refers to a choking sensation that occurs at night when the patient is supine.
      (2) Without the effect of gravity, fluid from the interstitial space moves into the vascular compartment.
      (3) This increases venous return to the right side of the heart and then to the failed left side of the heart.
      (4) The failed left heart cannot handle the excess load, and blood backs up into the lungs, producing dyspnea and pulmonary edema.
      (5) Dyspnea is relieved by standing or placing pillows under the head (called pillow orthopnea).
         (a) Both standing and raising the head on pillows increase gravity, which reduces venous return to the heart (decreases preload).
         (b) The number of pillows that causes symptomatic relief should be quantitated (e.g., three-pillow orthopnea is worse than one-pillow orthopnea).
   f. Serum B-type natriuretic peptide (BNP) is increased.
      (1) **Definition:** BNP is a cardiac neurohormone secreted from the ventricles when they are stretched because of volume overload (see Chapter 5).
      (2) BNP is useful in:
         (a) diagnosing LHF (BNP increased).
         (b) excluding LHF (BNP normal).
         (c) predicting survival (remains high; bad prognostic sign).
      (3) Serum atrial natriuretic peptide (ANP) is also increased in LHF because of left atrial dilation.

LHF: heart failure cells; alveolar MPs with hemosiderin

LHF: dyspnea

Dyspnea: cannot take full inspiration

LHF: pulmonary edema

Pulmonary edema: pulmonary capillary HP > OP

Cardiac asthma: peribronchiolar edema

Bibasilar inspiratory crackles (edema)

Rust-colored sputum

MPs with hemosiderin→ heart failure cells

Chest x-ray LHF

Congestion upper lungs (early)

Perihilar congestion ("bat-wing")

Fluffy alveolar infiltrates

Kerley lines (septal edema)

Air bronchograms

Left-sided S_3: 1st sign LHF

S_4: ↑LVEDP

LHF: functional MV regurgitation

Paroxysmal nocturnal dyspnea (PND)

Choking sensation at night with patient supine

Supine: ↑venous return to right/failed left side heart

Failed left heart → dyspnea, pulmonary edema

Dyspnea relieved: standing/pillows under head ("pillow orthopnea")

Pillows ↑gravitational effect → ↓venous return to right heart

↑Serum BNP

BNP: cardiac neurohormone

Released when ventricles stretched (volume overload)

Dx LHF (↑BNP)

Exclude LHF (normal BNP)

Predict survival (high bad sign)

↑Serum ANP: left atrial dilation in LHF

D. Right-sided heart failure (RHF)
1. **Definition:** RHF occurs when the RV cannot effectively pump venous blood into the lungs.
   a. Blood pools under pressure in the venous system (blood builds up behind the failed heart).
   b. RHF results in an increase in venous hydrostatic pressure.
2. Pathogenesis (Link 11-12)
   a. *One mechanism* involves an increase in right ventricular afterload caused by increased resistance to blood flow out of the RV into the lungs. This occurs because of increased pressure in the pulmonary vasculature (e.g., pulmonary artery [PA] and pulmonary capillaries). Examples: LHF (most common cause of RHF), PA HTN, PV stenosis, saddle embolus (see Chapters 5 and 17)
   b. A second mechanism is a decrease in right ventricular contraction. Examples: right ventricular infarction, myocarditis
   c. A *third mechanism* involves noncompliance of the RV (it cannot fill properly). Examples: restrictive cardiomyopathy (e.g., amyloidosis or glycogenosis), concentric RVH
   d. An increase in RV preload that increases work in pumping blood out of the RV into the PA is a *fourth mechanism*. Examples: TV and/or PV regurgitation, LV-to-RV shunt (e.g., ventricular septal defect [VSD])
3. Clinical and laboratory findings
   a. Distention of the internal jugular veins (JVs; Fig. 11-2 E; Link 11-9 right). Due to an increased volume of blood in the venous system behind the failed right ventricle.
   b. Tricuspid valve regurgitation. This is due to stretching of the tricuspid valve ring from right ventricle volume overload.
   c. Right-sided S₃ and S₄ heart sounds are present (summation gallop rhythm; Box 11-1). Both heart sounds are due to volume overload of the right ventricle.
   d. Painful hepatomegaly
      (1) Due to centrilobular hemorrhagic necrosis (CHN)
         (a) Systemic venous blood backs up into the hepatic veins and then into the central venules, which expand with blood and cause hepatic cell necrosis in zone III hepatocytes (see Chapter 2; see Fig. 19-5 B and Link 11-13).
         (b) Serum transaminases (aspartate aminotransferase [AST] and alanine aminotransferase [ALT] are markedly increased; see Chapter 19).
         (c) The increase in pressure is transmitted into the sinusoids of the liver and eventually the portal vein. An increase in portal vein (PV) pressure produces ascites (see Chapters 5 and 19).
      (2) Compression of the congested liver increases jugular neck vein distention (hepatojugular reflux).
   e. Dependent pitting edema (see Fig. 5-3 C; Link 11-14). Due to an increase in the venous hydrostatic pressure (HP; see Chapter 5).
   f. Cyanosis of the mucous membranes
      (1) Cyanosis (bluish discoloration of the skin) is more likely to occur in right-sided heart failure than LVHF.
      (2) Backup of blood in the venous system in RHF increases time that is available for peripheral tissue to extract O₂, which decreases O₂ saturation (SaO₂) enough to produce cyanosis (see Chapter 2).

E. High output failure (HOF)
1. **Definition.** High-output failure is a type of heart failure in which cardiac output (CO) is increased compared with values for the normal resting state, causing the heart to overwork and leading to heart failure.
2. Pathogenesis
   a. Increase in stroke volume (SV). Example: hyperthyroidism
   b. Decrease in blood viscosity. A decrease in blood viscosity decreases peripheral vascular resistance (PVR), which increases venous return to the heart. Example: severe anemia (e.g., sickle cell anemia)
   c. Vasodilation of the peripheral vascular resistant (PVR) arterioles
      (1) Vasodilation increases venous return to the heart. An analogy is opening all the flood gates in a dam to release water into a river.
      (2) Examples: thiamine deficiency (decreased adenosine triphosphate [ATP] synthesis; see Chapter 8), early phase of endotoxic shock (increased release of nitric oxide; see Chapter 5)

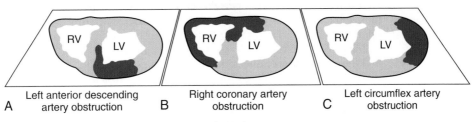

Posterior

A	B	C
Left anterior descending artery obstruction	Right coronary artery obstruction	Left circumflex artery obstruction

Anterior

11-3: Distribution of the coronary arteries. **A,** The distribution of an infarction in a left anterior descending coronary artery thrombosis. **B,** The distribution of an infarction in a right coronary artery thrombosis. **C,** The distribution of an infarction in a left circumflex coronary artery occlusion. *LV,* Left ventricle; *RV,* right ventricle. *(Modified from my friend Ivan Damjanov MD, PhD: Pathology for the Health-Related Professions, 2nd ed, Philadelphia, Saunders, 2000, p 154, Fig. 7-15.)*

    d. Arteriovenous fistula (Link 11-15)

       (1) **Definition:** Arteriovenous communications bypass the microcirculation (arterioles, capillaries, venules), causing increased venous return to the heart, ultimately resulting in heart failure.

       (2) Causes include trauma from a knife wound (most common cause), surgical shunt for hemodialysis, and mosaic bone in Paget disease (see Chapter 24).

IV. Ischemic Heart Disease (IHD)

  A. Definition. IHD is an imbalance between myocardial O_2 demand and supply from the CAs.

  B. Coronary artery (CA) blood flow

    1. CAs provide O_2 to cardiac muscle (Link 11-4).

      a. CAs normally fill during diastole.

      b. HR in excess of 180 beats/min limits filling of the CAs, potentially resulting in ischemia.

    2. Left anterior descending (LAD) CA (Fig. 11-3 A)

      a. Distribution of the LAD CA includes the anterior portion of the LV, anterior two-thirds of the interventricular septum (IVS), and the apex of the heart.

      b. LAD CA is the site for 40% to 50% of CA thromboses.

    3. Right coronary artery (RCA) (Fig. 11-3 B)

      a. Distribution of the RCA includes the:

       (1) posterobasal wall of the LV.

       (2) posterior third of the IVS. Sometimes perfused by the left circumflex CA.

       (3) RV (80% of individuals).

       (4) posteromedial papillary muscle in the LV.

       (5) atrioventricular and sinoatrial (SA) nodes.

      b. RCA is the site for 30% to 40% of CA thromboses.

    4. Left circumflex coronary artery (LCCA; Fig. 11-3 C); supplies the lateral wall of the LV in 80% of individuals and is the site for 15% to 20% of CA thromboses

    5. Slow reduction in blood flow (e.g., atherosclerotic narrowing of vessels) may lead to the formation of a collateral circulation. Well-established collateral circulation has a protective effect on preventing an acute myocardial infarction (AMI).

  C. Epidemiology of IHD

    1. IHD is the major COD in the United States.

      a. More common in men than women

      b. Incidence peaks in men after age 60 years and in women after age 70 years.

    2. Types of IHD include angina pectoris (AP; MC type), chronic ischemic heart disease (CIHD), sudden cardiac death (SCD), and AMI.

    3. Risk factors include:

      a. age.

       (1) Men ≥45 years old and women ≥55 years old are at risk.

       (2) Age is the most important risk factor for IHD.

      b. family history of premature coronary artery disease (CAD) or stroke.

      c. lipid abnormalities.

       (1) Low-density lipoprotein (LDL) >160 mg/dL

       (2) High-density lipoprotein (HDL) <40 mg/dL

       (3) Increased lipoprotein a (LPa) (see Chapter 10)

      d. smoking tobacco, hypertension (HTN), diabetes mellitus (DM)

Margin notes:

Arteriovenous fistula

Arteriovenous communications by-pass microcirculation

Knife wound, surgical shunt, mosaic bone Paget disease

Ischemic heart disease

IHD: imbalance in demand of O_2 and supply

CAs fill in diastole

Tachycardia ↓ diastole → ↓ filling CAs

LAD: Anterior portion LV; anterior 2/3^{rds} IVS; apex

LAD CA MC site CA thrombosis

RCA

Posterobasal wall LV

Posterior 1/3rd IVS

Right ventricle

Posteromedial papillary muscle LV

SA/AV nodes

LCCA

Lateral wall LV

Reduction CA blood flow → collateral circulation

Collateral circulation protective against AMI

Major COD in U.S.

Men > women

Angina pectoris MC IHD

CHID, SCD, AMI

Age; men ≥45 years old

Women ≥55 years old

Age most important risk factor IHD

Family Hx CAD/stroke

Lipid abnormalities

LDL >160 mg/dL

HDL <40 mg/dL

↑LPa

Smoking, HTN, DM

Angina pectoris

Substernal chest pain with/
without exertion

MC middle aged/older men

Women after menopause

Chronic angina pectoris

MC variant of angina

Imbalance myocardial O_2
supply and demand
(exercise/stress)

Causes chronic angina
pectoris

Fixed atherosclerotic CAD
MCC

One/more vessels
obstructed

Stenosis >70%

AV stenosis/HTN with
concentric LVH

Hypertrophic
cardiomyopathy

Cocaine-induced CA VC

Inadequate CA flow
reserve; endothelial
dysfunction

Subendocardial ischemia:
↓CA blood flow/concentric
hypertrophy

Exercise-induced substernal
chest pain 30 sec to 30 min

Intercourse, climbing stairs,
stress

SOB, pain left inner arm/
shoulder/jaw

Relieved by resting,
nitroglycerin

Stress test: ST-segment
depression >1 mm

Prinzmetal variant angina

Intermittent CA vasospasm
rest with/without CAAD

↑TXA_2, endothelin

Stress test: ST-segment
elevation

Unstable angina

Severe, fixed multivessel
disease; disrupted plaques
→ AMI

Multivessel CA disease/
disrupted plaques,
+/- platelet non-occlusive
thrombi

D. Angina pectoris (AP)
1. **Definition of AP:** Angina pectoris is substernal chest pain with or without exertion that is most often caused by coronary artery (CA) atherosclerosis.
2. Epidemiology
   a. Most common in middle-aged and older men
   b. Women are usually affected after menopause.
   c. Within 1 year of a diagnosis of stable angina, 10% to 20% of people will develop an AMI or unstable angina.
3. Chronic (stable) AP (chronic CAD).
   a. Chronic AP is the most common variant of angina.
   b. Fundamental problem in chronic AP is an imbalance between myocardial oxygen supply and demand. Symptoms are more likely to occur during periods of exercise or stress.
   c. Causes include:
      (1) fixed, atherosclerotic CAD (most common cause).
         (a) One or more vessels are obstructed.
         (b) Severity of stenosis is usually >70%.
      (2) Aortic valve (AV) stenosis or HTN with concentric LVH. The O_2 supply is *not* adequate for the thickened muscle wall.
      (3) Hypertropic cardiomyopathy (HCM) (see later discussion).
      (4) cocaine-induced CA vasoconstriction (VC).
      (5) inadequate CA flow reserve caused by endothelial dysfunction (i.e., insufficient vasodilatory response during exercise or stress).
   d. Pathogenesis includes subendocardial ischemia caused by decreased CA blood flow (most common cause) or a thick muscle wall (concentric hypertrophy).
   e. Clinical findings
      (1) Exercise-induced substernal chest pain lasting 30 seconds to 30 minutes
      (2) Other precipitating events include sexual intercourse, climbing stairs, eating a heavy meal, emotional stress, and cold temperature.
      (3) Often accompanied by shortness of breath (SOB), diaphoresis, numbness, and pain in the left inner arm, shoulder, or jaw
      (4) Relieved by resting or nitroglycerin
      (5) Stress test shows ST-segment depression >1 mm (Fig. 11-4).
4. Prinzmetal variant angina.
   a. **Definition:** Intermittent CA vasospasm at rest with or without superimposed coronary artery atherosclerotic disease (CAAD)
   b. Pathogenesis
      (1) In some cases, vasoconstriction may be caused by an increase in thromboxane A_2 (TXA_2) originating from platelets within a thrombus overlying an atherosclerotic plaque or, in 10% of cases, a thrombus *not* overlying an atherosclerotic plaque.
      (2) endothelin (vasoconstrictor).
   c. Stress test in Prinzmetal angina shows ST-segment elevation (transmural ischemia).
5. Unstable angina (UA).
   a. **Definition:** UA is a type of angina with severe, fixed multivessel CAD with disrupted atherosclerotic plaques that may progress to an AMI.
   b. Pathogenesis
      • Multivessel CAAD and disrupted plaques, with or without platelet non-occlusive thrombi

11-4: Electrocardiogram with ST-segment depression. Tracing in **A** is the patient at rest. *1*, The PQ junction (baseline reference); *2*, the J point, where the QRS complex joins the ST segment; *3*, the ST segment 80 msec from the PQ point. Tracing in **B** shows the amount of ST-segment depression measured 80 msec past the J point is 4 mm. *(From Goldman L, Ausiello D: Cecil's Textbook of Medicine, 23rd ed, Philadelphia, Saunders Elsevier, 2008, p 481, Fig. 70-2.)*

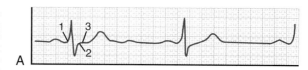

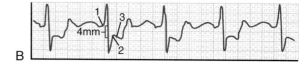

c. Clinical findings
   (1) Frequent bouts of chest pain occur at rest or with minimal exertion.
   (2) May progress to an AMI
6. Diagnostic tests for AP include:
   a. resting electrocardiogram (ECG).
   b. exercise test with ECG monitoring alone (without imaging).
   c. stress echocardiography (ECHO) or stress testing with myocardial perfusion imaging.
   d. computed tomography (CT) calcium scoring.
      (1) High scores (>75%) are associated with an increased risk of MI and death.
      (2) If the calcium score is intermediate or high, computed tomographic coronary angiography (CTCA) is the next step (Link 11-16).
   e. Coronary angiography confirms lesions demonstrated by CTCA. If angiography confirms the findings demonstrated by CTCA, an interventional cardiologist may proceed to angioplasty or stent, provide a referral for a revascularization bypass, or recommend close observation of the patient (Link 11-17).
   f. Magnetic resonance (MR) myocardial viability study is useful for demonstrating wall motion abnormalities and can differentiate a "stunned" myocardium (see previous discussion) from nonviable myocardium.
   g. Fluorodeoxyglucose positron emission tomography (FDG-PET) viability study can also be used to identify a "stunned" myocardium from a nonviable myocardium.

E. **Chronic ischemic heart disease (CIHD)**
   1. **Definition:** Refers to progressive CHF resulting from long-term ischemic damage to myocardial tissue
   2. Pathogenesis: caused by replacement of myocardial tissue with noncontractile scar tissue
   3. Clinical findings include:
      a. biventricular CHF (i.e., left and right-sided CHF).
      b. AP.
      c. evolution into a dilated cardiomyopathy.

F. **Acute myocardial infarction (AMI)**
   1. **Definition:** Refers to an acute onset of severe chest pain most often associated with occlusion of one or more CAs that leads to coagulation necrosis of myocardial tissue

The term **acute coronary artery syndromes (ACASs)** includes unstable angina (already discussed), non–ST-segment elevation myocardial infarction (NSTEMI) and ST-segment elevation myocardial infarction (STEMI). The common denominator in each of these syndromes is rupture of an atherosclerotic plaque leading to platelet aggregation and the formation of an intracoronary thrombosis (Link 11-18, *bottom*). Unlike chronic stable angina (previously discussed) in which symptoms occur with exertion, an ACAS is characterized by abrupt symptoms while at rest. Other symptoms include chest pain or pressure, shortness of breath (dyspnea), nausea, vomiting, diaphoresis (sweating), and radiation of the pain to the left arm, neck, or jaw.

2. Epidemiology
   a. Most common COD in adults in the United States
   b. Prominent in men between 40 and 65 years old
   c. At least 25% of AMIs are clinically unrecognized.
3. Pathogenesis
   a. Sequence for developing an AMI
      (1) An atheromatous plaque is suddenly disrupted (Fig. 10-5 B; Link 10-10).
      (2) Subendothelial collagen and thrombogenic necrotic material are exposed.
      (3) Platelets adhere to the exposed material and eventually form an occlusive platelet thrombus held together by fibrin.
   b. Role of throboxane A2 (TXA$_2$) in an AMI (see Chapter 15)
      (1) TXA$_2$ causes platelet aggregation, thus contributing to the formation of the platelet thrombus.
      (2) In addition, it acts as vasoconstrictor and causes vasospasm of the artery to reduce blood flow.
4. Less common causes AMI include:
   a. vasculitis (e.g., polyarteritis nodosa, Kawasaki disease; see Chapter 10).
   b. cocaine use (the CAs are normal).
   c. embolization of plaque material from the aorta (Ao) or CA.
   d. thrombosis syndromes (see Chapter 15). Examples of thrombosis syndromes: antithrombin III deficiency, polycythemia vera (PV)

Frequent bouts chest pain at rest/minimal exertion

May progress to AMI

Diagnostic tests

Resting ECG

Exercise test with ECG monitoring

Stress ECHO or stress with myocardial perfusion imaging

CT with calcium scoring

CTCA

Coronary angiography confirmatory

MR myocardial viability study: "stunned" vs nonviable myocardium

FDG-PET: "stunned" vs nonviable myocardium

CIHD

Progressive CHF due to ischemic myocardial damage

Muscle replaced by noncontractile scar tissue

Biventricular CHF

Angina pectoris

CHID → dilated cardiomyopathy

Acute myocardial infarction

Acute, severe chest pain; occlusion 1/more CAs → coagulation necrosis

ACAS

UA, NSTEMI, STEMI; ruptured plaque; thrombosis; symptoms at rest

MCC adult death in U.S.

Men 40–60 yrs old

25% AMI unrecognized

Sequence AMI

Disrupted atheromatous plaque

Collagen/thrombogenic necrotic debris exposed

Occlusive platelet thrombus

TXA$_2$ important in platelet thrombus

Polyarteritis nodosa, Kawasaki disease

Cocaine: AMI with normal CAs

Embolization Ao, CA

ATIII deficiency, PV

Revascularization
procedure, aortic dissection

STEMI

>80% have occlusion CA

Full thickness

New Q waves

↑Cardiac enzymes

High hospital mortality; low
reinfarction rate

NSTEMI

30%/40% have occlusion
CA

Subendocardium involved

Q waves absent

↑Cardiac enzymes

Low hospital mortality rate

High reinfarction rate
postdischarge

High 1-yr mortality rate

Ischemia/reperfusion injury
AMI

Reperfusion: spontaneous,
PCI, fibrinolytic Rx

May limit size infarction

Ischemic myocardial cells
not already irreversibly
damaged become so *after*
reperfusion

Timing reperfusion ischemic
tissue important

Myocardial stunning after
reperfusion is reversible

Contraction bands:
calcium-mediated sign
reperfusion.

Previously ischemic cells
become irreversibly
damaged.

Irreversible injury due to
superoxide FRs

Acute inflammation with
neutrophils

Neutrophils occlude
capillary channels

Neutrophils release
proteolytic enzymes/O₂ FRs

Apoptosis, platelet/
complement activation

First 24 hrs

No gross changes

Coagulation necrosis

Entry neutrophils

1 to 3 days

Pallor

Myocyte nuclei/striations
disappear

Abundant neutrophils; lysis

3 to 7 days

Red granulation tissue

MPs remove debris

Heart softest 3–7 days;
danger of rupture

   e. dissection of blood into the wall of a CA. Causes of dissection include revascularization procedures and aortic dissection (see Chapter 10).
 5. Types of AMI include:
    a. <u>ST</u> elevation <u>m</u>yocardial <u>i</u>nfarction (STEMI)
       (1) STEMI: full thickness; Q waves; cardiac enzymes increased
       (2) More than 80% have occlusion of a CA.
       (3) Refers to a full-thickness MI
       (4) New Q waves develop on ECG.
       (5) Cardiac enzymes are increased.
       (6) Associated with a high hospital mortality rate but low reinfarction rate after hospital discharge and a low 1-year mortality rate
    b. <u>Non-ST</u> elevation <u>m</u>yocardial <u>i</u>nfarction (NSTEMI)
       (1) Only 30% to 40% have occlusion of the CA.
       (2) Inner third of the myocardium (subendocardium) is involved.
       (3) Q waves are absent.
       (4) Cardiac enzymes are increased.
       (5) Associated with a low hospital mortality rate but a high reinfarction rate after hospital discharge and a high 1-year mortality rate
 6. Ischemia/reperfusion injury in AMI
    a. Reperfusion may occur spontaneously or, most commonly, after percutaneous coronary intervention (PCI) or thrombolytic (fibrinolytic) therapy.
       (1) Reperfusion may limit the size of the infarction by restoring blood flow (and thus oxygen supply) to previously ischemic tissue.
       (2) Reperfusion may have deleterious effects if ischemic myocardial cells that were *not* irreversibly injured are damaged by reperfusion (called reperfusion injury). Up to 50% of infarction size may be secondary to reperfusion injury.
    b. Effects of reperfusing ischemic tissue depend on when reperfusion occurs.
       (1) If reperfusion occurs <3 hours after cessation of blood flow, there is a greater chance of salvaging ischemic but *not* irreversibly damaged tissue.
          (a) Salvaged tissue is biochemically altered, which may interfere with normal function for several days or longer (called myocardial stunning) and predispose tissue to reperfusion dysrhythmias.
          (b) Reperfusion of previously irreversibly damaged cells results in their death and the formation of contraction bands due to the entry of Ca^{2+} into the cytosol, causing hypercontraction of the myocytes (Fig. 11-5; Link 11-19).
       (2) If reperfusion occurs >3 hours, there is a much greater chance that previously ischemic cells are irreversibly damaged (called reperfusion injury). Overall size of the infarction will increase.
    c. Mechanism of irreversible myocardial injury
       (1) Superoxide free radicals (FRs) are locally produced by xanthine oxidase and irreversibly damage myocytes.
       (2) Acute inflammation occurs with an infiltration of tissue by neutrophils (see Chapter 3).
          (a) Neutrophils occlude capillary lumens, which decreases blood flow to the ischemic tissue.
          (b) Neutrophils release proteolytic enzymes and increase the production of reactive O_2 species (see Chapter 2).
       (3) Other factors that contribute to irreversible myocardial injury include apoptosis (see Chapter 2) as well as platelet and complement system activation.
 7. Gross and microscopic (GM) findings in an AMI:
    a. during the first 24 hours.
       (1) No gross changes are evident until 24 hours.
       (2) Coagulation necrosis is present within 12 to 24 hours.
       (3) Neutrophils begin to enter the area of infarction from the periphery.
    b. from 1 to 3 days.
       (1) Pallor of the infarcted tissue is apparent.
       (2) Myocyte nuclei and striations disappear (Fig. 2-16 A).
       (3) Neutrophils are abundant and contribute to lysis of dead myocardial cells.
    c. during days 3 to 7.
       (1) Red granulation tissue surrounds the area of infarction.
       (2) Macrophages (MPs) begin to remove necrotic debris.
       (3) This period is the most dangerous time for myocardial rupture.

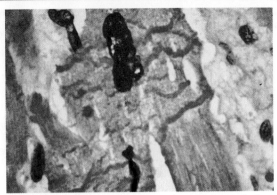

11-5: Contraction bands in cardiac myocytes after reperfusion. *(From my friend Ivan Damjanov MD, PhD: Linder J:* Anderson's Pathology, *10th ed, St. Louis, Mosby, 1996, p 374, Fig. 17.12.)*

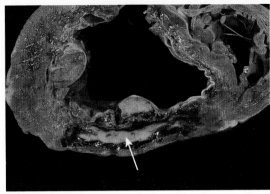

11-6: Acute myocardial infarction (day 7) in the posterior wall of the left ventricle. The yellow area *(arrow)* of necrosis is surrounded by a rim of dark, red granulation tissue. The area of necrosis produces the Q wave in an electrocardiogram *(From my friend Ivan Damjanov MD, PhD, Linder J:* Pathology: A Color Atlas, *St. Louis, Mosby, 2000, p 22, Fig. 1-47.)*

    d. from 7 to 10 days
        (1) Necrotic area is bright yellow (Fig. 11-6; see Fig. 2-16 B).
        (2) Granulation tissue (red rim around the yellow) and collagen formation are well developed.
    e. over the first 2 months
        (1) Infarcted tissue is replaced by white, patchy, noncontractile scar tissue.
        (2) As the amount of scar tissue increases, CIHD is likely to occur (see earlier).
8. Clinical findings of an AMI
    a. Sudden onset of severe, crushing retrosternal pain
        (1) Usually lasts >30 minutes.
        (2) *Not* relieved by nitroglycerin
        (3) Usually radiates down the inner left (most common) or right arm (less common), into the shoulders, or to the jaw or epigastrium (Link 11-20)
            (a) Nerves to the heart are T1 to T5.
            (b) Radiation to the inner arm and shoulder is in the T1 distribution.
            (c) Radiation to the epigastrium is in the T4 to T5 distribution.
        (4) Associated manifestations include sweating (diaphoresis), anxiety, and hypotension.
    b. Peak time of day for an AMI is 0800 to 1100 with a gradual decline from 1100 to 1800.
    c. "Silent" AMIs occur in ~20% of cases.
        (1) More likely in older adults and in individuals with diabetes mellitus (DM), who frequently have neuropathies and cannot feel pain
        (2) Also more likely in those with a high pain threshold
9. Complications of STEMI AMIs (Link 11-21)
    a. Cardiogenic shock occurs in ~7% of cases. Revascularization improves survival.
    b. Arrhythmias
        (1) Premature ventricular contractions (PVCs) are the most common arrhythmia.
        (2) Most common COD is ventricular fibrillation. Frequently associated with cardiogenic shock (see Chapter 5).
        (3) Heart block (Link 11-22). Incidence of 5% of inferior AMIs and in 3% of anterior AMIs
    c. Congestive heart failure (CHF). Typical onset within the first 24 hours
    d. Rupture (Link 11-22)
        (1) Most likely to occur between days 3 and 7 (range, 1–10 days)
        (2) Anterior wall rupture most common (Fig. 11-7)
            (a) Results in cardiac tamponade (Links 11-23 and 11-24)
            (b) Most commonly associated with thrombosis of the LAD CA
        (3) Posteromedial papillary muscle rupture or dysfunction
            (a) Most often associated with inferior AMI s caused by thrombosis of the right CA
            (b) Presents with an acute onset of MV regurgitation and left-sided heart failure (LHF)
        (4) IVS rupture.
            (a) Most often associated with a thrombosis in the LAD CA
            (b) Produces a left-to-right shunt, causing RHF (overloads the RV). Diagnosis is made by finding an increased O_2 saturation and pressure in the RV.

Margin notes:

7 to 10 days
Necrotic area bright yellow
Red rim granulation tissue
Collagen formation
Over first 2 months
Infarcted tissue → white scar tissue
↑↑Scar tissue → danger CIHD
Clinical findings AMI
Retrosternal pain >30 minutes
Pain *not* relieved by nitroglycerin
Radiation inner left arm → shoulders; jaw, epigastrium
Nerves to heart: T1–T5
Inner arm pain: T1 distribution
Epigastrium radiation: T4–T5 distribution
Diaphoresis, anxiety, hypotension
Peak time day: 0800 to 1100
"Silent" AMI
Elderly, DM patients: neuropathies (cannot feel pain)
Patients with high pain threshold
Cardiogenic shock
Arrhythmias
PVCs MC arrhythmia
Ventricular fibrillation MCC death
Heart block
Heart block inferior/anterior AMIs
CHF 1st 24 hours
Rupture
MC 3–7 days
Anterior wall rupture MC
Cardiac tamponade
MC with LAD thrombosis
Posteromedial papillary muscle: rupture/dysfunction
Inferior AMI; RCA thrombosis
Acute-onset MV regurgitation, LHF
IVS rupture
LAD thrombosis MCC
Left-to-right shunt → RHF → ↑O_2 saturation RV

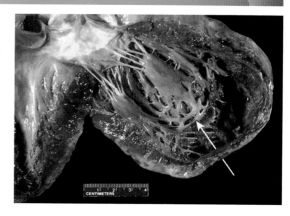

11-7: Acute myocardial infarction (day 7) in the posterior wall of the left ventricle with rupture. The yellow area *(arrow)* is surrounded by a rim of dark, red granulation tissue and is the location of the rupture site. *(From my friend Ivan Damjanov MD, PhD, Linder J: Pathology: A Color Atlas, St. Louis, Mosby, 2000, p 22, Fig. 1-47.)*

e. Mural thrombus
   (1) Occurs in ~10% of AMIs (Link 11-25).
   (2) Most often associated with thrombosis of the LAD CA
   (3) Danger of peripheral embolization (see Chapter 5).
f. Fibrinous pericarditis with or without effusion (see Fig. 3-8 C)
   (1) Most likely to occur during days 1–7 post STEMI
      (a) Presents with substernal chest pain that is relieved by leaning forward and aggravated by leaning backward
      (b) Precordial friction rub is present on auscultation (see later); caused by increased vessel permeability in the pericardium (exudate of acute inflammation [AI])
   (2) Autoimmune pericarditis (Dressler syndrome)
      (a) Typically occurs 1 to 8 weeks after the STEMI
      (b) Caused by autoantibodies directed against antigens within the damaged pericardial tissue (type II hypersensitivity reaction [HSR]; see Chapter 4).
      (c) Fever and a precordial friction rub are present.
g. Ventricular aneurysm (Fig. 11-8; Link 11-26)
   (1) Clinically recognized within 4 to 8 weeks after a STEMI; begins to develop in the first 48 hours
   (2) On physical exam, one detects a precordial bulge that is synchronous with systole. Blood fills up the aneurysm in systole, causing the anterior chest wall movement.
   (3) Complications
      (a) Systolic heart failure (SHF) occurs because of the lack of contractile tissue.
      (b) Clot material may embolize to distant sites.
      (c) Rupture is uncommon. Scar tissue has good tensile strength.
      (d) CHF is the most common COD.
h. Right ventricular AMI
   (1) Associated with RCA thrombosis
   (2) Occurs in one-third of inferior AMIs; clinically significant in 30% of cases
   (3) Clinical findings include hypotension, RHF, and preserved LV function.
10. Laboratory diagnosis of AMI (Fig. 11-9)
   a. Serial testing for creatine kinase isoenzyme MB (CK-MB)
      (1) CK-MB appears within 4 to 8 hours, peaks at 24 hours, and disappears within 1.5 to 3 days (Link 11-27).
         (a) Sensitivity and specificity are 95%.
         (b) May also be increased in myocarditis, muscular dystrophy, rhabdomyolysis (rupture of muscle), and polymyositis (PM). This decreases the test's specificity; however, they are *not* common disorders and are easy to differentiate from an AMI.
      (2) Reinfarction
         (a) **Definition:** Reinfarction refers to the reappearance of cardiac enzymes.
         (b) Reinfarction occurs in 10% of AMIs.
   b. Serial testing for cardiac troponins I (cTnI) and T (cTnT; Link 11-28).
      (1) Troponins normally regulate calcium-mediated muscle contraction.
      (2) cTnI and cTnT appear within 3 to 12 hours, peak at 24 hours, and disappear within 7 to 10 days (Link 11-27).

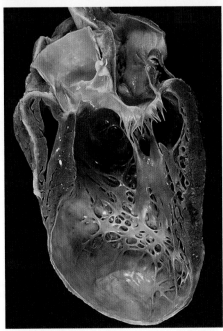

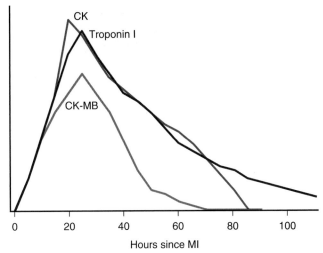

11-9: Typical rise and fall of cardiac biomarkers after an acute myocardial infarction (MI). *CK,* Creatine kinase; *CK-MB,* creatine kinase isoenzyme MB. *(From Carey WD:* Cleveland Clinic: Current Clinical Medicine, *2nd ed, St. Louis, Saunders Elsevier, 2010, p 67, Fig. 3.)*

11-8: Left ventricular aneurysm. The bulging aneurysm has a thin wall of scar tissue. There is very little functioning muscle in the left ventricle, so it is likely that this patient had chronic systolic heart failure and a very low ejection fraction. *(From my friend Ivan Damjanov MD, PhD, Linder J:* Pathology: A Color Atlas, *St. Louis, Mosby, 2000, p 24, Fig. 1-58.)*

   (a) Sensitivity of 84% to 96% and specificity of 80% to 95%

   (b) Troponins may also increase in NSTEMIs, unstable angina, pericarditis, myocarditis, left ventricular hypertrophy (LVH), CHF, and renal failure.

     • Decreases the test's specificity, which is evident in its wide range of specificity

     • Considered the gold standard for diagnosing an AMI

   (c) Troponins can also be used in diagnosing reinfarction. In patients in whom reinfarction is suspected, an immediate measurement of cTnI is recommended. A second sample should be obtained 3 to 6 hours later. If the cTn concentration in the second specimen is increased by 20% or more, then reinfarction is likely.

  (3) In most hospitals, troponins are primarily used to diagnose an AMI. As a practical point, irrespective of the time frames listed previously for the appearance of these markers, neither CK-MB nor troponins consistently appear in the blood within 6 hours of the ischemic event. Hence, serial studies are required to rule out an AMI.

  11. Correlation of ECG changes with pathologic changes (Fig. 11-10; Link 11-29 A, B)

    a. Inverted T waves: correlate with areas of ischemia at the periphery of the infarction

    b. Elevated ST segments: correlate with injured myocardial cells surrounding the area of necrosis

    c. New Q waves: correlate with the area of coagulation necrosis

  12. Classic ECG patterns in AMI

    a. Thrombosis of the LAD CA produces an anterior wall infarction: Q waves in leads V_1–V_2

    b. Anteroseptal AMI is caused by thrombosis of the proximal LAD CA: Q waves in leads V_1–V_2

    c. Anterolateral AMI is caused by a thrombosis of the mid-LAD or thrombosis of the circumflex CA: Q waves in leads V_4–V_6, I, aVL

    d. Lateral wall AMI is caused by thrombosis of the left circumflex CA: Q waves in leads I, aVL

    e. Inferior wall AMI is caused by a thrombosis of the RCA: Q waves in leads II, III, aVF

    f. Link 11-29 B shows the ECG findings in a subendocardial infarction. A subendocardial infarction (Link 11-30) is *not* related to a CA occlusion but rather to generalized hypoperfusion of the heart. Recall that the subendocardium receives the least amount of oxygenated blood from the CAs.

Lack specificity

cTnI, cTnT: gold standard for Dx AMI

Troponins diagnose reinfarction

Most hospitals use troponins

ECG findings in STEMI: inverted T waves, elevated ST segments, Q waves

Inverted T waves: ischemia at periphery of infarct

Elevated ST segments

Injured myocardium surrounding area of necrosis

New Q waves: area coagulation necrosis

Subendocardial infarction

Generalized hypoperfusion; *not* CA occlusion

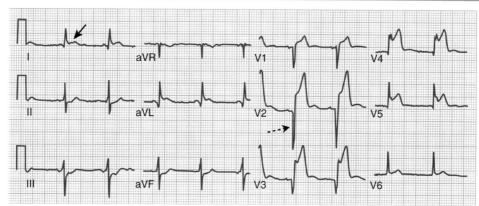

11-10: Electrocardiogram showing an acute anterior myocardial infarction. There is ST-segment elevation in lead 1 *(solid arrow)*, aVL, and V_1, to V_6. Q waves *(interrupted arrow)* are present in leads V_1 to V_4. *(From Goldman L, Ausiello D:* Cecil's Textbook of Medicine, *23rd ed, Philadelphia, Saunders Elsevier, 2008, p 502, Fig. 72-1.)*

<table>
<tr><td>

Sudden cardiac death

Unexpected death within 1 hr post symptoms

Documented/presumed cardiac cause

CIHD major cause

IHD most important risk factor

Obesity, glucose intolerance

↑Lipids, LVH, HTN

Smoking recent NSTEMI

Non-CA causes SCD

Cardiomyopathy

AV stenosis

MVP, cocaine, myocarditis, WWW

SCD children: MCC AV stenosis, cardiomyopathy, WPW

Pathogenesis SCD adults

Lethal arrhythmia MCC: ventricular tachycardia/ fibrillation

CAD *without* occlusive thrombus

Congenital heart disease

Fetal circulation

Chorionic villi: derived from fetus

Chorionic villi: primary site O₂ exchange.

UV: derived from villus vessels

UV: highest PO₂ fetal circulation

IVC: delivers blood to RA

RA blood shunted to LA via PFO

SVC → RA → RV

PA

PA → PDA → Ao

DA open due to PGE₂ (VD)

Fetal pulmonary arteries

Hypertrophied: chronic vc from ↓PO₂

Prevents blood from entering pulmonary capillaries/LA

</td></tr>
</table>

F. **Sudden cardiac death (SCD)**
1. **Definition:** Refers to sudden unexpected death that occurs within 1 hour of symptoms caused by documented or presumed cardiac cause
2. Epidemiology
   a. May be the first manifestation of ischemic heart disease (IHD)
   b. Approximately 70% of sudden natural deaths have a cardiac cause, and 80% of them are attributable to CIHD.
   c. Risk factors
      (1) IHD is the most important risk factor.
      (2) Other factors include obesity, glucose intolerance, hyperlipidemia, LVH, HTN, smoking, or a recent non–Q wave MI (NSTEMI).
   d. Non-CA causes of SCD syndrome include:
      (1) cardiomyopathy (all types; see later).
      (2) Aortic valve (AV) stenosis.
      (3) other causes: mitral valve prolapse (MVP), cocaine, myocarditis, conduction defects (Wolff-Parkinson-White [WPW] syndrome), prolonged QT interval.
   e. Causes of SCD in children include AV stenosis (most common cause), cardiomyopathies (usually hypertrophic type of cardiomyopathy), and WPW syndrome.
3. Pathogenesis of SCD in adults
   a. A lethal arrhythmia is responsible (e.g., ventricular tachycardia/fibrillation) in the majority of cases.
   b. Severe atherosclerotic CAD with disrupted plaques is present at autopsy. Occlusive CA thrombosis is *not* present at autopsy in most cases.

V. **Congenital Heart Disease (CHD)**
A. **Fetal circulation** (Fig. 11-11; Link 11-31).
1. Chorionic villi in the placenta (see Chapter 22). Derived from the fetus. Primary site for O₂ exchange. Umbilical vein is derived from the villus vessels.
2. Umbilical vein (UV)
   a. Vessel with the highest Po₂ in the fetal circulation
   b. *Exception* to the rule; vein, *not* the artery, has the highest Po₂
3. Inferior vena cava (IVC)
   a. Delivers blood into the right atrium (RA)
   b. Most of the blood in the RA is directly shunted into the LA through a patent foramen ovale (PFO; normal in a fetus).
4. Superior vena cava (SVC) blood. Most of the blood from the SVC is directed from the RA into the right ventricle (RV).
5. Pulmonary artery (PA) blood
   a. Blood from the PA is shunted through a patent ductus arteriosus (PDA) into the Ao. Bypasses fetal lungs. Ductus arteriosus (DA) is kept open by prostaglandin E₂, a vasodilator synthesized by the placenta.
   b. Fetal pulmonary arteries
      (1) Hypertrophied from chronic vasoconstriction caused by a decreased Po₂
      (2) Prevents blood from entering the pulmonary capillaries and the left atrium (LA)

6. Descending Ao
   a. Blood flows toward the placenta via two umbilical arteries; increased risk for congenital abnormalities in those with a single umbilical artery (see Chapter 6).
   b. Umbilical arteries have the lowest O_2 concentration. This is an exception to the rule that arteries have the highest O_2 concentration and veins the lowest O_2 concentration.
7. Changes in the fetal circulation at birth
   a. Ductus arteriosus (DA) closes.
      (1) Anatomic closure should occur within 2 to 8 weeks after birth.
      (2) Becomes the ligamentum arteriosum
   b. Gas exchange occurs in the lungs. PA opens up because of the increase in Pao_2.
   c. Foramen ovale (FO) functionally closes in 24 hours. DA closes after birth.

B. Congenital heart disease (CHD)
1. **Definition:** CHD refers to any defect involving the heart or the large arteries and veins at birth.
2. Epidemiology
   a. Most common heart disease in children
   b. Incidence is higher in premature than full-term newborns.
   c. *No* identifiable cause for CHD in ~90% of cases
   d. Most common known causes of CHD are:
      (1) multifactorial inheritance (85% of cases; see Chapter 6).
      (2) primary genetic factors (single-gene disorders, chromosome disorders; [see later], 10% of cases).
      (3) environmental factors (e.g., isotretinoin, alcohol, viruses [rubella], maternal factors; 3%–5% of cases [see later]).
   e. Examples of maternal risk factors include (see Chapter 6):
      (1) increased age (>45 years old).
      (2) previous child with CHD (1:50 chance of having a second child with CHD).
      (3) poorly controlled DM during pregnancy.
         (a) Associated with LV outflow obstruction (e.g., AV stenosis, hypertrophied IVS)
         (b) Associated with transposition of the great arteries and ventricular septal defect (VSD)
      (4) alcohol intake during pregnancy; associated with PV stenosis and VSD.
      (5) congenital infection (e.g., rubella) during pregnancy. Rubella infection is associated with PDA and PV stenosis.
      (6) aspirin intake; associated with the pulmonary HTN (PH) syndrome.
      (7) diphenylhydantoin intake; associated with AV stenosis and PV stenosis.
      (8) systemic lupus erythematosus (SLE); increased risk of complete heart block, pericarditis, and endomyocardial fibrosis.
   f. Spectrum of CHD includes:
      (1) valvular diseases (e.g., PV stenosis).
      (2) shunts (acyanotic and cyanotic types).
   g. Systemic complications of CHD
      (1) Secondary polycythemia (increased number of RBCs) with clubbing of the fingers may occur.
         (a) Occurs in cyanotic types of CHD
         (b) Decreased Pao_2 in cyanotic types of CHD stimulates the release of erythropoietin, which increases RBC production by the bone marrow.
      (2) Increased risk for developing infective endocarditis (IE) before or after corrective surgery
      (3) Metastatic abscesses may occur, particularly in cyanotic CHD.
3. Sao_2 findings that help distinguish cyanotic from noncyanotic shunts
   a. Left-sided to right-sided heart shunts
      (1) Oxygenated blood from the left side of the heart (Sao_2 95%) is mixed with unoxygenated blood on the right (Sao_2 75%).
      (2) Sao_2 is increased in the right side of the heart (step up) from 75% to 80% or more in affected chambers or vessels.
   b. Right-sided to left-sided heart shunts
      (1) Unoxygenated blood from the right side of the heart (Sao_2 75%) is mixed with oxygenated blood on the left side of the heart (Sao_2 95%).
      (2) Sao_2 is decreased in the left side of the heart (step down) from 95% to 80% or less in affected chambers or vessels.
         (a) Whether cyanosis occurs depends on how low the Sao_2 is in the left side of the heart.

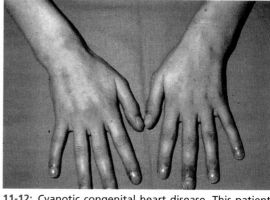

11-12: Cyanotic congenital heart disease. This patient with a ventricular septal defect had reversal of the shunt (Eisenmenger syndrome) and developed cyanosis and clubbing of the nails. *(From Grieg JD:* Color Atlas of Surgical Diagnosis, *London, Mosby-Wolfe, 1996, p 93, Fig. 14-1.)*

11-11: Fetal circulation. The umbilical veins have the highest oxygen content. The ductus venosus shunts most of the blood past the liver, and the foramen ovale and the ductus arteriosus act as shunts to bypass the pulmonary circulation. All of these shunts normally close at or shortly after birth, as do the umbilical vein and distal part of umbilical arteries. *Arrows* indicate blood flow. *(From Moore NA, Roy WA:* Rapid Review Cross and Developmental Anatomy, *3rd ed, Philadelphia, Mosby Elsevier, 2010, p 50, Fig. 2-30.)*

Diagram labels (Fig. 11-11): Superior vena cava, Lung, Foramen ovale, Right atrium, Inferior vena cava, Right hepatic vein, Liver, Portal vein, Umbilical vein, Umbilicus, Placenta, Umbilical arteries, Left hepatic vein, Internal iliac arteries, Urinary bladder, Kidney, Arch of aorta, Ductus arteriosus, Pulmonary trunk, Pulmonary veins, Left atrium, Ductus venosus, Descending aorta. High oxygen saturation, Medium oxygen saturation, Low oxygen saturation.

Margin notes:

SaO$_2$ is >85%: *no* cyanosis
SaO$_2$ <80%: cyanosis present
Left-sided to right-sided shunts
Volume overload right (*no* cyanosis)
PH: due to ↑blood flow PA
RVH: due to PH
PH ↑afterload RV must contract against
Concentric RVH
LVH: more blood returning to left heart
Eccentric type LVH (↑preload)
Shunt reversal due to PH and RVH
Eisenmenger syndrome: cyanosis/clubbing indicates shunt reversal
Tardive cyanosis (late-onset cyanosis)
Ventricular septal defect (VSD)
Defect membranous IVS: left-to-right shunt
VSD MC CHD
~25% CHD in children
Defect membranous portion of IVS MC

(b) If the SaO$_2$ is >85%, cyanosis is *not* present because this indicates that only a small volume of blood was shunted between the two sides of the heart.

(c) If the SaO$_2$ is <80%, cyanosis is present because this indicates that a large volume of blood was shunted between the two sides of the heart.

4. Left-sided to right-sided heart shunts

   a. Causes volume overload in the right side of the heart. Complications include:

    (1) PH caused by increased blood flow through the PA (more work than normal).

    (2) RVH due to PH. PH increases the afterload the RV must contract against to eject blood, causing concentric hypertrophy of the RV (concentric RVH).

    (3) LVH caused by more blood returning to the left heart than normal; increases LV volume (preload), producing an eccentric type of LVH.

    (4) reversal of the shunt due to PH and RVH causes the pressure in the right side of the heart to be greater than the pressure in the left side.

     (a) Signs of reversal of the shunt include cyanosis (called Eisenmenger syndrome) and clubbing of the fingers (Fig. 11-12).

     (b) Another term is tardive cyanosis (late-onset cyanosis).

   b. VSD (Fig. 11-13 A; Link 11-32).

    (1) **Definition:** Refers to a defect in the membranous portion of the IVS causing a left-to-right shunt

    (2) VSD is the most common CHD (30% of all CHDs).

    (3) Accounts for ~25% of CHD in children and ~10% of CHD in adults

    (4) Results from a defect in the membranous part of the IVS (75%–80% of cases), the muscular or trabecular part of the septum (5%–20% of cases), or less commonly, other sites

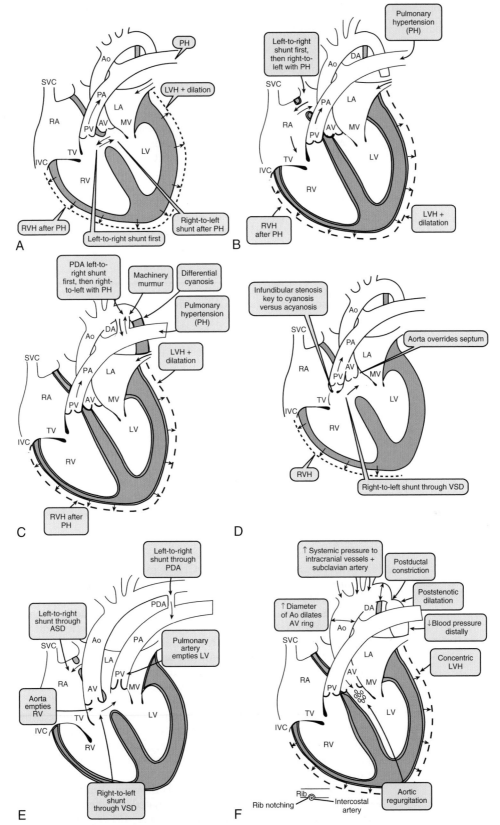

11-13: A, Ventricular septal defect (VSD). **B,** Atrial septal defect (ASD). **C,** Patent ductus arteriosus (PDA). **D,** Tetralogy of Fallot. **E,** Complete transposition of the great vessels. **F,** Postductal coarctation. *Ao,* Aorta; *AV,* aortic valve; *DA,* ductus arteriosus; *IVC,* inferior vena cava; *LA,* left atrium; *LV,* left ventricle; *LVH,* left ventricular hypertrophy; *MV,* mitral valve; *PA,* pulmonary artery; *PH,* pulmonary hypertension; *PV,* pulmonary valve; *RA,* right atrium; *RV,* right ventricle; *RVH,* right ventricular hypertrophy; *SVC,* superior vena cava; *TV,* tricuspid valve. *(**A–F** from Goljan EF: Star Series: Pathology, Philadelphia, Saunders, 1998.)*

LV → RV via patent IVS

↑Blood RV, PA

Step-up SaO$_2$ in RV and PA

Males = females

ASD, PDA, coarctation, subvalvular AV stenosis

Multiple VSDs in ToF

VSD: Cri du chat syndrome, fetal alcohol syndrome

Acquired VSD in AMI involving IVS

Harsh pansystolic murmur

30% to 50% spontaneously close

Lifetime risk IE 5% to 30%

Atrial septal defect (ASD)

Defect FO: left-to-right shunt

Females > males

MC CHD in adults

MCC patent foramen ovale

LA → RA via FO; overload right heart

Step-up SaO$_2$ in RA, RV, PA

Fetal alcohol syndrome, Down syndrome (primum type)

Soft midsystolic murmur

Wide/fixed split of S$_2$

↑Blood right heart takes longer for PV to close

Paradoxical embolism (venous clot in system circulation)

Persistence ductus arteriosus after birth

Patent ductus arteriosus (PDA)

DA connects PA with Ao

Fetus: normal for PDA to shunt blood from PA → Ao to by-pass lungs

Step-up SaO$_2$ in PA

Isolated defect 90% of cases

Congenital rubella, RDS, transposition, tetralogy

Continuous machinery murmur

Reversal of shunt if PH occurs

Unoxygenated blood below subclavian artery

Differential cyanosis (pink on top, blue on bottom)

Right-sided to left-sided shunts

Cyanotic CHD

Tetralogy of Fallot

(a) Blood flows from the LV into the RV through the patent IVS. This leads to an increased amount of blood in the RV and PA.

(b) Step-up (increased) Sao$_2$ in the RV and the PA

(5) Equal frequency in males and females

(6) Associations of VSD with other CHDs include atrial septal defect (ASD; 35% of cases), PDA (22%), coarctation of the Ao (COTA; 17% of cases), and subvalvular AV stenosis (4% of cases).

(7) Multiple VSDs are more likely to be associated with tetralogy of Fallot [ToF]).

(8) Associations of VSDs with other congenital diseases include cri du chat syndrome (see Chapter 6) and fetal alcohol syndrome (see Chapter 6).

(9) VSDs are acquired in an AMI when there is a rupture of the IVS.

(10) In a VSD, a harsh pansystolic murmur is present along the lower left sternal border.

(11) Spontaneously closes in 30% to 50% of cases. Criteria have been established as to whether corrective surgery is necessary.

(12) Lifetime risk for developing infective endocarditis (IE) ranges from 5% to 30%.

c. Atrial septal defect (ASD) (Fig. 11-13 B).

(1) **Definition:** Refers to a defect in the foramen ovale (FO) causing a left-to-right shunt

(2) Accounts for 8% to 10% of all CHDs

(3) Incidence is greater in females than in males.

(4) Most common CHD in adults

(5) Patent foramen ovale (PFO) (secundum type) is the most common cause in 80% of cases.

(a) Blood flows from the LA into the RA via the FO. This overloads the RA, RV, and PA.

(b) Step-up (increase) in SaO$_2$ in the RA, RV, and PA

(6) Associations of ASD with other CHDs include fetal alcohol syndrome (see Chapter 6) and Down syndrome (primum type in 25% of cases; see Chapter 6).

(7) ASDs are associated with a soft midsystolic murmur along the upper sternal border that is associated with increased PA blood flow.

(a) Characteristic wide and fixed split of the S$_2$ heart sound

(b) Because of increased blood in the right heart, it takes longer for the PV to close (S$_2$).

(8) Paradoxical embolism may occur (venous clot material enters the systemic circulation through the PFO; see Chapter 5).

(9) Criteria have been established by pediatric cardiologists as to whether surgical closure is required.

d. PDA (Fig. 11-13 C).

(1) **Definition:** Refers persistence after birth of communication between the PA and Ao

(2) A PDA accounts for 10% of all CHDs. In a fetus, the ductus arteriosus normally connects the PA with the Ao *below* the arch vessels (see Fig. 11-11). It is necessary because blood from the PA *cannot* enter into the fetal lungs for oxygenation and requires a shunt to bypass the lungs to empty its blood into the Ao.

(3) Note in Fig. 11-13 C that initially, there is a left-to-right shunt through the PDA (Ao to the PA; *left arrow*). This produces a step-up of SaO$_2$ in the PA because oxygenated blood from the Ao (higher pressure vessel) is entering the pulmonary arteries (normally carries venous blood to the lungs).

(4) A PDA is an isolated defect (*not* associated with other heart defects) in 90% of cases.

(5) PDA may be associated with congenital rubella, respiratory distress syndrome (caused by persistence of a decreased Pao$_2$), complete transposition of the great vessels (discussed later), and ToF (discussed later).

(6) Machinery murmur (harsh murmur) is heard continuously through systole and diastole.

(7) Reversal of the shunt may occur if PH develops from the increase in PA blood flow.

(a) In a reversal of the shunt, unoxygenated blood enters the Ao *below* the subclavian artery (Fig. 11-13 C, *right arrow*).

(b) Therefore, the child has a pink upper body and a cyanotic lower body, which is called differential cyanosis.

5. Right-sided to left-sided heart shunts

a. These shunts come under the heading of cyanotic CHD.

b. Complications of cyanotic CHD were discussed earlier.

c. ToF

(1) **Definition:** Refers to the presence of a VSD, infundibular pulmonic stenosis, RVH, and dextrorotation of the Ao

(2) Tetralogy is the most common cyanotic CHD after the age of 1 year (Fig. 11-13 D).

    (a) Accounts for 10% of all cases of CHD

    (b) Accounts for 50% to 70% of cyanotic CHD

    (c) Accounts for 85% of adults with cyanotic CHD

(3) Defects in ToF include (Link 11-33):

    (a) VSD.

    (b) infundibular (most common; narrowing of the outflow tract of the RV *below* the PV) or PV stenosis. Degree of PV stenosis determines whether the infant develops cyanosis or not after birth (see later).

    (c) RVH (RVH).

    (d) dextrorotated Ao (clockwise twist) with a right-sided aortic arch (25% of cases).

(4) Onset of cyanosis is usually after 3 months of age.

(5) Causes a harsh systolic crescendo/decrescendo murmur that results from RV outflow tract obstruction

(6) May be minimal infundibular PV stenosis or minimal PV stenosis

    (a) Leads to increased oxygenation of blood in the lungs

    (b) Less right-to-left shunting of blood through the VSD

    (c) Absence of cyanosis because the Sao_2 is >80%; acyanotic tetralogy

(7) May be severe infundibular stenosis or severe PV stenosis

    (a) Results in less oxygenation of blood in the lungs

    (b) Increased right-to-left shunting of blood through the VSD (more unoxygenated blood is entering the LV and going out the Ao)

    (c) Cyanosis is present because the Sao_2 is <80%.

    (d) Radiograph shows a "boot-shaped" heart (Link 11-34 A).

(8) Step-down (decrease) in Sao_2 in the LV and the Ao caused by the right-to-left shunting of unoxygenated blood

(9) Cardioprotective shunts increase oxygenation in ToF.

    (a) Presence of an ASD steps up the Sao_2 in the RA and RV; therefore, the blood that is shunting into the left side of the heart from the RV has a higher Sao_2.

    (b) PDA shunts unoxygenated blood from the Ao to the PA for oxygenation in the lungs.

(10) Tet spells (hypoxic spells)

    (a) Caused by a sudden increase in hypoxemia and cyanosis related to crying, fever, hypotension, anemia, or events that exacerbate right ventricular outflow obstruction

    (b) Squatting increases the PVR, causing temporary reversal of the right-to-left shunt to a left-to-right shunt (not shown in the schematic).

    (c) Unoxygenated blood in the RV is forced up into the PA for oxygenation.

d. Complete transposition of the great arteries (Fig. 11-13 E).

    (1) **Definition:** Complete transposition of the great arteries is an embryologic defect that results from abnormal formation of the truncal and aortopulmonary septa.

    (2) Defects that occur in complete transposition include Ao arising from the RV and the PA arising from the LV.

    (3) The LA and RA are normal (the vena cava empties into the RA, and the pulmonary vein empties into the LA).

    (4) Cardioprotective shunts that may occur in a complete transposition

        (a) An ASD steps up the Sao_2 in the RA. Increases Sao_2 in the RV for delivery to tissue via the transposed Ao.

        (b) A VSD shunts blood into the LV for oxygenation in the lungs via the transposed PA.

        (c) A PDA shunts blood into the transposed PA for oxygenation in the lungs.

    (5) Radiograph shows an "egg-shaped" heart (Link 11-34 B).

e. Other less common types of cyanotic CHD include:

    (1) total anomalous pulmonary venous return. **Definition:** The pulmonary vein empties oxygenated blood into the RA.

    (2) truncus arteriosus.

        • **Definition:** The Ao and the PA share a common trunk and intermix their blood.

Margin notes:

VSD, infundibular PS, RVH, dextrorotation Ao

MC cyanotic CHD after age 1 year

VSD

Infundibular pulmonic stenosis

Degree pulmonic stenosis correlates with cyanosis

RVH

Dextrorotation Ao

Cyanosis after 3 mo

Minimal infundibular/valve pulmonic stenosis: no cyanosis

Degree PV stenosis correlates with presence/absence of cyanosis

Severe infundibular/valve pulmonic stenosis: cyanosis

Severe PV stenosis → cyanosis; mild PV stenosis → no cyanosis

Step-down in Sao_2 in LV and Ao

Cardioprotective shunts: ASD, PDA

Tet spells (hypoxemic episode): squatting ↑PVR → reverses shunt → ↑Pao_2

Sudden increase hypoxemia/cyanosis

Squatting reverses shunt; ↑PVR

Complete transposition great arteries

Abnormal formation of truncal and aortopulmonary septa

Ao arising from RV, PA arising from LV

Transposition: Ao empties RV; PA empties LV; atria normal

Cardioprotective shunts in complete transposition

ASD

VSD

PDA

Egg-shaped heart

Total anomalous pulmonary venous return; oxygenated blood into RA

Truncus arteriosus

Ao and PA share common trunk

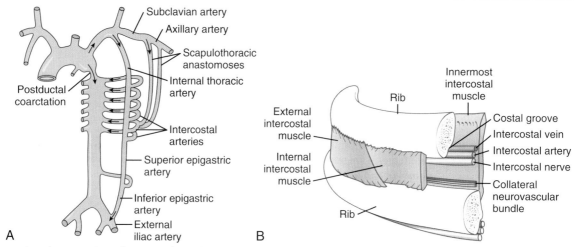

11-14: A, Postductal coarctation of aorta and resulting collateral circulation that is necessary to deliver blood into the descending aorta. *Arrows* show blood flow. **B,** Typical intercostal space. The neurovascular bundle lies between the internal intercostal and the innermost intercostal muscles near the superior border of the intercostal space. Increased pressure in the intercostal artery in the neurovascular bundle causes enlargement of the vessel and erosion of the costal groove, leading to a notch that is visible on chest radiography. *(A From Moore A, Roy W: Rapid Review Gross and Developmental Anatomy, 3rd ed, Philadelphia, Mosby Elsevier, 2010, p 49, Fig. 2.29; B from Moore A, Roy W: Rapid Review Gross and Developmental Anatomy, 3rd ed, Philadelphia, Mosby Elsevier, 2010, p 24, Fig. 2.2.)*

TV atresia	(3) TV atresia (the valve orifice fails to develop).
Usually and ASD with right-to-left shunt	(a) **Definition:** In TV atresia, the valve orifice fails to develop.
	(b) In addition to the TV atresia, there is usually an ASD with a right-to-left shunt.

C. Coarctation of the Ao (COTA; Fig. 11-14 A and B; see Fig. 11-13 F; Link 11-35).

Coarctation of Ao (COTA)

Obstruction Ao

Infantile preductal coarctation

MC coarctation

Constriction between subclavian artery and DA

VSD, Turner syndrome

Infants develop CHF if COTA *not* corrected

Adult coarctation

Children > adults

Constriction distal to ligamentum arteriosum

Volume/pressure blood increased in proximal branch vessels

↓Blood flow below constriction

Systolic ejection murmur

Bicuspid AV commonly present

↑Upper extremity SBP

Dilation of Ao: risk dissection

↑Cerebral blood flow (risk berry aneurysms)

Disparity between upper/ lower extremity blood pressure >10 mm Hg

Leg claudication: pain in calf/buttocks

HTN due to activation RAA system from ↓RBF

1. **Definition:** A coarctation is an obstruction of the Ao that is opposite the aortic end of the ductus arteriosus or ligamentum arteriosum.
2. Accounts for 6% to 8% of all CHDs
3. Infantile (preductal) coarctation
   a. This type of coarctation accounts for 70% of all coarctations.
   b. Constriction in the Ao is *between* the subclavian artery and the ductus arteriosus.
   c. Often associated with other congenital heart defects (e.g., VSD) and Turner syndrome
   d. Infants usually develop CHF and can die unless corrective surgery is performed.
4. Adult COTA
   a. Accounts for 30% of all coarctations
   b. Develops in children (most common) and adults (less common)
   c. Constriction of the Ao is *distal* to the ligamentum arteriosum (Fig. 11-13 F).
      (1) Blood flow into the proximally located branch vessels is increased, which increases the blood pressure in the upper extremity.
      (2) Blood flow below the constriction is decreased.
      (3) Constriction in the Ao produces a systolic ejection murmur posteriorly in the midthorax.
      (4) An additional defect that is often present is a bicuspid AV (50% of cases), which also produces a systolic ejection murmur along the sternal border.
   d. Clinical findings and possible complications proximal to the coarctation include:
      (1) increase in the upper extremity systolic blood pressure (SBP) caused by increased blood flow, particularly in the subclavian arteries.
      (2) dilation of the Ao, which increases the risk for developing an aortic dissection (occurs in 2%–6% of patients; see Chapter 10).
      (3) increase in cerebral blood flow, which increases the risk for developing saccular "berry" aneurysms (see Chapter 10 and Fig. 26-12 A).
   e. Clinical findings and possible complications distal to the coarctation include:
      (1) decrease in the SBP and pulse amplitude in the lower extremity (>10–mm Hg difference in blood pressure from the upper extremities).
      (2) leg claudication (pain in calf or buttocks when walking) may be present along with slight underdevelopment of the musculature compared with the upper body because of decreased blood flow distal to the coarctation.
      (3) decrease in renal blood flow (RBF), which activates the renin–angiotensin–aldosterone (RAA) system, causing HTN.

f. Development of collateral circulations in a coarctation (Fig. 11-14 A).

(1) Collaterals develop between the intercostal arteries (ICAs) above and below the constriction.

(a) Anterior intercostal arteries (AICA) arise from the internal thoracic artery (ITA).

(b) Posterior intercostal arteries (PICA) arise from the Ao.

(c) Increased pressure in the Ao extends into the subclavian artery → into the internal thoracic artery → into the AICAs, which stimulates the formation of a collateral circulation. PICAs with their increase in blood flow reverse the blood flow into the Ao.

(2) Collaterals develop between the superior epigastric artery and the inferior epigastric artery.

(a) Internal thoracic artery becomes the superior epigastric artery.

(b) Superior epigastric artery forms collaterals with the inferior epigastric artery, which is a branch of the external iliac artery.

(c) Reversal of blood flow in the inferior epigastric artery forces blood into the external iliac artery.

(3) Chest radiograph shows rib notching on the undersurface of the ribs (Fig. 11-14 B). Increased blood flow through the enlarged, pulsating ICA in the neurovascular bundle in the costal groove of the rib wears the bone away, producing rib notching.

g. Surgical removal of a coarctation corrects the HTN.

VI. **Acquired Valvular Heart Disease**

A. **Rheumatic fever (RF)**

1. **Definition:** An acute, noninfectious, inflammatory sequela to a group A β-hemolytic streptococcal *Streptococcus pyogenes* pharyngitis with joint, skin, subcutaneous (sc), neurologic, and cardiac symptoms appearing shortly after the infection

2. Epidemiology

a. First attack of acute RF usually occurs in children between 5 and 15 years of age.

b. Develops over 1 to 5 weeks (average, 20 days) after a group A streptococcal *(Streptococcus pyogenes)* pharyngitis

(1) Pharynx is the only site for infection leading to RF.

(2) Nephrogenic strains of group A streptococcus that produce poststreptococcal glomerulonephritis, lack the types of matrix (M) proteins (virulence factors) in their cell walls that are present in pharyngeal strains; hence, they never produce RF.

(3) Only 25% of patients have a positive pharyngeal culture for group A streptococcus.

c. Risk factors for developing streptococcal pharyngitis include:

(1) crowding and poverty. RF is common in impoverished countries.

(2) young age.

(3) living in Salt Lake City, Utah. For unexplained reasons, this area in the United States has the highest incidence and prevalence of RF.

d. Recurrent RF produces chronic valvular disease.

3. Pathogenesis of RF (Link 11-36)

a. Antibody-mediated disease that follows a group A streptococcal infection of the pharynx

b. Host develops antibodies against group A streptococcal M proteins.

(1) Antibodies that are produced cross-react with similar proteins in human tissue (called mimicry).

(2) Antibodies that are produced react against endocardium, myocardium (cardiac myosin and sarcolemmal membrane protein), as well as joints and skin.

(3) Type II antibody-mediated HSR (see Chapter 4)

4. Clinical findings (Link 11-36)

a. Migratory polyarthritis (~75% of cases)

(1) Most common initial presentation of acute RF

(2) Arthritis involves the large joints (knees), ankles, and wrists.

(3) *No* permanent joint damage

(4) Pain responds to aspirin (characteristic finding).

b. Carditis (~35% of cases)

(1) Most serious complication of RF

(2) Pancarditis that includes pericarditis, myocarditis, and endocarditis.

Collateral circulation in coarctation

Anterior and posterior intercostal arteries

AICA arise from ITA

PICA arise from Ao

Collaterals between superior epigastric artery in inferior epigastric artery

Pulsating intercostal artery → rib notching

Rheumatic fever

Noninfectious sequela group A *S. pyogenes* pharyngitis

Joint, skin/sc, neurologic, cardiac symptoms

1st attack: children 5 to 15 yrs old

1 to 5 wks post *S. pyogenes* pharyngitis

Pharyngeal cultures usually negative

Crowding, poverty

Young age

Salt Lake City, Utah

Recurrent RF → chronic valvular disease

Ab-mediated following group A strep pharyngeal infection

Abs against M proteins

M protein antibodies cross-react with human tissue (mimicry)

Abs against endocardium, myocardium, joints, skin

Type II HSR

Migratory polyarthritis

MC initial presentation

Knees, ankles, wrists

No permanent joint damage

Pain responds to aspirin

Carditis (35%)

Most serious complication

Pancarditis

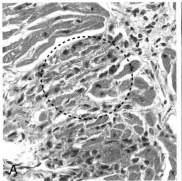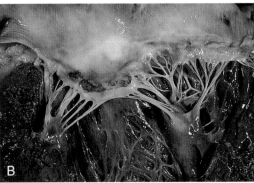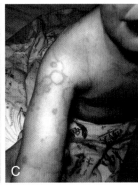

11-15: **A,** The Aschoff nodule in rheumatic fever is composed of an area of degenerate collagen surrounded by activated histiocytic cells *(interrupted circle)* and lymphoid cells. These lesions stimulate fibroblast proliferation and lead to scarring. **B,** Acute rheumatic fever. Uniform, verrucous sterile vegetations appear along the line of closure of the mitral valve. **C,** Erythema marginatum in a child with acute rheumatic fever. Note that most of the erythematous rash has a C-shaped appearance similar to the margin of the mitral valve. *(A from Stevens A, Lowe J, Scott I: Core Pathology, Mosby Elsevier, 3rd ed, 2009, p 187, Fig. 10.59; B from my friend Ivan Damjanov MD, PhD, Linder J: Pathology: A Color Atlas, St. Louis, Mosby, 2000, p 13, Fig. 1-22; C from Kliegman R: Nelson Textbook of Pediatrics, 19th ed, Philadelphia, Elsevier Saunders, 2011, p 922, Fig. 176.2, courtesy of Schachner LA, Hansen RC [eds]: Pediatric Dermatology, 3rd ed, St. Louis, Mosby, 2003, p 808.)*

Fibrinous pericarditis

Myocarditis: signs CHF

CHF MCC death in acute RF

Aschoff bodies (reactive histiocytes)

Endocarditis (inflammation valves)

MV MC: AV then TV

Sterile, verrucous vegetations

Embolism uncommon

MV and/or AV regurgitation

LHF (SHF type)

MV/AV stenosis in chronic RF

Subcutaneous nodules: extensor surface forearms

Centers have fibrinoid necrosis

Erythema marginatum

Circular/C-shaped areas erythema around normal skin

Sydenham chorea: involuntary movements

Late manifestation; reversible

Diagnose with revised Jones criteria

Major criteria: carditis, polyarthritis, chorea, EM, SC nodules

Minor criteria

Previous RF, arthralgia, fever

↑APRs (ESR, CRP, leukocytosis)

Prolonged PR interval

Lab findings

↑ASO titers

↑Anti-DNAase B titers

(3) Incidence declines with increasing age (30% incidence in adolescence vs 90% at 3 years of age).
(4) Fibrinous pericarditis presents with precordial chest pain with or without a friction rub.
(5) Myocarditis usually presents with signs of CHF.
  (a) CHF is the most common COD in acute RF.
  (b) Aschoff bodies are present in myocardial tissue (a postmortem finding; Fig. 11-15 A). Lesions have a central area of fibrinoid necrosis surrounded by Anitschkow cells (reactive histiocytes).
(6) Endocarditis refers to inflammation of cardiac valves.
  (a) Most commonly involves the MV, followed by the AV, followed by the TV.
  (b) Sterile, verrucous vegetations develop along the line of closure of the valve (Fig. 11-15 B). Embolism is uncommon.
  (c) MV regurgitation or AV regurgitation occurs depending on which valve is inflamed. LHF may occur (SHF).
  (d) Recurrent infection of the MV or AV over many years leads to stenosis of the respective valves.
  c. Subcutaneous nodules (~10% of cases) occur on the extensor surfaces of the forearms (Link 11-37).
    (1) Nodules are very similar to those seen in rheumatoid arthritis (RA).
    (2) Centers of the nodules have fibrinoid necrosis (see Chapter 2).
  d. Erythema marginatum (EM) presents as evanescent circular rings or C-shaped areas of erythema around normal skin (~10% of cases; Fig. 11-15 C).
  e. Sydenham chorea is characterized by reversible rapid, involuntary movements affecting all the muscles (~10% of cases). It is a late manifestation of acute RF.
5. Diagnosis of RF (revised Jones criteria)
  1. Two or more major manifestations or one major and two minor manifestations
  2. Major criteria include carditis, polyarthritis (joint swelling), chorea, erythema marginatum, and subcutaneous nodules.
  3. Minor criteria include:
    (1) previous RF, arthralgia (pain *without* joint swelling), fever.
    (2) increased acute phase reactants (APRs; see Chapter 3): increased erythrocyte sedimentation rate (ESR), increased C-reactive protein (CRP), absolute neutrophilic leukocytosis.
    (3) prolonged PR interval (first-degree heart block).
  4. Laboratory test findings include:
    (1) increased antistreptolysin O (ASO) titers >400 Todd units.
      (a) Titers peak at 4 to 5 weeks after streptococcal pharyngitis.
      (b) High titers are supportive but *not* diagnostic of acute RF.
    (2) increased anti–DNAase B titers (less reliable than ASO titers).

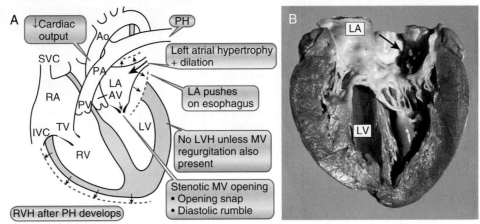

11-16: **A,** Mitral stenosis. Refer to the text for discussion. **B,** Mitral stenosis with left atrial thrombosis. This heart has been opened to show the left atrium (LA) and the left ventricle (LV), with the mitral valve (MV) between the two chambers. The valve and its chordae tendineae have been damaged by chronic rheumatic endocarditis, leading to thickening, dystrophic calcification and fusion of both valves. The combination of stasis in the dilated left atrium and coexisting atrial fibrillation has led to thrombus formation *(arrow)*. Atrial fibrillation increases the risk for systemic embolization. *Ao,* Aorta; *AV,* aortic valve; *IVC,* inferior vena cava; *LVH,* left ventricular hypertrophy; *PA,* pulmonary artery; *PH,* pulmonary hypertension; *PV,* pulmonary valve; *RA,* right atrium; *RV,* right ventricle; *RVH,* right ventricular hypertrophy; *SVC,* superior vena cava; *TV,* tricuspid valve. **(A** from Goljan EF: *Star Series:* Pathology, *Philadelphia, Saunders, 1998;* **B** from Stevens A, Lowe J, Scott I: Core Pathology, *Mosby Elsevier, 3rd ed, 2009, p 182, Fig. 10.50.)*

(3) positive throat culture. Evidence of a recent group A streptococcal infection is particularly significant if there is only one major criteria.

6. Clinical features of acute RF are summarized in Link 11-38.

B. Mitral valve stenosis

1. **Definition:** Refers to a narrowing of the MV orifice that causes the left atria to dilate as it works harder to pump blood across the narrowed orifice

2. Epidemiology
   a. Most commonly caused by recurrent attacks of RF
   b. Twice as common in women than men
   c. Clinically recognized in 50% of patients
   d. Pathophysiology
      (1) Narrowing of the MV orifice (<2.5 cm² [normal 4–6 cm²]; Fig. 11-16 A; Link 11-39)
      (2) LA becomes dilated and hypertrophied because of increased work in filling the LV during diastole.

3. Clinical findings
   a. Dyspnea (difficulty with breathing) and hemoptysis (coughing up blood) with rust-colored sputum (heart failure cells; Link 11-11). Caused by pulmonary capillary congestion and hemorrhage into the alveoli as blood builds up behind the LA.
   b. Atrial fibrillation (AF)
      (1) AF (irregularly irregular pulse) is a complication of left atrial dilation and hypertrophy.
      (2) Intraleft atrial thrombi develop from blood stasis (see Chapter 5; Fig. 11-16 B). Systemic embolization occurs in 80% of cases when AF is present.
   c. Pulmonary venous hypertension (HTN)
      (1) Caused by chronic backup of left atrial blood in the pulmonary vein
      (2) Pulmonary venous HTN leads to right-sided heart failure (RHF) and concentric RVH from the increase in afterload.
   d. Dysphagia (difficulty in swallowing) for solids
      (1) LA is the most posteriorly located chamber in the heart.
      (2) When markedly dilated, it compresses the esophagus, causing difficulty with swallowing solid food (dysphagia for solids).
   e. Signs of MV stenosis include an opening snap followed by an early to mid-diastolic rumble (Box 11-1).
      (1) LA must exert a lot of pressure to open valves that are fibrosed and dystrophically calcified.
      (2) Thickened MVs open with a snap. Blood from the LA, which should already have been emptied into the LV, rushes into the chamber, producing a mid-diastolic rumble.

Positive throat culture

↑ASO/DNase B titers; +throat culture

MV stenosis

Narrowing MV orifice → LA dilation

MCC recurrent attacks RF

Women > men

50% patients

Narrowing MV orifice

LA dilated/hypertrophied

Dyspnea, hemoptysis

Rust-colored sputum (heart failure cells)

Pulmonary capillary congestion/hemorrhage in alveoli

Atrial fibrillation

LA dilation/hypertrophy complication

LA thrombi (blood stasis)

Danger systemic embolization if AF present

Pulmonary venous HTN

Backup LA blood in PV

Pulmonary venous HTN → RHF → concentric RVH

Dysphagia for solids

LA posteriorly located

Dilated LA compresses esophagus

Dysphagia for solids

MV stenosis: opening snap → early/mid diastolic rumble

↑LA pressure to open fibrosed/calcified MV

Thickened MV opens with snap → then mid-diastolic rumble

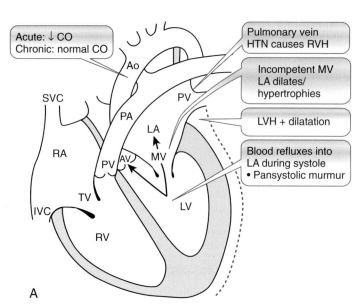

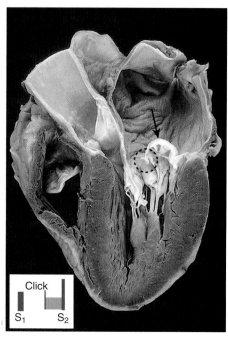

11-17: **A,** Mitral regurgitation. In systole, there is retrograde blood flow into the left atrium (LA), causing it to dilate and hypertrophy. The increased pressure in the LA transmits back into the pulmonary vein (pulmonary venous hypertension) and the right ventricle (RV) (concentric hypertrophy). Pulmonary congestion and edema are common findings. The cardiac output is decreased in acute mitral valve (MV) regurgitation but is normal in chronic MV regurgitation. **B,** MV prolapse. The *arrow* shows prolapse of the posterior mitral leaflet into the LA. The *interrupted circle* shows rupture of one of the chordae tendineae, which produced mitral regurgitation. *Ao,* Aorta; *AV,* aortic valve; *CO,* cardiac output; *HTN,* hypertension; *IVC,* inferior vena cava; *LA,* left atrium; *LV,* left ventricle; *LVH,* left ventricular hypertrophy; *PA,* pulmonary artery; *PH,* pulmonary hypertension; *PV,* pulmonary valve; *RA,* right atrium; *RVH,* right ventricular hypertrophy; *SVC,* superior vena cava; *TV,* tricuspid valve. (*A from Goljan EF: Star Series: Pathology. Philadelphia, Saunders, 1998; B from Kumar V, Fausto N, Abbas A: Robbins and Cotran Pathologic Basis of Disease, 7th ed, Philadelphia, Saunders, 2004, p 592, Fig. 12-23.*)

(3) Deep held inspiration for 3 to 5 seconds does *not* alter the intensity of the opening snap (OS) or mid-diastolic rumble (see Box 11-1).
4. Diagnosis of MV stenosis is confirmed by ECHO.
5. Treatment of MV stenosis is replacement of the valve (Link 11-40).

C. **Mitral valve regurgitation**
1. **Definition:** Refers to incompetence of the MV causing backward ejection of flow into the LA during LV systole
2. Epidemiology
   a. Causes
      (1) Mitral valve prolapse (MVP; most common cause)
      (2) Rupture or dysfunction of the posteromedial papillary muscle (e.g., posterior AMI; second most common cause)
      (3) Functional MV regurgitation (stretching of MV ring). Example: LHF
      (4) Infective endocarditis (IE) involving MV
      (5) Other causes: acute rheumatic fever (RF), dilated cardiomyopathy, myocarditis, Libman-Sacks endocarditis in systemic lupus erythematosus, and nonbacterial thrombotic endocarditis
   b. Pathophysiology of MV regurgitation (Fig. 11-17 A; Link 11-41)
      (1) Retrograde blood flow into the LA during systole.
         (a) In acute MV regurgitation, cardiac output (CO) is decreased.
         (b) If left uncorrected, the LA becomes dilated/hypertrophied because of the excess blood in the chamber.
            • Pulmonary venous pressure increases, leading to pulmonary vein HTN (PVH)
            • Pulmonary vein HTN leads to RVH and a potential for RHF
      (2) Volume overload occurs in the LV because there is more blood entering the LV in diastole (increase in preload) because of increased blood in the LA. An increase in preload in the LV produces eccentric LVH.
      (3) In chronic compensated MV regurgitation, the LA and LV have time to dilate and accommodate the regurgitant volume, which eventually normalizes the stroke volume (SV) and CO. LA pressure is often normal or only slightly elevated.

MV stenosis confirmed with ECHO

Rx: MV replacement

MV regurgitation

Retrograde blood flow into LA during LV systole

MVP MCC MV regurgitation

Rupture/dysfunction posteromedial papillary muscle; posterior AMI

Functional MV regurgitation: stretching MV ring (LHF)

Infective endocarditis

Retrograde blood flow into LA during systole

Acute: cardiac output decreased

Left uncorrected: LA dilated/hypertrophied

↑Pulmonary venous pressure → pulmonary vein HTN

PVH → RVH → RHF

↑Preload in LV→ eccentric LVH

Normalization SV/CO in chronic compensated MV regurgitation

(4) In the chronic decompensated phase of mitral regurgitation, muscle dysfunction occurs, which increases left ventricular and left atrial pressure. This ultimately leads to pulmonary edema and, potentially, cardiogenic shock.

3. Clinical findings in MV regurgitation include:
   a. dyspnea, inspiratory crackles (pulmonary edema), and cough from LHF (usually a systolic dysfunction type of heart failure).
   b. pansystolic murmur with S_3 and S_4 heart sounds (gallop rhythm; see Box 11-1). Deep held inspiration for 3 to 5 seconds does *not* alter the intensity of the murmur or the abnormal heart sounds.
4. Diagnosis is confirmed by echocardiography (ECHO).

D. **Mitral valve prolapse (MVP)**
   1. **Definition:** Refers to bulging of one or both of the MVs into the LA during left ventricular systole because of redundant valve tissue
   2. Epidemiology
      a. Most common MV lesion and cause of MV regurgitation. ECHO demonstrates MVP in 1% to 4% of the general population.
      b. More common in women than men. After age 50 years, it is more common in men.
      c. Prevalence of MVP in children and adolescents is 6% to 11%.
      d. Mean age of presentation is 9.9 years. Before age 20 years, the female-to-male ratio is 2 to 1. After age 20 years, the female-to-male ratio is equal.
      e. Commonly associated with Marfan, Ehlers-Danlos syndrome (EDS), and Klinefelter syndromes. It is also associated with anorexia nervosa, bulimia, osteogenic imperfecta, and autoimmune thyroid disease.
      f. Caused by defective embryogenesis in cells of mesenchymal origin
      g. Pathophysiology
         (1) Bulging of the anterior and/or posterior leaflets into the LA occurs during systole (Fig. 11-17 B; Link 11-42). It is analogous to air underneath a parachute, the latter representing the MV.
         (2) Redundancy of MV tissue is caused by an excess of dermatan sulfate in the MV leaflet (called myxomatous degeneration).
   3. Clinical findings
      a. Most patients are asymptomatic.
      b. Midsystolic click caused by sudden restraint by the chordae tendineae of the prolapsed MV during systole
      c. Mid to late systolic MV regurgitation murmur follows the click.
         (1) Decreased preload (decreased volume of blood in the LV) causes the click and murmur to move closer to the S_1 heart sound (length of systole is decreased). Examples of maneuvers or conditions that decrease preload include:
            (a) anxiety. Anxiety increases the heart rate (HR), which decreases the time for diastolic filling of the LV.
            (b) standing. Standing decreases venous return to the right side of the heart.
            (c) Valsalva maneuver (holding breath with the epiglottis closed). This maneuver produces an increase in positive intrathoracic pressure, which decreases venous return to the heart (compression of the vena cava and right side of the heart).
         (2) Increased preload (increase volume of blood in the LV) causes the click and murmur to move closer to the S_2 heart sound (the length of systole is increased). Examples of maneuvers or conditions that increase preload include:
            (a) reclining; increases venous return to the right side of the heart, which in turn increases the volume of blood in the left side of the heart.
            (b) squatting or sustained hand grip; increases peripheral vascular resistance (PVR), which impedes emptying of the LV; therefore, more blood is in the LV.
      d. Other clinical findings in MVP include palpitations, chest pain, and rupture of the chordae, producing acute MV regurgitation (Fig. 11-17 B).
   4. Diagnosis of MVP is confirmed by ECHO.

E. **Aortic valve (AV) stenosis**
   1. **Definition:** Aortic stenosis is obstruction to systolic blood flow from the LV into the Ao.
   2. Epidemiology
      a. Most common valve lesion of adults in Western countries
      b. Etiology of AV stenosis
         (1) Calcific AV stenosis is the most common cause of stenosis in persons >60 years old (Fig. 11-18 A; Link 11-43). Calcification may involve a normal or a congenital bicuspid AV (1%–2% of the population). Recall that the normal AV is tricuspid.

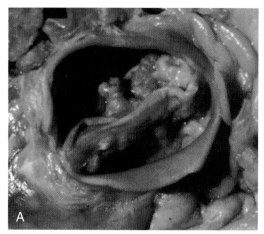

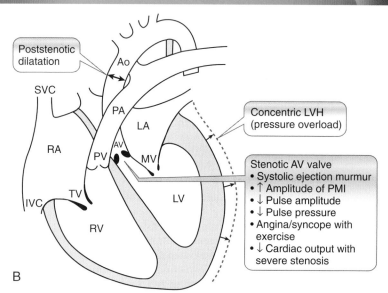

11-18: A, Aortic stenosis. The superior view shows a bicuspid aortic valve (normally tricuspid) with severe stenosis caused by fibrocalcific involvement of the three valve cusps. **B,** Aortic stenosis. The stenotic valve causes concentric hypertrophy of the left ventricle (LV). The pulse pressure is diminished, hence the pulse is diminished on physical examination. The cardiac output decreases with exercise, leading to syncope with exercise and angina. The latter is caused by decreased filling of the coronary arteries in diastole because of the increased heart rate from exercise. Less blood is delivered to the left ventricular muscle, and subendocardial ischemia leads to angina. *Ao,* Aorta; *AV,* aortic valve; *IVC,* inferior vena cava; *LA,* left atrium; *LVH,* left ventricular hypertrophy; *MV,* mitral valve; *PA,* pulmonary artery; *PH,* pulmonary hypertension; *PMI,* point of maximal impulse; *PV,* pulmonary valve; *RA,* right atrium; *RV,* right ventricle; *SVC,* superior vena cava; *TV,* tricuspid valve. *(A from my friend Ivan Damjanov MD, PhD, Linder J:* Anderson's Pathology, *10th ed, St. Louis, Mosby, 1996, p 1268, Fig. 45.6B; B from Goljan EF: Star Series: Pathology, Philadelphia, Saunders, 1998.)*

Congenital AV stenosis

Persons <30; 10% CHD

Obstruction level valve, below, or above

Associations with VSD, MV abnormalities, PDA

Age-related sclerosis, chronic RF

Normal AV orifice 3 cm²

Obstruction LV outflow in systole

Obstruction to LV outflow tract → concentric LVH

CO normal rest; ↓with exercise

Harsh systolic ejection murmur; radiation into neck

S₄ heart sound

↓Preload, ↓murmur intensity

↑Preload, ↑murmur intensity

Aortic stenosis: MC valvular lesion causing angina with exercise

Reduced filling CAs during diastole

Subendocardium receives less blood → subendocardial ischemia

MC valve lesion causing syncope with exercise

(2) Congenital AV stenosis

(a) Major cause of AV stenosis in persons <30 years of age; occurs of 10% of cases of congenital heart disease (CHD)

(b) Obstruction may occur at the level of the valve, below the valve, or above the valve.

(c) May be associated with a VSD, MV abnormalities, or PDA

(3) Other causes include age-related sclerosis of the AV (see later) and chronic RF is uncommon.

(4) Pathophysiology (Fig. 11-18 B)

(a) Normal AV orifice is 3 cm². Symptoms and signs appear when the orifice is <1 cm². Severe AV stenosis is present when the orifice is <0.5 cm².

(b) Obstruction of LV outflow during systole. Narrowing of the outflow tract results in obstruction of LV outflow during systole. Reduction in the AV orifice area produces concentric LVH and poststenotic dilation of the Ao caused by the jet stream of blood impacting on the wall of the vessel.

(c) At rest, the CO is normal; however, with exercise, it may be decreased, particularly with severe AV stenosis.

3. Clinical findings

a. Harsh systolic ejection murmur is heard in the right second intercostal space with radiation into the neck. Deep held inspiration for 3 to 5 seconds does *not* increase the intensity of the murmur (see Box 11-1).

b. Left-sided S₄ heart sound; caused by decreased compliance of the LV (see Box 11-1)

c. Decreasing preload lessens the volume of blood the LV must eject, causing the murmur intensity to decrease.

d. Increasing preload increases the volume the LV must eject, causing the murmur intensity to increase.

e. Angina may occur with exercise. AV stenosis is the MC valvular lesion causing angina with exercise.

(1) Decreased blood flow through the stenotic AV leads to reduced filling of the CAs during diastole.

(2) Subendocardium of the concentrically hypertrophied LV receives less blood, leading to subendocardial ischemia and angina.

f. Most common valve lesion associated with exercise-induced syncope. Decreased blood flow through the stenotic AV leads to decreased blood flow to the brain and syncope.

g. Hemolytic anemia (microangiopathic) with schistocytes and hemoglobinuria (hemoglobin in the urine) may occur (see Chapter 12).

    (1) Schistocytes are fragmented RBCs that occur when blood encounters a stenotic and dystrophically calcified AV.

    (2) Presence of schistocytes in the peripheral blood is an indication for AV replacement.

    (3) Fragmented and damaged RBCs release hemoglobin in the plasma, which enters the urine (hemoglobinuria), producing a pink discoloration of the urine (see Chapter 20).

h. Diminished pulse pressure (difference between the SBP and diastolic blood pressure [DBP]) is present with severe stenosis.

i. CO may be decreased in severe aortic stenosis.

4. Diagnosis of AV stenosis is confirmed by ECHO.

5. AV sclerosis

    a. **Definition:** AV sclerosis is a common asymptomatic condition in older adults that is generally detected either as a systolic ejection murmur on physical examination or as an incidental finding on ECHO.

    b. Epidemiology

        (1) Present in 26% to 29% of individuals ≥65 years of age

        (2) Prevalence increases with advancing age (e.g., 50% for those >80 years old).

    c. Clinical finding

        (1) May progress to calcific AV stenosis

        (2) Predictor of increased frequency of cardiovascular events and death (fatal AMI, sudden death)

F. Aortic valve (AV) regurgitation

1. **Definition:** AV regurgitation is retrograde blood flow into the LV during early diastole caused by an incompetent AV.

2. Epidemiology

    a. Most common cause of isolated AV regurgitation is aortic root dilation

    b. Other causes include:

        (1) IE (most common infectious cause of acute AV regurgitation).

        (2) chronic RF (most common cause of AV regurgitation in developing countries).

        (3) aortic dissection (see Chapter 10).

        (4) Coarctation of the aorta (COTA)

        (5) dilated AV ring, syphilitic aortitis (see Chapter 10), aortitis in ankylosing spondylitis (see Chapter 24), and Takayasu arteritis (see Chapter 10) or other less common causes.

    c. Pathophysiology (Fig. 11-19)

        (1) Incompetent closure of AV results in retrograde blood flow into the LV in diastole.

            (a) In acute AV regurgitation, this leads to a markedly increased LVEDP, normal left ventricular size, decreased SBP (decreased SV), normal to decreased pulse pressure (see Box 11-1), and decreased CO.

            (b) In chronic AV regurgitation, the LVEDP returns to normal, LV size is increased, SBP is increased, DBP is decreased (drop of arterial volume as blood drips back into the LV), pulse pressure is increased (see Box 11-1), and CO is normal.

        (2) Volume overload (increased preload) in the LV leads to eccentric (dilated) LVH.

3. Clinical findings

    a. Early diastolic murmur occurs because of blood flowing back into the LV right after the second heart sound.

        (1) S$_3$ and S$_4$ heart sounds are present (see Box 11-1).

        (2) Deep held inspiration for 3 to 5 seconds does *not* increase the intensity of the murmur or the abnormal heart sounds (see Box 11-1).

    b. In chronic AV regurgitation, signs of a hyperdynamic circulation are caused by a widened pulse pressure (see earlier); hyperdynamic signs include bounding pulses (Corrigan water-hammer pulse), head nodding with systole (de Musset sign), and pulsating nail bed with elevation of the nail (Quincke pulse).

    c. Austin Flint murmur

        (1) Occurs when the regurgitant blood in diastole from the incompetent AV hits the anterior MV leaflet, producing a diastolic murmur

        (2) Presence of this murmur is an indication for AV replacement.

    d. Normalization of the CO occurs in chronic aortic regurgitation.

4. Diagnosis of AV regurgitation is confirmed by ECHO.

Microangiopathic hemolytic anemia with schistocytes

Fragmented RBCs

Indication for AV replacement

Hemoglobinuria

Diminished pulse pressure

↓CO in severe AV stenosis

Aortic valve sclerosis

Asymptomatic condition in older adults; systolic ejection murmur

Prevalence increases with age

May progress to calcific aortic stenosis

Predictor ↑frequency cardiovascular events and mortality

Aortic valve regurgitation

Retrograde blood flow into LV early diastole

Isolated AV root dilation MCC AV regurgitation

IE MCC acute AV regurgitation

Chronic RF MCC AV regurgitation developing countries

Aortic dissection

Coarctation

Dilated AV ring; syphilitic/ankylosing spondylitis aortitis; Takayasu arteritis

Incompetent closure AV; retrograde blood flow into LV

Acute AV regurgitation

↑LVEDP, ↓SBP, normal/↓pulse pressure, ↓CO

Chronic AV regurgitation

Normal LVEDP, ↑SBP, ↓DBP, ↑pulse pressure, normal CO

Eccentric LVH

Early diastolic murmur

S$_3$, S$_4$

No ↑intensity with inspiration

Chronic AV regurgitation

Hyperdynamic circulation (widened pulse pressure)

Bounding pulses, head nodding, pulsating nail bed

Austin Flint murmur

Regurgitant blood in diastole → hits anterior MV leaflet → diastolic murmur

Sign for AV replacement

Normalization CO in chronic aortic regurgitation

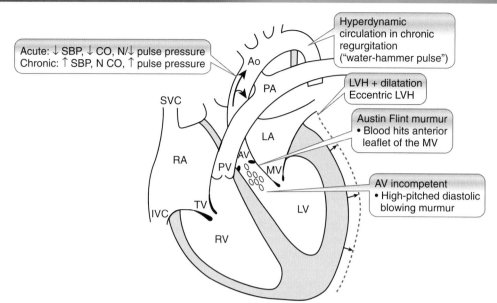

Acute: ↓ SBP, ↓ CO, N/↓ pulse pressure
Chronic: ↑ SBP, N CO, ↑ pulse pressure

Hyperdynamic circulation in chronic regurgitation ("water-hammer pulse")

LVH + dilatation Eccentric LVH

Austin Flint murmur
• Blood hits anterior leaflet of the MV

AV incompetent
• High-pitched diastolic blowing murmur

11-19: Aortic regurgitation. There is retrograde blood flow into the left ventricle (LV) caused by an incompetent valve or a dilated valve ring. Eventually, this volume overloads the LV, causing eccentric hypertrophy. In chronic compensated aortic regurgitation, the pulse pressure increases, causing signs of a hyperdynamic circulation. An additional diastolic murmur may occur from excess blood hitting the anterior leaflet of the mitral valve (Austin Flint murmur). *Ao,* Aorta; *AV,* aortic valve; *CO,* cardiac output; *IVC,* inferior vena cava; *LA,* left atrium; *LVH,* left ventricular hypertrophy; *MV,* mitral valve; *PA,* pulmonary artery; *PV,* pulmonary valve; *RA,* right atrium; *RV,* right ventricle; *SVC,* superior vena cava; *TV,* tricuspid valve. *(From Goljan EF: Star Series: Pathology, Philadelphia, Saunders, 1998.)*

Tricuspid valve regurgitation

Systole: retrograde blood flow into RA

Functional (stretching TV ring) in RHF; MCC in adults

CHD MCC adolescents/ young adults

IVDA: IE MCC TV regurgitation

PH, dilated cardiomyopathy, RV infarction, carcinoid heart disease

Retrograde blood flow into RA during systole

Stretching/damage to TV

RA dilation/hypertrophy → backup blood into venous system

Volume overload RV → eccentric RVH

Pulsating liver during systole

Congestive hepatomegaly

Dependent pitting edema

Ascites

Giant c-v wave in JVP

Pansystolic murmur

S₃/S₄ heart sounds

↑intensity with deep held inspiration

G. TV regurgitation
1. **Definition:** TV regurgitation is retrograde blood flow into the RA during systole caused by an incompetent TV.
2. Epidemiology
   a. Most common cause of TV regurgitation in the adult population is functional regurgitation caused by stretching of the valve ring in RHF.
   b. In adolescents and young adults, most cases are caused by CHD.
   c. Small degree of TV regurgitation (*not* clinically significant) occurs in ~70% of adults.
   d. In intravenous drug abusers (IVDAs), IE affecting the TV is the most common cause of regurgitation.
   e. Less common causes include PH, dilated cardiomyopathy, RV infarction, and carcinoid heart disease (see Chapter 18).
   f. Pathophysiology
      (1) Retrograde blood flow into the RA during systole is caused by stretching of the TV ring and/or damage to the TV (e.g., IE).
      (2) Causes right atrial dilation and hypertrophy and backup of blood into the venous system
      (3) Eccentric (dilated) RVH occurs because of volume overload (increased preload) of the RV.
3. Clinical findings include
   a. pulsating liver.
      (1) Blood backs up into the venous system and increases hepatic vein blood flow to the central venules, leading to an increase in pressure in the sinusoids and portal vein, causing pulsation of the liver during systole.
      (2) Causes congestive hepatomegaly ("nutmeg liver"; increased blood in central venules) similar to what occurs in RHF (Link 11-13)
   b. dependent pitting edema caused by increased venous hydrostatic pressure (see Chapter 5).
   c. ascites (increased fluid in the peritoneal cavity) caused by increased portal vein hydrostatic pressure (see Chapter 5).
   d. giant c-v wave is present in the jugular venous pulse (JVP; Box 11-1). This is a sign of severe TV regurgitation.
   e. pansystolic murmur that is heard best along the left parasternal border.
      (1) S₃ and S₄ heart sounds are present (Box 11-1).
      (2) Deep held inspiration for 3 to 5 seconds *increases* the intensity of the murmur and the abnormal heart sounds (Box 11-1).
4. Diagnosis of TV regurgitation is confirmed by ECHO.

H. PV stenosis
1. **Definition:** PV stenosis is obstruction to systolic blood flow from the RV into the PA.
2. Epidemiology
   a. Uncommon valve lesion
   b. Associated with CHD and carcinoid heart disease
3. Clinical findings
   a. Systolic ejection murmur is present in the left second intercostal space (Box 11-1).
   b. Right-sided S_4 heart sound caused by decreased compliance of the RV (Box 11-1).
   c. Concentric RVH is present because of contraction of the RV against an increased afterload at the level of the PV.
4. Diagnosis of PV stenosis is confirmed by ECHO.

I. PV regurgitation
1. **Definition:** PV regurgitation is retrograde blood flow into the RV during early diastole caused by an incompetent PV.
2. Epidemiology
   a. Most often a functional murmur from stretching of the PV ring. Example: PH (this is called a Graham Steell murmur)
   b. Pathophysiology. Volume overload of the RV leads to eccentric (dilated) RVH.
3. Clinical findings
   a. Diastolic murmur is heard after the second heart sound.
   b. Right-sided S_3 and S_4 heart sounds are present (Box 11-1).
   c. Extra heart sounds and murmur intensity increases with deep, held inspiration.
4. Diagnosis of PV regurgitation is confirmed by ECHO.

J. Carcinoid heart disease
1. **Definition:** Carcinoid heart disease is TV regurgitation and pulmonic stenosis caused by fibrosis of the valves by excess serotonin in the blood, typically secondary to liver metastasis from a primary carcinoid tumor of the small intestine.
2. Epidemiology (see Chapter 18)
   a. Serotonin, produced by the metastatic foci in the liver, gains access to the systemic circulation as follows: hepatic vein (HV) → IVC → right side of the heart.
   b. In the right side of the heart, serotonin causes fibrosis of the tricuspid and PVs, producing TV regurgitation and PV stenosis.

K. Infective endocarditis (IE)
1. **Definition:** IE is an infection of the endocardial surface of one or more valves or a septal defect in CHD.
2. Epidemiology
   a. Most frequently occurs in adults between 45 and 65 years of age
   b. Categories of IE include native valve endocarditis, acute and subacute; prosthetic valve endocarditis, early and late; IVDA endocarditis; and nosocomial (hospital-acquired endocarditis).
   c. Risk factors include:
      (1) DM, human immunodeficiency virus (HIV) infection.
      (2) poor dental hygiene, CHD (ASD, VSD, PDA).
      (3) MVP (20%–30% of cases of endocarditis), AV stenosis, bicuspid AV (predisposing factor if patient is >60 years old).
      (4) hemodialysis, prosthetic heart valve.
      (5) intravenous (IV) catheters, intravenous drug abuse (IVDA).
      (6) prior endocarditis.
   d. Microbial pathogens associated with IE
      (1) Acute endocarditis is most commonly caused by *Staphylococcus aureus* (usually methicillin-resistant strain), streptococcal species groups A through G, *Haemophilus influenzae,* and *Streptococcus pneumoniae.* AV is the most common valve involved.
      (2) Endocarditis in IVDAs is caused by *S. aureus* (most common), *Pseudomonas aeruginosa, Candida* spp., and enterococci.
      (3) Subacute endocarditis is most commonly caused by the viridans group of *Streptococcus* (most common overall pathogens causing endocarditis), *Streptococcus bovis,* enterococci, and *S. aureus.*
      (4) Endocarditis associated with artificial heart valves (early; <60 days) is caused by *Staphylococcus epidermidis* (coagulase negative; most common cause), *Candida* spp., and gram-negative bacilli.

Prosthetic valve IE late: *S. aureus*, enterococci, group D strep

Nosocomial: IV catheters: *S. aureus* MCC

Indwelling urinary catheters: enterococci MCC

IE ulcerative bowel lesions: *Streptococcus bovis*

Fungal: IVDA, ICU patients on broad-spectrum antibiotics

Dental procedures/poor dentition: *Streptococcus mutans*

Etiologic agent more important than type of endocarditis

Staphylococci/streptococci: most IE

Most valves involved left sided

Right-sided valves: IVDA

MV MC valve involved in IE

IVDA IE: TV/AV MC valves

Pathogenesis IE: turbulent blood flow damages valve

Viridans streptococci infect previously damaged valves

S. aureus infects normal/damaged valves

Vegetations destroy valve leaflet

Valve destruction → regurgitant murmurs

Fever most consistent sign in IE

IE MCC FUO

Fever, failure to thrive, arthralgias + RF

(5) Endocarditis associated with artificial heart valves (late; >60 days) is caused by *S. aureus*, enterococci, and group D streptococci.

(6) Nosocomial (hospital-acquired) endocarditis from IV catheters is most often caused by *S. aureus*. Enterococci are the most common cause in patients with indwelling urinary catheters.

(7) Endocarditis associated with ulcerative lesions in the colon (e.g., ulcerative colitis, colon cancer) is most commonly caused by *Streptococcus bovis* (*gallolyticus*).

(8) Fungal endocarditis is found in IVDAs and intensive care unit (ICU) patients who receive broad-spectrum antibiotics.

(9) Endocarditis associated with dental procedures on individuals with poor dentition is usually caused by *Streptococcus mutans*.

(10) The etiologic agent causing endocarditis is more important than classifying endocarditis into acute and subacute.

(11) *Staphylococci* and *streptococci* account for 80% to 90% of cases of IE.

e. Valves involved in IE
  (1) Most valves involved in IE are left sided (>90% of cases).
  (2) Right-sided valves with IE are usually associated with IVDA (inject veins with contaminated needles).
  (3) Mitral valve is the most common overall valve involved in IE.
  (4) TVs and AVs are the most common valves involved in IE caused by IV drug abuse.

f. Pathogenesis of IE (Link 11-44)
  (1) Turbulent blood flow damages the valve → adherence of fibrin and platelets to the areas of damage → trapping of circulating bacteria/fungi → proliferation of the pathogens + laying down of fibrin to encase the vegetation
  (2) *Viridans* group of streptococci infects previously damaged valves.
  (3) *S. aureus* infects normal or previously damaged valves.

g. Pathology of IE.
  (1) Vegetations destroy the valve leaflet and the chordae tendineae (Fig. 11-20 A; Link 11-45).
  (2) Valve destruction leads to regurgitation (insufficiency) murmurs.

3. Clinical findings (Links 11-46 and 11-47)
  a. Fever is the most consistent sign of IE (90% of cases).
    (1) IE is a common cause of fever of unknown origin (FUO; see Chapter 3).
    (2) Fever, fatigue and failure to thrive, arthralgias, and a positive rheumatoid factor (RF) are seen in 50% of cases.

11-20: A, Acute bacterial endocarditis. Large, friable, and irregular vegetation *(arrow)* is present on the margin of the mitral valve. Smaller vegetations are present along the line of closure of the valve. **B,** Roth spots. Note the areas of hemorrhage with white dots in the center *(white arrows)*. **C,** Splinter hemorrhages in the nail bed. Note the longitudinal red hemorrhages in the nail bed. These represent areas of microembolization. **D,** Osler nodes on the pads of the toes. These represent areas of microembolization of vegetation material and are usually painful. *(**A** from my friend Ivan Damjanov MD, PhD,* Linder J: Pathology: A Color Atlas, *St. Louis, Mosby, 2000, p 11, Fig. 1-16;* **B** *from Bouloux, P:* Self-Assessment Picture Tests Medicine, Vol. 1, *London, Mosby-Wolfe, 1997, p 63, Fig. 125;* **C** *from Swartz MH:* Textbook of Physical Diagnosis, *5th ed, Philadelphia, Saunders Elsevier, 2006, p 747, Fig. 8-10;* **D** *from Bouloux P:* Self-Assessment Picture Tests Medicine, Vol. 3, *London, Mosby-Wolfe, 1997, p 45, Fig. 89.)*

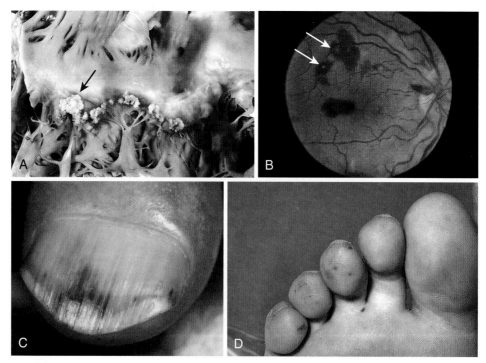

b. Immunocomplex (IC) vasculitis more likely occurs if IE is subacute. Examples: glomerulonephritis (nephritic type), Roth spot (irregular red area with central white dot; 2%–10% of cases; see Fig. 11-20 B)

c. Microembolization findings occur in >50% of cases.

    (1) Splinter hemorrhages are linear hemorrhages that are present in the nail beds (Fig. 11-20 C; Link 11-48; 15% of cases).

    (2) Janeway lesions are *painless* areas of hemorrhage on the palms and soles of the feet (10% of cases; Link 11-49).

    (3) Osler nodes are *painful* hemorrhagic nodules on the pads of the fingers or toes (Fig. 11-20D; Link 11-50; 10%–23% of cases). Although most references state that Osler nodes are an example of an IC vasculitis, more recent studies have contradicted that belief. Early biopsies frequently demonstrate bacteria within microabscesses *without* any evidence of a vasculitis, which favors microembolization as the *initial* process. However, as time progresses, the microabscess becomes sterile, and an immune-mediated vasculitis develops.

    (4) Infarctions may occur in different tissue sites (e.g., digits, brain).

    (5) Septic emboli produce metastatic abscesses and/or infarctions in different tissue sites in one-third of cases. If the brain is involved, it is usually in the distribution of the middle cerebral artery (MCA).

d. Heart murmurs (regurgitant types) may change in intensity because of microembolization and progressive damage to the valve (85% of cases).

e. Splenomegaly is present if IE is subacute.

4. Laboratory findings

a. Positive blood cultures are present in 80% of cases. Low percentage reflects the fact that many patients were already receiving antibiotics by the time that the cultures were drawn.

b. Neutrophilic leukocytosis occurs in acute IE.

c. Monocytosis occurs in subacute IE.

d. Mild anemia is most frequently caused by anemia of chronic disease (ACD; see Chapter 12).

5. Diagnosis

a. Three to five sets of blood cultures should be obtained within 60 to 90 minutes followed by the infusion of the appropriate antibiotic regimen.

b. ECHO or transesophageal echocardiography (TEE) is used to detect vegetations on the valves.

L. Libman-Sacks endocarditis

1. **Definition:** Libman-Sacks endocarditis is a nonbacterial type of endocarditis that is associated with SLE.

2. Occurs in 30% to 50% of patients with SLE

3. Sterile vegetations are located over the MV surface and chordae; produces valve deformity and MV regurgitation

M. Nonbacterial thrombotic endocarditis (NBTE; marantic endocarditis)

1. **Definition:** NBTE is a spectrum of noninfectious lesions of the heart valves that is most commonly seen in advanced malignancy.

2. Epidemiology

a. Paraneoplastic syndrome that occurs in 20% of cases of cancer (see Chapter 9). Paraneoplastic syndromes refer to distant effects of a tumor that are unrelated to metastasis.

b. Sterile, nondestructive vegetations are present on the MV. They are most often caused by the procoagulant effect of circulating mucin from mucin-producing tumors of the colon or pancreas.

3. Complications include embolization of vegetation material to distant sites and secondary infection of the vegetations.

VII. Myocardial and Pericardial Disorders

A. Myocarditis

1. **Definition:** Myocarditis refers to inflammation of the myocardial tissue; may be caused by either an infectious or non-infectious disease

2. Epidemiology

a. Major cause of sudden death (15%–20% of cases) in adults <40 years of age

b. Causes include:

    (1) microbial pathogens.

        (a) Viruses include adenovirus (most common), group B coxsackie viruses, HIV, parvovirus B19, and human herpesvirus 6.

Margin notes:

IC vasculitis: subacute endocarditis

Glomerulonephritis (nephritic), Roth spot in eyes

Microembolization >50%

Splinter hemorrhages nail beds

Janeway lesions (painless) palms/soles

Osler nodes painful nodules pads fingers/toes

Septic emboli may produce infarction

Septic emboli → metastatic abscesses (MCA distribution)

Changing heart murmurs

Splenomegaly (only subacute)

Positive blood culture majority cases

Neutrophilic leukocytosis acute

Monocytosis subacute

Mild ACD MC anemia

Blood cultures

ECHO, transesophageal echocardiography

Libman-Sacks endocarditis

Nonbacterial endocarditis associated with SLE

Valve deformity, MV regurgitation

NBTE

Noninfectious valvular disease in advanced malignancy

NBTE: paraneoplastic syndrome

Sterile vegetations MV; mucin-producing tumors

Embolization; 2° infection

Myocarditis

Inflammation myocardium; infectious/non-infectious

Major cause sudden death <40 years old

Microbial pathogens

Adenovirus MCC acute myocarditis U.S.

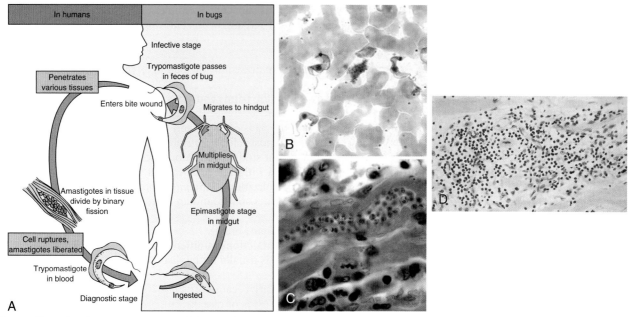

11-21: **A,** Life cycle of *Trypanosoma cruzi* (Chagas disease). The insect vector is a reduviid bug. **B,** Trypanosomes (trypomastigote) in the blood in Chagas disease. **C,** Amastigotes in cardiac tissue in Chagas disease. **D,** Viral myocarditis. The biopsy shows a lymphocytic infiltrate with dissolution of myocardial fibers. (**A** *from Murray PR, Rosenthal KS, Pfaller MA: Medical Microbiology, 6th ed, Philadelphia, Mosby Elsevier, 2009, p 851, Fig. 82.14;* **B** *and* **C** *from Kliegman R: Nelson Textbook of Pediatrics, 19th ed, Philadelphia, Elsevier Saunders, 2011, p 1193, Fig. 279.1;* **D** *from my friend Ivan Damjanov MD, PhD, Linder J: Pathology: A Color Atlas, St. Louis, Mosby, 2000, p 75, Fig. 1-28.*)

Bacteria (e.g., *Borrelia burgdorferi*)

Fungi (e.g., *Candida* spp.)

Parasites (e.g. *Trypanosoma*)

(b) Bacteria include *Borrelia burgdorferi, Mycoplasma* spp., and *Rickettsia rickettsia*.
(c) Fungi include *Candida, Mucor,* and *Aspergillus* spp.
(d) Parasites include *Trypanosoma cruzi* (Chagas disease; Fig. 11-21 A–C), *Trichinella spiralis,* and *Toxoplasma gondii*

American trypanosomiasis (Chagas disease) is caused by *Trypanosoma cruzi,* a protozoan (hemoflagellate). Transmission most commonly occurs through a bite around the eye or mouth that is contaminated with the feces of a reduviid bug (*Triatoma,* or kissing bug). Facial edema occurs near the bite site (called the Romaña sign) (Link 11-51). The flagellated trypomastigotes circulate in the blood, and the amastigotes (lack flagella) invade tissue. Common clinical findings are myocarditis causing chronic heart failure (most common COD) and arrhythmias; acquired achalasia, a motility disorder caused by destruction of ganglion cells in the lower esophageal sphincter; and acquired Hirschsprung disease (large bowel motility disorder) caused by destruction of ganglion cells in the rectosigmoid. The diagnosis is secured by finding trypomastigotes in the peripheral blood and/or amastigotes in tissue. Xenodiagnosis is used in some cases. An uninfected reduviid bug is allowed to feed on a patient, and after a short period of time, the intestine of the bug is examined for the parasite. Serologic tests are also available.

Chagas disease: MCC myocarditis leading to CHF in Central/South America

Myocarditis acute RF

Toxins: diphtheria, CO, black widow/scorpion venoms

Doxorubicin, daunorubicin, cocaine, alcohol

SLE, SS, Kawasaki disease, radiation

Sarcoidosis

Global enlargement heart/ chambers all dilated

Lymphocytic infiltrate/ necrosis

Fever, dyspnea, chest pain (MC)

Arrhythmias

(2) myocarditis in acute rheumatic fever (RF).
(3) toxins. Examples include diphtheria toxin, carbon monoxide (CO), and venom from black widows and scorpions.
(4) drugs. Examples include doxorubicin, cocaine, zidovudine, and sulfonamides.
(5) systemic and collagen vascular diseases. Examples of systemic and collagen vascular disease include SLE, systemic sclerosis (SS), and Kawasaki disease.
(6) radiation
(7) sarcoidosis (noninfectious granulomatous disease).
c. Pathology
(1) Global enlargement of the heart and dilation of all chambers
(2) Lymphocytic infiltrate with focal areas of necrosis is highly predictive of a viral myocarditis (Fig. 11-21 D; Link 11-52).
3. Clinical findings include:
a. dyspnea (difficulty with breathing; most common symptom).
b. fever (20% of cases), chest pain (35% of cases).
c. arrhythmias. A persistent tachycardia that is out of proportion to fever is a characteristic finding in myocarditis.

d. pericardial friction rub (see later), biventricular CHF with S_3 and S_4 heart sounds.

e. heart murmurs. Mitral valve regurgitation is the most common murmur and is caused by stretching of the MV ring from volume overload (increased preload) in the LV due to LHF. TV regurgitation caused by stretching of the TV ring is less common.

4. Diagnosis of myocarditis by ECHO and cardiac catheterization.

5. Laboratory findings include:

a. increased serum troponin T and/or I (a normal value does *not* exclude myocarditis).

b. increased serum CK-MB (a normal value does *not* exclude myocarditis).

c. detection of antibodies of the suspected pathogen.

6. Approximately 50% of patients die within 5 years.

B. Pericarditis

1. **Definition:** Pericarditis refers to inflammation (or infiltration by cancer) of the pericardium encasing the heart (epicardial surface, parietal surface).

2. Epidemiology

a. Causes include:

(1) idiopathic or viral in 80% to 90% of cases.

(2) infectious (similar to the pathogens producing myocarditis). Examples of infectious agents include adenovirus, coxsackievirus, bacterial (1%–2%), tuberculosis (TB) (4%–9%), amebic, HIV, and fungal.

(3) drug induced (procainamide, phenytoin, hydralazine, doxorubicin, mesalamine, adalimumab, cocaine).

(4) SLE (pericarditis with effusion is a common presentation), acute RF (ARF), post-MI pericarditis (Dressler syndrome; usually 2 weeks postinfarction), autoimmune pericarditis post-MI, systemic sclerosis (SS), uremia, postmediastinal radiation, iatrogenic (postpericardiotomy, postpacemaker lead), uremia, hypothyroidism, and metastasis (e.g., breast, lung, leukemia; Link 11-53).

b. Pathology of pericarditis and pericardial effusion.

(1) Fibrinous type of inflammation of the pericardial exudate (see Fig. 3-8 C; Link 11-54)

(a) A fibrinous exudate refers to inflammation that is caused by increased vessel permeability, with deposition of a fibrin-rich exudate on the surface of the tissue.

(b) Often accompanied by pericardial effusion (fluid in the pericardial sac; exudate)

(2) Dense scar tissue with dystrophic calcification may cause constrictive pericarditis.

3. Clinical findings include:

a. fever, tachycardia.

b. precordial chest pain that may radiate to the arms and back. Pain is relieved when leaning forward and increases when leaning back.

c. pericardial friction rub.

(1) Scratchy, three-component rub (systole, early, and late diastole). Best heard with the patient leaning forward. All three components are heard in ~50% of cases.

(2) Does *not* disappear when the person holds his or her breath, which distinguishes it from a pleural friction rub.

(3) Often accompanied by a pericardial effusion. **Pearl:** A young woman with a pericardial effusion most likely has SLE.

(a) Normal heart sounds are muffled. Fluid surrounding the heart makes heart sounds difficult to hear (Fig. 11-22 A).

(b) All pressures are equal in all chambers of the heart.

(c) CO is decreased because less blood is entering the right heart.

(d) Neck vein distention on inspiration (Kussmaul sign). In the normal state, the negative intrathoracic pressure on inspiration enhances the flow of blood from the vena cava (superior and inferior) into the RA. However, in a pericardial effusion, blood cannot easily enter the RA on inspiration because of fluid surrounding the heart. Therefore, some blood refluxes back into the JV on inspiration, causing distention of the JVs.

(e) Hypotension and pulsus paradoxus. On inspiration, there is a further increase in pressure of blood in the RV, which displaces the IVS to the left, causing a decrease in the volume of blood in the LV volume. This leads to a drop in the SBP that is >10 mm Hg (called pulsus paradoxus).

(f) Pericardial effusion triad is muffled heart sounds, JV distention on inspiration, and pulsus paradoxus.

Pericardial friction rub

Biventricular CHF (S_3/S_4)

Heart murmurs

MV regurgitation MC murmur

Dx: echocardiogram/catheterization

↑Serum troponin T and/or I

↑Serum CK-MB

Antibodies suspect pathogens

↑Mortality rate

Pericarditis

Pericardium inflammation (epicardial, parietal)

Idiopathic/viral 80% to 90% cases

Infections similar to myocarditis

Drugs: procainamide, doxorubicin

SLE, ARF, Dressler, autoimmune, SS, radiation, postpericardiotomy, uremia, metastasis

Fibrinous inflammation

Fibrinous inflammation

Pericardial effusion (exudate)

Healing with scar tissue/calcification

Fever, tachycardia

Precordial friction rub

Relief leaning forward, worse leaning back

Pericardial friction rub

3-Component rub

Does *not* disappear when holding breath

Pericardial effusion often present

Young woman: think SLE

Normal heart sounds muffled

All pressures all chambers equal

↓Cardiac output

Neck vein distention inspiration

Kussmaul sign

Hypotension, pulsus paradoxus

↓SBP >10 mm Hg on inspiration called pulsus paradoxus

Triad: muffled heart sounds, JV distention inspiration, pulsus paradoxus on inspiration

11-22: **A,** Hemopericardium. Note the "water bottle" configuration of the blood in the pericardial cavity. This was the result of a trauma. It may also occur in a rupture of the myocardium after acute myocardial infarction. **B,** Postero-anterior chest radiograph showing a pericardial effusion. Note the loss of the usual heart borders and the "water bottle" configuration. (*A from Klatt F: Robbins and Cotran Atlas of Pathology, Philadelphia, Saunders, 2006, p 52, Fig. 2-82; B courtesy of Sven Paulin, MD.*)

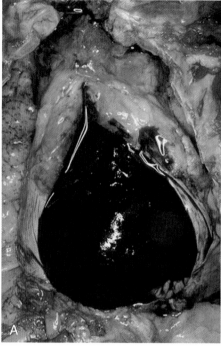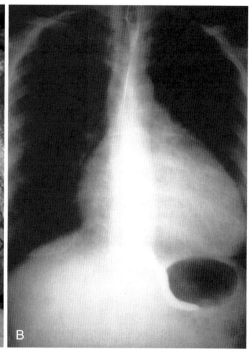

"Water bottle" configuration heart silhouette

Echocardiogram

ECG

Constrictive pericarditis

Scarring pericardial sac

Incomplete filling all chambers

TB MCC worldwide

Idiopathic/post open heart surgery in US

Pericardial calcification on x-ray

Incomplete filling from thickened pericardium

Pericardial knock

Calcification pericardium on x-ray/CT

Cardiomyopathy

Group diseases involving myocardium

Dilated, hypertrophic, restrictive

Dilated cardiomyopathy (nonischemic)

Ventricular dilation; ↓contractility; absence HTN, global ischemic disease

MC cardiomyopathy

MC cardiomyopathy young people

4. Diagnosis of pericardial effusion
   a. If an effusion is present, a chest radiograph shows a "water bottle" configuration (Fig. 11-22 B).
   b. ECHO is useful in detecting a pericardial effusion and in determining the amount of fluid.
   c. ECG in the acute phase shows PR-segment depression and diffuse ST-segment elevation in the precordial leads. Further changes occur in these segments as pericarditis progresses into an intermediate and late phase.
5. Constrictive pericarditis
   a. **Definition:** Constrictive pericarditis refers to scarring of the pericardial sac that limits the ability of the chambers in the heart to fill with blood.
   b. Epidemiology
      (1) TB is the most common cause of constrictive pericarditis worldwide.
      (2) Most cases in the United States are idiopathic or secondary to scarring from previous open heart surgery.
      (3) Pericardial calcification is seen on a chest radiograph in ~25% of cases.
      (4) Pathophysiology of constrictive pericarditis includes incomplete filling of the cardiac chambers caused by thickening of the parietal pericardium.
   c. Clinical findings. Pericardial knock is heard because of the ventricles hitting the thickened parietal pericardium.
   d. Chest radiography or computed tomography (CT) usually shows dystrophic calcification in the parietal pericardium (Link 11-55).

VIII. **Cardiomyopathy**
   A. **Definition and epidemiology of cardiomyopathy**
      1. The cardiomyopathies are a group of diseases that primarily involve the myocardium and produce myocardial dysfunction.
      2. Types of cardiomyopathy include dilated (congestive) cardiomyopathy, hypertrophic cardiomyopathy (HCM), and restrictive cardiomyopathy.
   B. **Dilated cardiomyopathy (nonischemic cardiomyopathy)**
      1. **Definition:** Dilated cardiomyopathy is a spectrum of heterogeneous myocardial disorders characterized by ventricular dilation and depressed myocardial contractility in the absence of abnormal loading conditions (e.g., HTN or valvular disease) or ischemic disease that is sufficient to cause global systolic impairment.
      2. Epidemiology
         a. Most common overall cardiomyopathy
         b. Most common cardiomyopathy in young people (accounts for 25% of cases)

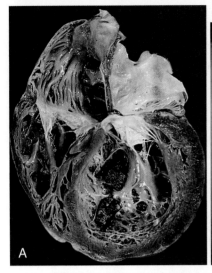
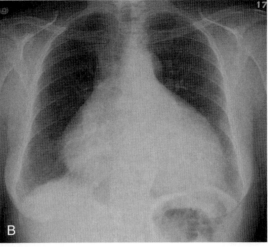

11-23: **A,** Dilated cardiomyopathy. Note the global enlargement of the heart and the dilated ventricle on the right and dilated atrium on the left. **B,** Dilated alcoholic cardiomyopathy. The cardiac silhouette is markedly enlarged, primarily as a result of biventricular enlargement. The patient had a long history of alcohol abuse. Dilated cardiomyopathy is frequently associated with biventricular heart failure. (**A** from my friend Ivan Damjanov MD, PhD, Linder J: Pathology: A Color Atlas, St. Louis, Mosby, 2000, p 17, Fig. 1-35; **B** from Herring W: Learning Radiology: Recognizing the Basics, 2nd ed, Philadelphia, Elsevier Saunders, 2012, p 79, Fig. 9.23.)

   c. Causes of dilated cardiomyopathy
     (1) CAD and idiopathic (unknown) are the most common causes.
     (2) Genetic types of cardiomyopathy account for 25% to 35% of cases.
     (3) Previous myocarditis (common cause)
     (4) Alcohol (15%–40% of cases)
       (a) May be either a result of direct toxic effect of alcohol or caused by thiamine deficiency associated with alcohol excess
       (b) In thiamine deficiency, there is a decrease in ATP (see Chapter 8), which is necessary for contraction of myocardial tissue.
     (5) Drugs (e.g., doxorubicin, daunorubicin, cyclophosphamide, and cocaine)
     (6) Postpartum state. Dilated cardiomyopathy may occur in the last trimester of pregnancy or up to 6 months postpartum.
     (7) Organic solvents ("glue sniffer's heart")
     (8) Endocrine disease in pregnancy, including acromegaly and myxedema heart in severe hypothyroidism
  3. Pathophysiology. Generalized decrease in contractility leading to global enlargement of the heart (Fig. 11-23 A; Link 11-56 B).
  4. Clinical findings include:
    a. global enlargement of the heart.
    b. signs and symptoms of LHF and RHF.
    c. narrow pulse pressure due to a decreased stroke volume (SV).
    d. presence of arrhythmias, such as bundle branch blocks (BBB); atrial and ventricular arrhythmias.
  5. Diagnosis
    a. ECHO shows an ejection fraction (EF) <45% (normal >55%).
    b. Chest x-ray shows global enlargement of the heart (Fig. 11-23 B).
C. Hypertrophic cardiomyopathy (HCM)
  1. **Definition:** HCM is a primary disorder of the cardiac muscle characterized by inappropriate myocardial hypertrophy of a nondilated LV in the absence of cardiovascular or systemic disease (i.e., hypertension, aortic stenosis).
  2. Epidemiology
    a. Second most common cardiomyopathy
    b. Most common cause of sudden death in young athletes
    c. Prevalence in the general population is 1 in 500.
    d. Familial form accounts for 60% to 70% of cases.
     (1) Autosomal dominant (AD) disease with nearly complete penetrance (see Chapter 6)
     (2) Primarily affects younger individuals
     (3) Most cases are caused by mutations of genes involved in the contractile process (e.g., β-myosin heavy chain [most common], troponin T, tropomyosin).
     (4) Familial screening of first-degree relatives with ECHO and ECG is mandatory.
    e. Sporadic form of HCM primarily occurs in older adults.
  3. Pathophysiology

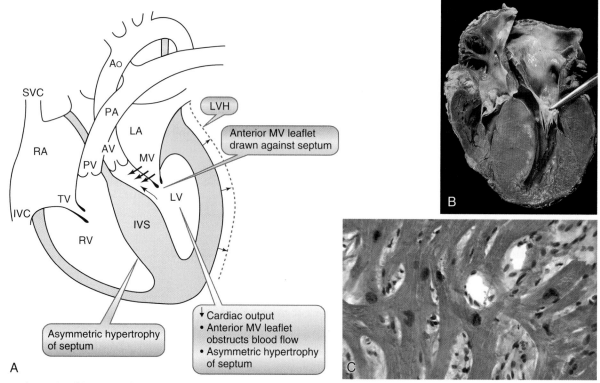

11-24: A, Schematic of hypertrophic cardiomyopathy. Note the asymmetric hypertrophy of the interventricular septum (IVS), causing it to obstruct the outflow tract. When systole occurs, the anterior leaflet is drawn against the septum, causing a marked decrease in blood flow. **B,** Hypertrophic cardiomyopathy. The heart shows asymmetric hypertrophy of the IVS *(black arrow)* with marked narrowing of the outflow tract. The histologic section of the conduction system in the septum **(C)** shows aberrant myofibers. *Ao,* Aorta; *AV,* aortic valve; *IVC,* inferior vena cava; *LA,* left atrium; *LV,* left ventricle; *LVH,* left ventricular hypertrophy; *MV,* mitral valve; *PA,* pulmonary artery; *PV,* pulmonary valve; *RA,* right atrium; *RV,* right ventricle; *SVC,* superior vena cava; *TV,* tricuspid valve. *(A from Goljan EF: Star Series: Pathology, Philadelphia, Saunders, 1998; B from Schoen FJ: Interventional and Surgical Cardiovascular Pathology: Clinical Correlations and Basic Principles, Philadelphia, Saunders, 1989; C from Kumar V, Abbas AK, Fausto N, Mitchell RN: Robbins Basic Pathology, 8th ed, Philadelphia, Saunders Elsevier, 2007, p 413, Fig. 11-25.)*

Hypertrophy of myocardium	a. Hypertrophy of the myocardium
IVS disproportionately thickened compared to free LV wall	(1) In particular, there is often a proportionately greater hypertrophy of the IVS compared with the free wall of the LV.
IVS hypertrophy may obstruct outflow tract	(2) Interventricular septal hypertrophy may mechanically obstruct blood flow through the LV outflow tract.
	(3) Most patients do *not have* obstruction of the LV outflow tract.
Obstruction outflow tract *below* AV	b. Obstruction to blood flow, if present, is located *below* the AV (Fig. 11-24 A, B; Link 11-56 C). As blood exits the LV, the *anterior leaflet* of the *MV* is drawn against the asymmetrically hypertrophied IVS, causing the obstruction.
Aberrant myofibers cause fatal arrhythmia, sudden death	c. Aberrant myofibers are present in the conduction system, which may cause fatal arrhythmias and sudden death (Fig. 11-24 C).
Noncompliant LV; diastolic dysfunction	d. Noncompliance of the LV. Muscle thickening restricts filling and produces diastolic dysfunction (decreased filling of the LV in diastole).
	4. Clinical findings
Harsh systolic ejection murmur	a. Harsh systolic ejection murmur, which is best heard along the left sternal border
Palpable double apical impulse	b. Palpable double apical impulse
Murmur intensity ↑ with ↓preload	c. Murmur intensity *increases* (obstruction worsens) with decreased preload (note that these changes are the opposite of those that occur with AV stenosis). Maneuvers that decrease preload (volume of blood in the ventricle) include standing up, Valsalva maneuver (increases positive intrathoracic pressure), and use of inotropic drugs (e.g., digitalis).
Preload changes are *opposite* those for AV stenosis	
Murmur intensity ↓ with ↑preload	d. Murmur intensity *decreases* (obstruction lessens) with increased preload (note that these changes are the opposite of those that occur with AV stenosis).
	(1) Maneuvers that increase preload include reclining, drugs decreasing cardiac contractility (e.g., β-blockers), sustained clenching of hands, and squatting.
	(2) Increasing the preload (more blood in the ventricle) opens the outflow track.

e. Angina or syncope may occur with exercise. This is similar in pathophysiology to what occurs in AV stenosis.

f. Sudden death from ventricular tachycardia or fibrillation may occur.

5. Diagnosis of HCM and screening for the disease is made with two-dimensional ECHO.

D. Restrictive cardiomyopathy

1. **Definition:** Restrictive cardiomyopathy is characterized by increased stiffness of the ventricular walls, causing impaired diastolic filling of the ventricles that leads to a precipitous rise in ventricular pressure with a small increase in volume.

2. Epidemiology (Link 11-56 D)

   a. Least common cardiomyopathy

   b. Most frequently caused by amyloidosis (most common), myocardial fibrosis after open heart surgery, and radiation

   c. Other causes include:

   (1) infiltrative diseases. Examples: Pompe glycogenosis, hemochromatosis

   (2) endocardial fibroelastosis in a child (Link 11-57). In this disease, there is thick fibroelastic tissue in the LV endocardium that prevents filling of the ventricle.

   (3) sarcoidosis. There is granulomatous inflammation in the myocardial tissue that prevents proper filling of the chambers.

   (4) SS. Fibrous tissue replaces the myocardial tissue, hence preventing proper filling of the chambers.

   d. Pathophysiology

   (1) Decrease in ventricular compliance leads to biventricular heart failure.

   (2) Complex neurohormonal mechanisms have been implicated.

   (3) Hallmark of the disease is a diastolic dysfunction type of LHF (DHF).

3. Clinical findings

   a. Progressive biventricular heart failure

   b. ECG is low voltage and has nonspecific ST-T wave changes.

4. Diagnosis. ECHO, cardiac catheterization, and endocardial biopsy are used.

IX. Tumors of the Heart

A. Epidemiology of tumors of the heart

1. Metastasis is more common than primary tumors. Example: extension of a primary lung cancer into the pericardium

2. Pericardium is the most common site for metastasis (Link 11-53); leads to pericarditis and effusions

3. Primary tumors or tumor-like conditions include cardiac myxoma and rhabdomyoma.

B. Cardiac myxoma

1. **Definition:** A cardiac myxoma is a primary, benign mesenchymal tumor of the heart.

2. Epidemiology/pathology

   a. Most common primary tumor of the heart in adults

   b. Approximately 90% arise from the LA (Fig. 11-25).

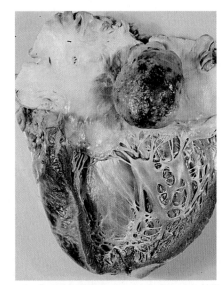

11-25: Cardiac myxoma in the left atrium. Note the large red mass in the left atrium. *(From my friend Ivan Damjanov MD, PhD, Linder J: Pathology: A Color Atlas, St. Louis, Mosby, 2000, p 27, Fig. 1-65A.)*

Angina/syncope with exercise similar to AV stenosis

Sudden death; ventricular tachycardia/fibrillation

Restrictive cardiomyopathy

Stiffness ventricular walls; impaired diastolic filling

Least common cardiomyopathy

Amyloidosis MCC

Open heart surgery, radiation

Infiltrative diseases

Pompe glycogenosis, hemochromatosis

Endocardial fibroelastosis

Thick fibroelastic tissue in LV

Sarcoidosis

Granulomatous inflammation myocardium

Systemic sclerosis

Fibrous tissue replaces myocardial tissue

↓Ventricular compliance

Biventricular heart failure

Complex neurohormonal mechanisms

DHF hallmark restrictive cardiomyopathy

Progressive biventricular heart failure

Characteristic low voltage ECG

Heart tumors

Metastasis > primary tumors

Pericardium MC site for metastasis

Pericarditis/effusions

Cardiac myxoma

Benign mesenchymal tumor of heart

MC adult primary heart tumor

MC in LA

Sessile or pedunculated

Pedunculated: may block MV orifice

Embolization; syncopal episodes

Dx: TEE

Rhabdomyoma

MC primary heart tumor infants/children

Association with tuberous sclerosis

Hamartoma of cardiac myocytes

    c. May be sessile or pedunculated

    d. If pedunculated, the tumor may have a "ball-valve" effect that blocks the MV orifice and prevents filling of the LV in diastole, simulating MV stenosis.

3. Clinical findings

    a. Nonspecific findings include fever (one of the causes of FUO; see Chapter 3), fatigue, malaise, and anemia.

    b. Complications of a cardiac myxoma include embolization and syncopal episodes (blocks the MV orifice).

4. Diagnosis. TEE is the most useful study for viewing the LA, which is the most posteriorly located chamber of the heart.

C. Rhabdomyoma

1. Most common primary tumor of the heart in infants and children. Major association with tuberous sclerosis (see Chapter 26)

2. Hamartoma (non-neoplastic) arising from cardiac myocytes

12 Red Blood Cell Disorders

ABBREVIATIONS

MC most common   MCC most common cause

I. Erythropoiesis

A. Erythropoiesis and erythropoietin

1. **Definition:** Erythropoiesis is the production of red blood cells (RBCs) in the bone marrow.

   a. Erythropoiesis is dependent on the release of erythropoietin (EPO) from the kidneys (Link 12-1).

   b. EPO is synthesized in the renal cortex by interstitial cells in the peritubular capillary bed.

   c. Stimuli for EPO release include:
   - hypoxemia ($\downarrow$arterial P_{O_2}), severe anemia, leftward shift of the O_2-dissociation curve (ODC), high altitude, and decreased O_2 saturation (S_{aO_2}; carbon monoxide poisoning, methemoglobinemia; see Chapter 2).

   d. Increased O_2 content suppresses EPO release (negative feedback; e.g., polycythemia vera).

Erythropoietin

RBC production in bone marrow
Renal cortex interstitial cells peritubular capillary bed

$\downarrow P_{aO_2}/\downarrow S_{aO_2}$, left-shifted ODC, high altitude
$\uparrow O_2$ content $\downarrow$EPO

> **EPO** increases the O_2-carrying capacity of blood by stimulating erythroid stem cells to divide (RBC hyperplasia; Fig. 12-1). Epoetin alfa, a form of EPO produced by recombinant DNA technology, is used in the treatment of anemia associated with renal failure, chronic disease, and chemotherapy. In addition, EPO has been used illicitly by endurance athletes to increase their oxygen-carrying capacity (and thus stamina) through increased RBC mass.

   e. EPO is ectopically produced in renal cell carcinoma and hepatocellular carcinoma (see Chapter 9).

2. During fetal development, hematopoiesis is first established in the yolk sac mesenchyme, later moves to the liver and spleen, and finally is limited to the bony skeleton (Link 12-2).
   - From infancy to adulthood, there is progressive restriction of productive marrow to the axial skeleton and proximal ends of the long bones.

Renal cell carcinoma, hepatocellular carcinoma

Yolk sac → liver/spleen → bony skeleton

Limited to axial skeleton → proximal ends long bones

B. Reticulocytes and the reticulocyte count

1. **Definition:** Reticulocytes are young RBCs containing RNA filaments in the cytoplasm.
   - Newly released RBCs from the bone marrow

2. Importance
   a. Peripheral blood markers of effective erythropoiesis in a person with anemia
   b. **Definition:** Effective erythropoiesis refers to an appropriate bone marrow response to anemia.
      - Correlates with an increase in the synthesis or release of reticulocytes from the bone marrow

3. Reticulocytes are easily identified in the peripheral blood with supravital stains.
   - Supravital stains detect the threadlike RNA filaments in the cytoplasm of immature RBCs (Fig. 12-2 A).

4. Reticulocyte becomes a mature RBC in 24 hours.
   - Maturation occurs with the help of splenic macrophages (MPs).

Contain RNA filaments

Peripheral marker effective erythropoiesis

Reticulocytes: RNA filaments present

Maturation to mature RBC 24 hrs

12-1: Morphology and lineage of hematopoietic cells. Pluripotent stem cells and colony-forming units (CFUs) are long-lived cells capable of replenishing the more differentiated functional and terminally differentiated cells. Erythropoietin (EPO) directly stimulates the erythroid CFU, leading to increased production of mature red blood cells. *(From Murray PR, Rosenthal KS, Pfaller MA: Medical Microbiology, 6th ed, Philadelphia, Mosby Elsevier, 2009, p 39, Fig. 7.1. Taken from Abbas K, et al: Cellular and Molecular Immunology, 5th ed, Philadelphia, WB Saunders, 2003.)*

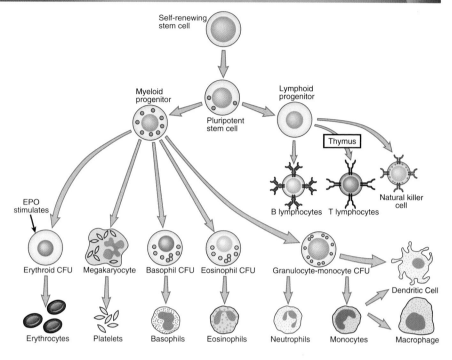

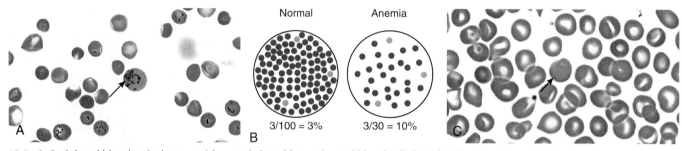

12-2: A, Peripheral blood reticulocytes with a methylene blue stain. Red blood cells (RBCs) with threadlike material in the cytosol represent residual RNA filaments and protein *(arrow)*. The patient has a hemolytic anemia; therefore, the number of reticulocytes is increased. **B,** Correction of the reticulocyte count for degree of anemia. Note that the normal reticulocyte count is 3% when 3 reticulocytes (pale blue RBCs) are expressed as a percentage of 100 RBCs in the microscopic field. However, the same 3 reticulocytes account for 10% of the RBCs in a patient with anemia, who has only 30 RBCs in the microscopic field. **C,** Polychromasia. The *arrow* indicates a blue discolored RBC without a central area of pallor. These cells are younger than reticulocytes and require anywhere from 2 to 3 days to become mature RBCs. *(A from Naeim F: Atlas of Bone Marrow and Blood Pathology, Philadelphia, Saunders, 2001, p 12, Fig. 1-15B; B from Goljan EF, Sloka KI: Rapid Review Laboratory Testing in Clinical Medicine, Philadelphia, Mosby Elsevier, 2008, p 146, Fig. 5-3; C from Naeim F: Atlas of Bone Marrow and Blood Pathology, Philadelphia, Saunders, 2001, Fig. 1-15A.)*

5. Reticulocyte count is reported as a percentage (normal, 0.5%–1.5%).
   a. **Definition:** A reticulocyte count is used to determine the number and/or percentage of reticulocytes in the peripheral blood in order to evaluate disorders that affect RBCs, such as anemia or bone marrow disorders. The purpose of the reticulocyte count is to evaluate the bone marrow (BM) response to anemia.

   Evaluate BM response to anemia

   b. Using the percentage reticulocyte count in anemia alone gives a falsely increased percentage (Fig. 12-2 B).
      (1) Clinician must correct the percentage of reticulocytes for the degree of anemia; called the reticulocyte index

   Correct reticulocyte count for degree of anemia

   Correction = Hct/45 × reticulocyte count

      (2) Reticulocyte index = (actual hematocrit [Hct]/45) × reticulocyte count, where 45 represents the normal Hct
      (3) Example calculation is as follows:
         (a) Hct, 30%; reticulocyte count, 5%
         (b) Reticulocyte index is 3% (30/45 × 5 = 3%).
   c. An additional correction is required if RBC polychromasia is present in the peripheral blood (see later).
      (1) Polychromatic RBCs are younger and larger than reticulocytes (Fig. 12-2 C).

(2) Appear in the peripheral blood when there is a very brisk hemolytic anemia (destruction of RBCS)
  - Also appear in the peripheral blood when "pushed out" by metastatic cancer invasion into bone
(3) Polychromatic RBCs require 2 to 3 days *before* becoming mature RBCs.
(4) When present, they falsely increase the initial reticulocyte count because they have RNA filaments and are incorrectly counted as "24-hour-old" reticulocytes.
(5) Correction for polychromasia is made by dividing the corrected reticulocyte count by 2.
(6) In the previous example, if polychromasia is present, the additional correction is 3%/2 = 1.5% (<2%).
(7) Importance of a reticulocyte index >2% in anemia (some authors use 3%)
  (a) Reticulocyte index >2% indicates a good BM response to anemia (called effective erythropoiesis).
  (b) Examples of effective erythropoiesis include:
    - increased reticulocyte count expected after treatment of iron deficiency with iron or the increased reticulocyte count seen in patients with a chronic hemolytic process (e.g., sickle cell anemia).
(8) Importance of a reticulocyte index <2% in anemia
  (a) Reticulocyte index of <2% indicates that there is a poor BM response to the anemia. This is called ineffective erythropoiesis.
  (b) Examples of ineffective erythropoiesis include:
    - untreated iron deficiency, anemia of chronic disease, folic acid deficiency, and aplastic anemia.
  (c) In the example calculation, the reticulocyte index of 3% initially appeared to be an appropriate response to the anemia (i.e., effective erythropoiesis); however, correction for polychromasia revealed a reticulocyte index of 1.5%, which is less than expected for the anemia (i.e., ineffective erythropoiesis). An example is the appearance of immature RBCs in the blood secondary to metastasis to the BM.

C. **Extramedullary hematopoiesis (EMH)**
  1. **Definition:** EMH refers to RBC, white blood cell (WBC), and platelet production that occurs *outside* the confines of the BM.
  2. Common sites for EMH are the liver and spleen (Link 12-2).
  3. Causes include:
    a. intrinsic BM disease (e.g., myelofibrosis [i.e., the BM is replaced by fibrous tissue]).
    b. accelerated erythropoiesis (e.g., severe hemolysis in sickle cell disease).
      (1) Erythroid hyperplasia expands the BM cavity.
      (2) A radiograph of the skull shows a "hair-on-end" appearance caused by expansion of the BM in the skull bones by RBC progenitors (Fig. 12-3).
  4. EMH produces hepatosplenomegaly (enlargement of the liver and spleen).

In fetuses, hematopoiesis (blood cell formation) begins in the yolk sac and subsequently moves to the liver and finally the BM by the fifth to sixth months of gestation (Link 12-3).

Marginal notes:
Polychromasia: original correction + 2

Reticulocyte index >2% → effective erythropoiesis

Reticulocyte index <2% → ineffective erythropoiesis

Erythropoiesis outside BM

EMH: most often occurs in liver and spleen

EMH: hepatosplenomegaly

Fetus: hematopoiesis begins in yolk sac

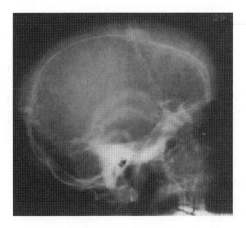

12-3: Lateral radiograph of the skull shows the typical "hair-on-end" appearance, with thinning of the cortical bone and widening of the marrow cavity from accelerated erythropoiesis (e.g., severe hemolysis in sickle cell disease). *(From Bouloux P: Self-Assessment Picture Tests Medicine, Vol. 1, London, Mosby-Wolfe, 1997, p 49, Fig. 97.)*

II. **Complete Blood Cell Count and Other Studies**

A. **Components of a complete blood cell (CBC) count** (Links 12-4 to 12-6)

1. Hemoglobin (Hb), Hct, RBC count
2. RBC indices, RBC distribution width (RDW)
3. WBC count with a differential count and platelet count
4. Evaluation of the peripheral blood morphology

B. **Hb, Hct, and RBC counts**

Factors affecting normal range: age, sex, and pregnancy

1. Factors affecting the normal range include age, sex, and pregnancy (see Chapter 1).
2. Anemia

a. **Definition:** Anemia refers to a decrease in Hb, Hct, or RBC concentration from any cause.

Pao_2/Sao_2 normal

b. Sao_2 and Pao_2 (partial pressure of arterial Po_2) are normal.
   • O_2 exchange in the lungs is normal; therefore, the Pao_2 and Sao_2 are normal.

↓O_2 content

c. O_2 content is decreased in anemia (see Chapter 2).
   (1) Recall that the O_2 content = (Hb g/dL × 1.34) × Sao_2 + Pao_2 × 0.003.
   (2) Note that if Hb is decreased, the O_2 content must also be decreased.

↓Production (hypoproliferative)

↑Destruction (hemolysis)

↑Acute blood loss (hemorrhage)

Sign of disease *not* a diagnosis

d. Mechanisms include:
   (1) decreased production of RBCs (hypoproliferative).
   (2) increased destruction of RBCs (hemolysis).
   (3) acute blood loss (hemorrhage).

e. Anemia is a sign of an underlying disease rather than a specific diagnosis.

f. General clinical findings include:
   (1) fatigue, dyspnea with exertion, inability to concentrate, and dizziness.
   (2) pulmonary valve flow murmur caused by decreased blood viscosity.
      • Indicates severe anemia (<5 g/dL).

Pallor skin/conjunctivae/palmar creases

   (3) pallor of the skin, conjunctivae (Link 12-7), and palmar creases.
      • Indicates severe anemia (<5 g/dL).

High-output heart failure due to ↓blood viscosity

   (4) high-output cardiac failure (see Chapter 11).
      • Caused by decreased blood viscosity in severe anemia (<5 g/dL)

C. **RBC indices**

MCV

Average volume RBCs

1. Mean corpuscular volume (MCV)

a. **Definition:** The MCV is the average volume of the RBCs.

b. Frequently used to classify anemia (Fig. 12-4) into a:

Microcytic <80 μm³
Normocytic 80–100 μm³
Macrocytic >100 μm³

   (1) microcytic anemia: MCV <80 μm^3.
   (2) normocytic anemia: MCV 80–100 μm^3.
   (3) macrocytic anemia: MCV >100 μm^3.

Average Hb concentration in RBCs

2. Mean corpuscular Hb concentration (MCHC)

a. **Definition:** MCHC is the average Hb concentration in RBCs.

↓MCHC → iron deficiency anemia

b. Clinical significance of a decreased MCHC
   (1) Correlates with decreased RBC synthesis of Hb (e.g., iron deficiency anemia)
   (2) Recognized by noting that the central area of pallor in a RBC is greater than normal because there is less Hb in the cell

MCHC: ↓microcytic anemias; ↑hereditary spherocytosis

      • This is called hypochromasia (compare Fig. 12-5 with Fig. 12-10 D).

c. Significance of an increased mean corpuscular Hb concentration
   (1) Correlates with the presence of spherical RBCs, which occurs in hereditary spherocytosis (HS)
      • Mature RBCs are biconcave disks (discussed later).
   (2) Spherocytes lack the central area of pallor that is present in a mature RBC.
      • Hematologists call this hyperchromasia (see Fig. 12-22 B).

3. RDW

Measure RBC size variation; anisocytosis

a. **Definition:** RDW is a measure of the variation in the size of the peripheral blood RBCs (i.e., small ones, big ones).
   (1) Size variation is called anisocytosis.
   (2) RDW value is only clinically significant if it is increased.

b. RDW is increased if RBCs are *not* uniformly the same size.
   • Example: peripheral blood shows a mixture of microcytic and normocytic cells (see Fig. 12-10 D)

c. RDW is most useful in distinguishing iron deficiency from other causes of a microcytic anemia (small RBCs).

MC microcytic anemia with ↑RDW

   (1) Iron deficiency is the most common microcytic anemia with an increased RDW.
      • RDW is increased because of a mixture of normocytic and microcytic RBCs in the peripheral blood.

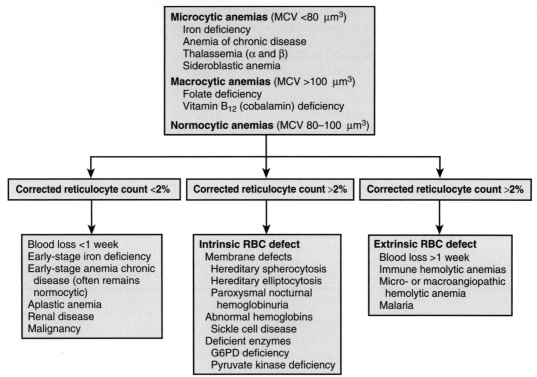

Microcytic anemias (MCV <80 μm^3)
  Iron deficiency
  Anemia of chronic disease
  Thalassemia (α and β)
  Sideroblastic anemia
Macrocytic anemias (MCV >100 μm^3)
  Folate deficiency
  Vitamin B_{12} (cobalamin) deficiency
Normocytic anemias (MCV 80–100 μm^3)

Corrected reticulocyte count <2%

Blood loss <1 week
Early-stage iron deficiency
Early-stage anemia chronic
  disease (often remains
  normocytic)
Aplastic anemia
Renal disease
Malignancy

Corrected reticulocyte count >2%

Intrinsic RBC defect
  Membrane defects
    Hereditary spherocytosis
    Hereditary elliptocytosis
    Paroxysmal nocturnal
      hemoglobinuria
  Abnormal hemoglobins
    Sickle cell disease
  Deficient enzymes
    G6PD deficiency
    Pyruvate kinase deficiency

Corrected reticulocyte count >2%

Extrinsic RBC defect
  Blood loss >1 week
  Immune hemolytic anemias
  Micro- or macroangiopathic
    hemolytic anemia
  Malaria

12-4: Classification of anemia using mean corpuscular volume (MCV). An intrinsic red blood cell (RBC) defect indicates a structural or biochemical flaw in the RBCs. An extrinsic RBC defect indicates that the RBCs are structurally normal, but that other factors cause the anemia. *G6PD,* Glucose-6-phosphate dehydrogenase.

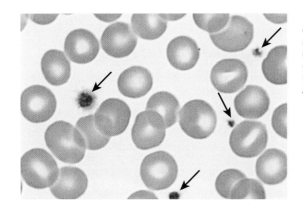

12-5: Normal peripheral blood smear showing red blood cells (RBCs). The RBCs are uniform in size, and the central areas of pallor are slightly less than half the total diameter of an RBC. The four dark objects *(arrows)* outside the RBCs are platelets. *(From Hoffbrand AV: Color Atlas: Clinical Hematology, 3rd ed, St. Louis, Mosby, 2000, p 22, Fig. 1-62.)*

(2) In other microcytic anemias, particularly anemia of chronic disease (ACD) and mild thalassemia, the RBCs appear more uniform and the RDW is normal.

D. Characteristics of mature RBCs (see Fig. 12-5)
  1. Mature RBCs are a biconcave disk (Link 12-8).
     a. Biconcave disk shape enhances gas exchange.
     b. This shape, along with the flexibility of the cytoskeleton, allows the RBC to deform readily, allowing them to squeeze through small capillaries.
     c. Biconcave shape is determined not only by the cytoskeleton but also by its electrolyte and water content and the lipid composition of the cell membrane.
  2. Mature RBCs lack mitochondria (mT); therefore, there is no citric acid cycle, β-oxidation of fatty acids, or ketone body synthesis.
  3. Mature RBCs lack a nucleus; therefore, they cannot synthesize DNA or RNA.
  4. RBCs use anaerobic glycolysis as their primary source of adenosine triphosphate (ATP).
     a. Lactic acid is the end product of RBC anaerobic metabolism.
     b. Lactic acid is converted by the liver into glucose via gluconeogenesis.
     c. Glucose derived from gluconeogenesis is used by RBCs to synthesize ATP.
  5. RBCs use the pentose phosphate pathway.

Biconcave disc

Enhances gas exchange

Enhances flexibility

Cytoskeleton/electrolyte/ water content/lipid composition

Lack mT/nucleus; no DNA/ RNA

Anaerobic glycolysis 1° source ATP

Anaerobic glycolysis; lactic acid end-product

Lactic acid → glucose in liver (gluconeogenesis)

RBC glucose from gluconeogenesis → ATP

GSH converts H_2O_2 to H_2O

a. Pathway synthesizes glutathione (GSH).
   (1) GSH is an antioxidant that converts hydrogen peroxide (H_2O_2) to water (see Chapter 2).
   (2) GSH also neutralizes acetaminophen free radicals (FRs).
b. Hydrogen peroxide is a product of oxidative metabolism in every living cell; therefore, this pathway must be functional to prevent destruction of RBCs by hydrogen peroxide.
6. Mature RBCs use the methemoglobin (metHb) reductase pathway (see Chapter 2).

MetHb reductase system reduces Fe^{3+} to Fe^{2+}

  a. Heme iron in methemoglobin is oxidized (Fe^{3+}); therefore, it *cannot* bind O_2.
  b. Methemoglobin reductase system converts oxidized iron back to its ferrous (Fe^{2+}) state so that it can bind O_2.
7. Mature RBCs use the Luebering-Rapoport pathway.

2,3-BPG → product of glycolytic cycle

  • Pathway synthesizes 2,3-bisphosphoglycerate (2,3-BPG), which is required for rightward shifting of the oxygen dissociation curve (ODC), leading to the release of O_2 to tissue (see Chapter 2).

RBCs lack HLAs

8. Mature RBCs lack human leukocyte antigens (HLAs) on their membranes (see Chapter 4).
9. Fate of senescent RBCs (Link 12-9)

Removed by splenic macrophages

  a. Normal RBC life span is 110 to 120 days in the peripheral blood.
  b. Senescent RBCs are phagocytosed in the cords of Billroth by splenic MPs.

UCB: end-product heme degradation by macrophages

  c. Heme degradation by the splenic MPs produces unconjugated bilirubin (UCB).
   • Most of the UCB that is normally present in blood derives from destruction of senescent RBCs.

E. WBC count and differential

A 100-cell differential count divides leukocytes by percentage (e.g., neutrophils, lymphocytes) and further subdivides neutrophils into segmented and band neutrophils. Multiplication of the percentage and the total WBC count gives the absolute number of a particular leukocyte. Example: lymphocytes 30%, total WBC count 10,000/mm³; absolute lymphocyte count is 0.30 × 10,000 = 3000 cells/mm³.

Platelets

Lack a nucleus

Pinch off megakaryocyte cytoplasm

Have HLAs

Ferritin

Soluble, iron-binding storage protein

F. Platelet count
1. Platelets lack a nucleus (anucleate).
2. Derived from cytoplasmic budding of megakaryocytes in the BM (see Fig. 15-1 B)
3. Unlike mature RBCs, they have HLAs on their membranes.

G. Iron studies (Fig. 12-6)
1. Serum ferritin
  a. **Definition:** Ferritin is a soluble iron-binding storage protein (see Chapter 2).

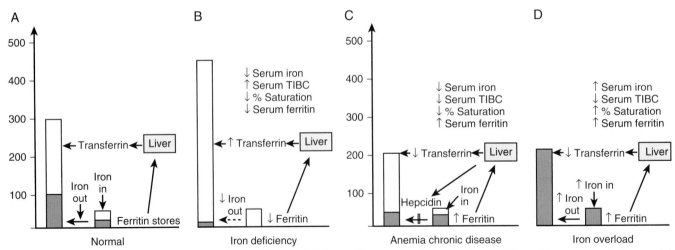

12-6: Iron studies in normal people (**A**) and those with iron deficiency (**B**), anemia of chronic disease (**C**), and iron-overload diseases (**D**). The column represents transferrin, the iron-binding protein. The *small box* represents bone marrow macrophage stores of ferritin. Note that iron comes into the macrophage and leaves the macrophage after attaching to transferrin via a ferroxidase reaction (not depicted). Every day an equal amount of iron goes into the macrophages and comes out of the macrophages. The iron coming into the macrophage derives from phagocytosis of senescent red blood cells and the degradation of heme into iron (binds to ferritin in the macrophage) + protoporphyrin, the latter converted to unconjugated bilirubin. Note that the amount of ferritin in the macrophages has a negative feedback on transferrin synthesis in the liver. If ferritin stores are decreased, the liver synthesizes more transferrin. If ferritin stores are increased, the liver synthesizes less transferrin. Refer to the text for discussion of the anemias. *TIBC*, Total iron-binding capacity.

(1) Synthesized by BM MPs and hepatocytes

(2) Ferritin keeps iron in a nontoxic form.

(3) MPs are the primary storage site for ferritin in the BM.

    (a) Refer to the *shaded area* in the small box in Figure 12-6 A.

    (b) Most of the iron in MPs comes from phagocytosis of senescent RBCs in the spleen.

(4) Serum levels directly correlate with ferritin stores in the MPs.

    • 1 µg/L of serum ferritin correlates with 8 mg of storage iron.

(5) Synthesis of ferritin in MPs (and hepatocytes) increases in inflammation.

    • Caused by the release of interleukin-6 (IL-6) (see Chapter 3)

  b. A decrease in serum ferritin is diagnostic of iron deficiency with or without anemia (Fig. 12-6 B).

  c. An increase in serum ferritin is present in ACD (Fig. 12-6 C) and iron overload disease (Fig. 12-6 D).

  d. Hemosiderin is an insoluble product of ferritin degradation in lysosomes (see Chapter 2).

    (1) Decreased and increased levels of hemosiderin correlate with changes in the ferritin stores in the BM MPs.

    (2) Hemosiderin is brown in hematoxylin and eosin–stained tissue and blue with the Prussian blue stain.

2. Serum iron

  a. **Definition:** Refers to the iron that is bound to transferrin in the circulating blood

    • Transferrin is synthesized by the liver and binds iron for transport in the bloodstream.

  b. Serum iron is the *shaded area* of the column in Figure 12-6 A.

    • Note that the normal serum iron level is ~100 µg/dL.

  c. Iron shown coming into the MPs in Figure 12-6 A is from the degradation of senescent MPs, *not* from transferrin.

    • The amount of iron coming into the MP is equal to the amount of iron that is leaving the MP to bind with transferrin.

  d. Decreased serum iron occurs in iron deficiency (Fig. 12-6 B) and ACD (Fig. 12-6 C).

  e. Increased serum iron occurs in iron overload diseases (see Fig. 12-6 D).

    • Examples of iron overload diseases include the sideroblastic anemias (see later) and hemochromatosis (see Chapter 19).

3. Serum total iron-binding capacity (TIBC)

  a. **Definition:** Correlates with the concentration of transferrin, the binding protein of iron

    (1) Height of the column in Figure 12-6 A correlates with serum transferrin and TIBC.

    (2) Note that the normal TIBC is ~300 µg/dL.

  b. Relationship of transferrin synthesis with ferritin stores in MPs

    (1) Inverse relationship between transferrin synthesis and ferritin stores in MPs

    (2) Decreased ferritin stores leads to increased liver synthesis of transferrin (Fig. 12-6 B).

    • Increase in transferrin and TIBC is present in iron deficiency.

    (3) Increased ferritin stores lead to decreased liver synthesis of transferrin (Fig. 12-6 C, D).

    • Decreases in transferrin and TIBC occur in ACD (Fig. 12-6 C) and iron overload disease (Fig. 12-6 D).

  c. Primary function of transferrin is to deliver ferric iron (Fe^{3+}) to erythroid precursors in the BM.

    • Iron on transferrin comes from the BM MPs and from the duodenum, the primary site for iron absorption.

4. Iron saturation (%)

  a. **Definition:** Refers to the percentage of binding sites on transferrin that are occupied by iron

    (1) Formula for calculating iron saturation is iron saturation (%) = serum iron/TIBC × 100.

    (2) In Figure 12-6 A, the normal percentage of saturation is 100/300 × 100, or 33%.

  b. Decreased iron saturation is present in iron deficiency (Fig. 12-6 B) and ACD (see Fig. 12-6 C).

  c. Increased iron saturation is present in iron overload diseases (Fig. 12-6 D).

H. Hb electrophoresis

1. Hb electrophoresis is used to detect hemoglobinopathies (Fig. 12-7), which include:

  a. abnormalities in globin chain structure (e.g., sickle cell disease).

  b. abnormalities in globin chain synthesis (e.g., thalassemia).

Margin notes:

BM macrophages/hepatocytes

Keeps iron in nontoxic form

MPs 1° storage site ferritin in BM

MP iron → phagocytosis senescent RBCs

Serum levels correlate ferritin stores in MPs

Synthesis ferritin MPs increases with inflammation (IL-6)

↓Serum ferritin → iron deficiency

↑Serum ferritin → ↑ACD, iron overload disease

Insoluble degradation product ferritin; Prussian blue +

Iron bound to transferrin

Serum iron ↓iron deficiency, ACD; ↑iron overload disease

↓TIBC = ↓transferrin; ↑TIBC = ↑transferrin

↓Ferritin stores/↑TIBC; ↑Ferritin stores/↓TIBC

Transferrin iron: from macrophages/duodenum

Iron saturation

↓Iron saturation: iron deficiency, ACD; ↑iron saturation: iron overload disease

	Pattern				Type of Anemia	Interpretation and Discussion
A.	A₂ — 2%	S	F — 1%	A — 97%	None	Normal Hb electrophoresis
B.	A₂ — 2%	S	F — 1%	A — 97%	Microcytic	α-Thal trait. Note that the proportion of the Hb types remains the same; however, the patient has a microcytic anemia.
C.	A₂ — 5%	S	F — 2%	A — 93%	Microcytic	β-Thal minor. Note that HbA is decreased because β-globin chain synthesis is decreased. There is a corresponding increase in HbA₂ and HbF.
D.	A₂ — 10%	S	F — 90%	A	Microcytic	β-Thal major. Note that there is no synthesis of HbA.
E.	A₂ — 2%	S — 45%	F — 1%	A — 52%	No anemia	Sickle cell trait. Note that there is not enough HbS to cause spontaneous sickling in the peripheral blood.
F.	A₂ — 2%	S — 90%	F — 8%	A	Normocytic	Sickle cell disease. Note that there is no HbA. There is enough HbS to cause spontaneous sickling.

12-7: Hemoglobin (Hb) electrophoresis in various hemoglobinopathies. See text for discussion. (*From Goljan E, Sloka K:* Rapid Review Laboratory Testing in Clinical Medicine, *St. Louis, Mosby Elsevier, 2008, p 159, Fig. 5-12.*)

Hb electrophoresis

HbA: 2α/2β
HbA₂: 2α/2δ
HbF: 2α/2γ

α, β, δ, γ microcytic anemia

Pathogenesis

Defects Hb synthesis; Hb = heme + globin chains

Iron deficiency, ACD, sideroblastic

α and β-Thalassemias

2. Types of normal Hb in adults that are detected by Hb electrophoresis include (Fig. 12-7 A):
   a. HbA, which has 2α/2β globin chains (97% in adults).
   b. HbA₂, which has 2α/2δ globin chains (2% in adults).
   c. HbF, which has 2α/2γ globin chains (1% in adults).
3. Examples of a few abnormal Hb detected by electrophoresis include:
   • sickle Hb, Hb H, and Hb Bart.

III. **Microcytic Anemias**
   A. **Types of microcytic anemia include:**
      1. iron deficiency (most common).
      2. ACD.
      3. thalassemia (thal; α and β).
      4. sideroblastic anemias (least common).
   B. **Pathogenesis** (Fig. 12-8)
      1. All microcytic anemias have a defect in Hb synthesis.
         • Hb = heme + globin chains
      2. Defects in heme synthesis (i.e., iron + protoporphyrin) include:
         • iron deficiency, ACD, and sideroblastic anemia.
      3. Defects in globin chain synthesis (i.e., α or β) include α- and β-thalassemia.

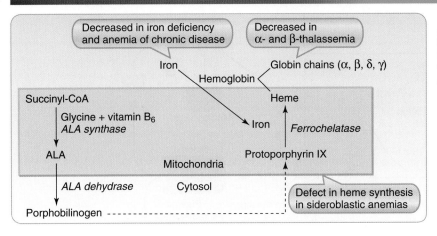

12-8: Pathophysiology of microcytic anemias. All microcytic anemias have a decrease in hemoglobin synthesis. A decrease in hemoglobin synthesis could be caused by a decrease in the synthesis of heme or a decrease in the synthesis of globin chains. *ALA*, Aminolevulinic acid.

C. Iron metabolism

1. Types of iron include:
   a. reduced Fe^{2+} (ferrous heme iron in meat).
   b. oxidized Fe^{3+} (ferric nonheme iron in plants).

2. Iron distribution
   a. Functional iron is present in Hb, enzymes, and myoglobin.
      Amount of functional iron in men is ~2500 mg and in women is ~2000 mg.
   b. Primarily stored as ferritin and hemosiderin in BM MPs.
      Amount of stored iron in men is ~1000 mg and 400 mg in women (decreased because of menses).
   c. Total iron stores in men is ~3500 mg and in women is ~2400 mg.

3. Iron absorption and regulation (Fig. 12-9; Link 12-10)
   a. Gastric acid frees elemental iron from heme (ferrous; Fe^{2+}) and nonheme products (ferric, Fe^{3+}).
      • Explains why achlorhydria (absence of stomach acid) decreases the availability of iron for absorption
   b. Iron from plants is in a nonheme or oxidized form (ferric, Fe^{3+}).
      (1) Nonheme (ferric) iron *cannot* be absorbed in the duodenum.
      (2) Nonheme (ferric) iron is converted by cytochrome B in the duodenal mucosa into reduced iron (Fe^{2+}), which can be reabsorbed.
      (3) Reduced iron is absorbed by divalent metal transporter 1 (DMT1) into the mucosal cell of the duodenum.
   c. Iron from meat and meat products is in a heme or reduced form (ferrous, Fe^{2+}).
      • Ferrous form of iron is directly absorbed in the duodenum by heme carrier protein 1.
   d. Absorbed iron is stored as mucosal ferritin or it enters the ferroportin 1 port and is immediately converted by hephaestin or ceruloplasmin to ferric iron (Fe^{3+}) so that it can bind to transferrin in the blood.
      • Transferrin transports iron to developing erythroid precursors in the marrow.
   e. Iron absorption is regulated.
      (1) Absorption of iron is dependent on total iron stores in the body, which are reflected by the amount of iron bound to transferrin.
      (2) Transferrin with iron binds to transferrin receptors in immature precursor cells of normal enterocytes, which serve as iron sensors in the duodenum.
      (3) *HFE* gene (hemochromatosis gene) protein product in the sensor cells acting with the transferrin receptor causes differentiation of these cells into mature enterocytes that absorb iron.
      (4) *HFE* protein product also regulates the production of hepcidin, a hormone synthesized in the liver.
         (a) Hepcidin is the "master" iron regulatory hormone that determines whether iron is absorbed or is not absorbed in the duodenum and whether iron is released from MPs or is not released.
         (b) A decreased level of transferrin-bound iron binding to transferrin receptors in enterocytes indicates iron depletion, which leads to reduced hepcidin synthesis in the liver.

Reduced Fe^{2+} (ferrous heme iron in meat)

Oxidized Fe^{3+} (ferric nonheme iron plants)

Hb, enzymes, myoglobin

Ferritin in BM MPs

Iron storage men > women

Heme (ferrous; Fe^{2+}); nonheme (ferric, Fe^{3+})

Acid frees elemental iron from heme/nonheme products

Plants: nonheme

Fe^{3+} cannot be reabsorbed

Fe^{2+} reabsorbed in duodenum

DMT1

Meat: Heme form

Fe^{2+} meat products directly reabsorbed

Iron bound to transferrin regulates iron absorption

HFE protein product + transferrin receptors differentiate sensor cells to enterocytes

HFE protein product: Regulates production of transferrin

Hepcidin master iron regulator

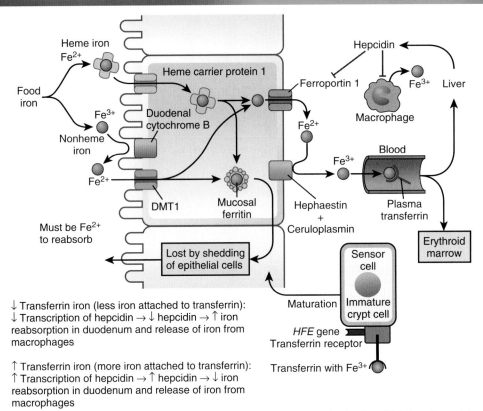

Food iron — Heme iron Fe²⁺

Heme carrier protein 1

Nonheme iron Fe³⁺

Fe²⁺

Must be Fe²⁺ to reabsorb

Duodenal cytochrome B

DMT1

Mucosal ferritin

Lost by shedding of epithelial cells

Ferroportin 1

Fe²⁺

Hephaestin + Ceruloplasmin

Hepcidin

Macrophage Fe³⁺ Liver

Fe³⁺ Blood

Plasma transferrin

Erythroid marrow

Sensor cell

Immature crypt cell

Maturation

HFE gene
Transferrin receptor

Transferrin with Fe³⁺

↓ Transferrin iron (less iron attached to transferrin):
↓ Transcription of hepcidin → ↓ hepcidin → ↑ iron reabsorption in duodenum and release of iron from macrophages

↑ Transferrin iron (more iron attached to transferrin):
↑ Transcription of hepcidin → ↑ hepcidin → ↓ iron reabsorption in duodenum and release of iron from macrophages

12-9: Iron absorption. The reabsorption of iron is dependent on total iron stores in the body, which is reflected in the amount of iron that is bound to transferrin. Transferrin with iron binds to immature precursor cells of normal enterocytes, which serve as iron sensors in the duodenum. The HFE hemochromatosis gene (*HFE* gene) protein product in these sensor cells acting together with the transferrin receptor causes the precursor cells to differentiate into mature enterocytes that can actively reabsorb iron. Absorptively active enterocytes absorb ferrous iron (Fe²⁺) directly via heme carrier protein 1 or through the divalent metal transporter (DMT1). Absorbed iron is either stored in the cytoplasm as mucosal ferritin or transferred to the ferroportin 1 port, where it is converted to ferric iron (Fe³⁺) by hephaestin and ceruloplasmin. Plasma transferrin then binds the iron and carries it to erythroid precursors in the bone marrow. The HFE protein also regulates the production of another protein called hepcidin, which is the "master" iron regulatory hormone. Hepcidin is produced by the liver and determines how much iron is absorbed from the diet and released from storage sites in the body. For example, if there is less transferrin iron bound to the receptor (decreased iron stores), then there is decreased transcription of hepcidin in the liver, and more iron is allowed to enter the circulation via the ferroportin 1 port to bind to transferrin and more iron is released from bone marrow macrophages to bind to transferrin. If there is increased transferrin iron bound to the receptor (excess iron stores), there is increased transcription of hepcidin, and iron is trapped in the mucosal cell because of downregulation of ferroportin 1. Furthermore, bone marrow macrophages cannot release iron (iron blockade). Enterocytes with excess iron are then shed, and the iron is lost in the stool. (*Modified from Kumar V, Fausto N, Abbas A, Aster J:* Robbins and Cotran Pathologic Basis of Disease, *8th ed, Philadelphia, Saunders Elsevier, 2010, p 661, Fig. 14-22; from my friend Ivan Damjanov MD, PhD:* Pathophysiology, *Philadelphia, Saunders Elsevier, 2009, p 69, Fig. 3-1.*)

↓T-bound iron → ↓hepcidin → ↑iron bound to T → ↑iron release from MPs

↑T-bound iron → ↑hepcidin → ↓iron bound to T → ↓iron release from MPs (iron blockade)

Menses, pregnancy, lactation, any anemia

- This upregulates ferroportin 1, causing more iron to be reabsorbed in the duodenum to bind to transferrin (T) and more iron to be released from BM MPs to bind to transferrin for erythropoiesis.
  (c) Increased level of transferrin-bound iron binding to transferrin receptors in enterocytes indicates iron excess, which leads to increased hepcidin synthesis in the liver.
    - Hepcidin downregulates ferroportin 1, causing iron accumulation in enterocytes, which are eventually shed into the bowel.
    - A reduced level of ferroportin 1 also inhibits the release of iron from BM MPs (less is available for binding to transferrin).
  4. Percentage of iron absorbed from the diet is increased (i.e., decreased hepcidin) in the following conditions:
    a. normal menstrual cycle.
    b. pregnancy and lactation.
    c. *any* anemia regardless of type.
  5. Definition and epidemiology of iron deficiency anemia (Link 12-11)
    a. **Definition:** Iron deficiency anemia is caused by insufficient iron for the normal synthesis of Hb.
    b. Epidemiology

TABLE 12-1   Causes of Iron Deficiency Anemia

CLASSIFICATION	CAUSES	DISCUSSION
Blood loss	Gastrointestinal loss	• Peptic ulcer in Meckel diverticulum (older children) • PUD (most common cause in adult men) • Hemorrhagic gastritis (e.g., NSAID) • Hookworm infestation • Polyps or colorectal cancer (most common cause in adults >50 yrs of age); associated with a positive test result for blood in stool
Increased utilization	Menorrhagia Pregnancy or lactation Infants and children	• Most common cause in women <50 yrs of age • Daily iron requirement is 3.4 mg in pregnancy and 2.5–3 mg in lactation; therefore, if a woman does not continue taking prenatal vitamins, she will become iron deficient. • Normal iron stores are ~400 mg. The net loss of iron in pregnancy is 500 mg; therefore, if a woman is *not* taking prenatal vitamins, she will become iron deficient. • Iron is required for tissue growth and expansion of blood volume in developing fetuses.
Decreased intake	Prematurity Infants and children Older adults	• Loss of iron each day a fetus is not in utero • Caused by blood loss from repeated phlebotomy for laboratory testing • Decreased intake of iron is the most common cause of iron deficiency in young children. • Restricted diets with very little meat intake decreases the intake of heme iron.
Decreased absorption	Celiac sprue Post–gastric surgery	• Absence of the villous surface in the duodenum decreases absorption of iron. • Rapid transit of food, which decreases iron absorption, and there is absent acid, which is required to release elemental iron from food.
Intravascular hemolysis	Microangiopathic hemolytic anemia	• Intravascular hemolysis produces a chronic loss of hemoglobin in the urine (hemoglobinuria), which ultimately leads to iron deficiency. • Paroxysmal nocturnal hemoglobinuria. Intravascular hemolysis of RBCs caused by complement destruction of RBCs at night

Hb, Hemoglobin; *NSAID,* nonsteroidal antiinflammatory drug; *PUD,* peptic ulcer disease; *RBC,* red blood cell.

(1) Most common overall anemia in the United States
(2) Most common nutritional deficiency worldwide
(3) Greatest prevalence of the anemia is found in:
    (a) toddlers aged 1 to 2 years.
       • Caused by inadequate intake of iron
    (b) females aged 12 to 49 years.
       • Caused by menstrual loss of iron
(4) Causes of iron deficiency are discussed in Table 12-1.
(5) Pathogenesis
    • Decreased synthesis of heme (iron + protoporphyrin) leads to a decreased synthesis of Hb (Fig. 12-8).

6. Clinical and laboratory findings
  a. Chronic iron deficiency is associated with:
    (1) esophageal web (Plummer-Vinson syndrome).
      • Esophageal web produces dysphagia (difficulty in swallowing) for solids but *not* liquids
    (2) achlorhydria.
      • Refers to the absence of hydrochloric acid in the stomach
    (3) glossitis and angular cheilosis.
      • Inflammation of the tongue and corner of the mouth, respectively
    (4) pallor of the conjunctivae and palmar skin creases (Fig. 12-10 A and B).
    (5) spoon nails (koilonychia; Fig. 12-10 C; Link 12-12).
    (6) craving (pica) for ice.
  b. Laboratory findings include:
    (1) decreased MCV.
    (2) decreased serum iron and iron saturation.
    (3) decreased serum ferritin.
    (4) increased TIBC and RDW.

Iron deficiency: MC overall anemia

Iron deficiency: MCC bleeding

Esophageal web, achlorhydria, glossitis/cheilosis, spoon nails

↓Iron, % saturation, ferritin; ↑TIBC, RDW

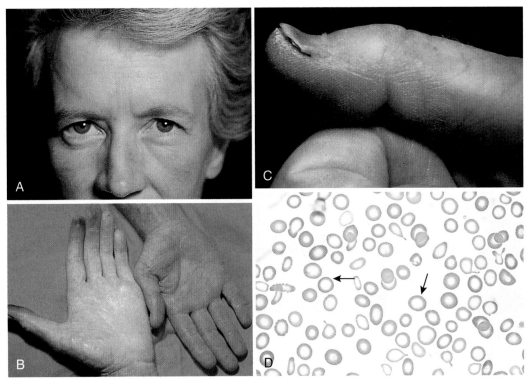

12-10: **A,** Note the generalized pallor of the face in this woman with severe anemia. **B,** Note the pallor of the hand in the patient with anemia *(left)* when compared with a normal hand *(right)*. **C,** Koilonychia. Note the spoon shape of the nail bed. **D,** Peripheral blood smear in iron deficiency anemia. The enlarged central area of pallor in the red blood cells (RBCs) *(arrows)* indicates a decrease in hemoglobin synthesis, which is characteristic of the microcytic anemias. The mean corpuscular hemoglobin concentration is decreased. Also note the size variation, which explains the increased RBC distribution width. *(A and B from Forbes C, Jackson W: Color Atlas and Text of Clinical Medicine, 3rd ed, London, Mosby, 2004, pp 405, 406, respectively, Figs. 10.3, 10.4, respectively; C from Savin JAA, Hunter JAA, Hepburn NC: Diagnosis in Color: Skin Signs in Clinical Medicine, London, Mosby-Wolfe, 1997, p 118, Fig. 4.60; D from Wickramasinghe SE, McCullough J: Blood and Bone Marrow Pathology, London, Churchill Livingstone, 2003, Fig. 11-6.)*

The **stages of iron deficiency** in sequence are as follows: absent iron stores; decreased serum ferritin; decreased serum iron, increased TIBC, and decreased iron saturation; normocytic normochromic anemia; and microcytic hypochromic anemia.

Stages of iron deficiency: all lab studies abnormal *before* anemia is present

(5) microcytic and normocytic cells with increased central area of pallor (Fig. 12-10 D).

(6) increased serum level of free erythrocyte protoporphyrin (FEP).
- Less iron to combine with protoporphyrin to form heme

(7) thrombocytosis (increased platelet count).
- (a) Common finding in chronic iron deficiency

Chronic iron deficiency; reactive phenomenon

- (b) Reactive phenomenon that increases the blood viscosity and prevents high-output heart failure (see Chapter 11)

(8) normal WBC count unless other disorders are present.
- Eosinophilia occurs in hookworm infestations.

D. Anemia of chronic disease (ACD)

Liver synthesis hepcidin in inflammation

1. **Definition:** ACD is a disorder of iron homeostasis promoted by liver synthesis of hepcidin in response to inflammation.

2. Epidemiology (Link 12-11)
- a. Most common anemia in hospitalized patients
- b. Second most common anemia after iron deficiency anemia

MC anemia in hospitalized patients

- c. Occurs in approximately 10% of men and women ages 65 to 85 years
- d. Occurs in >20% of adults older than 85 years
- e. Common causes include:
  - (1) chronic inflammation.
    - Examples: rheumatoid arthritis (RA), tuberculosis (TB), and Crohn disease
  - (2) alcoholism.
    - ACD is the most common anemia in alcoholism.

MC anemia in malignancy, alcohol excess

  - (3) malignancy.
    - ACD is the most common anemia in malignancy.

f. Pathogenesis

(1) Decreased heme synthesis (Fig. 12-8)

(2) Decreased renal production and/or impaired response to EPO

(3) Increased liver synthesis and release of hepcidin

(4) Hepcidin prevents the release of iron from enterocytes and MPs in the BM and other sites.

- This keeps iron away from pathogens (iron blockade), which use it for reproduction.

3. Laboratory findings include:

a. normal to decreased MCV.

(1) In some cases, ACD presents as a normocytic anemia.

(2) More likely to present as a microcytic anemia in the setting of severe active inflammatory conditions such as rheumatoid arthritis (RA) and Crohn disease

b. decreased serum iron, TIBC, and percent iron saturation.

c. increased serum ferritin.

d. increased serum FEP level.

- Because there is less iron available to combine with protoporphyrin to form heme

e. Hb rarely <9 g/dL.

f. increased BM iron in MPs.

E. Thalassemia (thal)

1. **Definition:** Genetic disease caused by a *decrease* in one or more of the globin chains in Hb

2. Epidemiology

a. Autosomal recessive (AR) disorder

b. α-Thalassemia is common in Southeast Asians, people who live on the African west coast, and in the black population (prevalence of 5%).

c. β-Thalassemia is common in blacks, Greeks (prevalence, 15%–30%), and Italians.

d. Definition/epidemiology of α-thalassemia

(1) **Definition:** Decrease in α-globin chain synthesis caused by α-globin chain gene deletions (Fig. 12-11)

- Four genes control α-globin chain synthesis (Fig. 12-11 A, left; Link 12-13 top left).

(2) One gene deletion produces a silent carrier (Link 12-13, top right).

- A silent carrier does *not* have anemia.

(3) Combination of two gene deletions is called α-thalassemia trait (see Fig. 12-11A right and B; Link 12-13 middle).

(4) Clinical and laboratory findings in α-thalassemia trait

(a) Produces a mild anemia with a normal to increased RBC count

- There is no consensus as to why the RBC count is normal to increased when the Hb and Hct are decreased; however, it is a very useful clinical finding.

(b) In the black population, it is associated with a loss of one gene on *each* chromosome (*trans: α/– α/–*; Fig. 12-11 A; Link 12-13, middle left).

(c) In the Southeast Asian population, it is associated with a loss of both genes on the *same* chromosome (*cis: –/– α/α*; Fig. 12-11 B; Link 12-13, middle right).

- Increased risk for developing more severe types of α-thalassemia, because one chromosome completely lacks α-globin genes.

↓Synthesis heme, ↓EPO synthesis/response, ↑hepcidin	
Iron blockade; prevents iron utilization by pathogens	
Sometimes normocytic	
↓Serum iron, TIBC, %saturation	
↑Serum ferritin	
↑Serum FEP	
Hb rarely <9 g/dL	
↑BM iron in MPs	
Decrease 1/more globin chains in Hb	
Autosomal recessive	
Blacks, Southeast Asians, African west coast	
Blacks, Greeks, Italians	
α-Globin chain gene deletions	
Four genes control α-globin chain synthesis	
Silent carrier 1 gene deletion	
α-Thal trait: 2 gene deletions	
Mild anemia; N/↑RBC count	
Black α-thal trait: trans α/– α/–	
Southeast Asian α-thal trait: cis –/– α/α; danger severe types	

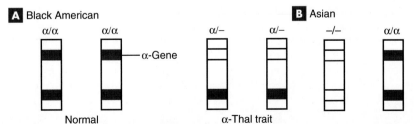

12-11: Gene deletions in α-thalassemia in the black population (**A**) and Asian population (**B**). Four α-genes are involved in α-globin chain synthesis (**A**, *left schematic*). The black population type is associated with a loss of one gene on each chromosome (transconfiguration: α/– α/–; schematic **A**, *right schematic*). This eliminates the possibility of developing severe types of α-thalassemia between members of the same race. In the Asian type (**B**), there is a loss of both genes on the same chromosome (cis configuration: –/– α/α). This poses an increased risk for developing more severe types of α-thalassemia (e.g., hemoglobin [Hb] H and Hb Barts disease) between members of the same race. *(From Goljan EF, Sloka KI: Rapid Review Laboratory Testing in Clinical Medicine, Philadelphia, Mosby Elsevier, 2008, p 158, Fig. 5-11.)*

HbH: 3 gene deletions

Hb Bart: 4 γ-chains; incompatible with life

- Combination of three gene deletions is called HbH (four β-chains) disease (Link 12-13, bottom left), which is associated with a severe hemolytic anemia. Excess β-chain inclusions cause MP destruction of RBCs (hemolytic anemia). Hb electrophoresis detects HbH.
- Combination of four gene deletions is called Hb Bart (four γ-chains) disease (Link 12-13, bottom right). Incompatible with life. Hb electrophoresis shows an increase in Hb Bart.

(d) Laboratory findings in α-thalassemia trait include:
- decreased MCV, Hb, and Hct.
- increased RBC count.
- MCV/RBC count ratio <13.
- target cells (look like a bull's eye) may or may not be present in the peripheral blood (Link 12-14).
- teardrop RBCs are inconsistently present (Link 12-14).

↓HbA, HbA₂, HbF (normal electrophoresis); ↑RBC count

- normal RDW, serum ferritin, serum FEP, and Hb electrophoresis (all Hbs are equally decreased).
- possible decrease in HbA₂.

The Hb electrophoresis is normal in α-thal trait because all Hb types require α-globin chains. The Hb concentration is decreased; however, the relative proportions of the normal Hbs remains the same (Fig. 12-7 B).

α-Thal trait: diagnosis of exclusion

Decrease in β-globin chain synthesis

Mild β-thal: DNA splicing defect; severe—stop codon

(e) α-Thalassemia trait is a diagnosis of exclusion.
- Usually, there is a family history of members with a mild microcytic anemia, a normal Hb electrophoresis, and normal iron study results.

3. Definition/epidemiology of β-thalassemia
a. **Definition:** Varying degrees of a decrease in β-globin chain synthesis (Fig. 12-8)
(1) Mild anemia is most often caused by DNA splicing defects.
(2) Severe anemia is caused by a nonsense mutation with formation of a stop codon (see Chapter 6).
- Stop codon causes premature termination of β-globin chain synthesis or absent β-globin chain synthesis.
b. Synthesis of α-, δ-, and γ-globin chains is normal.

Normal β-globin chain synthesis is designated β; some β-globin chain synthesis is designated β+; absence of β-globin chain synthesis is designated β°.

β-thal minor: β/β⁺

c. β-thalassemia minor (β/β⁺)
(1) Mild microcytic anemia
(2) MCV, Hb, and Hct are decreased.
(3) Increased RBC count
(4) MCV/RBC count ratio is <13.
(5) Target cells are consistently present in the peripheral blood (Fig. 12-12 A).

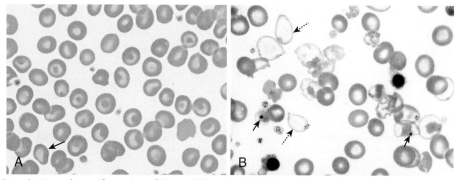

12-12: **A,** β-Thalassemia trait. Note the uniform size of the red blood cells (RBCs), which explains why the RBC distribution width is normal. Target cells are commonly seen in all hemoglobinopathies. The *arrow* points to a teardrop RBC. **B,** β-Thalassemia major. A few cells contain hardly any hemoglobin. What little is present is often precipitated at the membrane. Howell-Jolly bodies *(solid arrows;* nuclear remnants), poorly hemoglobinated nucleated RBCs (two nucleated cells), and a poorly hemoglobinated teardrop cell *(interrupted arrow)* are present. *(From McPherson R, Pincus M: Henry's Clinical Diagnosis and Management by Laboratory Methods, 21st ed, Philadelphia, Saunders, 2007, pp 587, 586, respectively, Figs. 31-27, 31-26, respectively.)*

(6) Teardrop RBCs are present (Fig. 12-12 B).
  - Teardrop RBC are caused by damage of the RBC membrane from removal of excess globin chains by splenic MPs.
(7) Normal RDW, serum ferritin, and serum FEP
  - Serum FEP is normal because heme synthesis is normal.
(8) Hb electrophoresis (Fig. 12-7 C)
  (a) HbA ($2\alpha/2\beta$) is decreased because β-globin chains are decreased.
  (b) Corresponding increase in HbA$_2$ ($2\alpha/2\delta$) and HbF ($2\alpha/2\gamma$)
(9) No treatment is available for β-thalassemia minor (β/β^+).

d. β-thalassemia major (Cooley anemia; β^o/β^o or β^o/β^+)
  (1) Results in a severe hemolytic anemia
    (a) RBCs with α-chain inclusions are removed by splenic MPs.
      - Marked increase in unconjugated bilirubin (UCB); jaundice. Recall that UCB is an end-product of MP destruction of RBCs. Iron is removed from heme to produce UCB, which binds to albumin in the blood. It is then converted in the liver to UCB (see Chapters 2 and 19).
    (b) RBCs with α-chain inclusions undergo apoptosis in the BM (called ineffective erythropoiesis).
  (2) EMH and accelerated erythropoiesis
    (a) EMH results in hepatosplenomegaly.
    (b) Radiographs of the skull show a hair-on-end appearance caused by accelerated erythropoiesis (Fig. 12-3).
  (3) RDW is increased because of increased size variation (Fig. 12-12 B).
  (4) Increase in reticulocytes, teardrop cells, Howell-Jolly (HJ) bodies (nuclear remnants), and nucleated RBCs (Fig. 12-12 B; Links 12-15 and 12-16)
  (5) Hb electrophoresis findings include (see Fig. 12-7 D):
    (a) *no* synthesis of HbA.
    (b) corresponding increase in HbA$_2$ and HbF.

F. Sideroblastic anemia
  1. **Definition:** Defect in heme synthesis *within* the mitochondria (mT) of developing RBCs in the BM (Fig. 12-8).
  2. Epidemiology
    a. Causes include:
      (1) chronic alcoholism (most common cause).
      (2) pyridoxine (vitamin B$_6$) deficiency.
      (3) lead (Pb) poisoning.
      (4) X-linked recessive (XR) disease (presents in childhood).
      (5) reversible sideroblastic anemia (alcohol, isoniazid [INH], chloramphenicol).
      (6) acquired idiopathic sideroblastic anemia (older individuals).
    b. Pathogenesis
      (1) Heme is the end-product of porphyrin synthesis.
      (2) Heme normally has a negative feedback relationship with δ-aminolevulinic acid (ALA) synthase.
      (3) Because there is a defect in heme synthesis in sideroblastic anemia, the iron within erythroid precursors is trapped within the mitochondria (location of heme synthesis). The accumulation of iron is what produces the ringed sideroblasts (Fig. 12-13).

Margin notes:

↓HbA; ↑RBC count, HbA$_2$, HbF; normal RDW; target/tear drop cells

β-thal minor: β/β^+

β-thal major: β^o/β^o or β^o/β^+

Severe hemolytic anemia; α-chain inclusions

EMH: extramedullary hematopoiesis

EMH; hair-on-end skull

No HbA; ↑HbA$_2$, HbF, RDW, reticulocytes

Defect heme synthesis within mt developing RBC

MCC chronic alcoholism

↓Pyridoxine, Pb poisoning, XR

Acquired idiopathic sideroblastic anemia older individuals

Iron accumulates in mT → ringed sideroblasts

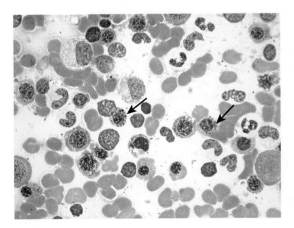

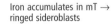

12-13: Ringed sideroblasts in a bone marrow aspirate. Dark blue iron granules around the nucleus of developing normoblasts *(arrows)* represent iron trapped within mitochondria and indicate a defect in mitochondrial heme synthesis (sideroblastic anemia). *(From Porwitt A, McCullough J, Erber WN:* Blood and Bone Marrow Pathology, *2nd ed, London, Churchill Livingstone Elsevier, 2011, p 402, Fig. 27.8C.)*

c. Sideroblastic anemia is classified as an iron-overload type of anemia.

Iron overload anemia

(1) Iron stores markedly increase in the BM MPs.

(2) Sideroblasts die in the BM (ineffective erythropoiesis).

Ineffective erythropoiesis

- They are phagocytosed by MPs, which leads to an excess in iron stores in the BM.

3. Chronic alcoholism

a. Alcohol is a mitochondrial toxin (poison).

Alcohol mT poison

- Alcohol damages heme biosynthetic pathways in the mitochondria.

b. Sideroblastic anemia is present in ~30% of hospitalized patients with chronic alcoholism.

4. Pyridoxine (vitamin B_6) deficiency

Pyridoxine cofactor δALA → rate-limiting reaction heme synthesis

INH MCC pyridoxine deficiency

a. Vitamin B_6 is a cofactor for ALA synthase, the rate-limiting reaction of heme synthesis in the mitochondria (Fig. 12-8).

b. INH therapy for tuberculosis is the most common cause of pyridoxine deficiency.

- INH (isoniazid) inactivates pyridoxine.

5. Lead (Pb) poisoning

a. Epidemiology

MC children 1–5 years

Pb crosses placenta

Uncommon

(1) Most common in children ages 1 to 5 years

(2) May occur in utero because lead crosses the placenta and enters the developing fetus

(3) Uncommon cause of sideroblastic anemia

(4) Causes include:

Pica (abnormal craving)

(a) pica (abnormal craving).

- This is a common cause of childhood lead poisoning in inner cities where there are apartments built *before* 1950, when lead-based paints were primarily used.
- Before 1978, lead-based paints were used for painting the exterior of homes.

(b) contact with pottery glazes (either commercial or homemade).

Paint, batteries, pottery glazes, radiator repair, moonshine

(c) working in a battery or ammunition factory.

(d) working as a radiator repair mechanic.

(e) air contamination from a smelter (form of extractive metallurgy).

(f) Other sources of lead include jewelry, moonshine, traditional medicines (e.g., Chinese tea), contaminated dietary supplements, lead plumbing, and imported toys (e.g., from China).

b. Lead denatures enzymes.

Denatures ferrochelatase, ALA dehydrase, ribonuclease

(1) Ferrochelatase is denatured (Fig. 12-8).

(a) Inhibits the incorporation of iron with protoporphyrin to form heme

(b) FEP, which is proximal to the enzyme block, is increased.

Denatures ALA dehydrase → ↑δALA

(2) ALA dehydrase is denatured.

- Causes an increase in ALA, which is proximal to the enzyme block

Coarse basophilic stippling (persistent ribosomes)

(3) Ribonuclease is denatured.

- Ribosomes cannot be degraded and therefore persist in the RBC, resulting in coarse basophilic stippling (Fig. 12-14 A).

Pb interferes with iron absorption/utilization

c. Lead interferes with iron absorption and utilization in heme pathways (see earlier discussion).

- Some authors state that the microcytosis in lead poisoning is caused by iron deficiency.

d. Clinical and laboratory findings include:

(1) colicky type of abdominal pain with constipation (children).

Abdominal colic/ constipation (child)

- Lead is visible in the gastrointestinal (GI) tract on plain abdominal radiographs (Fig. 12-14 B).

(2) encephalopathy (children).

(a) Cerebral edema and papilledema (swelling of the optic disk) are present.

- Lead damages capillary endothelium, causing leakage into the brain parenchyma.
- Lead also damages myelin and induces demyelination.

Encephalopathy: edema/ demyelination

(b) Disabilities may occur.

(3) Growth retardation (children)

Pb deposits in epiphyses; growth retardation

(a) Lead is deposited in the epiphysis of growing bone.

(b) Radiographs show increased density in the epiphyses (Fig. 12-14 C; Link 12-17).

(4) Peripheral neuropathy may occur in adults (children to a lesser extent).

- Examples of peripheral neuropathy: foot drop (peroneal nerve palsy), wrist drop (radial nerve palsy), and claw hand (ulnar nerve palsy)

Proximal renal tubular acidosis

(5) Nephrotoxic damage to proximal renal tubules (adults); proximal renal tubular acidosis

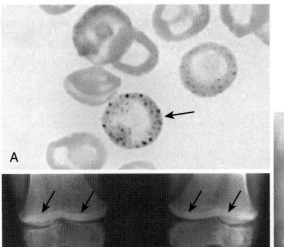

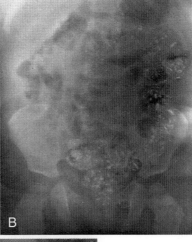

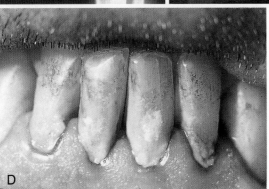

12-14: A, Peripheral blood with coarse basophilic stippling of red blood cells (RBCs) in lead poisoning. Note the mature RBC containing numerous dots representing ribosomes *(arrow)*. Lead denatures ribonuclease, hence the ribosomes persist in the cytoplasm. **B,** Abdominal radiograph showing numerous metallic foci representing lead chips. **C,** Bone radiograph showing densities (lead deposits; *arrows*) in the epiphysis of the distal femur and proximal tibia. **D,** Lead poisoning produces a blue line at the margin of the gum and teeth. *(**A** from Naeim F:* Atlas of Bone Marrow and Blood Pathology, *Philadelphia, Saunders, 2001, p 27, Fig. 2-22M;* **B** *and* **C** *from Katz D, Math K, Groskin S:* Radiology Secrets, *Philadelphia, Hanley & Belfus, 1998, p 310, Figs. 6 and Fig. 5, respectively;* **D** *from Forbes C, Jackson W:* Color Atlas and Text of Clinical Medicine, *3rd ed, London, Mosby, 2004, p 345, Fig. 8.27.)*

Tubular damage by lead causes **Fanconi syndrome.** The syndrome includes proximal renal tubular acidosis (loss of bicarbonate in urine), aminoaciduria, phosphaturia, and glucosuria.

(6) Lead line in the gums (Fig. 12-14 D)
- Usually occurs in adults who have preexisting gingivitis

(7) Reduced RBC survival time (? hemolytic anemia)

(8) Increased whole blood and urine lead levels
- These are the best screen and confirmatory tests for lead poisoning.

6. Laboratory findings in sideroblastic anemias include:
   a. increased serum iron, iron saturation, and ferritin.
   b. normal to decreased MCV and decreased TIBC.
   c. presence of ringed sideroblasts in a BM aspirate.

7. Summary table of microcytic anemias (Table 12-2)

IV. Macrocytic Anemias

A. Overview

- Macrocytic anemias are subdivided into megaloblastic anemias (enlarged hematopoietic cells caused by folic acid and/or vitamin B_{12} deficiency) and nonmegaloblastic anemia (e.g., macrocytosis related to alcohol intoxication).

B. Vitamin B_{12} (cobalamin) metabolism (Link 12-18)

1. Water-soluble vitamin present in meat, eggs, and dairy products

2. Parietal cells in the gastric mucosa synthesize intrinsic factor (IF) and hydrochloric acid (HCl).

Margin notes:

Peripheral neuropathy, nephrotoxic (proximal tubules), Pb line in gums

↑Whole blood/urine lead levels

Sideroblastic anemia

↑Serum iron, iron saturation, ferritin; N/↓MCV, ↓TIBC

Ringed sideroblasts BM aspirate

Only present in animal products

Synthesize IF/HCl

TABLE 12-2 Laboratory Findings in Microcytic Anemias

TEST	IRON DEFICIENCY	ANEMIA OF CHRONIC DISEASE	α-THAL/β-THAL MINOR	LEAD POISONING
MCV	↓	↓	↓	Normal to ↓
Serum iron	↓	↓	Normal	↑
TIBC	↑	↓	Normal	↓
Percent saturation	↓	↓	Normal	↑
Serum ferritin	↓	↑	Normal	↑
RDW	↑	Normal	Normal	Normal
RBC count	↓	↓	↑	↓
Hb electrophoresis	Normal	Normal	α-Thal trait: normal β-Thal trait: ↓HbA, ↑HbA$_2$/F	–
Ringed sideroblasts	None	None	None	+/– Present
Coarse basophilic stippling	None	None	None	Present

Hb, Hemoglobin; *MCV*, mean corpuscular volume; *RDW*, red blood cell distribution width; *Thal*, thalassemia; *TIBC*, total iron-binding capacity.

TABLE 12-3 Causes of Vitamin B$_{12}$ Deficiency

CLASSIFICATION	CAUSES	DISCUSSION
Decreased intake	• Pure vegan diet • Malnutrition	• Breastfed infants of pure vegans may develop deficiency. • Malnutrition may occur in older adult patients.
Impaired absorption	• ↓Intrinsic factor • ↓Gastric acid • ↓Terminal ileum absorption	• **Autoimmune destruction of parietal cells:** This occurs in pernicious anemia, the most common cause of vitamin B$_{12}$ deficiency. Gastric acid and intrinsic factor are both decreased, the former interfering with activation of pepsinogen and the latter the absorption of vitamin B$_{12}$ in the terminal ileum. • **Proton blockers** inhibit the synthesis of gastric acid. • **Gastrectomy** decreases both acid and intrinsic factor. • **Bacterial overgrowth:** Bacteria use available vitamin B$_{12}$. Bacterial overgrowth occurs in small bowel diverticulosis, blind loops, and defects in small bowel motility (e.g., diabetes mellitus; systemic sclerosis). • **Fish tapeworm:** The worms absorb more than 80% of the vitamin B$_{12}$ intake. • **Chronic pancreatitis:** Enzyme deficiency leads to inability to cleave R-binder from the vitamin B$_{12}$–R-binder complex. • **Crohn disease, celiac disease, small bowel resection involving the terminal ileum:** These disorders interfere with reabsorption of vitamin B$_{12}$.
Increased requirement	• Pregnancy/lactation	• Deficiency is more likely to occur in a pure vegan because their liver iron stores are depleted.

a. Gastric acid converts pepsinogen to pepsin.
b. Pepsin frees vitamin B$_{12}$ from ingested proteins.
3. Free vitamin B$_{12}$ binds to R-binders (haptocorrins) synthesized in salivary glands.

Binds to R-binder

• R-binders protect vitamin B$_{12}$ from acid destruction.

Cleave R-binder off B$_{12}$-IF complex

4. Pancreatic enzymes in the duodenum cleave off the R-binders.
• Vitamin B$_{12}$ binds to IF to form a complex.
5. Vitamin B$_{12}$–IF complex is absorbed in the terminal ileum.
6. Vitamin B$_{12}$ binds to transcobalamin II and enters the plasma.

Absorbed terminal ileum; 6–9-year supply liver

• Vitamin B$_{12}$ is delivered to metabolically active cells or stored in the liver (6- to 9-year supply).

Pernicious anemia MCC

C. **Causes of vitamin B$_{12}$ deficiency** (Table 12-3)
D. **Folic acid metabolism**
1. Polyglutamate form is present in green vegetables and animal proteins.
2. Converted to monoglutamates by intestinal conjugase in the jejunum

Conjugase → poly → mono; inhibited by phenytoin

• Intestinal conjugase is inhibited by phenytoin.
3. Monoglutamate is absorbed in the jejunum (active and passive transport).
a. Monoglutamate is converted to methyltetrahydrofolate (MTHF), the circulating form of folic acid.

Mono → MTHF

TABLE 12-4   Causes of Folic Acid Deficiency

CLASSIFICATION	CAUSES	DISCUSSION
Decreased intake	• Malnutrition • Infants and older adults • Chronic alcoholism • Goat milk	• Decreased intake is the most common cause of folic acid deficiency. • Alcoholics with a poor diet are likely to have folic acid deficiency (alcohol MCC). • Goat milk lacks folic acid unless it is fortified.
Malabsorption	• Celiac disease	• In celiac disease, villi in the jejunum may be destroyed, leading to folic acid deficiency.
Drug inhibition	• 5-Fluorouracil • Methotrexate, trimethoprim • Phenytoin • Oral contraceptives, alcohol	• Inhibits thymidylate synthase • Inhibit dihydrofolate reductase • Inhibits intestinal conjugase • Inhibit uptake of monoglutamate in jejunum • Alcohol also inhibits the release of folic acid from the liver.
Increased utilization	• Pregnancy and lactation • Disseminated malignancy • Severe hemolytic anemia	• Increased utilization of folic acid in DNA synthesis

b. Absorption of monoglutamate is blocked by alcohol and oral contraceptives (OCPs).

c. Liver contains only a 3- to 4-month supply of folic acid.

4. Main function of folic acid is the synthesis of deoxythymidine monophosphate (dTMP) in DNA

5. Both serum folate and RBC folate are used to diagnose folic acid deficiency. If the serum folate level is low, then the RBC folate is measured.

E. **Causes of folic acid deficiency** (Table 12-4)

F. **Pathogenesis of macrocytic anemia in folic acid and vitamin B$_{12}$ deficiency**

1. Impaired DNA synthesis delays nuclear maturation.

   a. Causes a block in cell division in all rapidly dividing cells, leading to large, nucleated hematopoietic cells with an open chromatin pattern

   • Cells that are affected include RBCs, leukocytes, megakaryocytes, and intestinal epithelium.

   b. Cellular RNA synthesis and protein synthesis are *not* affected.

   • Cytoplasmic volume continues to expand.

   c. Enlarged hematopoietic cells are called megaloblasts (Fig. 12-15).

2. Ineffective hematopoiesis is present in either or both deficiencies.

   a. Megaloblastic precursors outside the BM sinusoids are phagocytosed and destroyed by BM MPs.

   b. Megaloblastic precursors undergo apoptosis, causing pancytopenia (anemia, neutropenia, and thrombocytopenia).

G. **Vitamin B$_{12}$ and folic acid in conversion of homocysteine to methionine and in DNA synthesis** (Fig. 12-16)

Margin notes:
MG inhibited by alcohol/OCPs

Synthesis of dTMP

Alcohol MCC

Delayed nuclear maturation → megaloblasts

Megaloblast precursors destroyed by BM MPs

Apoptosis → pancytopenia

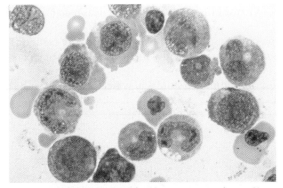

12-15: Megaloblasts in a bone marrow aspirate. Note the open chromatin pattern and enlarged nuclei of red blood cell and white blood cell precursors indicating a lack of nuclear maturation. (*From Goldman L, Ausiello D: Cecil's Medicine, 23rd ed, Philadelphia, Saunders Elsevier, 2008, p 1239, Fig. 170-4.*)

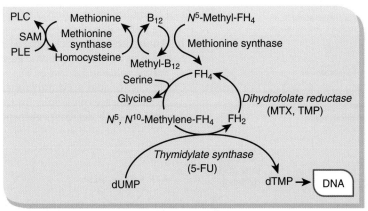

12-16: Vitamin B$_{12}$ and folic acid in DNA metabolism. See text for discussion. *dTMP*, Deoxythymidine monophosphate; *dUMP*, deoxyuridine monophosphate; *FH$_2$*, dihydrofolate; *FH$_4$*, tetrahydrofolate; *FU*, fluorouracil; *MTX*, methotrexate; *PLC*, phosphatidylcholine; *PLE*, phosphatidylethanol-amine; *SAM*, S-adenosylmethionine; *TMP*, trimethoprim. (*Modified from Pelley J, Goljan FF: Rapid Review Biochemistry, Philadelphia, Mosby, 2004, Fig. 4-3.*)

FA/FA derivatives → single carbon transfer reactions

1. Methionine synthase removes the methyl group (-$\underline{C}H_3$) from 5-methyltetrahydrofolate (N^5-methyl-FH_4), the circulating form of folic acid in the blood, to produce tetrahydrofolate (FH_4) and methyl-B_{12} (methylcobalamin).
   a. **Biochemistry pearl:** Folic acid (FA) and folic acid derivatives are important in single carbon transfer reactions from methyl groups (-$\underline{C}H_3$) and methylene groups (-$\underline{C}H_2$).
   b. Methionine synthase transfers the methyl group of methyl-B_{12} to homocysteine, which regenerates vitamin B_{12} (cobalamin) and releases the product methionine.

↓Vit B_{12} → false ↑ serum folic acid

↓FA/B12 → ↑homocysteine

   • Deficiency of vitamin B_{12} traps N^5-methyl-FH_4 in its circulating form, which falsely increases the serum folic acid in 30% of cases (MTHF trap).
   c. Deficiency of folic acid and/or vitamin B_{12} increases plasma homocysteine.

Folic acid deficiency is the most common cause of increased serum homocysteine levels in the United States. Homocysteine acts as an atherogenic factor by converting a stable atherosclerotic plaque into an unstable plaque that leads to thrombosis.

2. Tetrahydrofolate combines with serine to produce N^5,N^{10}-methylene-FH_4; glycine is a byproduct of the reaction.
   a. Tetrahydrofolate receives a methyl group (-$\underline{C}H_3$) from serine to produce N^5,N^{10}-methylene-tetrahydrofolate and glycine.
   b. In the conversion of N^5,N^{10}-methylene-FH_4 to dihydrofolate reductase (FH_2) by thymidylate synthase, the carbon from the methylene group is transferred to deoxyuridine monophosphate (dUMP) to produce dTMP.

Thymidylate synthase irreversibly inhibited by 5-FU

   • Thymidylate synthase is irreversibly inhibited by 5-fluorouracil (FU).
   c. Dihydrofolate (DHF) reductase converts dihydrofolate to tetrahydrofolate (FH_4).

DHF reductase inhibited by DHT (reversible), TMP

   • DHF reductase is inhibited by methotrexate (MTX) and trimethoprim (TMP).

H. Vitamin B_{12} in odd-chain fatty acid metabolism

Odd-chain FA metabolism

   1. Vitamin B_{12} is involved in odd-chain fatty acid metabolism, which explains the neurologic problems that are unique to vitamin B_{12} deficiency (Fig. 12-17).
   2. Propionyl CoA is converted to methylmalonyl CoA, which in turn is converted to succinyl CoA by methylmalonyl CoA mutase using vitamin B_{12} as a cofactor.
      a. When vitamin B_{12} is deficient, there is an increase in propionyl CoA and methylmalonyl CoA and their corresponding acids proximal to the enzyme block.
      b. Increase in serum propionic acid and methylmalonic acid is very useful in diagnosing vitamin B_{12} deficiency.

I. Clinical findings in vitamin B_{12} deficiency

PA MCC B_{12} deficiency

   1. Pernicious anemia (PA), the most common cause of vitamin B_{12} deficiency, has clinical findings that are *not* present in other causes of vitamin B_{12} listed in Table 12-3.
      a. Three antibodies (Abs) that are associated with the pathophysiology of pernicious anemia and its clinical findings include:

Ab against proton pump parietal cells

Ab block B_{12} binding to IF

      (1) antibodies directed against the proton pump in parietal cells (85%–90% of cases).
      (2) antibodies that block the binding of vitamin B_{12} to IF (60%–75% of cases).
         • These antibodies are the most specific test for pernicious anemia.

Ab prevent binding B_{12}-IF complexes ileal receptors

      (3) antibodies that prevent the binding of vitamin B_{12}–IF complexes to ileal receptors (30%–50% of cases).
      b. Antibodies that attack parietal cells in the body/fundus (type II hypersensitivity reaction) produce a chronic atrophic gastritis (CAG) that is associated with achlorhydria (lack of gastric acid) and a loss of IF.

CAG (↓acid, ↓IF)

Block release B_{12} from food

↓IF → ↓absorption B_{12} in terminal ileum

      (1) Loss of acid prevents proper digestion of food in the stomach, which interferes with the release of vitamin B_{12} from food.
      (2) Loss of IF decreases absorption of vitamin B_{12} in the terminal ileum.

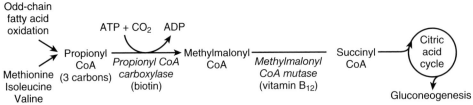

12-17: Odd-chain fatty acid metabolism. See text for discussion. *ADP*, Adenosine diphosphate; *ATP*, adenosine triphosphate. *(From Pelley J, Goljan E: Rapid Review Biochemistry, 2nd ed, Philadelphia, Mosby, 2007, p 117, Fig. 7-4.)*

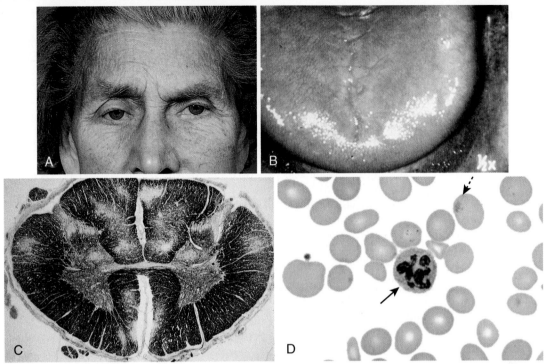

12-18: **A,** Typical lemon-yellow skin color of a woman with pernicious anemia and severe megaloblastic anemia. The color is from the combination of pallor (from anemia) and jaundice (from ineffective erythropoiesis). **B,** Glossitis caused by vitamin B_{12} deficiency in a patient with untreated pernicious anemia. There is atrophy of the papillae. An identical appearance occurs in folic acid deficiency because of impaired DNA synthesis in the mucosal epithelium. **C,** Subacute combined degeneration of the spinal cord. Note the pale areas of demyelination in the posterior columns and the lateral corticospinal tracts. **D,** Peripheral blood in megaloblastic anemia showing a hypersegmented neutrophil *(solid arrow)* with nine lobes. Neutrophils normally have less than five nuclear segments. Hypersegmented neutrophils are excellent markers of folate and vitamin B_{12} deficiency. The enlarged, egg-shaped red blood cells (macro-ovalocytes; *interrupted arrow*) characteristic of macrocytic anemias are associated with problems in DNA maturation. *(A from Forbes C, Jackson W: Color Atlas and Text of Clinical Medicine, 3rd ed, London, Mosby, 2004, p 413, Fig. 10.28; B from Taylor S, Raffles A: Diagnosis in Color Pediatrics, London, Mosby-Wolfe, 1997, p 209, Fig. 8-1; C from Wickramasinghe SN, McCullough J: Blood and Bone Marrow Pathology, London, Churchill Livingstone, 2003, p 237, Fig. 12-10B; D from Naeim F: Atlas of Bone Marrow and Blood Pathology, Philadelphia, WB Saunders, 2001, p 180, Fig. 14-10B.)*

(3) Achlorhydria leads to a corresponding increase in serum gastrin (hypergastrinemia; it has a negative feedback relationship with acid).

  Achlorhydria → ↑serum gastrin

(4) Intestinal metaplasia in chronic atrophic gastritis (CAG) (see Chapter 2) increases the risk for developing adenocarcinoma of the body/fundus.

  CAG → intestinal metaplasia → cancer body/fundus

c. Other antibodies associated with pernicious anemia also contribute to producing vitamin B_{12} deficiency.

d. Another clinical finding in pernicious anemia unrelated to the previously mentioned antibodies is a peculiar lemon yellow appearance of the skin (Fig. 12-18 A).

  Lemon yellow skin

e. PA is often associated with other autoimmune disease (e.g., type 1 diabetes mellitus [DM], Graves disease, Addison disease) and *Helicobacter pylori* infection.

  ↑Type I DM, Graves, Addison, *H. pylori* infection

2. Clinical problems associated with *all* causes of vitamin B_{12} deficiency include:

 a. glossitis associated with a smooth, sore tongue and atrophy of the papillae (Fig. 12-18 B).

 b. neurologic disease associated with demyelination.

  (1) Peripheral neuropathy with sensorimotor dysfunction

   Peripheral neuropathy

  (2) Subacute combined degeneration (demyelination) of spinal cord (Fig. 12-18 C), which includes:

   Subacute combined degeneration of spinal cord

   (a) posterior column (PC) dysfunction causing loss of vibratory sensation and proprioception (joint sense).

   (b) lateral corticospinal tract (LCST) dysfunction produces spasticity.

   (c) dorsal spinocerebellar tract (DSCT) dysfunction causes ataxia.

   Demyelination PC, LCST, DSCT

  (3) Dementia from involvement of the brain

   Dementia

  (4) Possible to have neurologic disease *without* anemia in 20% of patients

  (5) Mechanism for the demyelination is believed to be the lack of methyl-B_{12} for conversion of homocysteine to methionine (see Fig. 12-16). This results in decreased levels of methionine as well as decreased production of S-adenosyl-methionine (SAM; major methyl donor in the cell), which is needed for methylation of

   Macrocytic anemia + neurologic disease = vitamin B_{12} deficiency

phosphatidylethanolamine (PLE) to phosphatidylcholine (PLC) for incorporation into myelin.

- **Biochemistry pearl:** SAM is involved in the following methylation reactions: norepinephrine to epinephrine, guanidinoacetate to creatine, nucleotides to methylated nucleotides, and acetylserotonin to melanin.

J. **Laboratory findings**
   1. Serum vitamin B_{12} is decreased (<200 pg/mL).

   2. Increases in serum homocysteine (sensitive but *not* specific) and methylmalonic acid are seen in 95% of cases (sensitive and specific).
   3. MCV >110 fL is suggestive of vitamin B_{12} (or folic acid deficiency).
   4. Peripheral blood findings include:
      a. pancytopenia (stem cells destroyed in BM; RBCs, platelets, and WBCs decreased).
      b. oval (egg-shaped) macrocytes.
      c. hypersegmented neutrophils (Fig. 12-18 D).

      - Hypersegmented neutrophils have more than five nuclear lobes. They are a manifestation of the disparity between cytoplasmic maturation (normal) and nuclear maturation (abnormal). They have a high sensitivity and specificity for diagnosing megaloblastic anemias (vitamin B_{12} and folic acid deficiency).
   5. BM findings
      - Megaloblastic nucleated cells are present with a primitive open (lacy) chromatin pattern (Fig. 12-15).
   6. Schilling test localizes some of the causes of vitamin B_{12} deficiency.

      - Although it is *not* routinely performed anymore, it is a good review of causes of vitamin B_{12} deficiency.

The **Schilling test** is used to demonstrate the cause of impaired absorption of vitamin B_{12}. This is achieved indirectly by combining orally administered radioactive vitamin B_{12} with intrinsic factor (IF), with pancreatic extract, or alone after pretreatment with antibiotics followed by a 24-hour urine collection to measure radioactive vitamin B_{12}. Whereas a lack of absorption of radioactive vitamin B_{12} excludes a potential cause of impaired absorption, the presence of absorption confirms the cause of the impaired absorption. For example, if the combination of radioactive vitamin B_{12} and IF leads to an increase in radioactive vitamin B_{12} in the urine, the patient has pernicious anemia; if it does not, the diagnosis of pernicious anemia is excluded. Similarly, correction with pancreatic extract implicates chronic pancreatitis as the cause or bacterial overgrowth as the cause if antibiotics correct the absorption. If resection of the terminal ileum is the cause, there is no correction with adding IF, antibiotics, or pancreatic extract. To ensure that the oral radioactive vitamin B_{12} enters the kidney for excretion, the patient is given a massive intramuscular dose of nonradioactive vitamin B_{12} so that all available transcobalamin II sites are occupied by the vitamin B_{12}. Therefore, if radioactive vitamin B_{12} is absorbed in the terminal ileum, it cannot bind to transcobalamin II and must be excreted in the urine.

K. **Clinical findings in folic acid deficiency**

   1. Similar to vitamin B_{12} deficiency with the *exception* of subacute combined degeneration, which is more common in vitamin B_{12} deficiency
   2. Increased risk for open neural tube defects in the fetus if there is decreased maternal intake of folic acid *before* conception (see Fig. 26-4A, B, D, and E)

L. **Laboratory findings in folic acid deficiency**
   1. Peripheral blood and BM findings are similar to those for vitamin B_{12} deficiency.
   2. Serum folic acid and blood RBC folic acid levels are both decreased.

      a. RBC folic acid level is the best screening test; however, both tests are usually ordered at the same time.
      b. RBC folic acid best correlates with folic acid stores.

      - One-month supply of folic acid stored in the liver, hence the importance of having adequate amounts of folic acid in the diet
      c. Blood homocysteine is increased, and blood methylmalonic acid is normal.

It is important to distinguish folic acid deficiency from vitamin B_{12} deficiency. Pharmacologic doses of folic acid correct the hematologic findings in both folic acid and vitamin B_{12} deficiency; however, neurologic disease is *not* corrected.

M. **Comparison table of vitamin B_{12} and folic acid deficiency** (Table 12-5)
N. **Nonmegaloblastic macrocytosis**

   1. **Definition:** Nonmegaloblastic macrocytosis describes erythrocytes that are larger than normal but *not* caused by either vitamin B_{12} or folic acid deficiency.

TABLE 12-5 **Clinical and Laboratory Findings in Vitamin B$_{12}$ and Folic Acid Deficiencies**

LABORATORY AND CLINICAL FINDING	PERNICIOUS ANEMIA	OTHER VITAMIN B$_{12}$ DEFICIENCIES	FOLIC ACID DEFICIENCY
Achlorhydria	Present	Absent	Absent
Autoantibodies	Present	Absent	Absent
Chronic atrophic gastritis	Present	Absent	Absent
Gastric carcinoma risk	↑	None	None
Hypersegmented neutrophils	Present	Present	Present
Mean corpuscular volume	↑	↑	↑
Neurologic disease	Present	Present	None
Pancytopenia	Present	Present	Present
Plasma homocysteine	↑	↑	↑
Serum gastrin level	↑	Normal	Normal
Urine methylmalonic acid	↑	↑	Normal

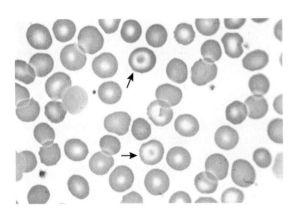

12-19: Round macrocytes and target cells in chronic alcoholism. Note the round macrocytes with target cell formation *(arrows)*. *(From Wickramasinghe SN, McCullough J: Blood and Bone Marrow Pathology, London, Churchill Livingstone, 2003, Fig. 6-2F.)*

2. Epidemiology
   a. General differences of nonmegaloblastic macrocytosis from megaloblastic macrocytic anemias include:
      (1) round macrocytes rather than oval or egg-shaped macrocytes.
      (2) absence of hypersegmented neutrophils in the peripheral blood.
      (3) normal numbers of leukocytes and platelets.
      (4) absence of glossitis and neuropathy.
      (5) absence of anemia in some cases.
   b. Alcohol excess is the most common cause for all types of the macrocytosis.
   c. Liver disease associated with alcohol is a common cause of nonmegaloblastic macrocytosis *without* anemia.
      (1) MCV range is 105 ± 10 μm^3.
      (2) Peripheral blood has thin, round, macrocytic target cells (Fig. 12-19).
         • Target cells are caused by excess RBC membrane lipid, which bunches up the membrane in the middle and causes the targetoid appearance.
      (3) Life span of the RBCs is *not* decreased.
   d. Direct toxic effect of alcohol on RBC precursors produces a nonmegaloblastic macrocytosis and mild anemia.
      (1) MCV ranges from 100 to 110 μm^3.
      (2) Vacuolization of RBC precursors is present in the BM.
      (3) Abstinence from alcohol reverses the macrocytosis and the anemia.
V. Normocytic Anemias: Corrected Reticulocyte Count or Index <2% (see Table 12-5)
   A. Acute blood loss
      1. **Definition:** Refers to blood loss from external or internal causes
      2. Epidemiology and causes
         a. External refers to blood loss outside the body.
            • Examples: open fractures, knife wounds

Round macrocytes, no hypersegmented neutrophils, no pancytopenia, +/–anemia

Round macrocytic target cells; no anemia

Vacuolization RBC precursors; reversal with abstinence from alcohol

Acute blood loss: external, internal

Correction <2%

Outside the body (open fracture)

Inside the body (ruptured spleen)

MCC hypovolemic shock

Hb, Hct, RBC count initially normal

Becomes apparent when plasma is replaced

IV normal saline immediately uncovers RBC deficit

Reticulocyte response 5–7 days after blood loss

Anemia normocytic *before* becoming microcytic

Serum ferritin useful; ↓iron deficiency, ↑ACD

Pancytopenia; marrow hypoplasia; retic index <2

15–25 yrs; > 60 yrs

Most cases idiopathic; drugs MC known cause

Immunologic destruction myeloid progenitor cells

Fever, bleeding, fatigue

Pancytopenia, reticulocyte index <2, hypocellular marrow

b. Internal blood loss refers to blood loss inside the body.
   • Examples: ruptured abdominal aortic aneurysm, ruptured spleen
   c. Acute blood loss is the most common cause of hypovolemic shock.
3. Clinical and laboratory findings in hypovolemic shock (see Chapter 5)
4. Hb, Hct, and RBC count are *initially* normal in acute blood loss because whole blood is lost.
   a. When plasma begins to be replaced by fluid from the interstitial space entering the vascular compartment, the RBC deficit becomes apparent, and the Hb, Hct, and RBC count decrease.
   b. If the patient is receiving intravenous (IV) normal saline (0.9%), the RBC deficit is immediately uncovered because the saline is "acting like" plasma.
   c. Usually takes 5 to 7 days *before* a reticulocyte response is observed in acute blood loss.
B. **Early iron deficiency or ACD**
1. In both iron deficiency and ACD, the anemia is normocytic *before* it becomes microcytic.
   • In ACD, it is microcytic in only 10% to 30% of cases, particularly if the anemia is caused by rheumatoid arthritis (RA) or Crohn disease.
2. Serum ferritin is most useful in distinguishing the two anemias because it is decreased in iron deficiency and increased in ACD.
C. **Aplastic anemia**
1. **Definition:** Syndrome of bone marrow (BM) failure characterized by peripheral pancytopenia (decreased RBCs, WBCs, platelets), a reticulocyte index <2, and marrow hypoplasia
2. Epidemiology
   a. Two peaks of presentation occur in aplastic anemia; one between 15 and 25 years of age and the other in patients >60 years old.
   b. Causes are discussed in Table 12-6.
      (1) Most cases are idiopathic.
      (2) Drugs are the most common known causes.
   c. Pathogenesis
      (1) Immunologic alterations occur, causing T-cell activation and release of cytokines that suppress or destroy the myeloid progenitor cells (see Fig. 12-1), leading to pancytopenia
      (2) Mutations in *TERT* (telomerase reverse transcriptase), the gene for the RNA component of telomerase, cause short telomerases in congenital aplastic anemia and some acquired causes of aplastic anemia.
3. Clinical findings include:
   a. fever caused by infection associated with neutropenia.
   b. bleeding caused by thrombocytopenia.
   c. fatigue caused by anemia.
4. Laboratory findings include:
   a. pancytopenia.
   b. reticulocytopenia (decreased reticulocytes; reticulocyte index <2).
   c. hypocellular BM (Fig. 12-20; Link 12-19).
      • Lymphocytes are present in the BM and peripheral blood because the pluripotential stem cell is proximal to the myeloid progenitor cells (see Fig. 12-1).

TABLE 12-6 Causes of Aplastic Anemia

CLASSIFICATION	EXAMPLES AND DISCUSSION
Idiopathic	• ~50%–70% of cases are idiopathic.
Drugs	• Most common known cause of aplastic anemia. • Dose-related causes are usually reversible (e.g., alkylating agents, antimetabolites). • Idiosyncratic reactions are frequently irreversible (e.g., chloramphenicol, phenylbutazone).
Chemical agents	• Toxic chemicals in industry and agriculture (e.g., benzene, insecticides such as DDT and parathion)
Infection	• May involve all hematopoietic cell lines (pancytopenia) or only erythroid cell line (pure RBC aplasia) • Examples– EBV, CMV, parvovirus, HCV
Physical agents	• Whole-body ionizing radiation (therapeutic or nuclear accident).
Miscellaneous	• Thymoma (may be associated with pure RBC aplasia) • Paroxysmal nocturnal hemoglobinuria
Fanconi anemia	• Most common congenital cause. It is characterized by short stature, genitourinary abnormalities, café-au-lait spots, microphthalmia (one or both eyes are abnormally small), mental retardation, skeletal anomalies, and aplastic anemia.

CMV, Cytomegalovirus; *EBV,* Epstein-Barr virus; *HCV,* hepatitis C virus; *RBC,* red blood cell.

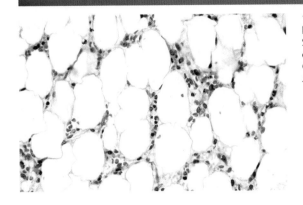

12-20: Bone marrow biopsy in aplastic anemia. The biopsy shows a marrow largely replaced by adipose cells. Scattered lymphocytes are present in between adipose cells. *(From Kumar V, Fausto N, Abbas A:* Robbins and Cotran Pathologic Basis of Disease, *7th ed, Philadelphia, Saunders, 2004, Fig. 13-27B.)*

5. Complete recovery from aplastic anemia occurs in <10% of cases.
   - BM transplantation is the treatment of choice in all patients <45 years of age with aplastic anemia when there is a human leucocyte antigen matched donor.
6. Pure RBC aplasia
   a. **Definition:** Uncommon type of aplasia that only involves suppression or destruction of RBC precursor cells (erythroid colony-forming unit; see Fig. 12-1)
   b. Causes include congenital problems (e.g., Diamond-Blackfan syndrome), thymomas, certain types of leukemia (e.g., B- and T-cell CLL), drugs (e.g., phenytoin, azathioprine, sulfonamides), and parvovirus (attaches to P antigen on the RBC membrane).
7. Transient erythroblastopenia of childhood (TEC)
   a. **Definition:** Idiopathic disorder of acquired RBC aplasia characterized by a gradual onset of pallor
   b. Epidemiology
      (1) Median age of presentation is 23 months.
      (2) Often a history of a previous viral illness
   c. Clinical findings
      - Except for pallor, the physical examination is otherwise unremarkable (absence of bruising, fever, lymphadenopathy, and hepatosplenomegaly).
   d. Laboratory findings
      - Normochromic normocytic anemia with a reticulocyte index <2
8. Diamond-Blackfan syndrome
   a. **Definition:** Genetic disorder that presents in childhood as a normocytic normochromic anemia with reticulocytopenia. Patients remain anemic throughout life.
   b. Epidemiology
      (1) The anemia presents during the first 6 months of life.
      (2) RBCs have fetal-like characteristics in that they have an increased MCV, increased levels of HbF, and the presence of i antigen on the RBC membrane (see Chapter 16).
      (3) Level of erythrocyte adenosine deaminase may be increased.

Biochemistry pearl: Adenosine deaminase is an enzyme that catalyzes the deamination of adenosine to inosine. It is a key enzyme in the degradation of nucleotides and purine salvage. The end-product of purine salvage is uric acid.

D. **Anemia in chronic renal failure (CRF)**
   1. **Definition:** Caused by a combination of a decrease in EPO and ACD (see previous discussion)
   2. Epidemiology
      - Anemia usually occurs when the creatinine clearance falls below 50 mL/min.
   3. Hematologic findings include:
      a. normocytic anemia.
      b. presence of burr cells in the peripheral blood (i.e., RBCs with undulating membranes).
      c. prolonged bleeding time because of a defect in platelet aggregation in the formation of a platelet thrombus (see Chapter 15).
         - Defect in platelet aggregation reversible with renal dialysis
E. **Malignancy; causes of anemia include:**
   1. ACD, which is the overall most common anemia in malignancy.

Margin notes:

Complete recovery <10%

Suppression/destruction erythroid colony-forming unit

Diamond-Blackfan syndrome, thymomas, leukemia, drugs, parvovirus

TEC

Idiopathic acquired RBC aplasia

History previous viral illness

Pallor + normochromic normocytic anemia retic index <2

Diamond-Blackfan syndrome

Genetic disease with reticulocytopenia childhood that persists

Presents first 6 mo of life

Fetal-like RBCs: ↑MCV, ↑HbF, i antigen

↑Adenosine deaminase

↑RBC adenosine deaminase

↓EPO + ACD

Creatinine clearance <50 mL/min

Burr cells in peripheral blood

↑Bleeding time → defect in platelet aggregation

Platelet dysfunction (reversible with dialysis), burr cells

ACD MC anemia

GI bleed

Metastasis to BM

NRBCs + immature myeloid cells

Cold IHA in CLL

RBC destruction before normal lifespan is over

Intrinsic (defect in RBC); e.g., spherocytosis

Extrinsic (factors outside RBC); e.g., IHA

Splenic/liver macrophage destruction RBCs

RBCs coated with IgG and/or C3b

RBCs abnormal shape (e.g., sickle cell)

Heinz body inclusions (G6PD)

↑UCB → jaundice

UCB end-product MP degradation Hb

2. GI bleeding (e.g., colorectal cancer), which produces a normocytic or microcytic anemia from the loss of iron.
3. Metastasis to the BM.
   a. Malignant cells displace normal marrow hematopoietic cells (e.g., myelocytes, nucleated RBCs [NRBCs]) into the peripheral blood (called a myelophthisic anemia).
   b. Presence of nucleated RBCs and immature myeloid cells in the peripheral blood is also called a leukoerythroblastic reaction (see Fig. 13-2).
4. Immune type of hemolytic anemia (discussed later).
   • Example: a cold type of immune hemolytic anemia (IHA) may occur in chronic lymphocytic leukemia (CLL)

VI. **Normocytic Anemias: Corrected Reticulocyte Count >2%** (see Table 12-5)
   A. **Definition:** Group of anemias in which RBCs are destroyed and removed from the bloodstream before their normal lifespan is over
   B. **Pathogenesis of hemolytic anemias**
      1. Intrinsic or extrinsic types of hemolytic anemia
         a. Intrinsic means that a defect in the RBC is causing the hemolytic anemia.
            • Examples: membrane defects (HS), abnormal Hb (sickle cell anemia), and enzyme deficiency (glucose-6-phosphate dehydrogenase [G6PD] deficiency)
         b. Extrinsic refers to factors outside the RBC that are causing the hemolytic anemia.
            • Examples: stenotic aortic valve (AV) damaging the RBCs and immune destruction of RBCs
      2. Mechanisms of RBC hemolysis (Fig. 12-21)
         a. Extravascular hemolysis
            (1) **Definition:** Refers to destruction of RBCs within splenic and/or liver macrophages (MPs)
            (2) Causes of RBC phagocytosis by MPs include:
               (a) RBCs coated by IgG with or without C3b.
                  • MPs have receptors for IgG and C3b.
               (b) Abnormally shaped RBCs (cannot reenter the peripheral circulation, e.g., spherocytes, sickle cells).
               (c) RBCs that contain inclusions that are recognized by MPs (e.g., Heinz bodies in G6PD deficiency).
            (3) Increase in serum unconjugated bilirubin (UCB), which produces jaundice if the bilirubin level is >2.5 mg/dL.
               • UCB is the end-product of MP degradation of Hb.

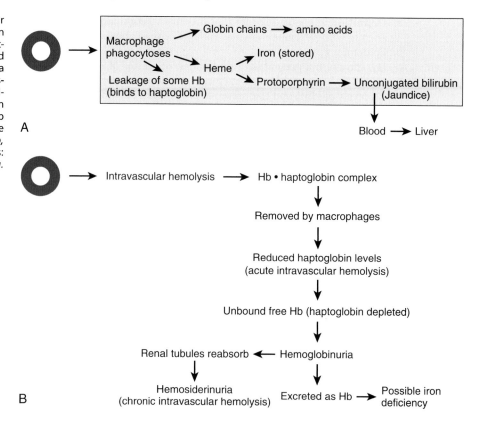

12-21: Extravascular (**A**) and intravascular (**B**) hemolysis of red blood cells (RBCs). In **extravascular hemolysis**, macrophage destruction of RBCs produces unconjugated hyperbilirubinemia and, in some cases, a decrease in serum haptoglobin. In **intravascular hemolysis**, hemoglobinuria, hemosiderinuria, and a decrease in serum haptoglobin are the key findings. There is some overlap in the two types of hemolysis, but these are the exception rather than the rule. *Hb,* Hemoglobin. *(From Goljan EF: Star Series: Pathology, Philadelphia, Saunders, 1998, Fig. 12-2.)*

(4) Serum lactate dehydrogenase (LDH) is increased from release of the enzyme into the peripheral blood from the hemolyzed RBCs.

↑LDH

(5) *May* be a decrease in serum haptoglobin if the RBC hemolysis is severe (see later discussion)

b. Intravascular hemolysis

(1) **Definition:** Refers to RBC hemolysis that occurs within the blood vessels

RBC hemolysis in blood vessels

(2) Causes include:

(a) enzyme deficiency (e.g., pyruvate kinase [PK] deficiency).

Enzyme deficiency (e.g., PK)

(b) complement destruction (e.g., IgM-mediated hemolysis; IgG-mediated in some cases).

Complement destruction

(c) mechanical damage (e.g., calcific aortic stenosis).

Mechanical damage (aortic stenosis)

(3) Laboratory findings include:

(a) increased plasma/urine Hb.

↑Plasma/urine Hb

(b) hemosiderinuria (proximal renal tubule cells convert iron in Hb into hemosiderin).

Hemosiderinuria

(c) decreased serum haptoglobin.

• Haptoglobin combines with Hb and is phagocytosed by MPs (see later discussion).

↓Serum haptoglobin

(d) increased serum LDH from the hemolyzed RBCs.

↑ Serum LDH

Haptoglobin is an acute phase reactant (see Chapter 3) that combines with hemoglobin (Hb) to form a complex that is phagocytosed and degraded by macrophage (MPs), causing a decrease in serum haptoglobin. The amount of Hb in the complexes may increase the unconjugated bilirubin (UCB) concentration, leading to jaundice. Because the serum UCB level must be >2.5 mg/dL to produce visible evidence of jaundice, the increase in UCB from MP removal of the haptoglobin–Hb complex may *not* be enough to cause jaundice. During active hemolysis of red blood cells, the rate of haptoglobin catabolism may exceed the liver's ability to synthesize it, resulting in a low to absent level in the blood. Because it is synthesized in the liver, primary liver disease (e.g., cirrhosis) may result in low levels. In addition, megaloblastic anemias (e.g., vitamin B$_{12}$ and folate deficiency) may result in decreased levels of haptoglobin caused by MP destruction and apoptosis of megaloblastic erythroid precursors in the BM. This reduces the test's specificity.

C. **Hereditary spherocytosis (HS)**

1. **Definition:** Genetic disorder with a defect in the RBC membrane causing an extravascular hemolytic anemia, jaundice, and splenomegaly

Genetic disorder; defect cell membrane

2. Epidemiology

a. Predominantly an autosomal dominant (AD) disorder

• Some cases are AR.

b. Common in people of Northern European descent

c. Intrinsic defect (something wrong with the RBC) that causes extravascular hemolysis

Intrinsic with extravascular hemolysis

d. Pathogenesis

(1) Membrane protein defect results in the loss of RBC membrane and volume, leading to spherocyte formation (Fig. 12-22 A; Link 12-20)

(a) A mutation in spectrin is the most common defect.

• Mutations in ankyrin, band 2 or band 3, account for other defects causing spherocytosis.

Spectrin MC mutation

(b) Microvesicles that form on the surface of the RBCs in the areas of membrane weakness are lost, causing the RBC to become a spherocyte (see Fig. 12-22 A; Link 12-21).

Microvesicle formation; loss K⁺ + H₂O (dehydrate cell) → spherocyte formation

(c) In addition, the membrane defect leads to a loss of both potassium and water, which produces cellular dehydration.

(d) Combination of microvesicle loss of cell membrane plus cellular dehydration yields spherocytes with a *decreased* surface to volume ratio.

Spherocyte: ↓surface to volume ratio

(2) Spherocytes are removed extravascularly by splenic MPs, producing a normocytic anemia.

3. Clinical findings

a. Jaundice commonly occurs because the splenic MPs destroy spherocytes. The resulting hemolysis leads to increased levels of UCB.

↑UCB → jaundice

(1) UCB is the end-product of heme degradation in the splenic or liver MPs (see Chapter 19).

(2) In newborns with HS, 30% to 50% develop a hemolytic anemia with unconjugated hyperbilirubinemia leading to jaundice.

b. Incidence of calcium bilirubinate gallstones is increased (see Fig. 19-9 C).

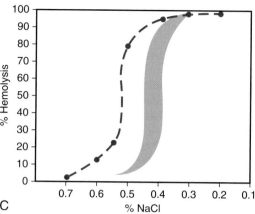

12-22: **A,** Schematic showing the formation of microvesicles on the red blood cell (RBC) membrane from areas of weakness in the RBC membrane. These are removed by macrophages in the spleen. Eventually, so much membrane has been lost that the RBC forms a spherocyte, which is phagocytosed and destroyed by splenic macrophages. **B,** Peripheral blood with spherocytes in hereditary spherocytosis. Numerous, round, dense RBCs without central areas of pallor represent spherocytes *(arrows).* The mean corpuscular hemoglobin concentration is increased. **C,** Osmotic fragility test. Comparison of RBC lysis in severe hereditary spherocytosis *(interrupted line)* and in normal blood *(shaded area).* The curve is shifted to the right of the normal range. **(A** *from Zitelli B, McIntire S, Nowalk A:* Zitelli and Davis' Atlas of Pediatric Physical Diagnosis, *6th ed, St. Louis, Saunders Elsevier, 2012, p 435, Fig. 11-14.* **B** *from my friend Ivan Damjanov, M.D., PhD, Linder J:* Pathology: A Color Atlas, *St. Louis, Mosby, 2000, p 75, Fig. 5-7;* **C** *from McPherson R, Pincus M:* Henry's Clinical Diagnosis and Management by Laboratory Methods, *22nd ed, Philadelphia, Saunders, 2011, p 573, Fig. 32-11.)*

Black calcium bilirubinate gallstones

        (1) Caused by increased liver conversion of excess amounts of UCB to water-soluble conjugated bilirubin (CB), which is excreted in the bile

        (2) CB is converted back to UCB in the gallbladder, and the UCB combines with calcium to form black calcium bilirubinate stones (see Fig. 19-9 C).

Splenomegaly (<u>work</u> hypertrophy)

    c. Splenomegaly (due to work hypertrophy from excessive RBC hemolysis) is present in 75% of cases.

  4. Laboratory findings include:

    a. normocytic anemia with spherocytosis (Fig. 12-22 B).

        • Other causes of spherocytosis include warm immune hemolytic anemia (IHA; discussed later) and ABO hemolytic disease of newborn.

↑MCHC

    b. increased mean corpuscular hemoglobin concentration (MCHC).

        (1) Caused by cellular dehydration from the loss of potassium and water by the spherocytes

        (2) HS is the only anemia with an increase in the MCHC. This is a useful finding in the diagnosis.

    c. increased RBC osmotic fragility (Fig. 12-22 C; Link 12-22)

↑RBC osmotic fragility (↓surface to volume ratio)

        (1) When compared with normal RBCs, there is increased osmotic fragility when spherocytes are placed in saline solutions of different tonicity. Spherocytes hemolyze in normal saline (0.7% NaCl).

        (2) Hemolysis is primarily caused by the decreased surface-to-volume ratio of spherocytes.

↑RDW

    d. increased RDW owing to the presence of both dense, round spherocytes and normal-sized RBCs.

D. Hereditary elliptocytosis

Genetic defect in cell membrane

  1. **Definition:** Genetic disorder with a defect in the RBC membrane leading to a shortened life span

  2. Epidemiology

AD disorder

    a. AD disorder

Mutations spectrin, band 4.1

    b. Most common mutations in the cell membrane are in spectrin and band 4.1.

Intrinsic defect with extravascular hemolysis

    c. Intrinsic defect (something wrong with the RBC) with extravascular hemolysis

  3. Clinical findings

    a. Majority of patients have *no* anemia or a mild hemolytic anemia.

    b. Splenomegaly is present (work hypertrophy).

  4. Laboratory findings

\>25% Elliptocytes in peripheral blood

    a. Elliptocytes account for >25% of the RBCs in the peripheral blood (Fig. 12-23).

↑Osmotic fragility

    b. RBC osmotic fragility is increased.

E. Paroxysmal nocturnal hemoglobinuria (PNH)

Intravascular hemolysis, vessel thrombosis, hemoglobinuria

  1. **Definition:** Rare, chronic, intravascular hemolysis causing vessel thrombosis and hemoglobinuria visible in the urine upon wakening

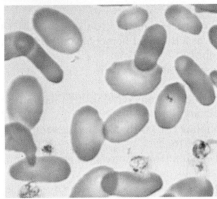

12-23: Peripheral blood with elliptocytes. In hereditary elliptocytosis, elliptocytes constitute more than 25% of the red blood cells, as in this smear. *(From my friend Ivan Damjanov, M.D., PhD, Linder J:* Pathology: A Color Atlas, *St. Louis, Mosby, 2000, Fig. 5-8A.)*

2. Epidemiology
   a. Intrinsic defect (something wrong with the RBC) with intravascular hemolysis
   b. Pathogenesis
      (1) Acquired stem cell disease with a somatic mutation after birth in the X chromosome gene *PIGA* (phosphatidylinositol glycan class A) in a myeloid stem cell clone
      (2) Mutation results in a defect in the anchoring of glycosyl phosphatidylinositol-anchored protein (GPI-AP) inhibitors of complement (CD55 [decay accelerating factor; DAF] and CD59) on the surface of RBCs, neutrophils, and platelets.
         • Inhibitors normally degrade C3 and C5 convertase on hematopoietic cell membranes, which prevents activation of the membrane attack complex (MAC) and subsequent lysis of RBCs, neutrophils, and platelets (pancytopenia).
      (3) Result is an intravascular, complement-mediated lysis of RBCs, neutrophils, and platelets, causing pancytopenia. MAC is *not* inhibited, causing lysis of the hematopoietic cells.

> Hemolysis occurs at night because the mild respiratory acidosis (retention of carbon dioxide) from sleeping enhances complement attachment to these blood cells. Some authors state that lysis occurs continuously and that the dark morning urine is caused by concentration of the urine overnight.

3. Clinical findings
   a. Iron deficiency is possible because of episodic hemoglobinuria (microcytic anemia) and the loss of iron in the urine.
   b. Increased incidence of vessel thrombosis (e.g., hepatic vein)
      • Caused by the release of aggregating agents from destroyed platelets (e.g., adenosine diphosphate)
   c. Increased risk for developing aplastic anemia and acute myeloblastic leukemia (AML; see Chapter 13)
4. Peripheral blood findings
   a. Normocytic anemia with pancytopenia (decrease in RBCs, platelets, and WBCs).
      • Anemia is microcytic if iron deficiency develops from hemoglobinuria.
   b. Negative leukocyte alkaline phosphatase (LAP) stain (see Chapter 13).
   c. Serum haptoglobin is decreased, and serum and urine Hb are increased.
5. Diagnosis
   a. The test of choice is flow cytometry for detecting granulocytes missing the anchor for the inhibitors of complement.
   b. Older tests for diagnosing PNH include:
      (1) screening test using the sucrose hemolysis test (sugar water test).
         • Sucrose enhances complement destruction of RBCs.
      (2) confirmatory test using the acidified serum test (Ham test).
         • Acidified serum activates the alternative pathway, causing hemolysis.
F. **Paroxysmal cold hemoglobinuria (PCH)**
   1. **Definition:** Rare hemolytic anemia caused by an IgG cold antibody that has bithermal activity.

Margin notes:

Intrinsic defect with intravascular hemolysis

Mutation X chromosome gene *PIGA* in myeloid stem cell clone

Defect anchoring inhibitors complement (CD55 [DAF], CD59)

Normally degrade C3/C5 convertase to prevent MAC activation

Intravascular hemolysis

Complement mediated pancytopenia

Nocturnal hemolysis due to respiratory acidosis enhancing complement destruction

Microcytic anemia loss iron in urine

Release platelet aggregating agents → vessel thrombosis

↑Risk AML, aplastic anemia

Normocytic/microcytic anemia; pancytopenia

Negative LAP stain

↓Haptoglobin; ↑serum/urine Hb

Flow cytometry detects missing anchors

Outdated tests: sucrose hemolysis test, acidified serum test

IgG cold antibody with bithermal activity

Extrinsic defect with intravascular hemolysis

Associated with syphilis

IgG cold antibody with bithermal activity; intravascular hemolysis

Ab binds to P antigen on RBCs

Cold→ Ab binds to RBCs, fixes C

Warm→ Ab detaches, activates C, intravascular hemolysis

Hemolytic anemia: warm to cold

Cold → hemoglobinuria

Severe pain

Raynaud phenomenon

Oliguria → renal failure

Resolves in warm temperature

Detect bithermal antibody

Genetic; multiorgan disease

Autosomal recessive

MC hemoglobinopathy in African descent

Intrinsic defect with extravascular hemolysis

Missense mutation: valine for glutamic acid

HbAS no anemia

HbSS severe anemia

Trait × trait: 25% normal, 50% trait, 25% disease

Protective against *P. falciparum*

ACS, stroke, infections

HbS aggregate/polymerize when deoxygenated

O$_2$ inhibits sickling

HbS >60% → sickle

HbAS <50% → no sickling peripheral blood

2. Epidemiology
   a. Extrinsic defect (something outside the RBC) with intravascular hemolysis
   b. Presents as a transient hemolytic anemia in children with measles, mumps, influenza, or chickenpox
   c. Often associated with syphilis
   d. Pathogenesis
      (1) IgG cold antibody develops that has bithermal activity (Donath-Landsteiner antibody).
      (2) Antibody (Ab) is directed against the P blood group antigen on surface of RBCs (see Chapter 16).
         (a) At cold temperatures, the antibody binds to the P antigen on RBCs and fixes complement (C).
         (b) At 37° C, it detaches from RBCs and activates complement, causing intravascular hemolysis.
      (3) Hemolysis usually occurs when the patient moves from a cold to a warm environment.
3. Clinical findings
   a. Within minutes after exposure to cold temperatures, the patient has fever, rigors, and chills followed by red to brown urine (hemoglobinuria).
   b. Back, leg, and abdominal pain are commonly present.
   c. May be associated with Raynaud phenomenon (bluish discoloration of the fingers and toes; see Chapter 10)
   d. Transient hepatosplenomegaly with jaundice may occur.
   e. Oliguria and renal failure may occur.
   f. Symptoms and hemoglobinuria usually resolve within hours, especially when moving into a warm environment.
4. Diagnosis
   • Special laboratory tests detect the bithermal antibody

G. Sickle cell disease
1. **Definition:** Genetic disease characterized by a chronic hemolytic state in which vasoocclusion in many organs is caused by sickle-shaped RBCs
2. Epidemiology of sickle cell disease
   a. AR disorder
   b. Most common hemoglobinopathy in individuals of African descent
      • Highest prevalence of sickle cell disease (~30%–40%) is in sub-Saharan Africa
   c. Intrinsic defect within the RBC that causes primarily extravascular hemolysis
      • Intravascular hemolysis of the sickle cells occurs to a small degree as well.
   d. Sickle cell disease (HbSS; homozygous state) is caused by a missense point mutation (see Chapter 6) with substitution of valine for glutamic acid at the sixth position of the β-globin chain.
   e. Heterozygote state (sickle cell trait, HbAS) has *no* anemia.
      • Sickle cell trait is present in ~10% of the black population.
   f. Homozygous condition (HbSS) produces a severe normocytic anemia.
   g. Using an example of a pedigree (Link 12-23) with two people with sickle cell trait, they will have a:
      (1) 25% chance of having a normal child.
      (2) 50% chance of having child with sickle cell trait.
      (3) 25% chance of having a child with sickle cell disease.
   h. Sickle cells are protective against *Plasmodium falciparum* malaria.
   i. Most life-threatening complications include acute chest syndrome (ACS), stroke, and infections.
3. Pathogenesis of sickle cell disease
   a. HbS molecules in the RBCs aggregate and polymerize into long, needle-like fibers when deoxygenated.
      (1) RBCs assume a sickle or boat-like shape (Fig. 12-24 A).
      (2) Oxygen inhibits sickling.
   b. Causes of sickling
      (1) Sickle HbS concentration >60% is the most important factor for sickling.
         • HbS concentration is too low in sickle cell trait (HbAS;<50%) to produce sickling in the peripheral blood (PB). However, it is low enough to produce sickling in various target organs in extreme hypoxic situations.

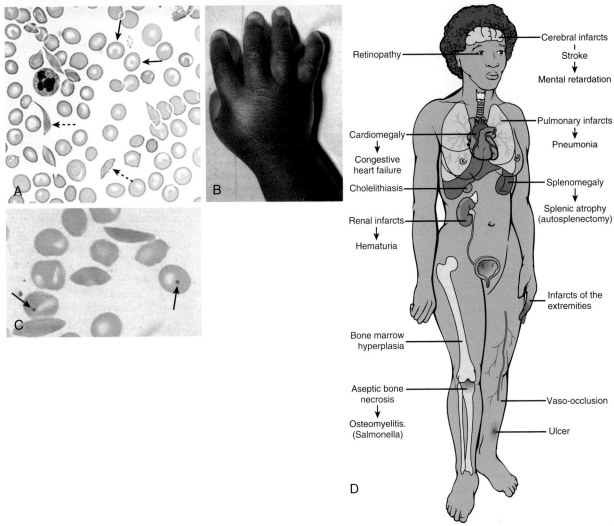

12-24: A, Peripheral blood with sickle cells *(interrupted arrows)* and target cells, showing the dense, boat-shaped sickle cells. Cells with a bull's-eye appearance are target cells *(solid arrows)*, which have excess red blood cell membrane that bulges in the center of the cell. **B,** Sickle cell anemia. This is the hand of young child with painful, swollen fingers (dactylitis) caused by infarction (aseptic necrosis) of the metacarpal bones. This acute syndrome rarely occurs after 2 years of age. **C,** Peripheral blood with sickle cells and Howell-Jolly (HJ) bodies. The three dense, boat-shaped sickle cells and the two cells containing a single dark, round inclusion *(arrows)* represent nuclear remnants. HJ bodies in sickle cell disease indicate splenic dysfunction. **D,** Clinicopathologic findings in sickle cell anemia. The findings are a consequence of infarctions, anemia, hemolysis, and recurrent infections. (*A from Hoffbrand AV: Color Atlas: Clinical Hematology, 3rd ed, St. Louis, Mosby, 2000, p 103, Fig. 5-85A; B from Forbes C, Jackson W: Color Atlas and Text of Clinical Medicine, 3rd ed, London, Mosby, 2004, p 419, Fig. 10.48; C from Henry JB: Clinical Diagnosis and Management by Laboratory Methods, 20th ed, Philadelphia, Saunders, 2001, Fig. 26-2A. D from my friend Ivan Damjanov MD, PhD: Pathology for the Health Professions, 4th ed, St. Louis, Saunders Elsevier, 2012, p 208, Fig. 9-10.*)

(2) Factors that increase the concentration of deoxyhemoglobin (deoxyHb) and increase the risk for sickling include:

    (a) acidosis, which shifts the oxygen dissociation curve (ODC) rightward, causing O_2 release from RBCs and leading to an increase in deoxyhemoglobin.

    (b) volume depletion, in which intracellular dehydration causes an increase in concentration of deoxyhemoglobin.

    (c) hypoxemia, in which a decrease in arterial Po_2 decreases the O_2 saturation of Hb, which increases the amount of deoxyhemoglobin.

c. Reversible and irreversible sickling

    (1) Initial sickling is reversible with administration of oxygen.

       • Oxygen inhibits sickling.

    (2) Recurrent sickling causes irreversible sickling because of membrane damage.

       (a) An influx of calcium ions cross-links membrane proteins, causing the egress of potassium (K^+) and water, leaving the cell dehydrated.

       (b) The number of irreversibly sickled cells correlates with the severity of hemolysis.

Acidosis → right-ward shift ODC

Volume depletion

Hypoxemia

Initial sickling reversible with O_2

Recurrent sickling → membrane damage → irreversible sickling

Removed by spleen/liver MPs

VOC → ischemic damage

↑Expression adhesion molecules

HbF prevents sickling

Sickling *not* present at birth
Hydroxyurea ↑HbF synthesis

Severe anemia, VOC: Occlusion of microcirculation

Dactylitis

Painful swelling hands/feet

Bone infarctions (aseptic necrosis)

MC presentation infants (6-9mth)

MC COD young people with HbSS

Pneumonia, bone infarction with fat embolism

Acute chest syndrome: MCC death in young people
Aseptic necrosis of femoral head

Dysfunctional by 1 year

HJ bodies sign splenic dysfunction

Loss MP function

Spleen fibrosed/smaller (autosplenectomy)

Impaired opsonization

Children: ↑risk
S. pneumoniae sepsis

S. pneumoniae sepsis, *Salmonella paratyphi* (MC) osteomyelitis

Aplastic RBC crisis

Sudden ↓RBCs

Parvovirus

(c) Irreversibly sickled cells are sequestered and are removed by MPs in the spleen and liver (extravascular hemolysis).

 d. Microvascular occlusions (vasoocclusive [VOC] crises; see later) produce ischemic damage.

  (1) Sickled cells are sticky because of increased expression of adhesion molecules on their surfaces; this enables them to stick to and damage endothelial cells in the microvasculature.

  (2) Microvascular occlusion leads to ischemic tissue injury.

 e. HbF prevents sickling (Link 12-24).

  (1) Increased HbF at birth prevents sickling in sickle cell disease (HbSS) until 5 to 6 months of age.

  (2) Hydroxyurea increases the synthesis of HbF.

  (3) HbF has a high affinity for O_2, which inhibits sickling.

4. Clinical findings in HbSS

 a. Key pathologic processes in sickle cell anemia include severe anemia and VOC crises.

 b. VOC crises occurs when the microcirculation is obstructed by sickled RBCs (readily adhere to endothelium), causing ischemic injury to the organ supplied and resultant pain.

  (1) Almost half of individuals with HbSS have VOC crises.

  (2) The frequency of these crises is variable but may be as many as six or more crises a year.

  (3) Examples of VOC crises include dactylitis and avascular necrosis of bone.

 c. Dactylitis (hand–foot syndrome)

  (1) **Definition:** Dactylitis refers to painful swelling of the hands (Fig. 12-24 B) and feet.

   (a) Pain is caused by infarctions (coagulation necrosis; see Chapter 2) in the metacarpal bones.

   (b) The term *aseptic necrosis* is also used to describe the bone changes.

  (2) Dactylitis occurs in infants (usually 6–9 months old) and is rarely seen after 2 years of age.

 d. Acute chest syndrome (ACS)

  (1) **Definition:** Refers to a segmental lung infiltrate that is associated with chest pain

  (2) Most common COD in young people with sickle cell disease

  (3) Precipitating factors include:

   (a) pneumonia.

    • *Streptococcus pneumoniae*, *Mycoplasma* spp., chlamydia, viruses

   (b) bone infarction with fat embolism.

  (4) Clinical findings include:

   • chest pain, wheezing, dyspnea, pleuritic chest pain (pain on inspiration), pleural effusion, and cough.

  (5) Arterial blood gas shows hypoxemia (decreased arterial PO_2).

  (6) Chest radiographs show lung infiltrates.

  (7) Other lung disorders in sickle cell disease include fat embolization from bone infarctions (see Chapter 5), restrictive lung disease, and pulmonary hypertension with cor pulmonale (right ventricular hypertrophy + pulmonary hypertension).

 e. Avascular necrosis of the femoral head may occur (see Chapter 24).

 f. Autosplenectomy (Link 12-25)

  (1) Initially, the spleen is enlarged but dysfunctional by age 10 to 12 months.

   • Nuclear remnants (HJ bodies) appear in RBCs, indicating loss of MP function in the spleen (Fig. 12-24 C).

  (2) Spleen is fibrosed and smaller in young adults.

   • Most authors refer to this stage as "autosplenectomy."

 g. Increased susceptibility to infections

  (1) Increased risk for infection is due to a dysfunctional spleen with impaired opsonization (antibody attachment) of encapsulated bacteria.

  (2) Children are at great risk for *S. pneumoniae* sepsis.

   (a) Common cause of death in children

   (b) Prophylactic penicillin is recommended.

  (3) Increased risk for osteomyelitis (infection of bone; see Chapter 24)

   • Osteomyelitis is most often caused by *Salmonella paratyphi* and less frequently to *Staphylococcus aureus*.

 h. Aplastic RBC crisis (decreased RBCs)

  (1) **Definition:** Refers to a sudden decrease in RBC progenitors in the BM

  (2) Most frequently associated with a parvovirus infection

(3) *No* reticulocytes (young RBCs) are present in the peripheral blood (reticulocytopenia).

   i. Sequestration crisis.

      (1) **Definition:** Associated with rapid splenic enlargement and entrapment of sickled RBCs causing a drop in the Hb and the number of circulating RBCs, resulting in hypovolemia (a decreased volume of blood)

      (2) Complication usually occurs in the first 2 years of life.

      (3) Reticulocytosis (increased reticulocytes) is present in the peripheral blood (this is different from an aplastic crisis where there is reticulocytopenia).

   j. Calcium bilirubinate gallstones (see previous discussion)

   k. Acute and chronic liver disease

   l. Strokes

      (1) Strokes may occur in children (usually between ages 2 and 5 years) as well as adults.

      (2) Common COD in children

      (3) Recurrence rate for strokes is 70%.

   m. Recurrent leg ulcers

     • Commonly above the medial or lateral malleolus

   n. Proliferative retinopathy

     • **Definition:** Increase in the number of new blood vessels in the retina; frequently leads to blindness

   o. End-stage renal failure occurs usually occurs after 40 years of age.

     • Other renal findings include hematuria, hyperuricemia, and hypertension.

5. Renal findings in sickle cell trait (HbAS; also in HbSS)

   a. Sickling occurs in peritubular capillaries in the medulla (Link 12-26).

     • O_2 tension is normally low enough in the medulla to induce sickling in both sickle cell trait and disease.

   b. Microhematuria (blood in the urine) occurs because of microinfarctions in the kidneys.

     • Always order a sickle cell screen in any black person with unexplained hematuria.

   c. Renal papillary necrosis (RPN) may occur (see Chapter 20).

     • Loss of renal papillae in the urine results in a loss of concentration and dilution of urine.

   d. Priapism (permanent erection) because of clogging of the vessels in the penis

   e. Cardiovascular findings include acute myocardial infarction and, less commonly, congestive heart failure.

6. Laboratory findings in sickle cell trait and disease

   a. Sickle cell screen

     • Sodium metabisulfite reduces O_2 tension, which induces sickling in a test tube.

   b. Hb electrophoresis (see Fig. 12-7 E, F)

      (1) HbAS (trait) profile: HbA, 55% to 60%; HbS, 40% to 45%

      (2) HbSS (disease) profile: HbS, 90% to 95%; HbF, 5% to 10%; no HbA

   c. Peripheral blood findings

      (1) Normal peripheral blood smear in HbAS

      (2) Sickle cells, target cells, NRBCs, and HJ bodies in HbSS (see Fig. 12-24 A; Link 12-27)

   d. Prenatal screening

     • Analysis of fetal DNA is used to detect the point mutation.

7. Preventive measures in sickle cell disease include:

   a. hydroxyurea to increase HbF.

   b. keep all routine immunizations current.

   c. pneumococcal vaccine to prevent *S. pneumoniae* infections.

   d. folic acid supplementation.

     • Folic acid is often decreased because accelerated erythropoiesis depletes its supply.

8. Overview of findings in sickle cell disease (Fig. 12-24 D; Link 12-28)

H. Glucose 6-phosphate dehydrogenase deficiency (G6PD)

1. **Definition:** Genetic type of hemolytic anemia caused by deficiency of G6PD, an early enzyme of the pentose phosphate pathway

2. Epidemiology

   a. Severity of hemolysis ranges from Class 1 (mild) to Class 5 (severe).

   b. X-linked recessive (XR) disorder

   c. Highest prevalence is in tropical Africa (most common location), the Middle East, Greece, Italy, and Asia.

Reticulocytopenia

Rapid splenic enlargement with entrapped blood → hypovolemia

First 2 yrs life

Reticulocytosis

Calcium bilirubinate gallstones

Strokes common in children; common COD in children

Recurrent leg ulcers around malleoli

Proliferative retinopathy → blindness

End-stage renal failure after 40 years old

Hematuria, ↑uric acid, HTN

Sickling in kidneys occurs in trait/disease

Microhematuria a key finding

RPN may occur; no concentration/dilution

Screen: sodium metabisulfite ↓O_2 tension, induces sickling

Close to equal amounts HbA and S

Mainly HbS and HbF

Normal HbAS

Sickle, target, NRBCs, HJ bodies

Prenatal screening: fetal DNA analysis

Hydroxyurea, immunizations, folic acid

Deficiency G6PD in pentose phosphate pathway

Severity Class 1 to 5

XR; MC in tropical Africa

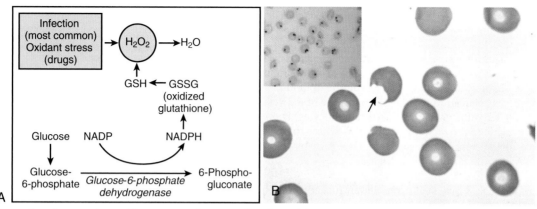

12-25: A, Pentose phosphate pathway. The enzyme glucose-6-phosphate dehydrogenase (G6PD) catalyzes the irreversible reaction that converts glucose 6-phosphate to 6-phosphogluconate. NADPH (reduced form of nicotinamide adenine dinucleotide phosphate [NADP]) is produced in this reaction and reduces oxidized glutathione (GSSG) to glutathione (GSH), which neutralizes peroxide and converts it to water. **B,** Peripheral blood smear with a bite cell and *inset* showing Heinz bodies in G6PD deficiency. The *arrow* shows a bite cell with part of the red blood cell membrane removed. The inset shows a peripheral blood smear with a supravital stain visualizing punctate inclusions representing denatured hemoglobin (Heinz bodies). *(A from Goljan EF: Pathology: Saunders Text and Review Series, Philadelphia, Saunders, 1998, Fig. 12-10; B from Kumar V, Fausto N, Abbas A: Robbins and Cotran Pathologic Basis of Disease, 7th ed, Philadelphia, Saunders, 2004, Fig. 13-8; inset from Wickramasinghe SN, McCullough J: Blood and Bone Marrow Pathology, London, Churchill Livingstone, 2003, Fig. 8-8. D, from my friend Ivan Damjanov MD, PhD: Pathology for the Health Professions, 4th ed, St. Louis, Saunders Elsevier, 2012, p 208, Fig. 9-10).*

Intrinsic defect, predominantly intravascular hemolysis

MC enzyme deficiency causing hemolysis

Mediterranean, black variants

Protective against *P. falciparum*

d. G6PD deficiency is an intrinsic defect with predominantly intravascular hemolysis.
  • Mild to moderate component of extravascular hemolysis as well
e. Most common enzyme deficiency causing hemolysis
f. Subtypes of G6PD deficiency include the Mediterranean variant and the black variant (occurs in 10% of blacks).
g. G6PD deficiency is protective against contracting *P. falciparum* malaria (hemolysis destroys RBCs with parasites).
3. Pathogenesis of hemolysis
  a. Decreased synthesis of the reduced form of nicotinamide adenine dinucleotide phosphate (NADPH) and GSH in the pentose phosphate pathway (Fig. 12-25 A).

↓Glutathione antioxidant against peroxide

Peroxide oxidizes Hb → Heinz bodies

Heinz bodies damage RBC membranes

   (1) GSH normally neutralizes hydrogen peroxide (H_2O_2), an oxidant product in RBC metabolism.
   (2) In G6PD deficiency, hydrogen peroxide (H_2O_2) oxidizes Hb (denatured Hb), which precipitates to form Heinz bodies (Fig. 12-25 B).
     (a) Heinz bodies damage the RBC membranes, causing intravascular hemolysis.
     (b) Heinz bodies removed from RBC membranes by splenic MPs produce bite cells (see Fig. 12-25B).
  b. Half-life of G6PD in the Mediterranean variant of G6PD deficiency is markedly reduced (<10% activity).

Enzyme half-life markedly reduced in old RBCs (<10% activity)

   (1) Enzyme is highest in young RBCs and lowest in older RBCs (old RBCs with the least amount of enzyme are preferentially destroyed).
     • In this variant, there are a lot more old RBCs that lack the enzyme.
   (2) Person has either a severe, chronic hemolytic anemia (class 5) or one with severe hemolysis associated only with an oxidant stress (see later).

Enzyme half-life moderately reduced in old RBCs (10% to 60% activity)

  c. Half-life of G6PD in the black variant is moderately reduced (10%–60% activity).
    • Produces an episodic type of hemolytic anemia *after* exposure to an oxidant stress.
  d. Oxidant stresses inducing hemolysis include:
   (1) infection (most common oxidant stress).

A **decrease in NADPH** impairs neutrophils and monocyte killing of bacteria by the O_2-dependent myeloperoxidase (MPO) system (see Chapter 3), which requires NADPH as a cofactor for NADPH oxidase. This explains why infection is the most important oxidant stress initiating hemolysis.

O_2-dependent MPO system dysfunctional; lack NADPH cofactor

Primaquine, dapsone, sulfonamides

Fava beans

Hemoglobinuria post oxidant stress

Jaundice in neonates/adults

   (2) drugs (e.g., primaquine, chloroquine, dapsone, sulfonamides, and nitrofurantoin).
   (3) fava beans (mainly in the Mediterranean variant).
4. Clinical findings
  a. Sudden onset of back pain with hemoglobinuria 2 to 3 days after an oxidant stress
  b. Jaundice is a possible finding in both neonates and adults.

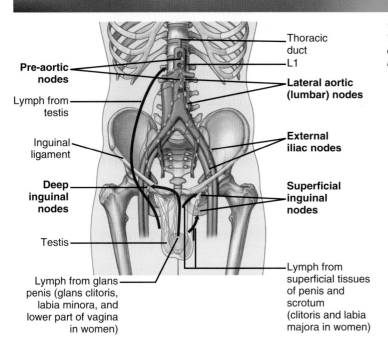

14-6: Lymphatic drainage of the perineum. *(From Drake RL, Vogl AW, Mitchell AWM: Gray's Anatomy for Students, 2nd ed, Philadelphia, Churchill Livingstone Elsevier, 2010, p 496, Fig. 5.79.)*

Thoracic duct
L1
Pre-aortic nodes
Lateral aortic (lumbar) nodes
Lymph from testis
External iliac nodes
Inguinal ligament
Deep inguinal nodes
Superficial inguinal nodes
Testis
Lymph from glans penis (glans clitoris, labia minora, and lower part of vagina in women)
Lymph from superficial tissues of penis and scrotum (clitoris and labia majora in women)

b. Examples include:
  (1) early stages of human immunodeficiency virus (HIV) infection.
  (2) other examples: rheumatoid arthritis (RA) and SLE
2. Paracortical hyperplasia
  a. **Definition:** T-cell antigenic response in the paracortex of lymph nodes
  b. Dermatopathic
    (1) **Definition:** Response that occurs in lymph nodes draining areas with a chronic dermatitis (e.g., psoriasis)
    (2) Epidemiology
      (a) Lymph nodes contain macrophages (MPs) with phagocytosis of melanin pigment.
      (b) Because of the black pigment, it is often confused with metastatic malignant melanoma.
  c. Other examples of paracortical hyperplasia include phenytoin and viral infections.
3. Mixed B- and T-cell hyperplasia
  a. Cat-scratch disease (Links 14-4 and 14-5)
    (1) **Definition:** Disorder characterized by fever and painful swelling of lymph nodes, caused by *B. henselae* resulting from the scratch or bite of a cat
    (2) Epidemiology
      (a) Granulomatous microabscesses are present in regional lymph nodes (e.g., axillary, cervical).
      (b) Most common cause of chronic unilateral regional lymphadenopathy in children. Cervical and axillary lymph nodes are most commonly involved. Other nodes that may be involved include the epitrochlear, preauricular, submandibular, and inguinal lymph nodes.
      (c) *B. henselae* is the etiologic agent. *B. henselae* IgM enzyme immunoassay (EIA) is the best test during the acute phase.
    (3) Clinical findings: Most patients do *not* recall a cat scratch. Kittens are usually the reservoir. Lymphadenopathy develops 1 to 2 weeks after the scratch.
    (4) Potential complications include prolonged fever of unknown etiology, Parinaud oculoglandular syndrome (conjunctivitis, ipsilateral preauricular lymphadenopathy), encephalitis, osteolytic bone lesions, neuroretinitis, hepatosplenomegaly, and erythema nodosum.
  b. Toxoplasmosis
    (1) **Definition:** Infection caused by the sporozoan *Toxoplasma gondii* that produces a mononucleosis-like syndrome with painful cervical lymphadenopathy.
    (2) Approximately 50% of the population has been infected by the sporozoan (Link 14-6). Infects the cervical lymph nodes producing painful lymphadenopathy.

Early HIV

RA, SLE

Paracortical hyperplasia

T-cell response paracortex

Dermatopathic

Nodal response to chronic dermatitis (psoriasis)

MPs with melanin pigment

Confused with melanoma

Phenytoin, viral infections

Mixed B-/T-cell hyperplasia

Cat-scratch disease

Painful lymphadenopathy due to *Bartonella henselae*

Granulomatous microabscesses

MCC chronic unilateral lymphadenopathy in children

Bartonella henselae; IgM EIA (acute phase)

Kittens are reservoir

Lymphadenopathy 1-2 weeks

Toxoplasmosis

Toxoplasma gondii (sporozoan)

Mono-like syndrome with painful cervical adenopathy

4. Other predominantly lymph node pathogens
   a. Tularemia
      (1) **Definition:** Rare infectious disease caused by the gram-negative rod *Francisella tularensis*. It may attack the skin, eyes, lymph nodes, and lungs.
      (2) Epidemiology
         (a) Zoonosis (infection transmitted from animals to humans) that is often seen in hunters and fur trappers
         (b) Reservoirs of the bacteria include rodents, deer, and rabbits (90%).
         (c) Transmission is by:
            • bites by *Dermacentor* ticks, skin contact with an animal hide (muskrat, rabbit, deer), and aerosol.
      (3) Ulceroglandular type of tularemia
         (a) Most common presentation of tularemia in the United States
         (b) Characterized by localized papular lesion that develops at the point of inoculation (tick bite) → ulceration of the papule → regional lymphadenitis (noncaseating granulomatous inflammation) → sepsis leading to dissemination throughout the body (e.g., spleen, liver)
   b. Plague
      (1) **Definition:** Potentially life-threatening infectious disease that is usually transmitted to humans by the bites of rodent fleas
      (2) Epidemiology
         (a) Caused by *Yersinia pestis,* a gram-negative facultative intracellular bacterium (Fig. 14-7 C)
         (b) *Yop* gene protein products inhibit phagocytosis of the bacterium and kill phagocytes.
         (c) Similar to all *Yersinia* species, it requires iron for growth.
      (3) Transmission
         (a) Bite of infected fleas that have bitten infected ground squirrels, prairie dogs, wood rats, or chipmunks, which are the reservoir of the bacterium
         (b) Droplet infection from a patient with the disease
      (4) Three main presentations of plague
         (a) Bubonic plague (most common presentation)
         (b) Septicemic plague (second most common presentation); Fig. 14-7 B
         (c) Pneumonic plague (transmits to others by aerosol [uncommon] or as a secondary complication of septicemic plague)
      (5) Bubonic plague mainly occurs in the Western United States (most commonly in Arizona, New Mexico, and Colorado).
         (a) Bubonic plaque may be limited to lymph node involvement or spread into the bloodstream (secondary septicemic plague), with or without spread to the lungs (secondary pneumonic plague).
         (b) Natural history
            • Organism enters the body at the site of a flea bite, usually the lower leg.
            • Infection spreads into the inguinal lymph nodes, where it produces buboes, which appear edematous and congested early in the disease.
            • Within the lymph nodes, there is massive proliferation of the organisms accompanied by an exudate *without* inflammatory cells, causing the nodes to swell to the size of hen's eggs (Fig. 14-7 A).
            • Eventually, the nodes exhibit hemorrhagic necrosis and vessel thrombosis with abscess formation, often leading to spontaneous rupture of the nodes.
            • Bacteria often escape from the nodes and enter the bloodstream (secondary septicemic phase), causing widespread necrosis within organs throughout the body. Disseminated intravascular coagulation (DIC) is a common complication in this phase. Endotoxemia produces septic shock (see Chapter 5).
         (c) If the lungs are involved (secondary pneumonic phase), hemorrhagic and necrotizing bronchopneumonia develops in all lobes, along with fibrinous pleuritis.
      (6) Clinical findings
         (a) Fever, chills, myalgia, arthralgia, headache, and prostration are the usual initial findings.
         (b) Septicemic plague findings are those of septic shock from endotoxemia. They include:
            • vomiting, abdominal pain, refractory hypotension, and renal failure.

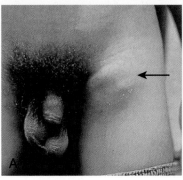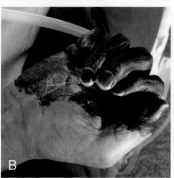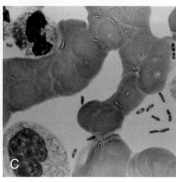

14-7: A, Swollen inguinal lymph nodes in a patient with bubonic plague. **B,** Hand of a patient with septicemic plague showing gangrene of the digits. The term "black plague" originated from this clinical finding. **C,** Wayson-stained blood smear of *Yersinia pestis* in a patient with septicemic plague. Note the characteristic bipolar staining of the gram-negative bacilli. *(A from Seidel H, Ball J, Dains, J, Benedict G: Mosby's Guide to Physical Examination, 6th ed, St. Louis, Mosby Elsevier, 2006, p 389; taken from Beeching, Nye, 1996. Bubonic plague. B and C from Goldman L, Schafer A: Goldman's Cecil Medicine, 25th ed, Philadelphia, Elsevier Saunders, 2016, p 1984, 1987 respectively, Figs. 312-1, 312-5, respectively. B courtesy of Centers for Disease Control and Prevention.)*

       (c) Pneumonic plague findings include:
- chest pain, dyspnea, and productive cough (Gram stain reveals numerous organisms). | Chest pain, dyspnea, productive cough

  c. Lymphatic filariasis | Lymphatic filariasis
    (1) **Definition:** Parasitic disease caused by microfilaria from the thread-like worms *Wucheria bancrofti* or *Brugia malayi* | Wucheria Bancroft/Brugia malayi
    (2) Epidemiology
      (a) Toxins released by the adult worms produce dilation of the lymphatics (lymphangiectasia). | Toxins → lymphangiectasia
      (b) Death of the adult worms causes lymphangitis. Worms infected with rickettsia-like bacteria release lipopolysaccharides, leading to further inflammation of the lymphatics. | Death of worms → lymphangitis
      (c) Transmission (Link 14-7)
- Bite of infected mosquito (*Anopheles* or *Culex*) | Bite *Anopheles* or *Culex* mosquito
- Microfilaria circulate in the bloodstream at night and enter into the lymphatics→ mature into adult worms that produce an inflammatory reaction resulting in lymphedema (elephantiasis) of the legs, scrotum, and so on. | Microfilaria circulate at night → adult worms → lymphedema

    (3) Laboratory diagnosis
      (a) Pronounced peripheral blood eosinophilia | Eosinophilia
      (b) Detect microfilaria in the blood at night; sheathed with nuclei that extend to the tail but *not* to the very tip of the tail (Link 14-8) | Microfilaria in blood at night
      (c) Indirect fluorescence (IF) and enzyme-linked immunosorbent assay (ELISA) detect antibodies in more than 95% of active cases and 70% of established cases. In addition, highly sensitive immunochromatographic card tests for circulating *Wucheria* antigen are available for immediate diagnosis. | ELISA, IF

  5. Sinus histiocytosis | Sinus histiocytosis
    a. **Definition:** Benign histicytic response that occurs in the sinuses of lymph nodes. Although nonspecific, this type of reactive change is commonly seen in lymph nodes that are draining a tumor. | Histiocytes nodal sinuses draining tumors
    b. Favorable sign in the axillary lymph nodes in breast cancer | Good prognostic sign in breast cancer

II. Non-Hodgkin's lymphoma (NHL; Table 14-1)
  A. Definition: Group of malignancies arising from cells of lymphocytic or histicytic origin and thus typically originate within lymphoid tissue in which most often appear (e.g., lymph nodes, tonsils, thymus, or Peyer patches) | Malignancy lymphoproliferative system

  B. Epidemiology
    1. Accounts for ~60% of adult lymphomas
- Greater than 80% are of B-cell origin and derive from the germinal follicle. | Majority B-cell origin
    2. Second most common cancer in AIDS | 2nd MC cancer AIDS
    3. Median age in adults is 65 to 70 years old. | 65–70 yrs old
    4. Slight male predominance | Slight male predominance
    5. Approximately one-third arise from extranodal sites. | One-third extranodal sites
      a. Extranodal sites include the stomach (most common), Peyer patches, anterior mediastinum (Link 14-9), and central nervous system (CNS; particularly in AIDS). | Stomach (MC), CNS, Peyer patches

TABLE 14-1 Common Types of B-Cell Non-Hodgkin Lymphoma

TYPE	EPIDEMIOLOGY	DESCRIPTION/IMMUNO-PHENOTYPE	CLINICAL FINDINGS
Burkitt lymphoma (see Fig. 14-8A and B; Link 14-11)	• 30% of children with NHL	• EBV relationship with t(8;14) "starry sky" appearance with neoplastic B cells (dark of night) and reactive histiocytes with phagocytic debris (stars)	• *American type:* GI tract, para-aortic nodes • *African type:* jaw • BM involvement • Leukemic phase common
Diffuse large B-cell lymphoma	• 50% of adults with NHL • Older adult and childhood populations	• Derives from the germinal center	• Localized disease with extranodal involvement: GI tract, brain (EBV association with AIDS)
Extranodal marginal zone lymphoma of MALT type	• 7.6% of lymphomas • Association with *Helicobacter pylori* gastritis	• Derives from MALT	• Low-grade malignant lymphoma of the stomach
Follicular lymphoma (Fig. 14-9, Link 14-12)	• 22% of adults with NHL • Older adults	• Derives from germinal center t(14;18), causing overexpression of *BCL-2* anti-apoptosis gene	• Generalized lymphadenopathy • BM involvement
Small lymphocytic lymphoma (SLL)	• 6.7% of lymphomas • Patients usually >60 yr of age	• Neoplasm of small, mature B lymphocytes • Deletion 13q14 • SLL if confined to lymph nodes • CLL if leukemic phase is present	• Generalized lymphadenopathy

BM, Bone marrow; *CLL,* Chronic lymphocytic leukemia; *EBV,* Epstein-Barr virus; *GI,* gastrointestinal; *MALT,* mucosa-associated lymphoid tissue; *NHL,* non-Hodgkin lymphoma.

Anterior mediastinum: SVC

Firm, fused together; "fish flesh" appearance

Low-grade/high-grade lymphomas

b. Anterior mediastinal sites can be associated with the superior vena caval syndrome (SVC; see Chapter 10).
6. Lymph nodes have a firm consistency and are fused together (Link 14-10). On cut section, they have a "fish flesh" appearance.
7. Classified into low- (indolent) and high-grade (aggressive) lymphomas
   a. Low-grade lymphomas include follicular lymphoma (grades 1 and 2), chronic lymphocytic leukemia (CLL), small lymphocytic leukemia (SLL), and most skin lymphomas.
   b. High-grade lymphomas include follicular lymphomas (grade 3B), diffuse large-cell lymphoma, mediastinal large B-cell lymphoma, peripheral T-cell lymphoma, mantle cell lymphoma, Burkitt lymphoma, and acute lymphoblastic lymphoma/leukemia.

Diffuse large cell lymphoma MC NHL

Childhood NHL

   c. Diffuse large-cell lymphoma is the overall most common type of NHL (30% of cases). The second most common type is follicular lymphoma (25% of cases).
8. Childhood NHL
   a. Peak age is 5 to 15 years.

Burkitt/SNCL MC 5-14

DLCL MC 15-19

NHL more aggressive children than adults

Abdomen MC site

   b. Whereas Burkitt and small, noncleaved cell lymphoma (SNCL) predominate among those in the 5- to 14-year-old age group, diffuse large-cell lymphomas (DLCLs) are more common among those 15 to 19 years of age.
   c. Generally more aggressive in children than adults
   d. As opposed to adults, most NHL that arises in childhood occur in extranodal sites (abdomen > mediastinal > outside head and neck region > Waldeyer ring, tonsils, or cervical > skin) and other sites.

The structures composing **Waldeyer ring** include the nasopharyngeal tonsils, lateral bands on the lateral walls of the oropharynx, and the lingual tonsils at the base of the tongue.

Waldeyer ring

Immunodeficiency syndromes

AIDS, immunosuppressive RX, viruses

EBV

   e. Associated with congenital immunodeficiency syndromes (see Chapter 4): Wiskott-Aldrich syndrome, ataxia-telangiectasia, X-linked lymphoproliferative syndrome, severe combined immunodeficiency, X-linked agammaglobulinemia, severe combined immunodeficiency, and Chediak-Higashi syndrome
   f. Other associations include AIDS, immunosuppressive therapy, and various viruses (see 9.a).
9. Risk factors include:
   a. viruses.
      (1) Epstein-Barr virus (EBV)

(a) Burkitt lymphoma
(b) Diffuse large B-cell lymphoma
(c) Primary CNS lymphoma (HIV)
  • Associated with AIDS
(2) Human T-cell lymphotropic virus (HTLV) type I
  • Adult T-cell lymphoma or leukemia
(3) Hepatitis C virus (HCV)
  • B-cell lymphoma
  b. *Helicobacter pylori.*
(1) Produces malignant lymphoma of the stomach (see Chapter 18)
  • Derives from mucosa-associated lymphoid tissue (MALT) in the stomach
(2) Treatment of peptic ulcer disease caused by *H. pylori* reduces the risk for developing this lymphoma.
  c. autoimmune disease.
(1) Sjögren syndrome
  • Salivary gland and gastrointestinal (GI) lymphomas
(2) Hashimoto thyroiditis
  • Malignant lymphoma arising within the thyroid gland
  d. immunodeficiency syndromes.
  • Chromosome instability syndromes (e.g., Bloom syndrome), AIDS
  e. immunosuppressive therapy that is used to prevent rejection in organ or bone marrow (BM) transplant patients.
  f. high-dose radiation that is used in the treatment of HL.
  g. chemical exposure (pesticides).
C. **Pathogenesis**
  1. Mutation produces a block at a specific stage in the development of B or T cells.
  2. Example of NHL is a follicular lymphoma with an accumulation of small cleaved B cells.
D. **B-cell lymphomas** (see Table 14-1; Fig. 14-8)
E. **T-cell lymphomas**
  1. Precursor T-cell lymphoblastic leukemia/lymphoma
  a. Accounts for 40% of childhood lymphomas
(1) Primarily involves the anterior mediastinal and cervical nodes
(2) BM and CNS involvement are common.
  b. Precursor T-cell lymphoblastic leukemia
  • Leukemic variant of T-cell lymphomas
  2. Mycosis fungoides (MV)
  a. **Definition:** Most common form of cutaneous T-cell lymphoma. It is characterized by infiltration of the skin by neoplastic CD4+ helper T (TH) cells.
  b. Epidemiology
  • Usually occur in adults 40 to 60 years of age
  c. Clinical findings
(1) Begins in the skin (rash to plaque to nodular masses)
  • Metastasizes to the lymph nodes, lung, liver, and spleen
(2) Groups of neoplastic cells that invade the epidermis are called Pautrier microabscesses (Link 14-13).
  d. Sézary syndrome
(1) Refers to the leukemic phase of mycosis fungoides
(2) Circulating malignant T cells are called Sézary cells.
F. **Tumor lysis syndrome**
  • **Definition:** Complication of NHL characterized by rapid cell breakdown leading to hyperuricemia, hyperkalemia, hyperphosphatemia, hypocalcemia, and acute renal failure (ARF)
G. **Survival statistics for NHL**
  • Survival rate varies with the type of NHL.
III. **Hodgkin lymphoma** (HL; Table 14-2)
A. **Definition:** A malignant lymphoma arising from germinal center B cells. It is characterized by the presence of multinucleated giant cells called Reed-Sternberg (RS) within a mixed inflammatory infiltrate.
B. **Epidemiology**
  1. Accounts for ~40% of adult lymphomas
  2. Age and sex differences in HL

Burkitt lymphoma

Diffuse large B-cell lymphoma

1° CNS lymphoma (HIV)

HTLV-I

Adult T-cell leukemia/ lymphoma

HCV: B-cell lymphoma

Low-grade malignant lymphoma stomach

Autoimmune disease

Sjögren syndrome

Salivary gland/GI lymphomas

Hashimoto thyroiditis → malignant lymphoma

Chromosome instability syndromes, AIDs

Immunosuppressive Rx

High-dose radiation

Pesticides

Mutation blocks B/T cells at specific stage of development

B-cell lymphomas

T-cell lymphomas

Common in children

Anterior mediastinum/ cervical nodes

BM/CNS commonly involved

Leukemic variant T-cell lymphoma

Mycosis fungiodes

Cutaneous CD4+ helper T (TH) cell lymphoma

Adults 40 to 60 years of age

Begins in skin

Metastasis nodes, lung, liver, spleen

Pautrier microabscesses (malignant T cells) in skin

Leukemic phase; Sézary cells (malignant T cells)

Tumor lysis syndrome

Complication NHL

↑Serum uric acid, K, phosphate; ↓calcium; ARF

~40% Adult lymphomas

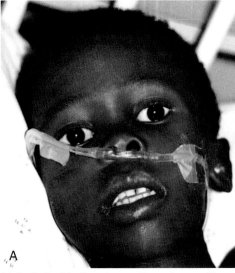

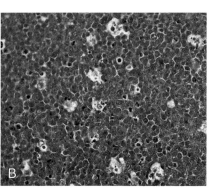

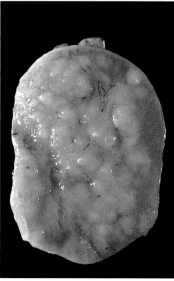

14-8: **A,** Burkitt lymphoma. Note the swelling of the jaw, a very characteristic location for this type of malignant lymphoma. **B,** Lymph node biopsy in Burkitt lymphoma. The lymph node is completely effaced with a monomorphic infiltrate of lymphocytes. Interspersed are clear spaces with reactive histiocytes containing phagocytic debris. At low power, the node has a "starry sky" appearance, with the stars represented by the reactive histiocytes. This type of lymphoma is associated with a t(8;14) translocation. *(A from Hoffbrand I, Pettit J, Vyas P: Color Atlas of Clinical Hematology, 4th ed, St. Louis, Mosby Elsevier, 2010, p 358, Fig. 19-82; B from Rosai J, Ackerman LV: Surgical Pathology, 9th ed, St. Louis, Mosby, 2004, p 1955, Fig. 21-103.)*

14-9: Follicular lymphoma. The neoplastic follicles bulge on the surface. *(From Rosai J. Rosai and Ackerman's Surgical Pathology, 10th ed, St. Louis, Mosby Elsevier, 2011, p 1825, Fig. 21.71. Courtesy of Dr. RA Cooke, Brisbane Australia, from Cooke RA, Stewar B: Colour Atlas of Anatomical Pathology. Edinburgh, Churchill Livingstone, 2004.)*

Males > females

Nodular sclerosing female dominant

Adults > children

Whites > blacks

Bimodal age distribution

15–34 years old

>50 years old

Younger age bracket than NHL

EBV association: e.g., mixed cellularity HL

HIV

Smokers

Defects in CMI; anergy

Lymphocyte rich classical

Nodular sclerosing classic (MC type)

Mixed cellularity classical

Lymphocyte depleted classical

Nodular lymphocyte predominant

Genetic susceptibility (children)

Activated NF-κB important in HL pathogenesis

Localized groups nodes; contiguous spread

a. More common in males (particularly in childhood) than females
   - *Exception*: Nodular sclerosing type is more common in females.
b. More common in adults than children
c. More common in whites than blacks
3. Bimodal age distribution in HL
   a. First large peak is 15 to 34 years old.
   b. Second smaller peak is >50 years old.
   c. Overall, tends to occur at younger ages than NHL
4. Most common site of initial involvement is the neck region.
5. EBV has been identified in certain types of HL (e.g., 60%–70% of cases of mixed cellularity HL).
6. Those infected with HIV infections have a higher incidence of HL relative to an uninfected population.
7. Increased risk in smokers
8. Defects may occur in cell-mediated immunity (CMI) in HL.
   - Example: defects in skin reactions to injection of common antigens (anergy; see Chapter 4)
9. Classification (see Table 14-2; Fig. 14-9)
   a. Lymphocyte rich classical
   b. Nodular sclerosing classical (most common type)
   c. Mixed cellularity classical
   d. Lymphocyte depleted classical
   e. Nodular lymphocyte predominant

C. Pathogenesis
1. Genetic susceptibility underlies HL in children.
2. Activation of the transcription factor NF-κB (nuclear factor kappa-light-chain-enhancer of activated B cells) is common in classical HL.
   a. NF-κB is activated by EBV or other factors.
   b. When activated, it turns on genes that promote proliferation of B cells.

D. Pathologic findings
1. Involves localized groups of nodes and has contiguous spread to other lymph node groups (Links 14-14 and 14-15)

TABLE 14-2   Types of Hodgkin Lymphoma (HL)

TYPE	EPIDEMIOLOGY AND CLINICAL FINDINGS	HISTOLOGIC FINDINGS
Lymphocyte-rich classical HL	• Accounts for 5% of cases • EBV association 40% of cases • Males greater than females • Older adults • Very good to excellent prognosis	• Classic RS cells are present • Reactive lymphocytes often completely efface the lymph node architecture
Nodular sclerosis classical HL (Fig. 14-10 B)	• Accounts for 70% of cases • Equal frequency in young adult men and women • EBV association infrequent • Usually involves anterior mediastinal nodes (seen on chest radiography) and either cervical or supraclavicular nodes • Excellent prognosis	• Classic RS cells infrequent • Lacunar type RS cells (called RS variants) present: monolobulated or multilobated nucleus, small nucleolus, abundant pale cytoplasm • Collagen separates nodular areas
Mixed cellularity classical HL	• Accounts for 20% of cases • Men >55 yr of age • EBV association (60%–70% of cases) • Type that most commonly occurs in HIV-positive patients (all are EBV positive) • Commonly affects abdominal lymph nodes and spleen • Advanced stage-disease and systemic signs are usually present • Overall prognosis is good	• Numerous classic RS cells • ↑Eosinophils, plasma cells, histiocytes
Lymphocyte-depleted classical HL	• Least common HL (<1% of cases) • Men >50 yr of age • EBV association, especially if associated with HIV-positive individuals • Most aggressive HL • Poorest survival statistics; usually present with advanced-stage disease	• RS cells are frequently present, some of which have bizarre features
Nodular lymphocyte–predominant HL	• "Nonclassical" type of HL • Accounts for 5% of cases • ~75% are male with one peak in children and the other with a median age of 30 to 40 yr • Good prognosis	• Classical RS cells infrequent • L&H cells or "popcorn" cells (nuclei resemble an exploded kernel of corn) are present; these cells are positive for B-cell antigens (CD19 and CD20) but are negative for CD15 and CD30

EBV, Epstein-Barr virus; *HL,* Hodgkin lymphoma; *L&H,* lymphocytic and histiocytic; *RS,* Reed-Sternberg.

    a. Most frequently involves cervical, supraclavicular, and anterior mediastinal lymph nodes. A mediastinal mass in a young person is most often HL.

    b. Cut section of involved lymph nodes has a bulging "fish-flesh" appearance.

  2. RS cell is present.

    a. RS cell is the neoplastic cell of HL.

      (1) Positive for CD15 and CD30

      (2) Most (not all) RS cell cells are of B-cell origin and are derived from lymph node germinal centers.

    b. Classic RS cell

      • Two mirror image nuclei, each with an eosinophilic nucleolus surrounded by a clear halo (Fig. 14-10 A; Links 14-16 to 14-18)

    c. RS variant: lacunar cell

      (1) *Not* a "classical" RS cell

      (2) Lacunar cells are nonlobulated or multinucleated cells with small nucleoli and abundant, pale cytoplasm.

      (3) Cell lies in a clear space, which is an artifact of fixation in formalin-fixed tissue.

      (4) Present in the nodular sclerosis type of HL (Fig. 14-10 B)

  3. Diagnosis

    • Presence of a classic RS cell is required to secure the diagnosis.

  4. Differences from NHL

    • HL less commonly involves Waldeyer tonsillar ring, mesenteric lymph nodes, and extranodal sites than NHL.

E. Clinical findings and prognosis

  1. Constitutional signs include:

    a. fever, unexplained weight loss, and night sweats (40% of cases).

    b. pruritus (itchy skin).

    c. Pel-Ebstein fever, an uncommon variant of fever.

      • Characterized by alternating bouts of fever followed by remissions

Margin notes:
Mediastinal mass young person MC HL
"Fish-flesh" appearance
RS cell neoplastic cell of HL
+CD15, +CD30
RS cell B cell origin (most cases)
Mirror image nuclei, eos nucleoli, clear halo
RS variant: lacunar cell
Not classical RS cell
Lacunar cell clear space
Nodular sclerosing HD
RS cell required to diagnose HL
HL: Waldeyer ring, mesenteric/extranodal sites
Fever, weight loss, night sweats
Pruritus
Pel-Ebstein fever
Alternating fever with remissions

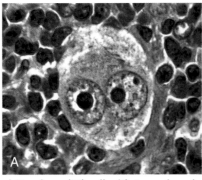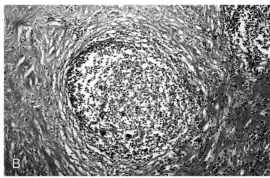

14-10: **A,** Classic Reed-Sternberg (RS) cell with two mirror image nuclei, each with reddish-purple nucleolus surrounded by a pale halo. **B,** Nodular-sclerosis classical Hodgkin lymphoma. The lymphoid nodule is encased by fibrous tissue. Note the clear spaces in the nodule within which are RS variants called lacunar cells (cytoplasm shrinks during formalin fixation). *(A from Rosai J: Rosai and Ackerman's Surgical Pathology, 10th ed, St. Louis, Mosby Elsevier, 2011, p 1808, Fig. 21.51. Courtesy of Dr. Fabio Facchetti, Brescia, Italy. B, from Rosai J, Ackerman LV: Surgical Pathology, 9th ed, St. Louis, Mosby, 2004, p 1924, Fig. 21-56.)*

2. Hematologic findings include:
    a. normocytic anemia (presenting symptom 40% of cases).
        - Anemia of chronic disease, immune hemolytic anemia
    b. painless enlargement of single groups of lymph nodes in the neck region.
        - Nodes become painful if the patient drinks alcohol.
3. Chest pain, cough, and dyspnea usually indicate the presence of a large mediastinal mass or metastasis to the lungs.
4. Primary factors that determine the prognosis.
    a. Clinical stage is more important than the type of HL.
    b. Majority have lymphadenopathy above the diaphragm (stages I and II), which correlates with an excellent prognosis.
5. Increased risk for developing second malignancies, usually acute myeloblastic leukemia (AML) or NHL.
    a. ↑Risk 2nd malignancies (AML, NHL)
    b. Increased risk is related to treatment with radiation and alkylating agents.

F. Prognosis and treatment
1. Majority are curable. Poor prognosis correlates with age >45 years, male gender, high stage, large mediastinal mass, and abnormal complete blood count (anemia, lymphopenia).
2. Radiotherapy and chemotherapy are used depending on the stage of the disease (Link 14-19).

IV. Histiocytosis Syndromes (Langerhans' Cell Histiocytosis [LCH])
A. Definition: Group of disorders characterized by infiltration and proliferation of cells of monocyte-MP or dendritic cell lineage. LCH (replacement term for histiocytosis X) is a multifaceted disorder that presents with isolated bone lesions (old term, *eosinophilic granuloma*), bone lesions with diabetes insipidus and exophthalmos (old term, *Hand-Schuller-Christian disease*), or bone lesions with disseminated disease (old term, *Letterer-Siwe disease*). Each will be discussed separately, with the understanding that they are now all part of LCH.
B. Epidemiology
1. Characteristics
    a. Histiocytes are CD1 positive and contain Birbeck granules (tennis racket appearance; Fig. 14-11 A).
    b. Birbeck granules are only visible with electron microscopy (EM).
2. Primarily occurs in children and young adults
C. Letterer-Siwe disease
1. Epidemiology
    - Malignant histiocytosis that usually occurs in children that are <2 years of age
2. Clinical findings
    a. Diffuse eczematous rash (Fig. 14-11 B)
    b. Multiple organs are involved.
    c. Lytic lesions occur in the skull, pelvis, and long bones.
3. Rapidly fatal
D. Hand-Schüller-Christian (HSC) disease
1. Epidemiology

Margin notes

Normocytic anemia

Painless lymph nodes neck region

Painful if alcohol ingested

Clinical stage > type HL

Majority nodes above diaphragm

↑Risk from Rx (radiation, chemo)

Majority curable

Histiocytosis syndromes

Monocyte/MP on dendritic cell origin

Histiocytes: CD1+; Birbeck granules (EM)

Letterer-Siwe disease

Children <2 years old

Diffuse eczematous rash

Multiple organ involvement

Lytic lesions skull, pelvis, long bones

Rapidly fatal

HSC disease

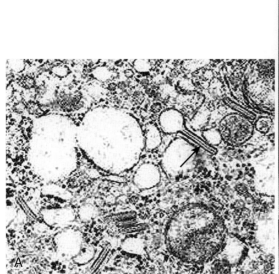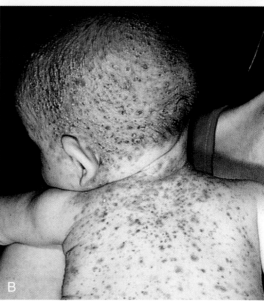

14-11: **A,** Electron micrograph showing racket-shaped Birbeck granules in a histiocyte. **B,** Child with Letterer-Siwe disease (Langerhans histiocytosis). Note the eczematous type rash over the body surface caused by malignant histiocytes infiltrating the skin and dermis. (*A courtesy William Meek, professor and vice chairman of Anatomy and Cell Biology, Oklahoma State University, Center for Health Sciences, Tulsa, OK; B from Kumar V, Fausto N, Abbas A:* Robbins and Cotran Pathologic Basis of Disease, *7th ed, Philadelphia, Saunders, 2004, p 1249, Fig. 25-18A.)*

a. Malignant histiocytosis — Malignant histiocytosis of children
b. Mainly affects children

2. Clinical findings
  a. General findings include:
    (1) fever. — Scalp, ear canals
    (2) localized rash on the scalp and in the ear canals. — Fever, localized rash
  b. Classic triad caused by infiltrative disease includes:
    (1) lytic lesions present in the skull and other sites (Link 14-20). — Lytic lesions skull, other sites
    (2) central diabetes insipidus (CDI) caused by invasion of the posterior pituitary stalk. — CDI
    (3) exophthalmos (bulging of eye) from infiltration of the orbit. — Exophthalmos
3. Intermediate prognosis

E. **Eosinophilic granuloma** — Eosinophilic granuloma
  1. Epidemiology
    a. Benign histiocytosis — Benign histiocytosis
    b. Occurs in adolescents and young adults — Adolescents, young adults
  2. Clinical findings
    a. Unifocal lytic lesions are present in the bone (skull, ribs, and femur) (Link 14-21). — Unifocal lytic lesions
    b. Bone pain and pathologic fractures are common. — Bone pain/fractures
  3. Prognosis is excellent.

V. **Mast Cell Disorders (Mastocytosis)** — Mast cell disorder
  A. **Definition:** Disorders that can occur in both children and adults. Increased numbers of mast cells can be present in the skin, lymph nodes, and internal organs (e.g., liver and spleen) and in the linings of the lung, stomach, and intestine — ↑Mast cells multiple locations
  B. **Overview of mast cell disorders**
    1. Epidemiology
      • Localized (urticaria pigmentosa and solitary mastocytoma) or systemic — Localized, systemic
    2. Mast cell release of histamine produces pruritus and swelling of tissue — Pruritus, swelling of tissue
  C. **Urticaria pigmentosa** — Urticaria pigmentosa
    1. Epidemiology
      a. Majority of persons with urticaria pigmentosa are children. — Majority are children
        • Urticaria pigmentosa resolves spontaneously.
      b. In adolescents and adults, urticaria pigmentosa is more likely to persist.
    2. Skin lesions
      a. Known as "freckles and hives" because of the appearance before and after scratching — "Freckles and hives"
      b. Multiple oval, red-brown, nonscaling macules (flat lesions) or papules are present. — Oval, red-brown, macules/papules

Scratching → erythema, swelling, pruritus

Darier sign

Dermatographism

Lesions remain hyperpigmented

Mast cells with metachromatic granules

Triggers: food, alcohol, drugs

Abdominal pain/diarrhea

Headaches with flushing

Anaphylactic reaction

↑Serum tryptase

Plasma cell dyscrasias

Monoclonal B-cell disorders; single M protein + light chain

Majority have IgG M protein: others suppressed

BJ protein

Free κ or λ light chains excreted in urine

Plasma cell malignancies, WM

SPE

Shows spike/quantitates M protein

Does *not* specify which M protein

Immunofixation

Characterizes M protein

Urine: Does *not* quantitate M protein

Identifies BJ protein

Does *not* specify κ or λ

Urine immunofixation

BJ protein κ or λ

Serum light chains

Detects, quantitates κ and λ

More sensitive than urine tests

MGUS

MM

Light chain

Solitary plasmocytosis

WM

HCD

c. Scratching of the lesions results in erythematous swelling and pruritus.
- Called the Darier sign
d. Dermatographism
- Dermal edema occurs when apparently normal skin is stroked with a pointed object.
e. Lesions remain hyperpigmented when they regress.
f. Skin biopsy shows mast cells with metachromatic granules that stain positive with toluidine blue and Giemsa stain.
3. Pruritus and flushing are triggered by foods, alcohol, or drugs (e.g., codeine).
4. Other findings include:
a. abdominal pain with diarrhea.
b. headaches with flushing of the skin.
c. anaphylactic reactions if envenomated by a bee, hornet, or wasp.
d. increased serum tryptase.

VI. **Plasma Cell Dyscrasias (Monoclonal Gammopathies [MGs])**
   A. **Overview of MGs (plasma cell dyscrasias)**
      1. **Definition:** Refers to a monoclonal B-cell disorder that is caused by an increase in a single immunoglobulin (M protein) and its corresponding light chain
      2. Epidemiology and clinical significance
         a. Majority of MGs are caused by an increase in IgG.
            - All other plasma cell clones are immunologically suppressed.
         b. Bence Jones (BJ) protein
            (1) **Definition:** Free κ or λ light chains that are excreted in urine
            (2) Associated with plasma cell malignancies and Waldenström macroglobulinemia (WM)
      3. Tests used to detect an MG
         a. Serum protein electrophoresis (SPE; see Chapter 3)
            (1) Useful in quantitating the M protein and shows a monoclonal spike (M protein; Fig. 14-12)
            (2) Does *not* specify which M protein is increased (e.g., IgG, IgA, IgM)
         b. Serum immunofixation electrophoresis
            (1) More sensitive than SPE and provides a characterization of the M protein (heavy and light chain subclass; e.g., IgGκ or IgGλ; IgMκ or IgMλ)
            (2) Does *not* quantitate the M protein
         c. Urine protein electrophoresis
            (1) Identifies BJ protein (free light chains) and quantitates the amount of light chains in the urine
            (2) Does *not* specify whether the light chains are κ or λ
         d. Urine immunofixation electrophoresis
            (1) Characterizes whether BJ protein is κ or λ
            (2) More sensitive in detecting BJ protein than the standard urine protein electrophoresis
         e. Serum for free light chains
            (1) Detects and quantitates κ and λ light chains in the serum
            (2) More sensitive for detecting light chains than any of the urine methodologies listed earlier
      4. Classification of MGs include: (Table 14-3)
         a. monoclonal gammopathy of undetermined significance (MGUS).
         b. multiple myeloma (MM).
         c. light chain amyloidosis.
         d. solitary plasmacytoma.
         e. WM.
         f. heavy chain disease (HCD).

14-12: Serum protein electrophoresis showing a schematic of a monoclonal gammopathy. *(From Goljan EF, Sloka KI: Rapid Review Laboratory Testing in Clinical Medicine, Philadelphia, Mosby Elsevier, 2008, p 284, Fig. 9-1C.)*

TABLE 14-3 Additional Plasma Cell Dyscrasias

TYPE	DISCUSSION
Monoclonal gammopathy of undetermined significance (MGUS)	• Most common monoclonal gammopathy (50%–65% of all monoclonal gammopathies) • MGUS is found in ~3% of individuals aged 50 yr • Small IgG M-spike in older adult patients (serum M protein ≤3 g/dL) • Plasma cells ≤10% in bone marrow • *No* serum or urine BJ protein or CRAB • 1% lifelong risk per year of progression to MM • *No* end-organ damage
Solitary skeletal plasmacytoma	• Accounts for 3%–5% of all monoclonal gammopathies • Twice as common in women • Single lytic lesion with clonal plasma cells in the following bone sites: vertebrae, ribs, pelvis • Small or no serum and urine M protein • Bone marrow is *not* consistent with MM • Normal skeletal survey • *No* end-organ damage • ~50% progress to MM over 4 to 5 yr
Extramedullary plasmacytoma	• Sites: upper respiratory tract (nasopharynx, sinuses, larynx) • Small or no serum and urine M protein • *No* malignant plasma cells in the bone marrow • Normal skeletal survey • *No* end-organ damage • Small percentage may develop MM
Lymphoplasmacytic lymphoma (Waldenström macroglobulinemia)	• Indolent B-cell lymphoplasmacytic lymphoma characterized by lymphoplasmacytic infiltration in the bone marrow or lymphatic tissue; M spike is caused by IgM • Primarily older mens (median age, 65 yr) • Main risk factor is MGUS • BJ protein is present (80% of cases) • Generalized lymphadenopathy (~30% of cases; *not* present in myeloma) • Anemia and bone marrow (no lytic lesions like myeloma), liver, and spleen involvement (hepatosplenomegaly; *not* common in myeloma) • Hyperviscosity syndrome caused by increased IgM: retinal hemorrhages, strokes, platelet aggregation defects; plasmapheresis important to remove IgM • Unlike MM, renal disease and amyloidosis are rare • Poor response to therapy • Median survival is 5 years. • Patients with a malignant lymphoma associated with an IgM M-spike but who do *not* meet the diagnostic criteria for Waldenström macroglobulinemia (<3 g M-spike) are classified as having lymphoplasmacytic lymphoma with an IgM M protein
Heavy-chain diseases	• M protein heavy chain *without* light chains • Absence of BJ protein • α-Heavy-chain disease: neoplastic infiltration of the jejunum, leading to malabsorption or localized upper respiratory tract disease • γ-Heavy-chain disease: presents as a lymphoma • μ-Heavy-chain disease: often associated with chronic lymphocytic leukemia or lymphoma
POEMS syndrome	• Paraneoplastic syndrome including **p**olyneuropathy, **o**rganomegaly, **e**ndocrinopathy, **m**onoclonal gammopathy, and **s**kin changes

BJ, Bence Jones; *CRAB,* calcium elevation, renal insufficiency, anemia, and bone lesions; *MM,* multiple myeloma.

B. **Multiple myeloma (MM)** (Links 14-22 to 14-25)

  1. **Definition:** Characterized by a clonal proliferation of malignant plasma cells in the BM and associated with a monoclonal protein in the bowel and urine

  2. Epidemiology

    a. Accounts for 10% of all hematologic malignancies

    b. Second most common hematologic malignancy

    c. Two times more common in blacks than whites

    d. Median age at onset is 68 years.

      • Rare before 40 years of age

    e. Male predominance

    f. Increased risk for developing MM if there is a history of radiation or benzene exposure

    g. M-spike in a SPE occurs in 80% to 90% of cases (Link 14-26).

      (1) IgGκ myeloma accounts for 70% of cases followed by IgA (20% of cases) and pure light chain myeloma (5%–10% of cases).

        • Serum M protein is >3g/dL.

      (2) Urinalysis for BJ protein is positive in 60% to 80% of cases.

Margin notes:

Multiple myeloma

Clonal proliferation malignant plasma cells in BM

2nd MC hematologic malignancy

Blacks > whites

Median age 68 years

Male predominance

Radiation, benzene exposure

M spike SPE 80%-90%

IgGκ MC type

IgG > IgA > light chain myeloma

Urine BJ + most cases

h. Evidence of end-organ damage in MM includes **c**alcium elevation (>11.5 mg/dL), **r**enal insufficiency (creatinine >2 mg/dL), **a**nemia (hemoglobin <10 g/dL), and **b**one lesions (osteopenia or lytic lesions). Mnemonic CRAB.
  i. Nonsecretory MM
    (1) Accounts for <2% of all cases
    (2) Absence of serum or urine M protein
    (3) BM plasma cells are >10%.
    (4) CRAB is present.
3. Pathogenesis
  a. Chromosome abnormalities (deletions, translocations) are present.
    • Detected with fluorescence in-situ hybridization (FISH) and have prognostic significance for detecting high-risk patients
  b. Possible evolution from normal plasma cells → MGUS → MM
4. Histologic findings
  a. Sheets of malignant plasma cells are present in a bone marrow aspirate or biopsy (Fig. 14-13 A; Link 14-27).
  b. Malignant plasma cells account for ≥10% of cells in the aspirate.
5. Skeletal system findings
  a. Bone pain occurs in ~60% of cases of MM.
    (1) "Punched-out" lytic lesions occur in the bone (Fig. 14-13 B and C).
      (a) Myeloma cells produce an inhibitor of osteoblast differentiation (DKK1).
      (b) Myeloma cells release interleukin-1 (IL-1; osteoclast activating factor), which activates osteoclasts.
    (2) Vertebrae are the most common sites of bone involvement.
    (3) Other sites include the ribs, skull, femur, and pelvis.
    (4) Pain commonly presents with pathologic fractures, particularly if rib lesions are present.
  b. Hypercalcemia (>11.5 mg/dL) is present in 25% of cases.
6. Renal findings
  a. Renal failure occurs in 50% of cases.
  b. Different renal presentations include:
    (1) proteinaceous tubular casts.
      (a) Casts are composed of BJ protein.
      (b) BJ protein is nephrotoxic and damages tubular epithelium.
      (c) Biopsy reveals an intratubular multinucleated giant cell reaction.

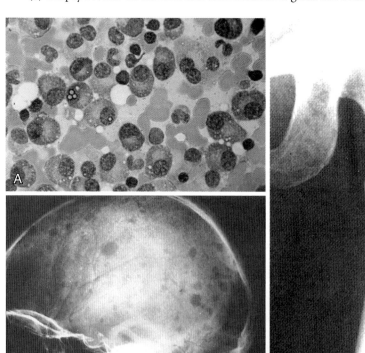

14-13: **A,** Malignant plasma cells in multiple myeloma (MM). The majority of malignant plasma cells show a dark blue cytoplasm, peripherally located nuclei, and perinuclear clearing. Occasional cells have vacuoles containing immunoglobulin. **B,** Radiograph of a skull showing multiple "punched-out" lytic lesions in MM. **C,** Multiple lytic lesions in the femur and pelvis in MM. (*A from Goldman L, Ausiello D: Cecil's Textbook of Medicine, 23rd ed, Philadelphia, Saunders Elsevier, 2008, p 1430, Fig. 198-4; B from my friend Ivan Damjanov, MD, PhD, Linder J: Anderson's Pathology, 10th ed, St. Louis, Mosby, 1996, p 1105, Fig. 41-61; C from Doherty M, George E: Self-Assessment Picture Tests in Medicine: Rheumatology, London, Mosby-Wolfe, 1995, p 7, Fig. 4.*)

(2) nephrocalcinosis.
    (a) Hypercalcemia leads to metastatic calcification of the tubular basement membranes in the collecting ducts (see Chapter 2).
    (b) Calcium deposits are a common cause of ARF in MM.
  (3) metastatic disease to interstitial tissue.
  (4) primary amyloidosis (10% of cases).
    • Light chains are converted into amyloid and produce a nephrotic syndrome (see Chapters 4 and 20).
7. Hematologic findings include:
  a. normocytic anemia with rouleaux (see Fig. 3-21).
  b. markedly increased erythrocyte sedimentation rate (ESR) (see Chapter 3).
  c. prolonged bleeding time (BT; see Chapter 15).
    (1) Defect in platelet aggregation
    (2) Dialysis restores the BT to normal.
8. Radiculopathy may occur from vertebral bone compression and vertebral fractures.
9. Recurrent infection leading to sepsis in tissue (bacteria and toxins) is a common cause of death.
  • Sepsis is commonly caused by *Haemophilus influenzae* or *Streptococcus pneumoniae* infection.
10. Prognosis
  • Median survival time is 5 years after diagnosis.

C. Other plasma cell dyscrasias (see Table 14-3)

VII. Spleen Disorders

A. Clinical anatomy and physiology
1. Red pulp of spleen
  • Contains the cords of Billroth with fixed MPs and sinusoids
2. White pulp of spleen
  • Contains B and T cells
3. Important functions include:
  a. blood filtration; MPs remove:
    (1) hematopoietic elements (e.g., senescent red blood cells [RBCs]).
    (2) intraerythrocytic parasites (e.g., malaria).
    (3) encapsulated bacteria (e.g., *S. pneumoniae*).
  b. antigen trapping and processing in MPs.
  c. reservoir for one-third of the peripheral blood platelet pool.
  d. site for extramedullary hematopoiesis (EMH; see Chapter 12).

B. Splenomegaly
1. Basic mechanisms and causes of splenomegaly
  a. "Work hypertrophy" caused by increased immune response; examples include:
    • infectious mononucleosis, subacute bacterial endocarditis, and malaria.
  b. Congestion; examples include:
    • splenic vein thrombosis and PH.
  c. RBC destruction work hypertrophy; examples include:
    • hereditary spherocytosis, pyruvate kinase deficiency, and β-thalassemia major.
  d. myeloproliferative disease (MPD); examples include:
    • polycythemia vera (PV), myelofibrosis (MF), and essential thrombocythemia (ET).
  e. neoplastic disease; examples include:
    • acute and chronic leukemias and malignant lymphoma.
  f. infiltrative disease; examples include:
    (1) primary and secondary amyloidosis, sarcoidosis, Gaucher disease, and Niemann-Pick disease.
    (2) Gaucher disease.
      (a) Autosomal recessive lysosomal storage disease with a deficiency of glucocerebrosidase and lysosomal accumulation of glucocerebrosides
      (b) MPs have a fibrillary appearance (Fig. 14-14 A).
    (3) Niemann-Pick disease
      (a) Autosomal recessive lysosomal storage disease with a deficiency of sphingomyelinase and lysosomal accumulation of sphingomyelin
      (b) MPs have a soap bubble appearance (Fig. 14-14 B).
2. Clinical findings include:
  a. left upper quadrant (LUQ) pain.
    • Pain may be caused by splenic infarctions causing friction rubs and a left-sided pleural effusion (Link 14-28) or by stretching of the capsule by an enlarged spleen.

Margin notes:

Hypercalcemia → metastatic calcification

Metastasis

Primary (AL) amyloidosis

Normocytic anemia/rouleaux

↑ESR

↑BT; defect platelet aggregation

Dialysis removes defect

Vertebral bone compression → radiculopathy

Infection → sepsis

Sepsis common COD

MGUS: MC monoclonal gammopathy

Red pulp: fixed MPs

B and T cells

MPs remove → senescent RBCs, malaria parasites, encapsulated bacteria

Antigen trapping

Reservoir for platelets

Site for EMH

Immune response work hypertrophy

Congestion

RBC destruction

MPD: PV, MF, ET

Neoplastic disease: leukemia, lymphoma

Infiltrative disease

Gaucher disease: ↓Glucocerebrosidase, ↑glucocerebroside, MPs fibrillary appearance

Niemann-Pick disease: ↓Sphingomyelinase, ↑sphingomyelin, MPs soap bubble appearance

LUQ pain; splenic infarcts, pleural effusiona (left)

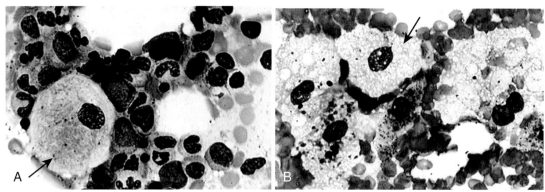

14-14: A, Gaucher disease. Note the fibrillary appearance of the cytoplasm in the macrophages *(arrow).* **B,** Niemann-Pick disease. Note the soap bubble appearance of the cytoplasm in the macrophages *(arrow). (A and B from Naeim F: Atlas of Bone Marrow and Blood Pathology, Philadelphia, Saunders, 2001, p 157, 159 respectively, Fig. 11-14B, 11-17B, respectively.)*

b. hypersplenism (see later discussion).

C. Spleen in portal hypertension (PH); increased portal vein pressure

Hypersplenism
Portal hypertension
Perisplenitis ("sugar-coated")

1. Gross findings
   • Spleen is covered by a thickened ("sugar-coated") capsule from perisplenitis.

Gamna-Gandy bodies: iron concretions in collagen

2. Microscopic findings
   • Calcium and iron concretions called Gamna-Gandy bodies are deposited in collagen.

Hypersplenism
Exaggeration normal function

D. Hypersplenism

1. **Definition:** An exaggerated state of splenic function
   • RBCs, white blood cells (WBCs), and platelets, either singly or in combination, are sequestered and destroyed.

Destruction RBCs, WBCs, platelets
MCC PH associated with cirrhosis

2. Most common cause is PH associated with cirrhosis of the liver (see Chapter 19).

Splenomegaly

3. Clinical findings include:
   a. splenomegaly.
   b. Peripheral blood cytopenias:

Peripheral blood cytopenias
Compensatory reactive BM hyperplasia

   • anemia, thrombocytopenia, and neutropenia, alone or in combination.
   c. compensatory reactive bone marrow hyperplasia.
   • Attempt by the marrow to replace lost hematopoietic cells.

Rx splenectomy

   d. correction of cytopenias with splenectomy.

Splenic dysfunction/ splenectomy

E. Splenic dysfunction and splenectomy

1. Signs of splenic dysfunction include:

HJ bodies nuclear remnants

   a. Howell-Jolly (HJ) bodies (nuclear remnants) in the peripheral blood RBCs (see Fig. 12-24 C).
   • With a functioning spleen, MPs would have removed RBCs with HJ bodies (nuclear remnants in RBCs).

Infection encapsulated pathogens
Streptococcus pneumoniae sepsis MC
Haemophilus/Salmonella/ Neisseria

   b. predisposition to infections by encapsulated pathogens.
   (1) Infections include septicemia, peritonitis, and osteomyelitis.
       (a) Pathogens include *S. pneumoniae* (most common), *Haemophilus influenzae, Salmonella* spp., and *Neisseria meningitidis.*
       (b) Immunization helps prevent infectious complications of splenic dysfunction.
   (2) Mechanisms causing infections by the pathogens just listed.

↓IgM synthesis → ↓C3b

       (a) Concentration of IgM drops, leading to a decrease in complement system activation (less C3b for opsonization).
           • Spleen is a site for IgM synthesis.

↓MP phagocytosis encapsulated pathogens
↓Tuftsin → ↓MP phagocytosis

       (b) Splenic MPs are *not* present in sufficient numbers to phagocytose the opsonized encapsulated pathogens.
       (c) Tuftsin, which is normally synthesized in the spleen, is lost.
           • Tuftsin activates receptors on MPs to increase their phagocytic activity.

Splenectomy
↑Risk for infection

2. Splenectomy
   a. Increases the risk for infections (see previous discussion)
   b. Hematologic findings include:

NRBCs
HJ bodies
Target cells
Thrombocytosis

   (1) nucleated RBCs (NRBCs).
   (2) HJ bodies.
   (3) target cells (excess membrane cannot be removed; Fig. 12-19).
   (4) thrombocytosis (increased platelet count in peripheral blood).
       • Platelets that would have been normally sequestered in the spleen are now circulating.

ABBREVIATIONS

MC most common   MCC most common cause

I. **Normal Hemostasis and Hemostasis Testing**
   A. **Definition** of hemostasis: Prevention of blood loss that requires the interaction of blood
      vessels, platelets, coagulation factors, and fibrinolytic agents
   B. **Factors preventing thrombus formation in small blood vessels**
      1. Small blood vessels include capillaries, venules, and arterioles.
      2. Thrombus formation is prevented by heparin-like molecules. Enhance antithrombin
         III (ATIII) activity, which neutralizes serine proteases, which include factors VII, IX,
         X, XI, and XII; thrombin (activated prothrombin).
      3. Prostaglandin (PG) I_2 (prostacyclin)
         a. Synthesized by intact endothelial cells (EC; see Chapter 3)
         b. PGH_2, the precursor PG, is converted by prostacyclin synthase to PGI_2.
            PGI_2 is a vasodilator (VD) and inhibits platelet aggregation.
      4. Proteins C and S
         a. Vitamin K–dependent coagulation factors
         b. Protein S acts a cofactor for protein C.
         c. Thrombin binds to thrombomodulin (TM) on the surface of ECs (Link 15-1).
            (1) Thrombin–TM complex activates protein C, which inhibits clotting by inactivating
                factors Va and VIIIa.
            (2) Demonstrates an *anticoagulant function* rather than a procoagulant function of
                thrombin
      5. Tissue plasminogen activator (tPA)
         a. Synthesized by ECs
         b. Activates plasminogen to release plasmin
         c. Plasmin degrades coagulation factors and lyses fibrin clots (thrombi).
   C. **Factors enhancing thrombus formation in small-vessel injury**
      1. Thromboxane A_2 (TXA_2)
         a. Synthesized by platelets
            (1) PGH_2 is converted into TXA_2 by TX synthase.
            (2) Aspirin *irreversibly* inhibits platelet (PLT) cyclooxygenase (COX; see Fig. 3-7).
                (a) Prevents the formation of PGH_2, the precursor for TXA_2
                (b) Platelets are functional 48 hours after discontinuing aspirin intake.
            (3) Other nonsteroidal antiinflammatory drugs (NSAIDs) *reversibly* inhibit platelet COX.
                Platelet function is restored 12 to 24 hours after discontinuing (DC) NSAIDs.
            (4) Prostacyclin synthase in ECs is minimally affected by NSAIDs.
         a. Functions of TXA_2 in hemostasis: vasoconstrictor (VC) and enhances platelet aggregation
      2. von Willebrand factor (vWF)
         a. Synthesized by ECs and megakaryocytes (MKCs) in the bone marrow (BM)
            (1) Synthesized in the Weibel-Palade bodies (WPBs) located in the ECs
            (2) Platelets carry some vWF in their α-granules (Fig. 15-1 A).

Prevention blood loss
Capillaries, venules,
arterioles
Thrombus prevention
Enhance ATIII activity
Neutralize activated serine
protease coagulation
factors
PGI_2 (prostacyclin)
Synthesized by ECs
PGH_2 converted to PGI_2
PGI_2: VD, inhibits platelet
aggregation
Proteins C/S
Vitamin K-dependent
Protein S cofactor for
protein C
Thrombin–TM complex
activates protein C →
inactivates Va/VIIIa
Anticoagulant function of
thrombin
tPA
Synthesized by ECs
Activates plasminogen to
release plasmin
Plasmin degrades
coagulation factors, lyses
fibrin clots
Factors enhancing thrombus
formation
TXA_2
Synthesized by platelets
PGH_2 converted to TXA_2: TX
synthase
Aspirin irreversibly inhibits
PLT COX
Prevents formation PGH_2
(precursor TXA_2)
Platelets functional 48 hrs
post discontinuing aspirin
NSAIDS reversibly inhibit
PLT COX

DC NSAIDs: plts function 12
to 24 hrs
Prostacyclin synthase ECs
minimally affected by
NSAIDS
TXA_2: VC; enhances platelet
aggregation
vWF
Synthesized by ECs/MKCs
(BM)
Synthesized in WPBs in ECs
vWF in PLT α-granules

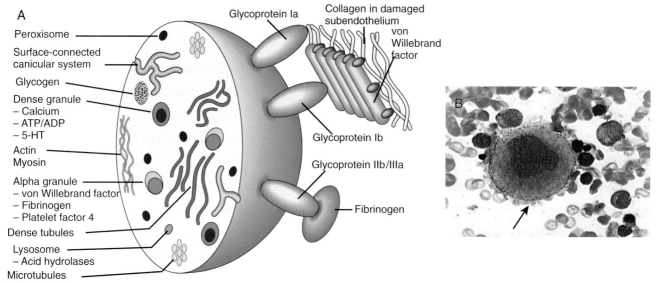

A

Peroxisome

Surface-connected
canicular system

Glycogen

Dense granule
– Calcium
– ATP/ADP
– 5-HT

Actin
Myosin

Alpha granule
– von Willebrand factor
– Fibrinogen
– Platelet factor 4

Dense tubules

Lysosome
– Acid hydrolases

Microtubules

Glycoprotein Ia

Collagen in damaged
subendothelium

von
Willebrand
factor

Glycoprotein Ib

Glycoprotein IIb/IIIa

Fibrinogen

B

15-1: **A,** Normal platelet structure. **B,** Megakaryocyte showing budding of platelets *(arrow)* along the periphery of the cell. *ADP,* Adenosine diphosphate; *ATP,* adenosine triphosphate; *5-HT,* 5-hydroxytryptamine, serotonin. **(A, from Walker BR, Colledge NR, Ralston SH, Penman ID:** Davidson's Principles and Practice of Medicine, *22nd ed, St. Louis, Churchill Livingstone Elsevier, 2014, p 998, Fig. 24.7.* **B,** *Photomicrograph courtesy William Meek, PhD, Professor of Anatomy and Cell Biology, Oklahoma State University, Center for Health Sciences, Tulsa, OK.)*

Functions vWF

Platelet adhesion molecule

Binds PLTs to exposed CG damaged small vessels

Stops bleeding damaged vessels

Platelet GpIb receptors bind vWF

vWF complexes with VIII:c: VIII:vWF

VIII:vWF prevents VIII:c degradation

↓VWF in VWD: also ↓VIII:c activity

b. Functions of vWF
 (1) Platelet adhesion molecule
   (a) Binds platelets to exposed collagen (CG) in small vessels so that a platelet thrombus is formed to stop bleeding from the damaged vessels
   (b) Platelets have glycoprotein (Gp) Ib receptors that bind to vWF, causing platelet adhesion to the damaged site (see Fig. 15-1 A).
 (2) vWF complexes with factor VIII coagulant (factor VIII:c) in the circulation (VIII:vWF)
   (a) These complexes prevent degradation of factor VIII:c in the circulation.
   (b) A decrease in vWF (e.g., von Willebrand disease [vWD]) secondarily decreases factor VIII:c activity.

Factor VIII:c is synthesized by the liver and reticuloendothelial tissues. When factor VIII:c is activated by thrombin, it dissociates from the factor VIII:vWF complex and performs its procoagulant function in the intrinsic coagulation cascade system.

Factor VIII:c: synthesized in liver + reticuloendothelial cells

Tissue thromboplastin (TT)

TT released from injured tissue

TT activates VII in extrinsic coagulation system

Derivation platelets

Cytoplasmic fragmentation of MKCs

Platelet location: PB, spleen

Platelets PB 8 to 10 days

Platelet receptors

GpIb (binds vWF)

GpIIb-IIIa (binds FNG)

Ticlopidine/clopidogrel

Inhibit PLT expression GpIIb-IIIa receptors Prevent FNG binding to receptor

Abciximab: directed against GpIIb-IIIa receptors

3. Tissue thromboplastin (TT; factor III)
 a. **Definition:** Noncirculating ubiquitous substance that is released from injured tissue
 b. Activates factor VII in the extrinsic coagulation system
4. Extrinsic and intrinsic coagulation systems are discussed later in the chapter.
D. Platelet structure and function
 1. Derivation of platelets
  a. Platelets are formed by cytoplasmic fragmentation of MKCs.
  b. Approximately 1000 to 3000 platelets are produced per MKC (Fig. 15-1 B).
 2. Locations of platelets
  a. Present in the peripheral blood (PB) and live for ~8 to 10 days
  b. Approximately one-third of the total platelet pool is stored in the spleen.
 3. Platelet receptors (Link 15-2).
  a. Gp receptors for vWF are designated GpIb (Fig. 15-1 A).
  b. Gp receptors for fibrinogen (FNG) are designated GpIIb-IIIa (Fig. 15-1 A).
   (1) Ticlopidine and clopidogrel
    (a) Both inhibit adenosine diphosphate (ADP)–induced expression of platelet GpIIb-IIIa receptors.
    (b) Prevent FNG binding to the receptor, which inhibits platelet aggregation
   (2) Abciximab: monoclonal antibody that is directed against the GpIIb-IIIa receptor, which prevents platelets from aggregating

4. Platelet factor 3 (PF3)
   a. Located on the platelet membrane
   b. Phospholipid substrate that is required for the clotting sequence
5. Platelet structure
   a. Contractile element called thrombosthenin helps in clot retraction. Thrombosthenin is deficient in Glanzmann disease.
   b. Dense bodies (Fig. 15-1 A) contain ADP, an aggregating agent, and calcium, a binding agent for vitamin K–dependent factors.
   c. α-Granules contain vWF, FNG, platelet-derived growth factor (PDGF), and PF4, which is a heparin-neutralizing factor.
6. Platelet functions
   a. Stabilize the vascular endothelial–cadherin complex at intercellular adherens junctions, particularly in postcapillary venules. This prevents leaking of red blood cells (RBCs) into the interstitial tissue.
      (1) The process is accomplished by platelet release of cytokines and growth factors stored within the platelet granules.
      (2) Stabilizing these junctions prevents the leakage of RBCs into the interstitium.
      (3) If the platelet count falls below critical levels, these junctions disassemble, causing extravasation of RBCs into the interstitium. This produces petechiae (a pinpoint area of hemorrhage), a hallmark of thrombocytopenia.
   b. Platelets are important in the formation of the hemostatic plug (fibrin thrombus) in small-vessel injury.
   c. PDGF in platelets stimulates smooth muscle hyperplasia. This is important in the pathogenesis of atherosclerosis (see Chapter 10).
E. **Coagulation system** (Fig. 15-2)
   1. The coagulation cascade consists of the extrinsic system (factor VII) and the intrinsic system (factors VIII, IX, XI, and XII).
   2. Extrinsic coagulation system
      a. Factor VII in the extrinsic system is activated (factor VIIa) by TT (factor III) released from damaged tissue.
      b. Factor VIIa activates factors IX and X, which are in the intrinsic system and the final common pathway, respectively (Fig. 15.2).
   3. Intrinsic coagulation system
      a. Factor XII (Hageman factor) in the intrinsic system is activated by exposed subendothelial CG and high-molecular-weight kininogen (HMWK).
      b. Functions of factor XIIa: activates factor XI, plasminogen (produces plasmin) and the kininogen system (produces kallikrein and bradykinin)

Margin notes:

PF3
Platelet membrane
Phospholipid required for clotting sequence
Platelet structure
Thrombosthenin contractile element
Deficient in Glanzmann disease
Dense bodies: ADP
ADP aggregating agent
Calcium binds K-dependent factors
α-Granules: vWF, FNG, PDGF, PF4
Platelet functions
Stabilize intercellular adherens junctions postcapillary venules
Platelet release cytokines/ growth factors
Prevents leaking RBCs into interstitium
↓Platelets → ↑RBC leakage → petechiae
Platelets: hemostatic plug small vessel injury
PDGF important in pathogenesis of atherosclerosis
Coagulation system
Extrinsic (VII)/intrinsic systems (VIII, IX, XI, XII)
Extrinsic system
VII activated by TT
Factor VIIa; activates factors IX/X (intrinsic system)
Intrinsic coagulation system
Factor XII (intrinsic system)
XII activation: CG, HMWK
XIIa: activates XI, plasminogen, kininogen system

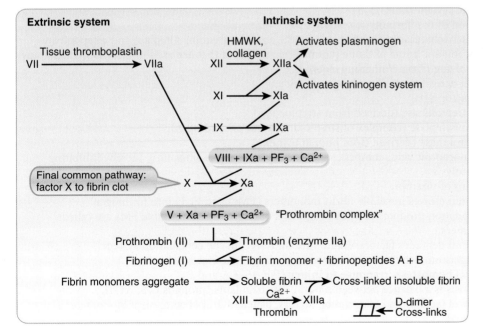

15-2: Coagulation cascade. Both the extrinsic and intrinsic coagulation systems use the final common pathway for the formation of a fibrin clot. See the text for a full discussion. *a*, Activated; *HMWK*, high-molecular-weight kininogen; *PF3*, platelet factor 3 (reaction accelerator).

c. Factors XIa and VIIa activate factor IX to form factor IXa (Fig. 15-2).
   (1) A four-component complex is formed (factors VIII and IXa, PF3, and calcium).
   (2) Calcium in the complex binds factor IXa, a vitamin K–dependent coagulation factor.
   (3) This complex is far more potent than factor VIIa alone in activating factor X.
4. Final common pathway
   a. The pathway includes factors V and Xa, prothrombin (II), and FNG (I).
   b. Prothrombin complex
      (1) The complex is a four-component system consisting of factor Xa, factor V, PF3 (phospholipid 3), and calcium.
      (2) Calcium binds factor Xa, a vitamin K–dependent coagulation factor.
      (3) Prothrombin complex cleaves prothrombin into thrombin (an enzyme).
   c. Functions of thrombin
      (1) Acts on FNG to produce FMs plus fibrinopeptides A and B.
      (2) Thrombin activates fibrin-stabilizing factor XIII → XIIIa, which converts soluble FMs to insoluble fibrin and enhances protein–protein cross-linking of insoluble fibrin to strengthen the fibrin clot. Cross-links are detected in the D-dimer assay (discussed later). Cross-links are analogous to links between tropocollagen molecules, which give CG its tensile strength.
      (3) Thrombin activates factor VIII:c in the intrinsic coagulation system.
      (4) Thrombin complexes with TM on ECs to activate protein C, which inactivates factors Va and VIIIa
5. Vitamin K–dependent factors include:
   a. procoagulant factors II, VII, IX, and X; anticoagulant protein C and protein S. The above factors are synthesized in the liver as nonfunctional precursor proteins.
   b. Function of vitamin K (see Chapter 8)
      (1) The majority of vitamin K is synthesized by colonic bacteria. After it is synthesized, vitamin K is activated in the liver by the enzyme epoxide reductase.
      (2) Activated vitamin K γ-carboxylates, each of the vitamin K–dependent factors. Carboxylated factors are now able to bind to calcium and PF3 in the cascade sequence.
6. Some of the coagulation factors are consumed in the formation of a fibrin clot. Consumed coagulation factors include FNG (factor I), factor V, factor VIII, and prothrombin (II).

When blood is drawn into a clot tube (no anticoagulant is added), a fibrin clot is formed. When the tube is spun down in a centrifuge, the supranate (the liquid lying above a layer of precipitated insoluble material) is called serum, which, unlike plasma, is missing FNG (factor I), prothrombin (factor II), factor V, and factor VIII. When blood is drawn into a tube that has an anticoagulant (e.g., heparin), a clot does not form. When the tube is spun down in a centrifuge, the supranate is called plasma and contains *all* of the coagulation factors.

F. **Fibrinolytic system** (Link 15-3)
   1. Activation of the fibrinolytic system
      a. tPA activates plasminogen to release the enzyme plasmin. Alteplase and reteplase are recombinant forms of tissue plasminogen activator that are used in thrombolytic therapy (dissolving fibrin containing clots).
      b. Other activators of plasminogen include:
         (1) factor XIIa.
         (2) streptokinase (derived from streptococci).
         (3) anistreplase (complex of streptokinase and plasminogen).
         (4) urokinase (derived from human urine).
      c. Aminocaproic acid: competitively blocks plasminogen activation, thereby inhibiting fibrinolysis
   2. Functions of plasmin
      a. Plasmin cleaves insoluble fibrin monomers (FMs) and FNG into fibrinogen degradation products (FDPs). Fragments of cross-linked insoluble FMs are called D-dimers.
      b. Plasmin degrades factors V and VIII, and FNG in the coagulation system.
   3. α₂-Antiplasmin, which is synthesized in the liver, inactivates plasmin
G. **Small-vessel hemostasis response to injury** (Fig. 15-3 A and B)
   1. Hemostasis is a balance between natural anticoagulants (proteins C/S, ATIII, fibrinolytic factors) and coagulation factors, platelets, and fibrinolysis inhibitors (Link 15-4).

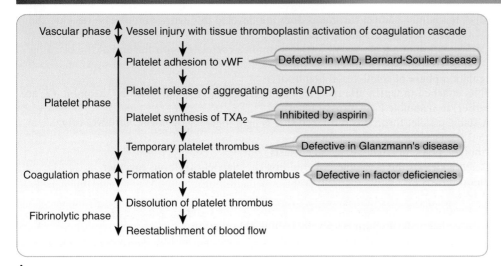

Vascular phase ⇅ Vessel injury with tissue thromboplastin activation of coagulation cascade

↓

Platelet phase

Platelet adhesion to vWF ◁ Defective in vWD, Bernard-Soulier disease

↓

Platelet release of aggregating agents (ADP)

↓

Platelet synthesis of TXA₂ ◁ Inhibited by aspirin

↓

Temporary platelet thrombus ◁ Defective in Glanzmann's disease

Coagulation phase ⇅ Formation of stable platelet thrombus ◁ Defective in factor deficiencies

↑

Dissolution of platelet thrombus

Fibrinolytic phase ↓

Reestablishment of blood flow

A

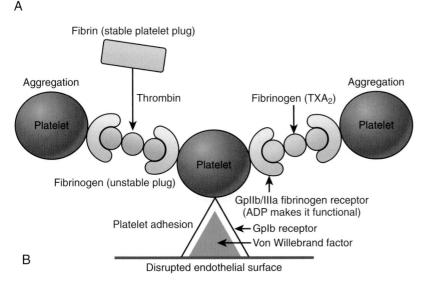

Fibrin (stable platelet plug)

Aggregation — Platelet

Thrombin

Fibrinogen (TXA₂)

Aggregation — Platelet

Platelet

Fibrinogen (unstable plug)

GpIIb/IIIa fibrinogen receptor (ADP makes it functional)

Platelet adhesion ← GpIb receptor

← Von Willebrand factor

Disrupted endothelial surface

B

15-3: A, Small-vessel hemostasis response to injury. A vascular phase, platelet phase, coagulation phase, and fibrinolytic phase are involved in small-vessel hemostasis with formation of a platelet thrombus. **B,** Platelet receptors and platelet aggregation. Disruption of the endothelial surface of small vessels exposes von Willebrand factor (vWF). This allows the glycoprotein (Gp) Ib receptor on the platelet to adhere to vWF on the endothelium, which is called platelet adhesion. The platelet releases preformed adenosine diphosphate (ADP) immediately after adhesion. ADP produces conformational changes in the GpIIb/IIIa fibrinogen receptor so that it is now able to bind to fibrinogen molecules. Thromboxane A₂ (TXA₂) is then synthesized de novo by the platelet. TXA₂ enhances fibrinogen attachment to the GpIIb/IIIa receptors on adjacent platelets, causing platelet aggregation and the formation of a temporary platelet thrombus. The platelet thrombus is unstable until thrombin, which is locally produced by activation of the coagulation system, converts fibrinogen to fibrin. This produces a stable platelet thrombus that stops bleeding from damaged small vessels. *vWD,* von Willebrand disease.

2. Sequence of small-vessel hemostasis includes vascular, platelet, coagulation, and fibrinolytic phases, in that order (see Fig. 15-3A; Links 15-5 and 15-6).

3. Vascular phase of small-vessel hemostasis (vessel injury)
   a. Transient vasoconstriction (VC) occurs directly after injury.
   b. Factor VII (extrinsic coagulation system) is locally activated by TT.
   c. Exposed CG activates factor XII (intrinsic coagulation system).

4. Platelet phase of small-vessel hemostasis
   a. Platelet adhesion
      (1) Platelet GpIb receptors adhere to exposed vWF in damaged ECs (Fig. 15-3 B).
      (2) Platelet adhesion is defective in vWD (no vWF is present) and Bernard-Soulier disease (absent GpIb receptor for vWF).
   b. Platelet release reaction
      (1) Platelets release ADP from dense bodies.
      (2) ADP produces conformational changes in the GpIIb-IIIa FNG receptor, which makes it functional for the next platelet phase.
   c. Platelet synthesis and release of TXA₂
      (1) TXA₂ is a vasoconstrictor, which reduces blood flow.
      (2) It is also a potent platelet aggregator that enhances the attachment of FNG to the now functional GpIIb-IIIa FNG receptors between FNG receptors on other platelets.
   d. Temporary platelet thrombus stops small-vessel bleeding (Fig. 15-3 A).
      (1) A temporary platelet thrombus is composed of numerous platelets held together by FNG, which makes it unstable and subject to rebleeding. By itself, FNG has no cohesive properties and cannot cause platelets to stick together.

Vascular>platelet>coagulation>fibrinolysis

Vascular phase hemostasis

Transient VC

Factor VII activated by TT

Exposed CG activates XII

Platelet phase hemostasis

Platelet adhesion

Platelet GpIb receptors adhere to vWF

Platelet release reaction

ADP from dense bodies

ADP conformation change GpIIb-IIIa FNG receptor

Platelet synthesis/release TXA₂

TXA₂ VC reduces blood flow

Potent platelet aggregator

Temporary platelet thrombus stops bleeding

Platelets held together by FNG (unstable)

(2) A temporary platelet thrombus does *not* develop in Glanzmann disease because the GpIIb-IIIa receptors are absent.

(3) Formation of a temporary platelet thrombus correlates with the end of the bleeding time (BT; discussed later).

5. Coagulation phase of small-vessel hemostasis
    a. FNG attached to GpIIb-IIIa receptors on other platelets is converted by thrombin (**T**; see earlier) to insoluble FMs (cross-linked).
    b. A stable platelet thrombus is formed that is held together by fibrin, *not* FNG (Fig. 15-3 B).

6. Fibrinolytic phase of small-vessel hemostasis
    a. Plasmin cleaves the insoluble FMs holding the platelet thrombus together.
    b. Blood flow is eventually reestablished.

H. Platelet tests

1. Platelet count
    a. The normal platelet count is 150,000 to 400,000 cells/mm^3.
    b. A normal platelet count does *not* guarantee normal platelet function. For example, a person taking aspirin has a normal platelet count, but the platelets are nonfunctional and cannot stop bleeding from injured small vessels.

2. BT
    a. **Definition:** The BT evaluates platelet function up to the formation of a temporary platelet thrombus (Link 15-7).
        (1) The normal reference interval for the BT is 1 to 9 minutes.
        (2) Many laboratories have discontinued using the BT because it is time intensive.
        (3) PFA (platelet function assay)-100 is an in vitro test that evaluates platelet function and has replaced the BT. In this test, blood is exposed to CG and ADP or CG and epinephrine (EPI), inducing a platelet plug to form.
    b. Disorders causing a prolonged BT are listed in Table 15-1.

3. Platelet aggregation tests (functional tests)
    a. Platelet aggregation tests evaluate platelet aggregation in response to the addition of aggregating reagents to a test tube.
    b. Aggregating agents that are used include ADP, EPI, CG, and ristocetin (RTC).

4. Tests for vWF: vWF mediates platelet adhesion to CG at sites of small-vessel injury.
    a. RTC cofactor activity (RCoA)
        (1) Evaluates vWF function
        (2) Abnormal functional assay occurs in:
            (a) classic vWD (deficiency of vWF).
            (b) Bernard-Soulier disease (absent GpIb vWF receptor for vWF).
    b. vWF antigen (vWFag) assay.
        (1) Measures the quantity of vWF that is present in serum regardless of function
        (2) vWFag is decreased in classic vWD.

I. Coagulation tests

1. Coagulation pathways (Fig. 15-4)
2. Prothrombin time (PT; Fig. 15-4)
    a. **Definition:** Evaluates the extrinsic coagulation system down to the formation of a fibrin clot in a test tube. Factors that are evaluated include VII, X, V, and II. Evaluation of factor I (FNG) is a separate test.
    b. The normal reference is 11 to 12.5 seconds; however, this varies in different laboratories. Only prolonged when a factor level is 30% to 40% of normal; hence, it is not a very sensitive test.
    c. International normalized ratio (INR)
        (1) **Definition:** The INR standardizes the PT when it is used to monitor warfarin anticoagulation therapy.
        (2) Results of the ratio are the same regardless of the reagents that are used to perform the test in any laboratory. A therapeutic INR is usually considered to be 2 to 3.5 in most institutions depending on the clinical situation.
    d. Uses of PT
        (1) Monitoring persons who are taking warfarin for anticoagulation to prevent small-vessel thrombosis
        (2) Evaluates liver synthetic function. An increased PT in a person with known liver disease indicates severe liver dysfunction (e.g., cirrhosis of the liver, chronic hepatitis).
        (3) Detect factor VII deficiency if the partial thromboplastin time (PTT) is normal

TABLE 15-1 Causes of Increased Bleeding Time

CAUSE	NATURE OF DEFECT	DISCUSSION
Aspirin or NSAIDs	• Platelet aggregation defect • Inhibition of platelet COX, which ultimately inhibits synthesis of TXA_2	• Normal platelet count
Bernard-Soulier syndrome	• Platelet adhesion defect • Autosomal recessive disease • Absent GpIb platelet receptors for vWF	• Thrombocytopenia, giant platelets • Lifelong bleeding problem
Glanzmann disease	• Platelet aggregation defect • Autosomal recessive disease • Absent GpIIb-IIIa fibrinogen receptors • Absent thrombosthenin (contractile protein)	• Lifelong bleeding problem
Renal failure	• Platelet aggregation defect • Inhibition of platelet phospholipid by toxic products	• Reversed with dialysis and DDAVP
Scurvy	• Vascular defect (perifollicular hemorrhages) • Caused by vitamin C deficiency • Defective collagen resulting from poor cross-linking of tropocollagen molecules	• May cause ecchymoses, hemarthroses, perifollicular hemorrhages, bleeding gums (Fig. 8-10 B)
Thrombocytopenia	• Decreased number of platelets	• Increased bleeding time when the platelet count is <90,000 cells/mm³
von Willebrand disease	• Platelet adhesion defect • Autosomal dominant disorder • Absent or defective vWF • Decreased factor VIII:c	• Combined platelet and coagulation factor disorder
Gray platelet syndrome	• Deficiency of α-granules (electron microscopy)	• Large, pale, platelets • Platelets aggregate with ristocetin
Storage pool disease	• Deficiency of dense bodies (electron microscopy	• Abnormal platelet aggregation test
Cardiopulmonary bypass	• Destruction of platelets in the bypass circuit and dysfunction from activation of the platelets	• 50% drop in platelet count is common postoperatively • Platelet dysfunction is a minor cause of postoperative bleeding • Platelet transfusion before surgery is *not* recommended

COX, Cyclooxygenase; *DDAVP,* desmopressin acetate; *Gp,* glycoprotein; *NSAID,* nonsteroidal antiinflammatory drug; *TXA₂,* thromboxane A₂; *vWF,* von Willebrand factor.

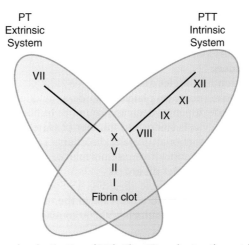

15-4: Prothrombin time (PT) and partial thromboplastin time (PTT). The PT evaluates the extrinsic system in sequential order factors VII, X, V, II, and I. The PTT evaluates the intrinsic system in sequential order factors XII, XI, IX, VIII, X, V, II, and I.

3. Activated partial thromboplastin time (aPTT; see Fig. 15-4)
   a. **Definition:** Evaluates the intrinsic coagulation system down to formation of a fibrin clot. Factors that are evaluated include XII, XI, IX, VIII, X, V, II, and I (separate test).
   b. A normal reference interval is 30 to 40 seconds; however, this may vary in different laboratories. Desired ranges for therapeutic anticoagulation are 1.5 to 2.5 times normal (e.g., 70 seconds). If the activated PTT is <50 seconds, the patient is *not* receiving

aPTT

Evaluates intrinsic coagulation system

Evaluates factors XII, XI, IX, VIII, X, V, II

therapeutic levels and needs more heparin. If the activated PTT is >100 seconds, it indicates that too much heparin is being given. The risk of serious spontaneous bleeding is high. The effects of heparin can be reversed immediately by the administration of protamine sulfate.

c. Uses of the PTT

(1) Monitor heparin anticoagulation therapy

(a) Heparin enhances ATIII activity. This prevents the formation of a thrombin clot in small vessels.

(b) PTT is *not* required to follow low-molecular-weight heparin (LMWH) therapy.

(2) The PTT detects factor deficiencies in the intrinsic coagulation system if the PT is normal.

Whether the patient is receiving heparin or warfarin anticoagulation therapy, both the PT and PTT are increased because both inhibit factors in the final common pathway. Experience has shown that whereas the PT performs better in monitoring warfarin, the PTT performs better in monitoring heparin.

J. Fibrinolytic system tests

1. **Definition:** Test for the presence of fibrin degradation products (FDPs) that are associated with plasmin degradation of fibrinogen or insoluble fibrin in fibrin clots.

2. D-Dimer assay

a. **Definition:** Detects cross-linked insoluble FMs (D-dimers) in a fibrin clot.

b. The assay does *not* detect FDPs because they are *not* cross-linked.

c. The assay has a high sensitivity (~95%) but poor specificity (50%).

(1) Specificity is low because of false positive test results that may occur in rheumatoid arthritis (RA) with high levels of rheumatoid factor (RF), liver disease, inflammation, pregnancy, malignancy, trauma, and advanced age.

(2) High sensitivity of the test is most useful in *excluding* fibrinolysis when the test result returns to negative because it is more likely to be a true negative rather than a false-negative test result.

d. D-Dimer testing is of clinical use when there is a suspicion for deep vein thrombosis (DVT), pulmonary thromboembolism (TE), and disseminated intravascular coagulation (DIC).

e. It is also used to follow thrombolytic therapy (dissolving thrombin clots) for coronary artery thrombosis, renal artery stenosis, stroke, and mesenteric venous thrombosis.

II. Platelet Disorders

A. Classification of platelet disorders

1. Quantitative (number) platelet disorders include:

a. thrombocytopenia (decreased number of platelets).

b. thrombocytosis (increased number of platelets).

2. Qualitative (functional) platelet disorders (Table 15-1). The number of platelets can be decreased (thrombocytopenia), normal, or increased (thrombocytosis).

B. Pathogenesis of platelet disorders

1. Thrombocytopenia (Table 15-2; Fig. 15-5; Links 15-8 to 15-13)

a. **Definition:** Refers to a decrease in the number of platelets to < 150,000 platelets/mm^3 (normal range in adults is 150,000 to 400,000 mm^3)

b. Pathogenesis includes:

(1) decreased production of platelets. Examples: aplastic anemia and leukemia

(2) increased destruction of platelets.

(a) Immune destruction. Examples: idiopathic thrombocytopenic purpura (ITP) and certain drugs.

(b) Nonimmune destruction. Examples: thrombotic thrombocytopenic purpura (TTP) and DIC

(3) sequestration (trapped) in the spleen. Example: hypersplenism in portal hypertension (HTN)

2. Thrombocytosis

a. **Definition:** An increase in the number of platelets that is greater than 400,000 platelets/mm^3

Margin notes:

Protamine sulfate reverses heparin effect

Uses PTT

Monitor heparin anticoagulation

Heparin enhances ATIII activity

PTT *not* for LMWH Rx

Evaluates intrinsic system factors if PT normal

PT/PTT increased warfarin/ heparin Rx; PT better for warfarin; PTT better for heparin

Fibrinolytic system tests

Fibrinogen degradation products

↑FDPs: plasmin lysis FNG/ fibrin in fibrin clots

D-Dimer assay

Detects cross-links between FMs

Does *not* detect FDPs

↑Sensitivity, ↓specificity

↑RF, liver disease, inflammation, pregnancy, trauma, old age

Useful in excluding fibrinolysis if negative

DVT

Pulmonary TE, DIC

Follow thrombolytic therapy

Platelet disorders

Thrombocytopenia (↓number)

Thrombocytosis (↑ number)

Functional disorders regardless of numbers

Platelets <150,000 platelets/mm^3

↓Production

Aplastic anemia, leukemia

Increased platelet destruction

Immune: ITP, drugs

Nonimmune destruction: TTP, DIC

Sequestration in spleen: hypersplenism

Thrombocytosis

Platelets >400,000 platelets/mm^3

TABLE 15-2 Disorders Producing Thrombocytopenia

DISEASE	COMMENTS
Acute immune thrombocytopenia (ITP; see Fig. 15-5; Link 15-8)	• Most common cause of thrombocytopenia in children 2 to 6 yr of age. Commonly affects women in the second or third decades of life. • IgG antibodies are directed against the GpIIb-IIIa receptors on platelets (type II hypersensitivity reaction). These antibodies can be detected in 80% of cases. • Abrupt onset, 1 to 3 wk after a viral infection. Patients present with epistaxis (nosebleed), easy bruising, and petechiae. Lymphadenopathy and splenomegaly are *not* present. • Secondary causes of ITP are associated with HIV, SLE, thyroid disease, chronic lymphocytic leukemia, malignant lymphoma, and solid tumors.
Chronic immune thrombocytopenia	• Most common cause of thrombocytopenia in adults. It is most common in women 20 to 40 yr of age. IgG antibodies are directed against the GpIIb-IIIa fibrinogen receptors (type II hypersensitivity reaction). • Insidious onset and presents with epistaxis, easy bruising, and petechiae • Newborn infants of mothers with chronic ITP may have transient thrombocytopenia caused by transplacental passage of IgG antibodies. • Secondary causes of chronic ITP: SLE, HIV, lymphoproliferative diseases
Neonatal alloimmune thrombocytopenia (NAIT)	• NAIT accounts for 20% of cases of thrombocytopenia in neonates. • Most common cause of isolated severe thrombocytopenia in the first week of life • Fetomaternal incompatibility for platelet-specific antigens (e.g., Pl^{A1}). Pl^{A1} is absent from 2% of the population; therefore, if a Pl^{A1}-negative mother is exposed to Pl^{A1}-positive platelets (paternal-inherited human platelet antigens, during pregnancy, or from a previous pregnancy or transfusion), she will develop IgG antibodies against the Pl^{A1} antigen. Transplacental passage of IgG antibodies targets fetal Pl^{A1}-positive platelets, leading to macrophage destruction of those platelets (type II hypersensitivity reaction). In the neonate, it may produce petechial hemorrhages in the first few days of life or CNS hemorrhages in severe cases. IgG antibodies against Pl^{A1} antigen and typing of fetal platelets for the antigen in the neonate can be used to confirm the diagnosis.
Posttransfusion purpura	• Primarily occurs in multiparous women because they are more likely to have been exposed to fetal blood from each of their pregnancies that may have contained fetal Pl^{A1}-positive platelets • If these women with IgG antibodies directed against Pl^{A1} antigen receive a blood transfusion with Pl^{A1}-positive platelets, they will develop a severe thrombocytopenia 7 to 10 days after the transfusion. Both the donor platelets and her Pl^{A1}-negative platelets are destroyed.
Heparin-induced thrombocytopenia (HIT; see Link 15-9)	• HIT is a common cause of thrombocytopenia in hospitalized patients. • Nonimmune type I variant of HIT is mild and occurs early in the course of heparin therapy and spontaneously resolves if heparin is continued. • Type II variant of HIT is immune mediated (Link 15-9). Produces a severe thrombocytopenia and vessel thrombosis 5 to 10 days after heparin therapy. Heparin attaches to PF4 (heparin neutralizing factor) on platelets. Then IgG antibodies attach to the heparin–PF4 complex and produce immune complexes that destroy the platelets. The complexes break free from platelets and damage endothelial cells, leading to activation of the coagulation system and vessel thrombosis. Confers a significant risk of in-hospital mortality. Heparin must be discontinued immediately, and thrombin antagonists should be used to prevent thrombosis. LMWH should *not* be used because of cross-reactivity.
Thrombotic thrombocytopenic purpura (TTP; see Links 15-10 to 15-12)	• TTP is most common in women in the fourth decade of life. 10% to 40% report a viral upper respiratory infection 2 weeks before onset of TTP. • Acquired or genetic deficiency in von Willebrand factor–cleaving metalloprotease (ADAMTS13) in endothelial cells. Absence of this enzyme results in an increase in circulating multimers of vWF that promote platelet activation and aggregation. Superimposed on this, is endothelial injury at arteriole–capillary junctions (? direct effect, production of neoantigens leading to production of autoantibodies) associated with drugs (e.g., cyclosporine, chemotherapy agents, oral contraceptives, ticlopidine, penicillin), the postpartum state, infection (e.g., HIV, *Streptococcus pneumoniae* sepsis), hypertension, autoimmune disease (e.g., SLE), malignancy (e.g., lymphoid leukemias, lymphomas), radiation, and bone marrow transplantation. • Platelets are consumed owing to production of numerous platelet thrombi that develop in the areas of endothelial injury at the arteriole–capillary junctions. • In 40% of cases, patients may have a clinical pentad including fever, thrombocytopenia, renal failure, MHA with schistocytes (damage by platelet thrombi; see Fig. 12-29), and CNS deficits. One or more of the findings in this pentad may be absent. • Recurrence rate is 20%–40% of cases. • Mortality rate is 10%–20%.
Hemolytic uremic syndrome (HUS; see Link 15-13)	• HUS primarily occurs in children <10 yr old. It may be epidemic, most commonly during the summer months in rural populations. • Most common cause of acute renal failure in children • Most often caused by *Escherichia coli* serotype O157:H7 • Activation of platelets and endothelial damage at the arteriole-capillary junctions may be related to the Shiga-like toxin and defects in complement regulatory proteins. Organisms proliferate in undercooked red meat, unpasteurized milk or milk products, water, fruits, and vegetables. • Other causes of HUS in children and adults are drugs (many of them are similar to those listed for TTP), non-Shiga toxin type infections (e.g., *Shigella, Salmonella, Yersinia, Campylobacter*, coxsackievirus, influenza virus), and complement disorders (e.g., defects in complement factor H [complement central protein], membrane cofactor protein, or factor I; these are the main causes in nondiarrheal atypical HUS). • Clinical findings are similar to TTP; however, CNS findings are less frequent. Bloody diarrhea occurs in 75% of cases. In HUS, there may be a clinical triad including thrombocytopenia (used up in forming thrombi at the arteriole–capillary junctions), acute renal failure, and microangiopathic hemolytic anemia (schistocytes; see Fig. 12-29). • Mortality rate is <5%.

CNS, Central nervous system; *DIC,* disseminated intravascular coagulation; *Gp,* glycoprotein; *LMWH,* low-molecular-weight heparin; *MHA,* microangiopathic hemolytic anemia; *PF4,* platelet factor 4; *Rx,* treatment; *SLE,* systemic lupus erythematosus; *vWF,* von Willebrand factor.

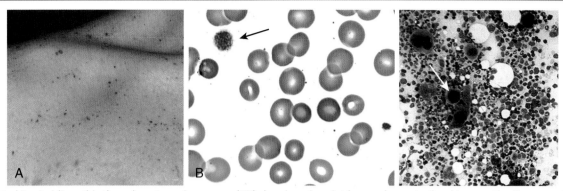

15-5: **A,** Petechiae in idiopathic thrombocytopenic purpura (ITP) showing pinpoint hemorrhages in the skin over the thorax and shoulders. Petechiae are most frequently caused by thrombocytopenia. When compressed, petechiae do not blanch with pressure. **B,** ITP. Peripheral smear *(left)* shows an overall decrease in platelets. The *arrow* shows a giant platelet. The bone marrow aspirate *(right)* shows an increase in immature megakaryocytes *(white arrow).* (*A* from Forbes C, Jackson W: Color Atlas and Text of Clinical Medicine, *3rd ed, London, Mosby, 2004, p 407, Fig. 10-10.* **B** from Kliegman RM, et al: Nelson Textbook of Pediatrics, *19th ed, St. Louis, Elsevier Saunders, 2011, p 2403, Fig. 484-3. Taken from Blanchette V, Bolton-Maggs P: Childhood immune thrombocytopenic purpura: diagnosis and management,* Pediatr Clin North Am *2008;55:393–420, Fig. 4.)*

TABLE 15-3   Clinical Findings in Platelet and Coagulation Disorders

CLINICAL FINDINGS	PLATELET DYSFUNCTION	COAGULATION FACTOR DEFICIENCY
Bleeding from superficial scratches	Yes	No
Petechiae	Yes (thrombocytopenia)	No
Late rebleeding	No	Yes
Hemarthroses	No	Yes (only very severe factor deficiencies)
Epistaxis, menorrhagia, gastrointestinal or genitourinary bleeding, easy bruising	Yes	Yes
Ecchymoses or purpura	Yes	Yes

1° Thrombocytosis

Essential thrombocythemia, PV

2° (Reactive) thrombocytosis

Chronic iron deficiency, malignancy, splenectomy

Qualitative disorders

Functional platelet defects

Acquired: aspirin, CRF

Hereditary: Glanzmann disease, Bernard-Soulier disease

Clinical findings platelet dysfunction

MC sign platelet dysfunction

Petechiae: MC caused by thrombocytopenia

Pinpoint hemorrhage

Ecchymoses: quarter size hemorrhage

RMSF, excessive BP cuff pressure

b. Pathogenesis
   (1) Primary thrombocytosis. Examples of primary thrombocytosis include essential thrombocythemia (Link 15-14) and polycythemia vera (PV; see Chapter 13).
   (2) Secondary (reactive) thrombocytosis. Examples of secondary (reactive) thrombocytosis include chronic iron deficiency, infections, splenectomy (platelet pool normally in the spleen is now circulating), and malignancy. This is a body mechanism to increase blood viscosity to prevent high-output cardiac failure (see Chapter 11).
3. Qualitative platelet disorders.
   a. **Definition:** A disorder in which the platelets do *not* function properly irrespective of the platelet number
   b. Pathogenesis includes:
      (1) acquired disorders (e.g., aspirin, chronic renal failure [CRF]).
      (2) hereditary disorders (e.g., Glanzmann disease, Bernard-Soulier disease).
C. **Clinical findings associated with platelet dysfunction** (Table 15-3).
   1. Epistaxis (nosebleeds) is the most common sign of platelet dysfunction. The Kiesselbach area is the most common site for bleeding in epistaxis (Fig. 15-6).
   2. Petechiae (Fig. 15-5 A) and multiple small ecchymoses (purpura) are most commonly caused by thrombocytopenia.
      a. Petechiae are pinpoint areas of hemorrhage in subcutaneous tissue (Link 15-15). RBCs leak through postcapillary venules in the endothelium.
      b. Ecchymoses are areas of bleeding that are the size of a quarter (Link 15-16).
      c. Other, less common causes of petechiae are seen in Rocky Mountain spotted fever (RMSF), in which rickettsiae invade ECs in small vessels causing them to rupture, and excessive mechanical compression (e.g., blood pressure cuff is pumped up too high). In the above examples, the petechiae are *not* caused by thrombocytopenia, but by localized damage of small vessels.

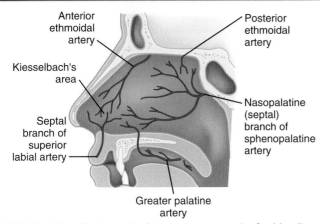

15-6: The Kiesselbach area is the most common site for bleeding in epistaxis. *(From Marx J: Rosen's Emergency Medicine Concepts and Clinical Practice, 7th ed, Philadelphia, Mosby Elsevier, 2010, p 884, Fig. 70-1.)*

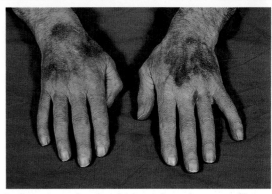

15-7: Senile purpura showing the large, irregular areas of hemorrhage on the backs of both hands. This benign condition primarily occurs in body areas that are frequently traumatized. It is caused by the normal vessel instability that is associated with aging. *(From Forbes C, Jackson W: Color Atlas and Text of Clinical Medicine, 3rd ed, London, Mosby, 2004, p 438, Fig. 10-101.)*

Ecchymoses (purpura; Link 15-16) are caused by a variety of disorders unrelated to thrombocytopenia. Palpable purpura (purpura that can be felt) is a sign of a small-vessel vasculitis (see Chapter 10) and not a problem with platelets. Because vasculitis is a type of acute inflammation, the lesions are palpable due to increased vessel permeability (tumor of acute inflammation). Ecchymoses are also present in scurvy (vitamin C deficiency) and are caused by vessel weakness related to lack of cross-bridges between tropocollagen molecules (see Chapter 8). Senile purpura is a normal finding in older adult patients and is caused by vessel instability that is normally associated with aging (Fig. 15-7). Ecchymoses (*not* associated with platelet dysfunction) develop in areas of trauma (e.g., back of the hands, shins).

3. Bleeding from superficial scratches. *No* temporary platelet thrombus is present to stop bleeding from injury to small vessels.
4. Other findings in platelet dysfunction include menorrhagia (excessive menstrual blood loss), hematuria (loss of RBCs in urine), bleeding from tooth extraction sites, easy bruising, and gastrointestinal (GI) and intracranial bleeding.

III. **Coagulation Disorders**
A. **Classification of coagulation disorders**
1. Acquired coagulation disorders. Single or multiple coagulation factor deficiencies may occur.
2. Hereditary coagulation disorders (e.g., hemophilia A): usually involve a single coagulation factor deficiency
B. **Pathogenesis**
1. Decreased production of coagulation factors. Examples: hemophilia A and cirrhosis (decreased synthesis of coagulation factors)
2. Pathologic inhibition of coagulation factors. Example: acquired circulating antibodies (inhibitors) against one or more coagulation factors
3. Excessive consumption of coagulation factors. Example: DIC
C. **Clinical findings** (see Table 15-3)
1. Late rebleeding after surgery or tooth extraction
   a. Lack of thrombin prevents formation of a stable platelet thrombus held together by fibrin.
   b. Temporary platelet thrombi are the only mechanical block preventing bleeding from the damaged small vessels. Moving around after surgery or rinsing the mouth out with water after a tooth extraction dislodges the temporary platelet thrombi (held together by FNG), leading to late rebleeding.
2. Findings in severe coagulation factor deficiencies include:
   a. hemarthroses (bleeding into joints; Links 15-17 to 15-19).
   b. retroperitoneal (refers to the space between the peritoneum and the posterior abdominal wall) and deep muscular bleeding (Link 15-18).
3. Clinical findings in coagulation factor deficiency that also occur in qualitative platelet disorders or thrombocytopenia (Table 15-3) include ecchymoses, epistaxis, menorrhagia, hematuria, bleeding from tooth extraction sites (Link 15-20), easy bruising, and GI and intracranial bleeding.

Senile purpura: vessel instability in elderly; occurs in areas of trauma

No temporary platelet thrombus

Menorrhagia, hematuria

Bleeding tooth extraction sites

Easy bruising

GI/intracranial bleeding

Coagulation disorders

Acquired

Single/multiple factor deficiencies

Hereditary disorder

Single factor deficiency

↓Production: hemophilia A, cirrhosis

Pathologic inhibition

Circulating antibodies against factors

Excessive consumption

DIC

Clinical findings

Late rebleeding: surgery, tooth extraction

Lack thrombin: *no* stable platelet thrombus

Only temporary platelet thrombi

Hemarthroses

Retroperitoneal/deep muscular bleeding

Overlap chemical findings coagulation/platelet disorders

Regarding clinical findings, there can be an overlap between those associated with a platelet disorder versus those associated with a disorder of the coagulation cascade. Note that bleeding from superficial scratches, however, is more likely to be a platelet problem than a coagulation deficiency.

Hemophilia A

X-linked recessive; ↓factor VIIIc

Male-dominant genetic disease

Females asymptomatic carriers

All sons affected males normal; all daughters carriers

Females are asymptomatic carriers; transmit to 50% of sons

Affected males have ↓VIII:c

↓VIII:c → ↓ activation factor X by activated factor VII

New mutation if *no* family Hx hemophilia

Females symptomatic rare but possible

Clinical: correlate VIII:c activity

Levels VIII:c never change
Mild: VIII:c 5% to 25%
Moderate: VIII:c 1% to 4%
Severe: VIII:c <1%
Bleeding: joints, skin, muscle

NB bleeding: circumcision, umbilical cord separation

D. **Hemophilia A**
1. **Definition:** X-linked recessive disorder caused by a deficiency of factor VIII coagulant (VIII:c). Rare cases are acquired.
2. Epidemiology
   a. X-linked recessive (see Chapter 6)
      (1) Male-dominant genetic disease found in all ethnic groups
      (2) Females are asymptomatic carriers.
      (3) All sons of affected males are normal, and all daughters are carriers (Fig. 6-12 C, middle).
      (4) Sons of female carriers have a 50:50 risk of disease (daughters have a 50:50 carrier risk; Fig. 6-12 C, left).
      (5) Affected males have a deficiency of factor VIII:c, a coagulation factor in the intrinsic coagulation system. Deficiency of VIII:c also decreases activation of factor X by activated factor VII because it is part of the factor VIII, IXa, PF3, calcium complex.
   b. If there is no family history of hemophilia and a person in that family has hemophilia, it is most likely caused by a new mutation (30% of cases).
   c. In rare cases, female carriers may have symptomatic disease.
      (1) Disease in affected females is caused by inactivation of more normal X chromosomes than X chromosomes with the mutation.
      (2) Females become "homozygous" for the abnormal X chromosome.
      (3) Another possibility is if a carrier female has children with an affected male (Fig. 6-12 C, right).
3. Clinical findings
   a. Signs and symptoms correlate with the level of factor VIII:c activity.
      (1) Levels of factor VIII:c never change in hemophilia A.
      (2) Mild disease occurs when factor VIII:c activity is 5% to 25% of normal.
      (3) Moderate disease occurs when factor VIII:c activity is 1% to 4% of normal.
      (4) Severe disease occurs when factor VIII:c activity is <1% of normal.
   b. Clinical features include spontaneous bleeding into joints (hemarthrosis; Links 15-17 and 15-19), skin, and muscle (Links 15-18 and 15-19).
   c. Bleeding problems may occur in male newborns (10%–15% of cases). Excessive bleeding may occur in male newborns after circumcision or umbilical cord separation. Only the temporary platelet plug is present to stop bleeding.

Hemophilia B (Christmas disease) is an X-linked recessive disorder involving a deficiency of factor IX. It is clinically indistinguishable from hemophilia A.

Hemophilia B: X-linked recessive; factor IX deficiency
↑aPTT
↓ VIII:c activity
Detection female carriers: DNA technology
Classic von Willebrand disease
AD disorder, ↓vWF
Functions vWF
Platelet adhesion; GpIb receptors adhere to vWF
Forms complex with VIII to prevent degradation
AD inheritance; males, females
vWD MC hereditary bleeding disorder
Several subtypes
Angiodysplasia: vascular malformations in bowel

4. Laboratory findings
   a. Activated PTT is increased.
   b. Factor VIII:c activity is decreased.
   c. Detection of female carriers is best accomplished with DNA technology.
E. **Classic vWD**
1. **Definition:** Autosomal dominant (AD) disorder with a deficiency of vWF
2. Functions of vWF
   a. Platelet adhesion. Platelet GpIb receptors adhere to exposed vWF in damaged ECs.
   b. Complexes with factor VIII in the peripheral blood, which protects factor VIII from degradation. If vWF is decreased, factor VIII may also be decreased.
3. Epidemiology
   a. AD disorder; therefore, it may occur in males and females.
   b. Most common hereditary bleeding disorder. Prevalence of vWD is 1 per 100 people.
   c. Several subtypes. Subtypes include types I (80%; only one discussed), IIA, IIB, and III vWD.
   d. Association with angiodysplasia (small vascular malformations in the bowel that tend to bleed) with vWD (Chapter 18). Persons who have angiodysplasia are more likely to bleed if they have vWD.

e. Severe aortic valve (AV) stenosis (see Chapter 11) may produce acquired vWD.
  (1) Large circulating multimeric complexes of vWF complexed with VIII:c are destroyed by the high shear stress in severe AV stenosis, which decreases both vWF and VIII:c (factor VIII: coagulant).
  (2) AV replacement corrects the problem.
f. People with blood group O have vWF factor levels lower than in people with non-O blood groups. Approximately 10% to 15% of blood group O people have subnormal levels of vWF. They do *not* always have a mutation of the *vWF* gene. There is an increased risk for bleeding if vWF is decreased.
4. Clinical findings vWD include:
  a. menorrhagia (80%; extremely common). Use of two pads or superabsorbent brands is routine. Stain through underclothes. Change pad or tampon every 30 to 120 minutes on heaviest days.
  b. postpartum hemorrhage (30%), bleeding after surgery (50%).
  c. easy bruising (80%).
  d. mucosal bleeding (hallmark of disease). Gingival bleeding (eruption of new teeth, flossing, tooth extraction [60%; Link 15-20]), epistaxis (50%), GI bleeding, rectal bleeding if hemorrhoids present.
5. Laboratory findings are variable (may require repeat testing).
  a. Increased aPTT is only present in 25% to 50% of cases; therefore, a normal PTT does *not* exclude the diagnosis of vWD.
  b. Increased BT is only present in 50% of cases; therefore, a normal BT does *not* exclude the diagnosis.
  c. Abnormal RTC cofactor activity assay
  d. Abnormal vWF antigen assay
  e. ↓Factor VIII:c activity
  f. Gene analysis is available to secure the diagnosis.
6. Desmopressin acetate (DDAVP) increases the release of vWF from WPBs, which in turn stabilizes circulating VIII:c by preventing its degradation. Oral contraceptive pills (OCPs) have a similar activity as DDAVP; however, their use is limited to women with vWD.

F. **Circulating anticoagulants (inhibitors).**
  1. **Definition:** Circulating antibodies that destroy specific coagulation factors
  2. Pathogenesis
    a. Coagulation factor or factors are immunologically destroyed by circulating antibodies.
    b. Most common antibody is directed against factor VIII:c. Factor VIII antibodies often occur postpartum or in patients with hemophilia receiving recombinant factor VIII.
  3. Clinical findings are similar to those with coagulation factor deficiencies caused by decreased production of coagulation factors.
  4. Laboratory findings
    a. Increased PT and/or increased PTT, depending on the factor deficiency. Tests do *not* differentiate immune destruction from decreased production of the coagulation factor.
    b. Mixing studies differentiate decreased production from increased destruction of a coagulation factor.
      (1) Normal plasma is mixed with patient plasma in a test tube.
      (2) *No* correction of the PT and/or the PTT indicates immune destruction of coagulation factors is present. Antibody is also destroying the coagulation factor in the normal plasma that is added to the test tube.
      (3) Correction of the PT and/or PTT indicates decreased production of coagulation factors.

G. **Vitamin K deficiency** (see Chapter 8)
H. **Hemostasis disorders in cirrhosis**
  1. Pathogenesis
    a. Decreased synthesis of most coagulation factors
      (1) Leads to multiple coagulation factor deficiencies
      (2) Decreased γ-carboxylation of vitamin K–dependent coagulation factors leads to lack of function of factors II, VII, IX, and X.
    b. Decreased synthesis of anticoagulants such as ATIII and proteins C and S
    c. Decreased synthesis of fibrinolytic agents (e.g., plasminogen)
    d. Decreased clearance of FNG/FDPs and D-dimers. This interferes with platelet aggregation and polymerization of fibrin.

Severe AV stenosis: acquired VWD

AV replacement corrects problem

Group O people may have ↓vWF levels; bleeding risk

vWD: combined platelet and coagulation factor disorder

Menorrhagia extremely common

Postpartum hemorrhage, bleed after surgery

Easy bruising

Mucosal bleeding hallmark

Epistaxis, GI/rectal bleeding

↑aPTT +/-

↑BT +/-

Abnormal RTC cofactor assay

Abnormal VWF antigen assay

↓VIII:c

Gene analysis

DDAVP releases vWF from WP bodies

OCP similar to DDAVP

Circulating anticoagulants (inhibitors)

Antibodies destroy specific coagulation factor(s)

Immunologic destruction

Factor VIII antibodies MC

Postpartum, hemophiliacs with recombinant Rx

Clinical findings similar to factor deficiencies

↑PT and/or PTT depending on factor deficiency

Mixing studies

Normal plasma mixed with patient plasma

PT and/or PTT *not* corrected with mixing study

Hemostasis disorders in cirrhosis

↓Synthesis coagulation factors

Multiple coagulation factor deficiencies

Lack function vitamin K–dependent factors

↓Synthesis ATIII, protein C/S

↓Synthesis plasminogen

↓Clearance FDPs, D-dimers

Interferes with PLT aggregation/polymerization of fibrin

↓Clearance tPA, ↓ synthesis α₂-antiplasmin

1°Fibrinolysis

↑PT, ↑PTT

↑FNG/FDPs, D-dimers

↑BT

DIC

Thrombohemorrhagic disorder

Fibrin thrombi: RBCs with trapped WBCs/platelets

Bleeding/anemia

Activation intrinsic and/or extrinsic coagulation system

Activation extrinsic system → release TT

Massive trauma

Hypovolemic/septic shock

Malignancies

Obstetrical problems

Pancreatitis, rattlesnake, ARDS

Activation intrinsic system

Gram-negative septicemia (*N. meningitidis*)

Gram-negative sepsis: MCC DIC

ICs (SLE)

Heat stroke, 3° burns

Fibrin thrombi in microcirculation

Thrombi obstruct blood flow (WF syndrome)

Consume coagulation factors (bleeding)

Trap platelets (bleeding)

MHA with schistocytes

2° Fibrinolysis: bleeding

↑PT, PTT

↓Serum FNG

Thrombocytopenia

Increased BT

D-Dimers most sensitive screen

Negative D-dimers *excludes* DIC

Normocytic anemia: bleeding skin, GI

Mechanical damage from MHA

Rx underlying disease most important

e. Decreased clearance of tPA and decreased synthesis of α₂-antiplasmin; may produce primary fibrinolysis (see Section IV)

2. Laboratory findings include:
   a. increased PT and PTT.
   b. increase in FNG/FDPs and D-dimers.
   c. increased BT.

I. **Disseminated intravascular coagulation (DIC)**
   1. Overview of DIC
      a. **Definition:** Disorder characterized by diffuse small-vessel thromboses and hemorrhage (thrombohemorrhagic disorder)
      b. Fibrin thrombi occlude the microcirculation throughout the body, producing widespread ischemic damage. Fibrin thrombi in the microcirculation are primarily composed of RBCs, with trapped leukocytes and platelets (see Chapter 5).
      c. Bleeding occurs from the GI tract, nose (epistaxis), and every puncture sites; may result in a normocytic anemia.
   2. Epidemiology (Link 15-21)
      a. Activation of the intrinsic and/or extrinsic coagulation system
         (1) Activation of the extrinsic system occurs by the release of TT from damaged tissue; examples include:
            (a) massive trauma (car accident; extensive surgery).
            (b) hypovolemic or cardiogenic shock (see Chapter 5).
            (c) malignancies (acute promyelocytic leukemia, adenocarcinomas [pancreas, prostate, lung, breast]).
            (d) obstetric problems (amniotic fluid embolism, abruptio placentae, toxemia of pregnancy, dead retained fetus).
            (e) acute pancreatitis, rattlesnake envenomation, acute respiratory distress syndrome (ARDS).
         (2) Activation of the intrinsic system is by activation of factor XII by surface contact with collagen secondary to injury to ECs; examples include:
            (a) Gram-negative septicemia (e.g., meningococcemia caused by *Neisseria meningitidis*; Link 15-22) with release of endotoxins (most common cause of DIC; >50% of cases; see Chapter 5).
            (b) deposition of immunocomplexes (ICs; e.g., systemic lupus erythematosus [SLE]).
            (c) severe temperature alterations (heatstroke, third-degree burns).
      b. With activation of either the intrinsic or extrinsic coagulation system, fibrin thrombi develop in the microcirculation; fibrin thrombi:
         (1) obstruct blood flow, causing ischemia and the potential for infarction (e.g., hemorrhagic infarction of the adrenal glands in Waterhouse-Friderichsen [WF] syndrome in *Neisseria meningitidis* sepsis; see Chapter 23).
         (2) consume coagulation factors (I, II, V, VIII), causing bleeding problems.
         (3) trap platelets, causing thrombocytopenia, which also contributes to bleeding. Petechiae and ecchymoses develop on the skin and mucous membranes.
         (4) damage circulating RBCs, producing microangiopathic hemolytic anemia (MHA) with schistocytes (see Chapter 12).
      c. Activation of the fibrinolytic system (secondary fibrinolysis) caused by activation of plasminogen by factor XII. FDPs interfere with platelet aggregation, which also contributes to bleeding.
   3. Laboratory findings
      a. Coagulation abnormalities in DIC include:
         (1) increase in the PT and PTT.
         (2) decrease in serum FNG.
      b. Platelet abnormalities in DIC include:
         (1) thrombocytopenia.
         (2) increased BT.
      c. Fibrinolysis abnormalities include the presence of FDPs and D-dimers. Negative D-dimers *excludes* DIC.
      d. Normocytic anemia in DIC is caused by:
         (1) extensive bleeding from the skin and GI tract.
         (2) mechanical damage to RBCs by fibrin thrombi, causing MHA with schistocytes (fragmented RBCs, see Chapter 12).
   4. Most important treatment is to correct the underlying cause of DIC!

IV. Fibrinolytic Disorders
A. Primary fibrinolysis
1. **Definition:** Disorder characterized by activation of the fibrinolytic system
2. Causes include:
   a. cardiopulmonary bypass (e.g., open heart surgery). Cardiopulmonary bypass causes a decrease in α_2-antiplasmin and an increase in tPA.
   b. radical prostatectomy. Surgery causes increased release of urokinase, which activates plasminogen.
   c. cirrhosis. Decrease in hepatic synthesis of α_2-antiplasmin.
3. Pathogenesis of primary fibrinolysis
   a. FDPs interfere with platelet aggregation.
   b. Plasmin degrades coagulation factors, causing multiple factor deficiencies.
4. Clinical findings include severe bleeding from multiple sites.
5. Laboratory findings include:
   a. increased PT and PTT caused by multiple coagulation factor deficiencies.
   b. increased BT caused by interference with platelet aggregation.
   c. positive test result for FDPs.
   d. *negative* D-dimer assay because *no* fibrin thrombi are present. D-dimer assay is positive in DIC.
   e. normal platelet count. Platelet count is decreased in DIC.
B. Secondary fibrinolysis
1. **Definition:** A compensatory fibrinolytic reaction usually associated with DIC
2. Increase in both FDPs and D-dimers. Recall that in primary fibrinolysis, D-dimers are *not* present.
3. Platelets are decreased (trapped in fibrin clots). Recall that in primary fibrinolysis, platelets are *not* decreased.
V. Summary of Laboratory Test Results in Hemostasis Disorders (Table 15-4)
VI. Thrombosis Syndromes
A. Acquired thrombosis syndromes
1. Antiphospholipid syndrome (APLS)
   a. **Definition:** APLS is an acquired thrombosis syndrome characterized by the clinical features associated with arterial and/or venous thrombosis. The hypercoagulable state is related to the presence of at least one type of antiphospholipid antibody (APA). The antibodies are directed against serum proteins bound to anionic phospholipids in endothelial tissue.
   b. Epidemiology
      (1) APLS is commonly associated with SLE. Approximately 40% of patients with SLE have APL antibodies; however, only 40% of these patients present with a thrombosis syndrome.
      (2) Other disease associations include rheumatoid arthritis (RA), Sjögren syndrome (SS), immune thrombocytopenic purpura (ITP), and HIV infection.
      (3) Most affected persons are young to middle-aged adults.
      (4) Both venous (most common) and arterial thrombi may occur.
      (5) Livedo reticularis is a characteristic finding (Link 15-23).

Fibrinolytic disorders

Primary fibrinolysis

Activation of fibrinolytic system

Cardiopulmonary bypass

$\downarrow \alpha_2$-antiplasmin, $\uparrow$TPA

Radical prostatectomy (urokinase)

Cirrhosis ($\downarrow$serum α_2-antiplasmin)

FDPs $\rightarrow$ $\downarrow$platelet aggregation

Multiple factor deficiencies (plasmin effect)

Bleeding multiple sites

$\uparrow$PT, PTT: factor deficiencies

$\uparrow$BT: interference with platelet aggregation

$\uparrow$FDPs

Negative D-dimers (*no* fibrin thrombi)

Normal platelet count

Secondary fibrinolysis

Compensatory reaction in DIC

$2°$ Fibrinolysis: $\uparrow$FDPs + D-dimers

$1°$ fibrinolysis: $\uparrow$FDPs *no* D-dimers

$2°$ fibrinolysis: $\downarrow$platelets (fibrin clots)

$1°$ fibrinolysis: platelets normal

Thrombosis syndromes

Acquired thrombosis syndromes

Antiphospholipid syndrome

Arterial and/or venous thrombi

Hypercoagulable state

APL ab directed against anionic phospholipids in endothelial tissue

Commonly associated with SLE

RA, SS, ITP, HIV infection

Young/middle-aged adults

Venous (MC) and arterial thrombi

TABLE 15-4 Laboratory Findings in Common Hemostasis Disorders

DISORDER	PLATELET COUNT	BLEEDING TIME	PT	PTT
Thrombocytopenia	$\downarrow$	$\uparrow$	Normal	Normal
von Willebrand disease	Normal	$\uparrow$	Normal	$\uparrow$
Hemophilia A	Normal	Normal	Normal	$\uparrow$
Disseminated intravascular coagulation	$\downarrow$	$\uparrow$	$\uparrow$	$\uparrow$
Primary fibrinolysis	Normal	$\uparrow$	$\uparrow$	$\uparrow$
Aspirin or NSAIDs	Normal	$\uparrow$	Normal	Normal
Warfarin or heparin	Normal	Normal	$\uparrow$	$\uparrow$

NSAID, Nonsteroidal antiinflammatory drug; *PT,* prothrombin time; *PTT,* partial thromboplastin time.

APAs: against − charge phospholipids

APA: ACA antibodies

False + syphilis serologic test
APA: LA
APA: Anti−β₂-Gp 1 antibody

APAs: venous thrombi > arterial thrombi

All APAs present, high titers, LA
↑Tissue factor release (infection, surgery)
Abnormal endothelium (vasculitis)
Atherosclerosis/DM, HTN, ↑lipids
Smoking, pregnancy, homocystinuria, OCPs
Hx previous thrombosis/ fetal loss
Clinical findings
Venous thrombosis: deep veins calf MC site
Veins (renal, hepatic, axillary, subclavian, retina, vc), placental bed thromboses
Livedo reticularis
Capillary thrombi with dilated venules
Arterial thrombosis sites
Cerebral arteries MC site
Coronary, renal, mesenteric, by-pass arteries
FP syphilis serology (ACA abs)
+RPR/VRDL but -FTA-ABS
LA present 80%
↑PTT *not* corrected with mixing studies
ACAs most sensitive/specific test
Anti-β₂-Gp 1 antibodies
Postoperative state
Malignancy
↑Coagulation factors
Reactive thrombosis
Release tumor procoagulants
↑Homocysteine: folic acid/ B₁₂ deficiency
OCPs: E ↑ coagulation factor synthesis, ↓ATIII
Hyperviscosity syndromes
PV, WM
Hereditary thrombosis syndromes
AD syndromes
DVT/PE early age
Venous thrombosis hepatic vein, dural sinuses

c. Pathogenesis
(1) APAs are directed against negatively charged phospholipids bound to plasma proteins.
(2) APAs include:
  (a) anticardiolipin antibody (ACA). Also reacts with the cardiolipin reagent in the rapid plasma reagin (RPR) test for syphilis, causing a false-positive syphilis serology.
  (b) lupus anticoagulant (LA).
  (c) anti−β_2-Gp 1 antibody.
(3) APAs produce arterial and venous thrombosis syndromes.
  (a) Venous thrombi are more common than arterial thrombi.
  (b) Possible mechanisms include resistance to protein C, impaired fibrinolysis, and EC injury with activation of platelets.
b. Factors that increase risk for thrombosis in a patient with APAs include:
(1) antibody characteristics: all three APL antibodies are present, high titers of antibody (>40 units), LA.
(2) increased release of tissue factor: infection, surgery.
(3) abnormal endothelium: vasculitis or inflammatory disease (e.g., SLE).
(4) atherosclerosis and risk factors (diabetes mellitus [DM], HTN, hyperlipidemia).
(5) prothrombotic risk factors: smoking, pregnancy, hereditary hypercoagulable disorders (e.g., homocystinuria), OCPs.
(6) history of previous thrombosis or fetal loss.
c. Clinical findings
(1) Venous thrombosis; vessels commonly involved include:
  (a) deep veins in the calf (most common site).
  (b) renal, hepatic, axillary, subclavian, and retinal veins; vena cava (vc); and the placental bed (recurrent spontaneous abortions).
  (c) skin (livedo reticularis; Link 15-23). Refers to a net-like discoloration of the skin that is caused by swelling of the venules owing to obstruction of capillaries by small blood clots.
(2) Arterial thrombosis sites include:
  (a) cerebral vessels (most common site; produces strokes).
  (b) coronary, renal, mesenteric, and bypass arteries.
d. Laboratory findings
(1) False-positive syphilis serologic test result
  (a) Occurs if ACAs are present
  (b) ACA antibodies react with beef cardiolipin in the test system for RPR and VDRL (Venereal Disease Research Laboratory); however, the FTA-ABS (fluorescent treponeme antibody-absorption) test result is negative.
(2) LA is present in >80% of cases. Produces an increased PTT that does *not* correct with mixing studies (see previous discussion).
(3) ACAs are present; most sensitive and specific test for the APLS.
(4) Anti−β_2-Gp 1 antibodies are present.
2. Other acquired causes of thrombosis include:
a. postoperative state with stasis of blood flow.
b. malignancy.
(1) Increased synthesis of coagulation factors in malignancy
(2) Reactive thrombocytosis may occur.
(3) Release of procoagulants from tumors, particularly pancreatic cancers
c. folic acid and/or vitamin B_{12} deficiency (see Chapter 12). Deficiency of either is accompanied by an increased plasma homocysteine level, which damages endothelial tissue. Hyperhomocysteinemia is associated with an increased risk for thrombosis.
d. OCPs. Estrogen (E) increases the synthesis of coagulation factors and decreases the concentration of AT III.
e. hyperviscosity syndromes (e.g., PV) (see Chapter 13) and Waldenström macroglobulinemia (WM; see Chapter 13).
B. Hereditary thrombosis syndromes
1. Epidemiology
a. Autosomal dominant (AD) syndromes
b. DVT and pulmonary emboli (PE) commonly occur at an early age.
c. Venous thromboses often occur in unusual places. Examples: hepatic vein and dural sinus.

2. Factor V Leiden
   a. **Definition:** Mutant form of factor V that *cannot* be degraded by activated protein C
   b. Most common hereditary thrombosis syndrome; occurs in 2% to 8% of the white population
   c. Heterozygotes for the disease have an increased risk for thrombosis by a factor of 5 to 10, but the risk for thrombosis in homozygotes is increased by a factor of 50 to 100.
3. Antithrombin III (ATIII) deficiency
   a. Normal functions of ATIII
      (1) ATIII activity is normally enhanced by heparin and heparin-like molecules.
      (2) Neutralizes activated serine proteases, which include factors II, VII, IX, X, XI, and XII.
   b. Therefore, when ATIII is deficient, the above factors are *not* neutralized and the person is thrombogenic.
   c. In ATIII deficiency, there is *no* increase in the PTT after injecting a *standard* dose of heparin because there is little or no ATIII to enhance. Will increase if greater doses of heparin are given. This is a major clinical clue that a person with a thrombosis syndrome has ATIII deficiency.
4. Proteins C and S deficiency.
   a. Pathogenesis of protein C and S deficiency
      (1) Recall that the *normal* function of protein C and S is to *inhibit* factors V and VIII.
      (2) Therefore, in patients with proteins C and/or S deficiency, the activated factors V and VIII are *not* inhibited; thus, these patients are hypercoagulable and at risk of thrombotic events.

There is a potential for heterozygote carriers of protein C deficiency to develop hemorrhagic skin necrosis when placed on warfarin. Heterozygote carriers have ~50% protein C activity. Protein C has a short half-life (~6 hours). When these patients are placed on warfarin, protein C activity falls to zero in 6 hours, causing a temporary hypercoagulable state because of increased activity of factors V and VIII. This causes cutaneous vessel thrombosis and concomitant hemorrhagic skin necrosis. This complication is *not* likely to occur in normal people.

Factor V Leiden

Mutant factor V; protein C *cannot* degrade

MC hereditary thrombosis syndrome

Heterozygotes/homozygotes at risk for thrombosis

ATIII deficiency

Normal ATIII functions

Enhanced by heparin/heparin-like molecules

Neutralizes activated II, VII, IX, X, XI, XII

Activated factors *not* neutralized in ATIII deficiency

Normal PTT after *standard* dose of heparin

Proteins C and S deficiency

Protein C/S *inhibit* factors V/VIII

Hemorrhagic skin necrosis: associated with warfarin therapy in protein C or S deficiency.

ABBREVIATIONS

MC most common   MCC most common cause

ABO antigens

Glycoproteins in RBC membranes

Group O

Group O: MC blood group

Group O: lack blood group antigens on RBC surface

Group O: anti-A IgM, anti-B IgM, anti-A IgG, anti-B IgG

I. ABO Blood Group Antigens
A. Definition of ABO blood group antigens
- ABO blood group antigens are glycoproteins that are attached to the red blood cell (RBC) surface as well as other tissues throughout the body (Link 16-1).

B. Blood group O characteristics
1. Blood group O is the most common blood group. *No* blood group antigens (A or B) are present on the RBC membrane.
2. All blood group O individuals have anti-A IgM and anti-B IgM natural antibodies (isohemagglutinins) in the serum (Link 16-1). They lack blood group antigens (A and B) on the surface of RBCs; therefore, the anti-A and anti-B antibodies cannot attach to the RBCs and destroy them. For unknown reasons, most blood group O individuals also have anti-A and anti-B IgG antibodies in their serum.

Blood group antibodies are natural antibodies that are synthesized in Peyer patches after birth. A and B antigens that are normally present in food are trapped by M cells, which are specialized epithelial cells that overlie Peyer patches. **M cells** transport the A and/or B antigens to B lymphocytes in Peyer patches, resulting in the development of natural antibodies against the antigens. Natural antibodies develop against antigens that are *not* present on the RBC, which explains why blood group O persons have antibodies against both A and B antigens.

M cells: A/B antigens in Peyer patches to B lymphocytes

Group O: duodenal ulcer risk

Group A: anti-B IgM

↑Gastric cancer risk

Group B: anti-A IgM

Group AB

Least common ABO blood group

Group AB: *no* natural antibodies

NBs: lack natural abs at birth

NBs: begin to develop abs 3-6 mths

Elderly frequently lose natural antibodies

3. Blood group O individuals have an increased incidence of duodenal ulcers. This may relate to the absence of A or B antigens on the mucosal cells, which have a protective effect on preventing acid injury.

C. Blood group A characteristics
1. Blood group A individuals have A antigens on the surface of RBCs and anti-B IgM natural antibodies in their serum (Link 16-1).
2. For unknown reasons, blood group A individuals have an increased incidence of gastric carcinoma.

D. Blood group B characteristics
- Blood group B individuals have B antigens on the surface of RBCs and anti-A IgM natural antibodies in their serum (Link 16-1).

E. Blood group AB characteristics
1. Least common of the ABO blood groups.
2. Blood group AB individuals have both blood group A and B antigens on the surface of RBCs and *no* natural antibodies (Link 16-1).

F. Newborns (NBs)
1. Newborns do *not* have natural antibodies in their serum at birth (Link 16-2).
2. They begin to develop these antibodies 3 to 6 months after birth.

G. Older adults
- Older adults frequently lose their natural antibodies.

	B	O	Father
Mother	A	AB	AO
	O	BO	**OO**

16-1: Possible phenotypes of children if the father is BO and the mother is AO. AB parents cannot have a blood group O child. O parents cannot have an A, B, or AB child. *(Adapted from Goljan EF: Star Series: Pathology, Philadelphia, Saunders, 1998.)*

	Forward Type		Back Type	
Blood group	Anti-A	Anti-B	A RBCs	B RBCs
O	−	−	+	+
A	+	−	−	+
B	−	+	+	−
AB	+	+	−	−

16-2: Forward and back type to identify ABO blood groups. Forward type identifies the blood group antigen by reacting test anti-A and anti-B antibodies against patient red blood cells (RBCs). Back type identifies the natural antibodies in the patient serum by reacting test blood group A RBCs and B RBCs against the patient serum. Refer to the text for discussion of the blood groups and their natural antibodies.

Older individuals may *not* have a hemolytic transfusion reaction (HTR) if they are transfused with the wrong blood group because they frequently lose their natural antibodies. However, this does *not* mean that older adults can safely receive blood from any blood group.

H. **Paternity issues in newborns**
   1. Blood group AB parents *cannot* have an O child.
   2. Blood group O parents *cannot* have an AB, A, or B child.
   3. Blood group A and B parents can have O children in the presence of AO and BO genotypes (Fig. 16-1).
I. **Determining an individual's ABO group in the laboratory**
   1. Forward type (Fig. 16-2; Link 16-3)
      a. **Definition:** Identifies an individual's blood group antigens; determined by placing an individual's RBCs into separate test tubes that contain either anti-A or anti-B test serum
      b. If an agglutination reaction occurs with anti-A test serum but *not* anti-B test serum, the individual is blood group A.
      c. If an agglutination reaction occurs with anti-B test serum but *not* anti-A test serum, the individual is blood group B.
      d. If an agglutination reaction occurs with anti-A test serum and anti-B test serum, the individual is blood group AB.
      e. If an agglutination reaction does *not* occur with either anti-A test serum or anti-B test serum, the individual is blood group O.
   2. Back type.
      a. **Definition:** Identifies the natural antibodies that are present in an individual's serum. Back type is determined by placing a sample of an individual's serum into test tubes that contain either A, B, or O test RBCs.
      b. If the serum agglutinates B test RBCs but *not* A test RBCs, the individual is blood group A, who normally have anti-B IgM natural antibodies.
      c. If the serum agglutinates A test RBCs but *not* B test RBCs, the individual is blood group B, who normally have anti-A-IgM natural antibodies.
      d. If the serum does *not* agglutinate either A test RBCs or B test RBCs, the individual is blood group AB, who do *not* have natural antibodies.
      e. If the serum agglutinates both A test RBCs and B test RBCs, the individual is blood group O, who normally have anti-A IgM and anti-B IgM natural antibodies.
   3. All possible genotypes for offspring of parents with each allelic contribution (Link 16-4)
II. **Rh and Non-Rh Antigen Systems**
   A. **Rh antigen system**
      1. Rh antigen system has three adjoining gene loci coding for D antigen (there is *no* d antigen), C and c antigen, and, E and e antigen.
      2. Rh antigen system has an autosomal codominant inheritance pattern.
         a. One of the sets of three Rh antigens from each parent is transmitted to each child (Fig. 16-3). The absence of D antigen on a chromosome is designated d even though the antigen does *not* exist.
         b. Possible Rh antigen profiles include DD, Dd, or dd; CC, Cc, or cc; or, EE, Ee, or ee.

Paternity issues

AB parents *cannot* have O child

O parents *cannot* have AB, A, B child

A and B parents → O children (AO and BO)

Forward type

Identifies blood group

Anti-A, anti-B test serum in tubes

Reaction anti-A: blood group A

Reaction anti-B: blood group B

Reaction anti-A and B: blood group AB

No reaction: blood group O

Back type

Back type identifies natural antibodies

A, B, O test RBCs in tubes

Rh antigen system

D, C, c, E, e; no d antigen

Autosomal codominant inheritance

Antigens: D, C, c, E, e

	cde	CDE	Father
Mother cDe	cDe/cde	cDe/CDE	
CDE	CDE/cde	CDE/CDE	

16-3: Possible Rh genotypes in children if the father is cde or CDE and the mother is cDE or CDE. *(Adapted from Goljan EF:* Star Series: Pathology, *Philadelphia, Saunders, 1998.)*

Rh+: D antigen +

Rh-: lack D antigen

Alloimmunization

Antibodies present against foreign RBC antigens

Abs against foreign antigen: called atypical

Atypical antibodies: may produce HTR

Patient has ab against foreign RBC ag; presence of ag produces HTR

Must receive blood lacking the antigen

Duffy (Fy) antigens

Binding site for *P. vivax*

Majority black population lack Fy antigen → protection *P. vivax* malaria

Parvovirus binds P antigen → pure RBC aplasia

I and i antigens

I, i antigens cold agglutinins, natural antigens on RBCs

Cold IHA

Anti-I cold IHA *M. pneumoniae* infection, anti-i mononucleosis

P antigen → PCH

Blood transfusion

Blood donors

Autologous transfusion

Transfusion with person's own blood

Safest transfusion

ABO, Rh type

ABS (indirect Coombs test)

ABS: detects atypical abs in donor blood

3. Individual who is Rh positive is D antigen positive.
   a. Approximately 85% of the population has D antigen.
   b. Individual who lacks the D antigen is considered Rh negative.
4. Testing for an individual's Rh phenotype
   a. Individuals RBCs are reacted with test antisera against each of the Rh antigens.
   b. Example: If an individual is positive for c, D, and E antigens but negative for C and e antigen, they have a DcE phenotype and most likely a DcE/DcE genotype (Link 16-5).

B. **Alloimmunization**
   1. **Definition:** The production of an antibody in the individual's serum that is directed against a foreign antigen that is *not* present on an individual's RBCs. For example, an individual may be exposed to an Rh antigen that he is lacking (e.g., D antigen) or a non-Rh antigen that he is lacking (e.g., Kell antigen).
   2. Antibodies that develop against foreign antigens are called *atypical* antibodies. An individual is considered to be *sensitized* if atypical antibodies are present in his or her serum.
   3. Clinical significance of alloimmunization
      a. Atypical antibodies may produce a life-threatening hemolytic transfusion reaction (HTR) during or shortly after a blood transfusion.
         (1) HTRs occur when blood containing a foreign RBC antigen (ag) is infused into an individual that has been previously sensitized against that antigen.
         (2) Example: An individual with anti-Kell antibodies in her serum is exposed to Kell antigen–positive RBCs in a blood transfusion and develops an HTR, leading to destruction of those transfused RBCs.
      b. If an individual has one or more atypical antibodies, he must receive blood with RBCs that are *lacking* the foreign RBC antigen(s) to which the individual has developed atypical antibodies. Example: An individual with anti-Kell antibodies must receive blood that is negative for the Kell RBC antigen.

C. **Clinically important non-Rh antigens**
   1. Duffy (Fy) antigens
      a. Fy antigens on RBCs are the binding site for infestation of RBCs by *Plasmodium vivax.*
      b. The majority of the black population lack the Fy antigen, which offers them protection from contracting *P. vivax* malaria.
   2. Parvoviruses bind to P antigens on RBCs, causing pure RBC aplasia (see Chapter 12).
   3. I and i antigen systems
      a. IgM antibodies (cold agglutinins) from an infection may develop against I or i antigens. They are natural antigens that are normally present on the surface of an individual's RBCs. When these antibodies react against the I or i antigens on the individual's RBCs, they produce a cold immune hemolytic anemia (IHA) with intravascular hemolysis (see Chapter 12).
      b. Two infections that may induce production of these antibodies, leading to a cold IHA, are infectious mononucleosis (may produce anti-i IgM antibodies) and *Mycoplasma pneumoniae* pneumonia (may produce anti-I IgM antibodies).
   4. A patient with P antigen on the surface of their RBCs may develop paroxysmal cold hemoglobinuria (PCH; see Chapter 12).

III. **Blood Transfusion Therapy**
   A. **Blood donors**
      1. Autologous transfusion
         a. **Definition:** The process of collection, storage, and reinfusion of a person's own blood
         b. Safest form of blood transfusion
      2. Tests normally performed in blood banks on donor blood include:
         a. group (ABO) and type (Rh).
         b. antibody screen (ABS; indirect Coombs test; see Chapter 12). The screen detects atypical RBC antibodies that may be present in the serum of the donor blood (e.g., anti-D, anti-Kell).

c. screening tests for infectious disease. Screening tests are available for syphilis, hepatitis B and C, HIV-1 and HIV-2, West Nile virus, and human T-lymphotropic virus type 1 (HTLV-1), to name a few.

Screening tests for infectious disease

There is a risk for **transmitting infection when transfusing blood** because there is an incubation period *before* specific antibodies are developed against the pathogen. The risk for developing an infection per unit of blood in the post–nucleic acid testing era has markedly reduced the risk for transmission of hepatitis B, hepatitis C, and HIV. The most common infectious agent transmitted by blood transfusion is cytomegalovirus (CMV), which is present in donor lymphocytes. Because a newborn's cellular immunity is *not* fully developed, a CMV infection would likely become disseminated. For this reason, a newborn must be transfused with either CMV-seronegative or leukocyte-reduced blood. The term "leukocyte-reduced" means that the blood unit was filtered to remove the WBCs (removal of WBCs from the unit removes the lymphocytes that might contain CMV).

NB transfusion: must give CMV-seronegative or leukocyte-reduced RBCs; CMV: MC pathogen transmitted by transfusion

B. **Patient crossmatch (CX) for a blood transfusion**
1. Components of a standard CX for an individual that is going to receive a blood transfusion include ABO group and Rh type, ABS to detect atypical RBC antibodies in the individual receiving the transfusion, direct Coombs test to identify atypical IgG antibodies on the persons RBCs, and the major CX.
2. Major CX
   a. **Definition:** Detects atypical antibodies in the individual receiving a blood transfusion that are directed against foreign antigens on donor RBCs from each individual RBC transfusion.
   b. Patient serum in a test tube is mixed with a sample of RBCs from a donor unit.
      (1) Each unit of donor blood must have a separate major CX.
      (2) Lack of RBC agglutination or hemolysis indicates a compatible CX (i.e., there are no atypical antibodies in the patient directed against donor RBC antigens).

Patient crossmatch
ABO, Rh type
ABS
Direct Coombs test
Major CX
Major CX: Patient serum + donor RBCs
Detects atypical abs in individual receiving blood
Each unit donor blood has separate major CX
Lack of agglutination → compatible CX

If a patient has a negative ABS to detect atypical RBC antibodies, the major CX should be compatible. However, a compatible CX does *not* guarantee that the recipient will *not* develop atypical antibodies, a transfusion reaction, or an infection.

Negative ABS ensures that major CX will be compatible.

3. Use of packed RBCs of blood group O for transfusion (Link 16-6)
   a. If absolutely necessary, blood group O packed RBCs (Table 16-1) can be transfused into any patient, regardless of the blood group.
   b. Blood group O RBCs lack A and B antigens; therefore, blood recipients with anti-A IgM and/or anti-B IgM natural antibodies *cannot* destroy the O RBCs.
   c. Blood group O individuals are considered universal donors.
   d. However, as a general rule, group A, B, and AB individuals should receive blood that matches their blood group.

O packed RBCs can be transfused into any person

Blood group O individuals universal donors
Group A, B, AB should receive blood matching their blood group

TABLE 16-1 Blood Components

COMPONENT	DISCUSSION
Packed RBCs	• Purpose: Increase O_2 transport to tissues. • Packed RBCs have less volume and a higher Hct than does whole blood. • Each unit of packed RBCs should raise the Hb by 1 g/dL and the Hct by 3%. • Lack of an increment implies a hemolytic transfusion reaction or continued blood loss in the patient. • *Yersinia enterocolitica,* a pathogen that thrives on iron, is the most common contaminant of stored blood.
Platelets	• Purpose: Stop medically significant bleeding related to thrombocytopenia or qualitative platelet defects (e.g., aspirin). • Platelets have HLA antigens and ABO antigens on their surfaces; however, they lack Rh antigens. • Each unit of platelets should raise the platelet count by 5000–10,000 cells/mm³. If the count is not increasing, they are most likely being consumed (e.g., DIC).
Fresh frozen plasma	• Purpose: treatment of multiple coagulation deficiencies (e.g., DIC, cirrhosis) or treatment of warfarin overanticoagulation if bleeding is life threatening. It contains previously γ-carboxylated vitamin K–dependent factors as well as all the other coagulation factors.
Cryoprecipitate	• Purpose: treatment of coagulation factor deficiencies involving fibrinogen or factor VIII (e.g., DIC) • Cryoprecipitate contains fibrinogen, factor VIII, and factor XIII. • Desmopressin acetate is used instead of cryoprecipitate in treating mild hemophilia A and vWD.

DIC, Disseminated intravascular coagulation; *Hb,* hemoglobin; *Hct,* hematocrit; *HLA,* human leukocyte antigen; *RBC,* red blood cell; *vWD,* von Willebrand disease.

4. Blood group AB patients can be transfused with blood from any blood group.
   a. Blood group AB patients lack natural antibodies in their serum.
   b. Blood group AB individuals are considered universal recipients.
   c. However, as a general rule, AB patients who require a transfusion should receive AB blood, if available.

Before blood is transfused into patients with T-cell deficiencies, it must be irradiated to kill donor lymphocytes. This prevents the patient from developing a graft-versus-host reaction (see Chapter 4) or a disseminated CMV infection. Criteria have been established for whether newborns should receive irradiated blood.

C. **Blood component therapy** (see Table 16-1)
D. **Blood transfusion reactions**
1. Allergic transfusion reactions
   a. **Definition:** Type I IgE-mediated hypersensitivity reaction (HSR) against proteins (allergens) present in the donor blood. Allergic reactions are the most common type of transfusion reaction.
   b. Pathophysiology
      (1) Because the patient has been previously sensitized to an allergen that is present in donor blood, IgE antibodies are already present on the patient's mast cells (see Chapter 4).
      (2) Exposure to the allergen from the donor blood leads to crosslinking of IgE antibodies specific for the allergen on the mast cell membranes in the patient.
      (3) Crosslinking of IgE antibodies triggers the release of mediators from the mast cells. Preformed mediators include histamine, eosinophil chemotactic factor, and serotonin.
   c. Clinical findings include:
      (1) urticaria with pruritus.
      (2) fever, tachycardia, wheezing.
      (3) potential for developing anaphylactic shock.
   d. Mild cases are treated with antihistamines.
   e. See Chapter 4 for a discussion of IgE-mediated allergic transfusion reactions in individuals who are deficient in IgA.
2. Febrile transfusion reaction
   a. **Definition:** Interaction between donor leukocytes and recipient anti–human leukocyte antigen (HLA) antibody leads to interleukin-1 (IL-1) release from donor leukocytes or recipient monocytes. IL-1 can then cause fever by stimulating prostaglandin E_2 production in the hypothalamus.
   b. Clinical findings in a febrile transfusion reaction include fever, chills, headache, and flushing.

Anti-HLA antibodies develop when individuals are exposed to foreign HLA antigens (e.g., leukocytes from a previous blood transfusion or organ transplant). Women commonly have these reactions owing to pregnancy, when there is an increased risk for exposure to fetal blood leukocytes during delivery or after a spontaneous abortion. Recall that there are *no* HLA antigens on RBCs.

3. Acute hemolytic transfusion reaction (HTR)
   a. Intravascular acute HTR (see Chapter 12)
      (1) Most frequently caused by ABO blood group incompatibility
      (2) Example: Group B person receives group A donor blood.
         (a) In this case, anti-A IgM in the recipient attaches to A positive donor RBCs, producing intravascular hemolysis.
         (b) Type II HSR
   b. Extravascular acute HTR (see Chapter 12)
      (1) Most frequently caused by an atypical IgG antibody in the recipient's blood that is reacting against a foreign antigen on donor RBCs
         (a) Rarely occurs because the recipient has had an ABS and major CX with the donor unit, which would have detected the atypical IgG antibody
         (b) In this type of HTR, splenic macrophages (MPs) phagocytose and destroy donor RBCs coated by the atypical IgG antibody (type II HSR).
      (2) Jaundice commonly occurs. Recall that unconjugated bilirubin (UCB) is the end-product of MP degradation of hemoglobin (Hb).

Margin notes (left column):

AB individuals universal recipients; lack isohemagglutinins

Group AB individuals: universal recipients

T cell deficiency: irradiate blood to prevent GVH, CMV

Allergic transfusion reactions

IgE-mediated; MC transfusion reaction

IgE ab on patient mast cells

Exposure to allergen: cross-links with IgE

Mast cell release histamine and preformed mediators

Urticaria/pruritus

Fever, tachycardia, wheezing

Potential for anaphylactic shock

Febrile transfusion reaction

Anti-HLA antibodies against donor leukocytes; type II HSR

Fever, chills, flushing

Anti-HLA antibodies: previous exposure to HLA antigens (blood transfusion, transplant)

Acute HTR

Intravascular HTR

MCC ABO blood group incompatibility

IgM-mediated destruction donor RBCs; type II HSR

Extravascular HTR

Atypical IgG ab reacts against foreign antigen on donor RBCs

ABS screen, major CX prevent this reaction

Splenic MPS phagocytose/ destroy RBC with IgG on their surface; type II HSR

Jaundice common

Individuals who have been infused with blood in the past may have been exposed to a foreign blood group antigen and developed atypical antibodies that are no longer circulating. In this case, the pretransfusion ABS result is negative. However, memory B cells are present, and reexposure to the foreign antigen causes them to produce antibodies, resulting in an extravascular hemolytic anemia. This reaction may occur within hours or as long as 3 to 10 days after the transfusion.

   c. Clinical findings in acute HTRs include fever, back pain, and hypotension.

   Acute HTR: fever, back pain, hypotension

   d. Potential complications in acute HTRs include disseminated intravascular coagulation (DIC; see Chapter 15) and acute renal failure (ARF).

   Complications: DIC, ARF

   e. Laboratory findings include:

   (1) positive direct Coombs test result on the recipient's RBCs (see Chapter 12).

   Positive direct Coombs test recipient RBCs

   (a) IgG antibody and/or C3b is coating the donor RBCs.

   Detection IgG and/or C3b on surface of donor RBCs

   (b) Positive direct Coombs test result is present in either intravascular or extravascular hemolysis.

   (2) positive indirect Coombs test result of the recipient's serum (see Chapter 12).

   Positive indirect Coombs test recipient's serum

   (a) Detects the atypical antibody in the recipient's serum

   Detects atypical ab in recipient's serum

   (b) Positive indirect Coombs test result is present in either intravascular or extravascular hemolysis.

   (3) *no* significant increase in Hb over pretransfusion levels; present in both intravascular and extravascular hemolysis.

   No significant increase in Hb (sign of hemolysis)

   (4) hemoglobinuria; mainly present in intravascular hemolysis.

   Hemoglobinuria (intravascular)

   (5) jaundice; mainly present in extravascular hemolysis.

   Jaundice (extravascular)

4. Actions that should be taken with a suspected transfusion reaction

   a. Immediately stop the blood transfusion.

   Stop blood transfusion!!!!

   b. Keep the intravenous (IV) line in place and infuse normal saline.

   Keep IV line open with normal saline

   c. Send the unit of blood back to the blood bank STAT for a transfusion reaction workup to identify the type of transfusion reaction.

   STAT transfusion reaction workup on unit

IV. Hemolytic Disease of the Newborn (HDN)

   Hemolytic disease of newborn

A. Definition of HDN

   • The transplacental passage of maternal IgG antibodies into the fetus, resulting in varying degrees of extravascular hemolytic anemia (EHA) with unconjugated hyperbilirubinemia (UCB) or intravascular hemolysis in the newborn depending on the type of hemolytic disease

   Transplacental passage maternal IgG abs into fetus → EHA with jaundice

B. ABO HDN (Fig. 16-4 A)

   ABO HDN

   1. **Definition:** Hemolysis of neonatal RBCs secondary to incompatibility between a type O mother and a type A or B newborn

   Incompatibility between O mother and A or B NB

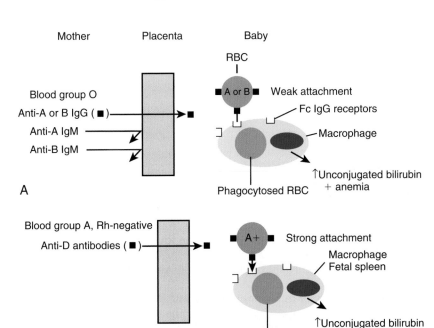

16-4: **A,** ABO hemolytic disease of the newborn (HDN). The mother is blood group O, and the baby is blood group A or B. Anti-A and anti-B IgG from the mother cross the placenta and attach to fetal blood group A or B red blood cells (RBCs). Sensitized RBCs are phagocytosed and destroyed by splenic macrophages (MPs), producing anemia and unconjugated hyperbilirubinemia (UCB). **B,** Rh HDN. The mother is Rh negative, and the baby is Rh positive. Anti–D IgG antibodies from a previously sensitized mother cross the placenta and attach to the fetal Rh-positive RBCs. Fetal RBCs are destroyed by lysozymes from MPs or natural killer cells (not shown), or they are phagocytosed and destroyed by MPs, producing anemia and UCB. *(From Goljan EF: Star Series: Pathology, Philadelphia, Saunders, 1998, Fig. 14-1.)*

2. Epidemiology
   a. Most common HDN. It is present in 20% to 25% of all pregnancies; however, only 10% of the neonates develop hemolysis to the degree that requires treatment.
   b. Mothers are blood group O and the fetus is either blood group A or B.
3. Pathogenesis
   a. Most blood group O individuals have anti-A IgG antibodies and anti-B IgG antibodies.
      (1) IgG anti-A and anti-B antibodies from the mother cross the placenta and attach to fetal blood group A or B RBCs.
         (a) IgG antibodies also attach to A and B antigens in other tissues; therefore, fewer antibodies attach to fetal A or B RBCs, which reduces the risk for hemolysis.
         (b) Because fetal expression of A and B antigen is poor, there are fewer attachment sites for the IgG antibodies, which also reduces the risk for hemolysis.
      (2) Fetal splenic MPs phagocytize antibody-coated RBCs, causing a mild hemolytic process possibly resulting in a mild anemia.
      (3) UCB is the end-product of extravascular hemolysis by the splenic MPs; however, it is readily metabolized by the placenta.
   b. ABO HDN may affect the firstborn or any future pregnancy in which ABO incompatibility exists. There is *no* natural protection against developing ABO hemolytic disease.
4. Clinical and laboratory findings
   a. Jaundice is *not* present at birth. Mild jaundice develops within the first 24 hours after birth.
      (1) Most common cause of jaundice in newborns during this period of time. A newborn liver *cannot* handle the excess bilirubin load because of low levels of glucuronosyltransferase, which is required for conversion of unconjugated to conjugated (water soluble) bilirubin for excretion in the urine.
      (2) Risk for developing severe hemolytic anemia requiring exchange transfusion and the risk for developing bilirubin encephalopathy (kernicterus) are very small compared with Rh HDN. This is true for the following reasons:
         (a) Most anti-A and anti-B antibodies are IgM, which *cannot* cross the placenta.
         (b) Anti-A and anti-B antibodies do *not* bind complement on the fetal RBC membrane.
         (c) A and B antigens in other tissues bind most of the anti-A and anti-B antibodies.
         (d) There are relatively few A and B antigen sites on fetal RBCs to bind the antibodies.
   b. Neonate liver and/or spleen may be slightly enlarged if the degree of RBC hemolysis requires RBC production in other sites (extramedullary erythropoiesis; see Chapter 12).
   c. In most cases, there is at most a mild normocytic anemia.
      (1) If hemolysis is severe, the Hb may be as low as 10 to 12 g/dL.
      (2) Reticulocytes may be increased depending on the severity of the anemia.
   d. Weakly positive direct Coombs test result on the fetal cord blood RBCs. Positive direct Coombs test result is caused by the presence of anti-A and/or anti-B IgG antibodies coating fetal A and/or B RBCs.
   e. Spherocytes are present in the cord blood peripheral smear. It is caused by fetal splenic MP removal of a portion of the RBC membrane in RBCs rather than complete destruction of the RBC after phagocytosis.
5. Treatment
   a. Jaundice is treated with phototherapy (discussed later).
   b. Exchange transfusion is sometimes indicated. In an exchange transfusion, the newborn's blood is removed and replaced with donor blood.

C. Rh HDN
1. **Definition:** Hemolysis of Rh-D antigen positive fetal RBCs caused by IgG Rh D antibodies acquired transplacentally from a sensitized RhD-negative mother
2. **Epidemiology:** uncommon because of preventive measures in Rh-negative women
3. Pathogenesis (Links 16-7 and 16-8)
   a. In Rh HDN, the mother is Rh (D antigen) negative, and the fetus is Rh (D antigen) positive.
   b. Exposure of the Rh-negative mother to Rh-positive fetal RBCs occurs as a result of an asymptomatic fetomaternal hemorrhage (fetal RBCs enter the mothers blood), usually at the time of delivery or less commonly during the third trimester when the cytotrophoblast in the placenta is absent (see Chapter 22 for a discussion of placental anatomy).

Margin notes:

ABO HDN most common HDN

Mother group O, fetus blood group A or B

Most O individuals have anti-A-IgG have anti-B-IgG abs

Maternal IgG anti-A/anti-B cross placenta → attach fetal A or B RBCs

IgG abs may also attach to A/B antigens other tissues

Fetal expression A/B antigen poor; less attachment sites for IgG abs

Fetal splenic MPs phagocytose ab-coated RBCs

Mild hemolytic anemia

↑UCB metabolized by placenta

May affect firstborn/subsequent ABO incompatible pregnancies

No natural protection against ABO HDN

Jaundice 1st 24 hours *after* birth

ABO HDN MCC jaundice in this time period

NB liver ↓ levels glucuronosyltransferase

Risk for severe anemia and kernicterus very small

Neonate liver/spleen may by slightly enlarged

ABO HDN: mild to no anemia

Weakly + direct Coombs test on fetal cord RBCs

Cord blood spherocytes: portion membrane removed by splenic MPs

Rx usually phototherapy

Exchange transfusion some cases

Rh HDN

Hemolysis RhD antigen + fetal RBCs by IgG-RhD abs from mother

Mother Rh (D antigen) negative, fetus Rh (D antigen positive

Mother exposed fetal Rh D antigen (delivery; 3rd trimester)

c. When a mother is exposed to D antigen, she develops anti-D IgG antibodies and is now sensitized for life. Because maternal exposure occurs in the first Rh-incompatible pregnancy, the firstborn child is *not* affected.

d. Subsequent Rh-incompatible pregnancies are at risk for developing Rh HDN (Fig. 16-4 B).

   (1) Anti-D IgG antibodies cross the placenta and strongly attach to fetal Rh-positive RBCs.

   (2) Sensitized fetal RBCs attach to Fc receptors for IgG on MPs in the reticuloendothelial system, particularly those in the spleen.

   (3) Numerous fetal RBCs are attached to these MPs, forming rosettes (fetal RBCs are arranged around the MP to form a cluster that looks like a flower).

       (a) Fetal RBCs are lysed by lysosomal enzymes released by the MPs and/or natural killer cells.

       (b) Fetal RBCs are phagocytosed and destroyed by the MPs. Spherocytes are *not* present because the whole RBC is phagocytosed.

   (4) MP destruction of fetal RBCs produces a severe anemia and an increase in UCB.

       (a) Prolonged hemolysis stimulates fetal erythropoiesis in the liver, spleen, bone marrow (normal sites for erythropoiesis in the fetus), and extramedullary sites, such as the skin and placenta. Hepatosplenomegaly may occur.

       (b) Placenta effectively metabolizes the UCB unless it is overwhelmed.

4. Clinical manifestations

   a. A wide spectrum of clinical manifestations may occur depending on the severity of the hemolysis.

   b. Hydrops fetalis is the most serious manifestation of Rh HDN (Fig. 16-5).

      (1) Marked erythropoiesis in the liver produces hepatic dysfunction manifested as a decrease in albumin synthesis. This decreases plasma oncotic pressure (see Chapter 5), which causes peripheral edema, ascites, and pleural effusions, hence the term *hydrops* (an abnormal collection of fluid).

      (2) Severe anemia produces high-output cardiac failure (see Chapter 11), leading to left-sided heart failure (LHF) with pulmonary edema and right-sided heart failure (RHF), with increased venous pressures contributing to peripheral edema and ascites.

Mother develops anti-D IgG antibodies (sensitized)

Rh HDN: firstborn child *not* affected

Subsequent Rh incompatible pregnancies at risk

Anti-D IgG crosses the placenta → attach to D antigen + fetal RBCs

Splenic MPs phagocytose sensitized fetal RBCs

MP rosettes

Fetal RBC with anti-D are destroyed by splenic MPs

↑MP destruction fetal RBCs → ↑serum UCB, severe anemia; no spherocytes

↑Fetal extramedullary hematopoiesis

Hepatosplenomegaly

Placenta effectively metabolizes UCB

Clinical findings parallel severity of hemolysis

Hydrops fetalis MC serious manifestation RhHDN

Hepatic dysfunction → ↓serum albumin synthesis

↓Plasma oncotic pressure → peripheral edema, ascites, effusions

Severe anemia → high-output cardiac failure → LHF (pulmonary edema)/RHF (peripheral edema, ascites

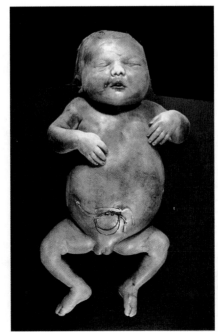

16-5: Hydrops fetalis (erythroblastosis fetalis) in a Rh hemolytic disease of the newborn. The swelling of the peripheral tissue is caused by edema from a decrease in serum albumin (decrease in oncotic pressure) and right-sided heart failure. The increased circumference of the abdomen is due to hepatosplenomegaly from extramedullary hematopoiesis and ascites. *(From my friend Ivan Damjanov, MD, PhD: Pathology for the Health-Related Professions, 2nd ed, Philadelphia, Saunders, 2000, p 60, Fig. 3-17.)*

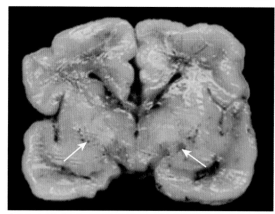

16-6: Cross-section of the brain of a newborn with kernicterus. *Arrows* depict yellow bilirubin pigment deposited in the basal ganglia. Bilirubin is toxic to neurons and produces long-term neurologic sequelae. *(From Kumar V, Fausto N, Abbas A: Robbins and Cotran Pathologic Basis of Disease, 7th ed, Philadelphia, Saunders, 2004.)*

Jaundice *after* birth (UCB)

UCB > in Rh HDN than ABO HDN

Most UCB is free unbound bilirubin

Low albumin levels (hepatic dysfunction)

Kernicterus (bilirubin >20 mg/dL)

Free unbound UCB → brain → kernicterus

Bilirubin neurotoxic; yellow discoloration of the brain

Degree anemia Rh HDN > ABO HDN

Reticulocytosis; accelerated erythropoiesis

↑Cord blood bilirubin

Direct/indirect Coombs test positive

No spherocytes; splenic MPs destroy entire RBC

Exchange transfusions

Removes antibodies/ corrects anemia/removes UCB

c. Jaundice (yellow discoloration of the skin) is a manifestation of the UCB.
   (1) Jaundice develops shortly *after* birth.
   (2) Level of UCB is much higher in Rh HDN than with ABO HDN.
       (a) Most of the UCB is *not* bound to albumin and circulates free in the blood.
       (b) Albumin levels are low because of hepatic dysfunction.
   (3) Increased risk for developing bilirubin encephalopathy (kernicterus), when bilirubin levels are >20 mg/dL.
       (a) Free, unbound, lipid-soluble UCB poses the greatest risk for bilirubin entry into the neonate brain through the poorly developed blood–brain barrier.
       (b) Bilirubin is neurotoxic and binds to lipids in the brain, imparting a yellow discoloration of the basal ganglia, thalamus, cerebellum, gray matter of the cerebral cortex, and spinal cord (Fig. 16-6, Link 16-9).
5. Laboratory findings
   a. Degree of anemia is more severe than with ABO HDN. Reticulocytosis and nucleated RBCs are commonly present in the peripheral blood. These are indicative of accelerated erythropoiesis.
   b. Cord blood bilirubin level is generally 3 to 5 mg/dL.
   c. Results of both direct and indirect Coombs tests on fetal cord RBCs are strongly positive.
   d. Spherocytes are *not* present in the cord blood because splenic MPs phagocytize the entire RBC.
6. Treatment of Rh HDN requires exchange transfusions.
   a. Newborn's blood is removed and replaced with fresh blood.
   b. Transfusion corrects the anemia and removes antibodies and UCB.

ABO incompatibility protects the mother from developing Rh sensitization. For example, in a mother who is O-Rh negative and carrying a fetus who is A-Rh positive, any A-Rh–positive fetal RBCs entering her circulation are destroyed by maternal anti-A IgM antibodies, thereby preventing Rh sensitization. ABO incompatibility is *not* protective if O-Rh–positive fetal RBCs enter the maternal circulation because anti-A or anti-B antibodies cannot destroy O RBCs.

ABO incompatibility: protects mother from Rh sensitization unless newborn is O+

Prevention anti-D globulin

Does *not* cross placenta

Protects mother from sensitization

Lasts ~3 mths in mother

Prevention of Rh HDN: Rh immune globulin (anti-D globulin)

7. Table 16-2 compares Rh HDN and ABO HDN.
8. Prevention of Rh HDN in Rh-negative mothers *without* anti-D.
   a. Women receive anti-D globulin (Rh immune globulin [RhoGAM]) during the 28th week of pregnancy.
   b. Does *not* cross the placenta
   c. Anti-D protects the mother from sensitization to fetal Rh-positive cells that may enter her circulation during the last trimester.
   d. Lasts ~3 months in the mother's blood
   e. Additional anti-D globulin is given to the mother after delivery if the baby is Rh positive.
9. Tests performed on sensitized (anti-D positive) women

TABLE 16-2   Comparison of Rh Hemolytic Disease of the Newborn and ABO Hemolytic Disease of the Newborn

CHARACTERISTICS	RH HEMOLYTIC DISEASE OF NEWBORN	ABO HEMOLYTIC DISEASE OF NEWBORN
Incidence	• Uncommon	• Common
Blood group association	• The mother can be any blood group.	• The mother must be group O, and the baby must be group A or B.
Rh association	• The mother must be Rh negative, and the baby must be Rh positive.	• ABO HDN is protective against Rh sensitization with the exception of an O Rh-positive baby.
Anemia at birth	• Frequent and often severe	• Mild to no anemia at birth • Severe anemia uncommon
Jaundice first 24 hr	• Frequent • Moderate to severe	• Mild
Hepatosplenomegaly	• Common • Sign of accelerated erythropoiesis causing EMH	• Uncommon
First pregnancy	• If the mother is Rh negative and has an Rh-positive baby, the baby is *not* affected, but the mother is at great risk for developing anti-D antibodies unless she receives anti-D globulin.	• The baby can be affected if the mother is blood group O and the baby is blood group A or B.
Later pregnancies	• If the mother has anti-D and the baby is Rh positive, the baby is at risk for Rh HDN.	• Each pregnancy is at risk for ABO HDN if the mother is blood group O.
Direct Coombs test on cord blood	• Strongly positive	• Weakly positive
Indirect Coombs test on cord blood	• Positive	• Usually positive
Spherocytes in the peripheral blood	• *Not* present (RBCs fully phagocytized)	• Present (part of the RBC membrane is removed by MPs)

EMH, Extramedullary hematopoiesis; *HDN,* hemolytic disease of the newborn; *MP,* macrophage; *RBC,* red blood cell.

Special tests (Kleihauer-Betke acid dilution technique) may be performed on the mother's blood to quantitate the amount of fetal RBCs that entered her circulation. This is important so that the appropriate of anti-D globulin is given. Anti-D globulin binds to the D antigen and either masks the antigenic sites or destroys the fetal RBCs to prevent the mother from developing an immune response against the D antigen. If the patient has already developed anti-D antibodies, there is *no* indication for giving the globulin because its main purpose is to prevent sensitization.

    a. Sequential antibody titers and periodic amniocentesis are used to monitor sensitized women.

    b. Amniotic fluid is submitted for spectrophotometric analysis to identify bilirubin pigment.

       (1) Bilirubin has absorbance at a wavelength of 450 nm.

       (2) Δ OD (optical density) 450 value is obtained on the amniotic fluid (AF). Δ OD 450 is the height of the bilirubin spike on the spectrophotometer reading from the baseline.

       (3) Δ OD 450 is sequentially plotted on a Liley chart (Link 16-10). The Liley chart correlates Δ OD 450 with the gestational age of the fetus.

       (4) Chart provides an indication of the severity of RBC hemolysis in the affected fetus.

       (5) Very severe cases at an early gestational age may require an in utero exchange transfusion.

D. Blue fluorescent light or sunlight

    1. Light is used as a treatment of jaundice in the newborn.

    2. UCB in the skin absorbs light energy from blue fluorescent light or sunlight.

    3. Photoisomerization converts the UCB to a nontoxic water-soluble dipyrrole (called lumirubin). Lumirubin is excreted in bile or urine.

Margin notes:

Kleihauer-Betke test detects fetal RBCs in maternal blood

Sequential ab titers; amniocentesis

Sensitized women: amniocentesis; bilirubin absorbance 450 nm

Δ OD 450 plotted on Liley chart

Chart correlates Δ OD 450 with gestational age

Indication degree severity RBC hemolysis

In utero exchange transfusion if severe

Rx jaundice in NB

UCB in skin: absorbs light energy (blue fluorescent light or sunlight)

Blue fluorescent light/ sunlight: converts UCB in skin to water-soluble dipyrrole

ABBREVIATIONS

Dx diagnosis	MC most common	R/O rule out
Hx history	MCC most common cause	

I. Overview of the Respiratory System (Links 17-1 to 17-5)

Human lung development is first marked by a longitudinal groove that appears on the ventral side of the primitive foregut 26 days after fertilization. This separates from the foregut, first at its caudal end, and then progressively forward until a connection is retained only at the cranial end. This bud then bifurcates and grows on either side of the foregut as the embryonic lungs, with successive branching giving rise to the lobar (about 33 days), segmental, and further divisions of the airways (Link 17-1 A). The developing lungs protrude into the coelomic cavity, the mesothelial lining of which forms from the mesoderm about the 14th day of gestation. With the development of the diaphragm and a pleuropericardial membrane the lungs become confined to the pleural cavities. Link 17-1 B shows the normal respiratory system divided into the upper, middle, and lower tract.

(Excerpt taken from Corrin B, Nicholson AG, Burke M, Rice A: *Pathology of the Lungs*, 3rd ed, St. Louis, Churchill Livingstone Elsevier, 2011, pp 39–40.)

Choanal atresia

Failure recanalization of nasal fossae

MC congenital anomaly of nose

MC unilateral, right-sided, females > males

Bony > membranous

Bilateral life-threatening

Nasal catheter blocked at birth

Other congenital anomalies likely

Newborn turns cyanotic when breast-feeding

Crying causes child to "pink up"

Nasal polyps

Non-neoplastic: nose mucous membrane, paranasal sinuses

Response to CI

Adults: MC associated with allergic rhinitis

Eosinophils in nasal smear

II. Symptoms and Signs of Respiratory Disease (Tables 17-1 and 17-2; Link 17-6)

III. Upper Airway Disorders

A. Choanal atresia

1. **Definition:** Congenital cause of nasal obstruction due to a blockage of the back of the nasal passage by bone or soft tissue (membrane) due to failure of recanalization of the nasal fossae during fetal development

2. Epidemiology
   a. Most common congenital anomaly of the nose
   b. More commonly unilateral and right-sided and affects females more than males
   c. More common bony (90%) than membranous (10%)
   d. Because infants are obligate nasal breathers, bilateral choanal atresia is life threatening.
   e. Suspected if a catheter cannot be passed into the nasopharynx at birth
   f. Approximately 50% to 70% affected infants have other congenital anomalies, particularly when bilateral.

3. Newborn turns cyanotic when breastfeeding. Crying causes the child to "pink up" again.

B. Nasal polyps

1. **Definition:** Non-neoplastic soft tissue masses arising mainly from the mucous membranes of the nose and paranasal sinuses. They develop as a response to chronic inflammation (CI).

2. Epidemiology
   a. In adults, are commonly associated with allergic rhinitis (IgE-mediated, see Chapter 4). Nasal smear shows numerous eosinophils.

TABLE 17-1   Common Symptoms of Respiratory Disease

SYMPTOM	CAUSES/DISCUSSION
Dyspnea	**Definition:** Difficulty with breathing Caused by stimulation of J receptors causing decrease in full inspiration Causes: • Decreased compliance (e.g., interstitial fibrosis) • Increased airway resistance (e.g., chronic bronchitis) • Chest bellows disease (e.g., obesity, kyphoscoliosis) • Interstitial inflammation/fluid accumulation (e.g., left-sided heart failure)
Cough	Cough receptors: located at bifurcations in airways, larynx, distal esophagus • Cough with a normal chest radiograph • Postnasal discharge is the most common cause Nocturnal cough with: • GERD: caused by acid reflux in tracheobronchial tree at night • Asthma: caused by bronchoconstriction Productive cough with: • Chronic bronchitis: caused by smoking cigarettes • Typical bacterial pneumonia • Bronchiectasis Drugs causing cough: • ACE inhibitors: inhibit degradation of bradykinin; causes mucosal swelling and irritation in tracheobronchial tree • Aspirin: causes an increase in LT C-D-E_4 (bronchoconstrictors)
Hemoptysis	Coughing up blood-tinged sputum Mechanisms: • Parenchymal necrosis • Bronchial or pulmonary vessel damage • Causes: chronic bronchitis (most common cause), pneumonia, bronchogenic carcinoma, TB, bronchiectasis, aspergilloma (fungus living in a cavitary lesion)

ACE, Angiotensin-converting enzyme; *GERD,* gastroesophageal reflux disease; *LT,* leukotriene; *TB,* tuberculosis.

TABLE 17-2   Signs of Respiratory Disease

SIGN	COMMENTS
Tachypnea	• Normal respiratory rate: 14–20 breaths/min in adults; up to 44 breaths/min in children • Tachypnea: rapid shallow breathing (>20 breaths/min) • Causes: restrictive lung disease; pleuritic chest pain; pulmonary embolus with infarction (key finding)
CHEST PALPATION	
Tracheal shift	• Pressure in pleural space shifts the trachea to the contralateral (opposite) side. Examples: large tension pneumothorax, large pleural effusion • Decreased volume in lung shifts the trachea to the ipsilateral (same) side. Examples: large spontaneous pneumothorax, resorption atelectasis
Vocal tactile fremitus	• Palpable thrill (vibration) transmitted through chest when patient says "E" or "1, 2, 3" or "99" • *Decreased* vocal tactile fremitus occurs with emphysema or asthma because there is trapping of air in the lungs leading to an increase in total lung capacity. This increases the AP diameter of the chest, which is visible with a lateral chest radiograph. • *Absent* vocal tactile fremitus with atelectasis (collapse of airways); large fluid effusion in the pleural cavity; excess air in the pleural space (tension pneumothorax) • *Increased* tactile fremitus: sound travels well through alveolar consolidations (e.g., lobar pneumonia where the alveoli are filled with pus; pulmonary edema where the alveoli are filled with a transudate)
Percussion	• *Dull* percussion with pleural effusion; examples: lung consolidation in lobar pneumonia; atelectasis (collapse of the alveoli caused by a lack of air) • *Hyperresonant* percussion: caused by increased air in the lungs or pleural cavity; examples: pneumothorax; asthma; emphysema
LUNG SOUNDS	
General breath sounds	• Origin for normal breath sounds: trachea • Mechanism: air velocity and turbulence induce vibrations in airway walls. • Sites modifying breath sound: terminal airway and alveolar disease modify breath sounds. Sounds heard with the stethoscope are produced in more central (hilar) regions and are altered in intensity and tonal quality as they pass through pulmonary tissue to the periphery. • Site for normal airway resistance: segmental bronchi (turbulent air flow) • Site for laminar airflow: begins at the bronchioles—"small airways" • Parallel branching: increases cross-sectional area of airways; converts turbulence into laminar airflow • Effects of inflammation of small airways (e.g., asthma, chronic bronchitis): air trapping, wheezing, increased airway resistance

Continued

TABLE 17-2   Signs of Respiratory Disease—cont'd

SIGN	COMMENTS

Tubular breath sounds	• Sound is like blowing air through a tube.
	• Tracheal breath sound: normal sound over lateral neck or suprasternal notch
	• Bronchial breath sounds: always an abnormal sound
	  • Loud, high-pitched sound with a peculiar hollow or tubular quality
	  • Expiratory sounds longer than inspiratory
	  • Significance: consolidation (e.g., lobar or bronchopneumonia)
	  • Mechanism: bronchi must be patent and *partially* collapsed
	  • Associated with an "air bronchogram": air-filled bronchi form silhouette against airless consolidated parenchyma
	
	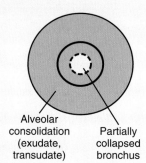
	
	Alveolar consolidation (exudate, transudate) Partially collapsed bronchus

Vesicular breath sounds	• Normal breath sounds: tracheal sounds that are modified (filtered) in alveoli • Sites: most lung fields *except* trachea and central bronchi • Inspiratory:expiratory ratio is 3:1 • Present in normal lungs, chronic bronchitis, emphysema • Diminished in: emphysema and asthma because of increased AP diameter • Absent in: pneumothorax; atelectasis; effusion
Bronchovesicular breath sounds	• Normal breath sounds heard over the main bronchi • Abnormal if heard in the lung periphery • Inspiratory and expiratory breath sounds are equal in length (1:1).
Adventitial sounds	Extra sounds that are normally absent in respiratory cycle
Crackles	• Crackles: usually heard on inspiration. • *Early and mid-inspiratory crackles*: caused by secretions in proximal large to medium-sized airways (e.g., chronic bronchitis); clear with coughing • *Late inspiratory crackles*: caused by reopening of distal airways partially occluded by increased interstitial pressure (e.g., interstitial fluid–pus, transudate in CHF). Do *not* clear with coughing. Vary from fine to coarse. • *Causes*: pulmonary edema; lobar pneumonia; interstitial fibrosis (e.g., sarcoidosis)

Wheezing	• Wheezing: high-pitched musical sound usually heard in expiration
	• Expiration is longer than inspiration.
	• Sometimes present during inspiration and expiration
	• Causes:
	  • Inflammation of segmental bronchi, small airways (e.g., asthma, chronic bronchitis)
	  • Pulmonary edema constricting airway (called cardiac asthma); pulmonary infarction (release of TXA_2 from platelets in embolus causes bronchoconstriction)

Rhonchi	• Low-pitched snoring sound heard during inspiration or expiration caused by secretions in large airways (bronchus, trachea) • Usually clear with coughing • Common in chronic bronchitis
Inspiratory stridor	• Inspiratory stridor: high-pitched inspiratory sound; sign of upper airway obstruction • Causes: epiglottitis (*Haemophilus influenzae*), croup (parainfluenza virus) • Inspiratory and expiratory stridor: sign of fixed upper airway obstruction (e.g., from cancer)
Pleural friction rub	• Pleural friction rub: two inflamed surfaces (pleural and parietal) rub against each other • Timing: rub is heard at the end of inspiration and in the early part of expiration. • Rub disappears: large effusions separate the inflamed surfaces. Holding the breath causes the rub to disappear. Recall that with a pericardial friction rub, holding the breath does *not* eliminate the pericardial friction rub. • Causes: pleuritis caused by cancer, infarction, pneumonia, serositis (SLE)
Grunting in newborns	• Labored breathing; sound created by rhythmic closure of the glottis • Always abnormal after 24 hr • Common finding in RDS
Transmitted voice sounds	• Bronchophony (sound of bronchi) • Normal lung: Spoken syllables or numbers (e.g., "99") are *indistinctly heard* with a stethoscope. • Alveolar consolidation: Syllables or numbers are heard louder and more distinctly with a stethoscope. • Whispered pectoriloquy (Latin for "voice of chest"): Clear and intelligible words (e.g., patient whispering "1, 2, 3") are heard with a stethoscope. • Egophony (Greek for "voice of goat"): patient saying "E" sounds like "A" with a stethoscope
Sputum findings (Link 17-6)	• Pulmonary edema: serous "frothy" pink sputum • Bronchitis, bacterial pneumonia: mucopurulent. If tinged with yellow, consider *Staphylococcus aureus*; tinged with green, think *Pseudomonas aeruginosa*; tinged with red, think *Serratia marcescens*

TABLE 17-2   Signs of Respiratory Disease—cont'd

SIGN	COMMENTS
Chest pain	**Adults:** • **Cardiac:** angina pectoris, Prinzmetal angina, unstable angina, coronary insufficiency, MI, nonobstructive-nonspastic angina, mitral valve prolapse, myocarditis • **Aortic:** aortic dissection • **Pleuropericardial:** pericarditis, pleurisy, pneumothorax, mediastinal emphysema • **Gastrointestinal:** hiatal hernia, reflux esophagitis, esophageal spasm, cholecystitis, peptic ulcer disease, pancreatitis • **Pulmonary:** pulmonary hypertension, pneumonia, pulmonary embolus, bronchial hyperreactivity, spontaneous or tension pneumothorax • **Musculoskeletal:** cervical radiculopathy, shoulder disorder or dysfunction, costochondritis, xiphodynia (painful xiphoid bone) • **Psychoneurotic:** illicit drug use (e.g., cocaine) **Children:** • **Idiopathic (most common cause; 45%):** musculoskeletal conditions; chest wall strain; costochondritis (10%–20%; often bilateral); direct trauma; carrying heavy books; slipping rib syndrome (refers to trauma to the costal cartilage of 8th to 10th ribs [these ribs do *not* attach to the sternum]). Pain is located under the ribs and in the upper abdominal quadrants. A popping sound is heard when actively moving. • **Respiratory:** asthma, cough, pneumonia, pneumothorax (radiation to shoulder), pleurodynia (coxsackievirus) • **Gastrointestinal:** gastroesophageal reflux (common), esophagitis, esophageal foreign body • **Psychogenic:** emotional stress • **Cardiac:** myocarditis or pericarditis, MI, precordial catch syndrome (slouched posture or bending related to exercise), coronary artery inflammation (Kawasaki disease), aortic valve stenosis, hypertrophic cardiomyopathy, hyperlipidemia, supraventricular tachycardia • **Hematopoietic:** sickle cell disease • **Medications:** tetracycline, doxycycline, swallowing tablets

AP, Anteroposterior; *CHF,* congestive heart failure; *MI,* myocardial infarction; *RDS,* respiratory distress syndrome; *SLE,* systemic lupus erythematosus; *TXA₂,* thromboxane A_2.

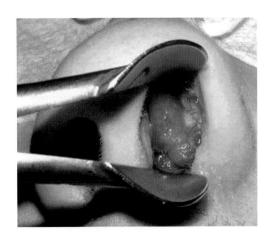

17-1: Nasal polyp. Note the gray-white mass in the left nasal cavity. *(From Swartz MH:* Textbook of Physical Diagnosis, *5th ed, Philadelphia, Saunders Elsevier, 2006, p 312, Fig. 11-24.)*

b. Triad asthma: asthma, nasal polyps, aspirin sensitivity

c. Nasal polyps are often associated with cystic fibrosis (CF; Fig. 17-1).

    (1) Thick secretions in cystic fibrosis cause inflammatory polyps to develop in the nose.

    (2) Sweat test to rule out cystic fibrosis is indicated whenever a child has a nasal polyp

d. May be associated with chronic sinusitis

C. Obstructive sleep apnea (OSA)

1. **Definition:** Characterized by excessive, loud snoring with intervals of breath cessation (apnea)

2. Epidemiology

    a. Obesity is the most common cause of OSA. Pharyngeal muscles collapse because of the weight of tissue in the neck.

    b. Other causes include tonsillar hypertrophy, nasal septum deviation, hypothyroidism, and acromegaly.

    c. Pathogenesis of OSA

        (1) Airway obstruction causes CO_2 retention (respiratory acidosis), leading to hypoxemia ($\downarrow PaO_2$ [partial pressure of O_2]; see Chapter 2).

        (2) Daytime somnolence often simulates narcolepsy.

3. Laboratory findings. PaO_2 and O_2 saturation (SaO_2) decrease, and the $PaCO_2$ (alveolar pressure of CO_2) increases (respiratory acidosis) during apneic episodes.

Asthma, nasal polyps, aspirin sensitivity

Often associated with CF

Thick secretions → inflammatory polyps

R/O CF with sweat test

Chronic sinusitis

Obstructive sleep apnea

Loud snoring → intervals with apnea

Obesity MCC OSA

Pharyngeal muscle collapse

Tonsillar hypertrophy, septum deviation, acromegaly, hypothyroidism

Respiratory acidosis → hypoxemia

Daytime somnolence simulates narcolepsy

$\downarrow PaO_2/SaO_2$, $\uparrow PaCO_2$

Complications

PH → RVH

↓PaO₂, ↑PaCO₂ VC SMCs PVs

Cor pulmonale (PH + RVH)

↓PaO₂ → ↑EPO →; 2° polycythemia

Nocturnal polysomnography confirmatory test

Rhinoscleroma

Chronic granulomatous disease

Klebsiella rhinoscleromatis

May involve other respiratory sites

Possible inherited predisposition

East Africa, Central/South America, Europe, Indian subcontinent

Catarrhal → granulomatous inflammation → fibrosis, scarring

Mikulicz cells: histocytes with intracellular bacilli

Rhinosporidiosis

Granulomatous disease; Rhinosporidium seeberi

Polypoid mass

Fungus vs aquatic protozoa

Granulomatous inflammation; sporangium-like structures

Water/soil reservoirs for pathogen

Sand workers, paddy cultivators, bathing stagnant water

Contact water/soil

Epistaxis, nasal obstruction, rhinorrhea

Sinusitis

Blockage sinus drainage into nasal cavity

Maxillary adults; ethmoid children

Acute sinusitis

Viral URI MCC sinusitis

Deviated nasal septum

Allergic rhinitis, barotrauma, smoking

Preceded by viral URI (rhinovirus); *S. pneumoniae* MC

Anaerobes, *S. aureus*

Mucor, Aspergillus

Diabetics: *Mucor* sinusitis

Fever

Nasal congestion +/- discharge

Pain/percussion tenderness over sinus

4. Complications
   a. Pulmonary hypertension (PH) may occur followed by right ventricular hypertrophy (RVH).
      (1) Hypoxemia and respiratory acidosis cause smooth muscle cells (SMCs) in the pulmonary vessels (PVs) to constrict, thus causing PH.
      (2) After PH develops, the right ventricle becomes hypertrophied.
      (3) A combination of PH and RVH is called cor pulmonale.
   b. Secondary polycythemia is commonly present in OSA. Hypoxemia stimulates the kidneys to release erythropoietin. Erythropoietin stimulates the red blood cell precursors within the bone marrow (RBC erythroid hyperplasia) to proliferate, causing secondary polycythemia (see Chapter 13).
5. Nocturnal polysomnography documents the periods of apnea during sleep (Link 17-7).

D. Rhinoscleroma
1. **Definition:** Chronic granulomatous disease involving the nose that is caused by a gram-negative, encapsulated bacillus called *Klebsiella rhinoscleromatis*
2. Epidemiology and clinical features
   a. Can also affect other sites within the respiratory tract
   b. Possible inherited predisposition leading to CI of the nasal passages
   c. Endemic in East Africa, Central and South America, Europe, and the Indian subcontinent
   d. Three stages: catarrhal (foul-smelling nasal discharge) → friable granulomatous masses in nasal passage leading to epistaxis (nosebleeds) and destruction of nasal cartilage → tissue fibrosis and scarring
   e. Histology shows granulomatous inflammation with multinucleated giant cells and epithelioid cells and Mikulicz cells (large histiocytes with intracellular bacilli).

E. Rhinosporidiosis
1. **Definition:** Granulomatous disease caused by *Rhinosporidium seeberi* that is characterized by a strawberry-like polypoid mass with tiny white dots that may affect the nose, nasopharynx, oropharynx, larynx, or conjunctiva
2. Epidemiology and clinical features
   a. Historically classified as a fungus but is now thought to be an aquatic protozoa
   b. Histologically, the tissue shows granulomatous inflammation with multinucleated giant cells and the presence of sporangium-like structures ("spore-containing" structures).
   c. Encountered in the Americas, Europe, Africa, and Asia with its greatest incidence in Sri Lanka and southern India
   d. Water and soil are thought to be reservoirs for the pathogen.
   e. Incidence of disease is highest among sand workers, paddy cultivators, and people bathing in stagnant waters; hence, the mode of transmission is thought to be contact with water and soil.
   f. Produces epistaxis, nasal obstruction, and rhinorrhea (runny nose)

F. Sinusitis
1. **Definition:** Acute or CI of the mucous membranes lining of one or more of the paranasal sinuses caused by blockage of sinus drainage into the nasal cavity
2. **Epidemiology:** In adults, sinusitis most often occurs in the maxillary sinus, but in children, it is most common in the ethmoid sinus.
3. Acute sinusitis; epidemiology, clinical
   a. Causes include:
      (1) viral upper respiratory infections (most common; URIs).
      (2) deviated nasal septum.
      (3) allergic rhinitis, barotrauma, and smoking cigarettes.
   b. Pathogens
      (1) Principal pathogens in descending order are *Streptococcus pneumoniae* (most common), nontypeable *Haemophilus influenzae,* and *Moraxella catarrhalis.* Acute bacterial sinusitis is usually preceded by a viral upper respiratory tract infection (rhinovirus [RV] most common), dental manipulation, or a flare of allergic rhinitis.
      (2) Other pathogens include anaerobes (chronic sinusitis), *Staphylococcus aureus* (nosocomial infections), and systemic fungi (e.g., *Mucor* or *Aspergillus* spp.). People with diabetes may have sinusitis caused by *Mucor* spp.
   c. Clinical findings include:
      (1) fever; nasal congestion with or without purulent discharge.
      (2) pain or percussion tenderness over the affected sinuses (Link 17-8).

(3) tooth pain (associated with maxillary sinusitis; Link 17-9), cough from postnasal discharge, and periorbital cellulitis (extension of an infection of the ethmoid sinus; Link 17-10). Risk of cavernous sinus thrombosis (CST; Link 17-11) with ethmoid sinusitis.

4. Chronic sinusitis
   a. **Definition:** CI of the paranasal sinuses that persists for at least 12 weeks
   b. Epidemiology and clinical findings
      (1) Defined by clinical symptoms (subjective) or endoscopic or radiologic changes (e.g., computed tomography [CT])
      (2) Most common symptoms include nasal congestion or blockage, facial pain and pressure to palpation or percussion, and diminished sensation of taste or smell. Other symptoms include cough, headache, throat discomfort (postnasal discharge), laryngeal irritation, hoarseness, halitosis (bad breath), and dental pain.
      (3) Endoscopy may reveal nasal polyps.
      (4) Anterior ethmoid sinuses are most commonly involved, followed by the maxillary, posterior ethmoid, sphenoid, and frontal sinuses.
      (5) Pathogens include *Staphylococcus epidermidis* (coagulase negative), *S. aureus* (coagulase positive), *Pseudomonas aeruginosa*, other gram-negative rods, anaerobes, and fungi (consider this pathogen if nasal polyps are present).
      (6) Asthma is present in 50% of patients without nasal polyps and 80% of patients with nasal polyps. Nasal secretions are likely to have eosinophils present, and peripheral blood eosinophilia is also likely present.
      (7) Because of thick secretions, patients with cystic fibrosis are likely to develop chronic sinusitis.
5. Diagnosis of sinusitis. CT is the most sensitive test (Fig. 17-2).
6. Recommendation is *not to* initially use antibiotics because most cases are viral and resolve within 2 weeks. If resolution does *not* occur, then antibiotics should be started.

G. **Nasopharyngeal (NP) carcinoma**
   1. **Definition:** Malignancy arising from the epithelial cells of the nasopharynx, which is located above the soft palate
   2. Epidemiology
      a. Most common malignant tumor of the nasopharynx; male dominant
      b. Increased in Chinese (common in adults) and African populations (common in children)
      c. In children, NP carcinoma is uncommon. Most cancers of the nasopharynx in children are rhabdomyosarcoma (malignancy of striated muscle) or malignant lymphomas.
      d. Pathogenesis: causal relationship with Epstein-Barr virus (EBV)
   3. Pathology findings include:
      a. squamous cell carcinoma (SCC), nonkeratinizing squamous carcinoma, or undifferentiated cancer (Link 17-12).
      b. Metastasizes to cervical lymph nodes is common (70% of cases).
   4. Clinical complications (Link 17-13). The 3-year survival rate is ~60%.

H. **Laryngeal carcinoma**
   1. **Definition:** Carcinoma involving the larynx (supraglottis, glottis, subglottis)
   2. Epidemiology
      a. Risk factors include:
         (1) cigarette smoking (most common cause).
         (2) alcohol (synergistic effect with smoking).
         (3) squamous papillomas and papillomatosis. Caused by human papillomavirus (HPV) types 6 and 11.
      b. Majority are located on the true vocal cords (Fig. 17-3; Link 17-14).
      c. Majority are keratinizing SCCs.
   3. Clinical findings include persistent hoarseness, often in association with painless cervical lymphadenopathy.

IV. **Atelectasis**
   A. **Definition of atelectasis**
      • Atelectasis is the loss of lung volume caused by inadequate expansion of the airspaces (collapse).
   B. **Resorption atelectasis** (Link 17-15 C)
      1. **Definition:** Airway obstruction causes the loss of preexisting air in the peripheral alveoli, leading to alveolar collapse.

Margin notes:

Painful teeth (maxillary sinusitis), cough, periorbital cellulitis (ethmoid sinusitis)

CST danger with ethmoid sinusitis

Chronic sinusitis

CI: chronic inflammation

CI at least 12 wks

Symptoms, CT changes

Nasal congestion/blockage

Cough, headache, hoarseness, halitosis

Nasal polyps

Anterior ethmoid sinus MC site

S. epidermidis coag neg; *S. aureus*, *P. aeruginosa*, anaerobes, fungi

Asthma 50%, asthma with polyps 80%

Eosinophilia

Cystic fibrosis: chronic sinusitis

CT most sensitive test

Nasopharyngeal carcinoma

Malignancy epithelial cells nasopharynx

MC malignant tumor nasopharynx

Male dominant

China, African populations

Children: rhabdomyosarcoma, malignant lymphomas

Association with EBV

SCC, nonkeratinizing SCC, undifferentiated

Cervical node metastasis

Laryngeal carcinoma

Supraglottis, glottis, subglottis

MCC cigarette smoking

Alcohol (synergism with smoking)

Papilloma, papillomatosis; HPV 6, 11

True vocal cord MC site; SCC

Keratinizing SCC MCC

Persistent hoarseness + cervical adenopathy

Atelectasis

Loss lung volume

Resorption atelectasis

Loss preexisting alveolar air

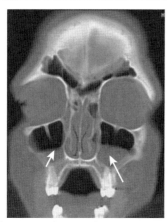

17-2: Computed tomography scan showing acute sinusitis. Note the fluid levels in the maxillary sinuses *(white arrows)*. *(From Carey WD: Cleveland Clinic: Current Clinical Medicine, 2nd ed, Philadelphia, Saunders Elsevier, 2010, p 39, Fig. 1.)*

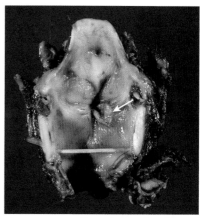

17-3: Laryngeal squamous cell carcinoma involving the right vocal cord *(arrow)*. *(From my friend Ivan Damjanov, MD, PhD, Linder J: Pathology: A Color Atlas, St. Louis, Mosby, 2000, p 47, Fig. 3-16.)*

Airway obstruction thick secretions

Bronchi, segmental bronchi, TBs

Mucus, aspiration, centrally located cancer

Absorption preexisting air → alveolar collapse

Collapse all/part of lung

MCC fever 24 to 36 hours postsurgery

Absent breath sounds, vocal/tactile fremitus

Dullness to percussion

Compression atelectasis

Air/fluid pleural cavity compresses small airways/alveoli

Tension pneumothorax

Pleural effusion

Surfactant

Phospholipids reduce surface tension

Prevents collapse on expiration

Type II pneumocytes: synthesize surfactant

Begins 28th wk gestation

Mostly lecithin

Cortisol/thyroxine ↑synthesis; insulin ↓synthesis

RDS in newborns

↓Surfactant in fetal lungs

Causes of RDS

Prematurity MCC

Poorly controlled maternal DM

Fetal hyperglycemia ↓ surfactant synthesis

2. Pathogenesis
   a. Airway obstruction by thick secretions prevents air from reaching the alveoli. Airway obstruction occurs in the bronchi, segmental bronchi, or terminal bronchioles (TBs).
   b. Causes of obstruction include mucus or mucopurulent plugs after surgery, aspiration of foreign material, and centrally located bronchogenic carcinoma (Link 17-15 C).
   c. After obstruction, the circulating blood in the pulmonary capillaries absorbs the preexisting air in the peripheral alveoli, leading to alveolar collapse and an airless state within a few hours.
   d. Airway collapse may involve all or part of a lung.
3. Clinical findings
   a. Most common cause are fever (*not* related to infection) and dyspnea (difficulty with breathing) within the first 24 to 36 hours after surgery
   b. Absence of breath sounds and vocal vibratory sensation (tactile fremitus)
   c. Dullness to percussion

C. **Compression atelectasis** (Link 17-15 B)
   1. **Definition:** Collapse of small airways and alveoli deep to the pleura that occurs when air or fluid in the pleural cavity is under increased pressure
   2. Examples include:
      a. tension pneumothorax, in which increased air pressure compresses the lung.
      b. large pleural effusion, in which increased fluid compresses the lung.

D. **Atelectasis caused by collapse (spontaneous pneumothorax;** Link 17-15 A; **discussed later)**

E. **Respiratory distress syndromes**
   1. Surfactant
      a. **Definition:** Surfactant is a mixture of phospholipids that reduces surface tension and counteracts the tendency for alveoli to collapse. Prevents collapse on expiration, when the collapsing pressure is greatest.
      b. Type II pneumocytes synthesize surfactant.
         (1) Surfactant is stored in lamellar bodies (Fig. 17-4 A; Link 17-16).
         (2) Synthesis of surfactant begins in the 28th week of gestation.
      c. Phosphatidylcholine (lecithin) is the major component.
      d. Synthesis is *increased* by cortisol and thyroxine and *decreased* by insulin.
   2. Respiratory distress syndrome (RDS) in newborns
      a. Etiology and pathogenesis
         (1) Decreased surfactant in the fetal lungs (Link 17-17)
         (2) Causes of the RDS include:
            (a) prematurity (most common cause).
            (b) poorly controlled diabetes in a mother with diabetes mellitus (DM). Hyperglycemia in the mother causes fetal hyperglycemia that in turn causes increased insulin release. The hyperinsulinemia decreases surfactant synthesis in the fetal lungs.

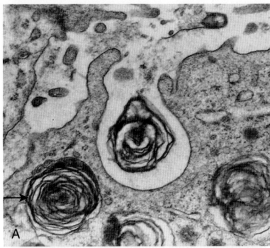
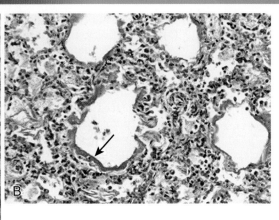
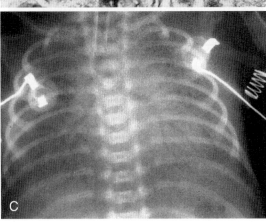

17-4: A, Electron micrograph of a type II pneumocyte showing a lamellar body *(arrow)* containing surfactant. **B,** Neonatal respiratory distress syndrome (RDS). Some of the dilated respiratory bronchioles and alveolar ducts are lined with a fibrin-rich membrane (hyaline membrane) *(arrow)*. The subjacent alveoli are collapsed. **C,** Chest radiograph in RDS. Note the fine, uniform granularity distributed throughout both lungs ("ground glass" appearance). *(A from Corrin B: Pathology of the lungs, London, Churchill Livingstone, 1999, p 15, Fig. 1-26; B from my friend Ivan Damjanov, MD, PhD: Pathology for the Health-Related Professions, 2nd ed, Philadelphia, Saunders, 2000, p 128, Fig. 5-25; C from Katz D, Math K, Groskin S: Radiology Secrets, Philadelphia, Hanley & Belfus, 1998, p 380, Fig. 2.)*

     (c) Cesarean section (C-section). Lack of the normal stress-induced increase in cortisol that is normally present in a vaginal delivery.

> Women who have to deliver their babies prematurely receive glucocorticoids to increase fetal surfactant synthesis, thereby reducing the potential for developing RDS. Good maternal glycemic control decreases the risk for RDS.

     (3) Widespread atelectasis results in massive intrapulmonary shunting (dead space).
          (a) Perfusion *without* ventilation (Link 17-17 middle; see Chapter 2)
          (b) Lungs are dark and airless (sink in water) (Link 17-18).
   b. Collapsed alveoli are lined by hyaline membranes (Fig. 17-4 B; Link 17-19). Membranes are derived from proteins leaking out of damaged pulmonary capillary vessels.
   c. Clinical findings in RDS include:
     (1) respiratory difficulty beginning within a few hours after birth.
     (2) grunting (Table 17-2).
     (3) tachypnea (rapid shallow breathing).
     (4) intercostal retractions (Link 17-20).
     (5) hypoxemia and respiratory acidosis.
   d. Diagnosis. Chest radiograph shows a "ground-glass" appearance (Fig. 17-4 C).
   e. Complications in RDS include:
     (1) superoxide free radical (FR) damage of the lungs from O_2 therapy. This may result in blindness and permanent damage to the small airways (bronchopulmonary dysplasia; Link 17-21).
     (2) intraventricular hemorrhage (see Fig. 6-36).
     (3) patent ductus arteriosus (PDA). Persistent hypoxemia prevents the ductus arteriosus from closing.
     (4) necrotizing enterocolitis (see Chapter 18, Links 18-153 and 18-154). Intestinal ischemia allows entry of gut bacteria into the intestinal wall.

Margin notes:

C-section: lack stress-induced ↑cortisol

Premature delivery → ↑maternal intake glucocorticoids → ↓risk for RDS

Massive atelectasis → ↑intrapulmonary shunting (dead space)

Perfusion *without* ventilation

Dark/airless fetal lungs

Alveoli lined by hyaline membranes

Grunting

Tachypnea

Intercostal retractions

Hypoxemia, resp acidosis

Ground-glass appearance

Superoxide FR damage

RDS O_2 complications: blindness, bronchopulmonary dysplasia

PDA (from hypoxemia)

Necrotizing enterocolitis

(5) hypoglycemia (a complication of poorly controlled maternal diabetes).
   (a) After delivery, excess insulin in the newborn decreases serum glucose, inducing seizures and damage to neurons.
   (b) Newborns born to women with poorly controlled diabetes may need to be given glucose to prevent hypoglycemia.

V. Acute Lung Injury

A. Pulmonary edema (see Chapters 5 and 11)

1. **Definition:** Accumulation of fluid in the alveoli of the lungs; results in poor alveolar gas exchange and breathing difficulties, making it difficult to breath (dyspnea) and exchange oxygen in the alveoli

2. Epidemiology
   a. May be caused by alterations in Starling pressure (transudate), which include:
      (1) increased hydrostatic pressure (HP) in the pulmonary capillaries. Etiologies include left-sided heart failure (LHF; most common cause of pulmonary edema), volume overload, and mitral stenosis. Edema fluid in the alveoli has a pink discoloration; no inflammatory cells are present (Link 17-22).
      (2) Decreased oncotic pressure (OP) from hypoalbuminemia; etiologies include nephrotic syndrome and hepatic cirrhosis
   b. Edema may also be due to microvascular or alveolar injury (exudate) caused by:
      (1) infections. Examples: sepsis, bronchopneumonia
      (2) aspiration. Examples: drowning (see Chapter 7) and gastric contents
      (3) drugs. Example: heroin use (see Chapter 7)
      (4) high altitude (see Chapters 2 and 7).
      (5) acute respiratory distress syndrome (ARDS; see the following).

B. ARDS

1. **Definition:** Noncardiogenic pulmonary edema resulting from acute alveolar-capillary damage. Sepsis and pneumonia are the most common causes.

2. Epidemiology
   a. Caused by direct injury to the lungs or systemic diseases
   b. Causes include gram-negative sepsis (>40% of cases), gastric aspiration (>30% of cases), severe trauma with shock (>20% of cases), and diffuse pulmonary infections (severe acute respiratory syndrome [SARS], hantavirus).
   c. Other causes include heroin overdose, smoke inhalation, acute pancreatitis, cardiopulmonary bypass, disseminated intravascular coagulation (DIC), and amniotic fluid or fat embolism.

3. Pathogenesis (Link 17-23)
   a. Acute damage occurs in the alveolar capillary walls and epithelial cells.
   b. Alveolar macrophages (MPs) and other cells release cytokines.
      (1) Cytokines are chemotactic to neutrophils.
      (2) Neutrophils transmigrate into the alveoli through pulmonary capillaries.
      (3) Capillary damage causes leakage of a protein-rich exudate, producing hyaline membranes.
      (4) Neutrophils damage type I and II pneumocytes. Decrease in surfactant causes atelectasis with intrapulmonary shunting.
   c. Late findings in ARDS include:
      (1) repair by type II pneumocytes.
      (2) progressive interstitial fibrosis (producing restrictive lung disease [RLD]).

4. Clinical findings include dyspnea or tachypnea and late inspiratory crackles.

5. Laboratory findings include:
   a. severe hypoxemia *not* responsive to O_2 therapy. PaO_2 is usually <50 mm Hg.
   b. pulmonary artery (PA) wedge pressure <18 mm Hg. It is important to distinguish ARDS from cardiogenic pulmonary edema, in which the PA wedge pressure is >18 mm Hg.
   c. respiratory acidosis or normal $PaCO_2$.
   d. increased alveolar-arterial (A-a) gradient caused by intrapulmonary shunting related to atelectasis and diffusion abnormalities related to hyaline membranes and an alveolar infiltrate.
   e. PaO_2/FiO_2 ratio ≥300 mm/Hg defines ARDS. PaO_2 is the arterial partial pressure of oxygen. FiO_2 is the fraction of the amount of oxygen a person is inhaling (room air, 0.21; nasal cannula, 0.24–0.44; Venturi mask, 0.24–0.50).
   f. chest radiography shows bilateral interstitial infiltrates initially and progression to widespread alveolar consolidation with air bronchograms (80%).

6. Resolution of ARDS is ultimately dependent on treatment of the underlying disease state.
7. Prognosis is poor (40%–50% mortality rate in ARDS). Mortality rate increases with age.

C. **Respiratory Failure in Children**
   1. **Definition:** Inadequate oxygenation to meet metabolic needs or inadequate excretion of CO_2
   2. Epidemiology
      a. Infants are at greater risk for development of respiratory failure than adults.
      b. Progression of respiratory distress to respiratory failure is faster than in adults. An infant's diaphragm is weaker and more easily fatigued than the diaphragm in adults. The caliber of airways in infants is small when compared with adults. Obstruction leads to hypoxemia and retention of CO_2. Pulse oximeter readings in infants may be inaccurate.
      c. Important signs to recognize in respiratory failure include increased respiratory rate (tachypnea) with distress (nasal flaring, grunting, intercostal muscle retraction, seesaw breathing) and cyanosis despite supplementary oxygen.

VI. **Pulmonary Infections**
   A. **Gram stain characteristics** (Link 17-24)
      1. Crystal violet iodine complex: stains both gram-positive and -negative cell walls
      2. Iodine: mordant that fixes crystal violet
      3. Alcohol
         a. Removes lipid from gram-negative bacteria, thereby losing the dye in the decolorization process
         b. Gram-positive organisms retain crystal violet.
      4. Safranin: counterstain that stains gram-negative organisms red
      5. Gram stain morphology
         a. Gram-positive cocci in clumps or clusters. Example: *Staphylococcus* spp.
         b. Gram-positive organisms that are lancet shaped, in pairs or chains. Examples: *S. pneumoniae* (*Pneumococcus* spp.), *Enterococcus* spp.
         c. Tiny gram-positive cocci: *Peptococcus* spp., *Peptostreptococcus* spp. (both are anaerobes)
         d. Gram-negative diplococci: *Neisseria* spp. ("coffee bean" shaped), *Moraxella* spp.
         e. Gram-negative fat rods: *Escherichia coli*, *Klebsiella* spp.
         f. Gram (−) thin rods. *Pseudomonas*, *Bacteroides* (anaerobe), *Haemophilus*, *Fusobacterium* (anaerobe)
         g. Large gram (+) rods. *Lactobacillus*, *Bacillus* species, *Clostridia*, *Corynebacteria* ("Chinese letters").
         h. Small gram (+) rods. *Listeria*, *Propionibacterium* (anaerobe), *Lactobacillus* (anaerobe in the vagina)
         i. Filamentous and branching gram (+) organisms.
            (1) *Nocardia* (aerobic and partially acid fast).
            (2) *Actinomyces* (anaerobe with sulfur granules; filamentous Gram +).

   B. **Pneumonia.**
      1. **Definition:** Inflammation of the pulmonary parenchyma that is usually caused by either a bacterial or viral infection. May involve the alveoli and/or interstitium in one or both lungs.
      2. Epidemiology
         a. Pneumonia may be acquired in the community or within a hospital or health care facility (sometimes called nosocomial).
         b. Clinical types of pneumonia include bronchopneumonia, lobar pneumonia, and interstitial pneumonia (Link 17-25, Link 17-26).
      3. Community-acquired pneumonia (CAP)
         a. Epidemiology
            (1) One of the top ten causes of death in the United States
            (2) Majority are caused by bacterial pathogens.
            (3) Most often caused by *S. pneumoniae* (20%–60% of cases; Fig. 17-5 A)
         b. Pathogenesis
            (1) Most commonly caused by microaspiration of oropharyngeal contents during sleep
            (2) Inhalation of aerosol drops ranging in size from 0.5 to 1 µm is the second most common cause of CAP.
            (3) Bloodstream infection is the *least* common cause of CAP.
         c. Bronchopneumonia (Links 17-25 A and 17-26 A)
            (1) **Definition:** Type of pneumonia that begins as an acute bronchitis with subsequent extension of the infection into surrounding alveoli

---

Margin notes:

Resolution: Rx underlying disease

Poor prognosis; ↑mortality with age

Inadequate oxygenation and/or excretion of CO_2

Progression respiratory distress to failure faster than adults

Caliber airways infants smaller/diaphragm weaker

↑Respiratory rate with distress, cyanosis

Crystal violet iodine: stains G+/- cell walls

Iodine fixes crystal violet

Alcohol

Removes lipid from cell wall Gram: lose dye

Gram + retain crystal violet

Safranin: counterstain (G− stain red)

Staphylococcus: G+ cocci clumps/clusters

Streptococcus: G+ lancet shaped, pairs/chains

Peptococcus/ Peptostreptococcus: tiny G+ cocci

Neisseria, Moraxella: gram − diplococci

E. coli, Klebsiella: gram − fat rods

Pseudomonas, Bacteroides, Haemophilus, Fusobacterium: Gram − thin rods

Lactobacillus, Bacillus: large Gram + rods

Listeria, Propionibacterium (anaerobe), *Lactobacillus* (anaerobe vagina): small Gram + rods

Filamentous/branching Gram +

Nocardia partial acid fast; Gram +

Actinomyces anaerobe sulfur granules; Gram +

Pneumonia

Lung inflammation alveoli and/or interstitium

Acquired in community/ hospital or health-care facility

Broncho-lobar-interstitial pneumonia

CAP

Top 10 COD in U.S.

Majority caused by bacteria

MCC S. pneumoniae

Microaspiration oropharyngeal contents during sleep

Inhalation aerosol drops

Bronchopneumonia

Acute bronchitis → local extension into parenchyma

17-5: A, Gram stain of *Streptococcus pneumoniae*. The sputum stain shows numerous lancet-shaped diplococci with the tapered ends pointing to each other. A few neutrophils contain phagocytosed bacteria. **B,** Bronchopneumonia showing patchy areas of consolidation *(arrows)* representing collections of neutrophils in the alveoli and bronchi. **C,** Lobar pneumonia. The lower lobe is uniformly consolidated. **D,** Posteroanterior radiograph of a right lower lobe pneumococcal pneumonia. Note the alveolar consolidation and the visible border of the right ventricle indicating that the middle lobe is not involved. *(A from Henry JB: Clinical Diagnosis and Management by Laboratory Methods, 20th ed, Philadelphia, Saunders, 2001, Plate 50-1; B from Kumar V, Fausto N, Abbas A: Robbins and Cotran Pathologic Basis of Disease, 7th ed, Philadelphia, Saunders, 2004, p 749, Fig. 15-33; C from Corrin B: Pathology of the Lungs, London, Churchill Livingstone, 2000, p 162, Fig. 5.2.5; D from Kliegman RM, Jenson HB, Behrman RE, Stanton BF: Nelson Textbook of Pediatrics, 18th ed, Philadelphia, Saunders Elsevier, 2007, p 1798, Fig. 397-2A.)*

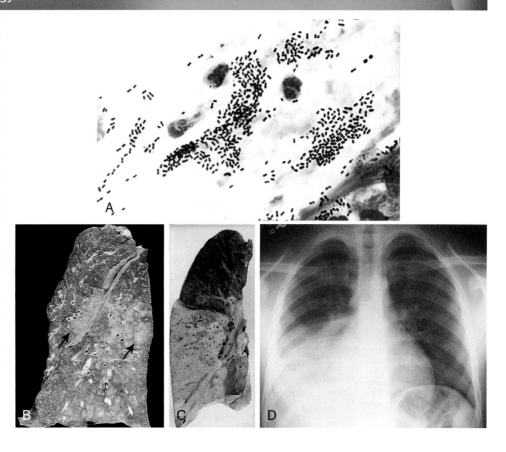

Lower lobes, right middle lobe

Patchy consolidation

Microabscesses in consolidation

Phagocytosis bacteria

Lobar pneumonia

Lobar consolidation

Abscess, empyema

Sepsis

High fever, productive cough

Chest pain inspiration

Tachycardia

Signs consolidation

Dullness to percussion

↑Vocal tactile fremitus

Late inspiratory crackles

Bronchial breath sounds, bronchophony/egophony

Chest x-ray gold standard screen

CT scan excellent

Chest x-ray: bronchopneumonia, lobar pneumonia

Gram stain 80% sensitivity

(2) Lower lobes or right middle lobe are most often involved.
(3) Lung has patchy areas of consolidation (firm, dense mass involving the alveoli; Fig. 17-5 B). Microabscesses containing neutrophils phagocytosing bacteria are present in the areas of consolidation.

d. Lobar pneumonia
   (1) **Definition:** A complete or near-complete consolidation of a lobe of the lung (Fig. 17-5 C; Link 17-25 B)
   (2) Complications include:
       (a) lung abscesses, empyema (pus in the pleural cavity).
       (b) sepsis (spread of infection into the blood).
   (3) Clinical findings include:
       (a) sudden onset of high fever with productive cough.
       (b) chest pain, usually on inspiration.
       (c) tachycardia (rapid heart rate).
       (d) signs of consolidation (alveolar exudate), which include (Tables 17-2 and 17-3):
           • dullness to percussion.
           • increased vocal tactile fremitus (vibratory sensation when the patient speaks). Sound is transmitted well through alveolar consolidations.
           • late inspiratory crackles.
           • bronchial breath sounds, bronchophony, and egophony.

e. Chest radiography is the gold standard screen.
   (1) Sensitivity ranges from 50% to 85%. Specificity is 93%.
   (2) Although chest radiography is most commonly used to diagnose pneumonia, it may miss small areas of consolidation in the alveoli. A CT scan is a far more sensitive test in identifying smaller areas of consolidation that would be missed with standard chest radiography. However, because of the expense of a CT scan, it is *not* recommended as the *first* step in evaluating a suspected pneumonia.
   (3) Chest radiography shows either patchy infiltrates (bronchopneumonia) or lobar consolidation (Fig. 17-5 D).

f. Laboratory findings in pneumonia
   (1) Gram stain has a sensitivity of 80%. More useful than culture; however, a culture is still obtained.

TABLE 17-3 Summary of Respiratory Microbial Pathogens

PATHOGEN	COMMENTS
	VIRUSES
Rhinovirus	• Most common cause of the common cold • Transmitted by hand to eye–nose contact • Other causes of colds: coronaviruses, adenoviruses, influenza C virus, coxsackievirus
Coxsackievirus	• Acute chest syndrome: fever with pleuritic chest pain • Diagnosis: PCR
Parainfluenza (see Fig. 17-6 A; Links 17-27 to 17-29)	• Most common cause of croup (laryngotracheobronchitis) in infants • Inspiratory stridor (upper airway obstruction) caused by submucosal edema in trachea; brassy cough; signs of respiratory distress • Anterior radiograph of neck shows "steeple sign," representing mucosal edema in the trachea (site of obstruction) (Links 17-27 and 17-28). • Bronchiolitis in infants. Multinucleated giant cells may be present on biopsies (Link 17-29). • Diagnosis: PCR
CMV (see Fig. 17-6 B; Link 17-30)	• Common pneumonia in immunocompromised hosts (e.g., bone marrow transplants, AIDS) • Enlarged alveolar macrophages or pneumocytes, contain eosinophilic intranuclear inclusions surrounded by a halo (Link 17-30) • Diagnosis: PCR
Influenzavirus (Link 17-31)	• Type A viruses are most often involved. • Hemagglutinins bind virus to cell receptors in the nasal passages (Link 17-31). • Neuraminidase dissolves mucus and facilitates release of viral particles (Link 17-31). • Influenza A produces worldwide epidemics. Pneumonia may be complicated by a superimposed bacterial pneumonia (usually *Staphylococcus aureus*). • Influenza B causes major outbreaks. • Antigen drift: minor mutation. Does *not* require new vaccine. • Antigen shift: major mutation in hemagglutinin or neuraminidase. A new vaccine is required. • Clinical: fever, headache, cough, myalgias, chest pain • Vaccination: mandatory for people >65 yr old and people with chronic illnesses • Associations: Reye syndrome with salicylate ingestion (see Chapter 19); Guillain-Barré syndrome (see Chapter 26) • Diagnosis: PCR
Rubeola (Link 17-32)	• Fever, cough, conjunctivitis, and excessive nasal mucus production • Koplik spots in the mouth *precede* onset of the rash. • Warthin-Finkeldey multinucleated giant cells are a characteristic finding (Link 17-32). • Diagnosis: PCR
RSV	• Most common cause of pneumonia and bronchiolitis (wheezing) in infants • Infections primarily occur in winter. • Causes otitis media in older children • Hand washing and use of gloves prevents nosocomial outbreaks in nurseries • Fusion protein causes cells to fuse, producing multinucleated giant cells. • Rapid diagnosis by detection of antigen in nasopharyngeal wash. PCR is also useful for diagnosis. • *Passive immunization* (high-risk children): Palivizumab (monoclonal antibody) reduces hospitalization rates between November and April.
SARS	• First transmitted to humans through contact with masked palm civets (China) and then from human-to-human contact through respiratory secretions (e.g., hospitals, families) • Develop severe respiratory infection • Diagnose with viral detection by PCR assay or detection of antibodies • Children: no therapy or vitamin A • Detection viral genome, PCR, ELISA
Hantavirus pulmonary syndrome	• Transmission: inhalation of urine or feces from deer mice in the Southwestern United States (desert areas) • Pulmonary syndrome: ARDS, hemorrhage, renal failure • Diagnosis: detect viral RNA in lung tissue • *No* effective treatment • High mortality rate • Diagnosis: PCR
Zika virus	• Spread mostly by the bite of an infected *Aedes* species of mosquito (*Aedes aegypti* and *Aedes albopictus*). Mosquitoes are aggressive during the daytime or at night. • Can be passed from a pregnant woman to her fetus. Infection during pregnancy can cause birth defects (microcephaly) and other brain defects. Can also be transmitted by sex and blood transfusion (likely but *not* yet confirmed). • Other problems are detected among fetuses and infants infected with the virus *before* birth, such as defects of the eye, hearing deficits, and impaired growth. • Symptoms include fever, rash, joint pain, conjunctivitis, myalgia, (muscle pain) and headache. Symptoms last for several days to a week. • Hospitalization is not usually required. Death is uncommon. • Recovery is the rule, and there is protection from future infections. • Increased risk for developing Guillain-Barré syndrome, a demyelination syndrome • Diagnostic testing of infant serum, cord blood, placenta, or umbilical cord specimens collected at birth. Antibody and PCR tests are available, as well as virus isolation testing. • *No* vaccine or medicine is available for preventing or treating the infection.

Continued

TABLE 17-3   Summary of Respiratory Microbial Pathogens—cont'd

PATHOGEN	COMMENTS
	BACTERIA
Chlamydia *Chlamydophila pneumoniae*	• Second most common cause of atypical pneumonia • Seroepidemiologic association with coronary artery disease • Associations with Alzheimer disease, asthma, and reactive arthritis have been proposed. • Diagnosis: PCR
Chlamydia trachomatis	• Newborn pneumonia (passage through birth canal) • Afebrile, staccato cough (choppy cough), conjunctivitis, and wheezing • Diagnosis: PCR
Mycoplasma pneumoniae	• Most common cause of interstitial pneumonia • Common in adolescents and military recruits (closed spaces) • Risk factor for Guillain-Barré syndrome (see Chapter 26) • Insidious onset with low-grade fever • Cold agglutinins in blood • Complications: bullous myringitis, cold autoimmune hemolytic anemia caused by anti-I IgM antibodies (see Chapter 12) • Diagnosis: PCR
Coxiella burnetii	• Usually transmitted without a vector • Contracted by dairy farmers, veterinarians • Associated with the birthing process of infected sheep, cattle, and goats and handling of milk or excrement • Atypical pneumonia, myocarditis, granulomatous hepatitis • Diagnosis: PCR
Bacteria gram+ *Streptococcus pneumoniae* (see Fig. 17-5 A)	• Gram-positive lancet-shaped diplococcus • Most common cause of typical community-acquired pneumonia (50%–75%) • Rapid onset, productive cough, signs of consolidation • Urine antigen test is an excellent screen.
Staphylococcus aureus (see Fig. 17-6 C; Links 17-33 to 17-35)	• Gram-positive cocci in clumps (Link 17-33) • Yellow sputum • Commonly superimposed on influenza pneumonia and measles pneumonia • Major lung pathogen in CF and IV drug abusers • Accounts for 3%–5% of community-acquired pneumonias • Hemorrhagic pulmonary edema, abscess formation, and pneumatoceles (thin-walled air-filled cysts that develop in the lung parenchyma, usually after pneumonia; Links 17-34 and 17-35) • Diagnosis: culture, antigen detection, PCR
Corynebacterium diphtheriae (see Fig. 17-6 D; Links 17-36 and 17-37)	• Gram-positive rod • Toxin inhibits protein synthesis by ADP ribosylation of elongation factor 2 involved in protein synthesis (Link 17-36). • Toxin also impairs β-oxidation of fatty acids in the heart (myocarditis with fatty change). • Toxin-induced pseudomembranous inflammation produces shaggy gray membranes in the oropharynx (Link 17-37) and trachea; toxic myocarditis (death). • Diagnosis: culture, PCR
Bacillus anthracis (see Fig. 17-6 E; Link 17-38)	• Gram-positive rod (Link 17-38) • Habitat: soil • Capsule inhibits phagocytosis • Exotoxins: protective antigen (PA), edema factor (EF; activates adenylate cyclase), and lethal factor (LF; inhibits a signal transduction protein involved in cell division). The toxins are nontoxic individually but form important toxins when combined. PA + EF forms edema toxin. PA + LF forms lethal toxin. These combinations are pathogenic. • Transmission: direct contact with animal skins or products (most commonly sheep and cattle) and entry of the organisms through abrasions or cuts; inhalation (use in germ warfare) • Cutaneous anthrax (90%–95% of cases): occurs through direct contact with infected or contaminated animal products. Resembles insect bite but eventually swells to form a black scab, or eschar, with a central area of necrosis (malignant pustule). If left untreated, death occurs in 20% of patients. • Pulmonary anthrax: "first sign of the disease is death." It is contracted by inhalation of spores that are present in contaminated hides or delivered by biological weapons. Produces a necrotizing pneumonia, meningitis, and pronounced splenomegaly. It disseminates throughout the rest of the body, leading to death. • Prevention: A vaccine is available for high-risk patients (e.g., veterinarians, soldiers entering developing countries). • Diagnosis: culture, PCR
Actinomyces israelii (see Fig. 18-3 F, G)	• Gram-positive filamentous bacteria. Strict anaerobe. Present in normal flora in the tonsils and adenoids. • Produces draining sinuses in the jaw, chest cavity, and abdomen. Pus contains sulfur granules (yellow specks) that contain the bacteria. • Diagnosis: gram stain, culture
Nocardia asteroides	• Gram-positive filamentous bacteria. Strict aerobe. Partially acid fast. • Produces granulomatous microabscesses in the lungs • Frequently disseminates to the CNS and kidneys • Diagnosis: culture, antibody detection

TABLE 17-3   Summary of Respiratory Microbial Pathogens—cont'd

PATHOGEN	COMMENTS
Bacteria gram-negative *Bordetella pertussis*	• Gram-negative rod • Pili attach to cilia in the upper respiratory tract. Toxin stimulates adenylate cyclase, which catalyzes the addition of ADP ribose to the inhibitory subunit of the G protein complex. Toxin also produces absolute lymphocytosis (normal-appearing lymphocytes) often in leukemoid reaction range. • Produces whooping cough. Transmitted by droplet infection. • Catarrhal phase: lasts 1–2 weeks. Mild coughing, rhinorrhea, and conjunctivitis. • Paroxysmal coughing phase: lasts 2–5 weeks. Characteristic 4–5 coughs in succession on expiration, followed by an inspiratory whoop. Absolute lymphocytosis may produce a leukemoid reaction (20,000–50,000 cells/mm³). Lymphocytes are normal in appearance. • Convalescence phase: lasts 1–2 weeks. Slow decline in coughing and lymphocytosis. • Complications: hemorrhage into skin, conjunctiva, bronchus, brain from coughing. Otitis media, meningoencephalitis (10%), rectal prolapse from coughing, and pneumonia. Pneumonia is the most common cause of death in children <3 yr old. Children <1 yr old have no protection from the mother's immunoglobulins. • Diagnosis: nasopharyngeal swabs using special cough plate; direct immunofluorescence of swab material
Haemophilus influenza (Link 17-39)	• Gram-negative rod • Common cause of sinusitis, otitis media, and conjunctivitis (pink eye) • Accounts for 3%–10% of community-acquired pneumonias • Inspiratory stridor may be caused by acute epiglottitis. • Swelling of the epiglottis produces a "thumbprint sign" on a lateral radiograph of the neck (Link 17-39). • Most common bacterial cause of acute exacerbation of preexisting COPD • Diagnosis: culture, antigen detection
Moraxella catarrhalis	• Gram-negative diplococcus • Common cause of typical pneumonia, especially in older adults • Second most common pathogen causing acute exacerbation of COPD • Common cause of chronic bronchitis, sinusitis, and otitis media
Pseudomonas aeruginosa	• Green sputum (pyocyanin pigment) • Water-loving bacteria most often transmitted by respirators • Most common cause of nosocomial pneumonia and death caused by pneumonia in CF • Pneumonia is often associated with infarction caused by vessel invasion by the bacteria
Klebsiella pneumoniae (Link 17-40)	• Gram-negative fat rod surrounded by a mucoid capsule • Common gram-negative organism causing lobar pneumonia and typical pneumonia in elderly patients in nursing homes • Common cause of pneumonia in alcoholics; however, *S. pneumoniae* is still the most common pneumonia in alcoholics • Typical pneumonia associated with blood-tinged, thick, mucoid sputum • Lobar consolidation and abscess formation (Link 17-40) are common. Presentation can be confused with tuberculosis.
Legionella pneumophila (Link 17-41)	• Gram-negative rod (requires IF stain [Link 17-41] or Dieterle silver stain to identify in tissue) • Water-loving bacterium (water coolers; mists in produce section of grocery stores; outdoor restaurants in summer; rain forests in zoos) • Risk factors: alcoholic, smoker, immunosuppression • Interstitial pneumonia associated with high fever, dry cough, flulike symptoms. Accounts for 2%–8% of adult community-acquired pneumonias. • May produce tubulointerstitial disease with destruction of the JG apparatus leading to hyporeninemic hypoaldosteronism (type IV renal tubular acidosis [hyponatremia, hyperkalemia, metabolic acidosis]). • Urine antigen test is an excellent screen.
Yersinia pestis	• Gram-negative rod • Cause of plague • Transmitted by bite of rat flea. Primary reservoir for the bacteria are ground squirrels in the Southwest. Also transmitted person to person by droplet infection. • Macrophages cannot kill bacteria because V and W antigens provide protection. • Three types of disease: bubonic (most common), pneumonic (transmitted by aerosol), and septicemic • Bubonic type: bite by rat flea that has recently bitten an infected ground squirrel. Infected lymph nodes enlarge (usually in the groin), mat together, and drain to the surface (buboes).
SYSTEMIC FUNGI	
Cryptococcus neoformans (see Fig. 17-6F; Links 17-42 to 17-44)	• Budding yeast with narrow-based buds. Surrounded by a thick capsule (Link 17-42). Forms pseudohyphae (Link 17-43). Found in pigeon excreta (around buildings, outside office windows, under bridges; Link 17-44). • Primary lung disease (40%): granulomatous inflammation with caseation. Do *not* have to be immunocompromised to acquire the disease.
Aspergillus fumigatus (see Fig. 17-6 G; Link 17-45)	• Fruiting body and narrow-angled (<45 degrees), branching septate hyphae (Link 17-45) • Aspergilloma: fungus ball (visible on radiography) may develop in a preexisting cavity in the lung (e.g., old TB site). Cause of massive hemoptysis (invades blood vessels). • Allergic bronchopulmonary aspergillosis: type I and type III HSRs. IgE levels increased and eosinophilia is present. There is intense inflammation of airways and mucus plugs in the terminal bronchioles. Repeated attacks may lead to bronchiectasis and interstitial lung disease. • Vessel invader: causes hemorrhagic infarctions and a necrotizing bronchopneumonia

Continued

TABLE 17-3   Summary of Respiratory Microbial Pathogens—cont'd

PATHOGEN	COMMENTS
Mucor spp. (Link 17-46)	• Wide-angled hyphae (>45 degrees) *without* septa (Link 17-46) • Clinical settings: diabetes mellitus, immunosuppressed patients • Vessel invader and produces hemorrhagic infarctions in the lung. • Invades the frontal lobes in patients with diabetic ketoacidosis (rhinocerebral mucormycosis)
Coccidioides immitis (see Fig. 17-6 H; Links 17-47 and 17-48)	• Contracted by inhaling arthrospores in dust while living or passing through arid desert areas in the Southwest (valley fever; southern Arizona, southern California). Increased infections after earthquakes (arthrospores are present in dust) (Link 17-47). • Spherules with endospores in tissues (Link 17-48) • Flulike symptoms and erythema nodosum (painful nodules on lower legs caused by inflammation of subcutaneous fat) • Granulomatous inflammation with caseous necrosis
Histoplasma capsulatum (see Fig. 17-6I and J; Links 17-49 to 17-51)	• Most common systemic fungal infection • Endemic in Ohio and central Mississippi river valleys • Contracted by inhalation of microconidia in dust contaminated with excreta from bats (increased incidence in cave explorers, spelunkers), starlings, or chickens (common in chicken farmers; Link 17-49) • Yeast forms are present in macrophages (Link 17-50). • Granulomatous inflammation with caseous necrosis • Simulates TB lung disease: produces coin lesions, consolidations, miliary spread, and cavitation (Link 17-51) • Marked dystrophic calcification of granulomas. Most common cause of multiple calcifications in the spleen seen on radiographs.
Blastomyces dermatitidis (see Fig. 17-6K; Links 17-52 and 17-53)	• Occurs in the Great Lakes region, central, and southeastern United States. Most often associated with fishing (most common), hunting, gardening, exposure to beaver dams (beavers are reservoirs for the fungus) (Link 17-52). • Yeasts have broad-based buds and nuclei (Link 17-53). • Male-dominant disease • Produces skin and lung disease. Skin lesions simulate squamous cell carcinoma. • Granulomatous inflammation with caseous necrosis
Pneumocystis jiroveci (see Fig. 4-16A; Link 17-54 to 17-56)	• Cysts (Link 17-54) and trophozoites are present in tissue. Cysts attach to type I pneumocytes in the lungs. • Similar to fungi but have *no* ergosterol in the plasma membrane • Primarily an opportunistic infection. Occurs when the CD_4 count is <200 cells/mm^3. • Common initial AIDS-defining infection • Predominantly produces pulmonary disease with dense consolidation and patchy areas of induration in the lungs (Link 17-54). Patients develop fever, dyspnea, and severe hypoxemia. Diffuse intraalveolar foamy exudates with cup-shaped cysts are best visualized with silver or Giemsa stains. • Chest radiography shows diffuse alveolar and interstitial infiltrates (Link 17-56)

ADP, adenosine diphosphate; *ARDS,* acute respiratory distress syndrome; *CF,* cystic fibrosis; *CMV,* cytomegalovirus; *CNS,* central nervous system; *COPD,* chronic obstructive pulmonary disease; ELISA, enzyme-linked immunoabsorbent assay; *EM,* electron microscopy; *HSR,* hypersensitivity reaction; *IF,* immunofluorescent; *IV,* intravenous; *JG,* juxtaglomerular; *PCR,* polymerase chain reaction; *RSV,* respiratory syncytial virus; *SARS,* severe acute respiratory syndrome; *TB,* tuberculosis.

Neutrophilic leukocytosis

Blood cultures

Interstitial pneumonia

Inflammation interstitial (not alveolar)

Mycoplasma pneumoniae: MCC interstitial pneumonia

Chlamydophila pneumoniae

RSV, influenza virus, adenovirus

C. trachomatis MCC in newborns

Inhalation (droplet infection)

Mononuclear infiltrate

Alveolar space clear

Insidious, low-grade fever

Nonproductive cough

Chest pain on inspiration

Flulike symptoms

No signs consolidation

(2) Neutrophilic leukocytosis is present.
(3) Blood cultures are positive in 20% of cases.
4. Interstitial types of pneumonia (old term, *atypical pneumonia*; Links 17-25 C and 17-26 B)
   a. **Definition:** Type of pneumonia in which inflammatory cells are present in the interstitium rather than the alveoli
   b. Epidemiology
      (1) Most commonly caused by *Mycoplasma pneumoniae* (7% of all pneumonias)
      (2) Other pathogens include:
         (a) *Chlamydophila pneumoniae*
         (b) viruses such as respiratory syncytial virus (RSV), influenzavirus, and adenovirus
         (c) *Chlamydia trachomatis* is the most common cause in newborns.
   c. Pathogenesis: contracted by inhalation (droplet infection)
   d. Histologic findings
      (1) Mononuclear infiltrate is present, rather than neutrophils (Links 17-25 C and 17-26 B).
      (2) Alveolar spaces are usually free of exudate (pus).
   e. Clinical findings include:
      (1) insidious onset of low-grade fever.
      (2) nonproductive cough.
      (3) chest pain on inspiration.
      (4) flulike symptoms, such as pharyngitis, laryngitis, myalgias (aching muscles), and headache.
      (5) *no* signs of consolidation on physical exam.

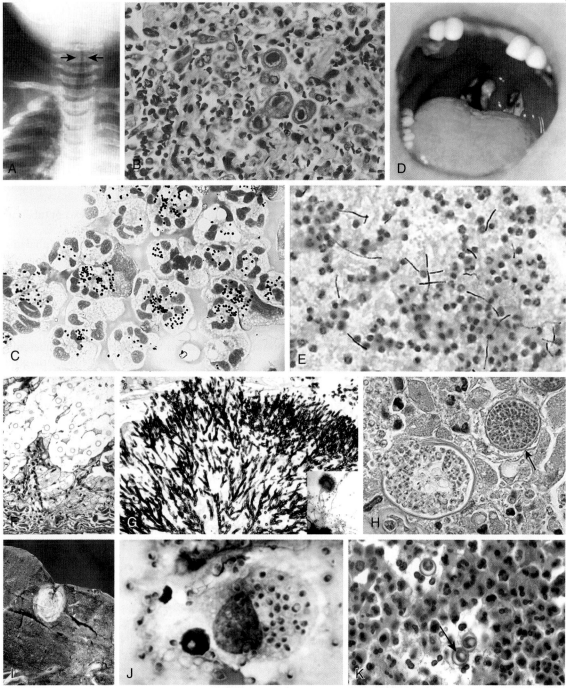

17-6: A, Parainfluenza virus producing laryngotracheobronchitis. Frontal radiograph showing narrowing of the trachea *(arrows)* producing the classic steeple sign. **B,** Cytomegalovirus. The enlarged nuclei of many of the type I pneumocytes contain large inclusions (eosinophilic staining with hematoxylin and eosin stain) surrounded by a clear halo. **C,** *Staphylococcus aureus.* Note the gram-positive cocci in clusters intermixed with neutrophils. **D,** Tonsillitis caused by *Corynebacterium diphtheriae.* Note the gray pseudomembrane covering the tonsils. **E,** *Bacillus anthracis.* Gram-positive rods. **F,** *Cryptococcus neoformans.* The yeast form produces a clear capsule without a visible nucleus. **G,** *Aspergillus fumigatus.* Lung biopsy stained with Gomori methenamine-silver shows septated hyphae and fruiting body *(inset).* **H,** *Coccidioides immitis.* Note the spherules containing endospores *(arrow).* **I,** *Histoplasma capsulatum.* Laminated granuloma at the lung periphery produces puckering of the pleural surface. **J,** *Histoplasma capsulatum.* Alveolar macrophage contains intracellular yeast forms. **K,** *Blastomyces dermatitidis.* Note the yeast forms with broad-based buds *(arrow). (**A** from Scholes MA, Ramakrishnan VR:* ENT Secrets, *4th ed, Philadelphia, Elsevier 2016, p. 327, Fig. 47.2B. Adapted from Duncan NO: Infections of the airway in children. Taken from Flint PW, Haughey BH, Lund VG, et al, editors:* Cummings Otolaryngology: Head & Neck Surgery, *5th ed, Philadelphia, 2010, Mosby, pp 2803-28011, Fig. 197-3;* **B** *from my friend Ivan Damjanov, MD, PhD, Linder J:* Pathology: A Color Atlas, *St. Louis, Mosby, 2000, p 56, Fig. 4-24;* **C** *from McPherson, R, Pincus, M:* Henry's Clinical Diagnosis and Management by Laboratory Methods, *22nd ed., Philadelphia, Saunders, 2011, p 1170, Fig. 57.2;* **D** *courtesy Franklin H. Top, Department of Hygiene and Preventive Medicine, State University of Iowa College of Medicine, Iowa City, IA, and Parke, Davis & Company's Therapeutic Notes;* **E** *and* **J** *from Murray PR, Rosenthal K, Pfaller M:* Medical Microbiology, *6th ed, Philadelphia, Mosby, 2009, Figs. 24-2, 73-10, respectively;* **F** *from Kradin RL:* Diagnostic Pathology of Infectious Disease, *Philadelpia, Saunders Elsevier, 2010, p 162, Fig. 7-84E;* **H** *from Klatt E:* Robbins and Cotran Atlas of Pathology, *Philadelphia, Saunders, 2006, pp 127, 126, Figs. 5-92, 5-91 on right, respectively.)*

5. Nosocomial pneumonia
   a. **Definition:** An infection that is acquired in a hospital or other type of health care facility that develops after the patient has been admitted for reasons other than the pneumonia
   b. Risk factors include:
      (1) ventilator: most common source of infection.
      (2) severe underlying disease, antibiotic therapy, and immunosuppression.
   c. Pathogens involved include:
      (1) gram-negative bacteria (account for >80% of nosocomial pneumonias). *P. aeruginosa* (ventilators), *Escherichia coli* (indwelling urinary catheters [IUCs])
      (2) Gram-positive bacteria (e.g., *S. aureus*; intravenous [IV] catheters)
6. Pneumonia is commonly seen in immunocompromised patients (e.g., AIDS and bone marrow transplantation). Common opportunistic infections include cytomegalovirus (CMV), *Pneumocystis jiroveci,* and *Aspergillus fumigatus.*
7. Table 17-3 summarizes important respiratory microbial pathogens except tuberculosis.
8. Tuberculosis
   a. **Definition:** Refers to disease caused by *Mycobacterium tuberculosis.* Inhalation of the organism results in an infection within the lungs. This infection, which is characterized by a granulomatous inflammatory host response, may be contained within the lung or disseminate throughout the body to any organ. Because the granulomas resemble millet seeds on gross examination and in radiographs, disseminated disease is referred to as "miliary tuberculosis."
   b. Epidemiology and pathogenesis
      (1) Contracted by inhalation of *M. tuberculosis* from a patient with tuberculosis
      (2) Organism resides in phagosomes within alveolar MPs. Mycobacteria produce a protein (cord factor) that prevents fusion of lysosomes with phagosome.
      (3) Characteristics of *M. tuberculosis*
         (a) Strict aerobe, acid-fast (because of mycolic acid in cell wall) (Links 17-57 and 17-58)
         (b) Virulence factor is cord factor.
            • **Definition:** Virulence factors are by-products produced by pathogens (i.e., bacteria, viruses, parasites, fungi) that contribute to the pathogenicity of the organism and enable them to colonize the human host (e.g., toxins, gas or acid, adhesion factors, capsules, degradative enzymes).
            • Cord factor helps induce granulomatous reactions in tuberculosis.
      (4) Screening for tuberculosis
         (a) Purified protein derivative (PPD; tuberculin skin test) intradermal skin test is the screening test for tuberculosis.
         (b) Does *not* distinguish active from inactive disease
      (5) Protein in cell wall is responsible for a positive PPD.
      (6) Drug resistance mechanisms involve:
         (a) chromosome mutations involving mycolic acid (MA).
         (b) chromosome mutations involving heme enzyme catalase peroxidase (KatG), the enzyme that is required to activate isoniazid (INH).
      (7) HIV increases risk for progression to active tuberculosis.
      (8) HIV increases risk for reactivation of tuberculosis.
      (9) HIV increases the mortality rate from tuberculosis.
      (10) Strains of tuberculosis that show resistance to INH and rifampin are known as multidrug-resistant tuberculosis.
      (11) Risk factors include: children > young adults; elderly; close contact with patients with active disease; overcrowding (homeless housing, prison, dormitories); chest radiography evidence of self-healed tuberculosis; smoking cigarettes; immunosuppression (ISP); leukemia/lymphoma; DM; chronic kidney disease (CKD); silicosis; malnutrition; vitamin A or D deficiency; recent measles in children.
   c. Primary tuberculosis
      (1) Subpleural location in the upper part of the lower lobes or lower part of the upper lobes (Fig. 17-7 A)
         (a) Ghon focus is an area of caseous necrosis (see Chapter 2) that is located in the periphery of the lung.
         (b) Ghon complex refers to involvement of both the lung as well as regional lymph nodes.
         (c) Patient usually asymptomatic.

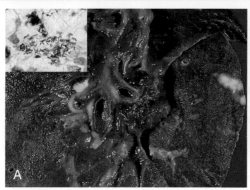
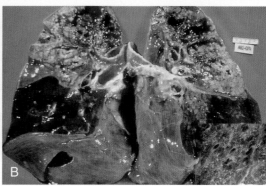

17-7: A, Primary tuberculosis. Note the tan-yellow subpleural granuloma with caseation necrosis and the tan-yellow area of caseation necrosis in the hilar lymph node in the mid-lung field. The two of these together is called a Ghon complex. The *inset* shows an acid-fast stain with numerous *Mycobacterium tuberculosis* organisms. **B,** Reactivation (secondary) tuberculosis. The apices of both lungs show gray-white areas of caseation necrosis and multiple areas of cavitation. *Inset* shows miliary tuberculosis. The lung is studded with numerous tubercles, each the size of a millet seed. *(A from Klatt E: Robbins and Cotran Atlas of Pathology, Philadelphia, Saunders, 2006, p 197, Fig. 8-4; inset from Hoffbrand AV: Color Atlas: Clinical Hematology, 3rd ed, St. Louis, Mosby, 2000, p 136, Fig. 7-85B; **B** from Kumar V, Fausto N, Abbas A: Robbins and Cotran Pathologic Basis of Disease, 7th ed, Philadelphia, Saunders, 2004, p 386, Fig. 8-32; **Inset** from Corrin B, Nicholson AG, Burke M, Rice A: Pathology of the Lungs, 3rd ed, St. Louis, Churchill Livingstone Elsevier, 2011, p 205, Fig. 5.3.12. Courtesy of Dr. M Kearney, Tromso, Norway.)*

(2) Ghon focus and complex usually resolve, producing a calcified granuloma or area of scar tissue; may be a nidus for secondary tuberculosis.

d. Secondary (reactivation) tuberculosis
  (1) Reactivation of a previous primary tuberculosis site
  (2) Involves one or both apices in upper lobes (Fig. 17-7 B). Massive cavitation may occur in reactivation tuberculosis (Links 17-59 and 17-60). Ventilation (oxygenation) is greatest in the upper lobes, where O_2 is greatest. This is a good site for a strict aerobe.
  (3) Release of cytokines from memory T cells results in a cavitary lesion (see Chapter 4).

e. Clinical findings include fever, drenching night sweats, and weight loss.

f. Complications include:
  (1) miliary spread in the lungs caused by invasion into the bronchus or lymphatics (Fig. 17-7 A).
  (2) miliary spread to extrapulmonary (EP) sites (see Fig. 17-7 B).
     (a) Spread is caused by invasion of pulmonary vein (PV) tributaries.
     (b) Cervical/mediastinal lymph nodes are the most common EP sites.
     (c) Kidney is a common EP site as well.
     (d) Adrenal involvement may result in Addison disease (hypocortisolism).
     (e) Lower intestine, peritoneum
     (f) Pericardial effusion, constrictive pericarditis (dystrophic calcification)
     (g) Meningeal disease
  (3) massive hemoptysis, bronchiectasis, scar carcinoma.
  (4) granulomatous hepatitis.
  (5) spread to vertebrae (Pott disease).

g. Diagnosis of tuberculosis
  (1) Bronchoalveolar lavage is best for staining and culture.
  (2) Sputum cultures, microscopy
  (3) Polymerase chain reaction (PCR), nucleic acid probes, nucleic acid sequencing (highly specific; highly sensitive if acid-fast smear is positive), interferon-γ release assays (IGRAs), QuantiFERON-TB t-gold standard test

Adenosine deaminase (ADA) test is *not* a diagnostic test, but it may be used along with other tests such as pleural fluid (PF) analysis, acid-fast bacillus (AFB) smear and culture, or tuberculosis molecular testing to help determine whether a person has a *M. tuberculosis* of the lining of the lungs (pleurae).

9. *Mycobacterium avium–intracellulare* complex (MAC)
  a. Atypical mycobacterium
  b. Composed of two species: *M. avium* and *M. intracellulare*

Margin notes:
Calcified granuloma
Possible nidus for 2° tuberculosis
Secondary (reactivation) tuberculosis
Reactivation from previous 1° site
One/both apices upper lobes; cavitation
↑Ventilation (oxygenation) upper lobes
Memory T cell cytokines → cavitation
Fever, drenching night sweats, weight loss
Complications
Miliary spread lungs (invasion bronchus/lymphatics)
Miliary spread EP sites
Invasion PV tributaries
Cervical/mediastinal nodes: MC EP sites
Kidney common EP site
Adrenal glands: possible Addison disease
Lower intestine, peritoneum
Pericardial effusion, constrictive pericarditis
Meningeal disease
Massive hemoptysis, bronchiectasis, scar cancer
Granulomatous hepatitis
Tuberculosis vertebrae
Dx of tuberculosis
Lavage
Sputum culture, microscopy
PCR, nucleic acid probes/sequencing, IGRAs
QuantiFERON-TB t-gold test

ADA test tuberculosis involving pleura
MAC
Atypical mycobacterium
M. avium/intracellulare

MC tuberculosis in AIDS

CD_4 T_H count <50 cells/mm^3

Infects elderly women

Right middle lobe syndrome (bronchiectasis, atelectasis)

"Tree in bud" opacities terminal bronchioles

Inhalation

Granulomatous inflammation +/- caseation

Lung abscess

Liquefactive necrosis

MCC aspiration oropharyngeal material

c. Most common tuberculosis in AIDS (immunosuppressed), where it often disseminates. This usually occurs when the CD_4 helper T cell (T_H) count falls to <50 cells/mm^3

d. Tends to infect older women

e. Commonly seen in the right middle lobe syndrome caused by bronchiectasis and chronic atelectasis. It also may involve small airways (Link 17-61).

f. Radiologically, the lesions are detected as "tree in bud" opacities, reflecting terminal bronchiolar infection.

10. Systemic fungal infections (Fig. 17-6 F to K)

a. Systemic fungal infections are contracted by inhalation of the pathogen.

b. Fungi initiate a granulomatous inflammatory reaction with or without caseation.

C. **Lung abscess**

1. **Definition:** Liquefactive necrosis of the lung tissue secondary to a microbial infection resulting in the formation of cavities that contains necrotic debris and inflammatory cells

2. Causes

a. Most often caused by aspiration of oropharyngeal material from the upper airway below the true vocal cords

b. An abnormality involving any phase of swallowing (functional or anatomic) can ultimately result in aspiration, leading to a lung abscess.

Four phases of swallowing. Bolus formation occurs in the **oral preparatory phase**. Transport of the bolus to the pharynx occurs in the **oral propulsive phase**. In the **pharyngeal phase**, the food bolus is transported from the pharynx into the esophagus. During this phase, the nasopharynx is closed, breathing stops, the vocal cords adduct (come together), the larynx rises, and the base of the tongue and pharyngeal muscles propel the bolus to the esophagus. In the **esophageal phase**, peristaltic contraction of the esophagus moves the bolus from the upper esophageal sphincter, into the body of the esophagus, through the lower esophageal sphincter, and into the stomach.

(Excerpted from Scholes MA, Ramakrishnan VR: *ENT Secrets*: 4th ed, St. Louis, Elsevier, 2016, p 338, Table 48-2. Four Phases of Swallowing.)

Swallowing
Oral preparatory, oral propulsive, pharyngeal phase, esophageal phase

Alcoholism, loss consciousness

Recent dental work

Aerobic/anaerobic strep

Staphylococcus, Prevotella

Fusobacterium, anaerobes (60%)

Complication bacterial pneumonia

Septic embolism from IE

Obstructive lung neoplasia (obstructed bronchus)

Vary size/location

Aspiration: superior segment right lower lobe

Spiking fever, productive cough, foul-smelling sputum

Cavitation/fluid level

Vascular lung lesions

Pulmonary thromboembolism

Blockage lung artery; thrombus deep veins lower leg

3rd MC cardiovascular COD

Majority from lower extremities

Deep calf veins → popliteal/femoral vein → embolize

Stasis blood flow, hypercoagulable states

Size determines vessel occluded

Saddle embolus (large)

(1) Risk factors for a lung abscess include alcoholism, loss of consciousness, and recent dental work.

(2) Microbial pathogens include aerobic and anaerobic streptococci, *Staphylococcus* spp., *Prevotella* spp., *Fusobacterium* spp., and anaerobes (present in 60% of cases).

c. May occur as a complication of bacterial pneumonia, particularly those caused by *S. aureus* and *Klebsiella pneumoniae*

d. Result of septic embolism due to infective endocarditis (IE; see Chapter 11)

e. Associated with obstructive lung neoplasia. Approximately 10% to 15% of lung abscesses occur distal to a cancer, causing bronchial obstruction.

3. Gross findings

a. Abscesses vary in size and location (Fig. 17-8 A).

b. Those caused by aspiration are primarily located on the right side (Box 17-1); superior segment, right lower lobe

4. Clinical findings

a. Spiking fever and productive cough (foul-smelling sputum) are common.

b. Chest imaging shows cavitation with an air-fluid level (Fig. 17-8 B).

VII. **Vascular Lung Lesions**

A. **Pulmonary embolism (PE)**

1. **Definition:** A sudden blockage in a pulmonary artery that is most often caused by an embolism of a thrombus usually located in the deep veins of the leg (most common) or other distant site (e.g., vena cava)

2. Epidemiology and pathogenesis (Link 17-62)

a. Third most common cardiovascular cause of death after acute myocardial infarction and stroke

b. Source

(1) Majority (90%) originate from the lower extremities

(2) Thrombi usually start in the calf veins and propagate into the popliteal and femoral vein, from which they embolize to the lungs.

c. Risk factors (see Chapter 5). Stasis of blood flow (e.g., prolonged bed rest) and hypercoagulable states (e.g., antithrombin deficiency) are the primary risk factors.

d. Size of the embolus determines the pulmonary vessel (PV) tributary that is occluded.

(1) Large emboli occlude the proximal portion of the pulmonary artery and are frequently called a saddle embolus (Fig. 17-9 A; Links 17-63, 17-64, and 17-65)

(2) Small emboli occlude medium-sized and small pulmonary arteries (PAs).

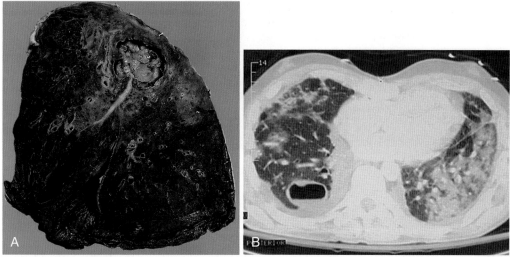

17-8: A, Lung abscess. Note the large abscess spanning the right upper and lower lobes. It is filled with necrotic material. **B,** Lung abscess. The chest computed tomography scan shows an abscess in the right lower lobe with an air-fluid level. (**A** *from Corrin B:* Pathology of the Lungs, *London, Churchill Livingstone, 2000, p 172, Fig. 5.5.16;* **B** *from Klatt E:* Robbins and Cotran Atlas of Pathology, *Philadelphia, Saunders, 2006, p 121, Fig. 5-74.)*

BOX 17-1   Aspiration Sites in the Lungs

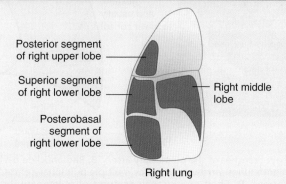

Right lung

Foreign material localizes to different portions of the lung, depending on the position of the patient. In the standing or sitting position, material localizes in the posterobasal segment of the right lower lobe; in the supine position, the superior segment of the right lower lobe; and in the right-sided position, the right middle lobe or the posterior segment of the right upper lobe. The most common aspiration site is the superior segment of the right lower lobe.

---

e. Potential consequences of PA occlusion include:
  (1) increase in PA pressure.
  (2) decrease in blood flow to the pulmonary parenchyma with the potential for developing a hemorrhagic infarction (see Chapter 2).
f. Approximately 8% to 10% of patients die within the first hour.

> Consequences pulmonary artery occlusion
> ↑PA pressure
> Potential for hemorrhagic infarction

In a patient with normal bronchial artery blood flow (originates from thoracic aorta and intercostal arteries [ICAs]) and ventilation, a pulmonary embolus produces a hemorrhagic infarction in ~10% of cases. However, if the patient has decreased bronchial artery blood flow (e.g., decreased cardiac output) or previously damaged lungs (e.g., obstructive lung disease), then occlusion of the PV will likely result in a hemorrhagic infarction, which significantly increases risk of morbidity and death.

> Bronchial arteries: arise from thoracic aorta and ICAs; Bronchial arteries: protect lungs from infarction

3. Pulmonary infarction is a red-blue, raised, wedge-shaped area that usually extends to the pleural surface (see Fig. 2-16 C).
  a. Pleural surface has a fibrinous exudate that produces a pleural friction rub on auscultation of the lungs. Hemorrhagic pleural effusion is usually present.

> Red-blue wedge shape extends to pleural surface
> Fibrinous pleural exudate → friction rub
> Hemorrhagic pleural effusion

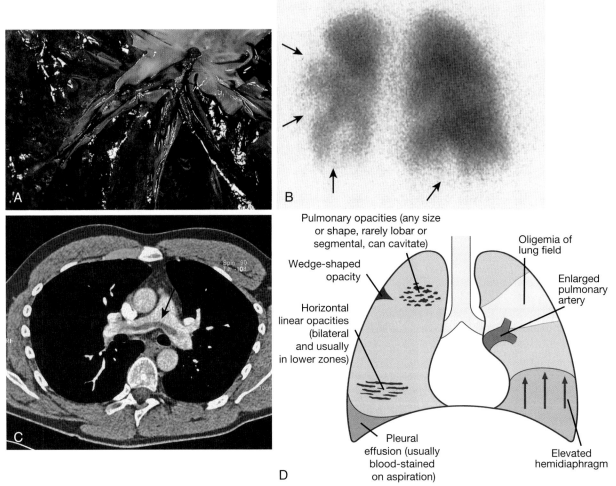

17-9: A, Saddle embolus occluding the main branches of the pulmonary artery. **B,** Radionuclide perfusion scan in the lung. The radionuclide scan shows multiple perfusion defects in both lungs *(arrows)* caused by multiple pulmonary emboli. **C,** Computed tomography pulmonary angiogram showing a saddle embolus *(arrow).* **D,** Chest radiographic features of pulmonary thromboembolism and infarction. *(A from my friend Ivan Damjanov, MD, PhD, Linder J: Pathology: A Color Atlas, St. Louis, Mosby, 2000, p 57, Fig. 4-26; B from Forbes C, Jackson W: Color Atlas and Text of Clinical Medicine, 2nd ed, London, Mosby, 2002, Fig. 4-49. C, From Walker BR, Colledge NR, Ralston SH, Penman ID: Davidson's Principles and Practice of Medicine, 22nd ed, St. Louis, Churchill Livingstone Elsevier, 2014, p 723, Fig. 19.69. D from Walker BR, Colledge NR, Ralston SH, Penman ID: Davidson's Principles and Practice of Medicine, 22nd ed, St. Louis, Churchill Livingstone Elsevier, 2014, p 722, Fig. 19.67.)*

MC site lower lobes; perfusion > ventilation

Saddle embolus →↑PA pressure → acute RV strain → sudden death

Dyspnea, tachypnea, fever

Pleuritic chest pain, friction rube, effusion

Expiratory wheezing

Respiratory alkalosis

PaO₂ <80 mm Hg

↑A-a gradient

↑D-dimers

Chest x-ray

Elevation ipsilateral hemidiaphragm

    b. Majority are located in the lower lobes because perfusion is greater than ventilation in the lower lobes.

4. Clinical findings

    a. If the patient has a saddle embolus, the sudden increase in PA pressure produces acute right ventricular (RV) strain and sudden death.

    b. Pulmonary infarction results in:

        (1) sudden onset of dyspnea (difficulty with breathing) and tachypnea (rapid breathing); fever.

        (2) pleuritic chest pain (pain on inspiration), friction rub, and percussion signs of an effusion.

        (3) expiratory wheezing caused by release of thromboxane A_2 (bronchoconstrictor) from platelets in the thromboembolus.

5. Laboratory findings include:

    a. respiratory alkalosis (arterial Pco_2 <33 mm Hg).

    b. Pao_2 <80 mm Hg (90% of cases; perfusion defect [see Chapter 2]).

    c. increase in A-a gradient (100% of cases; see Chapter 2).

    d. increase in D-dimers (see Chapter 15).

6. Diagnosis

    a. Chest radiography (Fig.17-9 D)

        (1) Elevation of the ipsilateral hemidiaphragm (most common finding)

(2) Pleural effusion (usually hemorrhagic) is frequently present.
(3) "Cut-off" sign is present in one or more PAs (Link 17-64 A).
(4) Hypovascularity behind the blocked vessel (Link 17-65)
(5) Hampton hump is present, which is a wedge-shaped area of consolidation.
  b. Perfusion radionuclide scan
  (1) Sensitivity, 77%; specificity, 98%
  (2) Because of the low sensitivity of the V/Q scan as an initial test for diagnosing a pulmonary embolus, the computed tomography pulmonary angiogram (CTPA [spiral CT]; Fig. 17-9 C) is frequently used as a screening test for the detection of PE because of the increased sensitivity (89%) and specificity (95%).
  (3) Ventilation scan is normal, but the perfusion scan findings are abnormal (see Fig. 17-9 B).
  c. Pulmonary angiogram is gold standard confirmatory test. However, it is expensive and is *not* available in smaller hospitals.
  d. D-dimer test result is usually positive (see Chapter 15).
  (1) Test is usually performed with ventilation/perfusion (V/Q) scan or CTPA.
  (2) Sensitivity of the test ranges from 85% to 98% for the diagnosis of a PE. Most useful in excluding a PE if the test result returns normal.
  (3) Specificity is poor.
  e. Cardiac troponins may be elevated because of RV dilation and myocardial injury.
  7. Prognosis of PE.
  a. Case fatality 1 month after diagnosis is 12%.
  b. Recurrence rate is ~6% during the first 6 months.
B. **Pulmonary arterial hypertension (PAH)**
  1. **Definition:** A mean PA pressure >25 mm Hg at rest
  2. Epidemiology and pathogenesis
  a. Primary PAH
  (1) Primary type is three times more common in women than men.
  (2) Generally occurs in younger patients (20–40 years old)
  (3) Genetic predisposition
  (4) Vascular hyperreactivity with proliferation of SMCs in the PVs.
  b. Secondary PAH
  (1) Caused by endothelial cell dysfunction (ECD) in which there is a loss of vasodilators (e.g., nitric oxide [NO]) and an increase in vasoconstrictors (e.g., endothelin)
  (2) Hypoxemia and respiratory acidosis stimulate vasoconstriction (VC) of PAs; causes SMC hyperplasia and hypertrophy (Link 17-66)
  (3) Causes of secondary PH include:
    (a) chronic hypoxemia. Examples: chronic lung disease, living at high altitude
    (b) chronic respiratory acidosis. Examples: chronic bronchitis (CB), OSA
    (c) loss of pulmonary vasculature, which increases the workload for remaining vessels. Examples: emphysema, recurrent pulmonary emboli
    (d) left-to-right cardiac shunts, which produces volume overloading of the pulmonary vasculature. Examples: ventricular septal defect (VSD), atrial septal defect (ASD), PDA
    (e) left-sided valvular disease in which there is a backup of blood into the pulmonary veins, causing pulmonary venous hypertension (PVH). Example: mitral valve stenosis
    (f) drugs. Examples: anorexigens (e.g., aminorex, fenfluramine), amphetamines
    (g) infections: HIV, schistosomiasis.
    (h) vascular impairment: sickle cell disease, chronic thromboembolic disease, pulmonary veno-occlusive disease.
    (i) miscellaneous: OSA, collagen vascular diseases (e.g., systemic sclerosis).
  3. Pathologic findings in pulmonary hypertension
  a. Atherosclerosis of main elastic PAs. Atherosclerosis is caused by increased pressure on the endothelium, leading to injury ("reaction to injury"; see Chapter 10; Link 17-67).
  b. Hyperplasia of myointimal cells (MICs) and SMCs in the pulmonary vasculature (Link 17-66)
  4. Clinical findings include:
  a. exertional dyspnea (most common presenting symptom), chest pain.
  b. accentuated P_2 (sign of PH).
  c. increased jugular venous pressure (JVP) with accentuated *a* wave (atrial contraction).

Left parasternal heave (RVH)

RHF due to cor pulmonale

Pedal pitting edema (LHF)

Catheterization

Chest x-ray

Enlarged PAs with tapering distal vessels

RV enlargement

ECG

Echocardiography

Paradoxic bulging IVS into LV during systole

Hypertrophy free wall RV

Estimates PA pressure

Cor pulmonale: PH + RVH → RHF

Goodpasture syndrome

Abs directed against BM pulmonary/glomerular capillaries

Hemoptysis, pulmonary hemorrhage, renal failure

Restrictive lung diseases

Obstructive vs RLD

Not directly measured: TLC, FRC, residual volume

TLC: Total amount air expanded lung

Residual volume: Volume left over post max expiration

TV: Volume air enters/leaves normal resp

FVC: Total volume air expelled post max inspiration

FEV$_1$: Amt air expelled 1 sec after max inspiration

Normal FEV$_1$/FVC: 4/5 L = 80%

   d. left parasternal heave (sign of RVH). Pulmonary hypertension imposes an increased afterload on the RV.
   e. right-sided heart failure (RHF) caused by cor pulmonale (see later).
   f. pedal pitting edema (LHF).
 5. Diagnosis includes:
   a. catheterization to measure pressures. Transthoracic Doppler echocardiography can also measure pressures.
   b. chest radiography.
     (1) Shows enlargement of the main PAs and rapid tapering of the distal vessels (Link 17-68)
     (2) Shows RV enlargement
   c. electrocardiogram (ECG): shows right axis deviation, RV enlargement, right atrial enlargement, and ST- and T-wave changes that reflect RV strain
   d. echocardiography.
     (1) Shows paradoxic bulging of the interventricular septum (IVS) into the left ventricle (LV) during systole caused by hypertrophy of the RV.
     (2) Shows hypertrophy of the RV free wall
     (3) Estimates PA pressure
 6. Cor pulmonale (Fig. 17-10; Link 17-69). Combination of PAH and RVH leading to right-sided heart failure (RHF).
  C. Goodpasture syndrome (see Chapter 20)
   1. Antibodies are directed against basement membrane (BM) in pulmonary capillaries and glomerular capillaries (type II hypersensitivity reaction [HSR]).
   2. Pulmonary hemorrhage with hemoptysis often precedes renal failure.
VIII. Restrictive Lung Diseases (RLDs)
  A. Spirometry (Fig. 17-11)
   1. Spirometry is helpful in distinguishing restrictive from obstructive lung disease.
   2. Important volumes and capacities
   a. Volumes *not* directly measured by spirometry include the total lung capacity (TLC), functional residual capacity (FRC), and residual volume.
     (1) TLC: total amount of air in a fully expanded lung
     (2) Residual volume: volume of air left over in the lung after maximal expiration
   b. Tidal volume (TV): volume of air that enters or leaves the lungs during normal quiet respiration
     (1) Forced vital capacity (FVC): total volume of air expelled after a maximal inspiration. Normal FVC is 5 L (see Fig. 17-11 A).
     (2) Forced expiratory volume in 1 second (FEV$_1$): amount of air expelled from the lungs in 1 second after a maximal inspiration. Normal FEV$_1$ is 4 L (see Fig. 17-11 A).
     (3) Ratio of FEV$_1$/FVC is normally 4/5, or 80%

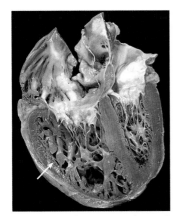

17-10: Cor pulmonale. Note the increased ventricular volume and hypertrophied muscle of the right ventricle *(arrow)*. The patient had pulmonary hypertension. *(From Kumar V, Fausto N, Abbas A, Aster J: Robbins and Cotran Pathologic Basis of Disease, 8th ed, Philadelphia, Saunders Elsevier, 2010, p 560, Fig. 12-21B.)*

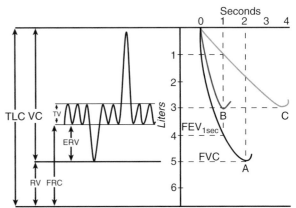

17-11: Spirometry showing normal lung volumes and capacities and forced expiratory volume in 1 second (FEV$_1$) and forced vital capacity (FVC) findings in a normal person (**A**), a person with restrictive lung disease (**B**), and a person with obstructive lung disease (**C**). *ERV,* Expiratory reserve volume; *RV,* residual volume; *TLC,* total lung capacity; *TV,* tidal volume; *VC,* vital capacity. *(From Goljan EF: Star Series: Pathology, Philadelphia, Saunders, 1998, p 229, Fig. 11.1.)*

B. Definition and epidemiology of RLD
1. **Definition:** Group of disorders characterized by a reduced TLC in the presence of a normal or reduced expiratory flow rate

RLD: ↓TLC

2. Epidemiology
   a. More common in men than women

Men > women

   b. Causes of RLD include:
      (1) chest wall disorders.

Chest wall disorders

         • Examples of chest wall disorders: pectum excavatum (Link 17-70), kyphoscoliosis (KS; outward curvature [kyphosis] and lateral curvature [scoliosis] of the spinal column; see Chapter 24; Link 17-71), pleural disease (e.g., mesothelioma), obesity (see Chapter 8).

Pectus excavatum, KS, pleural disease, obesity

      (2) acute or chronic interstitial lung diseases (CILDs; discussed later).
         (a) Acute interstitial lung disease (ILD; e.g., ARDS)

ARDS

         (b) Chronic interstitial lung disease, including:

CILD

            • fibrosing disorders (e.g., idiopathic pulmonary fibrosis [most common cause of RLD]; pneumoconiosis).
            • granulomatous disease (e.g., sarcoidosis).

Fibrosing/granulomatous disorders

C. Idiopathic pulmonary fibrosis (IPF)

Interstitial pulmonary fibrosis

1. Earliest manifestation is an alveolitis (inflammation limited to the alveolus; Link 17-72).
   • Leukocytes in the alveoli release cytokines, which stimulate fibrosis.

Alveolitis → interstitial fibrosis

2. Effects on the lungs include:
   a. decrease in lung compliance (stretch and expansion) on inspiration.

↓Lung compliance (expansion)

      (1) Decreased expansion of the lung parenchyma (less air in alveoli)

↓Expansion during inspiration

      (2) Damage to type I/II alveolar cells and endothelial cells

Damage type I/II alveolar cells, endothelial cells

         • Functional loss of alveolar and capillary units

Functional loss alveolar/capillary units

   b. increase in lung elasticity.

↑Lung elasticity

      • Recoil of the lung on expiration is increased.

↑Recoil on expiration

3. Clinical and laboratory findings include:
   a. dry cough and exertional dyspnea.

Dry cough, exertional dyspnea

   b. late inspiratory crackles in the lower lung fields.

Late inspiratory crackles

   c. potential for developing cor pulmonale (PH + RVH).

Potential for cor pulmonale

4. Pulmonary function test (PFT) findings and arterial blood gases (ABGs)
   a. All volumes and capacities are equally decreased.

Equal ↓ volumes/capacities

   b. Decreased FEV_1 (see Fig. 17-11 B)

↓FEV_1

      • Example: 3 L (normal 4 L)
   c. Decreased FVC (see Fig. 17-11 B)

↓FVC

      • Often the same value as the FEV_1 (3 L) because of increased lung elasticity
   d. Increased FEV_1/FVC ratio

↑FEV_1/FVC

      • Example: 3/3 = 100% (normal is 80%)
   e. Respiratory alkalosis (arterial PCO_2 <33 mm Hg) is present.

Respiratory alkalosis

   f. Decreased PaO_2 because of a diffusion defect in moving oxygen from the lungs into the pulmonary capillaries.

↓PaO_2; diffusion defect

5. Chest radiography findings in interstitial fibrosis

Diffuse reticulonodular infiltrates

   • Diffuse bilateral reticulonodular infiltrates throughout all lung fields

D. Pneumoconioses
1. **Definition:** Group of diseases of the lungs caused by the inhalation of mineral dust; leads to inflammation and interstitial fibrosis of the lungs

Inhalation of mineral dust

2. Epidemiology
   a. Mineral dust includes coal dust, silica, asbestos, and beryllium; accounts for ~25% of cases of chronic interstitial lung disease

Coal dust, silica, asbestos, beryllium

   b. Particle size determines the site of lung deposition of the mineral dust.
      (1) 1- to 5-μm particles reach the bifurcation of the respiratory bronchioles (RBs) and alveolar ducts.

1–5 μm reach bifurcation respiratory bronchioles/alveolar ducts

      (2) Particles smaller than 0.5-μm reach the alveoli and are phagocytized by alveolar MPs.

Particle size <0.5 μm alveoli

   c. Coal dust is the *least* fibrogenic particle.

Coal dust least fibrogenic

   d. Silica, asbestos, and beryllium are very fibrogenic.

Silica, asbestos, beryllium very fibrogenic

3. Coal worker's pneumoconiosis (CWP)

Coal worker's pneumoconiosis

   a. **Definition:** The inhalation of coal dust into the lungs

Inhalation coal dust

   b. Sources of coal dust (anthracotic pigment) include coal mines, large urban centers, and tobacco smoke.

Coal mines, urban areas, tobacco smoke

   c. Pulmonary anthracosis is usually asymptomatic.

17-12: A, Coal worker's pneumoconiosis. Note the heavy anthracotic pigment deposition in the fibrotic tissue. Subjacent alveoli are dilated. **B,** Silicosis. Note the nodular fibrotic mass in the lung. **C,** Asbestos body. The straight, golden-brown, beaded asbestos body represents an asbestos fiber coated by iron and protein. **D,** Malignant mesothelioma encases the lung and invades locally into the lung parenchyma. **E,** Sarcoid granuloma showing pink-staining epithelioid cells and foreign body type of multinucleated giant cells. **F,** Sarcoid nodules on the face (lupus pernio). On biopsy, these would contain noncaseating granulomas. *(A and B from Klatt E:* Robbins and Cotran Atlas of Pathology, *Philadelphia, Saunders, 2006, p 113, Figs. 5-48, 5-49, respectively; C from my friend Ivan Damjanov, MD, PhD, Linder J:* Pathology: A Color Atlas, *St. Louis, Mosby, 2000, p 65, Fig. 4-51B; D from Corrin B:* Pathology of the Lungs, *London, Churchill Livingstone, 2000, p 679, Fig. 14.8; E from Kumar V, Fausto N, Abbas A:* Robbins and Cotran Pathologic Basis of Disease, *7th ed, Philadelphia, Saunders, 2004, p 738, Fig. 15-23; F from Kliegman R:* Nelson Textbook of Pediatrics, *19th ed, Philadelphia, Elsevier Saunders, 2011, p 861, Fig. 159.2.)*

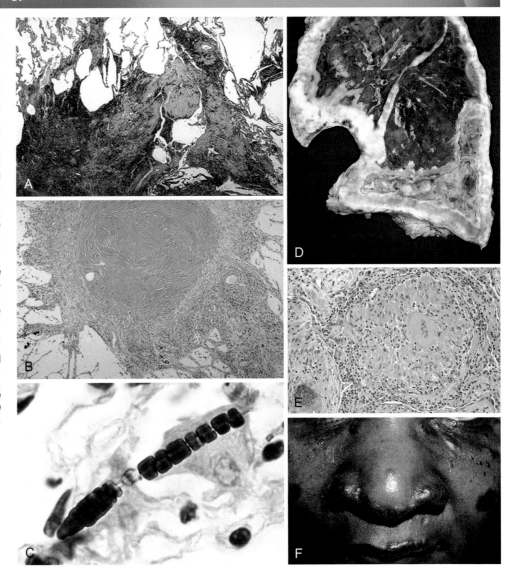

Black anthracotic pigment in interstitium; hilar nodes

Dust cells alveolar MPs with anthracotic pigment

Simple coal workers pneumoconiosis

SCWP opacities <1 cm

Centriacinar emphysema

Complicated coal worker pneumoconiosis

CWP opacities 1-2 cm; no necrotic centers

Crippling lung disease ("black lung")

No ↑risk tuberculosis, lung cancer

Cor pulmonale risk

Caplan syndrome: pneumoconiosis + cavitating rheumatoid nodules

Silicosis

Inhalation silica (quartz)

- Black anthracotic pigment is present in the interstitial tissue and hilar lymph nodes. Alveolar MPs with anthracotic pigment are called "dust cells."
  d. Simple coal worker's pneumoconiosis (SCWP)
  (1) **Definition:** Fibrotic opacities are smaller than 1 cm in the upper lobes and upper portions of the lower lobes
  (2) Coal deposits adjacent to respiratory bronchioles produce centriacinar (centrilobular) emphysema, which is a type of obstructive lung disease (discussed later).
  e. Complicated coal worker's pneumoconiosis (CWP; progressive massive fibrosis).
  (1) **Definition:** Characterized by the presence of fibrotic opacities larger than 1 to 2 cm with or without necrotic centers; usually located in the apices of the lung (Fig. 17-12 A; Links 17-74 and 17-75)
  (2) Crippling lung disease that is sometimes called "black lung" disease
  (3) Increased incidence of lung, colon, and urinary bladder cancer
  (4) *No* increased incidence of tuberculosis
  (5) Cor pulmonale may occur.
  (6) Caplan syndrome may occur (a combination of CWP plus large cavitating rheumatoid nodules in the lungs).
4. Silicosis
  a. **Definition:** The inhalation of silica (quartz) into the lungs
  b. Epidemiology

(1) Most common occupational disease in the world

(2) Quartz (crystalline silicone dioxide) is most often implicated as the cause of silicosis. Sources of silicone dioxide include foundries (casting metal), sandblasting, and working in mines.

   c. Pathogenesis

(1) Quartz is highly fibrogenic and primarily deposits in the upper lungs.

(2) Quartz activates and is cytolytic to alveolar MPs. Activated MPs release cytokines that stimulate fibrogenesis.

   d. Chest radiography findings in acute exposure show a "ground-glass" appearance in all lung fields.

   e. Chest radiography findings in chronic exposure show nodular opacities in the lungs.

(1) Nodules show concentric layers of collagen with or without central cavitation (Fig. 17-12 B; Link 17-76).

(2) "Egg-shell" calcifications are seen in the hilar lymph nodes: rim of dystrophic calcification in the lymph nodes that simulates an egg shell

   f. Complications of silicosis include:

(1) cor pulmonale, Caplan syndrome.

(2) increased risk for developing lung cancer and tuberculosis.

5. Asbestos-related disease (Link 17-77)

   a. Geometric forms of asbestos

(1) Serpentine

     (a) Curly and flexible asbestos fibers (e.g., chrysotile)

     (b) Produce interstitial fibrosis and lung cancer

(2) Amphibole

     (a) Straight and rigid asbestos fibers (e.g., crocidolite)

     (b) Produce interstitial fibrosis, lung cancer, and mesothelioma (cancer of the pleura)

(3) Deposition sites of asbestos include the respiratory bronchioles, alveolar ducts, and alveoli (respiratory unit)

   b. Sources of asbestos fibers include:

(1) insulation around pipes in old naval ships.

(2) roofing material, ceiling tiles, floor tiles used >20 years ago.

(3) demolition of old buildings.

(4) automobile shops (brakes in old cars had asbestos in brake pads).

   c. Appearance in tissue

(1) Asbestos fibers are coated by iron and protein (called ferruginous bodies).

     • MPs phagocytize and coat the fibers with ferritin (synthesized by MPs).

(2) Ferruginous bodies have a golden, beaded appearance in sputum or the in distal, small airways (Fig. 17-12 C; Links 17-78 to 17-80).

   d. Asbestos-related diseases include:

(1) benign pleural plaques.

     (a) Most common lesion associated with asbestosis; asymptomatic

     (b) Calcified plaques that are located on the pleura and the dome of the diaphragm (Links 7-81 A and 7-81 B)

     (c) *Not* a precursor lesion for developing a mesothelioma

(2) diffuse interstitial fibrosis with or without pleural effusions.

(3) primary bronchogenic carcinoma.

     (a) Risk further increases if the patient smokes cigarettes.

     (b) Latency period for developing bronchogenic carcinoma is ~20 years after exposure.

(4) Malignant mesothelioma of pleura

     (a) *No* etiologic relationship with smoking

     (b) Arises from the serosal cells lining the pleura

     (c) Encases and locally invades the subpleural lung tissue (Fig. 17-12 D; Link 17-81 C)

     (d) Latency period for developing a mesothelioma is 25 to 40 years after first exposure to asbestos.

(5) *No* increased risk for developing tuberculosis in asbestosis

   e. Additional complications of asbestos-related disease include cor pulmonale and Caplan syndrome.

6. Berylliosis

   a. **Definition:** A lung disease associated with inhalation of beryllium

   b. Beryllium is a metal (chemical element Be) that is stronger than steel and lighter than aluminum.

c. Exposure to beryllium may occur in aerospace industries and dentistry.

d. Produces a diffuse interstitial fibrosis with noncaseating granulomas

e. Increased risk for developing cor pulmonale and primary lung cancer

E. **Sarcoidosis**

1. **Definition:** Chronic, multisystem granulomatous disease characterized by the presence of noncaseating granulomas and chronic interstitial fibrosis in the lungs

2. Epidemiology

a. Most common noninfectious granulomatous disease

b. Accounts for ~25% of cases of chronic interstitial lung disease

c. Common in blacks and nonsmokers

d. More common in women than men

e. Incidence of sarcoidosis peaks between 20 to 39 years of age.

3. Pathogenesis

a. Disorder in immune regulation

- Major histocompatibility complex (*MHC*) genes and non-*MHC* genes have been located on the short arm of chromosome 6 that are genetic risk factors for sarcoidosis.

b. CD4 T$_H$ cells interact with unknown airborne antigens (e.g., mold or mildew, pesticides, mycobacterial KatG protein); causes the release of cytokines from the CD4 T$_H$ cells, resulting in the formation of noncaseating granulomas.

c. Diagnosis of exclusion. Clinician must rule out other granulomatous diseases (e.g., TB) before the diagnosis of sarcoidosis is made.

4. Overview of clinical features (Link 17-82)

5. Lung disease

a. Lungs are the primary target organ for sarcoidosis.

(1) Granulomas are located in the interstitium as well as mediastinal and hilar lymph nodes.

(2) Granulomas contain multinucleated giant cells (MGCs; Fig. 17-12 E; Link 17-83). Granulomas contain laminated calcium concretions (Schaumann bodies; Link 17-84) and stellate inclusions (called asteroid bodies; Link 17-85).

b. Dyspnea (difficulty with breathing) is the most common symptom.

6. Skin lesions

a. Nodular lesions containing noncaseating granulomas (Fig. 17-12 F)

b. Violaceous rash is often present on the nose and cheeks (called lupus pernio).

c. Erythema nodosum (EN) is present 10% of cases.

(1) Painful nodules located on the lower extremities (see Fig. 25-12 M)

(2) Biopsy shows inflammation of the subcutaneous fat.

7. Uveitis is a common lesion in the eye.

a. Uvea is the pigmented middle layer of the eye and consists of the choroid, ciliary body, and iris.

b. Clinical findings in uveitis include blurry vision, glaucoma, and corneal opacities.

8. Liver lesions

a. Granulomatous hepatitis is present.

b. Sarcoidosis is the most common noninfectious cause of hepatitis.

9. Other multisystem findings include:

a. enlarged salivary and lacrimal glands.

b. central diabetes insipidus (CDI; hypothalamic and posterior pituitary disease; see Chapter 5).

c. granulomas in the BM and spleen.

d. calcium renal stones and nephrocalcinosis (calcification of the BMs in renal tubules; see Chapter 20).

10. Laboratory findings include:

a. increased level of angiotensin-converting enzyme (ACE; 60% of cases). Nonspecific finding with poor sensitivity.

b. hypercalcemia (5% of cases). Increased synthesis of 1-α-hydroxylase in MPs in the granulomas (hypervitaminosis D; see Chapter 8).

c. Other findings include:

(1) polyclonal gammopathy (see Chapter 3).

(2) cutaneous anergy to common skin antigens (e.g., *Candida* spp.; see Chapter 4).

- Decreased total CD4 T$_H$ cell count caused by consumption of CD4 T$_H$ cells in granulomas and the loss of cells in alveolar secretions

(3) cranial nerve palsies, phalangeal bone cysts, arthropathies, peripheral neuropathy, cardiac arrhythmia, heart block, sudden death, meningitis, and splenomegaly.

11. Chest radiography

    a. Enlarged hilar and mediastinal lymph nodes (called "potato nodes"; Link 17-86) caused by granulomas

    b. Reticulonodular densities throughout the lung parenchyma

12. Prognosis: approximately 5% mortality rate (particularly black Americans)

F. Idiopathic pulmonary fibrosis (IPF)

1. **Definition:** Chronic, progressive fibrosing interstitial pneumonia of unknown cause occurring primarily in older adults. It is also called usual interstitial pneumonia (UIP).

2. Epidemiology

    a. Accounts for ~30% of cases of RLDs

    b. Possible autoimmune response to various agents

    c. More common in smoking men than in women

    d. Other causes: exposure to viruses (e.g., EBV), occupational dusts (metal or wood), chronic gastroesophageal reflux

    e. Usually occurs in individuals 40 to 70 years old

3. Pathogenesis

    a. Repeated cycles of alveolitis are triggered by an unknown agent.

    b. Release of cytokines produces interstitial fibrosis.

    c. Alveolar fibrosis leads to proximal dilation of the small airways.

      • Lungs have a honeycomb appearance (Links 17-87 to 17-89).

4. Clinical findings include:

    a. dyspnea with exertion.

    b. chronic, nonproductive cough.

    c. late inspiratory crackles.

5. Poor prognosis (median survival time, 3–5 years after diagnosis)

6. Other idiopathic interstitial pneumonias

    a. Nonspecific interstitial pneumonia (NSIP)

      (1) Similar to idiopathic pulmonary fibrosis; however, patients tend to be women and girls

      (2) Often associated with connective tissue disease, certain drugs, hypersensitivity pneumonitis, and HIV infection

      (3) Better prognosis than idiopathic pulmonary fibrosis

    b. Respiratory bronchiolitis interstitial pneumonia (RBIP)

      (1) More common in men and smokers

      (2) Usually presents in people 40 to 60 years of age

      (3) Cessation of smoking often leads to improvement.

    c. Desquamative interstitial pneumonia (DIP)

      (1) Misnomer, because the infiltrate consists of pigmented MPs rather than desquamated alveolar cells

      (2) Strong association with smoking (90% of cases)

      (3) Insidious onset of cough and dyspnea

      (4) Association with respiratory bronchiolitis and interstitial pneumonia (see earlier) is controversial.

    d. Cryptogenic organizing pneumonia ("bronchiolitis obliterans organizing pneumonia" [BOOP])

      (1) Clinical and radiologic type of pneumonia

      (2) Biopsy shows proliferation of immature bodies (Masson bodies; granulation tissue) and fibrous tissue in the bronchioles.

      (3) Response to systemic corticosteroids is excellent.

    e. Lymphocytic interstitial pneumonia (LIP)

      (1) More common in women than men

      (2) Broad age range from young to old. Most cases occur in middle age.

      (3) Slow onset

      (4) Both viruses and immune processes contribute. The viruses include EBV and, especially in children, HIV.

      (5) Prominent diffuse, alveolar infiltrate of lymphocytes and plasma cells and lymphoid follicles consisting of B cells

G. Collagen vascular diseases

1. Account for ~10% of cases of chronic interstitial lung disease

2. Systemic sclerosis (see Chapter 4)

    • Most common cause of death is lung disease.

Margin notes:

"Potato nodes"

Reticulonodular densities

IPF

Chronic fibrosing interstitial pneumonia; UIP

Smoking males > females

Viruses, dusts, chronic esophageal reflux

40 to 70 years old

Repeated cycles alveolitis

Cytokines → interstitial fibrosis

Fibrosis small airways → proximal dilation → honeycomb lungs

Dyspnea with exertion

Chronic nonproductive cough

Late inspiratory crackles

NSIP

Similar to idiopathic pulmonary fibrosis *except* more common in females

RBIP

Men, smokers

Cessation smoking shows improvement

DIP

Misnomer; pigmented MPs *not* alveolar cells

Smoking 90% cases

BOOP

Masson bodies (granulation tissue), fibrous tissue in bronchioles

LIP

Women > men

Middle age

EBV, HIV (children)

Lymphoid infiltrate, lymphoid follicles (B cells)

Collagen vascular diseases

Systemic sclerosis

MC COD lung disease

3. Systemic lupus erythematosus (SLE; see Chapter 4)

ILD 50%

Pleuritis/pleural effusions

a. ILD occurs in 50% of patients.
b. Pleuritis with pleural effusions are also commonly present.

Any unexplained pleural effusion in a young woman is SLE until proved otherwise. PF contains an inflammatory infiltrate (exudate); lupus erythematosus cells (neutrophils with phagocytosed DNA) are sometimes present. One of the key criteria for diagnosing SLE is the presence of serositis and pleuritic; a pleural effusion being a manifestation of this type of inflammation.

Pleural effusion young woman: consider SLE

Rheumatoid arthritis

Rheumatoid nodules + pneumoconiosis: Caplan syndrome

Interstitial fibrosis +/- rheumatoid nodules

Pleuritis with pleural effusions

Hypersensitivity pneumonitis

Extrinsic allergic alveolitis; known inhaled antigen

Does not involve IgE antibodies

Farmer's lung

Thermophilic actinomyces in moldy hay

1st exposure: IgG abs

2nd exposure: IgG + inhaled antigens; type III HSR

Chronic exposure granulomatous inflammation (type IV HSR)

Silo filler's disease

Inhalation oxides of plant material

Immediate dyspnea

Byssinosis

Inhalation particles cotton, linen, hemp, jute

Textile workers

Endotoxin in gram negative bacteria

Feel better on weekend

"Monday morning blues"

Bagassosis: sugar cane

Maple bark disease

Mushroom workers disease

Humidifier lung: contaminated fluids

Pigeon-breeder's lung: pigeon droppings

Furrier's lung: animal pelts

Drugs → interstitial fibrosis

Amiodarone

Bleomycin, busulfan

Cyclophosphamide

Methotrexate, methysergide

Nitrosourea, nitrofurantoin

4. Rheumatoid arthritis (RA; see Chapter 24)
   a. Rheumatoid nodules in lungs plus a pneumoconiosis is called Caplan syndrome.
   b. Pulmonary findings include:
      (1) Interstitial fibrosis with or without intrapulmonary rheumatoid nodules. Nodules often show cavitation.
      (2) Pleuritis is present with pleural effusions.

H. **Hypersensitivity pneumonitis**
   1. **Definition:** Extrinsic allergic alveolitis associated with exposure to a *known* inhaled antigen
      • Does *not* involve IgE antibodies (it is *not* a type I HSR) or have eosinophilia
   2. Overview of hypersensitivity pneumonitis (Link 17-90)
   3. Farmer's lung
      a. **Definition**: Hypersensitivity pneumonitis associated with exposure to *Saccharopolyspora rectivirgula* (thermophilic actinomycetes) in moldy hay
      b. First exposure
         • Patient develops precipitating IgG antibodies (present in serum).
      c. Second exposure
         (1) IgG antibodies combine with inhaled allergens to form immune complexes, which is a type III HSR.
         (2) Immunocomplexes produce an inflammatory reaction in lung tissue.
      d. Chronic exposure produces an additional component of granulomatous inflammation (type IV HSR).
   4. Silo filler's disease
      a. **Definition**: Hypersensitivity pneumonitis caused by inhalation of gases (oxides of nitrogen) from plant material
      b. Causes an immediate HSR associated with dyspnea
   5. Byssinosis
      a. **Definition**: Form of occupational asthma with inhalation of particles of cotton, linen, hemp, or jute (fiber in rope and burlap)
      b. Epidemiology
         (1) Occurs in workers in textile factories
         (2) May be associated with exposure to bacterial endotoxin from gram-negative bacteria growing on the cotton
      c. Clinical findings
         (1) Dyspnea develops on exposure to the previous products.
         (2) Workers feel better over the weekend (no exposure to antigens).
            • Depression occurs when returning to work on Monday ("Monday morning blues").
   6. Other HSRs include:
      a. bagassosis (source of antigen is sugar cane).
      b. maple bark disease (source of antigen is maple bark, particularly when collecting maple syrup).
      c. mushroom worker's disease (source of antigen is mushrooms).
      d. humidifier lung (source of antigen is contaminated fluid).
      e. pigeon-breeder's lung (pigeon droppings [coops, under bridges]).
      f. furrier's lung (animal pelts).

I. **Drugs associated with interstitial fibrosis include:**
   1. amiodarone.
   2. bleomycin and busulfan.
   3. cyclophosphamide.
   4. methotrexate and methysergide.
   5. nitrosourea and nitrofurantoin.

J. Radiation-induced lung disease (see Chapter 7)
1. Acute pneumonitis may occur 1 to 6 months after radiation therapy.
2. Clinical findings in radiation-induced lung disease include:
   a. fever and dyspnea.
   b. pleural effusions.
3. Some patients develop chronic radiation pneumonitis.
4. Chest radiography shows infiltrates.

IX. Chronic Obstructive Pulmonary Disease (COPD)
A. Definition: Progressive, largely irreversible obstruction to airflow out of the lungs
B. Epidemiology
1. Cigarette smoking is the principal cause of COPD (see Chapter 7).
2. Greater than 10% of the population older than 45 years of age has airflow obstruction.
3. Majority of patients with COPD have both emphysema (air space destruction) and CB (chronic bronchitis; conducting airway inflammation).
C. Emphysema
1. **Definition:** Permanent enlargement of all or part of the respiratory unit
   • Respiratory unit includes respiratory bronchioles, alveolar ducts, and alveoli.
2. Epidemiology
   a. Causes
      (1) Smoking cigarettes is the most common cause of emphysema.
      (2) α_1-Antitrypsin (AAT) deficiency is a cause of emphysema.
   b. Types of emphysema associated with smoking or loss of AAT include:
      (1) centriacinar (centrilobular) emphysema.
      (2) panacinar emphysema.
3. Pathogenesis
   a. Increased compliance (ability to stretch) and decreased elasticity (lung recoil) of the respiratory unit
      (1) Imbalance between elastase and antielastases (e.g., AAT)
      (2) Imbalance between oxidants (FRs) and antioxidants (e.g., glutathione)
      (3) Elastase and antioxidants derive from neutrophils and MPs.
      (4) Net effect of the presence of elastases, and FRs is the destruction of elastic tissue
   b. Cigarette smoke is chemotactic to neutrophils and MPs. Neutrophils and MPs accumulate in the respiratory unit and release FRs and elastases.
   c. FRs in cigarette smoke inactivate AAT and antioxidants (functional AAT).
   d. Normal function of elastic tissue
      (1) Elastic fibers attach to the outside wall of the small airways (Fig. 17-13 A).
      (2) Elastic fibers apply radial traction to keep the airway lumens open.
   e. Destruction of the elastic tissue causes in these sites results in the loss of radial traction; small airways collapse, particularly on expiration
   f. Sites of elastic tissue destruction in emphysema include:
      (1) distal terminal bronchiole at its junction with the respiratory bronchioles.
      (2) all or part of the respiratory unit.

Sidebar notes (right margin):
Radiation-induced lung disease

1-6 mths after radiation

Fever, dyspnea

Pleural effusions

COPD

Progressive, irreversible outflow obstruction to airflow

MCC cigarette smoking

Emphysema targets air space, CB target conducting airways

Permanent enlargement all/part respiratory unit

Respiratory bronchioles, alveolar ducts, alveoli

Smoking cigarettes: MCC emphysema

AAT deficiency

Centriacinar (centrilobular)

Panacinar

↑Compliance/↓elasticity

Imbalance elastase and α_1-anti-trypsin

Imbalance oxidants/antioxidants

Neutrophils/MPs

Net effect → destruction elastic tissue

Chemotactic to neutrophils/MPs

FRs inactivate AAT/antioxidants

Functional AAT deficiency

Normal function elastic tissue

Attach to outside wall small airways

Apply radial traction: keep airway lumens open

Loss radial traction in respiratory unit

Collapse on expiration

Distal TB/RB junction

All/part of respiratory unit

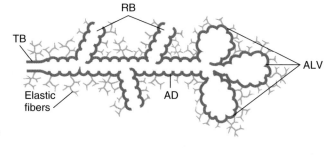

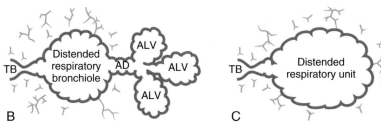

17-13: Types of emphysema. **A,** Schematic shows a normal distal airway, including a terminal bronchiole (TB) leading into the respiratory unit consisting of a respiratory bronchiole (RB), alveolar duct (AD), and alveoli (ALV). Elastic fibers apply radial traction to keep these airways open. **B,** Centriacinar (centrilobular) emphysema is characterized by trapping of air in the respiratory bronchioles. Note how the elastic fibers of the distal TB are destroyed, causing obstruction to airflow. This causes the trapped air to distend the RBs, whose elastic tissue support is destroyed. **C,** Panacinar emphysema is characterized by trapping of air in the entire respiratory unit behind the collapsed TB.

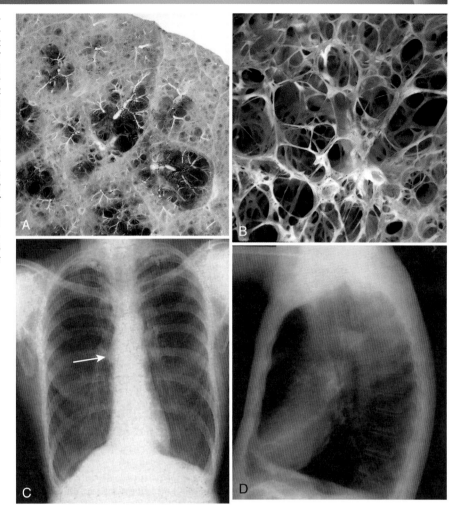

17-14: **A,** Centriacinar (centrilobular emphysema). The enlarged spaces in the lung parenchyma are air-filled respiratory bronchioles that have lost their elastic tissue support. **B,** Panacinar emphysema. The enlarged spaces in the lung parenchyma are air-filled respiratory bronchioles, alveolar ducts, and alveoli that have lost their elastic tissue support. **C,** Chest radiograph in emphysema showing a vertically oriented heart *(arrow)* and depressed diaphragm. **D,** Radiograph of the thorax in a patient with emphysema. There are an increase in lung volume, darkness of the lungs (increased air relative to tissue), and an increase in space between the sternum and the heart. *(A and B reproduced by permission of the late Professor B.E. Heard, Brompton, UK; C from Forbes C, Jackson W: Color Atlas and Text of Clinical Medicine, 2nd ed, London, Mosby, 2002, p 186, Fig. 4-94; D from Goldman L, Schafer AI: Cecil's Medicine, 24th ed, Philadelphia, Saunders Elsevier, 2012, p 540, Fig. 88-3B.)*

Air trapping behind collapsed distal TBs

Trapped air distends parts of respiratory unit without elastic tissue

Centriacinar (-lobular) emphysema

Upper lobes; destruction elastic tissue distal TBs, RBs

MC emphysema in smokers

Primarily involves upper lobes

Distal TB/RB elastic tissue destroyed

Distention RBs

↑Residual volume, TLC

Panacinar emphysema

Lower lobes; destruction all/ part respiratory unit

Genetic/acquired AAT deficiency

AAT synthesized in liver

AD disorder

g. Site of obstruction and air trapping in emphysema
  (1) During expiration, the distal terminal bronchioles collapse. This prevents egress (exit) of air from the respiratory unit.
  (2) Trapped air distends the parts of the respiratory unit that have lost their elastic tissue support.
4. Centriacinar (centrilobular) emphysema
  a. **Definition:** Type of emphysema that preferentially involves the upper lobes and is characterized by destruction of the elastic tissue in the distal terminal bronchioles and respiratory bronchioles
  b. Epidemiology: most common type of emphysema in smokers
  c. Pathogenesis
    (1) Primarily involves the apical segments of the upper lobes.
    (2) Specifically, the distal terminal bronchioles and the respiratory bronchioles (Figs. 17-13 B and 17-14 A; Link 17-91 B) are the sites of elastic tissue destruction.
    (3) Air trapped behind the collapsed distal terminal bronchioles distends the respiratory bronchioles.
      • Trapped air increases the residual volume and TLC.
5. Panacinar emphysema
  a. **Definition:** Type of emphysema that preferentially involves the lower lobes and is characterized by destruction of the elastic tissue in all or parts of the respiratory unit
  b. Epidemiology
    (1) Associated with AAT deficiency; may be either a genetic or acquired deficiency (e.g., cigarette smoke inactivates AAT). AAT is synthesized in the liver.
    (2) Genetic type of AAT deficiency that is an autosomal dominant (AD) disorder
      (a) Alleles of AAT (protease) activity are designated M, normal; S, intermediate; Z, marked decrease; and null, absent (rare).

(b) Phenotypes
- MM, MS, and MZ have no increased risk.
- MS has a mildly increased risk.
- ZZ has an increased risk for emphysema and a potential for liver disease as well in 10% of cases.

(3) Emphysema develops at an earlier age in the genetic type compared with the acquired type.

c. Pathogenesis
(1) Distal terminal bronchioles and all or parts of the respiratory unit are the sites of elastic tissue destruction (Figs. 17-13 C and 17-14 B; Link 17-91 C).
(2) Air trapped behind the collapsed terminal bronchioles distends all or part of the respiratory unit.

d. Laboratory findings. Absence of α_1-globulin peaks in serum protein electrophoresis (SPE; see Chapter 3 discussion of SPE).

6. Clinical findings in centriacinar and panacinar emphysema
a. Premature lung disease (occurs at 30–40 years of age in smokers and at age 50–60 years in nonsmokers)
b. Progressive dyspnea and hyperventilation (respiratory alkalosis)
(1) Dyspnea is severe and occurs *early* in the disease.
(2) Hypoxemia occurs *late* in the disease because it takes time for destruction of respiratory units.
(3) Sometimes patients are called "pink puffers" because of their color and the way they breathe through pursed lips on expiration (Links 17-92 A and 17-93 A).
c. Centriacinar (centrilobular) emphysema frequently coexists with CB (see later) because both conditions are associated with smoking cigarettes.
d. Breath sounds are diminished because of hyperinflation of the lungs.
e. Cor pulmonale (PH + RVH) is uncommon.

7. Chest radiography in emphysema (Fig. 17-14 C and D)
a. Lung fields are hyperlucent (lung is less dense than normal).
b. Increased anteroposterior (AP) diameter because the RV is increased
c. Vertically oriented heart
d. Both diaphragms are depressed because of the hyperinflated lungs.
(1) Hyperinflated lungs (increased TLC) push the spleen and the liver down, giving the false impression of splenomegaly and hepatomegaly.
(2) Percussion of the upper and lower borders of the spleen and liver reveals that the spleen and liver are of normal size.

8. PFTs and ABGs
a. Increased TLC caused by an increase in the residual volume
b. FEV_1 is decreased (e.g., 1 L vs 4 L; see Fig. 17-11 C).
c. FVC is decreased (e.g., 3 L vs 5 L; see Fig. 17-11 C).
- FEV1/FVC ratio is decreased (e.g., 1/3 = 33%).
d. Decreased PaO_2 develops *late* in the disease.
- Destruction of the capillary bed matches the destruction of the respiratory unit it is associated with.
e. Arterial PCO_2 is normal to decreased (respiratory alkalosis; "pink puffer").

9. Other types of emphysema that are unrelated to smoking or AAT deficiency include:
a. paraseptal emphysema.
(1) Localized disease in a subpleural location. Destruction of lung tissue primarily targets the alveolar ducts and alveoli.
(2) Does *not* produce obstructive airway disease
(3) Increased incidence of spontaneous pneumothorax caused by rupture of subpleural blebs (discussed later)
b. irregular emphysema.
(1) Localized disease that is associated with scar tissue
(2) Does *not* produce obstructive airway disease

D. Chronic bronchitis
1. **Definition:** The presence of a productive cough for at least 3 months for 2 consecutive years
2. Epidemiology
a. Causes include:
(1) smoking cigarettes (most common).
(2) Cystic fibrosis.

Phenotypes

MM, MS, MZ no ↑risk

MS mild ↑risk

ZZ has ↑risk emphysema; possible liver disease

Earlier onset emphysema in genetic type

Distal TB, all/parts respiratory unit elastic tissue

Air distends all/part respiratory unit

Panacinar emphysema: no α_1-globulin peak SPE

Centriacinar/panacinar emphysema

Premature disease if smoker; later if nonsmoker

Dyspnea, hyperventilation (respiratory alkalosis)

Dyspnea severe *early* in disease

Hypoxemia late in disease

"Pink puffers"

Centriacinar emphysema can coexist with CB

Diminished breath sounds

Cor pulmonale uncommon

Chest radiograph emphysema

Hyperlucency

↑AP diameter

Vertically oriented heart

Both diaphragms depressed

False impression hepatomegaly/ splenomegaly

Percussion of borders essential

PFTs, ABGs

↑TLC due to ↑residual volume

↓FEV_1

↓FEV_1/FVC

↓PaO_2 late in disease

Normal to ↓arterial PCO_2 (respiratory alkalosis; "pink puffer")

Paraseptal emphysema

Subpleural location

Targets alveolar ducts/ alveoli

Does *not* produce obstructive airway disease

↑Risk spontaneous pneumothorax

Irregular emphysema

Localized disease associated with scar tissue

No obstructive airway disease

Chronic bronchitis

Productive cough 3 mths, 2 consecutive years

Smoking cigarettes: MCC

Cystic fibrosis

Hypersecretion mucus

Mucus plugs obstruct airflow

Fibrosis segmental bronchi/bronchioles

↑Secretion submucosal mucus glands trachea; bronchi

Productive cough

Acute/chronic inflammation

Loss ciliated epithelium; replaced by squamous metaplasia

Mucus plugs bronchioles → retain CO_2 (respiratory acidosis)

Goblet cell metaplasia

CI, fibrosis narrows lumens

   b. Pathogenesis includes:
     (1) hypersecretion of mucus in the bronchus and its subdivisions.
     (2) obstruction to airflow from mucus plugs located in the segmental bronchi and proximal bronchioles.
     (3) irreversible fibrosis in chronically inflamed segmental bronchi and bronchioles.
   c. Changes that occur in the bronchi include:
     (1) hypersecretion of submucosal mucus-secreting glands in the trachea and bronchi. Primarily responsible for sputum overproduction (i.e., productive cough).
     (2) acute inflammation (neutrophils) that is often superimposed on chronic inflammation (CI).
     (3) loss of ciliated epithelium and the presence of squamous metaplasia (see Chapter 2).
   d. Changes that occur in the bronchioles include:
     (1) mucus plugs in lumens (block the exodus of CO_2, causing respiratory acidosis).
     (2) goblet cell metaplasia (goblet cells are *not* normally present in the bronchus).
     (3) CI and fibrosis that narrows the lumen.
  3. Clinical findings include:

Turbulent airflow in the bronchus and its subdivisions is converted to laminar airflow primarily in the nonrespiratory bronchioles (<1 mm diameter). These bronchioles undergo parallel branching, which reduces airway resistance and spreads air out over a large cross-sectional area. In CB, mucus plugs located in the small diameter segmental bronchi and proximal nonrespiratory bronchioles allow air to move around them on inspiration (airways expand). However, on expiration when airway diameter is reduced, the mucus plugs decrease the exodus of CO_2 arising from the distally located branching airways. This results in respiratory acidosis (see Chapter 5). Furthermore, expiratory wheezing may also occur as air under pressure is forced past these areas of obstruction.

Productive cough

Dyspnea *late*

Hypoxemia/respiratory acidosis early

Cyanosis from ↓O_2 saturation: O_2 saturation is decreased from hypoxemia (see Chapter 2).

"Blue bloaters"

Stocky or obese

Expiratory wheezes, sibilant rhonchi

↑Risk cor pulmonale

Large, horizontally oriented heart

↑Bronchial markings

CB: chronic respiratory acidosis/hypoxemia

Slight ↑TLC, residual volume

Chronic respiratory acidosis

$PaCO_2$ >45 mmHg

Serum bicarbonate >30 mEq/L (compensation)

Early moderate/severe hypoxemia

Asthma

Cough, wheezing, dyspnea

    a. productive cough.
    b. dyspnea that occurs *late* in the disease (reverse of emphysema).
    c. hypoxemia and respiratory acidosis occur *early* in the disease (reverse of emphysema).
    d. cyanosis of the skin and mucous membranes (see Chapter 2 discussion of cyanosis) (Links 17-92 B and 17-93 B).
      • Patients are called "blue bloaters" because of the presence of cyanosis of the skin and mucous membranes.
    e. tendency for the patient to be stocky or obese.
    f. presence of expiratory wheezing and sibilant rhonchi.
    g. increased risk for cor pulmonale.
  4. Chest radiograph findings include:
    a. large, horizontally oriented heart.
    b. increased bronchial markings.
  5. PFTs and ABG findings include:
    a. less of an increase in TLC and residual volume than emphysema.
    b. chronic respiratory acidosis (see Chapter 5).
     (1) Arterial PCO_2 is >45 mm Hg.
     (2) Serum bicarbonate is >30 mEq/L (compensatory metabolic alkalosis).
    c. moderate to severe hypoxemia that occurs *early* in the disease.
  6. A summary of findings in emphysema and CB is found in Table 17-4.
 E. Asthma
  1. **Definition:** A chronic inflammatory respiratory condition of the airways that is characterized by episodes of cough, wheezing, and dyspnea

TABLE 17-4　Comparison of Emphysema and Chronic Bronchitis

PARAMETER	EMPHYSEMA	CHRONIC BRONCHITIS
PaO_2	Decreased	Decreased
$PaCO_2$	Normal to decreased	Increased
pH	Normal to increased	Decreased
Cyanosis	Absent	Present
Habitus	Thin	Stocky
Cor pulmonale	Rare	Common
Onset of hypoxemia	Late	Early
Onset of dyspnea	Early	Late

2. Epidemiology
   a. In most cases, it is an episodic and reversible airway disease.
   b. Approximately 80% of individuals with asthma have an allergic diathesis (atopy) and positive skin test results for allergens.
   c. Characterized by increased sensitivity of the airways to constrict in response to nonspecific stimulation (hyperreactive airways)
   d. Primarily targets the bronchi and its subdivisions and the nonrespiratory bronchioles
   e. Most common chronic respiratory disease in children
     (1) More common in children than adults
     (2) Majority (50%–80%) develop symptoms *before* 5 years of age
   f. Extrinsic and intrinsic types of asthma
3. Extrinsic asthma
   a. **Definition:** A type I HSR caused by exposure to extrinsic allergens
   b. Pathogenesis (Link 17-94)
     (1) Typically develops in children with an atopic family history to allergies
     (2) See Chapter 4 for mediator reactions involved with initial sensitization to an inhaled allergen.
   c. Histologic changes in bronchi include (Links 17-95 and 17-96):
     (1) thickening of the BM.
     (2) edema and a mixed inflammatory infiltrate.
     (3) hypertrophy of submucosal glands.
     (4) Hypertrophy and hyperplasia of SMCs
   d. Histologic changes in the bronchioles include:
     (1) formation of spiral-shaped mucus plugs.
       (a) Contain shed epithelial cells called Curschmann spirals.
       (b) Result of the pathologic effect of major basic protein (MBP) and cationic protein
     (2) presence of crystalline granules in eosinophils that coalesce to form Charcot-Leyden crystals.
     (3) patchy loss of epithelial cells, goblet cell metaplasia.
     (4) thick BMs.
     (5) SMC hypertrophy and hyperplasia.
   e. Clinical findings include:
     (1) episodic expiratory wheezing (inspiratory as well when severe).
     (2) nocturnal cough.
     (3) increased AP diameter caused by air trapping and an increase in respiratory volume.
   f. Laboratory findings
     (1) Patients initially develop respiratory alkalosis because they work hard at expelling air through the inflamed airways (hyperventilate).
       (a) May progress into respiratory acidosis if bronchospasm is *not* relieved Sequence of respiratory alkalosis → normal pH → respiratory acidosis ($\uparrow PaCO_2$, $\downarrow PaO_2$ [hypoxemia])
       (b) Normal pH or respiratory acidosis is an indication for intubation and mechanical ventilation.
     (2) FEV_1 is the best measure of the severity of the asthma. Less expensive measurements include the peak expiratory flow rate (PEFR) and peak flow meters.
     (3) Eosinophilia is frequently present.
     (4) Results of various skin tests are positive for specific allergens.
4. Intrinsic asthma
   a. **Definition:** A nonimmune type of asthma that is *not* associated with allergens
   b. Causes include:
     (1) viral respiratory infections. Examples: parainfluenza virus (PIV), RSV.
     (2) air pollutants. Refer to ozone (O_3) and other pollutants in Chapter 7 (Table 7-5).
     (3) aspirin or nonsteroidal antiinflammatory drug (NSAID) sensitivity.
       (a) Above drugs block cyclooxygenase (COX) activity and therefore inhibit formation of prostaglandins and thromboxanes (Fig. 3-7).
       (b) Leaves the lipoxygenase pathway open for production of leukotrienes (bronchoconstrictors [BCs]).
     (4) stress, exercise, and cigarette smoke.
F. **Bronchiectasis**
  1. **Definition:** Permanent dilation of the bronchi and bronchioles secondary to destruction of airway cartilage and elastic tissue arising as a result of recurrent airway infection and inflammation

---

Margin notes:

Episodic, reversible most cases

Atopy in majority

Hyperreactive airways

Targets bronchi + subdivisions; non-RBs

MC chronic resp disease children

Children > adults

Symptoms *before* 5 yrs of age

Extrinsic/intrinsic types

Type I HSR: allergens

Children with atopic family Hx allergies

Histology bronchi

Thickening BM

Edema, mixed infiltrate

Hypertrophy submuc glands

Hypertrophy/-plasia SMCs

Spiral-shaped mucus plugs

Curschmann spirals (shed epithelial cells)

MBP, cationic protein

Charcot-Leyden crystals from eosinophils

Patchy loss endothelial cells, goblet cell metaplasia

Thick BMs

SMC hypertrophy/-plasia

Expiratory wheezing

Nocturnal cough

$\uparrow$AP diameter; air trapping ($\uparrow$RV)

Initial respiratory alkalosis

Progression to respiratory acidosis + hypoxemia

Normal pH/respiratory acidosis intubate

FEV_1 best indicator severity

Eosinophilia

Skin tests + for specific allergens

Intrinsic asthma

Nonimmune asthma

Viruses (PIV, RSV)

Air pollutants (ozone)

Aspirin, NSAIDs

Block COX activity

Lipoxy pathway releases leukotrienes (BCs)

Stress, exercise, cigarette smoke

Bronchiectasis

Permanent dilation bronchi/bronchioles

MCC bronchiectasis U.S.;
Tuberculosis MCC
worldwide

Infections

Tuberculosis MCC
worldwide

MAC, adenovirus, *S. aureus,*
H. influenza

"Tree-in-bud" sign

CT: centrilobular nodules
with linear branching

Usually endobronchial
spread of infection

Bronchiolitis (CMV,
obliterative bronchiolitis)

Bronchioles with pus/
exudate: aspiration,
Mycobacteria

Bronchiectasis with mucus
plugging (CF)

Bronchovascular interstitial
infiltration (sarcoid)

Bronchogenic carcinoma;
distal bronchiectasis

Primary ciliary dyskinesia

Absent dynein arm in cilia

Dynein arm contains ATPase
required for cilia movement

Allergic bronchopulmonary
aspergillosis

Pertussis immunization
↓incidence bronchiectasis

MC in lower lobes

Saccular bronchi/ioles filled
with pus

Dilated airways to periphery

Productive cough (cupfuls)

Hemoptysis; often massive

Digital clubbing

Cor pulmonale

Cystic fibrosis

AR, dysfunction exocrine
glands

2. Epidemiology
   a. Causes include:
      (1) Cystic fibrosis. Most common cause of bronchiectasis in the United States.
      (2) infections.
          (a) Tuberculosis is the most common cause worldwide.
          (b) MAC (typically involves the right middle lobe and lingula), adenovirus,
              S. aureus, and *H. influenzae.*
          (c) "Tree-in-bud" sign.
              • **Definition:** The CT appearance of multiple areas of centrilobular nodules
                with a linear branching pattern. It usually represents endobronchial spread of
                infection. It is *not* identified on plain lung radiographs.
              • Occurs as a result of a number of processes, including bronchiolitis (e.g., CMV
                pneumonitis, obliterative bronchiolitis), bronchioles filled with pus or exudate
                (e.g., aspiration bronchopneumonia, tuberculosis, atypical *Mycobacteria*
                infection), bronchiectasis with mucus plugging (e.g., cystic fibrosis), and
                bronchovascular interstitial infiltration (e.g., sarcoidosis, lymphoma)
      (3) bronchial obstruction. Example: A proximally located bronchogenic carcinoma
          occludes the lumen, resulting in bronchiectasis distal to the cancer.
      (4) primary ciliary dyskinesia.
          (a) Dynein arm in cilia is absent.
          (b) Dynein arm contains ATPase (adenosine triphosphatase) for movement of the
              cilia.
      (5) allergic bronchopulmonary aspergillosis (see Table 17-3).
   b. Protection from pertussis infection by immunizations has decreased the incidence of
      bronchiectasis
3. Gross findings
   a. Most commonly occurs in the lower lobes
   b. Dilated cylindrical and saccular bronchi and bronchioles are filled with pus (Fig. 17-15
      A, B; Links 17-97 and 17-98).
      (1) Dilated airways extend to the lung periphery.
      (2) Dilations are tube-like and/or saccular.
4. Clinical findings include:
   a. cough productive of copious sputum (often cupfuls).
   b. hemoptysis (coughing up blood) that is sometimes massive.
   c. digital clubbing.
   d. cor pulmonale (PH + RVH).
5. Chest radiography and CT scan findings in bronchiectasis show crowded bronchial
   markings that extend to the lung periphery (see Fig. 17-15 B; Links 17-97 and 17-98).
6. Cystic fibrosis
   a. **Definition:** Autosomal recessive, multisystem disease associated with dysfunction of
      the exocrine glands (e.g., sweat glands, pancreatic glands)

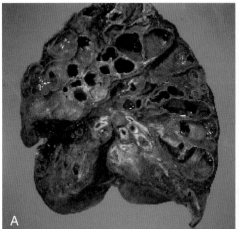
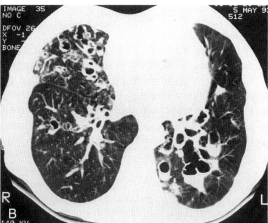

17-15: A, Bronchiectasis showing dilated airways filled with pus. **B,** Computed tomography scan showing bronchiectasis in both lungs.
Note the dilated airways with cystic to saccular appearance. (**A** *from Corrin B:* Pathology of the Lungs, *London, Churchill Livingstone,*
1999, p 85, Fig. 3-5; **B** *from Goldman L, Ausiello D:* Cecil's Textbook of Medicine, *23rd ed, Philadelphia, Saunders Elsevier, 2008, p 633,*
Fig. 90-2.)

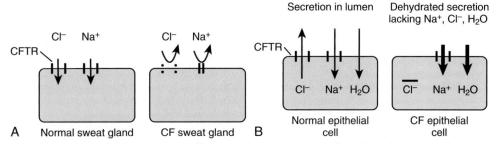

17-16: Schematic showing the normal function of cystic fibrosis transmembrane regulator *(CFTR)* in sweat glands **(A)** and epithelial cells **(B)** and what happens in cystic fibrosis (CF). Note that in sweat glands, CFTR normally increases chloride ion reabsorption and, indirectly, sodium reabsorption. Absence of CFTR in CF leads to a loss of both sodium and chloride ions. In epithelial cells, CFTR normally pumps chloride ions into secretions to maintain their viscosity, but in CF, absence of CFTR leads to absence of chloride in secretions and, indirectly, a loss of sodium and water from secretions, causing them to be less viscous (dehydrated).

    b. Epidemiology

        (1) Primarily affects whites (>98% of cases); uncommon in Asians and blacks

        (2) Most common fatal hereditary disorder in whites in the United States

        (3) Median age of diagnosis is ~5 months

        (4) Median survival time is 30 years of age.

        (5) Carrier frequency is 1 in 32 in United States.

    c. Pathogenesis

        (1) Most common mutation is a three-nucleotide deletion on chromosome 7 that normally codes for phenylalanine (70% of cases)

        (2) Mutation causes defective protein folding in the cystic fibrosis transmembrane conductance regulator (CFTR)

            (a) CFTR is normally regulated by cyclic adenosine monophosphate (cAMP)–dependent phosphorylation and by intracellular adenosine triphosphate (ATP).

            (b) Function in cells is to regulate chloride ion permeability in sweat glands and other secretions (Fig. 17-16 A, B, *left*).

        (3) Defective CFTR is degraded in the Golgi apparatus.

        (4) Loss of the CFTR causes decreased Cl⁻ reabsorption in the sweat glands and other exocrine glands (Fig. 17-16 A right schematic); basis of the chloride sweat test, which is used to diagnose cystic fibrosis

        (5) Effect of loss of CFTR in other secretions (Fig. 17-16 B, *right schematic*)

            (a) Increased Na^+ and water reabsorption from luminal secretions

            (b) Decreased Cl⁻ secretion out of epithelial cells into the luminal secretions

            (c) Net effect of these electrolyte alterations is dehydration of body secretions caused by a lack of NaCl (Link 17-99). Secretions are dehydrated (thickened) in bronchioles (Link 17-100), pancreatic ducts, bile ducts, meconium, cervix, and seminal fluid.

    d. Clinical findings include:

        (1) nasal polyps in children (25% of cases) (see Fig. 17-1).

        (2) heat exhaustion (caused by a loss of sodium-containing fluid from the skin).

        (3) respiratory infections or failure.

            (a) Most common cause of death from cystic fibrosis

            (b) *P. aeruginosa* is the most common respiratory pathogen. Chronic mucoid *Pseudomonas* infection is common. Other common pathogens include *S. aureus*, *H. influenzae*, *Burkholderia* spp., and *Aspergillus* spp.

            (c) Bronchiectasis is responsible for coughing up copious amounts of pus (Link 17-101); major cause of morbidity and mortality in children

            (d) Pulmonary hypertension (PH) occurs followed by cor pulmonale (PH plus RVH).

        (4) pneumothorax (20% of cases) (caused by rupture of blebs that develop from lung infections).

        (5) hemoptysis (coughing up blood).

        (6) malabsorption (80% of cases). Dehydrated pancreatic secretions block the pancreatic ducts, leading to chronic pancreatitis with destruction of pancreatic parenchyma. This causes a deficiency of the exocrine secretions necessary to digestion and potentially in the destruction of islet cells causing type 1 DM (20% of cases).

        (7) infertility in men (95% of cases): atresia (absence of a normal opening) of the vas deferens.

(8) infertility in females (20% of cases). Thick cervical mucus prevents sperm penetration.

(9) meconium ileus (20% of cases; Link 17-102). Type of small bowel (SB) obstruction in newborns (thick meconium; see Chapter 18).

(10) rectal prolapse caused by straining at stool.

(11) gallstones (>50% of cases).
  (a) Usually occur in older cystic fibrosis patients
  (b) Caused by stasis of thickened bile
  (c) Common bile duct (CBD) obstruction occurs in 15% to 20% of cases of cystic fibrosis (obstructive jaundice).

(12) Secondary biliary cirrhosis often occurs because of obstruction of bile ductules by thick secretions (Links 17-103 and 17-104).

(13) Malnutrition and poor growth in children

e. Screening tests in infants show an increase in serum immunoreactive trypsin (IRT).

f. Sweat chloride test findings (see Fig. 17-16) diagnostic for cystic fibrosis include:
  (1) sweat chloride >40 mmol/L in infants.
  (2) sweat chloride >60 mmol/L in children and adults.

g. Genotyping available.

X. **Lung Tumors**

A. **Epidemiology**

1. Primary lung cancer is the most common fatal cancer in both men and women worldwide. It accounts for >30% of cancer deaths in men and for >25% of cancer deaths in women.

2. Incidence is declining in men but increasing in women.

3. Peak incidence is at 55 to 65 years of age.

4. Black men have the highest incidence rates.

5. Risk factors include:
  a. cigarette smoking.
    (1) Most common cause of lung cancer
    (2) Tobacco smoking accounts for 80% to 90% of cases and secondhand smoke for 3% to 5% of cases.
    (3) Risk increases with quantity and duration of smoking.
    (4) Men who smoke have a greater risk for lung cancer than women who smoke.
    (5) Non–smoking-related lung cancer is more common in women than men.
  b. radon gas (uranium mining).
  c. asbestos and coal dust.
  d. certain metals: chromium, cadmium, beryllium, and arsenic.
  e. ionizing radiation, air pollution, and a history of tuberculosis.

6. Molecular genetics in lung cancer
  a. Most common oncogenes associated with lung cancer include *KRAS, MYC* family, *HER-2*, and *BCL-2, EGFR* (epidermal growth factor receptor).
  b. Most common suppressor genes are *p53* (most common), *RB1*, and *p16*.

7. Primary lung cancers are classified as small cell or non–small cell (most common) cancers (Link 17-105). Non–small cell accounts for 60% to 80% of cases, and small cell cancers account for 15% to 20% of cases.

8. Common sites for metastasis include:
  a. hilar lymph nodes most common site.
  b. adrenal gland (50% of cases), liver (30% of cases), brain (20% of cases), bone (usually osteolytic).

B. **Tumors and tumor-like disorders** (Table 17-5)

A **solitary pulmonary nodule** or coin lesion is the term applied to a peripheral lung nodule <5 cm. Causes of a solitary pulmonary nodule in descending order include granulomas (e.g., tuberculosis, histoplasmosis), malignancy (usually primary cancer), and bronchial (chondroid) hamartoma. Patients <35 years old have a 1% risk of a solitary coin lesion representing a malignancy, but patients ≥50 years old have a 50% to 60% risk of malignancy, usually a primary cancer. In evaluating solitary coin lesions, comparing previous chest radiographs for changes in size of the nodule is the most important initial step.

C. **Metastatic cancer**

1. Epidemiology
  a. Most common lung cancer
  b. Cancers that are most often responsible for metastasis include:

TABLE 17-5   Tumors and Tumor-Like Disorders of the Lung

TYPE OF TUMOR OR DISORDER	LOCATION IN LUNG	COMMENTS
Adenocarcinoma (see Fig. 17-17E and F; Links 17-106 B and 17-107 to 17-110)	Peripheral	• Most common primary cancer (35%–40%) • Most common cancer in nonsmokers • Weakest smoking relationship • More common in women than men • Grow slowly but metastasize early • High frequency of *KRAS* mutations • Scar carcinomas: develop in scars (e.g., old tuberculous granuloma). *No* relationship to smoking. • Alveolar carcinoma in situ (formerly called bronchioloalveolar carcinoma) (Links 17-109 and 17-110): derives from Clara cells (nonciliated epithelium (most common), mucin-secreting bronchiolar cells or type II pneumocytes. Accounts for 5% of primary lung cancers. Malignant cells spread along alveolar walls (look like pegs). Radiologically mimics lobar pneumonia. *No* relationship to smoking.
Squamous cell carcinoma (see Fig. 17-17A, C; Link 17-106 A, Links 17-111 and 17-112)	Central	• Account for 20%–30% of primary cancers • More common in men than women • Strong association with cigarette smoking • Tends to cavitate • High frequency of *p53* mutations • May ectopically secrete PTH-related protein (peptide)
Small cell carcinoma (see Fig. 17-17B, C; Link 17-113 to 17-115)	Central	• Accounts for 15%–20% of primary cancers • Slightly more common in men than women • Strong association with cigarette smoking • Arise from neuroendocrine cells (Kulchitsky cells); neurosecretory granules are noted on EM • High frequency of *p53*, *RB1* mutations • Rapidly growing cancer that metastasizes early • May ectopically secrete ADH or ACTH
Large cell carcinoma (Link 17-116)	Central or peripheral	• Accounts for 10%–15% of primary cancers • More common in men than women • Undifferentiated cancer (adenocarcinoma or squamous cell carcinoma) that metastasizes early • Strong relationship with smoking
Bronchial carcinoid (Link 17-117)	Central or peripheral	• Accounts for 1%–5% of primary lung cancers • Most common primary lung tumor in children • *No* sex predilection or association with smoking • Usually present in persons <40 yr old • Low-grade cancer of neuroendocrine origin • Intraluminal mass that penetrates bronchial wall and fans out (sometimes called "iceberg" tumor) • Approximately 20% locally metastasize • Present with hemoptysis (most common), cough, carcinoid syndrome (<1%) • Does *not* have to metastasize to the liver to have signs of carcinoid syndrome (e.g., flushing).
Carcinoma metastatic to the lung (see Fig. 17-18 A to C; Links 17-118 to 17-120)	Multifocal	• More common than primary cancer • Sites of metastasis: parenchyma (most common), pleura or pleural space, endobronchial mucosa, and lymphatics (causes dyspnea)
Bronchial hamartoma (Link 17-121)	Peripheral (90%) Central (10%)	• Non-neoplastic proliferation of cartilage and adipose tissue • Appears as solitary "coin" lesion on chest radiography"; popcorn" calcifications

ACTH, Adrenocorticotropic hormone; *ADH,* antidiuretic hormone; *EM,* electron microscopy; *PTH,* parathyroid hormone.

    (1) primary breast cancer: most common cause.
    (2) colon cancer and renal cell carcinoma.
  2. Sites of lung metastasis include:
    a. parenchyma (Fig. 17-18; Links 17-118 and 17-119).
    b. pleura and pleural space (malignant effusions).
    c. lymphatics (causes severe dyspnea; Link 17-120).
  3. Dyspnea is the most common symptom.
D. Clinical findings for primary lung cancer include (Link 17-122):
  1. cough: most common symptom (75% of cases) for primary lung cancer.
  2. weight loss (40% of cases).
  3. chest pain (30% of cases).
  4. hemoptysis (coughing up blood; 25%–30% of cases); usually centrally located cancers.

Breast cancer MCC

Colon, renal cancers common

Parenchyma

Pleura/pleural space

Lymphatics

Dyspnea MC symptom

Cough MC symptom

Weight loss

Chest pain

Hemoptysis (usually centrally located)

17-17: A, Sputum cytology in squamous cell carcinoma. Note the orange-staining, keratinized squamous carcinoma cells with irregular, hyperchromatic nuclei *(arrow).* **B,** Fine-needle aspirate of a lymph node with metastatic small cell carcinoma of lung. Note the cluster of cells with hyperchromatic nuclei and scant cytoplasm. **C,** Carcinoma arising in a central bronchus and extending into the lumen. Possibilities include squamous cell carcinoma or small cell carcinoma of the lung. Note that the lumen is obstructed by gray-white tumor, causing distal bronchiectasis *(solid arrow)* and obstructive pneumonia *(interrupted arrow).* **D,** Chest radiograph of bronchogenic carcinoma presenting as a central right hilar mass *(arrow).* **E,** Peripheral adenocarcinoma with scar retracting the pleural surface (scar carcinoma). The black pigment is anthracotic pigment. **F,** Chest radiograph of bronchogenic carcinoma presenting as a mass in the periphery of the right upper lobe *(arrow). (A and B from Kumar V, Fausto N, Abbas A: Robbins and Cotran Pathologic Basis of Disease, 7th ed, Philadelphia, Saunders, 2004, p 760, Figs. 15-43A, 15-43B, respectively; C and E from Corrin B: Pathology of the Lungs, London, Churchill Livingstone, 1999, pp 463, 412, Figs. 13-1.5, 13-1.13B, respectively; D and F from Grieg JD: Color Atlas of Surgical Diagnosis, London, Mosby-Wolfe, 1996, pp 90, 89, Figs. 13-7, 13-6, respectively.)*

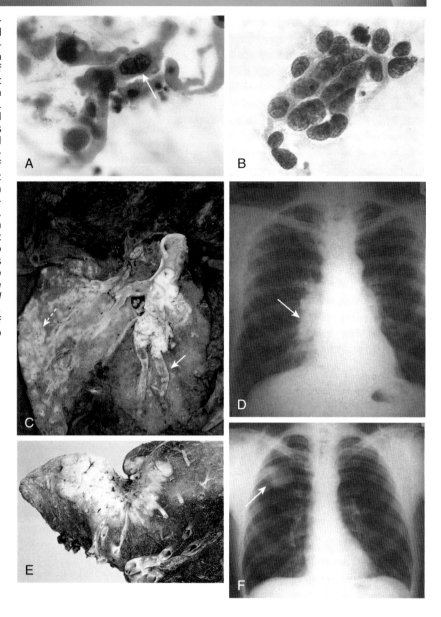

Dyspnea

SCC at apex

Destruction SCSG

Ipsilateral lid lag, miosis, anhydrosis

Shoulder pain

Digital clubbing

Muscle weakness

Ab against calcium channel

Small cell carcinoma

Ectopic hormone secretion

Chest x-ray

Central: SCC, small cell carcinoma

Peripheral: adenocarcinoma, scar carcinoma

5. dyspnea.
6. Pancoast tumor (superior sulcus tumor)
   a. Tumor is usually a primary SCC located at the extreme apex of the lung.
   b. Destruction of superior cervical sympathetic ganglion (SCSG) produces Horner syndrome (Fig. 17-19 A), which includes ipsilateral eyelid lag, miosis (pinpoint pupil), and ipsilateral anhydrosis (lack of sweating).
   c. Shoulder pain is commonly present.
7. Superior vena cava syndrome (see Chapter 9; Fig. 17-19 B)
8. Paraneoplastic syndromes include (see Chapter 9):
   a. digital clubbing: caused by reactive periosteal changes in the underlying bone (see Fig. 9-16 A, B).
   b. muscle weakness (Eaton-Lambert syndrome).
      (1) Antibody directed against calcium channel in muscle
      (2) Usually associated with small cell carcinoma
   c. ectopic hormone secretion (see paraneoplastic syndromes).

E. Diagnosis of lung cancer
1. Chest radiography (Fig. 17-17 D)
   a. Central masses include squamous cell carcinoma (SCC) and small cell carcinoma.
   b. Peripheral masses include adenocarcinoma and scar carcinoma (*not* a specific histologic type of lung cancer but rather one that appears to have arisen in an area of scarring [usually adenocarcinoma]).

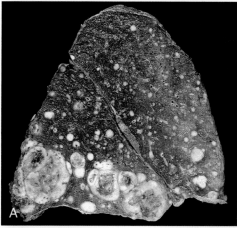
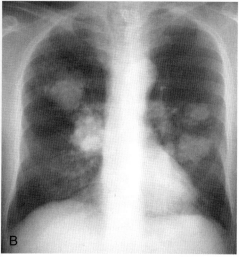
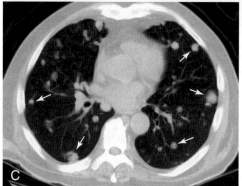

17-18: A, Metastatic renal cell carcinoma showing multiple nodular lesions scattered throughout the lung parenchyma. **B,** Chest radiograph showing multiple metastatic nodules throughout both lung fields. **C,** Computed tomography image showing multiple discrete metastatic nodules in the lungs *(arrows)* from a colon adenocarcinoma. *(**A** from Kumar V, Fausto N, Abbas A: Robbins and Cotran Pathologic Basis of Disease, 7th ed, Philadelphia, Saunders, 2004, p 766, Fig. 15-47; **B** from Goldman L, Ausiello D: Cecil's Textbook of Medicine, 23rd ed, Philadelphia, Saunders Elsevier, 2008, p 600, Fig. 84-9; **C** from Herring W: Learning Radiology: Recognizing the Basics, 2nd ed, Philadelphia, Elsevier Saunders, 2012, p 25, Fig. 3.18A.)*

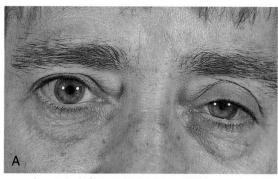
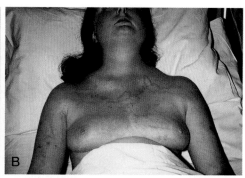

17-19: A, Horner syndrome in left eye. Note the eyelid lag and miotic pupil on the left compared with the right eye. **B,** Superior vena caval syndrome. Note the swelling of the face and neck and development of the collateral circulation in the veins on the chest wall. *(**A** from Bouloux P: Self-Assessment Picture Tests: Medicine, Vol. 1, London, Mosby-Wolfe, 1997, p 38, Fig. 75; **B** from Forbes CD, Jackson WF: Color Atlas and Text of Clinical Medicine, 3rd ed Mosby, 2003 p 193, Fig. 4.163.)*

   c. Chest radiography sensitivity is 74%, and specificity is 91%. *Not* a good screen for cancer.
2. CT scan has a sensitivity of 94% and a specificity of 73%; therefore, it is a better screen than chest radiography for lung cancer.
3. Sputum cytologic examination, fine-needle aspiration (FNA), and bronchoscopy with lavage are commonly used.
4. New techniques for early detection include:
   a. low-dose spiral (helical) CT scan
   b. positron emission tomography (PET) with 18F-fluorodeoxyglucose is superior to CT in detecting mediastinal and distal metastases in non–small cell cancers. Use of PET-CT is very useful for preoperative staging of non–small cell cancers.
   c. Molecular markers in sputum
F. Prognosis for lung cancer
   • Non–small cell cancers fare better than small cell carcinomas.

CT best screening test

Sputum cytology, FNA, bronchoscopy with lavage

Low-dose spiral (helical) CT scan

PET scans are superior to CT scans

Molecular markers in sputum

Non-small cell fare better than small cell carcinoma

A **solitary pulmonary nodule** or coin lesion is the term applied to a peripheral lung nodule ≤3 cm. If >3 cm, it is called a mass, of which 90% are malignant. Causes of a solitary pulmonary nodule in descending order include granulomas (60%; e.g., tuberculosis, histoplasmosis, coccidioidomycosis [Link 17-123]), malignancy (40%; usually primary cancer), and bronchial (chondroid) hamartoma. Patients <35 years old have a 1% risk of a solitary coin lesion representing a malignancy, but patients ≥50 years old have a 50% to 60% risk of malignancy, usually a primary cancer. In evaluating solitary coin lesions, comparing previous chest radiographs for changes in size of the nodule is the most important initial step. PET is useful in defining the metabolic activity of the nodule. Malignant tumors have an increased rate of uptake compared with benign lesions or normal tissue. False-negative results can occur with small tumors (<1 cm) with low metabolic activity (e.g., bronchial carcinoid). However, active infections, granulomatous infections can have an increased uptake (false positives). The PET scan has a sensitivity of 97% and specificity of 82%. Solitary coin lesions have various calcification patterns, some of which are suggestive of benign disorders, but others suggest malignancy (Link 17-124). CT scans are useful in identifying these lesions (Link 17-125). If the doubling time of the nodule is 25 to 450 days, it suggests a malignant process. If the doubling time is less than 25 days or more than 450 days, it suggests a benign process.

Granuloma MC solitary pulmonary nodule

Metastatic cancer in older patients

Primary disease in younger patients

Anterior mediastinum MC site

Neurogenic tumors posterior; MC primary mediastinal mass

Malignant in children: neuroblastoma

Benign in adults: ganglioneuroma

Thymoma anterior mediastinum

Pericardial cyst middle mediastinum

Lymphoma anterior mediastinum

Nodular sclerosing HL

Teratoma anterior mediastinum

Majority benign

Thymoma

Mediastinal tumor epithelial cells

Anterior mediastinum

Majority benign

Epithelium neoplastic *not* lymphoid tissue

Majority express symptoms myasthenia gravis

Myasthenia gravis: follicular B-cell hyperplasia in thymus

Hypogammaglobulinemia

Pure RBC aplasia

↑Incidence autoimmune disease

Mediastinitis

Acute/Cl mediastinal connective tissue

Chronic = sclerosing mediastinitis

Acute: head/neck infection heart/lung surgery, esophageal perforation

Sclerosing mediastinitis commonly due to *Histoplasma*

XI. **Mediastinum and Pleural Disorders**
   A. **Mediastinal masses** (Links 17-126 to 17-128)
      1. Epidemiology
         a. Usually metastatic primary lung cancer in older patients
         b. Usually primary disease in younger patients
         c. Anterior mediastinum is the most common site (>50% of cases; Link 17-128).
         d. Most common primary mediastinal masses, in descending order, include (Links 17-126 and 17-127):
            (1) neurogenic tumors.
               (a) Located in the posterior mediastinum
               (b) Usually malignant in children. Example: neuroblastoma
               (c) Usually benign in adults. Example: ganglioneuroma
            (2) thymoma (anterior mediastinum; see later).
            (3) pericardial cyst: located in the middle mediastinum.
            (4) malignant lymphomas.
               (a) Located in the anterior mediastinum
               (b) Usually a nodular sclerosing Hodgkin lymphoma (HL) in a woman (see Chapter 14).
            (5) teratoma (see Chapter 9).
               (a) Located in the anterior mediastinum
               (b) Majority are benign cystic teratomas.
               (c) Small percentage of teratomas are malignant.
      2. Thymoma
         a. **Definition:** Mediastinal tumor originating from the epithelial cells of the thymus.
         b. Epidemiology
            (1) Located in the anterior mediastinum
            (2) Benign in 70% of cases and malignant in 30% of cases.
         c. Epithelium is the neoplastic component, *not* the lymphoid tissue.
         d. Majority express systemic symptoms of myasthenia gravis, which include muscle weakness, ptosis (drooping of the eyelids), and problems with swallowing liquids and solids (see Chapter 24).
            (1) Fewer than 15% of patients with myasthenia have a thymoma.
            (2) Majority (65%–75%) have follicular B-cell hyperplasia in the thymus. It is the site for synthesis of anti–acetylcholine receptor antibodies.
         e. Other thymoma associations include hypogammaglobulinemia, pure RBC aplasia (see Chapter 12), and an increased incidence of autoimmune disease (e.g., Graves disease).
      3. Mediastinitis
         a. **Definition:** An acute or chronic infection of the mediastinal connective tissue that fills the interpleural spaces and surrounds the mediastinal organs (airways, vessels, heart). Chronic mediastinitis is called sclerosing mediastinitis because of increased formation of connective tissue in the mediastinum.
         b. Epidemiology
            (1) Acute mediastinitis is most frequently associated with head and neck infections, cardiothoracic surgery, or esophageal perforation.
            (2) *Histoplasma capsulatum* is frequently associated with excessive fibrous tissue formation and is the most common predisposing factor for the development of sclerosing mediastinitis.

(a) Fibrous tissue entraps the airways, producing postobstructive pneumonia; thoracic duct, producing the thoracic duct syndrome; heart, producing constrictive pericarditis; superior vena cava (SVC), producing the superior vena cava syndrome; PA, producing RHF; and pulmonary vein, producing LHF.

(b) Other pathogens associated with sclerosing mediastinitis include tuberculosis, *Nocardia* spp., and actinomycosis.

c. Clinical findings of acute mediastinitis include fever, chest pain, and respiratory distress as well as signs of acute inflammation if it is associated with cardiothoracic surgery (e.g., sternal wound erythema and pus).

d. Clinical findings in chronic mediastinitis (sclerosing mediastinitis) are usually asymptomatic until fibrosis entraps airways (postobstructive pneumonia), the thoracic duct (thoracic duct syndrome), the heart (constrictive pericarditis), or the superior vena cava (superior vena cava syndrome) or causes obstruction of the PA or pulmonary veins.

4. Diagnosis of mediastinitis
   a. Chest radiography shows widening of the mediastinum, abscess formation, and gas bubbles.
   b. CT is important in assessing the extent of mediastinal involvement and is useful in detecting dystrophic calcification, which is often missed with a chest radiography.
   c. CTA shows vascular occlusion in sclerosing mediastinitis.
   d. Magnetic resonance imaging (MRI) is most useful in evaluating the extent of disease and vascular involvement in sclerosing mediastinitis; however, it is less useful in identifying dystrophic calcification than CT.

B. Pleural effusions
   1. Movement of pleural fluid
      a. Fluid moves from the parietal pleura to the pleural space to the lungs. Parietal pleura → pleural space → lungs (Link 17-129).
      b. Movement of PF depends on the balance of Starling pressures (see Chapter 5).

Normally, the parietal capillary hydrostatic pressure (HP) is greater than the visceral capillary HP. Under normal circumstances, small amounts of fluid in the pleural spaces are exchanged by the fluid coming in from the systemic capillaries. At the same time, the fluid is drained from the pleural space entering into the pulmonary lymphatics and the venous system of the lungs. A pleural effusion forms if more fluid enters the pleural space than is drained.

(Excerpt modified from my friend Ivan Damjanov, MD, PhD: *Pathophysiology*, St. Louis, Saunders Elsevier, 2009, p 183.)

---

2. Etiology and pathogenesis include:
   a. increased HP in the visceral pleura. Example: congestive heart failure (CHF)
   b. decreased osmotic pressures (OP). Example: nephrotic syndrome
   c. increased permeability of capillaries within the visceral pleura. Examples: pulmonary infarction, pneumonia
   d. metastasis to the pleura. Example: metastatic breast cancer
3. Types of pleural effusions include:
   a. transudates (see Chapter 5).
      (1) **Definition:** Ultrafiltrate of plasma caused by an alteration in Starling pressures
      (2) Examples include:
         (a) increased HP in congestive heart failure (CHF).
         (b) decreased OP in the nephrotic syndrome or cirrhosis.
   b. exudates (see Chapter 3).
      (1) **Definition:** Collection of protein-rich and cell-rich (usually neutrophils) fluid; caused by increased vessel permeability in acute inflammation
      (2) Examples: pneumonia, tuberculosis (common), infarction, metastasis (common)
   c. chylous effusions (Link 17-130).
      (1) Type of an effusion usually associated with an interruption of the thoracic duct
      (2) Causes of chylous effusions include;
         (a) malignancy (most common cause; e.g., malignant lymphoma 75% of cases). Tumor blocks the lymphatic drainage.
         (b) trauma. Example: iatrogenic tear occurring during surgery
      (3) Turbid, milky appearance caused by the presence of chylomicrons (Link 17-130)

Margin notes:

Fibrous tissue airway, thoracic duct, heart, SVC, pulmonary artery/vein

Tuberculosis, *Nocardia*, actinomycosis

Acute: fever, chest pain, respiratory distress (CT surgery)

Chronic: varied symptoms/sign depending on structures entrapped

Dx mediastinitis

Chest x-ray: widening mediastinum, abscess, gas bubbles

CT: extent, dystrophic calcification

CT angiography: vascular occlusion

MRI useful in evaluating extent of disease

Pleural effusions

Parietal pleura → pleural space → lungs

↑HP: CHF

↓OP: nephrotic syndrome

↑Vessel permeability

Pulmonary infarction, pneumonia

Pleural metastasis

Breast cancer

CHF: MCC pleural effusion

Alteration Starling pressures

↑HP: CHF

↓OP: nephrotic syndrome/cirrhosis

↑Protein/inflammatory cells

↑Vessel permeability

PF exudate: tuberculosis/malignancy common

Interruption thoracic duct

Malignant lymphoma MCC

Trauma

Iatrogenic tear during surgery

Milky; chylomicrons with TG

Supranate

↑PF triglyceride

Pseudochylous: CH + necrotic debris

Rheumatoid lung disease

PF LDH, protein, ratios

pH >7.4 transudate

pH <7.4 exudate

Dullness to percussion

Absent breath sounds

Absent tactile fremitus

Contralateral shift trachea

Blunting costophrenic angle

Obscuration of diaphragm

Pleuritis

Inflammation parietal/ visceral pleura

Visceral pleura does *not* have pain receptors

Viruses MCC (e.g., coxsackievirus)

(a) Chylomicrons are lipoproteins that contain diet-derived triglyceride (TG; see Chapter 10).

(b) Chylomicrons form a supranate (floating on the surface) in a test tube after refrigeration.

(4) PF TG that is >110 mg/dL is diagnostic.

d. Pseudochylous effusions also have a turbid, milky appearance.

(1) Caused by inflammation with an increased amount of necrotic debris. PF cholesterol (*not* TG) is increased.

(2) Most commonly caused by rheumatoid lung disease (see Chapter 24)

4. Laboratory distinction of transudates versus exudates in the PF (see Table 17-6)

a. PF and serum concentrations of lactate dehydrogenase (LDH) and ratios of PF protein to serum protein and PF LDH to serum LDH are useful in making a distinction between a transudate and exudate.

b. Test sensitivity is 99%, and test specificity is 98% if at least one of the above three criteria for an exudate is present.

c. An additional criterion for distinguishing a transudate and exudate involves measuring the pH of the fluid.

(1) pH >7.4 indicates a transudate.

(2) pH <7.4 indicates an exudate.

5. Clinical findings in pleural effusions include dullness to percussion, absent breath sounds, absent vocal tactile fremitus, and contralateral shift of the trachea with large effusions.

6. Chest radiography findings with pleural effusions include (Fig. 17-20; Link 17-131):

a. blunting of the costophrenic angle.

b. obscuration of the diaphragm.

C. Pleuritis

1. **Definition:** Inflammation of the pleura

2. Epidemiology

a. Visceral pleura (lining lungs) is *not* innervated by pain receptors (nociceptors). Inflammation of the periphery of the lung parenchyma results in inflammation of the parietal pleura causing pain (called empyema; Links 17-132 left and 17-133).

b. Viruses are the most common cause of pleurisy. Examples include coxsackievirus, RSV, EBV, adenovirus, CMV, PIV, and influenza virus.

TABLE 17-6   Pleural Fluid Transudates Versus Exudates

COMPONENT	TRANSUDATE	EXUDATE
PF protein/serum protein	<0.5	>0.5
PF LDH/serum LDH	<0.6	>0.6
PF LDH	<200 U/L	>200 U/L

LDH, Lactate dehydrogenase; *PF*, pleural fluid.

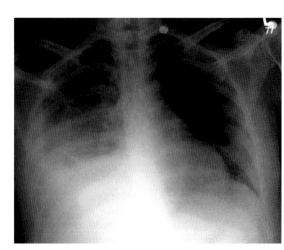

17-20: Frontal chest radiograph showing a right pleural effusion. Note the blunting of the right costophrenic angle and obscuration of the right hemidiaphragm. (*From Pretorius ES, Solomon JA:* Radiology Secrets, *2nd ed, Philadelphia, Mosby, 2006, p 539, Fig. 66-2A.*)

c. Bacterial causes include *Streptococcus pneumoniae*, *S. aureus*, *Legionella pneumophila*, and tuberculosis, to name a few.

d. Fungal causes include coccidioidomycosis and histoplasmosis, to name a few.

e. Rheumatologic diseases (e.g., SLE)

f. Malignancy of the lung (e.g., adenocarcinoma) or pleura (mesothelioma; metastatic disease)

g. Trauma from a rib fracture, pulmonary infarction, uremia

3. Clinical findings in pleurisy

a. Sharp chest pain or "catch," particularly on inspiration when the pleura is stretched

b. Chest pain when coughing, movements of the chest wall or trunk

c. May be accompanied by a pleural effusion

D. Pleural effusions

1. Movement of PF

a. Fluid moves from the parietal pleura to the pleural space to the lungs. Parietal pleura → pleural space → lungs (Link 17-129)

b. Movement of PF depends on the balance of Starling pressures (see Chapter 5).

Normally, the parietal capillary HP is greater than the visceral capillary HP. Under normal circumstances, small amounts of fluid in the pleural spaces are exchanged by the fluid coming in from the systemic capillaries. At the same time, the fluid is drained from the pleural space entering into the pulmonary lymphatics and the venous system of the lungs. A pleural effusion forms if more fluid enters the pleural space than is drained.

(Excerpt modified from my friend Ivan Damjanov, MD, PhD: *Pathophysiology*, Philadelphia, Saunders Elsevier, 2009, p 183.)

2. Etiology and pathogenesis include:

a. increased HP in the visceral pleura. Example: CHF.

b. decreased OP (albumin). Example: nephrotic syndrome

c. increased permeability of capillaries within the visceral pleura. Examples: pulmonary infarction, pneumonia

d. metastasis to the pleura. Example: metastatic breast cancer

3. Types of pleural effusions include:

a. transudates (see Chapter 5).

(1) **Definition:** Ultrafiltrate of plasma caused by an alteration in Starling pressures

(2) Examples include:

(a) increased HP in CHF (overall most common cause of a pleural effusion).

(b) decreased OP in the nephrotic syndrome/cirrhosis.

b. exudates (see Chapter 3)

(1) **Definition:** Collection of protein-rich and cell-rich (usually neutrophils) fluid; caused by increased vessel permeability in acute inflammation

(2) Examples: pneumonia, tuberculosis (common), infarction, metastasis (common)

c. chylous effusions.

(1) Type of an effusion is usually associated with an interruption of the thoracic duct

(2) Causes of a chylous effusions include:

(a) malignancy (most common cause; e.g., malignant lymphoma 75% of cases). Tumor blocks the lymphatic drainage.

(b) trauma. Example: iatrogenic tear occurring during surgery

(3) Turbid, milky appearance because of the presence of chylomicrons (Link 17-130).

(a) Chylomicrons are lipoproteins that contain diet-derived TG (see Chapter 10).

(b) Chylomicrons form a supranate (floating on the surface) in a test tube after refrigeration.

(4) PF TG that is >110 mg/dL is diagnostic.

d. Pseudochylous effusions also have a turbid, milky appearance.

(1) Caused by inflammation with an increased amount of necrotic debris

(2) PF cholesterol (*not* triglyceride) is increased.

(3) Most commonly caused by rheumatoid lung disease (see Chapter 24).

4. Laboratory distinction of transudates versus exudates in the PF (see Table 17-6)

a. PF and serum concentrations of LDH and ratios of PF protein to serum protein and PF LDH to serum LDH are useful in making a distinction between a transudate and exudate.

Margin notes:

S. pneumoniae

Coccidioidomycosis, histoplasmosis

SLE

Malignancy

Rib fracture, infarction, uremia

Sharp chest pain on inspiration

Pleural effusion may be present

Parietal pleura → pleural space → lungs

↑HP: CHF

↓OP: nephrotic syndrome

↑Vessel permeability

Pulmonary infarction, pneumonia

Pleural metastasis

Breast cancer

Transudates

Alteration Starling pressures

↑HP: CHF

CHF: MCC pleural effusion

↓OP: nephrotic syndrome/cirrhosis

↑Protein/inflammatory cells

↑Vessel permeability

PF exudate: tuberculosis/malignancy common

Chylous effusion

Interruption thoracic duct

Malignant lymphoma MCC

Trauma

Iatrogenic tear during surgery

Milky; chylomicrons with TG

Supranate

↑PF triglyceride

Pseudochylous: turbid, milky

Inflammation + necrotic debris

Pseudochylous: ↑PF CH

Rheumatoid lung disease

PF LDH, protein, ratios

b. Test sensitivity is 99%, and test specificity is 98% if at least one of the previous three criteria for an exudate is present.

c. An additional criterion for distinguishing a transudate and exudate involves measuring the pH of the fluid.

(1) pH >7.4 indicates a transudate.

(2) pH <7.4 indicates an exudate.

5. Clinical findings in pleural effusions include dullness to percussion, absent breath sounds, absent vocal tactile fremitus, and contralateral shift of the trachea (only large effusions shift the trachea).

6. Chest radiography findings with pleural effusions include (see Fig. 17-20; Link 17-131):

a. blunting of the costophrenic angle.

b. obscuration of the diaphragm.

E. **Pleural diseases** (see Fig. 17-20; Links 17-132 and 17-133)

F. **Spontaneous pneumothorax**

1. **Definition:** A spontaneous accumulation of air in the pleural space that causes the lung to collapse

2. Epidemiology

a. *Not* associated with a precipitating event

b. More common in men than women

c. Commonly seen in tall, thin, young men aged 20 to 40 years

d. Risk for developing a spontaneous pneumothorax increases with smoking, family history, Marfan syndrome, and homocystinuria.

e. Approximate 25% recurrence rate within 2 years

3. Causes include:

a. rupture of an apical subpleural bleb or blebs (most common primary cause).

(1) Bleb formation is secondary to high negative intrapleural pressure.

(2) Most patients with these blebs are male smokers between 30 and 40 years old.

b. COPD. Most common secondary cause of a spontaneous pneumothorax.

c. associated with a paraseptal emphysema (see previous discussion).

d. Marfan syndrome (see Chapter 10).

e. scuba diving (see Chapter 7).

f. insertion of a subclavian catheter. Always order chest radiography after insertion!

4. Pathogenesis (Link 17-134 top)

a. Rupture of a subpleural or intrapleural bleb produces a hole in the pleura.

b. This results in loss of the negative intrathoracic pressure in the pleural cavity that is required to keep the lung inflated. Pleural cavity pressure is now the *same* as the atmospheric pressure. This causes either a portion of the lung or the entire lung to collapse.

5. Clinical findings

a. Sudden onset of dyspnea with a pleuritic type of chest pain (pain on inspiration; 90% of cases).

b. Physical examination reveals a tympanitic percussion note, absent breath sound on the affected side, and a tracheal shift to the side of the collapse if there is total lung collapse.

6. Upright chest radiography findings include a white visceral pleural line (pleural edge) and absence of vessel markings peripheral to the line.

G. **Tension pneumothorax**

1. **Definition:** A lung laceration that allows a progressive build-up of air to occur within the pleural space caused by a laceration in the lung parenchyma

2. Causes include penetrating trauma to the lungs (e.g., knife wound) or rupture of a tension pneumatocyst (seen with *S. aureus* pneumonias).

3. Pathogenesis

a. Flaplike pleural tear (check valve) allows air into the pleural cavity but *prevents* it from exiting (Link 17-134 bottom). It is similar to filling a tire up with air (air goes in but does *not* come out).

b. Pleural cavity pressure increases with each inspiration.

c. Increased pressure produces compression atelectasis.

4. Clinical findings

a. Sudden onset of severe dyspnea and pleuritic chest pain.

b. Physical examination findings

(1) Tympanitic percussion note and absent breath sounds.

---

pH >7.4 transudate

pH <7.4 exudate

Dullness to percussion

Absent breath sounds

Absent tactile fremitus

Contralateral shift trachea

Blunting costophrenic angle

Obscuration of diaphragm

Spontaneous pneumothorax

Air in pleural space → lung collapses

No precipitating event

Men > women

Tall, thin, young men

↑Risk with smoking, family Hx, Marfan syndrome

↑Recurrence rate

Rupture apical subpleural bleb

Blebs 2°high – intrathoracic pressures

Male smokers 30-40 yrs old

COPD MC 2° cause

Paraseptal emphysema

Marfan syndrome

Scuba diving

Insertion subclavian catheter

Rupture bleb → hole in pleura

Loss – intrathoracic pressure

Portion or total lung collapses

Sudden onset dyspnea/ pleuritic chest pain

Tympany to percussion

Absent breath sounds

Tracheal shift to side of collapse (ipsilateral)

Pleural line

Absence vessel markings

Tension pneumothorax

Lung laceration; accumulation air in pleural space

Penetrating trauma (knife)

Rupture tension pneumatocyst (*S. aureus*)

Flap similar to check valve (air in not out)

↑Intrapleural cavity pressure with inspiration

Compression atelectasis

Sudden onset dyspnea, pleuritic chest pain

Tympanic percussion note, absent breath sounds

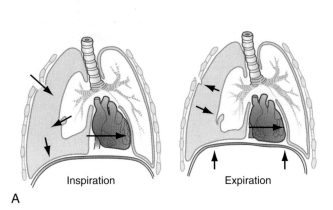
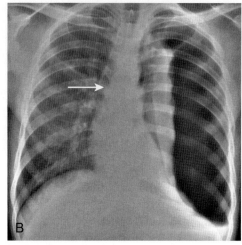

17-21: A, Tension pneumothorax with total collapse of the right lung and shift of mediastinal structures to the left. Air passes into the pleural cavity on inspiration and is trapped there on expiration. **B,** Left tension pneumothorax. Note the margin of the lung in the left pleural cavity and the tracheal deviation to the right *(arrow). (A from Marx J: Rosen's Emergency Medicine Concepts and Clinical Practice, 7th ed, Philadelphia, Mosby Elsevier, 2010, p 940, Fig. 75.1; B from Goldman L, Ausiello D: Cecil's Textbook of Medicine, 23rd ed, Philadelphia, Saunders Elsevier, 2008, p 601, Fig. 84-11.)*

(2) If large enough, the air pressure within the pleural cavity will cause deviation of the trachea to the contralateral side (Fig. 17-21; Link 17-134, *bottom*). This decreases venous return to the heart if the pneumothorax is located on the left side.

5. Chest radiography findings show (see Fig. 17-21):
    a. deviation of the trachea away from the side of the tension pneumothorax.
    b. shift of the mediastinum away from the side of the tension pneumothorax.
    c. depression of the hemidiaphragm on the side of the tension pneumothorax.

Trachea deviates to contralateral side

Left tension pneumothorax compromises venous return

Deviation trachea contralateral side

Shift mediastinum contralateral side

Depression hemidiaphragm on ipsilateral side

18 Gastrointestinal Disorders

ABBREVIATIONS

MC most common	MCC most common cause

I. Overview of the Gastrointestinal (GI) System (Fig. 18-1; Links 18-1 and 18-2)

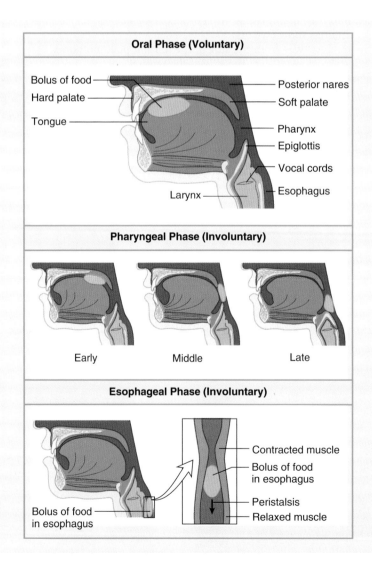

Oral Phase (Voluntary)

Bolus of food
Hard palate
Tongue
Posterior nares
Soft palate
Pharynx
Epiglottis
Vocal cords
Esophagus
Larynx

Pharyngeal Phase (Involuntary)

Early   Middle   Late

Esophageal Phase (Involuntary)

Contracted muscle
Bolus of food
in esophagus
Peristalsis
Relaxed muscle
Bolus of food
in esophagus

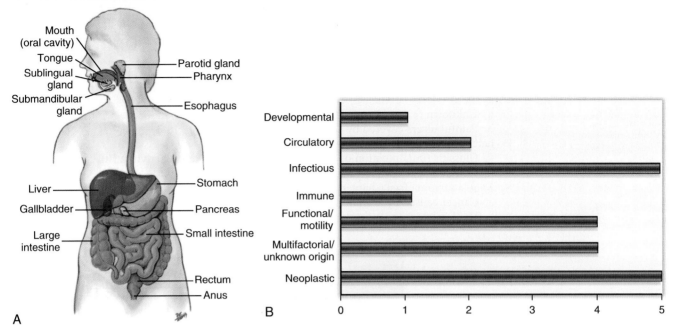

18-1: A, Anatomy of the gastrointestinal system. The gastrointestinal system is divided into an upper and lower portion. **B,** Relative clinical significance of various gastrointestinal diseases grouped by their cause. (**A,** *From my friend Ivan Damjanov, MD, PhD:* Pathology for the Health Professions, *Saunders Elsevier 4th ed, 2012, p 229, Fig. 10-1 A, B. Taken from Applegate EJ:* The Anatomy and Physiology Learning System, *4th ed, Philadelphia, 2011, Saunders.* **B,** *From my friend Ivan Damjanov, MD, PhD:* Pathophysiology, *Saunders Elsevier, 2009, p 237, Fig. 7-1).*

Swallowing occurs in three phases. In the voluntary or oral phase, the tongue presses food against the hard palate, forcing it toward the pharynx. In the involuntary or pharyngeal phase, peristalsis forces the bolus between the tonsils. Respirations cease, the airway is covered, and the esophagus is stretched open. In the involuntary esophageal phase, relaxation of the upper esophageal sphincter allows peristalsis to move the bolus down the esophagus.

(From Carroll RG: Elsevier's Integrated Physiology, St. Louis, Mosby Elsevier, 2007, p 144, Fig. 12-3).

II. Oral Cavity, Salivary Gland, and Neck Disorders

A. Cleft lip and palate

1. **Definition:** A cleft lip is an opening in the upper lip that can extend into the base of the nostril. A cleft palate is an opening in the roof of the mouth.

2. Epidemiology

   a. Most common congenital disorders of the oral cavity

      (1) Occurs in ~1:800 live births

      (2) Etiology is multifactorial, with 30 to 40% of cases associated with genetic factors; subsequent siblings at increased risk (3% of cases).

      (3) Higher frequency in Native Americans, those of Asian and Latin American descent; lowest frequency in blacks

      (4) Caused by failure of fusion between the medial nasal prominence and the maxillary prominence, the lateral nasal prominence, or both

      (5) Cleft lip and palate occur in 50% of cases.

      (6) Cleft palate alone occurs in 35% of cases (Fig. 18-2; Link 18-3). It is more common in females than males.

      (7) Cleft lip alone occurs in 15% of cases. It is more common in males than females.

      (8) May be unilateral or bilateral

      (9) Common syndrome associations include Pierre Robin sequence, Apert syndrome, Treacher Collins syndrome, and 22q11 deletion syndromes (DiGeorge complex syndrome).

      (10) May be diagnosed prenatally by ultrasound (US; >21 weeks' gestation)

   b. Complications include:

      (1) malocclusion (imperfect positioning of the teeth when the jaws are closed).

      (2) eustachian tube dysfunction (e.g., chronic otitis media).

Cleft lip opening upper lip

Cleft palate opening roof mouth

MC congenital disorder oral cavity

1:800 live births

Multifactorial, genetic

Native Americans, Asian, Latin American descent

Lowest frequency blacks

Failure fusion facial processes

Cleft lip/palate 50%

Palate alone 35%; females > males

Lip alone 15% of cases; males > females

Unilateral or bilateral

Prenatally diagnosed by US

Malocclusion

Eustachian tube dysfunction

(3) speech problems.

(4) reflux saliva and food into nasopharynx (NP).

   3. Treatment is surgery.

B. Common infections in the oral cavity (Table 18-1)

C. Oral manifestation of human immunodeficiency (HIV) include:

   1. candidiasis (Fig. 18-3 J). Most common oral infection.

   2. aphthous ulcers (stomatitis; canker sores; Link 18-14).

      a. Unknown origin (virus versus immunologic). Often stress induced

      b. Painful ulcers covered by a shaggy gray membrane (Fig. 18-4)

   3. hairy leukoplakia (Fig. 18-3 B).

      • Glossitis (inflammation of the tongue) caused by Epstein-Barr virus (EBV). Commonly seen as a pre-AIDS lesion.

   4. Kaposi sarcoma (see Chapters 4 and 9).

      a. Cancer caused by human herpesvirus 8 (HHV-8)

      b. Hard palate is the most common location

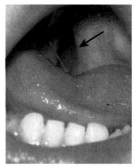

18-2: Cleft palate. Note the defect in the palate *(arrow)*. *(From Grieg JD:* Color Atlas of Surgical Diagnosis, *London, Mosby-Wolfe, 1996, p 68, Fig. 10-7.)*

TABLE 18-1 Infections of the Oral Cavity

INFECTION	PATHOGEN	FEATURES
		VIRAL
Exudative tonsillitis (Fig. 18-3A)	Viruses: most cases	Culture is necessary to differentiate bacterial versus viral infection.
Hairy leukoplakia (Fig. 18-3B, Link 18-4)	EBV	• Glossitis associated with bilateral white excrescences on lateral border of tongue. • Pre-AIDS–defining lesion (see Chapter 4).
Herpes labialis (gingivostomatitis) (Fig. 18-3C; Link 18-5)	HSV type 1	• Recurrent vesicular lesions on the lips (virus remains dormant in cranial sensory ganglia). • Reactivated by stress, sunlight, and menses.
Mumps (Fig. 18-3D)	Paramyxovirus	• Bilateral parotitis (70%) with increased serum amylase. • Complications: meningoencephalitis, unilateral orchitis or oophoritis, pancreatitis.
Herpangina (Fig. 18-3E)	Coxsackievirus	• Occurs in children. • Typically occurs in epidemics during the summer. • Painful vesicles or small white papules occur on an erythematous base typically at the junction of the soft and hard palate.
Hand-foot-and-mouth disease	Coxsackievirus	• Occurs in young children. • Vesicles located in mouth and distal extremities.
		BACTERIAL
Cervicofacial actinomycosis (Figs. 18-3F, G; Link 18-6, Link 18-7, Link 18-8)	*Actinomyces israelii*	• Draining sinus tract from facial or cervical area. • "Sulfur granules" in pus contain gram-positive, branching filamentous anaerobic bacteria. • Often follows extraction of an abscessed tooth.
Diphtheria	*Corynebacterium diphtheria*	• Gram positive rod. • Toxin produces "shaggy" gray pseudomembrane in posterior pharynx and upper airways. • Prominent cervical lymphadenopathy ("bull-neck" appearance). • Toxin-induced myocarditis is a common cause of death.

TABLE 18-1   Infections of the Oral Cavity—cont'd

INFECTION	PATHOGEN	FEATURES
Tonsillitis (Link 18-9)	*Streptococcus pyogenes*	• Gram-positive coccus. • Swollen, erythematous tonsils with punctuate areas of white pus (Link 18-9). • Peritonsillar abscess is a complication of tonsillitis. Infection extends into the surrounding soft tissue. The uvula deviates to the contralateral side. "Hot potato" voice. Foul-smelling breath. Stiff neck. • Computerized tomography (CT) scanning best delineates the space and detect small lymph nodes in this area that should normally disappear between the ages of 4 or 5 years.
Retropharyngeal abscess (Link 18-10)	• Group A, β-hemolytic streptococcus (*Streptococcus pyogenes*) • *Staphylococcus aureus* • *Haemophilus influenza*. • Anaerobes	• Retropharyngeal space is located in the tissues in the back of the throat behind the posterior pharyngeal wall. • Presents fever, stiff neck, drooling, difficulty with breathing (airway obstruction), croup-like cough. • Infection may extend into prevertebral space and mediastinum (mediastinitis).
Ludwig angina	• Aerobic/anaerobic *Streptococcus* gram positive coccus) • *Eikenella corrodens* (microaerophilic gram-negative rod)	• Cellulitis involving the submaxillary and sublingual space. Follows fascial planes and may spread into pharynx, carotid sheath, and superior mediastinum. • Causes: dental extraction (most common), trauma to floor of mouth.
Pharyngitis	*Streptococcus pyogenes*	• Gram-positive coccus. • Associated with tonsillitis. • Potential for acute rheumatic fever and glomerulonephritis (immunologic).
Scarlet fever (Link 18-11)	*Streptococcus pyogenes*	• Gram-positive coccus. • Pharyngitis, tonsillitis, glossitis (inflammation of tongue). • Erythrogenic toxin produces desquamating, sandpaper-like rash on skin and tongue (initially white and then strawberry colored). • Increased risk for nephritic type of glomerulonephritis (immune-mediated). • Nephritogenic strains pose *no* risk for acute rheumatic fever
Sialadenitis	*Staphylococcus aureus*	• Bacterial inflammation of major salivary gland. • Secondary to a calculus, which obstructs the duct in postoperative patients.
Congenital syphilis (Fig. 18-3H; Link 18-12)	*Treponema pallidum* (spirochete)	Abnormalities involving incisors (notched and tapered like a peg) and molar teeth (resemble mulberries).
Acute necrotizing gingivitis (Vincent angina) (Fig. 18-3I)	Anaerobes: *Prevotella, Fusobacterium;* spirochetes	• Anaerobic bacterial infection of gingiva. • Necrosis of interdental papilla with punched-out lesions covered by a grayish pseudomembrane.
FUNGAL		
Oral thrush (Fig. 18-3J; Link 18-13)	*Candida albicans* (yeast)	• May occur in neonates, immunocompromised patients (common pre-AIDS–defining lesion), diabetes mellitus, and after antibiotic therapy. • Angular cheilitis (Link 18-13): inflammation of one or both corners of the mouth. Infections include *Candida albicans* and *Staphylococcus aureus*. It may also be a feature of allergic eczema.

EBV, Epstein-Barr virus; *HSV,* herpes simplex virus; *TMP-SMX,* trimethoprim–sulfamethoxazole.

D. **Dental caries**
1. **Definition:** Refers to tooth decay; caused by specific types of bacteria that produce acid, which in turn destroys the tooth enamel
2. Caused by *Streptococcus mutans*, which produces acid from sucrose fermentation. Acid erodes the enamel and exposes the underlying dentine (Links 18-15 and 18-16).
3. Fluoride prevents dental caries (see Chapter 8). Excess fluoride causes a chalky discoloration of the teeth (fluorosis).
E. **Noninfectious ulcerations in the oral cavity**
1. Pemphigus vulgaris (PV) and mucous membrane pemphigoid (pemphigoid). Both are immunologic skin disorders and are discussed in Chapter 25.
2. Erythema multiforme (see Chapter 25)
    a. Hypersensitivity reaction (HSR) against *Mycoplasma* or drugs (e.g., sulfonamides)
    b. Called Stevens-Johnson syndrome when it involves the mouth
3. Aphthous ulcers (stomatitis [inflammation of mucous membrane of the mouth]); Fig. 18-4; Link 18-14)
4. Behçet syndrome

Dental caries

Bacterial destruction enamel

Caused by *Streptococcus mutans*

Fluoride preventive

Chalky discoloration

Noninfectious ulcerations

PV, pemphigoid

Immunologic disorders

Erythema multiforme

Hypersensitivity reaction against *Mycoplasma*, drugs

Stevens-Johnson syndrome if involves mouth

Aphthous ulcers: stomatitis

Behcet syndrome

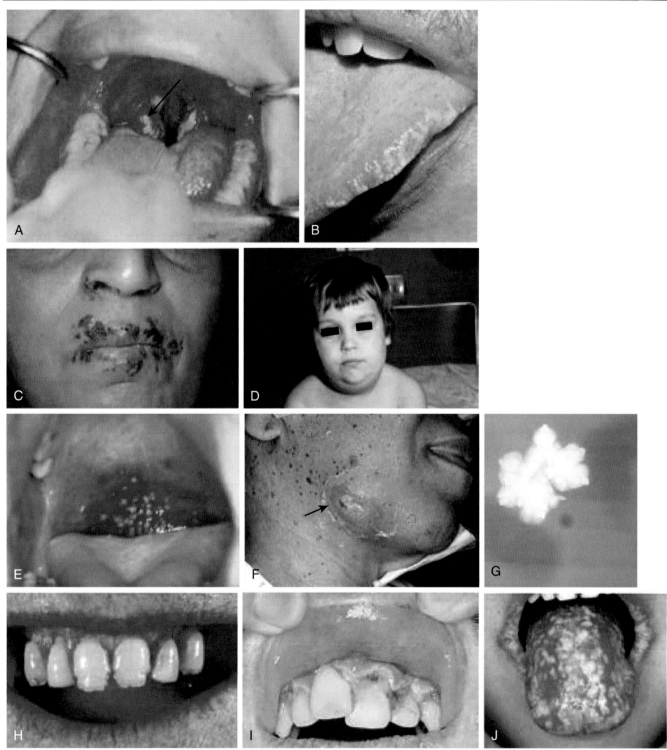

18-3: **A,** Exudative tonsillitis. Note the gray-white pus in the tonsillar crypts *(arrow)*. **B,** Hairy leukoplakia along the lateral border of the tongue. It is a glossitis caused by Epstein-Barr virus and is a pre-AIDS–defining lesion. **C,** Herpes simplex type 1. Note the clusters of vesicles around the vermilion border of the upper and lower lips. **D,** Child with mumps. Note the parotid gland swelling. **E,** Herpangina caused by coxsackievirus. Note the multiple white papules on an erythematous base located at the junction of the soft and hard palate. **F,** Cervicofacial actinomycosis. Note the draining sinus tract. **G,** Sulfur granule of Actinomyces. **H,** Notched teeth in congenital syphilis. **I,** Acute necrotizing gingivitis. Note the necrosis of interdental papilla with lesions covered by a grayish pseudomembrane. **J,** Oral thrush. Note the extensive white "curd-like" plaque that can be wiped off leaving an erythematous base. *(A, courtesy Edward L. Applebaum, MD, Department of Otolaryngology, University of Illinois, Urbana, Illinois; B, from Lookingbill D, Marks J:* Principles of Dermatology, *3rd ed, Philadelphia, Saunders, 2000, p 338, Fig. 23-7; C, from Swartz MH:* Textbook of Physical Diagnosis, *5th ed, Philadelphia, Saunders Elsevier, 2006, p 333, Fig. 12-10; D from Kliegman, R:* Nelson Textbook of Pediatrics, *19th ed, Philadelphia, Elsevier Saunders 2011, p 1080, Fig. 240.3l; from the Centers for Disease Control and Prevention: Public health image library [PHIL] [website]. http://phil.cdc.gov/phil/home. asp. Accessed March 8, 2011; E, from Cohen J, Opal SM, Powderly WG:* Infectious Diseases, *3rd ed, St. Louis, Mosby Elsevier, 2010, p 362, Fig. 32.12; F and G, from Murray PR, Rosenthal KS, Pfaller MA:* Medical Microbiology, *6th ed, Philadelphia, Mosby Elsevier, 2009, pp 394, 393 respectively, Figs. 40.5, 40.2, respectively; Hm from Bouloux P:* Self-Assessment Picture Tests: Medicine, *Vol. 1, London, Mosby-Wolfe, 1997, p 11, Fig. 21; I from Cohen J, Opal SM, Powderly WG:* Infectious Diseases, *3rd ed, St. Louis, Mosby Elsevier, 2010, p 361, Fig. 32.9, courtesy Professor I. Brook; J from Grieg JD:* Color Atlas of Surgical Diagnosis, *London, Mosby-Wolfe, 1996, p 65, Fig. 10-1.)*

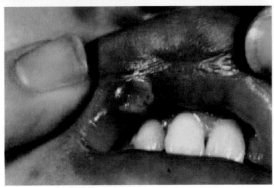

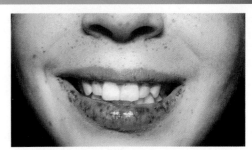

18-5: Peutz-Jeghers syndrome. Note the melanin pigmentation on the lips. *(From Swartz MH:* Textbook of Physical Diagnosis, *5th ed, Philadelphia, Saunders Elsevier, 2006, p 334, Fig. 12-12.)*

18-4: Aphthous ulcer. Note the ulcerated surface on the lip covered by a shaggy gray exudate. *(From Bouloux P:* Self-Assessment Picture Tests: Medicine, *vol. 1, London, Mosby-Wolfe, 1997, p 35, Fig. 69.)*

a. **Definition:** Rare small-vessel vasculitis that has a characteristic triad of recurring crops of aphthous ulcers in the mouth, genital ulcers, and inflammation in the uvea of the eye (uveitis)

b. Epidemiology
   (1) Caused by a combination of environmental and genetic factors; human leukocyte antigen (HLA)-B51, HLA-B27 associations (see Chapter 5)
   (2) May be triggered by herpes simplex virus (HSV) or parvovirus
   (3) High incidence in Turkey and in eastern Mediterranean countries

c. Pathophysiology: type of immune complex small vessel vasculitis (type III HSR; see Chapter 10)

d. Clinical findings include:
   (1) recurrent aphthous ulcers and genital ulcerations.
   (2) uveitis (inflammation of the uvea [pigmented area of the eye]), erythema nodosum (EN; painful nodules on the lower legs).
   (3) attacks that last 1 to 4 weeks.

F. **Pigmentation abnormalities in the oral cavity**
   1. Peutz-Jeghers syndrome (see Section IV): melanin pigmentation of the lips and oral mucosa (Fig. 18-5; Link 18-17)
   2. Addison disease (Fig. 23-15 A)
      a. **Definition:** Characterized by hypocortisolism caused by autoimmune destruction of the adrenal cortex that is associated with increased levels of adrenocorticotropic hormone (ACTH) via a negative feedback relationship with cortisol ($\downarrow$cortisol $\rightarrow$ $\uparrow$ ACTH)
      b. Increased ACTH stimulates melanocytes in the buccal mucosa and skin, causing increased melanin pigmentation in these locations.
   3. Lead poisoning (see Chapter 12). Lead deposits along the gingival margins in adults with gingivitis (see Fig. 12-14 D).

G. **Tooth discoloration**
   1. Tetracycline
      a. Drug discolors newly formed teeth (Link 18-18).
      b. *Not* recommended for use in children <12 years of age
   2. Fluoride: Excess fluoride produces mottled teeth with a chalky white discoloration.
   3. Congenital erythropoietic porphyria
      a. **Definition:** Rare autosomal recessive porphyria caused by a deficiency of uroporphyrinogen III synthase that leads to an accumulation of porphyrins that deposit in the skin, teeth, and other organs
      b. Porphyrin deposits in the teeth give them a reddish-brown discoloration.

H. **Macroglossia (enlarged tongue); causes include:**
   1. myxedema. Severe type of primary hypothyroidism (see Chapter 23).
   2. Down syndrome (see Chapter 6).
   3. acromegaly (excess growth hormone and insulin growth factor I; see Chapter 23).
   4. systemic amyloidosis (see Chapter 4).
   5. mucosal neuromas in multiple endocrine neoplasia (MEN) syndrome IIb (see Chapter 23).

Small-vessel vasculitis

Triad: aphthous ulcers, genital ulcers, uveitis

Environmental/genetic (HLA)

Triggers: HSV, parvovirus

Type III HSR small-vessel vasculitis

Recurrent aphthous ulcers, genital ulcers

Uveitis, EN

Attacks last 1 to 4 wks

Pigmentation abnormalities

Melanin lips/oral mucosa

Addison disease

Autoimmune destruction adrenal cortex; $\downarrow$cortisol $\rightarrow$ $\uparrow$ACTH

$\uparrow$ACTH $\rightarrow$ stimulates melanocytes

Tooth discoloration

Tetracycline

Discolors newly formed teeth

Fluoride chalky discoloration teeth

Congenital erythropoietic porphyria

Hereditary porphyria: defects in heme group

Porphyrins deposit skin, other organs

Teeth reddish-brown discoloration

Macroglossia

Myxedema: severe primary hypothyroidism

Down syndrome

Acromegaly

Systemic amyloidosis

Mucosal neuromas: MEN IIb

I. **Glossitis (inflammation of tongue)**
1. **Definition:** A sore, beefy red tongue with or without papillary atrophy (Link 18-19)
2. Causes include:
   a. long-standing iron deficiency (see Chapter 12).
   b. vitamin B₁₂ and/or folate (folic acid) deficiency (see Chapter 12).
   c. scurvy (vitamin C deficiency; Chapter 8).
   d. pellagra (niacin deficiency; Chapter 8).
   e. scarlet fever (Table 18-1; see Chapter 25).
   f. EBV-associated hairy leukoplakia (Fig. 18-3B).
3. Geographic tongue (benign migratory glossitis)
   a. **Definition:** Benign, asymptomatic condition characterized by well-defined areas of atrophy of filiform papillae bordered by white arcs of normal or hyperplastic filiform papillae (Link 18-20)
   b. Epidemiology
      (1) Present in 2% of the normal population
      (2) Areas change over a period of time, hence the name *migratory glossitis*

J. **Mucoceles**
1. **Definition:** Benign mucous cysts of the oral mucosa
2. Epidemiology
   a. Present as soft, white to blue, solitary asymptomatic lesions, usually on the mucous surface of the lower lip; less common on the gingivae, tongue, or buccal mucosa (Link 18-21)
   b. Usually <1 cm in diameter and contain a clear to white viscous fluid
   c. Result of minor trauma (lip biting) causing rupture of a mucous duct draining a minor salivary gland with and extravasation of sialomucin into the tissues
   d. Occasionally, lesions may rupture spontaneously, although this is usually followed by eventual recurrence.

K. **Pyogenic granuloma** (see Table 10-2; Fig. 10-14 E; Link 10-31)

L. **Temporomandibular Joint (TMJ) Dysfunction**
1. **Definition:** Pain and dysfunction of the muscles of mastication and the TMJs, which connect the mandible to the skull
2. Epidemiology and clinical findings
   a. Three groups of disorders include muscle disorders with myofascial pain (most common); disc displacement with or without reduction (second most common); and arthralgia, arthritis, arthrosis (degenerative disease; third most common).
   b. Pain must relate to jaw movements and mastication (chewing).
   c. Tenderness to palpation of the joint or muscles
   d. Usually there is a sudden change in the occlusion of the teeth.

M. **Leukoplakia and erythroplakia**
1. Definitions
   a. Leukoplakia literally means "white patch" (Fig. 18-6 A; Link 18-22).
   b. Erythroplakia is a red patch (Fig. 18-6 B; Link 18-23).
   c. Combination of leukoplakia and erythroplakia is called leukoerythroplakia.
2. Epidemiology
   a. Initially show squamous hyperplasia of the epidermis
      (1) May progress into squamous dysplasia → squamous cell carcinoma (SCC) in-situ → invasive SCC
      (2) Leukoplakia may progress to oral cancer in ~30% of cases.
      (3) Erythroplakia may progress to oral cancer in ~60% of cases.
   b. Locations include:
      (1) vermilion border lower lip (most common site).
      (2) buccal mucosa, hard and soft palates, or floor of the mouth.
   c. Causes include:
      (1) chronic irritation (e.g., dentures).
      (2) all forms of tobacco use.
      (3) alcohol abuse.
      (4) HPV.
   d. Always biopsy these lesions because of the high risk for progression to oral cancer.

N. **Lichen planus** (see Chapter 25)
1. **Definition:** Immune condition that can affect the skin, hair, nails and mucous membranes
2. Epidemiology

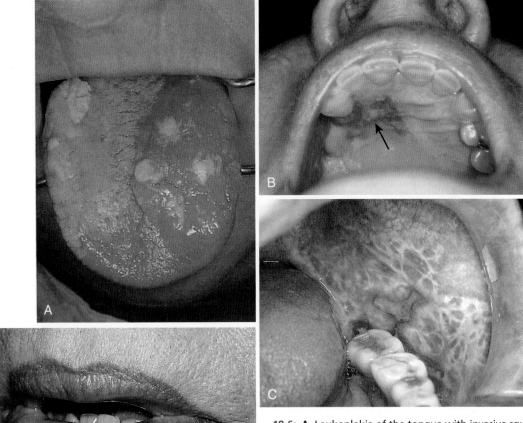

18-6: A, Leukoplakia of the tongue with invasive squamous cell carcinoma (SCC). Discrete raised white patches are evident on both sides of the tongue. **B,** Erythroplakia. Note the raised erythematous area *(arrow)* on the palate. **C,** Wickham striae on the buccal mucosa in a patient with lichen planus. Note the fine, white, lacy lesions. **D,** SCC on the lower lip. *(A from Forbes C, Jackson W: Color Atlas and Text of Clinical Medicine, 2nd ed, London, Mosby, 2002, p 362, Fig. 8-28; B and C from Goldman L, Ausiello D: Cecil's Textbook of Medicine, 23rd ed, Philadelphia, Saunders Elsevier, 2008, pp 1451, 2870, respectively, figs. 200-2, 451-4, respectively; D from Swartz M: Textbook of Physical Diagnosis: History and Examination, 5th ed, Philadelphia, Saunders Elsevier, 2006, p 158, Fig. 8.29.)*

    a. Often associated with Wickham striae on the buccal mucosa. Striae have a fine, white, lacy appearance (Fig. 18-6 C).

    b. Associated with SCC in the oral cavity

O. Dentigerous cyst

  1. **Definition:** Cysts that derive from epithelial elements of dental origin (odontogenic origin)

  2. Epidemiology

    a. Associated with the crown of an unerupted or impacted third molar

    b. Associated with ameloblastomas in 15% to 30% of cases (discussed later)

P. Benign tumors of the oral cavity (excluding salivary glands)

  1. Squamous papilloma

    a. **Definition:** A small, benign wartlike growth on the mucous membrane that is derived from squamous epithelium in the oral cavity

    b. Epidemiology

      (1) Most common benign tumor of oral cavity

      (2) May occur on the tongue, gingiva, palate, or lips

  2. Ameloblastoma

    a. **Definition:** Benign tumor that may arise from odontogenic epithelium (ameloblasts) or a dentigerous cyst that is located in the mandible

    b. Epidemiology

      (1) Most common odontogenic tumor

      (2) Produces a radiolucency in bone that has a "soap bubble" appearance in the mandible

      (3) Locally invasive but does *not* metastasize

Wickham striae white/lacy

Association squamous dysplasia/SCC

Dentigerous cyst

Odontogenic origin

Crown unerupted/impacted 3rd molar

Association with ameloblastoma

Squamous papilloma

Benign wartlike growth mucous membrane

MC benign tumor oral cavity

Tongue, gingiva, palate, lips

Ameloblastoma

Benign tumor: odontogenic epithelium or dentigerous cyst

MC odontogenic tumor

"Soap bubble" radiolucency in mandible

Locally invasive; does *not* metastasize

Q. Malignant tumors of the oral cavity (excluding salivary glands); epidemiology

1. Majority (>90%) are well-differentiated SCCs.
2. More common in men than women
3. Risk factors for malignant tumors of the oral cavity include:
   a. human papillomavirus (HPV), particularly those associated with tumors arising in at the base of the tongue and in the tonsillar region. Other sites are more often associated with tobacco products (see later).
   b. use of tobacco products, including pipe tobacco, cigarettes, chewing tobacco, and betel nut in Asian countries (40% of cancers). Incidence is declining in the United States.
   c. alcohol abuse (synergistic with smoking). Incidence is declining in the United States.
      (1) Synergism (combined effect) between smoking and alcohol excess means that the combined risk is greater than the risk of either individually.
      (2) Combination increases the relative risk for developing cancer 30-fold.
   d. chronic irritation from dentures.
   e. lichen planus (see previous; Chapter 25).
4. SCC most common oral cancer
   a. Cancer sites in descending order include the:
      (1) lower lip (vermilion border; >90%) more common than upper lip; Fig. 18-6 D; Link 18-24).
         (a) Lip cancer accounts for 15% to 30% of all cancer within the oral cavity.
         (b) Vermilion border of the lips is exposed to external environmental factors (ultraviolet [UV] radiation).
      (2) floor of the mouth (Link 18-25).
      (3) lateral border of the tongue (20%–30%).
   b. Tonsillar node (superior jugular node) is the most lymph node site for metastasis.
5. Verrucous carcinoma
   a. Variant of a well-differentiated SCC
   b. Oral cavity is its most common location, although it has been reported in the larynx, nasal cavity, esophagus, penis, anorectal region, vulva, vagina, uterine cervix, and skin (particularly the sole of the foot).
   c. Wartlike appearance; associated with smokeless tobacco (chewing tobacco or snuff dipping; Link 18-26)
   d. Most patients are older men.
   e. Large fungating tumor that tends to become infected and slowly invades contiguous structures
   f. May grow through the soft tissues of the cheek, penetrate into the mandible or maxilla, and/or invade perineural spaces
   g. Regional lymph node metastases are exceedingly rare.
6. Basal cell carcinoma (BCC)
   a. Most common cancer of the upper lip. SCC is more often located on the lower lip.
   b. Associated with exposure to UVB light

R. Salivary gland disorders

1. Sialolithiasis
   a. **Definition:** Stones that develop in the major ducts of submaxillary (most common site), sublingual, and parotid glands
   b. Epidemiology
      (1) Saliva in submaxillary glands is more saturated with calcium, hence the greater predisposition for calcium stones in this gland (Link 18-27).
      (2) Calculi block secretions, causing swelling of the distal SG tissue.
      (3) Persistent obstruction may cause inflammation and scarring, leading to destruction of the gland. Stones may occur in SG ducts as a reaction to inflammation (sialadenitis).
2. Sialadenitis
   a. **Definition:** Acute or chronic inflammation of a major SG
   b. Epidemiology
      (1) Acute sialadenitis can be localized to one SG (usually parotid or submaxillary gland) or be the expression of a systemic infection.
         (a) Viral sialadenitis can be caused by paramyxovirus (mumps), EBV, coxsackievirus, influenza, and parainfluenza viruses.
         (b) Suppurative sialadenitis (pus) is most often caused by *Staphylococcus aureus*, *Streptococcus* spp., and gram-negative bacteria.
         (c) Volume depletion, malnutrition, immunosuppression, and sialolithiasis are risk factors.

(2) Chronic sialadenitis of a major SG is usually asymptomatic.

    (a) Mild lymphocytic infiltration is the rule accompanied by atrophy, fibrosis, and stones.

    (b) Some cases are more common in women with rheumatoid arthritis (RA; immune related).

3. Sjögren syndrome (see Chapter 24)
4. Female-dominant autoimmune disease associated with RA

  a. Autoimmune destruction of the minor SGs and lacrimal glands

  b. Biopsy of the lip is commonly used to secured the diagnosis.

5. Salivary gland tumors

  a. Epidemiology

    (1) Parotid gland is the most common site. Major SG tumors are more likely to be benign.

    (2) Minor SG tumors are more likely to be malignant.

  b. Pleomorphic adenoma (mixed tumor)

    (1) **Definition:** A benign SG tumor that has epithelial cells (ECs), myoepithelial cells (MECs), and a stromal (mesenchymal) component

    (2) Epidemiology

      (a) Most common benign tumor of the major and minor SGs

      (b) Parotid gland most common site (Link 18-28 A)

      (c) Female-dominant tumor

      (d) Painless, moveable mass that is located at the angle of the jaw (Fig. 18-7). It obscures the angle of the jaw.

      (e) Histologic exam reveals ECs intermixed with a myxomatous (loose connective tissue embedded with mucus) and a cartilaginous (cartilage-containing) stroma (Link 18-28 B).

      (f) Projections of tumor through the capsule increase risk of recurrence.

      (g) May transform into a malignant tumor. Facial nerve involvement is a sign of malignancy.

  c. Warthin tumor (papillary cystadenoma lymphomatosum)

    (1) **Definition:** Benign cystic tumor found almost exclusively in the parotid gland. Contains abundant lymphocytes and germinal centers (lymph node–like stroma)

    (2) Epidemiology

      (a) Male dominant

      (b) Smokers have an increased risk for developing these tumors.

      (c) Within cystic spaces (*white*) are glands lined by *red* epithelium underlying, which is benign lymphoid tissue (*blue*). The term "red-white-blue" tumor has been used (Link 18-29).

      (d) Malignant transformation is rare.

  d. Adenoid cystic carcinoma

    (1) **Definition:** Slow-growing malignant neoplasm of the major and minor SGs with a tendency for nerve invasion

Margin notes

Usually asymptomatic

Lymphocytes, atrophy, fibrosis, stones

Sjögren syndrome

Autoimmune; RA association

Immune destruction minor salivary/lacrimal glands

Bx lip for Dx

Parotid gland MC site

Major gland tumors usually benign

Minor gland tumors usually malignant

Pleomorphic adenoma

Mixed tumor

ECs, MECs, stroma

MC major/minor salivary gland tumor

Parotid MC site

Female dominant

Painless, moveable, obscures angle of jaw

ECs mixed with myxomatous/cartilaginous stroma

↑Recurrence; extension thru capsule

May become malignant; facial nerve involvement

Warthin tumor

Benign cystic parotid gland tumor

Lymphocytes, germinal centers

Male dominant

Smokers ↑risk

"Red-white-blue" tumor

Malignant transformation rare

Adenoid cystic carcinoma

Slow growing malignancy; nerve invasion

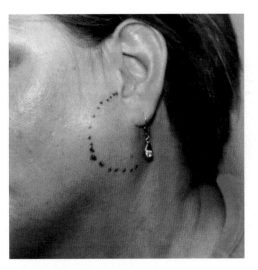

18-7: Pleomorphic adenoma of the parotid gland. Note the swelling at the angle of the jaw. *(From Townsend C: Sabiston Textbook of Surgery, 18th ed, Philadelphia, Saunders Elsevier, 2008, p 836, Fig. 33-16A.)*

(2) Epidemiology
    (a) Most common cancer of minor SGs
    (b) Contain nests and columns of cells arranged concentrically around glandlike spaces (pseudocysts; Link 18-30 A)
    (c) Perineural invasion is common (Link 18-30 B). Facial nerve palsy is a sign of malignancy.

  e. Mucoepidermoid carcinoma
    (1) **Definition:** Most common malignant salivary gland tumor characterized by numerous mucin-filled spaces and malignant squamous epithelium with or without keratinization
    (2) Epidemiology
      (a) Most commonly located in the parotid gland
      (b) Mixture of neoplastic squamous cells and mucus-filled spaces

S. Neck disorders (excluding thyroid gland)
  1. Lingual thyroid
    a. **Definition:** Normal thyroid tissue located at the base of the tongue
    b. Epidemiology
      (1) Caused by a failed descent of the thyroid anlage from the base of the tongue (Fig. 18-8 A and B)
      (2) In most cases, it represents all of the thyroid tissue.
    c. Clinical findings include:
      (1) dysphagia for solids (difficulty in swallowing solids).
      (2) presence of a mass lesion at the base of the tongue. An ^{123}I scan locates the lingual thyroid and identifies any other thyroid tissue that is present in other organ sites (e.g., functioning thyroid tissue in a cystic teratoma of the ovary).
  2. Thyroglossal duct cyst
    a. **Definition:** A cystic midline mass that is close to or within the hyoid bone (Fig. 18-8 C)
    b. Epidemiology
      (1) Usually diagnosed clinically but can also be diagnosed by US
      (2) Most common nonodontogenic cyst in the neck

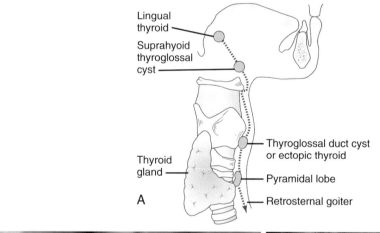
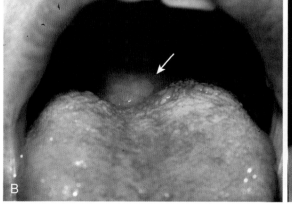
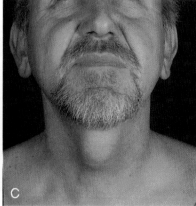

18-8: A, The *broken blue line* shows the course of the thyroglossal duct. *Blue circles* indicate possible sites of ectopic thyroid tissue and thyroglossal duct remnants. The *arrow* shows the direction of thyroid migration. **B,** Lingual thyroid. Note the mass lesion at the base of the tongue (*white arrow*). An ^{123}I uptake study will show uptake by the thyroid tissue and identifies any other thyroid tissue that is present. **C,** Person with a midline thyroglossal duct cyst. (*A from Moore A, Roy W: Rapid Review Gross and Developmental Anatomy, 3rd ed, Mosby Elsevier, 2010, p 221, Fig. 7-18; B and C from Bouloux P: Self-Assessment Picture Tests: Medicine, vol. 1, London, Mosby-Wolfe, 1997, pp 7, 52, respectively, Figs. 14, 103, respectively.*)

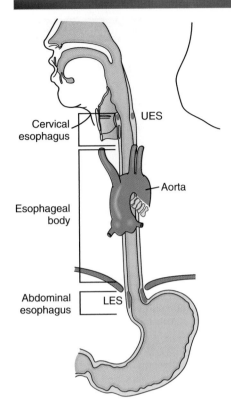

18-9: Anatomy of the esophagus showing the upper esophageal sphincter (UES) and the lower esophageal sphincter (LES). *(From Ashar BH, Miller RG, Sisso SD: The Johns Hopkins Internal Medicine Board Review, 4th ed, Elsevier, 2012, p 199, Fig. 26-1.)*

Cervical esophagus

UES

Aorta

Esophageal body

Abdominal esophagus

LES

   (3) Anomalous development and migration of the thyroid gland during the fourth through eighth weeks of gestation
   (4) Most common complications are infection and malignancy (thyroid).
  3. Branchial cleft cyst.
    a. **Definition:** Congenital cyst located on the lateral side of the neck most commonly caused by failure of obliteration of the second branchial cleft in embryonic development (Link 18-31)
    b. Epidemiology
      (1) Deep in the anterior border of the sternocleiodomastoid muscle
      (2) May be unilateral or bilateral
      (3) May open onto the skin surface or drain into the pharynx
III. Esophageal Disorders
  A. Overview of Anatomy (Fig. 18-9)
    1. Upper one-third of esophagus has striated muscle.
    2. Middle one-third has striated and smooth muscle.
    3. Distal one-third has smooth muscle.
  B. Physiology of Swallowing (Box 18-1)
  C. Signs and symptoms of esophageal disease include:
    1. heartburn.
      a. **Definition:** A burning sensation in the lower chest that is worsened by bending or lying down
      b. Most commonly caused by gastroesophageal reflux disease (GERD; discussed later)
    2. dysphagia (difficulty swallowing) for solids alone (Link 18-32).
      a. Symptom of an obstructive lesion in the esophagus
      b. Examples: esophageal cancer, esophageal web, and esophageal stricture
    3. dysphagia for solids and liquids.
      a. Symptom of a motility disorder
      b. Oropharyngeal (upper esophageal) dysphagia is a striated muscle dysmotility.
        • Examples: dermatomyositis/polymyositis (DM, PM), myasthenia gravis (MG), amyotrophic lateral sclerosis (ALS), and stroke (cerebrovascular accident [CVA]; 25% of cases). In CVAs, oropharyngeal dysphagia is a risk factor for aspiration and pneumonia.
      c. Lower esophageal dysphagia is a smooth muscle cell (SMC) dysmotility.

Anomalous development/ migration

Infection/malignancy (thyroid)

Branchial cleft cyst

Lateral neck; 2nd branchial cleft

Anterior border sternocleidomastoid muscle

Unilateral or bilateral

Sinus on skin surface or into pharynx

Esophageal disorders

Upper 1/3rd esophagus striated muscle

Middle: striated/smooth muscle

Distal: smooth muscle

S/S esophageal disease

Heartburn

Burning sensation lower chest

MCC GERD

Dysphagia: difficulty swallowing solids alone

Solids alone: obstructive lesion

Cancer, web, stricture

Dysphagia solids and liquids

Motility disorder

Oropharyngeal dysphagia; skeletal muscle

DM/PM, MG, ALS, CVA

Lower esophageal dysphagia: SMC dysmotility

BOX 18-1   Normal Swallowing and Movement of Food Through the Esophagus to the Stomach

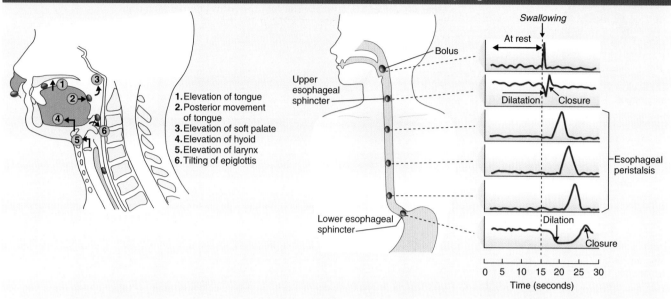

1. Elevation of tongue
2. Posterior movement of tongue
3. Elevation of soft palate
4. Elevation of hyoid
5. Elevation of larynx
6. Tilting of epiglottis

The initial processing of the food begins with chewing and swallowing. The movements of the upper gastrointestinal tract participate in the processing and digestion of food. This can be broken down into several phases as follows: Ingestion. Intake of food occurs in most instances by voluntary opening of the mouth and biting of solid food or sucking of fluids. Chewing (mastication). Breakdown of solid food into smaller morsels is accomplished by coordinated movements of the jaws, known as chewing. It is in part based on voluntary movements and in part on a chewing reflex coordinated from the centers in the brainstem. It involves a coordinated action of masticatory muscles such as the masseter, medial pterygoid, and temporalis muscle. Swallowing (deglutition). Food that has been reduced to smaller morsels is swallowed. Swallowing has three phases: an initial voluntary phase (oral phase, which involves the swallowing reflex), followed by two involuntary phases (pharyngeal and esophageal phases). The swallowing reflex (left schematic) involves a sequential contraction and relaxation of several muscles in the mouth and throat. The sequence of events is listed numerically from 1 to 6 in the schematic. Swallowing has three phases: an initial voluntary phase (oral phase), followed by two involuntary phases (pharyngeal and esophageal phases; right schematic). During the voluntary phase the tongue forms a bolus and pushes it into the oropharynx. Pharyngeal phase. Once the bolus enters the oropharynx, it activates the swallowing center in the medulla and lower pons, which propels the food into the esophagus. At the same time the reflex leads to the closure of the glottis and vocal cords so that the food does not enter into the respiratory system. Esophageal phase. Once the bolus has entered into the esophagus it is propelled caudally by esophageal peristalsis. Two forms of peristalsis are recognized: primary and secondary. Primary peristalsis, which is initiated by swallowing, is under the control of the vagus nerve, emerging from the swallowing centers in the medulla. As soon as food enters the esophagus, the upper esophageal sphincter contracts, preventing the regurgitation of the food. The peristaltic waves of primary peristalsis are slow, and when a person is eating in an erect position the food drops faster due to gravity rather than to peristaltic propulsion. It should be noticed that the vagus nerve controls both the striated muscle in the upper esophagus and the smooth muscle cells. Vagotomy abolishes the primary esophageal reflex. Secondary peristalsis, which is initiated by the entry of food into the esophagus, is mediated by intramural mechanical stretch receptors. It is coordinated by intramural nerves, and vagotomy does *not* abolish it. This type peristalsis leads to the opening of the lower esophageal sphincter, and it persists until the food is passed to the stomach. Once the food has passed into the stomach the lower esophageal sphincter contracts, preventing reflux from the stomach.

Excerpt and figures taken from my friend Ivan Damjanov, MD, PhD: *Pathophysiology,* Saunders Elsevier, 2009, p 245, 246 respectively; Figs. 7-6, 7, respectively)

SS, CREST, achalasia

Eosinophilic esophagitis
MCC dysphagia in child

- Examples: systemic sclerosis (SS), CREST syndrome (c̲alcinosis/c̲entromere antibodies, R̲aynaud phenomenon, e̲sophageal dysmotility, s̲clerodactyly, t̲elangiectasia), and achalasia
  d. The most common cause of dysphagia in children is eosinophilic esophagitis.

Eosinophilic esophagitis is increasing in incidence and recognition. It is thought to be an allergic condition in which an increase in tissue eosinophils leads to remodeling of the esophagus and decreased distensibility, manifested by the development of rings and strictures. Esophageal biopsy shows >15 eosinophils per high-powered field. Endoscopy shows circumferential rings, longitudinal fissures, and white plaques, the latter representing eosinophilic abscesses.

TE fistula

D. Overview of Common Esophageal Disorders
E. Tracheoesophageal (TE) Fistula

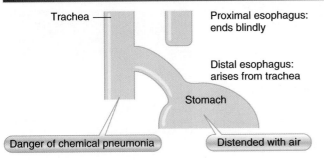

Trachea

Proximal esophagus: ends blindly

Distal esophagus: arises from trachea

Stomach

Danger of chemical pneumonia

Distended with air

18-10: Tracheoesophageal fistula. The proximal esophagus ends blindly, and the distal esophagus arises from the trachea. The stomach is distended with air owing to communication of the esophagus with the trachea.

1. **Definition:** Abnormal connection between the trachea and esophagus
2. Epidemiology
   a. Most common congenital anomaly of the esophagus
   b. Characteristics of the most common type (87%) of TE fistula include:
      (1) esophageal atresia (proximal esophagus that ends blindly; Fig. 18-10; Link 18-33 A).
      (2) distal esophagus that arises from the trachea.
   c. Risk factors include advanced maternal age, smoking, and obesity.
3. Clinical findings include:
   a. maternal polyhydramnios (excess amniotic fluid [AF]). AF is normally swallowed by the baby and absorbed in the small intestine. Esophageal atresia prevents the AF from reaching the small intestine for absorption, hence the accumulation of AF (polyhydramnios).
   b. abdominal distention in the newborn (NB). Air in the stomach comes from a tracheal fistula connecting the trachea with the distal esophagus.
   c. frothing and bubbling around the mouth at birth.
   d. difficulty with feeding at birth.
      (1) Food is regurgitated out of the mouth.
      (2) Newborn develops chemical pneumonia from aspiration (inhaling materials such as vomitus, food, or liquid).
   e. VATER syndrome; components include:
      (1) <u>v</u>ertebral abnormalities.
      (2) <u>a</u>norectal abnormalities (usually anal atresia).
      (3) <u>TE</u> fistula.
      (4) <u>r</u>enal disease and absent <u>r</u>adius.
   f. VA<u>C</u>TER<u>L</u> syndrome. Same as VATER syndrome *except* <u>C</u> stands for cardiac and <u>L</u> stands for limb abnormalities.
F. **Plummer-Vinson syndrome** (see Chapter 12)
   1. **Definition:** Intermittent dysphagia for solids caused by an esophageal web or stricture
   2. Epidemiology and pathogenesis
      a. Caused by chronic iron deficiency
         (1) Iron is important in the maturation of epithelial tissue.
         (2) Lack of iron impairs maturation of the squamous epithelium, causing the formation of a web or stricture.
      b. Leukoplakia occurs in the oral cavity oral and esophagus; increased risk for developing SCC.
G. **Esophageal diverticulum**
   1. Types of diverticulum
      a. True diverticulum. **Definition:** Outpouching lined by mucosa, submucosa, muscularis propria, and adventitia.
      b. False, or pulsion diverticulum. **Definition:** Pulsion type of diverticulum is located in upper esophagus, where the area of weakness is the cricopharyngeus muscle (Fig. 18-11 A, B).
   2. Zenker diverticulum of upper esophagus
      a. **Definition:** Pulsion type is located in upper esophagus, where the area of weakness is the cricopharyngeus muscle (Fig. 18-11 A, B).
      b. Clinical findings include:
         (1) painful swallowing.
         (2) halitosis (bad breath) caused by entrapped food in the diverticulum.
         (3) regurgitation of undigested food.
         (4) risk for developing esophageal diverticulitis (DTS).

Connection between trachea and esophagus

MC congenital esophageal anomaly

Proximal esophagus ends blindly

Distal esophagus arises from trachea

Risk factors: advanced maternal age, smoking, obesity

Maternal polyhydramnios

Stomach distention/feeding problem

Frothing/bubbling

Food regurgitation at birth

Chemical pneumonia

VATER syndrome

Vertebral abnormalities

Anorectal abnormalities

TE fistula

Renal disease, absent radius

VACTERL

Addition Limb abnormality

Plummer-Vinson syndrome

Dysphagia solids; esophageal web/stricture

Chronic iron deficiency

↓Iron: impairs squamous epithelium maturation → web

Leukoplakia mouth/ esophagus; ↑risk SCC

Esophageal diverticulum

True diverticulum

All layers

False/pulsion diverticulum

Zenker diverticulum

Weakness cricopharyngeus muscle

Painful swallowing

Halitosis; food trapped in diverticulum

Regurgitation undigested food

Esophageal diverticulitis risk

18-11: A, Schematic of a Zenker diverticulum (pulsion diverticulum). The area of weakness is the cricopharyngeus muscle. **B,** Solid white arrow shows dye in the diverticular sac. *(A from Townsend C:* Sabiston Textbook of Surgery, *18th ed, Philadelphia, Saunders Elsevier, 2008, p 1061, Fig. 41-20; B from Herring W:* Learning Radiology: Recognizing the Basics, *2nd ed, Philadelphia, Elsevier Saunders, 2012, p 175, Fig. 18.3A.)*

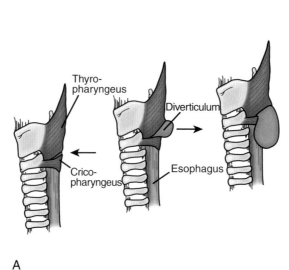

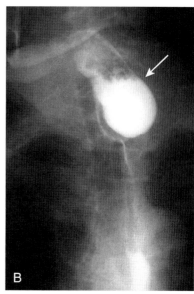

A

B

Hernias at hiatus

Sliding hiatal hernia

GEJ above diaphragm; fundus thru diaphragm

MC hiatal hernia

Risk increases with age

Women > men

Sigmoid diverticulosis, esophagitis

Duodenal ulcers, gallstones

Clinical findings

Heartburn leaning over/ lying down

Nocturnal epigastric distress

Bowel sounds left lung base

Hematemesis

Ulceration/stricture

Paraesophageal

GEJ at level of diaphragm; fundus +/− into thoracic cavity

Bleeding/strangulation

H. Hernias at the hiatus

1. **Definition** of a sliding hiatal hernia (HH): Type of HH in which the gastroesophageal junction (GEJ) migrates through the hiatus into the posterior mediastinum as a result of laxity of the phrenoesophageal ligament. The fundus cardia of the stomach slides upward through the diaphragm (Link 18-33 B, *left*).

2. Epidemiology
   a. Most common type of HH (95%)
   b. Found in 50% of persons >50 years old. Risk of developing a HH increases with age.
   c. More common in women than men
   d. Other associations with HH include sigmoid diverticulosis, esophagitis, duodenal ulcers, sigmoid diverticulosis, and gallstones.

3. Clinical findings include:
   a. heartburn that gets worse when leaning over or lying down.
   b. nocturnal epigastric distress from acid reflux.
   c. bowel sounds are heard over the left lung base.
   d. less common but severe problems include:
      (1) hematemesis (vomiting blood).
      (2) ulceration, stricture.

4. Definition of paraesophageal hernia (1%; Link 18-33 B, *right*):
   a. Uncommon type of hernia in which the GEJ remains at the level of the diaphragm and the gastric fundus +/− body bulges into the thoracic cavity
   b. Danger of bleeding and strangulation

A **pleuroperitoneal diaphragmatic hernia** (Bochdalek hernia) accounts for 90% of the hernias seen in newborns (Fig. 18-12; Link 18-34). The visceral contents extend through the posterolateral part of the diaphragm on the left into the chest cavity, causing severe respiratory distress at birth. Loops of bowel are present in the left pleural cavity on radiographs.

Bochdalek hernia: defect left diaphragm; bowel in left pleural cavity; NB respiratory difficulty

Gastroesophageal reflux (GERD)

Reflux gastric acid/bile into distal esophagus

Pregnancy (80%)

Hiatal hernia often present

Smoking/alcohol

Caffeine, fatty foods, chocolate

Pregnancy, obesity, hiatal hernia

Transient LES relaxation

I. Gastroesophageal reflux disease (GERD)

1. **Definition:** Reflux of gastric acid and bile into the distal esophagus, causing heartburn

2. Epidemiology
   a. Approximately 10% to 20% of adults have GERD daily.
   b. Approximately 80% of pregnant women have GERD.
   c. HH is present in ~70% of people with GERD.
   d. Risk factors for GERD include smoking, alcohol, caffeine, fatty foods, chocolate, pregnancy, obesity, and HH.

3. Pathogenesis of GERD; most common causes include:
   a. transient relaxation of lower esophageal sphincter (LES); causes reflux of acid bile into the distal esophagus (Fig. 18-13 A; Links 18-35 and 18-36).

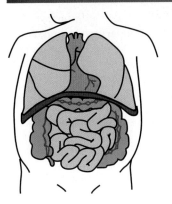 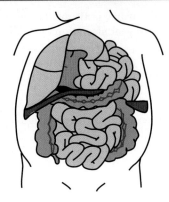

Normal diaphragm

Bochdalek diaphragmatic defect

A   B

18-12: Pleuroperitoneal diaphragmatic hernia (Bochdalek hernia). The visceral contents extend through the posterolateral part of the diaphragm on the left into the chest cavity causing respiratory distress at birth. *(From Kliegman, R:* Nelson Textbook of Pediatrics, *19th ed, Philadelphia, Elsevier Saunders, 2011, p 594, Fig. 95.10.)*

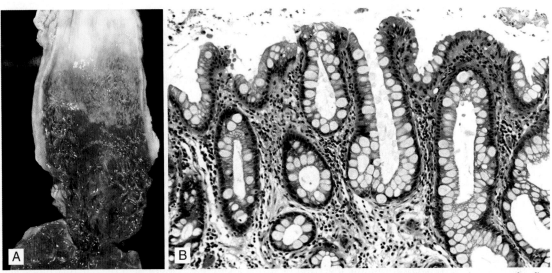

18-13: A, Gross appearance of reflux esophagitis. Marked hyperemia with focal hemorrhage is present in the area of reflux. **B,** Barrett's esophagus. This biopsy specimen came from the distal esophagus and shows intestinal metaplasia with numerous goblet cells replacing squamous epithelium. *(A from Rosai J:* Rosai and Ackerman's Surgical Pathology, *9th ed, St. Louis, Mosby, 2004, p 619, Fig. 11.7; B from Iacobuzio-Donahue CA, Montgomery E, Goldblum JR:* Gastrointestinal and Liver Pathology, *2nd ed, Saunders Elsevier, 2012, p 44, Fig. 2-12.)*

    b. reduced LES pressure caused by HH.

    c. *Helicobacter pylori* (HP) has *no* role in the pathogenesis of GERD.

4. Clinical findings in GERD include:

    a. retrosternal noncardiac chest pain caused by heartburn and regurgitation are the most common complaints.

      (1) Heartburn is characterized by a painful retrosternal burning sensation that may last several minutes.

      (2) Regurgitation refers to the backflow of gastric contents into the mouth that is not associated with retching or vomiting (called "water brash"; sour fluid or almost tasteless saliva in the mouth; see later). Retching refers to gastric and esophageal movement of vomiting *without* oral expulsion of vomitus.

    b. dysphagia triggered by esophageal spasm (40% of patients with long-standing GERD).

    c. odynophagia: painful swallowing described as sharp or lancinating pain behind the sternum.

    d. nocturnal cough, nocturnal asthma (vagus nerve mediated bronchoconstriction).

    e. chronic laryngitis (acid injury to vocal cords).

    f. acid injury to the enamel (also common in bulimia nervosa).

    g. water brash: sudden appearance of slightly sour or salty fluid in the mouth; vagus nerve–mediated secretions from the salivary glands in response to acid reflux.

5. Complications of GERD include sinusitis, otitis media, chronic obstructive pulmonary disease (COPD), esophagitis, esophageal ulceration or stricture, pulmonary aspiration, and Barrett esophagus (see later).

6. Diagnostic tests that are available if the presentation is *atypical* include:
   a. 24-hour esophageal pH monitoring. Sensitivity and specificity are 80% and 90%, respectively.
   b. esophageal endoscopy.
   c. manometry (measurement of pressure in the esophagus). Lower esophageal sphincter (LES) pressure is <10 mm Hg.

J. Barrett esophagus
1. **Definition:** Glandular (intestinal) metaplasia (conversion of squamous epithelium to glandular epithelium) in the distal esophagus that is secondary to chronic mucosal irritation caused by GERD
2. Epidemiology
   a. Found in 5% to 15% of patients with GERD
   b. More common in white men >50 years of age
   c. Gastric-type columnar cells as well as small intestinal type goblet cells are present (see Figs. 2-15 F and 18-13 B; Link 18-37).
3. Complications include:
   a. ulceration with stricture formation (most common complication).
   b. glandular dysplasia with increased risk for the development of an adenocarcinoma within the distal esophagus (see later).

K. Infectious esophagitis
1. Usually a complication of immunosuppression (e.g., AIDS)
2. Pathogens that are involved include:
   a. *herpes simplex* virus (HSV; Link 18-38).
      (1) Type I or II HSV.
      (2) Endoscopy shows ulcers and/or vesicles.
      (3) Biopsies show multinucleated squamous cells (SCs) with intranuclear inclusions (Fig. 18-14 A).
   b. cytomegalovirus (CMV). Large cells with eosinophilic intranuclear inclusions (Fig. 18-14 B).
   c. *Candida*. Yeasts and pseudohyphae (extended yeast forms) are present (Links 18-39 and 18-40).
3. Infectious esophagitis presents with painful swallowing (i.e., odynophagia).

L. Corrosive esophagitis
1. **Definition:** The ingestion of strong alkali (e.g., lye) or acid (e.g., hydrochloric acid [HCl])
2. Complications include stricture formation, perforation, and SCC.

M. Esophageal varices
1. **Definition:** Dilated distal esophageal submucosal (left gastric) veins; complication of portal hypertension most commonly associated with cirrhosis of the liver (Fig. 18-15; Links

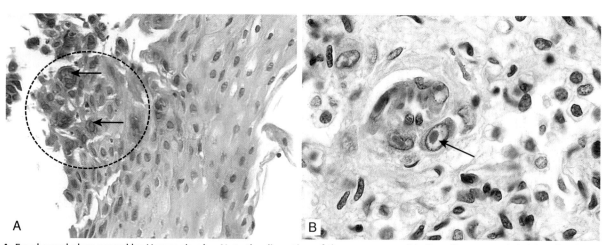

18-14: A, Esophageal ulcer caused by *Herpes simplex*. Note the disruption of the squamous epithelium *(interrupted circle)* and multinucleation with many of the nuclei exhibiting nuclear clearing and the presence of small inclusions *(arrows)*. Many of the nuclei have tiny inclusions in them *(black arrows)*. **B,** Cytomegalovirus (CMV) infection. Note the enlarged nucleus *(arrow)*, nuclear clearing and eosinophilic inclusion representing the virus. *(From King TS: Elsevier's Integrated Pathology, Mosby Elsevier, 2007, p 70, Fig. 3-10 A, B.)*

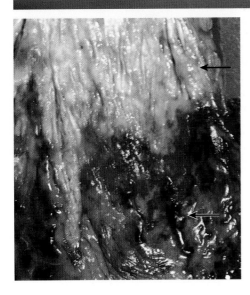

18-15: Esophageal varices, showing linear-oriented dilated and tortuous veins *(arrows)* in the submucosa of the distal esophagus. *(From Morson BC: Colour Atlas of Gastrointestinal Pathology, London, Harvey Miller Ltd, 1988, p 33, Fig. 1.54.)*

18-41 and 18-42). Left gastric vein drains blood from the distal esophagus and proximal stomach into the portal vein.

2. Epidemiology
   a. Alcohol abuse is the most common cause.
   b. Rupture of esophageal varices is the most common cause of death secondary to cirrhosis of the liver.
3. Most common clinical finding of esophageal varices is rupture with massive hematemesis (vomiting blood)
4. Diagnosis is made by endoscopy.

N. Mallory-Weiss syndrome
   1. **Definition:** A mucosal tear in the proximal stomach and distal esophagus that is caused by severe retching, most often associated with alcoholism or bulimia (self-induced vomiting)
   2. Severe retching → vomiting blood

O. Boerhaave syndrome
   1. **Definition:** Rupture of the distal esophagus
   2. Causes include endoscopy (~75% of cases) and retching (e.g., bulimia).
   3. Complications of Boerhaave syndrome include:
      a. pneumomediastinum, in which air dissects subcutaneously into the anterior mediastinum. A crunching sound (Hamman sign) is heard on auscultation.
      b. pleural effusion contains food, acid, and amylase (an enzyme from the mouth).

P. Motor disorders of the esophagus

Manometry is used to measure intraluminal pressure and assess coordination of contraction in the esophagus via a catheter. Two types of manometry are conventional and high-resolution manometry, the former having wider sensors and the latter shorter sensors to analyze pressure patterns.

---

   1. SS (90% esophageal involvement) and CREST syndrome (see Chapter 4)
   2. Achalasia (Links 18-33 C and 18-43)
      a. **Definition:** Motility disorder characterized by incomplete relaxation of the LES and lack of peristalsis of the esophageal smooth muscle producing a functional obstruction of the esophagus
      b. Epidemiology
         (1) Most common neuromuscular disorder of the esophagus
         (2) Bimodal age distribution
            (a) Occurs in those 20 to 40 years old
            (b) Also occurs after 60 years of age
         (3) Men and women are equally affected.
         (4) Risk factor for esophageal cancer (SCC)

Margin notes:

Alcohol MCC

Rupture MC COD cirrhosis

Massive hematemesis

Endoscopy Dx

Mallory-Weiss syndrome

Mucosal tear proximal stomach/distal esophagus

Severe retching → vomiting blood

Boerhaave syndrome

Rupture distal esophagus

Endoscopy MCC

Retching (bulimia)

Pneumomediastinum

Hamman sign

Pleural effusion: food, acid, amylase

Motor disorders of esophagus

Manometry: measures intraluminal esophageal pressure

Systemic sclerosis

Achalasia: motility disorder

Incomplete relaxation LES

Lack peristalsis esophageal smooth muscle (functional obstruction)

MC neuromuscular disorder esophagus

Bimodal age distribution

Men = women

Esophageal cancer risk

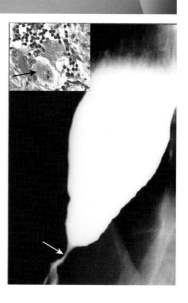

18-16: Barium study of the esophagus in achalasia. Note the dilated esophagus ending in a narrowed esophagogastric junction ("birds-beak" appearance) *(white arrow)*. The esophagus proximal to the lower esophageal sphincter is dilated. The **inset** shows the myenteric plexus with T lymphocytes (dark cells) destroying ganglia in the myenteric plexus *(black arrow)*. *(From Kliegman R: Nelson Textbook of Pediatrics, 19th ed, Philadelphia, Elsevier Saunders, 2011, p 1265, Fig. 313.1. Inset from Iacobuzio-Donahue CA, Montgomery E, Goldblum JR: Gastrointestinal and Liver Pathology, Saunders Elsevier 2nd ed, 2012, p 13, Fig. 1-18.)*

LES relaxation NO, VIP

Achalasia: incomplete relaxation LES

Loss MP/loss GCs (T cell destruction)

Loss PGIN containing NO/VIP

PGENs spared → cholinergic stimulation → ↑LES pressure

Dilation/loss peristalsis proximal to LES

Chagas disease: achalasia, myocarditis

Clinical findings

Dysphagia solids/liquids

Nocturnal regurg undigested food

Chest pain/heartburn

Nocturnal cough

Dx achalasia

Beak-like tapering distal esophagus

Absent peristalsis; manometry gold standard

Absent gastric bubble

Diffuse esophageal spasm

Uncoordinated contractions of normal amplitude

Chest pain aggravated by stress

Dysphagia solids/liquids

GERD in most cases

"Corkscrew" esophagus

Lower esophageal pressure > 35 mm Hg

Nutcracker esophagus

Coordinated contractions; extremely high esophageal pressure

Chest pain, dysphagia solids/liquids, GERD

c. Pathogenesis
(1) Normal relaxation of the smooth muscle in the LES is caused by nitric oxide (NO) and vasoactive intestinal peptide (VIP).
(2) In achalasia, there is incomplete relaxation of the LES.
(a) Loss of myenteric (Auerbach) plexus (MP) and loss of ganglion cells (GCs) are associated with a patchy inflammatory (autoimmune) response consisting primarily of T cells. End result is a selective loss of postganglionic inhibitory neurons (PGINs) containing NO and VIP.
(b) Postganglionic excitatory neurons (PGENs) are spared; therefore, cholinergic stimulation is unopposed, leading to high resting LES pressure.
(3) Dilation and a loss of peristalsis in the esophagus proximal to the LES
(4) Acquired cause of achalasia is Chagas disease, in which there is destruction of GCs by amastigotes (lack flagella) producing achalasia and myocarditis (see Fig. 11-21).
d. Clinical findings in achalasia include:
(1) dysphagia for solids and liquids most common complaint (70%–90%).
(2) nocturnal regurgitation of undigested food without an acid taste (75%).
(3) chest pain and heartburn (50%).
(4) nocturnal cough from aspiration.
e. Diagnosis of achalasia
(1) Barium study shows a dilated, aperistaltic esophagus with a beak-like tapering at distal end and dilation of the esophagus (Fig. 18-16; Link 18-43).
(2) Fluoroscopy shows a lack of peristalsis. High-resolution manometry (HRM) is the gold standard for diagnosing achalasia. It shows detailed colored pressure recordings from the pharynx to the stomach.
(3) Chest radiography shows an absent gastric bubble.
3. Diffuse esophageal spasm
a. **Definition:** Characterized by uncoordinated contractions that are of normal amplitude (pressure) and involve the entire esophagus
b. Epidemiology
(1) Can present as chest pain that is aggravated by stress
(2) Associated with dysphagia for solids and liquids and chest pain
(3) GERD is present in 70% of cases.
c. Barium swallow reveals a "corkscrew" esophagus (Link 18-44).
d. Lower esophageal pressure is >35 mm Hg.
4. Nutcracker esophagus (hypertensive peristalsis; "jackhammer" esophagus)
a. **Definition:** Condition in which the muscle contractions are coordinated but are too strong (high amplitude or pressure), causing severe chest pain
b. Epidemiology
(1) Symptoms include chest pain, difficulty with swallowing, dysphagia for both solids and liquids, and GERD.

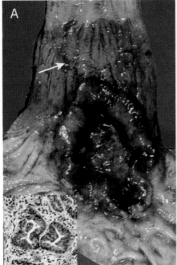
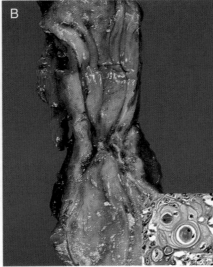
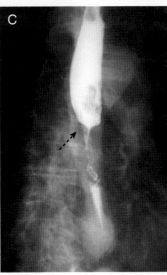

18-17: A, Distal esophageal adenocarcinoma. Note the ulcerated mass with raised margins. There is a background of Barrett's esophagus *(arrow)*. The inset shows a well-differentiated adenocarcinoma with glands lined by hyperchromatic glandular cells. **B,** Midesophagus squamous cell carcinoma (SCC). Note the elevated nodular mass with a central area of ulceration. The inset shows a keratinizing SCC with bright red keratin pearls. **C,** Radiograph showing an annular constricting SCC of the mid-esophagus (dotted black arrow). The tumor encircles and obstructs the normal lumen. *(**A, A inset, B inset** from Iacobuzio-Donahue CA, Montgomery E, Goldblum JR:* Gastrointestinal and Liver Pathology, *2nd ed, Saunders Elsevier, 2012, pp 54, 55, 59, respectively; inset Figs. 2-24, 26, 32, respectively. **B** from Rosai J, Ackerman LV:* Surgical Pathology, *9th ed, St. Louis, Mosby, 2004, p 626, Fig. 11-14C. Inset from **C** from Herring W:* Learning Radiology Recognizing the Basics, *2nd ed, Philadelphia, Elsevier Saunders, 2012, p 175, Fig. 18.4A.)*

    (2) Primarily diagnosed with manometry, which demonstrates the high esophageal pressure

Q. Esophageal tumors

1. Leiomyoma
   a. **Definition:** Benign tumor of smooth muscle
   b. Most common benign tumor of the esophagus
2. Incidence of esophageal cancer has plateaued.
3. Adenocarcinoma of distal esophagus (Fig. 18-17 A; Links 18-45 to 18-47)
   a. Most common primary cancer of the esophagus in the United States
   b. Peak age, 65–75 years old
   c. Male: female ratio, 4 : 1
   d. Adenocarcinoma greater in white men than black men
   e. Risk factors include:
      (1) Barrett esophagus is the most common predisposing cause for this cancer.
      (2) smoking may increase the risk, particularly if Barrett esophagus is present.
      (3) obesity, HH, diets lacking fresh fruit and vegetables, high-fat diet from red meats.
      (4) chronic GERD.
      (5) bisphosphonates (used in treating osteoporosis).
   f. Dysphagia is indicative of a poor diagnosis.
4. Squamous cell carcinoma (SCC) of the esophagus
   a. Epidemiology
      (1) Most common primary cancer in developing countries from the Caspian Sea to Northern China
      (2) More common in blacks than whites
      (3) Occurs in men more often than women
      (4) Risk factors include:
         (a) smoking: most common cause.
         (b) alcohol abuse, lye strictures.
         (c) achalasia and Plummer-Vinson syndrome.
         (d) nitrates converted to nitrites (South Asia, China); bisphosphonates.
         (e) long exposure to extremely hot tea.
         (f) radiation-induced strictures.
         (g) fungal toxins in pickled vegetables.
         (h) HPV.

Manometry shows high esophageal pressure

Esophageal tumors

Leiomyoma

Benign tumor smooth muscle

MC benign tumor esophagus

Adenocarcinoma MC 1° cancer distal esophagus U.S.

65-75 yrs old

M/F 4:1

White > black men

Barrett esophagus MC predisposing cause

Smoking

Obesity, HH, ↓fruit/ vegetable, ↑ fat in diet

Chronic GERD

Bisphosphonates

Dysphagia poor prognosis

SCC

MC cancer developing countries

Blacks > whites

Men > women

Smoking MCC

Alcohol, lye strictures

Achalasia, PV

Nitrates to nitrites; bisphosphonates

Hot tea

Radiation-induced strictures

Fungal toxins pickled vegetables

HPV

Middle 3rd MC site

Local nodes first

Dysphagia solids; poor prognosis

Weight loss short duration

Enlarged supraclavicular nodes

Dry cough, hemoptysis; trachea invasion

Invasion recurrent laryngeal nerve

Odynophagia (proximal)

Ectopic production PTH-related peptide

Endoscopy, biopsy

G cells gastrin → acid from parietal cells

D cells somatostatin (inhibits gastrin)

Goblet cells: protective mucus

Gastrin, Ach stimulate H⁺ secretion by parietal cells

Histamine: stimulates H⁺ secretion by parietal cells

Gastric fundus/body: parietal cells → acid; pepsinogen

CCs → pepsinogen → pepsin

Gastric acid secretion Vagus nerve: stimulate H⁺/K⁺ ATPase

Histamine: stimulates H⁺ secretion by parietal cells

Gastrin: stimulates H⁺/K⁺ ATPase (acid production/secretion)

Hematemesis: vomiting blood

PUD MCC

Varices, hemorrhagic gastritis

Melena: dark, tarry stools

Hb + acid → hematin (black stool)

GI bleed proximal to DJJ; 4th part duodenum

Angiography, technetium 99M-RBC study

Vomiting

(5) Locations include:
  (a) upper third (~15%).
  (b) middle third (~50%) (Fig. 18-17 B, C; Links 18-48 and 18-49).
  (c) lower third (~35%).
(6) Cancer spreads to local nodes first and then to the liver and lungs.
  b. Clinical findings include:
  (1) dysphagia for solids initially; indicative of a poor prognosis.
  (2) rapid weight loss.
  (3) painless enlarged supraclavicular nodes.
  (4) dry cough and hemoptysis. Findings suggest tracheal invasion by the cancer.
  (5) hoarseness. Indicates invasion of the recurrent laryngeal nerve.
  (6) odynophagia if proximal (painful swallowing).
  (7) hypercalcemia. Ectopic production of parathyroid hormone–related peptide, which also occurs in SCC of the lungs (see Chapters 9 and 17).
  c. Diagnosis secured by endoscopy with biopsy
  d. Overall 5-year survival rate is 15%.

IV. Stomach Disorders
  A. Overview of stomach anatomy and physiology (Links 18-50 to 18-53)
    1. Pyloric glands in antrum
      a. G cells contain gastrin, which stimulate acid release from parietal cells.
      b. D cells contain somatostatin, which inhibits gastrin release.
      c. Goblet cells contain mucus, which produces a protective coating over the stomach mucosa.
      d. Histamine is secreted by endocrine-type cells in the gastric mucosa in the H⁺ secreting regions of the stomach. Along with gastrin and acetylcholine (Ach), histamine stimulates H⁺ secretion by the gastric parietal cells.
    2. Gastric fundus and body contain glands that secrete acid (parietal cells) and pepsinogen (chief cells; CCs), which is cleaved into pepsin by HCl (chief cells; CCs), which is cleaved into pepsin by hydrochloric acid (HCl). In excess amounts, pepsin can damage the gastric mucosa.
    3. Gastric acid secretion
      a. Vagus nerve → release Ach → stimulate H⁺/K⁺ ATPase → acid production/secretion
      b. Histamine → stimulates H⁺ secretion by parietal cells
      c. Gastrin → stimulates H⁺/K⁺ ATPase → acid production/secretion
  B. Signs and symptoms of stomach disease include:
    1. hematemesis (vomiting blood).
      a. Most commonly caused by peptic ulcer disease (PUD)
      b. Other causes of hematemesis include esophageal varices and hemorrhagic gastritis.
    2. melena (dark, tarry stools).
      a. Hemoglobin (Hb) is converted into hematin (black pigment) by gastric acid.
      b. Signifies a bleed proximal to the duodenojejunal junction (DJJ; 90% of cases)
        (1) Anatomically, the DJJ is the fourth part of the duodenum.
        (2) Surrounded by a peritoneal fold containing muscle fibers called the ligament of Treitz
      c. In addition to endoscopy, radiologic tests that can be used to identify the site of bleeding include a technetium 99M-RBC study and catheter angiography. Barium studies have no role in the initial evaluation of acute GI bleeding.
    3. vomiting.

A **gastric analysis** includes measurement of basal acid output (BAO), maximal acid output (MAO), and the BAO/MAO ratio. BAO is the acid output of gastric juice collected via a nasogastric tube over a 1-hour period on an empty stomach (normally <5 mEq/hr). MAO is the acid output of gastric juice that is collected over 1 hour after pentagastrin stimulation. Normally, the MAO is 5 to 20 mEq/hr. The normal BAO/MAO ratio is 0.20:1.

Measures BAO and MAO

HPS

Narrow passage between stomach and small intestine

Males > females

Acquired complication chronic DUD

Greater 90% sporadic

  C. Hypertrophic pyloric stenosis (HPS)
    1. **Definition:** A narrowing of the passage between the distal stomach and the proximal duodenum of the small intestine caused by hypertrophy of muscle
    2. Epidemiology
      a. More common in males than females (4:1 ratio)
      b. Acquired pyloric obstruction is a complication of chronic duodenal ulcer disease (DUD) with pyloric scarring.
      c. More than 90% are sporadic.

d. A total of 7% to 10% of cases are familial. Mother who had HPS as an infant increases the risk HPS in offspring (19% for boys and 7% for girls). Offspring of a father with history of HPS as an infant are also at an increased risk (5% for boys and 2.5% for girls).

3. Pathophysiology
   a. Caused by progressive hypertrophy of the circular muscles in the pyloric sphincter (PS). HPS is *not* present at birth but may occur in 2-week- to 2-month-old infants.
   b. Deficiency of nitric oxide (NO) synthase in muscle precipitates the disease. It results in a decrease in NO, a vasodilator.

4. Clinical findings include:
   a. projectile vomiting of fluid that is *not* bile stained.
   b. palpation of the hypertrophied pylorus in the epigastrium (70% of cases). The hypertrophied pylorus is sometimes called an "olive."
   c. visible hyperperistalsis.

5. Radiograph shows narrow pyloric channel ("string sign"; Link 18-54). Do *not* confuse this string sign with the one that is present in the terminal ileum in Crohn disease (CD).

D. Gastric acid secretion overview

Margin notes:
7% to 10% familial

Hypertrophy PS muscles
Not present at birth; 2 wks to 2 mths

↓NO synthase in muscle → ↓NO, vasodilator

Projectile vomiting *not* bile stained

"Olive"
Visible hyperperistalsis

"String sign"

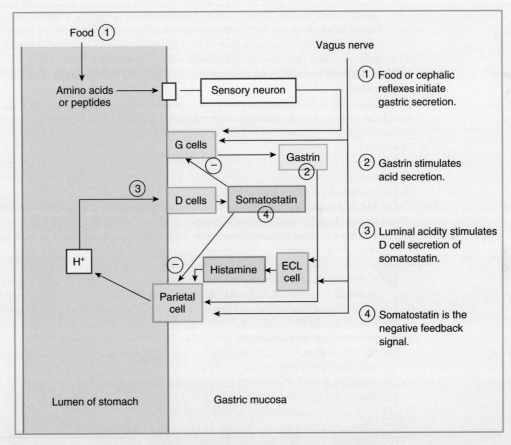

Gastric acid secretion is regulated by neural, endocrine, and paracrine agents. Gastric acid secretion by the parietal cell is under complex regulation. The enterochromaffin-like (ECL) cell releases histamine that stimulates acid secretion. Both the hormone gastrin and the neurotransmitter acetylcholine (Ach) can stimulate the ECL cell to release histamine and can directly stimulate the parietal cell to secrete acid. Gastrin is released by amino acids or peptides in the lumen of the stomach, and Ach is released by nervous system reflexes. Excess acid in the lumen of the stomach causes D cells to release somatostatin, which inhibits both gastrin release and parietal cell acid secretion.

(Schematic and description from Carroll RG: *Elsevier's Integrated Physiology,* St. Louis, Mosby Elsevier, 2007, p 150, Fig. 12-8.)

E. Gastroparesis
   1. **Definition:** Decreased gastric motility and emptying of the stomach in the absence of mechanical obstruction
   2. Epidemiology

Margin notes:
Gastroparesis
↓Gastric motility/emptying (absence mechanical obstruction)

Primarily occurs in women

DM, vagotomy, anorexia/bulimia, MS, drugs

Early satiety, bloating

Vomiting undigested food after eating

Acute gastritis

Hemorrhagic erosions/ulcers

Breach mucosal epithelium

Breach mucosa→ deeper

NSAIDs MCC; alcohol 2nd

HP, CMV (AIDS), smoking

Stress related

Trauma, burns, sepsis, CNS injury

Burns (Curling), CNS injury (Cushing)

Uremia, *Anisakis*

Hematemesis, melena, iron deficiency

Chronic gastritis

Chronic inflammation, intestinal metaplasia

MCC HP; autoimmune gastritis

HP chronic gastritis

Spiral gram– flagellated G – rod

Corkscrew motility for penetration

Humans principal reservoir

Childhood infection

Infects antrum; neutrophils infiltrate mucosal cells

MC transmission: fecal–oral route

HP attaches to O group receptors

Not invasive

Urease, proteases, cytotoxins

Urease → ammonia

Secretion products → chronic gastritis, PUD

Poor sanitation

Tests for HP

IgG antibody test

Urea breath test

Stool antigen test

Urease test gastric Bx gold standard

Gastric biopsy/histologic exam

Gastric acid ↑/slightly ↓

Serum gastrin (N/↓

a. Affects 3% of the population. Of these, 75% are women averaging 34 years of age.
b. May be a complication of autonomic neuropathy (e.g., diabetes mellitus [DM], previous vagotomy), multiple sclerosis (MS), Parkinson disease, hypothyroidism, drugs (e.g., anticholinergics, proton pump inhibitors, calcium channel blockers), anorexia nervosa, or bulimia nervosa
3. Clinical findings include:
a. early satiety (feeling full after eating small amount) and bloating.
b. vomiting of undigested food a few hours after eating.

F. Acute gastritis
1. **Definition:** Inflammation of the stomach mucosa associated with hemorrhage caused by erosions, ulcers, or both
a. Erosions are a breach in the epithelium of the mucosa (Link 18-55).
b. Ulcers are a breach in the mucosa with extension into the submucosa or deeper (Link 18-55).
2. Causes include:
a. nonsteroidal antiinflammatory drugs (NSAIDs) are the most common cause.
b. alcohol (second most common cause), Heliocobacter pylori (HP; see later), CMV (AIDS), smoking.
c. stress-related ulcers.
• Occur in patients with severe trauma, burns, sepsis, central nervous system (CNS) injury (Link 18-56). Those occurring with severe burns or trauma are sometimes called Curling ulcers, while those associated with CNS injury are called Cushing ulcers. Hemorrhagic gastritis involves all of the gastric mucosa (Link 18-57).
d. uremia, *Anisakis* (worm associated with eating raw fish).
3. Clinical findings include hematemesis, melena, and iron deficiency.

G. Chronic gastritis
1. **Definition:** Chronic inflammation of the gastric mucosa with a loss of the normal gastric glandular cells and replacement by intestinal-type epithelium (intestinal metaplasia), pylorus-type glands, and fibrous connective tissue
2. Epidemiology
a. Most common cause is HP (90% of cases) and the remainder by autoimmune gastritis (10% of cases).
b. HP-associated chronic gastritis
(1) HP is a spiral, gram-negative flagellated rod that has corkscrew motility for penetrating the gastric mucus layer.
(2) Humans are the principal reservoir. In the United States, 40% to 60% of individuals older than 60 years of age are infected.
(3) Infection most likely occurs in childhood.
(4) Colonizes mucus layer lining within the antrum (less commonly cardia) of the stomach (Fig. 18-18 A; Links 18-58 to 18-60). Neutrophils are the primary inflammatory infiltrate and are noted within the lamina propria as well as the mucosal cells themselves (characteristic finding). They may also extend into the pits to produce crypt abscesses.
(5) Most commonly transmitted by the fecal–oral route (the organism is passed in stools and can live in water)
(6) Attaches to blood group O receptors on mucosal cells
(7) *Not* an invasive bacterium
(8) Produces urease, proteases, and cytotoxins
(9) Urease converts amino groups in proteins to ammonia.
(10) Secretion products produce chronic gastritis and PUD.
(11) Common in areas of poor sanitation
(12) Tests to identify HP are highly sensitive and specific.
(a) IgG antibody test is useful for diagnosis (specificity, 93%–98%) and documenting eradication (sensitivity, 88%–99%).
(b) Urea breath test: sensitivity is 90% to 97%, and specificity is 90% to 100%.
(c) Stool antigen test. Less expensive than the urea breath test. Sensitivity is 90%, and specificity is 97% to 98%.
(d) Tests to detect urease in a gastric biopsy (Clo-test). Sensitivity is 89% to 98%, and specificity is 93% to 98%. Considered by most to be the gold standard test.
(e) Gastric biopsy with histologic exam. Sensitivity is 93% to 99%, and specificity is 95% to 99%.
(13) Gastric acid production is increased to slightly decreased. Serum gastrin levels are normal to decreased.

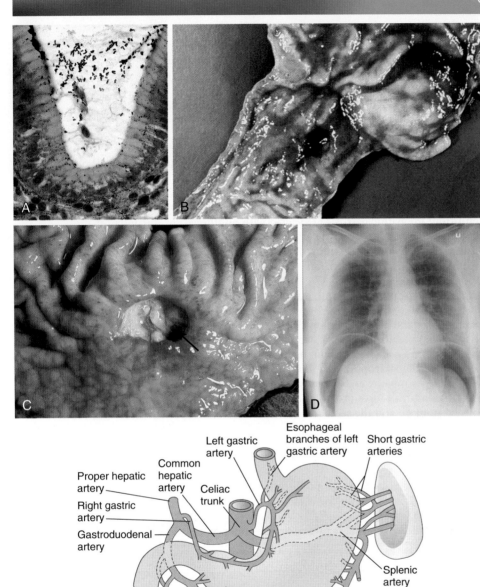

18-18: A, Silver stain showing *Helicobacter pylori* organisms in the mucus layer lining the gastric epithelial cells. **B,** Duodenal ulcer in the first part of the duodenum. **C,** Chronic gastric ulcer. Note the sharply delimited peptic ulcer with converging folds of normal gastric mucosa in the upper half. The base of the ulcer contains white necrotic debris and a bleeding site is note in the right lower quadrant (black arrow). **D,** Plain abdominal radiograph in a supine patient with a perforated peptic ulcer. Note the presence of air under both diaphragms. **E,** Schematic of arterial system in the stomach. The gastroduodenal artery and the right gastric artery are eroded for bleeding from a duodenal ulcer and gastric ulcer, respectively. *(A from Kumar V, Fausto N, Abbas A: Robbins and Cotran Pathologic Basis of Disease, 7th ed, Philadelphia, Saunders, 2004, p 815, Fig. 17-15; B from my friend Ivan Damjanov, MD, PhD, Linder J: Anderson's Pathology, 10th ed, St. Louis, Mosby, 1996, p 1680, Fig. 53.21B; C, From Rosai J: Rosai and Ackerman's Surgical Pathology, 10th ed, Mosby Elsevier, 2011, p 621, Fig. 11.30B; D from Goldman L, Ausiello D: Cecil's Textbook of Medicine, 23rd ed, Philadelphia, Saunders Elsevier, 2008, p 1015, Fig. 142-3; E from Moore A, Roy W: Rapid Review Gross and Developmental Anatomy, 3rd ed, Philadelphia, Mosby Elsevier, 2010, p 73, Fig. 3-15.)*

(14) Other disease associations with HP that are discussed later include DU and gastric ulcers (GUs); adenocarcinoma; and low-grade B-cell <u>m</u>ucosa-<u>a</u>ssociated <u>l</u>ymphoid <u>t</u>issue (MALT) lymphoma.

c. Autoimmune chronic gastritis

(1) Accounts for 10% of chronic gastritis

(2) Primarily involves the body of the stomach

(3) Loss of parietal cells is caused by CD_4-T cells directed against parietal cell components and H^+/K^+-ATPase (proton pump) is the principle cause of autoimmune chronic gastritis, a type IV HSR.

(4) In addition, antibodies are directed against the H^+/K^+-ATPase (PP, proton pump) and intrinsic factor (IF). Antibodies are present in ~80% of cases; a type II HSR.

(5) Sequelae include pernicious anemia (PA; vitamin B_{12} deficiency caused by loss of IF), glandular atrophy, hyperplasia of neuroendocrine cells (danger for increasing one's risk of carcinoid tumor), and adenocarcinoma.

(6) Other autoimmune associations include Hashimoto thyroiditis (HT), Graves disease, and DM.

(7) Gastric acid levels are decreased and serum gastrin levels are increased.

DUs/GUs

Adenocarcinoma

Low grade MALToma

Autoimmune chronic gastritis

10% Chronic gastritis

Body of stomach

CD_4-T helper cell destruction parietal cells

Type IV HSR

Abs against PP/IF

Type II HSR

PA, atrophy, adenocarcinoma, carcinoid tumor

HT, Graves, DM

↓Gastric acid, ↑gastrin

d. Microscopic findings in chronic gastritis
   (1) Chronic inflammatory infiltrate involving the lamina propria
   (2) Intestinal metaplasia (similar Barrett esophagus): precursor lesion for adenocarcinoma

H. Other types of gastritis
1. Lymphocytic gastritis
   a. **Definition:** Type of chronic gastritis associated with increased intraepithelial T lymphocytes with or without foveolar hyperplasia, erosions, or ulcers
   b. Epidemiology
      (1) Primarily affects women
      (2) Type of gastritis associated with hypersensitivity to gliadin or other unknown agents (40%) or autoimmune diseases
      (3) Clinical associations include celiac disease (sprue) and Ménétrier disease (see later).
2. Granulomatous gastritis
   a. **Definition:** Idiopathic gastritis associated with multifocal chronic inflammation with epithelioid granulomas
   b. Epidemiology: Causes include sarcoidosis, Crohn's disease (CD), drug reactions, infections (fungal, Mycobacterium, spirochetal), and vasculitis.
3. Eosinophilic gastritis
   a. **Definition:** Type of gastritis with eosinophilic inflammation involving the gastric antrum and pylorus
   b. Epidemiology and clinical findings
      (1) Etiologies include idiopathic food allergy, parasitic disease, and drug allergy.
      (2) Clinical findings include pain, nausea or vomiting, weight loss, and anemia.

I. Ménétrier disease (hypertrophic lymphocytic gastritis)
1. **Definition:** A gastropathy associated with overexpression of transforming growth factor α (TGF-α) that in turn causes proliferation of the mucus-producing cells; results in giant rugal folds in the stomach and the secretion of excess amounts of protein-rich mucus (Link 18-61).
2. Epidemiology
   a. Mucus secretions contain protein and thus hypoproteinemia may occur (protein-losing enteropathy).
   b. Atrophy of parietal cells, which produces resulting in achlorhydria (lack of HCl).
   c. Increased risk for developing gastric adenocarcinoma

J. Peptic ulcer disease (PUD)
1. **Definition:** An ulceration that is present in the stomach and/or duodenum caused by an imbalance between protective and damaging factors in the mucosa
2. Epidemiology
   a. Most often caused by HP (70% of cases). In other parts of the world, >90% of cases are caused by HP.
   b. Lifetime prevalence of PUD is 5% to 10%.
   c. Eradication of HP reduces the recurrence of PUD.
   d. Protective factors to prevent PUD include mucous-bicarbonate barrier, microcirculation, prostaglandins (PGEs), growth factors, and increased cell turnover.
   e. Factors that increase the risk for PUD include advanced age (>70 years), excess pepsin, excess acid, NSAIDs; low-dose aspirin), ischemia or hypoxia, bile acids, delayed gastric emptying, hypercalcemia, drugs, alcohol, and infections (HP, viruses).
   f. Duodenal ulcers (DU) are more common than gastric ulcers (GU). Incidence of bleeding is the same for both ulcers.
   g. Locations of the ulcers
      (1) DUs occur in the first portion of the duodenum (>90% of cases; Fig. 18-18 B).
      (2) GUs occur in the lesser curvature near the incisura angularis (bend in the lesser curvature near the end of the pylorus; Fig. 18-18C; Link 18-62). Fewer than 3% are malignant. Fig. 18-18 D shows a perforation of GU with air located underneath the diaphragms. Perforation also may occur with a DU. Pain is referred to the shoulders.
      (3) Figure 18-18 E shows a schematic of the arterial system of the stomach and the most common location for a gastric and DU.
   h. Recurrence rate for untreated PUD is ~60% of cases in nonsmokers and >70% in smokers.
   i. Epigastric pain is the most common symptom.
3. Gross appearance of ulcers
   a. Ulcers are clean, sharply demarcated, and slightly elevated around the edges (Link 18-62).
   b. Most GUs are benign. A small percentage may be malignant, which is the reason why they are biopsied.

TABLE 18-2 Comparison of Gastric Ulcers and Duodenal Ulcers

FEATURE	GASTRIC ULCERS	DUODENAL ULCERS
Percentage of ulcer cases	25%	75%
Epidemiology	• Male/female ratio 1:1 • Smoking may delay healing. • Risk for developing gastric cancer (increased risk with blood group A individuals). • Risk factors: *Helicobacter pylori* (most common), chronic intake of NSAIDs (synergism with *H. pylori*), moderate alcohol consumption	• Male/female ratio 1:1. • Risk increased with MEN I. • Smoking may delay healing. • Risk factors: *H. pylori* (most common), chronic intake of NSAIDs, type O blood group (lack blood group antigens that are protective to the mucosal surface).
Helicobacter pylori association	Duodenal ulcer > gastric ulcer	Duodenal ulcer > gastric ulcer
Pathogenesis	• Defective mucosal barrier caused by *H. pylori*. • Mucosal ischemia (reduced PGE; normally a vasodilator), bile reflux, delayed gastric emptying. • BAO and MAO normal to decreased.	• Defective mucosal barrier caused by *H. pylori*. • Increased acid production (increased parietal cell mass). • BAO and MAO both increased.
Location	Single ulcer on lesser curvature of antrum (same location for cancer) (Fig. 18-18 C)	Single ulcer on anterior portion of first part of duodenum (Fig. 18-18 B). Followed by single ulcer on posterior portion (danger of perforation into pancreas and pancreatitis).
Complications	• Bleeding (most commonly ulceration of left gastric artery; Fig. 18-18 E). Bleeding spontaneously ceases in 80% of cases. • Perforation (air under diaphragm, pain radiates to left or right shoulder; Fig. 18-18 D).	• Bleeding (anterior ulcer; most commonly ulceration of gastroduodenal artery (Fig. 18-18E). Bleeding spontaneously ceases in 80% of cases. • Perforation (anterior ulcer). Air under diaphragm. Pain radiates to left or right shoulder. • Gastric outlet obstruction, pancreatitis (posterior ulcer).
Clinical findings	Epigastric pain *exacerbated* by eating.	Epigastric pain *relieved* by eating.
Diagnosis	• Endoscopy: 90%–95% accuracy. • Must biopsy gastric ulcers (1%–4% malignant). • Upper GI barium study: identify 70%–80% PUD.	• Endoscopy: 90%–95% accuracy. • *No* need to biopsy because never malignant • Upper GI barium study: identify 70%–80% PUD.

BAO, Basal acid output; *COPD*, chronic obstructive pulmonary disease; *GI*, gastrointestinal; *MAO*, maximal acid output; *MEN*, multiple endocrine neoplasia; *NSAIDs*, nonsteroidal antiinflammatory drugs; *PGE*, prostaglandin E; *PUD*, peptic ulcer disease.

      c. DUs are *rarely* malignant; hence, they are usually *not* biopsied.

      d. Four layers in sequence are noted in histologic sections of ulcers. Necrotic debris → inflammation with a predominance of neutrophils → granulation tissue (repair tissue) → fibrosis.

    4. Comparison of gastric and DUs is presented in Table 18-2.

    5. Complications of PUD (Link 18-63)

K. Zollinger-Ellison (ZE) syndrome

    1. **Definition:** Gastrin-secreting tumor in the duodenum or pancreas that causes overproduction of gastric acid, resulting in recurrent PUD

    2. Epidemiology

      a. Tumors are often (~two-thirds of cases) malignant.

        (1) Gastrin secretion increases the parietal cell mass in the stomach; net result is parietal cell hyperplasia.

        (2) More than 50% of the tumors are locally invasive.

      b. Majority of the tumors are located in the duodenum (60% of cases); most of the remainder are located in the pancreatic islet cells (30% of cases).

      c. Syndrome is sporadic in two-thirds of cases and is associated with multiple endocrine neoplasia (MEN) type I in one-third of cases, where the tumors tend to be multiple.

      d. Ulcers are usually single and located in the usual locations; however, multiple ulcers may occur.

      e. Findings that are suggestive of ZE syndrome include:

        (1) presence of multiple peptic ulcers.

        (2) ulcers that are resistant to standard therapy (Rx).

        (3) ulcer that is located distal to the first portion of the duodenum.

Margin notes:

DUs *rarely* malignant

Necrotic debris, neutrophil inflammation

Granulation tissue, fibrosis

Zollinger-Ellison syndrome

Gastrin-secreting tumor islet cells/duodenum/ pancreas → peptic ulcer(s)

Frequently malignant

↑Gastrin → ↑parietal cell mass in stomach → parietal cell hyperplasia

Majority are locally invasive

Duodenum > pancreas (islet cells)

Sporadic 2/3rds cases

One-third MEN type I association

Single usually/multiple ulcers

Zollinger-Ellison syndrome

Multiple peptic ulcers

Ulcers resistant to Rx

Ulcer distal to 1st portion duodenum

(4) peptic ulcers plus diarrhea.

(5) family history of parathyroid or pituitary tumors (MEN type I syndrome).

(6) PUD in a patient *without* HP or a history of taking NSAIDs.

3. Clinical findings include:
   a. epigastric pain (most common complaint; upper abdomen immediately below the ribs) with weight loss.
   b. heartburn from GERD (60% of cases).
   c. peptic ulceration. Most are solitary DUs rather than multiple ulcers.
   d. acid hypersecretion with diarrhea.
   e. maldigestion (incomplete digestion) of food. Acid interferes with normal pancreatic enzyme activity.

4. Laboratory findings include:
   a. serum gastrin level >1000 pg/mL (best screen).
   b. increased basal acid output (BAO), maximal acid output (MAO), and BAO/MAO ratio.
   c. secretin stimulation test (provocative test) shows increased serum gastrin (>200 pg/mL).

5. Radiolabeled octreotide is used to localize the tumor(s).

L. Gastric polyps

1. **Definition:** Small, sessile or raised growths arising from the gastric mucosa
2. Epidemiology
   a. Some cases may be a complication of chronic gastritis and achlorhydria.
   b. Types of polyps include fundic gland polyp, hyperplastic polyp, and adenomatous polyp (gastric adenoma).
3. Fundic polyp (50%)
   a. Most common, gastric polyp
   b. Sporadic or associated with familial polyposis
   c. Association with the use of proton pump inhibitors, ZE syndrome, and familial polyposis. In the latter association, the polyps may develop dysplastic features.
   d. Occur in the body and fundus of the stomach
   e. Usually multiple with polypoid projections. Key feature is the presence of microcysts lined by fundic epithelium.
4. Hyperplastic polyp
   a. Second most common type of gastric polyp (40%; Link 18-64); frequently multiple if associated atrophic gastritis
   b. Benign non-neoplastic polyps that have a natural history that is different from hyperplastic polyps from the colon. They share some molecular alterations that are similar to adenomatous polyps (see later).
   c. Rarely, they may undergo progression to dysplasia to cancer.
5. Gastric adenoma (adenomatous polyp; 10%). Benign neoplastic polyp with the potential for malignant transformation (Link 18-65).

M. Leiomyoma

1. **Definition:** Benign gastrointestinal stromal tumor (GIST) arising from the smooth muscle layer of the stomach wall (muscularis propria); usually <3 cm in diameter
2. Epidemiology
   a. Most common benign GIST in the stomach (60%). The next most common site is the small intestine (30%). Less common sites include the rectum, colon, and esophagus.
   b. Presents as a submucosal lesion or, less commonly, as a pedunculated lesion on a stalk that is (may be ulcerated and/or bleeding).
   c. Approximately 20% to 25% of gastric GIST tumors become clinically aggressive (develop increased numbers of mitotic figures) and develop into a leiomyosarcoma.

N. Primary gastric adenocarcinomas

1. **Definition**: Type of cancers arising from glandular cells in the stomach
2. Epidemiology
   a. Incidence within the United States decreased 85% during the 20th century.
   b. Highest incidence of stomach cancer is in Asia (Republic of Korea, Mongolia, Japan), Latin America, and the Caribbean. Lowest incidence is in Africa and Northern America. Scandinavian countries have a higher incidence than the United States.
   c. Increased incidence in those with blood group A (reason is unknown)
3. Intestinal type of gastric adenocarcinoma
   a. Most common type of gastric carcinoma
   b. Risk factors include:
      (1) intestinal metaplasia associated with chronic gastritis caused by HP is the most important risk factor. Progression to gastric adenocarcinoma (called the Correa

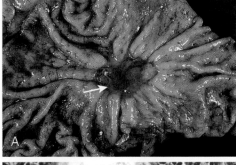

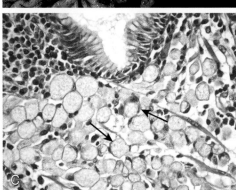

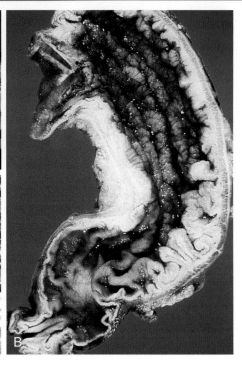

18-19: **A**, Gastric adenocarcinoma of the ulcerative type. Notice that it is very similar in appearance to a chronic gastric ulcer, hence, the importance of biopsy. The border of the ulcer is irregular and not as sharply delineated as a chronic peptic ulcer. In addition, blood, not necrotic debris is present in the base of the ulcer. **B**, Typical gross appearance of diffuse carcinoma of so-called linitis plastica type. Practically the entire wall of the stomach is involved by tumor. Note the prominence of rugal folds. **C**, Diffuse type of gastric adenocarcinoma with signet ring carcinoma cells *(arrows)*. Mucin produced by the cancer cells pushes the nucleus to the periphery. *(A, B from Rosai J: Rosai and Ackerman's Surgical Pathology, 10th, 9th ed, respectively, St. Louis, Mosby, 2011,2004, pp 628, 664, respectively; Fig. 11.44, 11.47, respectively; C from Kumar V, Fausto N, Abbas A: Robbins and Cotran Pathologic Basis of Disease, 7th ed, Philadelphia, Saunders, 2004, p 825, 17-27B.)*

cascade) is as follows: HP infection → chronic gastritis → atrophic gastritis → intestinal metaplasia → dysplasia → gastric cancer.

    (2) nitrosamines, smoked foods (Japan), diets lacking fruits and vegetables.

    (3) Autoimmune chronic gastritis (ACG) caused by pernicious anemia (PA).

    (4) Ménétrier disease.

  c. Grossly, intestinal type gastric adenocarcinoma are often exophytic with or without ulceration (Fig. 18-19A; Links 18-66 to 18-69).

  d. Locations of the intestinal type of gastric adenocarcinoma include the lesser curvature of the pylorus and antrum (50%–60% of cases) and cardia (25% of cases), body, and fundus.

4. Diffuse type of gastric adenocarcinoma

  a. Incidence has remained unchanged for this type of gastric adenocarcinoma.

  b. Male:female ratio is 3:2. *No* causal relationship with HP.

  c. Diffuse infiltration of malignant cells throughout the stomach wall (Fig. 18-19 B; Link 18-70 A).

    (1) Old terms are "linitis plastica" and "leather bottle stomach."

    (2) Stomach lacks peristalsis.

    (3) Signet ring cells diffusely infiltrate the stomach wall (Fig. 18-19 C; Link 18-70 B).

    (4) Associated with Krukenberg tumors of the ovaries. Refers to the hematogenous spread of signet ring cells from the stomach to the ovaries (see Chapters 9 and 22). It is *not* an example of seeding.

5. Clinical findings in primary gastric adenocarcinoma include:

  a. cachexia (wasting) and weight loss (most common finding in 70%–80% of cases).

  b. epigastric pain or abdominal mass (30%–50% of cases).

  c. vomiting, often with melena (20%–40% of cases).

  d. metastasis to the left supraclavicular node (Virchow node).

  e. paraneoplastic skin lesions (see Chapter 9) including acanthosis nigricans (see Fig. 25-10 B) and appearance of multiple seborrheic keratoses (Leser-Trélat sign; see Fig. 25-10 A).

  f. metastasis to the umbilicus (Sister Mary Joseph nodule); metastasis to left supraclavicular node (Virchow node), metastasis to left axillary node (Irish node). Other common metastatic sites include the liver, lung, and ovaries.

  g. Approximately 10% to 15% overall 5-year survival rate

6. Primary gastric lymphoma

  a. Stomach is the most common site for extranodal lymphomas (lymphoma that does *not* originate from the lymph node).

Nitrosamines
Smoked foods (Japan)
Diets lacking fruits/vegetables
ACG due to PA
Ménétrier disease
Polypoid/ulcerated
MC site lesser curvature pylorus/antrum
Cardia, body/fundus less common
Diffuse gastric adenocarcinoma
Incidence unchanged
M:F 3:2
No relationship with *H. pylori*
Diffuse infiltration
"Linitis plastica," "leather bottle stomach"
Lacks peristalsis
Signet ring cells
Krukenberg tumor both ovaries
Hematogenous spread
Clinical findings
Cachexia/weight loss MC finding
Epigastric pain, abdominal mass
Vomiting often with melena
Metastasis left supraclavicular (Virchow) node
Acanthosis nigricans
Seborrheic keratoses: Leser-Trélat sign
Metastasis to umbilicus (Sister Mary Joseph nodule)
Supraclavicular node (Virchow node)
Left axillary node (Irish node)
Liver, lung, ovaries
Poor survival rate
Primary gastric lymphoma
Stomach MC site for extranodal lymphomas

b. Low-grade B-cell lymphoma is the most common extranodal gastric lymphoma.
(1) Causal relationship with HP-induced chronic atrophic gastritis
(2) Lymphoma derives from MALT.
(3) 50% cure rate if the HP chronic atrophic gastritis is treated
c. Other lymphoma types: high-grade B- or T-cell lymphoma (see Chapter 14).
7. Gastric carcinoid tumor is discussed under Small Bowel Malignancy.
O. **Causes of upper GI bleeding** (Link 18-71)
V. **Small Bowel and Large Bowel Disorders**
A. **Signs and symptoms of small bowel disease (SBD)**
1. Colicky pain
a. **Definition:** Pain followed by a pain-free interval that is accompanied by constipation and inability to pass gas
b. Symptom of bowel obstruction. Bowel obstruction is more common in the small bowel (SB; smaller caliber lumen) than the large bowel (LB; larger caliber lumen)
c. Example of bowel obstruction: bowel adhesions from a previous surgery
2. Diarrhea
a. **Definition:** The passage of >250 g of liquid stool per day
b. Could be a sign of infection, malabsorption, or osmotic and secretory diarrhea
c. If bloody, it may be a sign of infarction, volvulus, or dysentery.
3. Anemia in SBD could be caused by malabsorption of iron, folic acid, or vitamin B_{12}.
B. **Signs and symptoms of large bowel disease**
1. Diarrhea
a. **Definition:** The passage of >250 g of liquid stool per day
b. Causes include infection and malabsorption as well as osmotic and secretory processes.
c. If bloody, it may be a sign of infarction or dysentery.
2. Dysentery
a. **Definition:** Bloody diarrhea with mucus
b. Usually a sign of infection
3. Pain occurs in inflammatory bowel disease (IBD), ischemic colitis, diverticulitis (DTS), appendicitis (APS), and peritonitis (PTS).
4. Tenesmus
a. **Definition:** The continued feeling of needing to pass stool despite having emptied the rectal vault through defecation
b. Commonly present in ulcerative colitis (UC)
5. Lower GI bleeding
a. **Definition:** The presence of bright red blood in the stool
b. Causes of lower GI bleeding (Link 18-72)
6. Iron deficiency. Possible causes include polyps or colorectal cancer.
7. Hematochezia
a. **Definition:** The passage of bright red blood per anus usually in or with stools
b. Causes include sigmoid diverticulosis (most common) and angiodysplasia.
8. Black mucosa (melanosis coli)
a. **Definition:** The presence of a black mucosa caused by chronic use of laxatives with senna and rhubarb derivatives
b. Bowel is black because of an increase in submucosal macrophages (MPs) containing lipofuscin pigment (Link 18-73).
C. **Diarrheal diseases (excluding malabsorption)**
1. Types of diarrhea
a. Acute diarrhea is defined as diarrhea for <3 weeks, and chronic diarrhea is defined as diarrhea for >4 weeks.
b. Subdivided into include invasive, osmotic, and secretory types of diarrhea (Table 18-3)
2. Important screening tests for diarrhea include:
a. fecal smear for leukocytes (e.g., invasive diarrhea; Link 18-74).
b. calculation of the stool osmotic gap (SOG).
(1) 300 mOsm/kg (value used to represent normal POsm [see Chapter 5]) − 2 × (random stool Na^+ + random stool K^+)
(2) Osmotic gap <50 mOsm/kg from POsm is a secretory diarrhea (characterized by a loss of isotonic fluid; e.g., cholera). Indicates that the diarrheal fluid POsm approximates the normal POsm.

TABLE 18-3 Types of Diarrhea

TYPE	CHARACTERISTICS	CAUSES	SCREENING TESTS
Invasive	• Pathogens invade enterocytes. • Low-volume diarrhea • Diarrhea with blood and leukocytes (i.e., dysentery)	• *Shigella* spp. • *Campylobacter jejuni* • *Entamoeba histolytica*	• Fecal smear for leukocytes: positive in most cases. • Order stool culture, stool for O&P, stool antigens.

Secretory	• Loss of isotonic fluid
	• High-volume diarrhea
	• Mechanisms:
	  • Laxatives
	  • Enterotoxins stimulate Cl⁻ channels regulated by cAMP and cGMP.
	  • Serotonin increases bowel motility.
	• Absence of inflammation in bowel mucosa.
		• Laxatives: danger of melanosis coli (black bowel syndrome) with use of laxatives.
		• Production of enterotoxins: *Vibrio cholerae*, enterotoxigenic *E. coli*
		• Increased serotonin: carcinoid syndrome.
			• Fecal smear for leukocytes: negative
			• Increased 5-HIAA: carcinoid syndrome.
			• Stool osmotic gap <50 mOsm/kg.

Osmotic	• Osmotically active substance is drawing hypotonic salt solution out of bowel. • High-volume diarrhea • No inflammation in bowel mucosa	• Disaccharidase deficiency • Ingestion of poorly absorbable solutes (e.g., magnesium sulfate laxatives)	• Fecal smear for leukocytes: negative • Stool osmotic gap >100 mOsm/kg

cAMP, Cyclic adenosine monophosphate; *cGMP*, cyclic guanosine monophosphate; *5-HIAA*, 5-hydroxyindoleacetic acid; *O&P*, ova and parasites.

(3) Osmotic gap >100 mOsm/kg from POsm is an osmotic diarrhea (e.g., lactase deficiency, certain laxatives). Indicates a hypotonic loss of stool caused by the presence of osmotically active substances.

Osmotic: SOG >100 mOsm/kg from POsm

Osmotic: hypotonic loss stool

Lactase deficiency is a common genetic defect in Native Americans, Asians, and blacks. Colonic anaerobes degrade undigested lactose into lactic acid and H_2 gas, leading to abdominal distention with explosive diarrhea. Treatment is to avoid dairy products.

3. Overview of bacterial diarrhea that may be caused by an ingested toxin (Link 18-75)
4. Table 18-4 is a summary table of microbial pathogens causing diarrhea (Fig. 18-20; Links 18-76 to 18-100).

Disaccharidase deficiency in brush border; avoid dairy products

D. Overview of digestion of carbohydrates, protein, and fat (Links 18-101 to 18-104)
E. Malabsorption

Malabsorption

1. **Definition:** Chronic diarrhea with increased fecal excretion of fat (called steatorrhea). Concurrent deficiencies of fat-soluble vitamins, minerals, carbohydrates (carbs), and proteins are commonly present.

Chronic diarrhea with fatty stools (steatorrhea)

Deficiencies protein, carbs, minerals, fat soluble vitamins

2. Epidemiology of fat malabsorption

Epidemiology

a. The three main causes of fat malabsorption are pancreatic insufficiency, bile salt/acid deficiency, and small bowel disease (SBD).

Pancreatic insufficiency, bile salt/acid deficiency, SBD

b. Pancreatic insufficiency

Pancreatic insufficiency

(1) **Definition:** Condition characterized by deficiency of the exocrine pancreatic enzymes (e.g., lipase, trypsin), resulting in the inability of the small bowel to digest food properly

Exocrine pancreatic enzyme deficiency

(2) Epidemiology

(a) Most often caused by chronic pancreatitis. Chronic pancreatitis is most commonly caused by alcohol in adults and cystic fibrosis in children (see Chapter 19).

Chronic pancreatitis MCC; alcohol, cystic fibrosis

(b) Dietary triglycerides (TGs) *cannot* be hydrolyzed into monoglycerides (MGs) and fatty acids (FAs) caused by a deficiency of pancreatic lipase (see Chapter 8). Undigested fats produce a fatty stool, which is called steatorrhea.

Lipase normally hydrolyzes TG to MGs + FAs

Undigested fats produce fatty stool (steatorrhea)

(3) Maldigestion of proteins also occurs in pancreatic insufficiency, caused by diminished production of pancreatic trypsin. Undigested meat fibers are in present in the stool.

Maldigestion proteins

↓Pancreatic trypsin

Undigested meat fibers in stool

(4) Carbohydrate absorption is *not* affected because the presence of amylase from SGs, and disaccharidases from the brush border of the small intestinal epithelium are still functioning in those with pancreatic insufficiency.

Carbohydrates *not* affected; salivary amylase, brush border disaccharidases

c. Bile salt/acid deficiency

Bile salt/acid deficiency

TABLE 18-4   Microbial Pathogens Causing Diarrhea and Other Miscellaneous Diseases

PATHOGEN	DISCUSSION
	VIRUSES
Cytomegalovirus	Common cause of diarrhea in AIDS when CD4 T_H cell count <50–100 cells/mm³.
Norovirus (Norwalk) virus	• Most common cause of adult gastroenteritis. • Fecal-oral transmission. • Common infection on cruise ships • Nausea, vomiting, diarrhea that resolves in 12–24 hours. • Occasionally can be fatal.
Rotavirus	• Most common cause of childhood diarrhea; particularly occurs in winter months. • Fecal-oral transmission. • Damages ion transport pump in small intestine; secretory diarrhea. • Rotazyme test on stool establishes diagnosis. • Rotavirus vaccine highly effective in prevention. Oral vaccine.
	BACTERIA
Campylobacter jejuni (Fig. 18-20 A; Link 18-76)	• Curved or S-shaped gram-negative rod. • Transmission fecal-oral (animal to human) via contaminated water, poultry, or unpasteurized milk. • Animal reservoirs: cattle, chicken, puppies (common source for children). • Most common food-borne illness and invasive enterocolitis in the United States. • Invasive and secretory enterocolitis: dysentery (bloody diarrhea) with crypt abscesses and ulcers resembling ulcerative colitis. • High fever and cramping abdominal pain. • Organisms in stool with blood and leukocytes. • Complications: Guillain-Barré syndrome (antibodies cross-react with neurons), hemolytic uremic syndrome, and HLA-B27 positive seronegative spondyloarthropathy. • Diagnosis: culture, stool antigen, serology.
Bacillus cereus	• Gram positive rod • Enterotoxins are virulence factors. • Preformed enterotoxin similar to cholera in that it adds adenosine diphosphate-ribose (ADP-ribosylation) to a G protein which stimulates adenylate cyclase. Increases cAMP in enterocytes causing secretory type of diarrhea. • Transmission: reheated fried rice or tacos with rice. • Two syndromes: nausea and vomiting within 4 hrs of eating. Watery diarrhea after 18 hours. • Gram positive rods in stool. • *No* Rx.
Clostridium botulinum (Link 18-77)	• Gram-positive rod. • **Adult food poisoning** with preformed toxin (blocks release of acetylcholine in presynaptic terminal of neuromuscular junction in autonomic nervous system). Causes descending paralysis, mydriasis, dry mouth. • **Infant food poisoning** often contracted by eating spores in honey (lack protective bacteria until 1 year of age). Spores → bacteria producing toxins. Floppy baby with constipation.
Clostridium difficile (see Fig. 3-8 D; Fig. 18-20 B, Link 18-78, Link 18-79)	• Gram-positive rod. • Person-to-person induced in 30% of cases. Normally present in 3% of people. Carrier rate increases to >20% in hospitalized patients (related to fecal-oral contamination and contact with spores in environment to a lesser extent). • Associated with **pseudomembranous colitis**. Most common cause of nosocomial diarrhea, antibiotic-induced diarrhea, and health care–associated diarrhea. Secretory type of diarrhea. • Antibiotic-induced in 65%–90% of cases. Antibiotics (e.g., ampicillin, quinolones, clindamycin) cause overgrowth of toxin-producing *C. difficile* in colon. Antibiotics increase gastrointestinal reabsorption of toxins A and B from the bacterial cell membrane. Toxins release proinflammatory mediators and cytokines that attract neutrophils and stimulate excess fluid secretion (watery diarrhea). • Pseudomembrane covers colon mucosa. Membranes composed of cellular debris, leukocytes, fibrin, and mucin. • Nonspecific lab findings: neutrophilic leukocytosis with left shift, fecal leukocytes, and decreased serum albumin. • Cytotoxin assay of diarrheal (not solid) stool has greater specificity (75%–100%) than culture of stool (75%–80%) for securing the diagnosis. Glutamate dehydrogenase antigen test is also used and has excellent sensitivity and specificity (enzyme is present in all strains of *C. difficile*).
Clostridium perfringens	• Gram-positive rod. • **Food poisoning:** Heat resistant spores survive cooking and germinate in food. Organisms proliferate rapidly in reheated foods (meat dishes like beef and turkey. Enterotoxin (superantigen similar to *Staphylococcus aureus*) is the virulence factor. • Produced during spore formation in the gut. Self-limited.
Escherichia coli	• Gram-negative rod. • **ETEC (Enterotoxigenic *Escherichia coli*):** certain strains produce toxin that activate adenylate or guanylate cyclase, causing secretory diarrhea (traveler's diarrhea, no fever, no bowel inflammation, accounts for 60% of cases). Other causes include *Campylobacter, Salmonella, Shigella*. • **STEC (O157:H7 serotype; Shiga toxin-producing" *E. coli*):** contracted by eating undercooked beef, bean sprouts, undercooked cookies. Produces gastroenteritis with bloody diarrhea and hemolytic uremic syndrome (HUS in 8% of cases. See Chapter 15). Antibiotics are *not* recommended. May enhance toxin release. • Diagnosis: DNA assays, enzyme immunoassays for toxin.
Listeria monocytogenes	• Small gram-positive rod with tumbling motility and β-hemolysis. • Virulence factors: actin rockets allow organism to move from cell to cell. Listeriolysin O degrades cell membranes. • Transmission: eating contaminated, ready to eat foods, soft cheeses, unpasteurized milk or cheese, hot dogs.

TABLE 18-4 Microbial Pathogens Causing Diarrhea and Other Miscellaneous Diseases—cont'd

PATHOGEN	DISCUSSION
Mycobacterium avium-intracellulare complex (MAC) (Link 18-80)	• Acid-fast rods. • Causes diarrhea with malabsorption in AIDS (CD4 count <50 cells/mm³). • Foamy macrophages in lamina propria simulate Whipple disease.
Mycobacterium tuberculosis	• Acid-fast organisms are swallowed from a primary focus in the lung. • Invade Peyer patches. • Circumferential spread in lymphatics leads to stricture formation in the bowel and obstruction.
Salmonella spp. (Link 18-81, Link 18-82)	• Gram-negative rod. • Pathogenic *Salmonella*: *S. typhi*, *S. paratyphi*, *S. enteritidis*. • Animal reservoirs: turtles, hamsters, lizards. • **Salmonella enteritidis enterocolitis:** Second most common food-borne illness in United States. Contracted by eating unpasteurized or undercooked egg products, raw milk and milk products, drinking contaminated water, or improper washing of the hands after handling the previously mentioned animal reservoirs (animal to human). • **Typhoid fever caused by Salmonella typhi** (Link 18-81): • Week 1: invades Peyer patches (Link 18-82) and produces sepsis (blood culture best for diagnosis). • Week 2: diarrhea (positive stool culture). Classic triad of bradycardia, neutropenia, splenomegaly. • Treatment may increase frequency of carrier states. • Chronic carrier state caused by gallbladder disease: cholecystectomy.
Shigella dysenteriae and *Shigella sonnei*	• Gram-negative rod. • *No* animal reservoirs. • Highly infectious (human to human transmission). Children in day care centers, psychiatric hospitals, homosexual men, and crowded conditions. Four F's: food, feces, flies, fingers. • Mucosal ulceration, pseudomembranous inflammation in rectosigmoid, dysentery. Bloody diarrhea. • Positive fecal smear for leukocytes. • Association with HLA-B27 positive seronegative spondyloarthropathy.
Staphylococcus aureus	• Gram-positive coccus in clumps. • **Food poisoning** with preformed toxin. Culture food, *not* stool. • **Gastroenteritis** occurs in 1–6 hours after eating. • Self-limited.
Vibrio cholerae (Link 18-83)	• Gram-negative comma-shaped rod. • Enterotoxin stimulates adenylate cyclase in the small bowel. • Contracted by drinking contaminated water or eating contaminated seafood, especially crustaceans. • *No* bowel inflammation. "Rice-water" stool.
Vibrio parahemolyticus	• Gram-negative rod. • Transmission: ingestion of raw or undercooked seafood (oysters). • Enterotoxin similar to *V. cholerae* and invasion. • Severe watery diarrhea.
Yersinia enterocolitica	• Gram-negative coccobacillus with bipolar staining. • Enterocolitis in children; mesenteric lymphadenitis (granulomatous microabscesses) that simulates acute appendicitis. • Association with HLA-B27 positive seronegative spondyloarthropathy.
PROTOZOA	
Balantidium coli (Link 18-84, Link 18-85)	• Protozoan (ciliate). Largest protozoan. • Fecal-oral transmission. Ingestion of cysts in food or water. • Produces colonic ulcers with bloody diarrhea.
Cryptosporidium parvum (Fig. 18-20 C; Link 18-86, Link 18-87, Link 18-88)	• Protozoan (sporozoa). • Fecal-oral transmission: ingestion of oocysts in food or water. • Responsible for outbreaks of diarrhea in water supply (e.g., Milwaukee, Wisconsin and diarrhea in children who are in close contact (e.g., daycare). • Most common cause of diarrhea in AIDS and diarrhea from swimming in municipal swimming pools. • Diagnosis: stool antigen test (sensitivity/specificity 98%). Oocysts are partially acid-fast.
Isospora belli (Link 18-89, Link 18-90)	• Protozoa (sporozoa). • Fecal-oral transmission: oocysts are the infective form of the protozoa. • Common pathogen in AIDS diarrhea. • Isospora oocysts are partially acid-fast. • Cyclospora can contaminate raspberries. Cyclospora oocysts are partially acid-fast. • Microsporidia spores are not partially acid-fast.
Entamoeba histolytica (Fig. 18-20 D, Link 18-91, Link 18-92, Link 18-93)	• Protozoa (amoeba). • Transmitted by ingestion of cysts in food and water. • Infective forms: cysts, trophozoites. • Cysts are non-motile and are present in formed stool. • Trophozoites are motile and are present in diarrhea fluid. They characteristically phagocytose red blood cells. • Dysentery (bloody diarrhea). Cysts excyst in the cecum and become trophozoites in the cecum. Trophozoites release powerful cytolytic agents that produce flask-shaped ulcers. Trophozoites can penetrate portal vein tributaries and drain into the liver to produce a liver abscess ("anchovy paste" abscess). Trophozoites can penetrate hepatic vein tributaries and produce widespread systemic disease. • Diagnosis: stool antigen test (sensitivity/specificity 100%).

Continued

TABLE 18-4 Microbial Pathogens Causing Diarrhea and Other Miscellaneous Diseases—cont'd

PATHOGEN	DISCUSSION
Giardia lamblia (Fig. 18-20 E; Link 18-94, Link 18-95)	• Protozoa (flagellate). • Most common protozoal cause of diarrhea in United States. • Fecal-oral transmission by ingestion of cysts in food and water. Reservoirs for Giardia that contaminate water supplies include beavers, voles, and muskrats. • Common in day care centers, psychiatric hospitals, hikers, water supplies (chlorination does not kill the cysts), men who have sex with men (anal-oral contact), IgA deficiency, and common variable immunodeficiency. • Produces acute and chronic diarrhea with malabsorption. Cysts are in formed stool, while trophozoites are in loose stools. • Diagnosis: stool antigen test (sensitivity/specificity 100%).
HELMINTHS	
Anisakis simplex	• Intestinal nematode. • Transmission: eating raw fish (i.e., sushi, sashimi) or pickled herring. • Larvae penetrate gastric and intestinal mucosa. • Produces cramping abdominal pain, epigastric distress with nausea, vomiting, and diarrhea a few hours after eating. • Diagnosis: endoscopy, IgE antibody test.
Enterobius vermicularis (Fig. 18-20 F; Link 18-96, Link 18-97)	• Intestinal nematode. • Fecal-oral transmission by ingestion of eggs (infective form). • Most common helminth in the United States. Most contagious round worm infection worldwide. • Eggs deposited in anus by adult worms cause pruritus ani, restless sleep. • Other infections: urethritis in girls, vulvovaginitis, salpingitis (fallopian tube infection), peritonitis, and appendicitis. • No eosinophilia because adult worms are not invasive.
Trichuris trichiura (Fig. 18-20 G, H)	• Intestinal nematode (whipworm). • Fecal oral transmission by ingestion of eggs (infective form). • Produces diarrhea. Can produce rectal prolapse in children. • Diagnosis: stool for ova and parasites, eosinophilia.
Ascaris lumbricoides (Fig. 18-20 I, J; Link 18-98)	• Largest intestinal nematode. • Fecal oral transmission by ingestion of eggs (infective form). • Larval phase through lungs: cough, pneumonitis, eosinophilia (invasion of tissue). • Bowel obstruction or common bile duct obstruction in adult phase. No eosinophilia (no invasion of tissue).
Necator americanus	• Intestinal nematode (hookworm). • Transmission by direct penetration or autoinfection. Filariform larvae are the infected form. • Adults attach to villi, resulting in blood loss and iron deficiency.
Strongyloides stercoralis (Fig. 18-20 K; Link 18-99, Link 18-100)	• Intestinal nematode • Transmission: filariform larvae in soil penetrate the feet → larval phase through the lungs → swallowed and molt into adults that enter the intestinal mucosa and lay eggs → eggs hatch into rhabditiform larvae, which enter the intestinal lumen and are passed in the stool (no eggs in stool) → develop into filariform larvae (infective form) in the soil • Autoinfection may occur if filariform larvae in the intestine penetrate the mucosa and migrate to the lungs to repeat the cycle • In immunocompromised patients (e.g., AIDS), massive reinfection occurs with dissemination throughout the body (hyperinfection). • Produces abdominal pain and diarrhea. Can penetrate skin and migrate throughout the body (wheezing and cough with pulmonary involvement). Infected for life!
Diphyllobothrium latum	• Intestinal cestode (tapeworm). • Transmission: ingest larvae (sparganum) in lake trout (Great Lakes). • Produce diarrhea with or without vitamin B_{12} deficiency. Preferential uptake of vitamin B_{12} by the worm. • Diagnosis: eggs in the stool.
Hymenolepis nana	• Intestinal cestode. • Dwarf tapeworm. Common parasite of house mice. Found worldwide. • Fecal-oral transmission by ingestion of the egg. • Eggs hatch in the small intestine → oncosphere burrows into villi and develops into cysticercoid larva → larva breaks out into the bowel lumen to become an adult worm. • Asymptomatic or may have abdominal pain and diarrhea.
Hymenolepis diminuta	• Intestinal cestode. • Common parasite in rats. Infected rats have droppings with eggs. Flour beetles or moths ingest the eggs, and cysticercoid larvae develop in these arthropods. Humans ingest the infected beetles/flour moths in the flour and larvae develop into adult worms in the human intestine. • Asymptomatic or have abdominal pain or diarrhea.

ETEC, Enterotoxigenic *Escherichia coli*; *STEC*, Shiga toxin *E. coli*; *TMP-SMX*, trimethoprim-sulfamethoxazole.

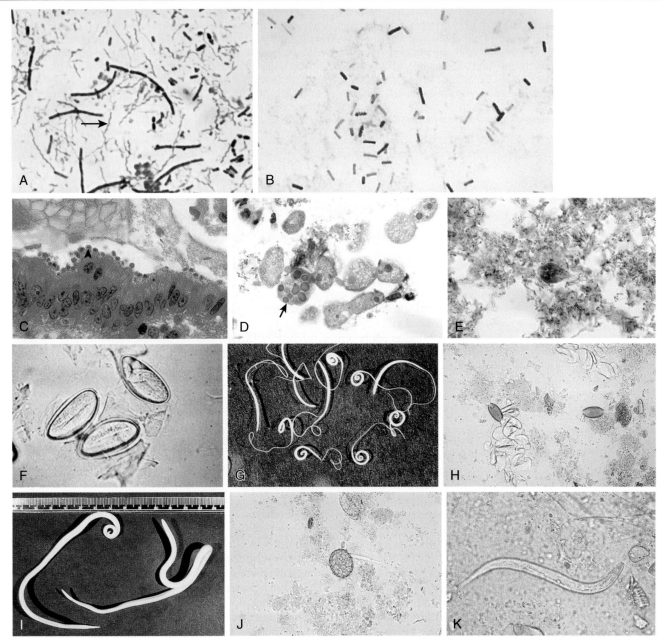

18-20: A, *Campylobacter jejuni.* Note the curved gram-negative rods. **B,** *Clostridium difficile.* Gram-positive rods. **C,** Cryptosporidiosis. Note the small round oocysts of Cryptosporidium parvum lining the luminal surface of the small intestine. **D,** *Entamoeba histolytica* trophozoites showing erythrophagocytosis *(arrow).* **E,** Giardia lamblia with two nuclei and flagella. **F,** Embryonated eggs of *Enterobius vermicularis.* **G,** Adult whipworms, *Trichuris trichiura.* Note females with straight tails and males with coiled tails. **H,** Eggs of *T. trichiura* (×400). The eggs are barrel shaped and have two prominent polar plugs at the ends. Internally, an unsegmented ovum is present. **I,** Adult female and male *Ascaris lumbricoides,* the large human roundworm. **J,** Fertile, unembryonated egg of Ascaris lumbricoides (×400). **K,** *Strongyloides stercoralis.* Larvae in stool sample. No eggs are in the stool with Strongyloides infections. *(A from Murray PR, Shea YR: Medical Microbiology, 6th ed, Philadelphia, Mosby, 2009, Fig. 32-1; B and K from Murray PR, Shea YR: Medical Microbiology, 2nd ed, St. Louis, Mosby, 2002, pp 402, 887, respectively, Figs. 40-1, 84-9, respectively; C from Klatt E: Robbins and Cotran Atlas of Pathology, Philadelphia, Saunders, 2006, p 175, Fig. 7-69; D, E, and G to J from McPherson RA: Henry's Clinical Diagnosis and Management by Laboratory Methods, 22nd ed, Philadelphia, Saunders, 2011, Figs. 62-11C, 62-14C, 62-17D, 62-17E, 62-17F, 62-17G, respectively; F from Hart P, Shears CT: Color Atlas of Medical Microbiology, St. Louis, Mosby, 1996, p 271, Fig. 446.)*

Bile salts are primarily used to emulsify fatty acids and monoacylglycerol and package them into micelles, along with fat-soluble vitamins, phospholipids, and cholesteryl esters, for reabsorption by villi in the small bowel. **Primary bile acids** (e.g., cholic acid and chenodeoxycholic acid) are synthesized in the liver from cholesterol. Primary bile acids are conjugated before secretion in the bile with taurine (taurochenodeoxycholic acid) or glycine (glycocholic acid). Bile acid synthesis is inhibited by bile acids (negative feedback) and stimulated by cholesterol. Intestinal bacteria alter bile acids in the small intestine to produce **secondary bile acids**. Bile acids are converted into deoxycholic and lithocholic acid (glycine and taurine are removed). The enterohepatic circulation in the terminal ileum recycles about 95% of bile acids back to the liver. Secretion of reabsorbed bile acids is preceded by conjugation with taurine and glycine. Bile salt deficiency leads to malabsorption of fat and fat-soluble vitamins.

(From Pelley JW, Goljan EF: *Rapid Review Biochemistry*, 3rd ed, St. Louis, Mosby Elsevier, 2011, pp 89-90.)

About 70% to 80% of cholesterol is converted to bile acids; primary bile salts from liver, secondary bile salts from intestinal bacteria

Causes bile salt/acid deficiency

Inadequate liver synthesis bile salts/acids

Intrahepatic bile duct obstruction

Bacterial overgrowth small intestine

Excess binding bile salts

Terminal ileal disease

Bile salts/acids form micelles

MGs, FAs, fat-soluble vitamins, CH esters

Micelles *not* formed in bile salt deficiency

SBD causes

Damage villi → cannot reabsorb micelles

↓ApoB48 → ↓formation chylo

↓ApoB48/lymphatic blockage → ↓ chylo to blood

Steatorrhea (fatty stools)

↓A, D, E, K vitamins

↓Folic acid/B_{12}

Combined anemias

Ascites/pitting edema: hypoproteinemia ↓OP

Fermentation by intestinal bacteria

Urinary D-xylose test

↓Urinary D-xylose levels → carb malabsorption

Protein malabsorption

Small intestine bacterial overgrowth

↓AAT clearance, abnormal albumin scintigraphy

General tests fat malabsorption

Quantitative stool for fat

(1) Causes of bile salt deficiency
    (a) inadequate synthesis of bile salts/acids from cholesterol in the liver (e.g., cirrhosis).
    (b) intrahepatic/extrahepatic blockage of bile. Examples: primary biliary cirrhosis (PBC), stone in common bile duct.
    (c) bacterial overgrowth in the small bowel with destruction of bile salts or acids. Examples: small bowel diverticula, autonomic neuropathy
    (d) excess binding of bile salts. Example: cholestyramine
    (e) terminal ileal disease. Examples: Crohn's disease, resection terminal ileum
(2) Bile salts/acid normally produce micelles to enhance reabsorption of fats by the small intestinal villi.
    (a) Micelles contain monoglycerides (MGs), FAs, fat-soluble vitamins, and cholesterol (CH) esters. Note that all the fat-soluble vitamins (vitamins A, D, E, and K) are packaged in micelles along with the products of fat digestion; hence, any disease producing maldigestion of fats also produces deficiencies of all the fat-soluble vitamins.
    (b) In bile salt deficiency, micelles are *not* formed, which produces a fatty stool (steatorrhea).
  d. Pathophysiology of SBD causing malabsorption
    (1) Damage to the villi (e.g., celiac disease)
        (a) Villi increase the absorptive surface of the small intestine. Villi are required to reabsorb micelles into the enterocytes.
        (b) Loss of the villi leads to the loss of micelles in the stool (steatorrhea).
    (2) Apoprotein B48 (apoB48) in enterocytes is important in resynthesizing TGs and packaging them into chylomicrons. Loss of enterocytes or deficiency of apoB48 reduces the formation of chylomicrons (chylo).
    (3) ApoB48 is also important in transporting chylomicrons into the lymphatics. Deficiency of apoB48 or lymphatic blockage in the intestinal cells (e.g., Whipple disease; discussed later) decreases chylomicron transportation into the blood.
3. Clinical findings in malabsorption include:
  a. steatorrhea. Excessive, large, sticky stools that float.
  b. fat-soluble vitamin deficiencies (see Chapter 8). Fat-soluble vitamins are A, D, E, and K.
  c. water-soluble vitamin deficiencies, particularly folic acid and vitamin B_{12} (see Chapter 8).
  d. combined anemias (see Chapter 12). Examples: folic acid or vitamin B_{12} deficiency and iron deficiency (duodenum involved in celiac disease)
  e. ascites and pitting edema (see Chapter 5): caused by hypoproteinemia and a decrease in oncotic pressure (OP; see Chapter 5).
  f. carbohydrate malabsorption.
    (1) Fermentation of undigested carbohydrates by intestinal bacteria.
    (2) Urinary D-xylose test is useful to diagnose carbohydrate malabsorption. After the patient ingests D-xylose, urinary D-xylose levels are measured. If the levels are decreased, then carbohydrate (carb) malabsorption is present.
    (3) Lactose intolerance caused by lactase deficiency has previously been discussed.
  g. protein malabsorption.
    (1) Most likely caused by small intestine bacterial overgrowth
    (2) Alpha-1-antitrypsin (AAT) clearance or 99mTc-albumin gamma camera scintigraphy is useful in securing the diagnosis.
4. General screening tests for fat malabsorption
  a. Quantitative stool for fat
    (1) Test requires a 72-hour collection of stool.
    (2) Positive test result >6 g fat/24 hours.

b. Qualitative stool for fat
   (1) Sudan III stain used to identify fat in stool.
   (2) Test lacks sensitivity.
c. Serum beta carotene. Beta carotene is a precursor for fat-soluble retinoic acid (vitamin A; see Chapter 8). It is decreased in fat malabsorption.
d. D-Xylose screening test.
   (1) Xylose does *not* require pancreatic enzymes for absorption.
   (2) Lack of absorption of orally administered xylose indicates SBD as the cause of fat malabsorption.

5. Tests to evaluate pancreatic insufficiency as a cause of malabsorption.
   a. Serum immunoreactive trypsin (SIT)
      (1) Trypsin is a specific enzyme in the pancreas.
      (2) Concentration of trypsin is decreased in chronic pancreatitis.
      (3) Concentration of trypsin is increased in *early* cystic fibrosis (CF), and then it eventually decreases when chronic pancreatitis is present.
   b. Fecal elastase and chymotrypsin levels are also useful (levels would be low) in distinguishing pancreatic versus intestinal causes of fat malabsorption.
   c. Computed tomography (CT) scan of the pancreas shows dystrophic calcification. It is a sign of chronic pancreatitis. Best test for chronic pancreatitis.
   d. Functional tests for pancreatic insufficiency
      (1) Secretin stimulation test (requires instrumentation): tests the ability of the pancreas to secrete fluids and electrolytes
      (2) Bentiromide test: tests the ability of pancreatic chymotrypsin to cleave orally administered bentiromide to *para*-aminobenzoic acid (measured in urine)

6. Tests for bile salt deficiency. Quantitative stool for bile acids. Total serum bile acids are decreased in liver disease (e.g., cirrhosis).

7. Tests for bacterial overgrowth
   a. Endoscopic jejunal aspirate culture
   b. Lactulose-H_2 test: measures H_2 in the breath
   c. Bile breath test (oral radioactive test). Conjugated bile acid labeled with carbon 14 is swallowed and the amount of radioactively labeled carbon dioxide in the breath is measured at hourly intervals. Increased CO_2 in the breath indicates bacterial overgrowth.
   d. ^{14}C-xylose: most sensitive and specific test; measures $^{14}CO_2$ in the breath

8. Celiac disease
   a. **Definition:** A chronic autoimmune disease characterized by malabsorption and diarrhea associated with the ingestion of gluten-containing products
   b. Epidemiology
      (1) Prevalence is 1 in 200 individuals in the United States.
      (2) Inappropriate immune response to gluten in wheat and protein products in rye or barley products
      (3) Particularly affects the second portion of the duodenum and proximal jejunum
      (4) Common in whites and uncommon in blacks and Asians
      (5) Occurs at any age. Highest incidence is in infancy. Identified with the first introduction to gluten products. Increased risk if infant is exposed to gluten in the first 3 months of life.
      (6) Frequent association with pregnancy in third decade
      (7) Frequent association with the elderly population in seventh decade
      (8) Other disease associations that commonly occur in celiac disease include:
         (a) dermatitis herpetiformis (greatest association).
         (b) autoimmune disease. Examples: hyperthyroidism (see Chapter 23), primary biliary cirrhosis (see Chapter 19), autoimmune hepatitis (see Chapter 19)
         (c) type 1 DM (see Chapter 23). Celiac disease imposes a greater risk for developing retinopathy and nephropathy. Celiac disease and type 1 DM share common alleles.
         (d) IgA deficiency (2%–5%; see Chapter 4).
         (e) Down syndrome and Turner syndrome (see Chapter 6).
         (f) small bowel (SB) lymphoma.
   c. Pathogenesis
      (1) Multiorgan autoimmune disease
      (2) Inappropriate T-cell and IgA-mediated response against gluten in genetically predisposed persons; associations with HLA-DQ2 (95% of cases) or HLA-DQ8 (5% of cases)

18-21: A, Normal villus in the small intestine. **B,** Celiac disease showing subtotal atrophy of the villi, lengthening of the crypts, and a heavy chronic inflammatory infiltrate in the lamina propria. **C,** Dermatitis herpetiformis showing vesicles with erythema on the extensor surface of the forearm. Presence of this lesion has a strong association with underlying celiac disease. **D,** Whipple disease. Note the foamy macrophages in the lamina propria and the flattened villi. (*A from my friend Ivan Damjanov, MD, PhD, Linder J: Pathology: A Color Atlas, St. Louis, Mosby, 2000, p 128, Fig. 7-25B; B from my friend Ivan Damjanov, MD, PhD, Linder J: Pathology: A Color Atlas, St. Louis, Mosby, 2000, p 128, Fig. 7-25A; C from Savin JAA, Hunter JAA, Hepburn NC: Diagnosis in Color: Skin Signs in Clinical Medicine, London, Mosby-Wolfe, 1997, p 92, Fig. 3.25; D from Morson BC: Colour Atlas of Gastrointestinal Pathology, London, Harvey Miller Ltd, Saunders, 1988, p 119, Fig. 4.50.*)

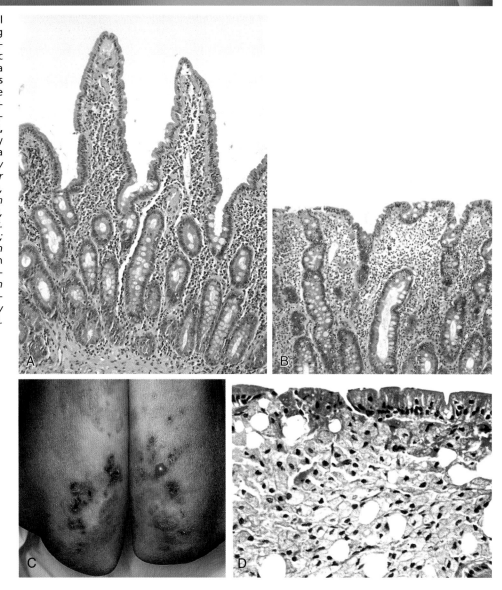

(3) Timing and dose when gluten is introduced in the diet are important.

(4) Tissue transglutaminase (tTG; deaminating enzyme) in the lamina propria has a pivotal role in producing celiac disease.

- *tTG has pivotal role*

  (a) It deaminates mucosa-absorbed gluten to produce deaminated and negatively charged gluten peptides (deaminated gluten peptides [DGPs]).

- *tTG deaminates gluten →DGPs*

  (b) DGPs stimulate the immune system; phagocytosed by antigen-processing cells in the lamina propria

- *DGPs stimulate immune system*

  - Presented in complex with HLA-DQ2 (90%) or HLA-DQ8 to gluten-specific CD_4 helper T cells
  - CD_4 T cells produce cytokines that release matrix proteases, causing cell death and degradation of the endothelial cells, resulting in the loss of the villous surface in the small intestine (Fig. 18-21 A and B; Links 18-105 [normal villus] and 18-106 [celiac disease]).

d. Important diagnostic antibodies include:

(1) anti-tTG IgA antibodies.

- *Anti-tTG IgA antibodies*
- *Excellent sensitivity/specificity*

  (a) Sensitivity is 90% to 98%, and specificity is 95% to 97%.

  (b) Excellent screening test as well as a test to confirm celiac disease

(2) antiendomysial (EMA) IgA antibodies.

- *Anti-EMA IgA antibodies*
- *Excellent sensitivity/specificity*

  (a) Sensitivity is 85% to 98%, and specificity is 97% to 100%.

  (b) Excellent screening test as well as a test to confirm celiac disease

(3) antigliadin IgA, IgG antibodies.

    (a) Sensitivity and specificity are 80% and 85%, respectively.

    (b) Moderately good screening test

  e. Clinical findings in celiac disease include steatorrhea, weight loss, and failure to thrive in infants and children.

    (1) pallor caused by anemia (often combined anemias); iron deficiency in 50% of patients (duodenal involvement); folic acid deficiency (jejunal involvement)

    (2) Dermatitis herpetiformis (Fig. 18-21 C; Link 18-107)

      (a) Considered to be a form of celiac disease

      (b) Villous atrophy occurs in 75% of cases with or without diarrhea.

    (3) findings related to water-soluble and fat-soluble vitamin deficiencies (see Chapter 8)

    (4) other systemic findings in celiac disease:

      (a) bone: osteomalacia (vitamin D deficiency).

      (b) CNS: seizures, depression.

      (c) reproductive: delayed puberty, miscarriages, infertility.

  f. Diagnosis includes:

    (1) presence of the diagnostic antibodies discussed earlier.

    (2) increased total serum IgA levels. Very useful test if antibody tests are *not* conclusive. If levels are *not* increased, then celiac disease can be ruled out.

    (3) endoscopic biopsy showing:

      (a) flattened villi, particularly in the duodenum and jejunum and hyperplastic glands with intense lymphocytic infiltration (Fig. 18-21 B; Link 18-106).

      (b) gold standard for diagnosing celiac disease is to see restitution of the villi after gluten is eliminated from the diet.

  g. Treatment is a lifelong complete gluten-free diet.

9. Whipple disease

  a. **Definition:** Rare, systemic infectious disease caused by the gram-positive bacterium *Tropheryma whipplei*, which produces malabsorption of fats and carbohydrates and other systemic findings

  b. Epidemiology

    (1) Occurs in men more commonly than women

    (2) Peak incidence in middle age

    (3) *Tropheryma whipplei* can be identified by a polymerase chain reaction (PCR) amplification of a species-specific sequence of bacterial DNA. It can also be identified by electron microscopy (EM; Link 18-108).

    (4) Microscopic findings include:

      (a) blunting of the villi.

      (b) Presence of foamy periodic acid–Schiff (PAS)–positive MPs in the lamina propria (Fig. 18-21 D). MPs obstruct the lymphatics and the reabsorption of chylomicrons leading to fat malabsorption.

    (5) Clinical findings include steatorrhea (fatty stools), fever, recurrent polyarthritis, generalized painful lymphadenopathy, and increased skin pigmentation.

10. Tropical sprue

  a. **Definition:** Uncommon cause of chronic diarrhea and malabsorption that is acquired by residing in or traveling to a tropical or subtropical area

  b. Epidemiology

    (1) Locations: Caribbean, Central/South America, India/southeast Asia

    (2) Fecal–oral contamination in water and foods

    (3) Infectious agents are implicated (e.g., *Klebsiella, Escherichia coli, Enterobacter* spp.).

    (4) Defective intestinal barrier, repeated bouts of diarrhea in early childhood, and chronic exposure to fecal bacteria (see previous) have been implicated.

    (5) Upper small intestine is predominantly but *not* exclusively affected (e.g., terminal ileum may be involved).

    (6) Decreased reabsorption of folic acid (reabsorbed in the jejunum) and vitamin B_{12} if the terminal ileum is involved.

  c. Biopsies show flattening of the villi in areas of involvement.

  d. Macrocytic anemia (folic acid/vitamin B_{12} deficiency) with hypersegmented neutrophils.

11. Consequences of malabsorption (Links 18-109 and 18-110)

F. Bowel obstruction

1. **Definition:** Blockage that keeps food or liquid from passing through the small intestine or large intestine (colon)

Marginal notes:

Anti-gliadin IgA, IgG antibodies

Moderately useful

Steatorrhea, weight loss

Failure to thrive infants/children

Combined anemias

Dermatitis herpetiformis

Form of celiac disease

Villous atrophy with/without diarrhea

Water/fat soluble deficiencies

Bone: osteomalacia

CNS: seizures, depression

Reproductive: delayed puberty, miscarriages, infertility

Diagnostic abs

↑Total serum IgA

Endoscopy Bx

Flattened villi; hyperplastic glands; lymphocytic infiltration

Normal glands post gluten free diet

Lifelong gluten free diet

Whipple disease

Tropheryma whipplei; G+ rod

Men > women

Middle age

PCR, EM

Blunting of villi

Foamy MPs

Foamy MPs block lymphatics → ↓chylomicron reabsorption

Steatorrhea, fever

Recurrent polyarthritis

Painful nodes, ↑skin pigmentation

Tropical sprue

Chronic diarrhea; tropical/subtropical

Caribbean, Central/South America, India/SE Asia

Fecal–oral contamination water/foods

Infectious agents implicated

Defective intestinal barrier, childhood diarrhea, chronic exposure fecal bacteria

Upper small intestine affected

↓Reabsorption folic acid, B_{12} (if terminal ileum involved)

Bx: flattening of villi

Macrocytic anemia

Bowel obstruction

Blockage food/liquid distal to obstruction

2. Epidemiology
   a. Causes of obstruction are listed and discussed in Table 18-5 and Links 18-111.
   b. Small bowel (SB) is the most common site for obstruction. This is related to the small lumen of the small bowel compared with the diameter of the large bowel.

SB: MC site for obstruction

TABLE 18-5   Small and Large Bowel Obstruction

ETIOLOGIC DISORDER	DISCUSSION
Adhesions (Fig. 18-22 B)	• Most common cause of small bowel obstruction (60% of cases). • Adhesions from previous surgery (most common), metastasis to the small bowel (second most common cause), endometriosis, and radiation.
Crohn disease	• Lumen in terminal ileum is narrow because of full-thickness inflammation of the bowel wall. • Serosal adhesions from bowel to bowel also cause obstruction.
Duodenal atresia (Fig. 18-22 C)	• First part of the duodenum has *not* developed thus passage of food bolus is impaired. Atresia refers to absence or abnormal narrowing of an opening. • Caused by extrinsic compression by abnormal neighboring structures (e.g., annular pancreas) or congenital bands with malrotation. Accounts for 25% to 40% of all cases of intestinal atresia. • Failed recanalization of the intestinal lumen during 4th and 5th week of gestation. • Approximately 50% of infants are premature. • Other congenital abnormalities may be present such as congenital heart disease (30%), malrotation (20% to 30%), annular pancreas (30%), to name a few. • Maternal history of polyhydramnios (excessive amniotic fluid) is present in 50% of cases caused by inadequate absorption of amniotic fluid in the distal intestine (see Chapter 22). • Vomiting of bile-stained fluid (bilious vomiting) *without* abdominal distension within the first day of life. Recall that in infantile hypertrophic pyloric stenosis, projectile vomiting is *not* bile-stained (non-bilious vomiting) and peristaltic waves are visible. • Jaundice is present in ~30% of cases. • Plain abdominal radiograph shows a distended stomach with a "double-bubble" gas shadow, with a gas shadow in the stomach and proximal duodenum and absence of gas in the distal bowel.
Gallstone ileus	• Occurs in elderly women with chronic cholecystitis and cholelithiasis. • Fistula develops between gallbladder and small bowel. Stone passes into small bowel and lodges at the ileocecal valve causing obstruction. • Radiograph shows air in the biliary tree.
Hirschsprung disease (Figs 18-22 D, E, F; Links 18-113, 18-114, 18-115, 18-116, 18-117)	• Incidence is 1 case for 5000 live births. • Male dominant (80% of cases). Increased risk (10%) in trisomy 21 (Down syndrome). • Approximately 10% of children have a family history of Hirschsprung disease. • Approximately 80% of cases are caused by genetic mutations that are autosomal dominant with incomplete penetrance. • Usually involves the distal sigmoid colon and rectum (75%). The proximal uninvolved bowel is dilated and has peristalsis. • Pathogenesis: Most commonly caused by failure of migration of parasympathetic ganglion cells from the neural crest. The ganglion cells in the myenteric plexus of Auerbach and the submucosal plexus of Meissner are part of the enteric nervous system. Their absence interrupts the expression of the parasympathetic nerves causing inhibition of relaxation of the affected muscles. The affected bowel remains contracted with a loss of peristalsis in the involved segment. In addition, there is a loss of the rectosphincteric reflex; therefore, a bolus of stool in the rectum does *not* result in relaxation of the internal anal sphincter. This results in the absence of stool in the rectal vault (key physical diagnosis finding). • Hirschsprung disease is an example of a functional obstruction rather than an anatomic obstruction of the bowel. • Acquired Hirschsprung disease occurs in Chagas disease, secondary to destruction of ganglion cells by amastigotes. • Clinical findings in newborns: vomiting (most common), abdominal distention, chronic constipation, and failure to pass meconium within 48 hrs after birth. • Clinical findings in older infants and children: chronic constipation, abdominal distention, vomiting, history of problems with stooling since birth, poor weight gain, alternating signs of obstruction with diarrhea, and, absence of significant encopresis (involuntary defecation). • Rectal exam reveals an increased rectal sphincter tone and an absence of stool on the examining finger. After the digital exam, there is usually an explosive bowel movement. The absence of stool in the rectal vault is a very important differential point from other causes of chronic constipation. • Complications: enterocolitis may occur in the dilated bowel causing perforation, which is the most common cause of death. • Diagnosis can be made with barium enema, rectal suction, surgical full-thickness biopsy, or anorectal manometry (pressure readings). The initial test of choice is the unprepared barium enema. The biopsy shows absence of ganglion cells as well as nerve cell hypertrophy. In addition, there is increased acetylcholinesterase with special staining.
Indirect inguinal hernia	• Second most common cause of small bowel obstruction (Table 18-6). • Small bowel becomes trapped in the inguinal canal.

TABLE 18-5   Small and Large Bowel Obstruction—cont'd

ETIOLOGIC DISORDER	DISCUSSION
Femoral hernia	• Highest rate of bowel incarceration (Table 18-6).
Intussusception (Fig. 18-22 G; Link 18-118, Link 18-119, Link 18-120, Link 18-121)	• Peak incidence ages 1–5. • In children, the terminal ileum invaginates into the cecum. Hyper-plastic lymphoid tissue in Peyer patches that project into the lumen serves as the nidus for the intussusception. Rarely seen in association with rotavirus oral vaccine. • Combination of obstruction and ischemia with a potential for infarction and perforation. • Clinical findings: colicky pain with bloody diarrhea ("currant jelly" stool; classic but not common finding). Up to 75% of children do *not* have bleeding. An oblong mass is palpated in the midepigastrium (Dance sign). Usually self-reduces without intervention. May require air reduction under fluoroscopy or ultrasound. • In adults, a polyp or cancer is more often the nidus for intussusception. • Ultrasound is the preferred method for diagnosis in many hospitals. • Color Doppler is useful evaluate for a lack of blood flow indicating ischemic injury.
Meconium ileus (Link 18-122, Link 18-123)	• Complication of newborn with cystic fibrosis (see Chapter 17). • Meconium lacks NaCl and obstructs the bowel lumen.
Volvulus (Fig. 18-22 H; Link 18-124, Link 18-125)	• Bowel twists around mesenteric root producing obstruction and strangulation. • Sigmoid colon is most common site in elderly. • Cecum is the most common site in young adults. • Risk factors: chronic constipation (most common), pregnancy, and, laxative abuse.

3. Radiographic findings in small bowel obstruction include:
   a. bowel distention, air-fluid (a-f) levels with a step-ladder appearance, and absence of air distal to the obstruction (Fig. 18-22 A; Links 18-111, 18-112, 18-113, 18-114, 18-115, 18-116, 18-117, 18-118, 18-119, 18-120, 18-121, 18-122, 18-123, 18-124, and 18-125). Upright chest films are important to look for air under the diaphragms, indicating a perforation.
   b. CT is the definitive test for a suspected small bowel obstruction. The hallmark is identification of a transitional zone (junction of normal and obstructed bowel) unless the site of obstruction is at the ileocecal valve. In this case, the entire small bowel is dilated.
4. Clinical findings in bowel obstruction include:
   a. colicky pain. Colicky pain is severe pain that alternates with pain-free intervals.
   b. abdominal distention, *no* rebound tenderness, tympanitic to percussion, high-pitched tinkling sounds (stethoscope).
5. Treatment is surgery.
G. **Hernias**
   1. **Definition:** A bulge or protrusion of an organ through the structure or muscle in which it resides
   2. Mechanisms predisposing to acquired hernias include:
      a. increased intraabdominal pressure (e.g., coughing, heavy weight lifting).
      b. structural weakness in the abdominal wall.
   3. Types of hernias are listed and discussed in Table 18-6 (Fig. 18-23; Links 18-126, 18-127, and 18-128).
H. **Vascular Disorders in the Bowel**
   1. Blood supply of the small and large bowel
      a. Areas of bowel supplied by the superior mesenteric artery (SMA; Fig. 18-24 A) include most of the small bowel (*not* shown in the schematic) and ascending and transverse colon up to the left colic flexure (splenic flexure; circle in figure).
      b. SMA and inferior mesenteric artery (IMA) overlap at the splenic flexure. Recall that the splenic flexure is a watershed area and is thus susceptible to infarction (see Chapter 2).
      c. Areas of the bowel supplied by the IMA include the descending and sigmoid colons (Fig. 18-24 A), proximal rectum (not shown), and the upper half of the anal canal (not shown).
   2. Types of bowel infarctions include:
      a. transmural infarction.
         (1) Full-thickness hemorrhagic infarction; usually involves all or part of the small bowel (Link 18-129)
         (2) Usually caused by thrombosis of the SMA
      b. mural and mucosal infarction. Usually occurs in hypoperfusion states (e.g., shock).
   3. Causes of acute ischemia involving the small bowel include:

Bowel distention, a-f levels, absence air distal to obstruction

CT definitive test: detect transition zone

Pain alternating with pain-free intervals; sign bowel obstruction

No rebound tenderness, tympanitic

High-pitched tinkling sounds

Hernias

Bulge/protrusion thru structure/muscle

↑Intraabdominal pressure

Structural weakness abdominal wall

Indirect inguinal hernia MC hernia

Vascular disorders

Blood supply small/large bowel

Most SB, ascending/transverse colon to splenic flexure

SMA/IMA overlap at splenic flexure

Splenic flexure watershed area; danger infarction

IMA: descending/sigmoid colon

IMA: proximal rectum

IMA: upper ½ anal canal

Transmural infarction

Full-thickness hemorrhagic infarction

All/part of SB

MCC SMA thrombosis

Mural/mucosal infarctions: hypoperfusion (shock)

Acute ischemia SB

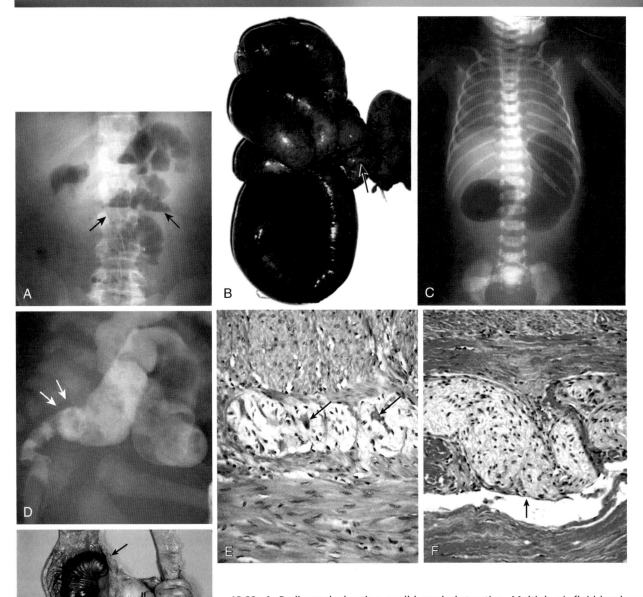

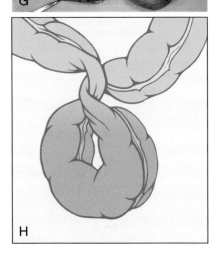

18-22: **A,** Radiograph showing small bowel obstruction. Multiple air-fluid levels are present *(arrows)* in dilated small bowel. There is absence of air distal to the obstruction. **B,** Strangulation of loops of small bowel caused by adhesions *(arrow).* The bowel is dilated and its serosal surface is congested indicating an early stage of infarction. **C,** Duodenal atresia. Plain film of the abdomen showing a dilated stomach (right of the vertebra) and duodenal bulb (left of the vertebra; "double bubble" sign) in a patient with duodenal atresia. **D,** Hirschsprung disease. The barium enema demonstrates the zone of transition *(arrows)* from the dilated proximal normal colon to the reduced caliber of the distal aganglionic colon. **E,** Normal ganglion cells (GCs; *arrows*) in the myenteric plexus of the colon. **F,** Hirschsprung disease. Absence of GCs in the myenteric plexus and thick myenteric fibers *(arrow).* **G,** Ileocecal intussusception. The beginning of the intussusception is the ileum labeled IL. A large sausage-shaped mass covered by hemorrhagic mucosal membrane with patchy necrosis is noted in the lumen of the cecum and ascending colon. This represents the intussuscepted ileum. The apex of the intussusception is located by the arrow. A length of mesentery has also been drawn into the ascending colon sufficient to cause obstruction of the vessels causing infarction and necrosis of the intussuscepted ileum. **H,** Schematic of sigmoid volvulus. Note how the bowel twists around itself producing obstruction and strangulation. *(A from Katz DS:* Radiology Secrets, *Philadelphia, Hanley & Belfus, 1998, p 117, Fig. 25-1; B, E, F, and G from Morson BC:* Colour Atlas of Gastrointestinal Pathology, *London, Harvey Miller Ltd, 1988, pp 108, 176, 176, 107, respectively, Figs. 4.29, 6.9, 6.10, 4.26 respectively; C from Zitelli B, McIntire S, Nowalk A:* Zitelli and Davis' Atlas of Pediatric Physical Diagnosis, *6th ed, Saunders Elsevier, 2012, p 665, Fig. 17.63. D from Townsend C:* Sabiston Textbook of Surgery, *18th ed, Philadelphia, Saunders Elsevier, 2008, p 2065, Fig. 71-13; H from Kumar V, Abbas AK, Fausto N, Mitchell RN:* Robbins Basic Pathology, *8th ed, Philadelphia, Saunders Elsevier, 2007, p 605, Fig. 15-26.)*

TABLE 18-6   Hernias

HERNIA	DISCUSSION
Direct hernia (Fig. 18-23A; Link 18-126A)	• Single layer of transversalis is stretched in the floor of the triangle of Hesselbach. • Medial border of triangle is rectus sheath, lateral border is inferior epigastric artery, inferior border is inguinal ligament. • Hernia bulges through floor of triangle of Hesselbach. Bulge disappears when patient reclines. • Small bowel cannot enter scrotal sac; therefore, there is *no* obstruction or incarceration.
Indirect (inguinal hernia) (Fig. 18-23B; Link 18-126B)	• Most common hernia. • Pathogenesis in children: persistence of peritoneal connection between inguinal canal and tunica vaginalis. Highest in premature infants. Six time more common in male than females. Right-sided hernias are predominant (60%). Inguinal, scrotal, or labial bulge on exam. A useful clinical finding is the "silk glove sign," which refers to a thickening "smoothness" of the spermatic cord. May be associated with an undescended testis. • Pathogenesis in adults: protrusion of new peritoneal process into inguinal canal. • Small bowel passes through internal inguinal ring and may enter scrotal sac. • Bowel directly hits the examining finger within the inguinal canal. • Complications: entrapped in inguinal canal (incarceration) or strangulated obstruction (hemorrhagic infarction). Incarcerated means there is still a good blood supply, whereas strangulated means that the herniated structures (bowel, omentum) have lost their blood supply because of anatomic constriction at the neck of the hernia. • Inguinal hernia (particularly in children) plus a hydrocele indicates an open processus vaginalis.
Femoral (Link 18-126C)	• Most common in women. • Bulge located below inguinal ligament. • Highest rate of incarceration of small bowel. In children, 15% to 20% are incarcerated.
Umbilical (Fig. 18-23 C: Link 18-127, Link 18-128)	• Most common hernia in adults with ascites (cirrhosis), pregnancy, or obesity. • Most common hernia in black newborns (6 to 10 times more common than in white newborns). • More common in trisomy 13, 18, and 21. • More common with hypothyroidism. • Peritoneal protrusion extends into a fascial defect containing remnants of umbilical cord. Covered by skin and subcutaneous tissue. • Majority close spontaneously by the second year. • Incarceration more likely in adults than children.
Ventral (incisional hernia)	• Hernia develops in weakened area of previous surgical excision. • Obesity most common cause.

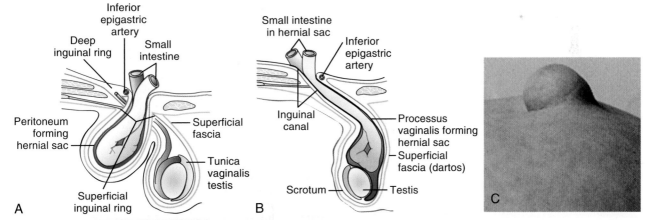

18-23: **A**, Schematic of direct inguinal hernia. See Table 18-6 for discussion. **B**, Schematic of indirect inguinal hernia. See Table 18-6 for discussion. **C**, Umbilical hernia. See Table 18-6 for discussion. *(A and B from Moore NA, Roy WA: Rapid Review Gross and Developmental Anatomy, 2nd ed, Philadelphia, Mosby Elsevier, 2007, p 69, Fig. 3-5A; C from Taylor S, Raffles A: Diagnosis in Color Pediatrics, London, Mosby-Wolfe, 1997, Fig. 1.103.)*

a. acute mesenteric ischemia (50% of cases).
  (1) Caused by embolism from the left side of the heart to the SMA
    (a) Atrial fibrillation (AF) is the most common predisposing arrhythmia that leads to thrombosis in the left atrium and then embolism from the left atrium, through the left ventricle and out into the systemic arterial circulation.
    (b) The SMA has the greatest velocity of blood flow and the most acute angle off the aorta of all the arteries originating from the abdominal aorta; hence, the predisposition for emboli to enter that artery.
  (2) thrombosis of the SMA (Fig. 18-24 B).

Acute mesenteric ischemia MCC SB ischemia

Embolism left side heart to SMA

AF MC arrhythmia → systemic embolism

SMA anatomy favors embolization

SMA thrombosis

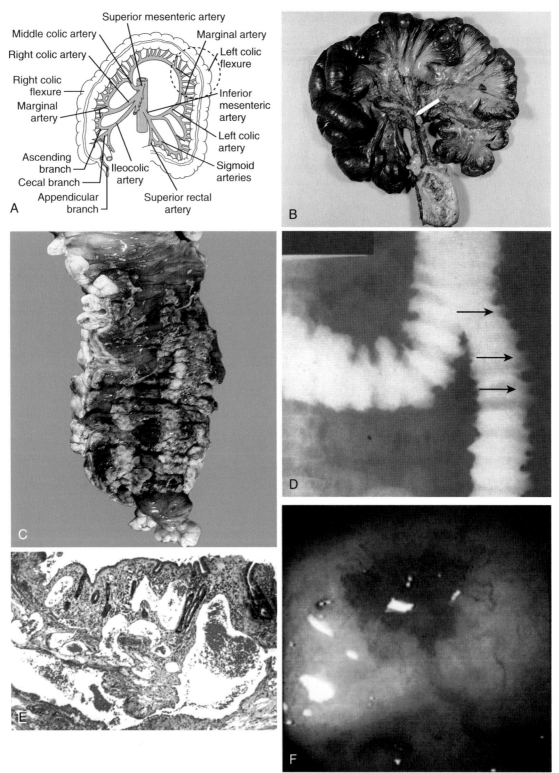

18-24: A, Schematic of arteries of the large intestine. The superior mesenteric artery (SMA) supplies most of the small bowel, the ascending and transverse colon up to the left colic flexure (splenic flexure; interrupted circle). The inferior mesenteric artery (IMA) supplies the descending and sigmoid colons, proximal rectum (not shown), and upper half of the anal canal (not shown). Note that the colon has the benefit of two blood supplies (SMA and IMA), whereas the small intestine only has one major blood supply (SMA). This explains why the small bowel is more likely to have ischemia damage than the large bowel. **B,** Hemorrhagic infarction of small bowel, showing the diffuse dark discoloration of the small bowel. Arrow shows a thrombosed SMA attached to the aorta. **C,** Ischemic colitis in the splenic flexure. The mucosa is markedly hyperemic and covered by a fibrinopurulent exudate. **D,** Single contrast barium enema showing "thumbprinting" of the colonic mucosa *(arrows)* in the region of the splenic flexure in ischemic colitis. **E,** Angiodysplasia of the cecum with dilated venules in the mucosa/submucosa. **F,** Colonoscopic view of the cecum showing an area of mucosal bleeding from a ruptured telangiectatic vessel in angiodysplasia. *(A from Moore A, Roy W: Rapid Review Gross and Developmental Anatomy, 3rd ed, Philadelphia, Mosby Elsevier, 2010, p 76, Fig. 3-21; B from my friend Ivan Damjanov, MD, PhD, Linder J: Pathology: A Color Atlas, St. Louis, Mosby, 2000, p 124, Fig. 7-8; C from Rosai J: Rosai and Ackerman's Surgical Pathology, 9th ed, St. Louis, Mosby, 2004, p 790, Fig. 11.170; courtesy Dr. RA Cooke, Brisbane, Australia; from Cooke RA, Stewart B: Colour Atlas of Anatomical Pathology. Edinburgh, Churchill Livingstone, 2004; D and F from Grieg JD: Color Atlas of Surgical Diagnosis, London, Mosby-Wolfe, 1996, p 202, Figs. 26-9, 26-8, respectively; E from Morson BC: Colour Atlas of Gastrointestinal Pathology, London, Harvey Miller Ltd, 1988, p 178, Fig. 6.14.)*

b. nonocclusive ischemia (25% of cases); causes include hypotension secondary to heart failure (most common), hypovolemic shock, and digitalis (?vasospasm).

c. superior mesenteric vein (SMV) thrombosis (25% of cases; Link 18-112).

(1) Occurs in the thrombosis states

(2) Examples of thrombosis states include polycythemia vera (PV; see Chapter 13), antiphospholipid syndrome (APLS), and protein C deficiency (see Chapter 15).

d. extension of renal cell carcinoma (RCC) into the inferior vena cava (IVC).

4. Clinical and laboratory findings of small bowel infarction include:

a. sudden onset of diffuse abdominal pain. Pain is disproportionate to the physical findings.

b. bowel distention, bloody diarrhea, absent bowel sounds (ileus), absence or rebound tenderness (peritonitis) early in infarction.

c. profound neutrophilic leukocytosis, positive stool guaiac.

5. Radiographic findings in small bowel infarction include:

a. "thumbprint sign" caused by edema in the bowel wall.

b. bowel distention with air-fluid levels similar to bowel obstruction.

c. CT/computed tomography angiography (CTA) has the greatest sensitivity for the diagnosis of a small bowel infarction.

6. Ischemic colitis

a. **Definition:** An inflammatory condition of the large intestine that develops when there is insufficient blood flow to the colon leading to ischemic injury. It is characteristically associated with severe pain and possible hemorrhage.

b. Typically occurs in at the splenic flexure of the large bowel (Fig. 18-24 C), which is a watershed area between the vascular distribution of the SMA and the IMA (see Chapter 2)

c. Atherosclerotic narrowing of the SMA causes mesenteric angina.

(1) **Definition:** Mesenteric angina is severe pain that occurs in the right upper quadrant (RUQ; splenic flexure) shortly after eating.

(2) Patient often loses weight for fear of pain related to eating.

d. Clinical findings include:

(1) history compatible with mesenteric angina.

(2) pain localized to the left upper quadrant (LUQ; splenic flexure; Fig. 18-24 A, *circle*). Pain is out of proportion to the physical findings.

(3) bloody diarrhea caused by mucosal or mural infarction.

(4) barium study that shows thumbprinting of the colonic mucosa (Fig. 18-24 D). Thumbprinting is caused by mucosal edema.

e. Normal repair of the infarction site may result in fibrosis, a common cause of ischemic strictures and colonic obstruction.

7. Angiodysplasia

a. **Definition:** Dilation of the mucosal and submucosal venules (vascular ectasia), typically in the cecum and right colon (Figs. 18-24 E and F)

b. Epidemiology

(1) Usually occurs in older individuals; vascular ectasias (dilation) in the cecum increase with age

(2) Increased wall stress in the cecum stretches the venules. Recall that the cecum has an increased diameter, and according to the law of Laplace, increased diameter increases wall stress.

c. Hematochezia is the most common clinical presentation. A significant amount of blood may be lost. Vascular ectasias are more likely to bleed if the patient has autosomal dominant von Willebrand disease (vWD) or acquired vWD caused by calcific aortic stenosis (see Chapter 15). In aortic stenosis, multimers of von Willebrand factor are destroyed by hitting the calcified plaques in the stenotic valve producing acquired vWD.

d. Diagnosis of angiodysplasia is made with colonoscopy and angiography. Bleeding often subsides after aortic stenosis is corrected.

I. **Small bowel diverticula**

1. Meckel diverticulum

a. **Definition:** A terminal ileum diverticulum, which is located two feet proximal to the ileocecal valve (left lower quadrant; LLQ)

b. Epidemiology

(1) Omphalomesenteric (vitelline) duct remnant (Link 18-130 E). Note: Link 18-130 shows other abnormalities resulting from persistence of the omphalomesenteric duct that are *not* discussed.

Nonocclusive ischemia

Hypotension 2nd heart failure MC

Hypovolemic shock

Digitalis

SMV thrombosis

Thrombosis states

PV, APLS

Protein C deficiency

RCC into IVC

Sudden diffuse abdominal pain

Bowel distention, bloody diarrhea

Ileus

Absence peritonitis

Neutrophilic leukocytosis

+ Stool guaiac

Radiographic findings

"Thumbprint sign": edema bowel wall

Distention; air-fluid levels

CT/CTA best for DX

Ischemic colitis

Insufficient blood flow to colon

Severe pain, possible hemorrhage

Splenic flexure: watershed area

Atherosclerosis SMA

Mesenteric angina: pain RUQ after eating

Fear of pain from eating

LUQ pain

Bloody diarrhea

Thumbprinting (mucosal edema)

Possible ischemic strictures

Angiodysplasia

Vascular ectasia (submucosal venules) cecum/right colon

Elderly; vascular ectasias increase with age

↑Wall stress stretches venules

Angiodysplasia: 2nd MCC hematochezia

Acquired VWD

Colonoscopy/angiography

Bleeding subsides if aortic stenosis corrected

Small bowel diverticula

Meckel diverticulum

Terminal ileum diverticulum

2 feet proximal to ileocecal valve (LLQ)

Omphalomesenteric duct remnant

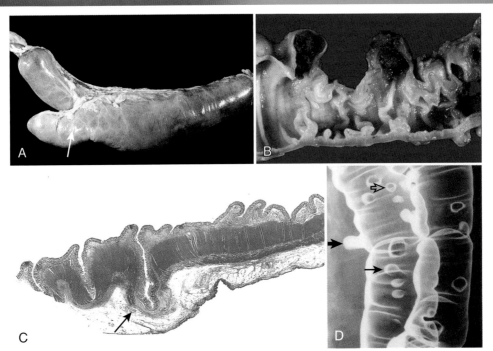

18-25: A, Meckel diverticulum located on the antimesenteric side of the small intestine (white arrow). Mesenteric fat is located on the superior aspect of the small bowel. **B,** Gross section of sigmoid colon showing pulsion diverticula with fecal material (fecaliths). **C,** Whole mount of colon with a diverticulum (arrow shows a blood vessel). **D,** Double contrast barium enema showing numerous diverticula. The solid thick black arrow shows a barium-filled diverticulum. The thin solid black arrow shows a small pool of barium resembling a meniscus. The open arrow shows a diverticulum with no barium in the lumen. (*A from Kumar V, Fausto N, Abbas A:* Robbins and Cotran Pathologic Basis of Disease, *7th ed, Philadelphia, Saunders, 2004, p 830, Fig. 17-31; B from Klatt E:* Robbins and Cotran Atlas of Pathology, *Philadelphia, Saunders, 2006, p 183, Fig. 7-94; C from Rosai J:* Rosai and Ackerman's Surgical Pathology, *9th ed, St. Louis, Mosby, 2004, p 781, Fig. 11.157; D from Pretorius ES, Solomon JA:* Radiology Secrets Plus, *3rd ed, Philadelphia, Mosby Elsevier, 2011, p 129, Fig. 16.20.)*

True diverticulum (all layers)

2″, 2 feet, 2% symptomatic

Pancreatic rests → peptic ulcer (bleeding)

Fecal material umbilical area

Persistence vitelline duct

GI bleed MC sign

Iron deficiency NBs/young child

S/S 1st, 2nd yr life

Diverticulitis

Mimics acute appendicitis

Dx ^{99m}Tc nuclear scan

(2) True diverticulum in that all layers are present from mucosa to serosa (Fig. 18-25 A; Links 18-130 E [Meckel diverticulum] and 18-131)
(3) Mnemonic: 2 inches long, 2 feet from the ileocecal valve, 2% of the population, 2% are symptomatic
(4) May contain pancreatic rests and heterotopic gastric mucosa, increasing the risk for bleeding
c. Clinical findings in a Meckel diverticulum include:
  (1) presence of fecal material in the umbilical area in a newborn infant, caused by the persistence of the omphalomesenteric duct (vitelline duct; Link 18-130).
  (2) GI bleeding, the most common sign.
    (a) Common cause of iron deficiency in newborns and young children.
    (b) Symptoms and signs usually arise during the first and second years of life.
  (3) Diverticulitis (acute inflammation of the diverticulum). It is clinically impossible to distinguish Meckel diverticulitis from appendicitis.
d. Diagnosis of a Meckel diverticulum is secured with a ^{99m}Tc nuclear scan, which identifies parietal cells in ectopic gastric mucosa in the diverticulum (Link 18-132).
e. Treatment is surgery.

An omphalocele is a type of abdominal wall defect in which the intestines, liver, and occasionally other organs remain outside of the abdomen in a sac caused by a defect in the development of the muscles of the abdominal wall (Link 18-133).

Abdominal wall defect: intestines, liver, other organs

Mucosal herniation thru areas weakness; pulsion diverticulum

Duodenum MC site; wide-mouthed diverticula (SS)

2. Small bowel diverticula (Link 18-134)
  a. **Definition:** Herniations of mucosa and submucosa through areas of weakness in the muscularis layer in the small bowel wall. *No* muscular covering. Often called a false (pulsion) diverticulum because they do not have all layers of the bowel.
  b. Epidemiology
    • Duodenum is the most common site in the small bowel for diverticula. Wide-mouthed diverticula (large opening) suggests the diagnosis of SS.

c. Complications of small bowel diverticula include:

(1) diverticulitis (inflammation).

(2) perforation leading to peritonitis (inflammation of the parietal peritoneum; discussed later).

(3) bacterial overgrowth: may produce bile salt and/or vitamin B_{12} deficiency.

d. Treatment is surgery.

J. **Sigmoid colon diverticular disease** (Links 18-135 and 18-136)

1. **Definition**: Herniations of mucosa and submucosa through areas of weakness in the muscularis layer in the large bowel wall

2. Epidemiology

a. Incidence in the general public of sigmoid diverticular disease is 35% to 50%.

b. Incidence increases with age (typically sixth decade or older).

c. Most common site is the left colon (95%). The sigmoid colon is the most common site for diverticula in the entire GI tract.

d. Diverticula are located on the mesenteric border where the vasa recta penetrates the muscle wall (Fig. 18-25 B and C).

e. Pain with diverticulosis is caused by perforation from the diverticulum. The resulting leakage may be minimal and contained within the pericolic fat or extensive and involve the mesentery or other organs.

f. Most common cause of a lower GI bleed (most often from diverticula in the right colon)

g. Associations of sigmoid colon diverticular disease include Marfan syndrome, Ehlers-Danlos syndrome (EDS), and adult polycystic kidney disease (APKD)

h. Pathogenesis

(1) Straining with defecation caused by a low-fiber diet with increased constipation

(2) Area of weakness is where vasa recta penetrate the muscular propria (Fig. 18-25 C; Links 18-135 and 18-136). Diverticula are juxtaposed to the vasa recta, thus markedly increasing the risk for significant bleeding into the colon.

3. Clinical findings

a. Diverticulitis is the most common complication.

(1) Caused by stool that is impacted (fecalith) in the diverticulum sac (Fig. 18-25 B); produces ulceration and ischemia (compression of the vasa recta).

(2) Clinical findings include:

(a) fever (only with diverticulitis).

(b) diarrhea initially followed by constipation.

(c) LLQ pain ("left-sided appendicitis") with rebound tenderness to palpation.

(d) palpation of a tender mass in some cases.

(e) microscopic bleeding common (gross bleeding uncommon).

(3) Diverticulitis is diagnosed with a CT scan (best test) or with a double-contrast barium enema (Fig. 18-25 D).

(a) Increased risk for perforation and abscess formation

(b) Diverticulitis is the most common cause of fistula formation (connection between hollow structures).

Colovesical fistula (connection between the large bowel and the bladder) is a common fistula in the GI tract. Associated findings include pneumaturia (air in urine) and recurrent urinary tract infections. Diverticulitis is the most common cause of this fistula and others between subjacent bowel loops.

b. Sigmoid diverticulosis *without* inflammation

(1) Clinical finding in sigmoid diverticulosis (*not* –itis) is painless bleeding resulting in hematochezia. Can result in massive blood loss. Sigmoid diverticulosis is the most common cause of hematochezia.

(2) Usually caused by erosion of a juxtaposed vessel by a fecalith (hardened impacted stool; like a "stone"). Bleeding stops spontaneously in 60% of cases. Scarring of the juxtaposed vessel in recurrent attacks of diverticulitis prevents bleeding.

c. Consequences of sigmoid diverticular disease are summarized in Links 18-137 and 18-138.

K. **Inflammatory bowel disease (IBD)**

1. Ulcerative colitis (UC) (Table 18-7)

a. **Definition:** Chronic relapsing ulceroinflammatory disease of undetermined etiology that starts in the rectum and extends into the colon for a variable distance

---

Diverticulitis

Perforation/peritonitis

Bacterial overgrowth

Bile salt/B_{12} deficiency

Sigmoid colon diverticular disease

Herniation mucosa/submucosa thru muscularis layer

Incidence ↑ with age

Left colon MC site

Located mesenteric border

Pain = perforation

MCC lower GI bleed

Marfan syndrome, EDS, APKD

Low fiber diet; constipation

Weakness: vasa recta penetrates muscularis propria

Marked risk for bleeding

Diverticulitis MC complication

Stool impacted in diverticulum → ulceration, ischemia

Fever (diverticulitis *not* –osis)

Diarrhea → constipation

"Left-sided appendicitis," rebound tenderness

Tender mass LLQ

Microscopic bleeding common

CT best test

Risk perforation/abscess

Fistula formation

Sigmoid diverticulitis: CT scan best for Dx

Diverticulosis MCC hematochezia

Erosion by fecalith

Bleeding stops spontaneously (60%)

Inflammatory bowel disease

Ulcerative colitis

Ulceroinflammatory disease; starts in rectum → proximal colon

TABLE 18-7   Comparison of Ulcerative Colitis and Crohn Disease

FEATURE	ULCERATIVE COLITIS (UC)	CROHN DISEASE (CD)
Epidemiology	• Most common IBD. • More common in whites than blacks • No sex predilection • Occurs between ages 15 and 40 yrs and 50 and 80 yrs. • Higher prevalence in Ashkenazi Jewish descendants. • Lower incidence in current smokers and other nicotine users. Increased risk for ex-smokers. • Lower incidence if previous patient had appendectomy prior to <20 years of age. • Infection with non-typhoid strains of *Salmonella* or *Campylobacter jejuni* associated with greater risk in the following year. • Increased risk if patient has autoimmune disease.	• More common in whites than blacks, in Jews than non-Jews. • No sex predilection. • Smoking is a risk factor. • Bimodal (3rd and 5th decades).
Extent	Mucosal and submucosal.	Transmural (Fig. 18-26 C)
Location	• Mainly rectum (usually begins in this location). • Extends in continuity into left colon (may involve entire colon; pancolitis). • Does *not* involve other areas of GI tract. Rarely, there may be "back-wash ileitis."	• Terminal ileum alone (30% of cases; Fig. 18-26 E; Link 18-143), ileum and colon (50% of cases), colon alone (20% of cases). • Involves other areas of GI tract (mouth to anus).
Gross features	• Ulceration and hemorrhage (Fig. 18-26 A). • Inflammatory pseudopolyps (Fig. 18-26 B; Link 18-139). • *No* adhesions.	• Thick bowel wall and narrow lumen (leads to obstruction). • Aphthous ulcers in bowel (early sign; Link 18-144). • Skip lesions, strictures, fistulas, bowel adhesions. • Deep linear ulcers with cobblestone pattern (Links 18-145 and 18-146). Pseudo-polyps are present. • Fat creeping around serosa.
Microscopic features	• Ulcers and crypt abscesses containing neutrophils (Link 18-140). • Dysplasia (Link 18-141) or cancer may be present.	• Noncaseating granulomas (60% of cases; Link 18-147), lymphoid aggregates (Fig. 18-26). • Dysplasia or cancer less likely than ulcerative colitis.
Clinical findings	• Recurrent left-sided abdominal cramping with bloody diarrhea and mucus. Abdominal pain is not severe. • Fever, tenesmus, weight loss. • Proctitis (inflammation or rectum and anus). • Toxic megacolon (up to 10% of patients). Mortality rate 50%. • No fistulas. • Overall risk for colorectal cancer is 2% to 5%. • Extra-gastrointestinal findings: *primary sclerosing cholangitis (UC > CD), *primary biliary cirrhosis (UC > CD), erythema nodosum, iritis/uveitis (CD > UC), pyoderma gangrenosum (Link 18-142), HLA-B27 positive arthritis. • p-ANCA antibodies 60% of cases. • Elevated C-reactive protein (CRP), ESR, and thrombocytosis are common.	• Severe recurrent right lower quadrant colicky pain (obstruction) with non-bloody diarrhea and weight loss. • Bleeding occurs only with colon or anal involvement (fistulas, abscesses, perianal tags [Link 18-148]). • Aphthous ulcers in mouth. • Overall risk for colorectal cancer in Crohn disease with extensive colon involvement is 2% to 5%. Small bowel cancer risk is also increased. • Extragastrointestinal findings: erythema nodosum, sacroiliitis (HLA-B27 association), pyoderma gangrenosum (Link 18-142), iritis (CD > UC), *primary sclerosing cholangitis (UC > CD). • p-ANCA antibodies 60% of cases. • Anti-*Saccharomyces cerevisiae* antibodies (80% of cases). The test for anti-*Saccharomyces cerevisiae* (yeast) antibodies (ASCA) is used to help distinguish between Crohn disease (CD) and ulcerative colitis (UC). • Elevated C-reactive protein (CRP), ESR, and thrombocytosis are common.
Radiography	"Lead pipe" or "tubular" appearance in chronic disease. Tubular appearance results from the loss of haustral folds.	"String" sign in terminal ileum from luminal narrowing by inflammation (Fig. 18-26 G), fistulas. Skip lesion are present.
Complications	• Toxic megacolon (hypotonic and distended bowel; fever, tachycardia, leukocytosis, anemia). • Adenocarcinoma: greatest risks are pancolitis, early onset, duration of disease >10 years).	• Anal fistulas to skin, bowel, or vagina (Fig. 18-26 F), obstruction, colon cancer (UC > CD). • Calcium oxalate renal calculi (increased reabsorption of oxalate through inflamed mucosa). • Malabsorption caused by bile salt deficiency. • Macrocytic anemia caused by vitamin B_{12} deficiency if the terminal ileum is involved.

*All patients with primary sclerosing cholangitis and primary biliary cirrhosis should be screened for inflammatory bowel disease by colonoscopy.
ANCA, Anti-neutrophil cytoplasmic antibodies; *ESR,* erythrocyte sedimentation rate; *GI,* gastrointestinal.

b. Epidemiology
(1) Most common IBD
(2) Ulcerations are in continuity (Fig. 18-26 A). Ulcerations are limited to the mucosa and submucosa of rectum and colon (Fig. 18-26 B; Link 18-143). Crypt abscesses are commonly present (Link 18-140). Mucosal dysplasia may be present.

MC IBD

Ulcerations in continuity

Ulcerations limited to mucosa/submucosa rectum/colon

Mucosal dysplasia

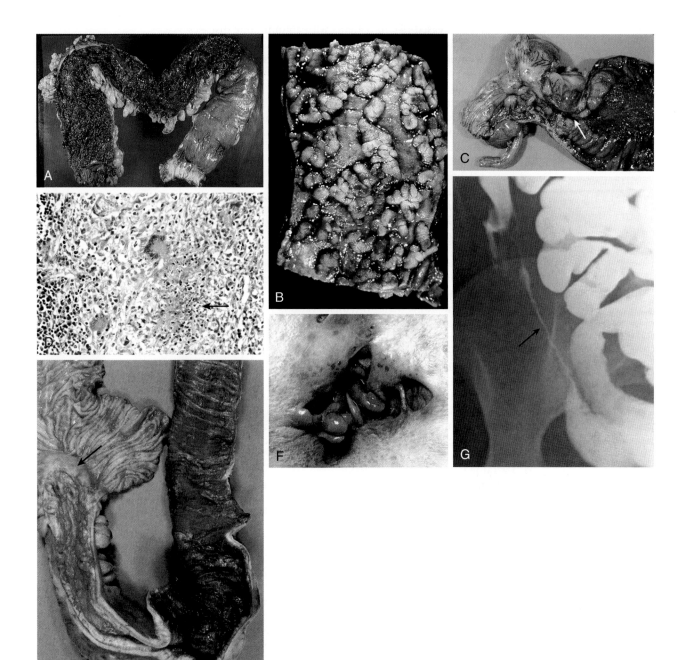

18-26: A, Ulcerative colitis (UC). The colon shows diffuse ulceration of the mucosal surface. **B,** UC. Note the linear ulcers and islands of residual mucosa called pseudopolyps. **C,** Crohn disease (CD), showing a resection of the terminal ileum with attached cecum and appendix; the appendix is to the left. The thickened terminal ileal wall (transmural inflammation) causes the narrowing *(arrow)* at the junction of the ileum and the cecum. The proximal ileum is dilated (caused by obstruction), and the ileal mucosa has a cobblestone appearance caused by linear ulcerations (aphthous ulcers) that cut into the underlying submucosa. **D,** CD granuloma with central necrosis (arrow; not caseation) and multinucleated giant cells. **E,** CD with stricture and proximal ulceration (arrow; ileocecal valve). **F,** CD of the anus. Note the fistulas and ulcerations and edematous tags. **G,** CD. The terminal ileum (solid black arrow) is markedly narrowed (string sign) and stands apart from other loops of small bowel. (*A and C from my friend Ivan Damjanov, MD, PhD:* Pathology for the Health-Related Professions, *2nd ed, Philadelphia, Saunders, 2000, p 271, Figs. 10-10A, 10-10B, respectively;* **B,** *from Rosai J:* Rosai and Ackerman's Surgical Pathology, *9th ed, St. Louis, Mosby, 2004, p 784, Fig. 11.161B;* **D, E,** *and* **F** *from Morson BC:* Colour Atlas of Gastrointestinal Pathology, *London, Harvey Miller Ltd, 1988, pp 126, 121, 272, respectively, Figs. 4.67, 4.53, 7.9, respectively;* **G** *from Herring W:* Learning Radiology Recognizing the Basics, *2nd ed, Philadelphia, Elsevier Saunders, 2012, p 179, Fig. 18.12A.*)

(3) Most common between ages 15 and 40 years with a second peak between 50 and 80 years

(4) Infection with nontyphoid strains of *Salmonella* or *Campylobacter jejuni* is associated with a greater risk for developing the disease in the following year.

(5) Higher prevalence in Ashkenazi Jewish descendants

(6) Abnormalities in humoral and cellular adaptive immunity are present.

(7) Decreased risk in current smokers and increased risk for ex-smokers

(8) Increased risk in patients with autoimmune diseases

2. Crohn's disease (CD)
   a. **Definition:** Chronic granulomatous, ulceroconstrictive disease of unknown etiology that most commonly involves the terminal ileum and has discontinuous spread that may involve any part of the GI tract
   b. Epidemiology
      (1) Characterized by transmural inflammation (from mucosa to serosa; Fig. 18-26 C)
      (2) Noncaseating granulomas are a hallmark of the disease (60% of cases; Fig. 18-26 D)
      (3) Most common in whites and those of Jewish descent; bimodal peak in the 3rd to 5th decade of life
      (4) Immune system dysfunction (increased risk in patients with other autoimmune diseases)
      (5) Smoking increases risk.

3. Indeterminate colitis (10%); features of UC and CD

4. Table 18-7 summarizes the key features of UC and CD. Systemic complications of IBD are summarized in Link 18-149.

L. Other types of colitis
   1. Lymphocytic colitis
      a. **Definition:** Chronic colitis typified by increased intraepithelial lymphocytes and surface damage (Link 18-150)
      b. Epidemiology: Male-to-females ratio is 1:1. Mean age of onset is 43 years.
      c. Clinical
         (1) Chronic, nonbloody watery diarrhea (95%)
         (2) Weight loss (91%), abdominal pain (40%), urgency (29%), and nocturnal diarrhea (22%)
   2. Collagenous colitis
      a. **Definition:** Chronic colitis typified by increased intraepithelial lymphocytes and an irregular band of subepithelial collagen (Link 18-151)
      b. Epidemiology: Male-to-females ratio is 7:5 to 15:1. Mean age of onset is 51 years.
      c. Clinical is the same listed for lymphocytic colitis *except* signs are worse in collagenous colitis.

M. Irritable bowel syndrome (IBS)
   1. **Definition:** A chronic functional colonic motility disorder manifested by recurrent abdominal pain and bloating
   2. Epidemiology (Link 18-152)
      a. Intrinsic colonic motility disorder
         (1) Possible loss of tolerance to normal GI flora
         (2) Genetic factors may be involved.
         (3) Environmental triggers (e.g., food, coffee) commonly aggravate the disease.
      b. Most common functional bowel disorder
      c. Responsible for >50% of referrals to gastroenterologists; second leading cause of work absenteeism
      d. Occurs more often in females than males
      e. Bacterial overgrowth in the small bowel may be present in some cases.
      f. Risk factors for irritable bowel syndrome include history of childhood sexual abuse; domestic abuse in women; increased stress, depression, and personality disorder; and postinfectious gastroenteritis.
      g. Motility disturbance (slower myoelectric rhythm in colon)
      h. Abnormal sensitivity to rectal distention
   3. Patients may have constipation (most common), diarrhea (never nocturnal), or intermittent episodes of the two.
      a. Abdominal pain and bloating are usually relieved by defecation. Abdominal pain is central and below the area of the stomach or in the LLQ (above the left lower hip).
      b. Stools are commonly accompanied by mucus.
      c. Abnormal defecation includes straining and a sense of incomplete evacuation.
      d. C-reactive protein is normal, which rules out inflammation.

4. Flexible sigmoidoscopy or colonoscopy results are normal.

5. Radiologic study results are normal.

N. Necrotizing enterocolitis (NEC)

1. **Definition:** A disease of unknown origin that primarily affects premature infants and is manifested by a spectrum ranging from abdominal distention with hematochezia to a fulminant septic shock–like picture with transmural necrosis of the entire GI tract

2. Epidemiology

   a. Most common life-threatening emergency of the GI tract in the newborn period and the most common abdominal surgical emergency of the newborn period

   b. Affects premature infants in 90% of cases, typically after the onset of enteral alimentation during convalescence from common cardiopulmonary disorders associated with prematurity (e.g., patent ductus arteriosus, respiratory distress syndrome)

   c. Major risk factors include low birth weight (LBW), sepsis, congenital heart disease (CHD), respiratory distress syndrome (RDS), and maternal cocaine abuse.

   d. Cause of NEC is most likely multifactorial; however, prematurity is the greatest risk factor.

   e. Various degrees of mucosal or transmural necrosis of the intestine may occur along with marked distention of the bowel (Links 18-153 and 18-154).

   f. Colonization of the gut by bacteria is somehow involved in the pathogenesis.

   g. Another factor is the volume of milk fed to infants. Large-volume milk feedings that are increased too rapidly during feeding schedules may place undue stress on a previously injured or immature intestine.

   h. In 20% to 30% of cases, blood cultures have been positive for *Staphylococcus epidermidis* followed by gram-negative bacilli such as *E. coli* and *Klebsiella* spp.

   i. Probiotics appear to have reduced the incidence of NEC but not the mortality rates in infants who develop NEC.

   j. Distal part of the ileum and the proximal segment of colon are most frequently involved.

3. Clinical: abdominal distention, vomiting, bloody stools, temperature lability, apnea, and bradycardia

O. Pneumatosis cystoides intestinalis

1. **Definition:** The presence of gas in the bowel wall

2. Epidemiology

   a. Ominous finding in ischemia of the bowel

   b. Primary pneumatosis intestinalis (15% of cases) is a benign idiopathic condition characterized by the presence of multiple thin-walled cysts in the submucosa or subserosa of the colon.

   c. Secondary pneumatosis intestinalis (85% of cases) is associated with COPD (e.g., cystic fibrosis, emphysema), as well as with obstructive and necrotic GI disease, particularly NEC.

   d. Chronic inflammation, crypt abscesses, granulomas, and cysts lined by multinucleated giant cells (MGCs) mimic CD. Gas is generated from the lumen of the bowel or within inflamed crypts (Link 18-155).

P. Peritonitis

1. **Definition:** Refers to inflammation of the peritoneum; characteristically painful.

2. Epidemiology

   a. Subdivided into spontaneous peritonitis and secondary peritonitis. The latter is either localized (abscess) or diffuse if there has been a breach in the abdominal viscera (perforation, postoperative, posttraumatic).

   b. Clinical conditions commonly associated with peritonitis include tuboovarian abscess (*Neisseria gonorrhoeae*), ruptured ectopic pregnancy (EP; sterile peritonitis caused by blood), ruptured ovarian cyst (sterile peritonitis), acute diverticulitis, acute appendicitis, acute cholecystitis, ruptured hepatic adenoma (HA), hepatocellular carcinoma (HCC), and ruptured spleen, to name a few conditions.

   c. Majority of pathogens are gram-negative bacteria (e.g., *E. coli*, *Enterobacter*, *Klebsiella*). Common gram-positive bacteria are enterococci, staphylococci, or streptococci. Common anaerobes are *Bacteroides fragilis* and *Clostridium* species.

3. Spontaneous bacterial peritonitis

   a. **Definition:** Refers to a peritonitis that is associated with ascites in a patient with cirrhosis of the liver

   b. Epidemiology

      (1) Prevalence in cirrhotic patients admitted to the hospital is 10% to 30%.

      (2) Males are affected more than females.

Colonoscopy normal

Radiologic studies normal

Necrotizing enterocolitis

Primarily affects premature infants

MC NB life-threatening/ surgical emergency GI tract

Premature infants (90%)

LBW, sepsis, CHD, RDS, maternal cocaine abuse

Multifactorial; prematurity greatest risk factor

Mucosal to transmural necrosis

Gut colonization

Large volume milk feeding

S. epidermidis MC sepsis

Probiotics helpful

Distal ileum, proximal colon MC sites

Distention, vomiting, bloody stools

Temperature lability, apnea, bradycardia

Pneumatosis cystoides intestinalis

Gas in bowel wall

Ominous finding in bowel ischemia

Primary 15%

Secondary 85%: COPD, NEC

Chronic inflammation, crypt abscesses, granulomas, cysts lined by MGCs

Peritonitis

Inflammation peritoneum

Spontaneous, 2nd peritonitis (localized, diffuse)

Tuboovarian abscess, ruptured EP

Ruptured ovarian cyst

Acute diverticulitis, appendicitis, cholecystitis

Ruptured hepatic adenoma/ spleen, HCC

Majority G- bacteria

E. coli, Enterobacter, Klebsiella

Enterococci, staphylococci

B. fragilis, *Clostridium* spp.

Spontaneous bacterial peritonitis

Peritonitis, ascites due to cirrhosis

Males > females

Ascitic fluid: ↓albumin, ↓bacterial opsonins

Transmigration bacteria thru bowel wall → ascitic fluid

E. coli adults, Streptococcus pneumoniae children

Fever, diffuse abdominal pain, rebound tenderness

Peritoneal fluid WBC count >250 cells/mm³

Small bowel malignancy

Least common GI site for malignancy

Adenocarcinoma; duodenum MC site

Carcinoid tumor

Neuroendocrine malignancy; NSGs (EM)

MC SB tumor; malignant neuroendocrine tumors

Size/depth invasion determine metastasis risk

Foregut: stomach; hindgut:rectum rarely metastasize

Midgut: terminal ileal carcinoid invade/ metastasize

Appendix MC site

Rarely metastasize

Small bowel

Terminal ileum; metastasize to liver

Tumors produce bioactive compounds (e.g., serotonin)

Compounds delivered by PV to liver

Serotonin → 5-HIAA → excreted in urine

No signs/symptoms carcinoid syndrome

(3) Low protein content (low albumin levels) and low levels of bacterial opsonins in ascitic fluid increase the risk for infection.

(4) Bacteria transmigrate through the bowel wall into the ascitic fluid. *E. coli* is the most common pathogen in adults and *Streptococcus pneumoniae* is the most common pathogen in children. Polymicrobial infections are usually associated with bowel perforation.

4. Clinical findings include fever, generalized abdominal pain, and rebound tenderness.

5. Laboratory findings reveal a peritoneal fluid WBC count >250 cells/mm³ with >25% of the cells representing neutrophils.

Q. Small bowel malignancy

1. Epidemiology. Small bowel is the *least* common site in the GI tract for a primary malignancy.

2. Primary adenocarcinoma of the small bowel. Duodenum is the most common site for the cancer.

3. Carcinoid tumor

   a. **Definition:** Slow-growing neuroendocrine cancer that contains neurosecretory granules (NSG) visible by electron microscopy (EM), may arise in many sites throughout the body (e.g., lung, small bowel, colon, appendix, rectum)

   b. Epidemiology

   (1) Most common small bowel malignancy. Malignant neuroendocrine tumor.

   (2) Metastatic potential correlates with their size and depth of invasion.

      (a) Size >2 cm increases their risk for metastasis.

      (b) If depth of invasion is ~50% of the bowel thickness, there is an increased risk for metastasis.

   (3) Foregut (e.g., stomach) and hindgut (e.g., rectum) carcinoid tumors invade but *rarely* metastasize.

   (4) Midgut carcinoid tumors (e.g., terminal ileum) commonly invade and metastasize.

   c. Common locations for carcinoid tumors in the GI tract include the:

   (1) vermiform appendix (Fig. 18-27A).

      (a) Most common site in the GI tract (40% of cases).

      (b) Usually <2 cm, and thus at low risk of metastasizing to the liver.

   (2) small bowel (20% of cases).

      (a) Majority occur in the terminal ileum (15%).

      (b) Commonly metastasize to the liver.

   (3) In the previous locations, the tumor produces bioactive compounds (e.g., serotonin).

      (a) Compounds are delivered to the liver by the portal vein (PV), which empties into the sinusoids. Compounds include amines and peptides secreted from neuroendocrine cells (serotonin, bradykinin, histamine).

      (b) Serotonin is taken up by hepatocytes and is metabolized to 5-hydroxy-indoleacetic acid (5-HIAA). 5-HIAA is excreted in the urine.

      (c) Serotonin is completely metabolized and does *not* enter the systemic circulation. *No* signs or symptoms of carcinoid syndrome.

   (4) Less common locations for carcinoid tumors in the GI tract include esophagus, stomach, colon (collectively represent 10% of cases), and rectum (15%). In addition, carcinoid tumor may involve the bronchus (12%).

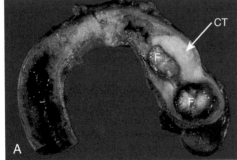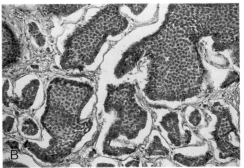

18-27: A, Carcinoid tumor (CT) of the vermiform appendix. Note the yellow mass in the wall of the appendix *(arrow)*. The lumen contains fecaliths (F). **B,** Microscopic section of a carcinoid tumor showing well-circumscribed islands of similar appearing cells with dark nuclei and surrounded by clear cytoplasm. *(A, From Grieg JD:* Color Atlas of Surgical Diagnosis, *London, Mosby-Wolfe, 1996, p 196, Fig. 25-20. B, From Rosai J:* Rosai and Ackerman's Surgical Pathology, *Mosby Elsevier 10ᵗʰ ed, 2011, p 690, Fig. 11.109B).*

(5) Grossly, carcinoid tumors have a bright yellow color. Serotonin induces a fibroblastic response that may produce obstruction, particularly in the terminal ileum (Link 18-156). Histologically, the tumor cells have round-to-ovoid nuclei and eosinophilic cytoplasm and exhibit a "nested" growth pattern (Fig. 18-27B; Link 18-157).

d. Carcinoid syndrome
   (1) **Definition:** Constellation of clinical findings caused by the endogenous secretion of serotonin by a carcinoid tumor. Characteristic findings include red-purple flushing of the skin and diarrhea.
   (2) Epidemiology
       (a) Within the GI tract, the carcinoid tumors that are most likely to cause the carcinoid syndrome are those involving the terminal ileum. Serotonin induces a fibroblastic reaction in the bowel, which may lead to obstruction.
       (b) Liver metastasis from these tumors *must* occur to produce the syndrome.
       (c) Serotonin is secreted by metastatic tumor nodules in the liver.
       (d) Serotonin entering hepatic vein (HV) tributaries then accesses the systemic circulation, leading to the signs and symptoms of the carcinoid syndrome.
       (e) Bronchial carcinoids, though uncommon, may cause the carcinoid syndrome in the absence of hepatic metastasis.
   (3) Clinical findings
       (a) Clinical findings are caused by serotonin and other bioactive compounds (e.g., histamine, bradykinin, kallikrein).
       (b) Flushing of the skin occurs in 75%–90% of cases (Link 18-158). Caused by vasodilation, may be triggered by emotion, alcohol, as well as some foods.
       (c) Diarrhea occurs in >70% of cases). Caused by increased bowel motility induced by serotonin.
       (d) Intermittent wheezing and dyspnea may occur in 25% of cases. Caused by bronchoconstriction.
       (e) Facial telangiectasia (dilated vessels) may be present.
       (f) Tricuspid regurgitation and pulmonary stenosis may occur. Serotonin increases collagen production in the right-sided heart valves (see Chapter 11).
   (4) Diagnosis
       (a) Increase in urinary 5-hydroxyindoleacetic acid (HIAA).
       (b) Computerized tomography (CT scan) is useful in the detection of hepatic metastasis.
       (c) Scanning techniques are available to detect primary location and metastasis sites. Radiolabeled octreotide scan visualizes previously undetected or metastatic lesions.
4. Malignant lymphoma in bowel (see Chapter 14).
   a. Usually arises from lymphoid tissue in Peyer patches of the terminal ileum.
   b. Usually arises from B cells (e.g., Burkitt lymphoma).

R. **Small and large bowel polyps**
   1. **Definition:** Polyps are abnormal tissue growths of tissue arising from the mucosa; that may be sessile (flat; sessile) or pedunculated (on a stalk).
   2. Non-neoplastic (hamartomatous) polyps in the small and/or large bowel
      a. Hamartomas are characterized by disorganized tissue indigenous to particular site.
      b. Hyperplastic polyp (Fig. 18-28A; Link 18-159)
         (1) Most common adult polyp. They are hamartomas (non-neoplastic).
         (2) Majority are located in the sigmoid colon. Typically occur in 6th to 7th decade.
         (3) *No* malignant potential or association with polyposis syndromes (see Chapter 9).
         (4) Histologically, they have a "sawtooth" appearance with goblet cells in the mucosa.
      c. Juvenile (retention) polyps
         (1) **Definition:** A type of hamartomatous polyp that most commonly occurs in children < 5 years of age.
         (2) Most common overall colon polyp in children.
         (3) Most commonly located in the rectum. Sometimes prolapse out of the rectum and bleed.
         (4) Solitary polyp with a smooth surface and enlarged cystic spaces on cut section (Link 18-160).
         (5) Primary polyp in juvenile polyposis, which is an autosomal dominant (AD) disease or nonhereditary.
         (6) Primary polyp in Cronkhite-Canada (C-C) syndrome, which is a nonhereditary polyposis syndrome also associated with ectodermal abnormalities of the nails.

Bright yellow; "nested" growth pattern

Carcinoid syndrome

Red-purple flushing skin/diarrhea

Terminal ilium MC site: produce serotonin

Liver metastasis necessary for syndrome

Serotonin secreted by metastatic nodules

Serotonin enters HV tributaries → systemic circulation

Syndrome may occur in bronchial location

Metastasis unnecessary

Serotonin, histamine, bradykinin, kallikrein

Flushing skin most cases

Diarrhea most cases

↑Bowel motility

Intermittent wheezing; bronchoconstriction

Facial telangiectasia

Tricuspid regurgitation, pulmonic stenosis

↑Urine HIAA

CT detects liver metastasis

Radiolabeled octreotide scan

Malignant lymphoma bowel

Lymphoid tissue: Peyer patches in terminal ileum

B cell origin: Burkitt lymphoma

Small/large bowel polyps

Sessile, stalk

Disorganized tissue

Hyperplastic polyp

MC adult polyp

Hamartomatous polyp

Majority sigmoid colon

6th to 7th decade

No malignant potential

No association with polyposis syndromes

"Sawtooth" appearance

Juvenile retention polyps

Hamartomatous polyp MC children < 5 yrs old

MC colon polyp children

MC in rectum

Prolapse/bleed

Smooth surface, cystic spaces

Primary polyp in juvenile polyposis (AD or non-hereditary)

Primary polyp C-C syndrome

18-28: **A,** Hyperplastic polyps. Arrows show numerous sessile (no stalk) polyps. **B,** Tubular adenoma. The head of the stalked polyp has a lobulated, mushroom-like appearance. The arrow points to the stalk. **C,** Villous adenoma. Note the large cauliflower-like mass in the rectosigmoid. These tumors secrete mucus rich in potassium and protein. **D,** Villous adenoma. The cut surface of a villous adenoma shows leaf-like villous processes. **E,** Familial polyposis. Note the numerous small, sessile polyps. These were present in the entire large bowel. **F,** Adenocarcinoma of the sigmoid colon. Resection of the rectosigmoid shows an annular and ulcerating growth, causing a stricture. **G,** Spot radiograph from a single contrast phase of a double contrast barium enema showing an adenocarcinoma of the rectum with circumferential narrowing of the lumen ("apple core" lesion). (**A** and **E** from Rosai J, Ackerman LV: Surgical Pathology, 9th ed, St. Louis, Mosby, 2004, pp 805, 802, respectively, Figs. 11.201, 11-195, respectively; **B** from my friend Ivan Damjanov, MD, PhD, Linder J: Pathology: A Color Atlas, St. Louis, Mosby, 2000, p 138, Fig. 7-55; **C** and **D** from Morson BC: Colour Atlas of Gastrointestinal Pathology, London, Harvey Miller Ltd, 1988, p 229, Figs. 6.117, 6.118, respectively; **F** from my friend Ivan Damjanov, MD, PhD: Pathology for the Health-Related Professions, 2nd ed, Philadelphia, Saunders, 2000, p 272, Fig. 10-21B; **G** from Pretorius ES, Solomon JA: Radiology Secrets, 2nd ed, St. Louis, Mosby, 2006, p 125, Fig. 15-9.)

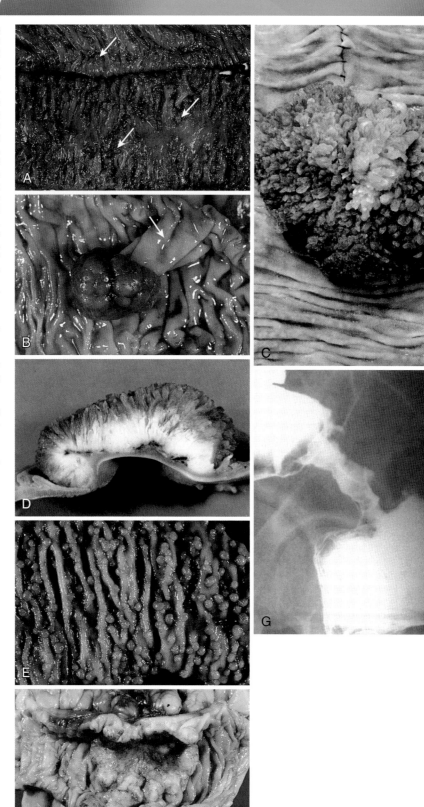

d. Peutz-Jeghers polyposis (PJP)
  (1) **Definition:** Autosomal dominant (AD) disease with hamartomatous polyps
  (2) Median age 15 years old
  (3) Hamartomatous polyps in stomach, small bowel (SB; MC site), colon, and rectum
  (4) Clinical findings:
    (a) mucosal pigmentation of the buccal mucosa and lips (see Fig. 18-5).
    (b) increased risk (>50%) for colorectal, breast, lung, pancreatic, and thyroid cancer.

3. Adenomatous polyps (tubular adenomas)
  a. **Definition:** Refer to benign neoplastic polyps that, though benign, exhibit dysplastic features histologically and thus have a variable degree of malignant potential
  b. Epidemiology. Premalignant dysplastic colonic polyps that increase with age and have an equal sex incidence
  c. Adenomatous polyp (tubular adenoma; Link 18-161 left; Link 18-162)
    (1) Most common colonic polyp (60% of cases). Frequency increases with age.
    (2) Locations: 40% in right colon, 40% in left colon, and 20% in rectum
    (3) Blacks have a lower prevalence than do whites.
    (4) Usually a stalked polyp that looks like a mushroom (Fig. 18-28B). On histologic examination, they show a complex branching of glands, which is called adenomatous change by pathologists (see Fig. 9-1A).
  d. Tubulovillous adenoma (TVA; 20%–30% of polyps)
    (1) Usually a stalked polyp
    (2) Histologically, they have adenomatous and villous change (similar to small bowel villi).
  e. Villous adenoma (VA; 10% of polyps)
    (1) Sessile polyp (*no* stalk) with primarily a villous (finger-like fronds) component (Fig. 18-28C, D; Link 18-161 right-side schematic)
    (2) Rectosigmoid location and secrete excessive amounts of a protein and potassium-rich mucus. Large tumors can produce hypoalbuminemia and hypokalemia.
  f. Serrated polyposis syndrome
    (1) Characterized by the presence of serrated polyps (Link 18-163)
    (2) Larger than hyperplastic polyps. They may display dysplastic features similar to that seen in adenomatous polyps. They may develop into an adenocarcinoma. Histologic features that distinguish them from a hyperplastic polyp should be confirmed by experts because of their association with colorectal cancer. World Health Organization criteria are available to assist with the diagnosis.
  g. Risk factors for malignancy in adenomas include:
    (1) size >2 cm (40% risk of malignancy).
    (2) presence of multiple polyps.
    (3) polyps with an increased villous component. Villous adenomas have a 30% to 40% risk for malignancy.
  h. Familial polyposis (FP) epidemiology (Fig. 18-28E, Fig. 18-29; Link 18-164)
    (1) Autosomal dominant (AD) disease with complete penetrance
      (a) All patients develop tubular adenomas and cancer (complete penetrance).
      (b) Polyps begin to develop between 10 and 20 years of age.
    (2) Pathogenesis: Inactivation of adenomatous polyposis coli (APC) suppressor gene (see Chapter 9)

Peutz-Jeghers polyposis

AD hamartomatous polyp SB

Median age 15

Stomach, SB (MC site), colon, rectum

Buccal mucosa/lip pigmentaion

↑Risk colorectal, breast, lung, pancreatic, thyroid cancers

Adenomatous polyps

Benign neoplastic polyps with variable malignant potential

↑With age; equal sex incidence

Tubular adenoma

MC colonic polyp

Frequency increases with age

Majority left/right colon

Blacks < whites

"Mushroom"

Complex branching of glands

Tubulovillous adenoma

TVA stalked polyp

Adenomatous/villous change

Villous adenoma

Sessile polyp; finger-like fronds

Rectosigmoid location; ↑mucus secretion

Possible hypoproteinemia/hypokalemia

Serrated polyposis syndrome

Serrated polyps

Serrated polyposis syndrome: ↑risk colorectal cancer

Risk for malignancy

Adenoma >2 cm

Multiple polyps

Villous component greatest malignancy risk

Familial polyposis

AD; complete penetrance

All develop adenomas/cancer

Polyps begin 10-20 yrs age

Inactivation APC suppressor gene

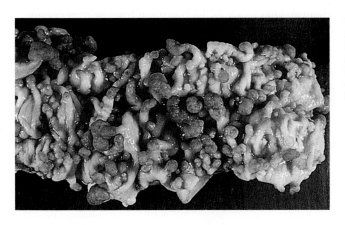

18-29: Familial polyposis. This segment of colon shows numerous adenomatous polyps. *(From Ashar BH, Miller RG, Sisso SD: The Johns Hopkins Internal Medicine Board Review, 4th ed, Elsevier, 2012, p 441, Fig. 52.2. Taken from Skarin AT, Shaffer K, Wieczorek T [eds]: Atlas of Diagnostic Oncology, ed 3, St. Louis, Mosby, 2003, p 152. In Abeloff MD, Armitage JO, Niederhuber JE, et al: Clinical Oncology, ed 3, Philadelphia, Churchill Livingstone, 2004, Fig. 80-7.)*

Malignant transformation
35-40 yrs of age

CHRPE/desmoid tumor
association

Aggressive tumors anterior
abdominal wall

Gardner syndrome

AD polyposis syndrome; risk
CC

Benign osteomas, desmoid
tumors

Turcot syndrome

AR polyposis syndrome; CC
risk

Malignant brain tumors

Lynch syndrome

(3) Clinical findings
    (a) Malignant transformation usually occurs between 35 and 40 years of age.
    (b) Prophylactic colectomy is recommended.
    (c) Associated with congenital hypertrophy of retinal pigment epithelium (CHRPE) and desmoid tumors. Desmoid tumors are locally aggressive tumors of the anterior abdominal wall and are composed of fibrous tissue.
(4) Gardner syndrome
    (a) Autosomal dominant polyposis syndrome has an increased risk for developing colorectal cancer (CC).
    (b) Additional findings include benign osteomas (benign tumor composed of bone; see Chapter 24) and desmoid tumors.
(5) Turcot syndrome
    (a) Autosomal recessive (AR) polyposis syndrome with an increased risk for colorectal cancer (CC).
    (b) Associated with malignant brain tumors (astrocytoma and medullo-blastoma; see Chapter 26).
(6) Lynch syndrome (HNPCC, or hereditary nonpolyposis colorectal cancer).

Autosomal dominant polyposis syndrome associated with an increased risk of cancers involving the colon, rectum, and other sites including endometrial [2nd MC cancer], ovarian, stomach, small intestine, hepatobiliary tract, upper urinary tract, brain, and skin.

AD, risk other cancers
(endometrial)

Colon cancer

3rd MC cancer/cancer-
related death men/women

Incidence decreasing
(screening tests)

Peak incidence 7th decade

50% flexible
sigmoidoscopy/90%
colonoscopy

Risk factors

Age >50 yrs, smoking,
obesity

Inactivity, heavy alcohol
intake

HPSs

HNPCC

Family cancer syndrome

1st degree relatives with
colon cancer

IBD; UC > CD

Dietary factors (low fiber
diet, ↑saturated fats

↓Intake of vegetables

Type 2 DM

Hx pelvic radiation,
previous endometrial/
ovarian cancer

Aspirin/NSAIDs ?protective
effect

Smoking

Carcinogenesis

Adenoma-carcinoma
sequence

APC, KRAS, p53 genes

APC/MMR gene mutations
for sporadic cancers

Germline mutations *APC*
gene → FAP

Germline mutations *MMR*
genes → HNPCC cancer

CI, MIS, hypermethylation
→ colorectal cancer

S. Colon cancer
1. Epidemiology
    a. Third most common cancer-related death in men and women
    b. Third most common cancer in men and women
    c. Incidence rates have been decreasing, caused by an increase in screening with the fecal occult blood test and colonoscopy (allows visualization of the entire colon).
    d. Peak incidence of colon cancer is in the seventh decade (60–69 years old).
    e. Approximately 50% of rectal cancers are detected by digital rectal examination.
    f. Approximately 50% of colon cancers are detected by flexible sigmoidoscopy and 90% by colonoscopy.
    g. Risk factors include:
      (1) age >50 years, cigarette smoking, obesity, decreased activity, heavy alcohol intake.
      (2) hereditary polyposis syndromes (HPS; see previous).
      (3) hereditary nonpolyposis colon cancer (HNPCC/ see Chapter 9).
      (4) family cancer syndrome (see Chapter 9), first-degree relatives with colon cancer.
      (5) IBD. UC greater risk than CD.
      (6) dietary factors. Low-fiber diet, increased intake of saturated fats, and reduced intake of vegetables (see Chapter 8).
      (7) type 2 DM.
      (8) history of pelvic radiation, previous endometrial or ovarian cancer.
    h. Aspirin and NSAIDs may have a protective effect.
    i. smoking. Even though it may be protective, it is *not* recommended.
2. Carcinogenesis
    a. Adenoma-carcinoma sequence
      (1) Sequence-specific genetic abnormalities result in the transition from normal colonic mucosa to invasive carcinoma. Normal colon → mucosa at risk → adenomas → carcinoma.
      (2) Genes that are involved include *APC, KRAS,* and *p53.* Telomerase is involved in the carcinoma part of the sequence.
    b. Mutations involving adenomatous polyposis coli (*APC*) account for 80% of sporadic colon cancers, whereas, mutations involving mismatch repair (*MMR*) genes account for 15% of sporadic colon cancers (see Chapter 9).
    c. Germline mutations in adenomatous polyposis coli (*APC*) gene cause familial adenomatous polyposis (FAP).
    d. Germline mutations of *MMR* genes cause hereditary nonpolyposis colon cancer (Lynch syndrome; see Chapter 9).
    e. Various molecular pathways may lead to colorectal cancer (CC). These involve chromosome instability (CI; most cases), microsatellite instability (MIS), and

hypermethylation of the *CpG dinucleotide in tumor suppressor genes causing inactivation of these genes. *p indicates a phosphodiester bond connecting the C (cytosine) and G (guanine). The latter two pathways are involved with serrated adenoma transformation into colorectal cancer.

3. Specific locations of colon cancer in descending order are the sigmoid colon (23.6%), rectum (22.1%), cecum (12.5%), transverse colon (11%), ascending colon (9%), rectosigmoid junction (8.6%), and descending colon (6.1%).

4. Morphologic features of colon cancer (Link 18-165 A,B, C, Link 18-166)
   a. Screening tests include:
      (1) fecal occult blood (guaiac) test (FOBT).
         (a) *Not very* sensitive (15%–30%) or specific for colon cancer
         (b) Does *not* distinguish Hb from myoglobin
      (2) fecal immunochemical test. Antibodies to detect globin.
      (3) Fecal DNA test
         (a) Human DNA is extracted from stool.
         (b) Test detects DNA alteration in genes associated with colon cancer (e.g., *p53, KRAS, APC, BAT26* [involved in microsatellite instability]).
         (c) Much greater sensitivity than the previously mentioned tests for detecting cancer (51% versus 13%).
   b. Colonoscopy includes:
      (1) standard colonoscopy with biopsy.
      (2) computed tomography (CT) colonoscopy. More sensitive and specific than colonoscopy with biopsy.

5. Clinical findings in colon cancer
   a. Majority are adenocarcinomas (glandular; see Link 18-165A).
   b. Most common clinical finding is abdominal pain (44%). Other signs include change in bowel habits, melena, hematochezia. Symptoms include weight loss and weakness.
   c. Left-sided colon cancer
      (1) Tend to have signs of obstruction
         (a) Bowel diameter is smaller than the right colon.
         (b) Lesions have an annular, "napkin ring" appearance (Fig. 18-28F, G; Link 18-165B).
      (2) More likely to have a change in bowel habits (obtained by history) including:
         (a) constipation and diarrhea with or without bleeding.
         (b) bright red blood that coats the stool.
      (3) Increased incidence of *Streptococcus bovis* endocarditis (see Chapter 11)
   d. Right-sided colon cancer
      (1) Tend to bleed
         (a) Bowel diameter is greater than the left colon.
         (b) Tumors may be polypoid (Link 18-165C; Link 18-166, left) or ulcerated (Link 165B; Link 18-166, *arrow*) in appearance. Bleeding often occurs whether the tumor is polypoid or ulcerated. Obstruction occurs in those that invade around the circumference of the colon (Link 18-165B).
      (2) Blood is often mixed in with stool if they are located in the proximal portion of the sigmoid colon. Blood is more likely to cover the surface of the stool when located in the anorectal region.
      (3) Iron deficiency may occur if excessive amounts of blood are lost in the stool.

6. Sites of metastasis include liver (most common), lungs, bone, and brain.

7. Prevention
   a. Aspirin and other nonsteroidal antiinflammatory drugs (NSAIDs). Decrease the incidence of colorectal adenomas (possible precursors to cancer).
   b. annual/biennial fecal occult blood test (FOBT).
   c. fecal DNA testing.
   d. dietary alterations including decreasing fat intake to 30% of total calories; increasing fiber; and increasing the intake of fruits and vegetables.
   e. stop cigarette smoking.

8. Prognosis
   a. Survival rate depends on the stage of the disease. Overall 5-year survival rate is ~65%.
   b. Serum carcinoembryonic antigen (CEA) is used to detect recurrences. Serum CEA should be measured prior to surgery and then followed postoperatively as an increased in CEA may indicate tumor recurrence.

Marginal notes:

Sigmoid colon MC site

Screening tests

FOBT *not* sensitive/specific

Does *not* distinguish Hb from myoglobin

Fecal immunochemical test: abs detect globin

Fecal DNA test

Human DNA extracted from stool

Fecal DNA test: more sensitive than FOBT

Colonoscopy

CT colonoscopy highest sensitivity Dx colon cancer

Majority adenocarcinoma

Abdominal pain MC sign

Left-sided colon cancer

Tend to obstruct

Bowel diameter < right colon

"Napkin ring" appearance

Change in bowel habits

Constipation/diarrhea with/without bleeding

Bright red blood coats stool

↑S. bovis endocarditis

Right-sided colon cancer

Tend to bleed

Bowel diameter > left colon

Bleeding, obstruction may occur

Blood mixed with stool proximal sigmoid

Blood coats stool in anorectal cancers

Iron deficiency occurs if excessive blood is lost

Liver MC site metastasis

Aspirin, NSAIDs

FOBT

Fecal DNA testing

↓Fat intake, ↑Fiber

↑Fruits/vegetables

Stop cigarette smoking

Survival depends on stage

CEA useful to detect recurrences

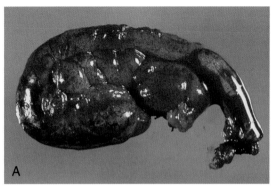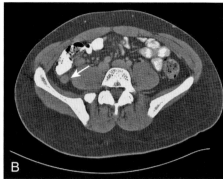

18-30: **A,** Acute appendicitis showing erythema and vascular congestion of the serosal surface of the appendix. **B,** Abdominal CT shows a cross-section of an enlarged, fluid-filled retrocecal appendix *(arrow)*, with appendicitis in the right lower quadrant. The wall of the appendix is thickened. *(**A,** From my friend Ivan Damjanov, MD, PhD, Linder J: Pathology: A Color Atlas, St. Louis, Mosby, 2000, p 131, Fig. 7-30. **B,** From Grossman ZD, Katz DS, Alberico RA, et al.: Cost-Effective Diagnostic Imaging: The Clinician's Guide, 4th ed, Mosby Elsevier, 2006, p 68, Fig. 10-1).*

Acute appendicitis

Fecalith obstruction; lymphoid hyperplasia

MC abdominal surgical emergency

Pathogenesis children

Lymphoid hyperplasia post viral infection

Adult → fecalith obstruction appendix

Seeds, parasites, neoplasms, bacterial infections

E. coli MCC

Initial periumbilical pain

C fiber irritation

Pain referred to midline

Fever

Pain *precedes* nausea/ vomiting

T12 skin hypersensitivity

Pain shifts to RLQ 12-18 hrs

Aδ fibers localize pain

Rebound tenderness RLQ

Pain with right thigh extension

RLQ pain with palpation LLQ

T. Acute appendicitis

1. **Definition:** Refers to acute inflammation of the vermiform appendix, usually as a result of a bacterial infection, associated with obstruction of the lumen by a fecalith (hard stool; adults) or lymphoid hyperplasia (children)
2. Epidemiology
   a. Occurs in 10% of the population
   b. Most common abdominal surgical emergency
3. Pathogenesis in children
   a. Usually associated with lymphoid hyperplasia (60% of cases) often secondary to a viral infection. Other causes include a fecalith or inspissated enteric material blocking the appendiceal orifice.
   b. Examples: adenovirus, measles virus infection or immunization.
4. Pathogenesis in adults
   a. Fecalith (hard stool) obstructs the proximal lumen of the appendix (30% to 35%; similar to the pathogenesis of acute diverticulitis) (Fig. 18-30A). Increased intraluminal pressure from the obstruction causes mucosal ischemia and infarction. There is also decreased bacterial clearance from the appendiceal lumen, with subsequent bacterial overgrowth, inflammation, infection, infarction, and pain. Protracted obstruction may result in perforation.
   b. Other causes of acute appendicitis (4% of cases) include seeds (sunflower, persimmons), pinworm infection, bacterial infections (e.g., *Yersinia, Salmonella, Shigella*), and neoplasms (carcinoid tumor; 1%).
   c. Primary pathogens are *Escherichia coli* (most common aerobe; 77%), *Strepto-coccus viridans* (43%), group D streptococcus (27%), and *Bacteroides fragilis* (most common anaerobe; 80%).
5. Clinical findings in sequence include:
   a. initial colicky periumbilical pain (50% of cases).
      (1) Caused by irritation of unmyelinated afferent C fibers on the *visceral* peritoneal surface
      (2) Pain is referred to the midline.
   b. fever. Very important sign for identifying appendicitis in children with abdominal pain.
   c. nausea, vomiting, and fever. Pain *precedes* nausea and vomiting.
   d. cutaneous hyperesthesia (excessive hypersensitivity of skin) at level of T12 (level of umbilicus).
   e. pain shifts to the right lower quadrant (RLQ) in 24 to 36 hours. Right lower quadrant tenderness (sensitivity 65–100%, specificity 1–92%)
      (1) Caused by irritation of Aδ fibers on the *parietal* peritoneum. Localizes pain to the exact location in the right lower quadrant.
      (2) Rebound tenderness at McBurney point (sensitivity 50%–94%, specificity 75%–86%).
      (3) Pain with right thigh extension (psoas sign; sensitivity 13%–42%, specificity 42%–79%).
      (4) Right lower quadrant (RLQ) pain with palpation of the left lower quadrant (Rovsing sign; sensitivity 7%–68%, specificity 58%–96%).

f. Flexion and then internal rotation of the right hip stretches the right obturator internus muscle causing pain (obturator sign; sensitivity 8%, specificity 94%)

g. Signs of a lower urinary tract (LUT) infection may occur, which include increased frequency and dysuria (painful urination).

h. Laboratory findings include:

(1) neutrophilic leukocytosis with left shift (90% of cases; see Chapters 3 and 13).

(2) abnormal urinalysis with increased protein, hematuria (RBCs in the urine), pyuria (neutrophils in the urine).

6. Retrocecal appendicitis

a. Inflamed appendix is located behind the cecum.

b. Radiograph shows a sentinel loop in the right lower quadrant (RLQ), caused by a localized ileus (lack of motility) from the subjacent appendicitis.

7. Complications of appendicitis include:

a. periappendiceal abscess with or without perforation.

(1) Most common complication

(2) May develop into a subphrenic abscess, an accumulation of pus between the diaphragm, liver, and spleen. Usually caused by *Bacteroides fragilis*.

b. pylephlebitis.

(1) **Definition:** Infection of the portal vein (PV)

(2) Poses a danger for developing portal vein thrombosis (PVT; see Chapter 19)

(3) Radiograph shows gas in the portal vein.

c. Subphrenic abscess.

(1) Usually presents with persistent postoperative fever.

(2) Diaphragm is fixed on the right with associated right-sided pleural effusion.

(3) Tenderness over the lateral seventh and eighth ribs.

(4) Diagnosis can be made using US, computerized tomography, or a gallium scan.

8. Diagnosis of acute appendicitis

a. Clinical examination.

b. Abdominal computed tomography (CT) is the best test after both oral and intravenous contrast medium (Fig. 18-30B). Sensitivity is 90% and specificity is 94%,

c. Ultrasonography (*not* recommended). Sensitivity is 75% and specificity is 90%.

Many disorders mimic appendicitis including viral gastroenteritis, ruptured follicular cyst, ruptured ectopic pregnancy, mesenteric lymphadenitis, and Meckel diverticulitis.

VI. Anorectal Disorders

A. Signs and symptoms of anorectal disease include:

1. bleeding, caused by internal hemorrhoids (IHs; painless; MCC) and anorectal cancer, infection, fissure.

2. pain, caused by anal fissure or thrombosed external hemorrhoids

3. pruritus (e.g., pinworms), anal fistula (e.g., CD).

B. Anorectal Disorders

1. Internal hemorrhoids

a. **Definition:** Refers to dilated superior hemorrhoidal veins (SHVs) in the mucosa and submucosa located *above* the pectinate line (superior plexus; Fig. 18-31A; Link 18-167B)

b. Epidemiology: causes include:

(1) straining at stool (most common cause). Straining is often associated with constipation and a low-fiber diet.

(2) pregnancy, obesity.

(3) anal intercourse, portal hypertension.

c. Clinical findings

(1) Often prolapses out of the rectum (Fig. 18-31B; Link 18-167B)

(2) Commonly pass bright red blood with the stool. Blood coats the stool. Bleeding is usually painless.

In an adult, never assume that blood coating the stool is caused by an internal hemorrhoid. Other causes include colorectal and anal cancer; therefore further investigation is necessary.

Anal pruritus and soiling of underwear is commonly present.

Margin notes:

Flexion right hip/internal rotation

Signs LUT infection some cases

Neutrophilic leukocytosis

UA: ↑protein, hematuria, pyuria

Retrocecal appendicitis

Appendix behind cecum

Sentinel loop (ileus)

Complications of appendicitis

Periappendiceal abscess +/− perforation

MC complication

Subphrenic abscess

Bacteroides fragilis

Pylephlebitis

Infection PV

Danger PVT

Gas PV

Subphrenic abscess

Persistent postoperative fever

Diaphragm fixed on right; right pleural effusion

Diagnosis of acute appendicitis

Clinical examination

Acute appendicitis diagnosis: spiral CT or plain CT with rectal contrast

Ultrasonography

Anorectal disorders

Signs/symptoms anorectal disease

Bleeding: internal hemorrhoids MCC

Anorectal cancer, infection, fissure

Pain: anal fissure, thrombosed EHs

Pruritus: pinworms

Anal fistula: CD

Anorectal disorders

Internal hemorrhoids

Dilated SHVs

MCC straining at stool

Constipation, low-fiber diet

Pregnancy, obesity

Anal intercourse, portal hypertension

Prolapse out of rectum

Blood coats stool

Painless bleeding

Anal pruritus/soiling underwear

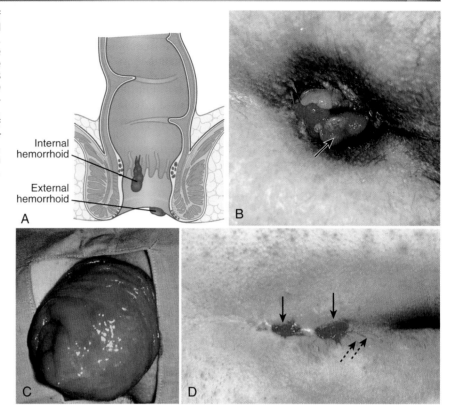

18-31: A, Schematic showing formation of internal and external hemorrhoids. **B,** Prolapsed internal hemorrhoids *(arrow)*. **C,** Rectal prolapse. Note the hyperemic mucosal surface of the rectum. **D,** Pilonidal sinus with pits in skin crease of natal cleft (solid arrows) from which hairs protrude (interrupted arrows). *(A from Kliegman R: Nelson Textbook of Pediatrics, 19th ed, Philadelphia, Elsevier Saunders, 2011, p 1361, Fig. 336.5; B and D from Morson BC: Colour Atlas of Gastrointestinal Pathology, London, Harvey Miller Ltd, 1988, pp 275, 290, respectively, Figs. 7.16, 7.50, respectively; C from Townsend C: Sabiston Textbook of Surgery, 18th ed, Philadelphia, Saunders Elsevier, 2008, p 1418, Fig. 50-64.)*

Internal hemorrhoid

External hemorrhoid

External hemorrhoids

Dilated inferior hemorrhoidal veins

Painful thrombosis MC complication

Rectal prolapse

Protrusion rectum thru anus

Weak rectal support

Child: whooping cough, trichuriasis, cystic fibrosis (early sign)

Elderly straining at stool

Heavy squats weight lifters

Pilonidal sinus/abscess

Cyst/abscess deep gluteal folds

Hair/debris traumatically buried

Intermittent/constant anal itching

Males > females

Internal hemorrhoids common

Pinworms, *Candida,* VDs

Irritants

2. External hemorrhoids (EHs)
   a. **Definition:** Refer to dilated inferior hemorrhoidal veins that are located *below* the pectinate line (inferior plexus; Fig. 18-31A)
   b. Painful thrombosis is the most common complication (Link 18-167A; Link 18-168).
3. Rectal prolapse
   a. **Definition:** Refers to protrusion of the rectum through the anus (Fig. 18-31C; Link 18-169)
   b. Epidemiology
      (1) Caused by weak rectal support mechanisms
      (2) Causes of rectal prolapse in children <2 years old include whooping cough (*Bordetella pertussis*), trichuriasis, caused by *Trichuris trichiura* (whipworm), and cystic fibrosis (straining at stool associated with dehydrated fecal matter).
         • Common early sign in infants with cystic fibrosis
      (3) Common in the elderly caused by straining at stool
      (4) May occur with the increase in intraabdominal pressure associated with heavy weightlifting (e.g., squats in weight lifters)
4. Pilonidal sinus and abscess
   a. **Definition:** Small cyst or abscess that occurs in the deep gluteal fold that is filled with hair and debris (Fig. 18-31D).
   b. Epidemiology
      (1) Hair/debris is traumatically buried into the sinus usually after sitting for a long time.
      (2) Presents as a painful sacrococcygeal mass with purulent drainage
5. Pruritus ani
   a. **Definition:** Refers to intermittent or constant itching of the anus
   b. Epidemiology
      (1) More common in males than females
      (2) Occurs in 1% to 5% of the population
      (3) Causes of pruritus ani include:
         (a) anorectal conditions: internal hemorrhoids (common), fissures, anal incontinence, diarrhea, and cancer.
         (b) infections: pinworm, *Candida,* and venereal diseases (VDs).
         (c) local irritants: soap, underwear, obesity, coffee, beer, and acidic foods.

(d) dermatologic disease: psoriasis and atopic dermatitis.

(e) Diabetes mellitus (DM).

6. Anorectal abscess with fistula

    a. **Definition:** Refers to an anorectal abscess with an inflammatory tract (fistual) with an external opening in the perianal skin and an internal opening in the anal canal at the dentate line (Link 18-170).

    b. Epidemiology

       (1) Occurs in all ages

       (2) Associated with constipation

       (3) Pediatric population

          (a) More common in infants in first 6 to 8 months of life

          (b) Occurs in boys more often than girls

       (4) Etiology

          (a) Nonspecific cryptoglandular (epithelium lining the anal canal) infection is the most common cause.

          (b) IBD, with CD being more common than UC

          (c) Secondary to trauma from an episiotomy, prostatectomy, or anal intercourse

          (d) Secondary to anal carcinoma or treatment for anal carcinoma

7. Anal fissure

    a. **Definition:** Refers to a tear in the epithelial mucosa of the anal canal from the dentate line to the anal verge

    b. Epidemiology

       (1) Accounts for >10% of anal complaints

       (2) More common in men than women

       (3) Common in women before and after childbirth

       (4) Most common cause of rectal bleeding infants

       (5) Causes of anal fissures include:

          (a) passage of hard stool. Once the fissure is formed, it is perpetuated by bowel movements.

          (b) frequent stooling or diarrhea.

          (c) infections, including HSV, human immunodeficiency virus, CMV, sexually transmitted disease (e.g., syphilis, gonorrhea), IBD (e.g., CD, UC).

    c. Clinical findings of anal fissures

       (1) Fissures usually in the midline (90% posterior). A posterior fissure (90% of cases) and/or ulcer is located between the anal verge and the dentate line. Lateral anal fissures may also occur (Link 18-171). Consider CD if the fissure is *not* midline.

       (2) Location is marked by an anal tag at the anal verge.

       (3) Prominent proximal anal papilla

       (4) Sharp burning exacerbated by stooling

       (5) Bright red blood may be seen coating the stool, in the toilet water, or on the toilet paper.

8. Anal carcinoma

    a. Basaloid (epidermoid or cloacogenic) carcinoma

       (1) Most common type

       (2) Located in the transitional zone (TZ) above the dentate line. Female dominant.

    b. Squamous cell carcinoma (SCC)

       (1) Located in the anal canal

       (2) Majority occur in men who have sex with men. HPV 16 and 18 association.

Margin notes:

Psoriasis, atopic dermatitis

DM

External opening skin; internal opening anal canal

All ages

Constipation

Infants

Boys > girls

Cryptglandular infection MCC

CD > UC

Episiotomy, prostatectomy, anal intercourse

Anal carcinoma or Rx

Anal fissure

Tear anal mucosa anal canal

Men > women

Women before/after childbirth

MCC infant rectal bleeding

Firm bowel movements

Frequent stooling/diarrhea

Infections, IBD

Most are midline fissures

Consider CD if fissure *not* midline

Anal tag marks location

Sharp burning with stooling

Blood on toilet paper

Anal carcinoma

Basaloid carcinoma MC type

TZ above dentate line

Female dominant

SCC

Anal canal

Men-sex-men

HPV 16/18

ABBREVIATIONS

MC most common	MCC most common cause	COD cause of death

I. **Overview of the Liver and Biliary System** (Links 19-1, 19-2, 19-3, 19-4, and 19-5)

II. **Laboratory Evaluation of Liver Cell Injury**

   A. **Bilirubin metabolism and jaundice**

     1. Bilirubin metabolism in sequence (Fig. 19-1 A)

       a. Unconjugated bilirubin (UCB)

         (1) Senescent red blood cells (RBCs) are phagocytosed by splenic macrophages (MPs).

         (2) UCB is the end-product of heme (iron + protoporphyrin) degradation in MPs. UCB is lipid soluble (indirect bilirubin).

       b. UCB combines with albumin in the blood.

         (1) UCB is taken up by hepatocytes.

         (2) Conjugated to glucuronic acid by uridine glucuronosyltransferase (UGT) to produce conjugated bilirubin (CB). CB is water soluble (direct bilirubin).

       c. CB is secreted into the intrahepatic bile ducts.

         (1) Temporarily stored in the gallbladder

         (2) CB enters the duodenum via the common bile duct (CBD).

       d. Intestinal bacteria convert CB to urobilinogen (UBG; some use the term *stercobilinogen*).

         (1) UBG is spontaneously oxidized to urobilin (stercobilin).

         (2) Urobilin produces the brown color of stool.

       e. Approximately 20% of the UBG in the intestine is recycled to the liver (90%; enterohepatic circulation) and kidneys (10%).

     2. Jaundice

       a. **Definition:** A yellowish discoloration of the sclera in the eyes, skin, and mucous membranes caused by an excess of UCB, CB, or both

       b. Epidemiology

         (1) First noticed in the sclera (Fig. 19-1 B) because it has a high affinity for bilirubin

         (2) Classification of causes of jaundice is based on the percentage of CB (Table 19-1).

           (a) Percent CB = CB/total bilirubin.

           (b) %CB <20% defines unconjugated hyperbilirubinemia, which is caused by increased production of UCB (e.g., extravascular hemolytic anemias [EHAs; e.g., hereditary spherocytosis]; see Chapter 12) or decreased liver uptake and/or conjugation of UCB (e.g., physiologic jaundice of the newborn).

           (c) % CB between 20% and 50% defines mixed hyperbilirubinemia, which are primarily caused by hepatitis, which causes problems with uptake, conjugation, and secretion of bilirubin into the bile.

Bilirubin metabolism/jaundice

Unconjugated bilirubin

Senescent RBCs phagocytosed splenic MPs

UCB end-product heme degradation

UCB lipid soluble (indirect bilirubin)

UCB combines with albumin

Liver uptake UCB

UGT → converts UCB to CB

CB water soluble; direct bilirubin

CB secreted into liver bile ducts

CB temporarily stored in gallbladder

CB→ CBD → duodenum

Bacteria: CB → UBG

UBG → urobilin

Urobilin produces stool color

UBG: 20% recycled liver/kidneys

Jaundice

Yellow discoloration skin/sclera

Jaundice ↑UCB and/or CB

Sclera first site jaundice

%CB = CB/total bilirubin

%CB <20% = unconjugated hyperbilirubinemia

EHA, ↓uptake/conjugation UCB

%CB 20%–50% = mixed hyperbilirubinemia; hepatitis

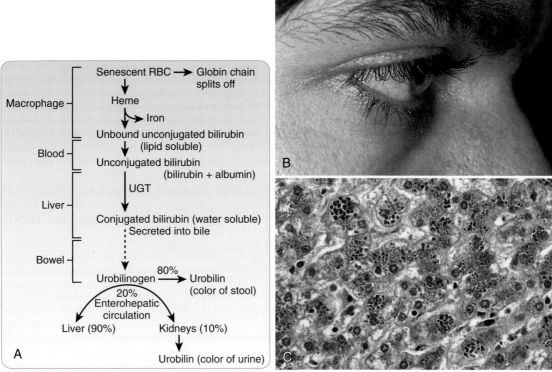

19-1: A, Bilirubin metabolism. Refer to the text for discussion. **B,** Scleral icterus. Note the yellowish discoloration of the sclera. **C,** Pigment in lysosomes in Dubin-Johnson syndrome. *RBC,* Red blood cell; *UGT,* uridine glucuronosyltransferase. (*B from Savin J, Hunter JA, Hepburn NC:* Diagnosis in Color: Skin Signs in Clinical Medicine, *London, Mosby-Wolfe, 1997, Fig. 6.28: **C** from MacSween R, Burt A, Portmann B, Ishak K, Scheuer P, Anthony P:* Pathology of the Liver, *4th ed, London, Churchill Livingstone, 2002, p 221, Fig. 4.91.*)

TABLE 19-1 Causes of Jaundice

TYPE OF HYPERBILIRUBINEMIA	URINE BILIRUBIN	URINE UBG	EXAMPLES OF DISORDERS
CB <20% (ALL UCB)			
Increased production of UCB	Absent	↑	Extravascular hemolytic anemias: e.g., hereditary spherocytosis, Rh and ABO hemolytic disease of newborn, warm autoimmune hemolytic anemia
Decreased uptake or conjugation of UCB	Absent	*Not* useful	• Gilbert syndrome (familial nonhemolytic jaundice): common autosomal dominant defect with incomplete penetrance defect. Occurs in >5% of the population; males > females. Second most common jaundice (hepatitis is the most common). Most common hereditary cause of jaundice. Impaired UGT activity (70%–75% decrease in activity). Jaundice occurs with fasting, volume depletion, stress, menses. Serum UCB is rarely >5 mg/dL. All other liver function tests are normal. Liver biopsy is *not* necessary. *No* treatment required. • Crigler-Najjar syndromes: rare autosomal disorders with decreased to absent UGT. Type I is autosomal recessive and has *no* UGT activity; incompatible with life (liver transplantation necessary). Type II is autosomal dominant and is associated with decreased levels of UGT. • Physiologic jaundice of newborn: begins on day 3 of life. Caused by the inability of the newborn liver to handle the bilirubin load associated with the normal destruction of fetal RBCs within macrophages. • Breast milk jaundice: caused by pregnane-3α,20α-diol, which inhibits UGT. Does *not* require treatment.
MIXED			
CB 20%–50%	↑	↑	Viral hepatitis: defect in uptake, conjugation of UCB, and secretion of CB
OBSTRUCTIVE			
CB >50%	↑	Absent	• Decreased intrahepatic bile flow (obstructive jaundice) • Drug induced (e.g., oral contraceptive pills) • Primary biliary cholangitis (discussed later) • Dubin-Johnson syndrome: autosomal recessive disorder caused by impaired secretion of conjugated bilirubin into intrahepatic bile ducts (mutation in an apical canalicular membrane protein responsible for excretion of bilirubin). Black pigment is present in lysosomes in hepatocytes (? etiology; Fig. 19-1 C). • Rotor syndrome: Autosomal recessive disorder similar to Dubin-Johnson syndrome but *without* black pigment in hepatocytes • Decreased extrahepatic bile flow • Gallstone in CBD. Carcinoma of the head of pancreas causing compression of the common bile duct.

CB, Conjugated bilirubin; *CBD,* common bile duct; *HDN,* hemolytic disease of newborn; *OCP,* oral contraceptive pill; *UBG,* urobilinogen; *UCB,* unconjugated bilirubin; *UGT,* uridine glucuronosyltransferase.

%CB >50% = unconjugated hyperbilirubinemia; stone blocking CBD

Viral hepatitis: MCC jaundice

Gilbert disease: 2nd MCC jaundice; fasting ↑UCB

Prodrome, jaundice, recovery

Fever

Painful hepatomegaly

Distaste alcohol/cigarettes

Transaminases peak *before* jaundice

Atypical lymphocytosis

Jaundice

Uncommon in HCV
↑UB/urine UBG
Jaundice resolves

Lymphocytes

Apoptosis

Persistent inflammation/ fibrosis unfavorable

HAV: MC viral cause jaundice

Hepatitis A virus

MCC viral hepatitis

HAV: anti-HAV IgM indicates infection; anti-HAV IgG indicates recovery/vaccination

Hepatitis B virus

Appears 2–8 wks; 1st antigen

Persists 4 mths post recovery

HBeAg/HBV-DNA infective particles

Nonprotective ab

Persists in "window phase"
Anti-HBc IgG by 6 mths

Anti-HBs protective ab
Marker of immunization

HBsAg >6 months = chronic HBV

HBsAg, anti-HBc IgG ("healthy chronic carrier")
HBV DNA, HBeAg absent
Still contagious

HBsAg, HBeAg, HBV-DNA, anti-HBc IgG

↑Risk cirrhosis/HCC
Chronic active hepatitis risk for HCC

(d) % CB >50% defines obstructive liver disease caused by intrahepatic disease (e.g., cirrhosis) or extrahepatic disease (e.g., a gallstone blocking the CBD).

(3) Box 19-1 shows schematics of the pathophysiology of each of the major causes of jaundice (Link 19-6). Viral hepatitis is the MCC of hepatitis.

B. **Summary of liver function tests** (Table 19-2; Links 19-7 and 19-8)

C. **Summary of laboratory findings in selective liver disorders** (Table 19-3)

III. **Viral Hepatitis**

A. **Phases of acute viral hepatitis**

1. Prodrome: characterized by:
   a. fever, painful hepatomegaly (caused by stretching of the capsule of the liver).
   b. distaste for alcohol or cigarettes.
   c. steady increase in serum transaminases (AST and ALT). Transaminases peak just *before* jaundice occurs.
   d. atypical lymphocytosis (antigenically-stimulated lymphocytes; see Chapter 14).

2. jaundice
   a. Variable finding depending on the type of hepatitis (e.g., hepatitis C [HCV], where jaundice is uncommon)
   b. Increased urine bilirubin (UB) and urine UBG

3. recovery. Jaundice resolves in this phase.

B. **Microscopic findings in acute viral hepatitis**

1. Lymphocytes infiltrate the parenchyma and destroy hepatocytes (Link 19-9). Apoptosis of hepatocytes is prominent throughout the liver parenchyma (Councilman bodies; Link 19-9).

2. Persistent inflammation and fibrosis is an unfavorable sign. Sign of chronic hepatitis progressing to postnecrotic cirrhosis.

C. **Epidemiology and clinical findings of viral hepatitis** (A, B, C, D, E types; Table 19-4)

D. **Serologic studies in viral hepatitis** (A, B, C, D, E)

1. Hepatitis A virus (HAV) (Fig. 19-2 A; Link 19-15)
   a. Most common cause of viral hepatitis
   b. Anti-HAV IgM indicates active infection.
   c. Anti-HAV IgG indicates recovery from infection or previous vaccination.
      • Protective antibody

2. Hepatitis B virus (HBV) (Fig. 19-2 B and Table 19-5; Link 19-16)
   a. Acute hepatitis B serology (Link 19-17 A)
      (1) Hepatitis B surface antigen (HBsAg)
         (a) Appears within 2 to 8 weeks after exposure; first marker of infection
         (b) Persists up to 4 months in acute hepatitis. Presence of HBsAg for longer than 6 months defines chronic hepatitis B.
      (2) Hepatitis B e antigen (HBeAg) and HBV-DNA
         (a) Infective particles
         (b) Appear *after* HBsAg and disappear *before* HBsAg
      (3) Anti-HBV core antibody IgM (anti-HBc IgM)
         (a) Nonprotective antibody that remains positive in acute infections
         (b) Persists during "window phase" or "serologic gap" when HBsAg, HBV DNA, and HBeAg are absent
         (c) Converts entirely to anti-HBc IgG by 6 months
      (4) Anti-HBV surface antibody (anti-HBs)
         (a) Protective antibody
         (b) Marker of immunization after HBV vaccination
   b. Chronic HBV serology (Link 19-17 B)
      (1) Defined as the persistence of HBsAg for longer than 6 months. All of the anti-HBc IgM converts to anti-HBc IgG by 6 months.
      (2) "Healthy" chronic carrier
         (a) HBsAg and anti-HBc IgG are *both* present.
         (b) HBV DNA and HBeAg are *absent*.
         (c) Patient is still contagious but at a much lower risk.
      (3) Infective chronic carrier
         (a) HBsAg, anti-HBc IgG, and infective particles (DNA and e antigen) are all present.
         (b) Increased risk for developing postnecrotic cirrhosis and hepatocellular carcinoma (HCC; discussed later)
         (c) Chronic active hepatitis is also a risk for HCC.

BOX 19-1   Common Causes of Jaundice

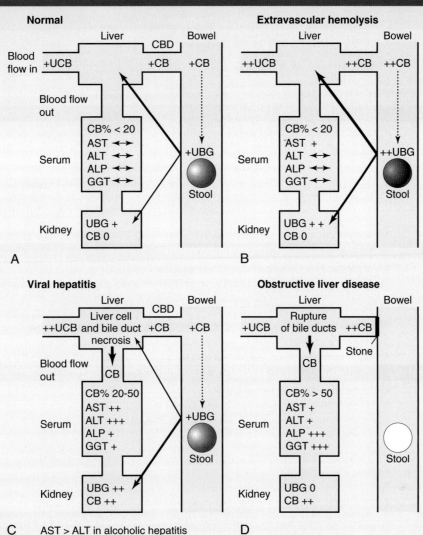

In this discussion, the symbol + is used to indicate degrees of magnitude. Normal bilirubin metabolism (A) shows liver uptake of lipid-soluble unconjugated bilirubin (UCB) and its conjugation with glucuronic acid by uridine glucuronosyltransferase producing water-soluble conjugated bilirubin (CB). CB is secreted into the common bile duct (CBD) and is emptied into the bowel. Intestinal bacteria convert CB to urobilinogen (UBG, stercobilinogen), which is spontaneously oxidized to the pigment urobilin. Urobilin is responsible for the color of stool. A small percentage of UBG is reabsorbed into the blood. Most of it enters the liver (large arrow) and a small percentage (small arrow) enters the urine (UBG). Urobilin is responsible for the color of urine. All of the normal bilirubin in blood is UCB (CB% <20%) primarily from macrophage destruction of senescent red blood cells (RBCs). UCB does not enter urine because it is attached to albumin in the blood and is soluble in lipid, not water. CB is never a normal finding in urine because it does not have contact with blood in its metabolism.

In extravascular hemolysis (B) (e.g., hereditary spherocytosis), increased macrophage production of UCB causes an increase in serum UCB (++) (CB% <20%). There is a corresponding increase in uptake and conjugation of UCB, conjugation to CB (++), and conversion of CB in the bowel to UBG (++). This causes darkening of the stool. There is a greater percentage of UBG recycled back to the liver (wide arrow) and urine (wide arrow). The increase in urine UBG (++), darkens the color of urine. Because RBCs contain the enzyme aspartate aminotransferase (AST), hemolysis of RBCs causes an increase in serum AST. Alanine aminotransferase (ALT), alkaline phosphatase (ALP), and γ-glutamyltransferase (GGT) levels are normal.

In viral hepatitis (C), there is generalized liver dysfunction involving uptake and conjugation of UCB, secretion of CB into bile ducts, and recycling of UBG. Serum UCB is increased (++) owing to a decrease in uptake and conjugation. Serum and urine CB are increased (++) because of liver cell necrosis and disruption of bile ductules between hepatocytes. Urine UBG is increased (++) because UBG is redirected from the liver (smaller arrow) to the kidneys (larger arrow). Because there is an increase in serum UCB and CB, there is a mixed hyperbilirubinemia with a CB% of 20% to 50%. In viral hepatitis, ALT is higher (+++) than AST (++) and there is a slight increase in ALP and GGT (+). In alcoholic hepatitis, AST is greater than ALT because alcohol damages mitochondria, which is where AST is normally located.

In obstructive liver disease (D), an increase in serum and urine CB (++) is caused by obstruction of intrahepatic or extrahepatic bile flow (stone in the CBD in this case). This causes increased pressure in the intrahepatic bile ductules, leading to rupture and egress of CB into sinusoidal blood. There is absence of UBG in the stool (light colored) and urine. CB% >50% and there is a marked increase in serum ALP and GGT (+++) and only a slight increase in serum AST and ALT (+).

TABLE 19-2 Liver Function Tests

TEST	DISCUSSION
	LIVER CELL NECROSIS
Serum alanine transaminase (ALT)	• Specific enzyme for liver cell necrosis • Present in the cytoplasm • ALT > AST: viral hepatitis
Serum aspartate transaminase (AST)	• Present in mitochondria • Alcohol damages mitochondria: AST > ALT indicates alcoholic hepatitis
	CHOLESTASIS
Serum γ-glutamyl-transferase (GGT)	• Present in bile duct epithelial cells • Increased in intrahepatic (bile ducts in the liver) or extrahepatic obstruction to bile flow (common bile duct obstruction) where there is compression of the bile duct epithelium causing release of GGT • Induction of cytochrome P450 system (e.g., alcohol): increases GGT (see Chapter 2)
Serum alkaline phosphatase (ALP) 5' Nucleotidase	• Normal GGT and increased ALP: source of ALP is outside the liver (e.g., osteoblastic activity in bone. Osteoblasts contain ALP.) • Increased GGT and ALP: liver cholestasis (bile duct obstruction). GGT and ALP are synthesized by bile duct epithelium; hence, both are increased • Facilitates the hydrolysis of the phosphate group from 5'-nucleotides, resulting in corresponding nucleosides
	BILIRUBIN EXCRETION
CB <20%	Unconjugated hyperbilirubinemia: e.g., extravascular hemolytic anemias (e.g., hereditary spherocytosis)
CB 20%–50%	Mixed hyperbilirubinemia (e.g., viral hepatitis)
CB >50%	Conjugated hyperbilirubinemia (e.g., bile duct obstruction)
Urine bilirubin	Bilirubinuria: viral hepatitis, intrahepatic or extrahepatic obstruction of bile ducts
Urine UBG	• Increased urine UBG: extravascular hemolytic anemias, viral hepatitis • Absent urine UBG: liver cholestasis (keeps conjugated bilirubin from entering the small intestine)
	HEPATOCYTE FUNCTION
Serum albumin	• Albumin is synthesized by the liver • Hypoalbuminemia: indicates severe liver disease (e.g., cirrhosis)
Prothrombin time (PT)	• Majority of coagulation factors are synthesized in the liver • Increased serum PT: severe liver disease
Factor V	Decreased in severe liver disease
Blood urea nitrogen (BUN)	• Urea cycle is present in the liver • Decreased serum BUN: cirrhosis, fulminant hepatitis
Serum ammonia	• Ammonia is metabolized in the urea cycle in the liver. • Ammonia derives from metabolism of amino acids and from the release of ammonia from amino acids by bacterial ureases in the bowel. It is reabsorbed from the bowel and enters the liver urea cycle, where it is converted into urea and excreted in the urine. If the liver is markedly damaged (e.g., cirrhosis, Reye syndrome), serum ammonia levels increase and contribute to hepatic encephalopathy (discussed later).
	IMMUNE FUNCTION
Serum IgM	Increased in primary biliary cholangitis (marker for the disease)
Anti-mitochondrial antibody	Primary biliary cholangitis (antibody important in causing the disease)
Anti–smooth muscle antibody	Autoimmune hepatitis
Antinuclear antibody (ANA)	Autoimmune hepatitis
	TUMOR MARKER
α-Fetoprotein (AFP)	Marker for hepatocellular carcinoma

CB, Conjugated bilirubin; *UBG,* urobilinogen.

TABLE 19-3 Summary of Laboratory Findings in Selected Liver Disorders*

DISEASE	% CB	AST	ALT	ALP	GGT	UB	URINE UBG
Normal						Absent	↑
Viral hepatitis	20–50	↑↑↑	↑↑↑↑	↑	↑	↑↑	↑↑
Alcoholic hepatitis	20–50	↑↑	↑	↑	↑↑↑	↑↑	↑↑
Cholestasis	>5%	↑	↑↑	↑↑↑	↑↑↑	↑↑↑	Absent
Extravascular hemolysis	<20	↑↑RBCs†	N	N	N	Absent	↑↑

*Arrows represent degree of magnitude.
†RBCs contain AST.
ALP, Alkaline phosphatase; *ALT,* alanine aminotransferase; *AST,* aspartate aminotransferase; *CB,* conjugated bilirubin; *GGT,* γ-glutamyltransferase; *UB,* urine bilirubin; *UBG,* urobilinogen.
From Goljan EF, Sloka KI: *Rapid Review Laboratory Testing in Clinical Medicine,* Philadelphia, Mosby, 2008, Table 9-20, p 312.

TABLE 19-4   Viral Hepatitis: Clinical Findings

VIRUS	DISCUSSION
Hepatitis A (HAV)	• Incubation, 15–50 days (average, 30 days) • RNA virus • Transmission: oral–fecal yes, sexual uncommon, blood uncommon, vertical no (transmission of a pathogen from mother to baby immediately before and after birth) • Chronic infection: no • Second most common reported acute hepatitis in United States • Most preventable infection in travelers (immunize with vaccine) • Increased incidence in children or employees in daycare centers, prisons, travelers to developing countries, men who have sex with men (anal intercourse), and parents adopting children from other countries • Virus replicates in the liver and is shed in high concentrations in feces from 2 weeks before to 1 week after the onset of clinical illness. Virus is cytotoxic to liver cells (Link 19-10). • Adults more likely to be symptomatic than children • Clinical: jaundice >70% of cases (most common hepatitis producing jaundice) • Fever, nausea or vomiting, abdominal pain • Majority recover. *No* carrier state. *No* chronic hepatitis. • Passive immunization: immunoglobulin (passive transfer of antibodies) for preexposure prophylaxis and postexposure prophylaxis • Active immunization: protective antibodies in 1 month. Recommended for all travelers to high-risk countries and all children >1 years old. • Serology discussed in III.D
Hepatitis B (HBV)	• Incubation, 30–180 days • DNA virus • Transmission: oral, yes; fecal, no; sexual, yes; blood, yes; saliva, yes; vertical transmission via pregnancy and breastfeeding, yes • Chronic infection: yes • Primarily spread via blood (IVDA 40%–60% of cases), accidental needlestick (1%–40% chance of developing HBV; most common mechanism for HBV in health care workers) • Most common reported acute hepatitis in the United States; second most common cause of fulminant hepatitis • Immunologic destruction of the virus via a type IV hypersensitivity reaction (Link 19-11) • Clinical: variable fever, profound malaise, painful hepatomegaly (87% of cases), serum sickness prodrome (15%–20% of cases), immunocomplex disease (HBsAg + antibody), vasculitis (PAN), urticaria, polyarthritis, membranous glomerulopathy • Recovery in >90% of immunocompetent patients; 1–2% develop chronic hepatitis • Hepatocytes have a "ground-glass" appearance caused by hypertrophy of the smooth endoplasmic reticulum related to excess HBsAg (Link 19-12) • Newborns and immunodeficient patients are more likely to develop chronic hepatitis (>90% of cases) • Complications: fulminant hepatitis 7% of cases; hepatocellular carcinoma secondary to chronic active hepatitis or postnecrotic cirrhosis • Prevention: immunization with recombinant vaccine • Serology discussed in III.D
Hepatitis C (HCV)	• Incubation, 2–26 weeks (average, 6–7 weeks) • RNA virus • Transmission: oral, yes; fecal, no; sexual, uncommon (unless multiple partners are involved); blood, yes, vertical uncommon (5%). Most common cause of hepatitis caused by IVDA (60%–70% of cases; >90% of persons with HIV from IVDA are infected with HCV). Hemophiliacs transfused *before* 1987. Accidental needlestick (1%–6% chance of developing HCV). Tattoo. • Chronic infection: most common chronic blood-borne infection in the United States • Third most common acute hepatitis in the United States • Most common indication for liver transplantation in the United States • Posttransfusion hepatitis is rare because of screening. • Clinical: mild hepatitis (70%–80% subclinical); jaundice uncommon (80% are anicteric) • Chronic hepatitis in 85% of cases if *not* treated. 20% develop postnecrotic cirrhosis. Histology shows "interphase hepatitis (old term, "piecemeal necrosis") in the portal triads (Link 19-13). Fatty change may also be present (only viral hepatitis with fatty change; Link 19-14). • Other clinical associations: type I membranoproliferative glomerulonephritis, alcohol excess, porphyria cutanea tarda, lichen planus, B-cell malignant lymphoma, cryoglobulinemia • Complications: HCC secondary to postnecrotic cirrhosis (1%–3% risk per year for developing HCC) • Prevention: *no* preventive vaccine available • Serology discussed in III.D
Hepatitis D (HDV)	• Incubation, variable • Incomplete RNA virus that requires HBsAg to replicate • Transmission: fecal, no; oral, unknown; vertical, yes; sexual, yes; blood, yes • Accounts for <1% of acute hepatitis in the United States • Chronic state less likely with co-infection (HBV and HDV exposure at same time; Link 19-19) than superinfection (HBV carrier exposed to blood containing HDV; Link 19-20). Cytolytic virus, so fulminant hepatitis may occur. • Chronic infection develops in 60%–85% of people infected • Prevention: immunization with recombinant vaccine for HBV • Serology discussed in III.D
Hepatitis E (HEV)	• Incubation, 15–45 days • RNA virus. • Transmission: oral, unknown; fecal, yes; sexual, unknown; blood, no; vertical, no • Occurs primarily in developing countries (increasing in the United States). • Mainly produces acute hepatitis • Chronic rarely in immunocompromised patients • Fulminant hepatitis may develop in pregnant women • Serology discussed in III.D (Link 19-21)

HBsAg, Hepatitis B surface antigen; *HCC*, hepatocellular carcinoma; *IFN*, interferon; *IVDA*, intravenous drug abuse; *MPGN*, membranoproliferative glomerulonephritis; *PAN*, polyarteritis nodosa; *PCT*, porphyria cutanea tarda.

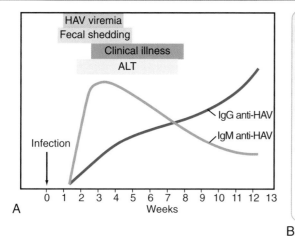
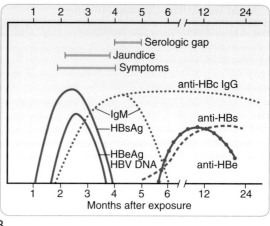

19-2: **A,** Clinical course and serologic markers in hepatitis A. **B,** Serologic markers in hepatitis B. ALT, Alanine aminotransferase; *Anti-HBc,* anti-HBV core antigen; *anti-HBe,* anti-HBV e antigen; *anti-HBs,* anti-HBV surface antibody; *HBsAg,* hepatitis B surface antigen; *HBeAg,* hepatitis B e antigen; *HAV,* hepatitis A virus; *HBV,* hepatitis B virus; *IgG,* immunoglobulin G; *IgM,* immunoglobulin M. (*A from Mandell GL, Bennett JE, Dolin R: Principles and Practice of Infectious Diseases, 7th ed, Philadelphia, Elsevier, Churchill Livingstone, 2010, p 1582, Fig. 115.4A.*)

TABLE 19-5 Serologic Studies in Hepatitis B Virus

HBSAG	HBEAG HBV DNA	ANTI-HBC IGM	ANTI-HBC IGG	ANTI-HBS	INTERPRETATION
+	−	−	−	−	Earliest phase of acute HBV
+	+	+	−	−	Acute infection
−	−	+	−	−	Window phase, or serologic gap
−	−	−	+	+	Recovered from HBV
−	−	−	−	+	Immunized
+	−	−	+	−	"Healthy" carrier
+	+	−	+	−	Infective carrier

Anti-HBc, Core antibody; *anti-HBs,* surface antibody; *HBeAg,* e antigen; *HBsAg,* surface antigen; *HBV,* hepatitis B virus.

Hepatitis C virus

Screen with EIA (infection/recovery)

Anti-HCV IgG active infection or recovery

Not protective

RIBA confirmatory test

HCV RNA PCR: viral load

HCV RNA PCR: gold standard test for DX

+RIBA, +HCV RNA PCR: active infection

+RIBA, −HCV RNA PCR: cure

Hepatitis D virus

Anti-HDV IgM/IgG active infection

Anti-HDV-IgG not protective

HCV, HDV: no protective antibodies

Coinfection same time; superinfection later date

Hepatitis E virus

3. Hepatitis C virus (HCV)
   a. Screen with enzyme immunoassay (EIA).
      (1) Presence of anti-HCV IgG indicates active infection or recovery (Link 19-18 A). Sensitivity of the test is >97%.
      (2) Does *not* differentiate among acute, chronic, or resolved infection
      (3) *Not* a protective antibody
   b. Confirmatory tests include:
      (1) recombinant immunoblot assay (RIBA).
         (a) Must be ordered if the EIA is positive
         (b) More specific but less sensitive than the EIA
      (2) HCV RNA using polymerase chain reaction (PCR) detects the viral load.
         (a) Gold standard test for diagnosing hepatitis C and diagnosing chronic HCV (Link 19-18 B [chronic HCV]).
         (b) Detects the virus as early as 1 to 2 weeks after infection
         (c) Used to monitor patients on antiviral therapy to indicate a cure from HCV
      (3) Positive RIBA and HCV RNA PCR indicates active infection.
      (4) A positive RIBA and a negative HCV RNA PCR indicates cure after treatment.
4. Hepatitis D virus (HDV)
   a. Presence of anti-HDV IgM or IgG indicates active infection.
   b. Anti-HDV-IgG is *not* a protective antibody.
   c. Chronic state may occur.
   d. Coinfection (same time) with HBV and superinfection (later date) with HBV (Links 19-19 and 19-20).
5. Hepatitis E virus (HEV)

a. Presence of anti-HEV IgM indicates active infection (Link 19-21).

b. Anti-HEV IgG indicates recovery (protective antibody).

6. Comparison table of hepatitis A, B, C, D, and E (Link 19-22)

E. **Other laboratory test findings in viral hepatitis** (see Box 19-1 C)

1. Mixed hyperbilirubinemia ($\uparrow$UCB + CB; CB 20%–50%)

a. Uptake/conjugation of UCB is decreased.

b. CB accesses the blood via damaged bile ductules.

2. Increased urine UBG and urine bilirubin

a. CB is water soluble and is filtered by the kidneys.

b. Urobilinogen (UBG) that is recycled back from the intestine to the inflamed liver (90%), and 10% is redirected to the kidneys.

3. Increased serum transaminases

a. Serum alanine aminotransferase (ALT) is greater than serum aspartate aminotransferase (AST). Serum ALT is more specific for liver cell necrosis than serum AST.

b. Serum ALT is the last liver enzyme to return to normal.

IV. **Other Inflammatory Liver Disorders**

A. **Summary of important infectious diseases** (Table 19-6; Fig. 19-3)

B. **Autoimmune hepatitis**

1. **Definition:** Type of liver inflammation characterized by hepatitis on histologic exam, autoantibodies, and hypergammaglobulinemia; negative viral serologies

Margin notes:
Anti-HEV IgM active infection

Anti-HEV IgG recovered (protective)

$\downarrow$Uptake/conjugation of UCB

Viral hepatitis: urine UBG ++, urine bilirubin ++

CB water soluble → kidneys

UBG recycled liver/kidneys

ALT > AST

ALT more specific for necrosis than AST

Serum ALT last enzyme to return to normal

Autoimmune hepatitis

Immune destruction; negative viral serologies

TABLE 19-6 Infectious Diseases of the Liver

DISEASE	PATHOGEN(S)	CHARACTERISTICS
Ascending cholangitis (Link 19-23)	*Escherichia coli*	• Inflammation of bile ducts (cholangitis) from concurrent biliary infection and duct obstruction (e.g., stone) • Life-threatening disease • Triad of fever, jaundice, RUQ pain • Most common cause of multiple liver abscesses
Liver abscess (Link 19-24)	*Escherichia coli, Bacteroides fragilis, Enterococcus faecalis*	• Two major types are pyogenic or amebic (see later) • Majority are in the right lobe and solitary. • Gram-negative aerobes (50%–70%): *E. coli* (most common), *Klebsiella* spp., *Proteus* spp. • Gram-positive aerobes (25%): *Streptococcus faecalis*, β-streptococci • Anaerobes (40%–50%): *Fusobacterium nucleatum*, *Bacteroides* spp. • Causes: ascending cholangitis (most common; 35%), intraabdominal infection (e.g., spread via the portal vein, diverticulitis, bowel perforation), direct extension (e.g., empyema of gallbladder, subphrenic abscess), hematogenous spread (e.g., bacterial endocarditis) • Clinical: spiking, intermittent fever, RUQ or right costovertebral angle tenderness. Jaundice is uncommon. Pronounced elevation alkaline phosphatase (90%). • Diagnosis: ultrasound (least expensive), CT scan
Granulomatous hepatitis	*Mycobacterium tuberculosis, Histoplasma capsulatum*	Sign of miliary spread (see Chapter 17)
Spontaneous peritonitis (see text discussion)	*Escherichia coli* in adults, *Streptococcus pneumoniae* in children.	Develops in ascites (e.g., cirrhosis, nephrotic syndrome)
Leptospirosis (Fig. 19-3 A; Link 19-25)	*Leptospira interrogans*	• Gram-negative rod; tightly wound spirochetes • Crook at the end resembles a shepherd's staff • Reservoirs: rats, dogs (most common); spirochetes are excreted in urine • Transmission: swimming in contaminated water (ponds in farms; rivers, particularly if they are rising after a rain because infected animals urinate near rivers), farmers near rivers, miners, people who work with sewage • Biphasic disease (Weil disease) • **Septicemic phase:** fever, jaundice, hemorrhagic diathesis, renal failure (interstitial nephritis), conjunctivitis and photophobia, meningitis; phase is terminated by the appearance of antibodies (beginning of immune phase) • **Immune phase:** presence of numerous organisms in the urine; urine is best examined by dark field microscopy • Diagnosis: serum enzyme immunoassay, 90% sensitive; urine test for detecting antigen is also available

Continued

TABLE 19-6   Infectious Diseases of the Liver—cont'd

DISEASE	PATHOGEN(S)	CHARACTERISTICS
Amebiasis (Fig. 19-3 B; Links 19-26 and 19-27)	*Entamoeba histolytica*	• Protozoan (amoeba) • Most common cause of a liver abscess worldwide (*not* in the United States) • Usually produces a right lobe abscess
Clonorchiasis (Link 19-28)	*Clonorchis sinensis* (Chinese liver fluke)	• Intestinal fluke (trematode) • Nonschistosomal life cycle: egg (human) → ciliated miracidial larva → infects snail (1st intermediate host) → produce fork-tailed cercarial larvae → infect a second intermediate host (fish in clonorchiasis) → form infective metacercariae → man ingests the 2nd intermediate host → develops disease • Contracted by ingesting encysted larvae in fish; larvae enter CBD and become adults • May produce cholangiocarcinoma
Schistosomiasis (Fig. 19-3 C, D; Link 19-29)	*Schistosoma mansoni*	• Fluke (trematode) • Schistosomal life cycle: egg (human) → ciliated miracidial larva → infects snail (first intermediate host) → produce fork-tailed cercarial larvae → penetrate skin in human → produce disease • *Schistosoma* mansoni: larvae in the superior mesenteric vein enter into the portal vein, where they develop into adult worms that deposit eggs to which the host develops an inflammatory response marked by concentric fibrosis ("pipestem cirrhosis") in the vessel wall. *S. japonicum* also produces pipestem cirrhosis, though it more commonly invades the urinary bladder vessels and produces squamous cancer of the bladder. • Complications of cirrhosis: portal hypertension, ascites, esophageal varices
Echinococcosis (hydatid cyst; Fig. 19-3 E, Links 19-30 and 19-31)	*Echinococcus granulosus* (sheepherder's disease)	• Intestinal tapeworm (cestode) • Single or multiple cysts contain larval forms; cysts often present in the liver (most common site), lungs, and brain. • Eggs develop into a larval form only; larval form only develops into an adult, which lays eggs • The infected sheep is the intermediate host (larval form is in the liver cyst). The dog eats the liver of a dead sheep and becomes the definitive host because the larvae develop into adults, which produce eggs. The human who accidentally ingests the embryonated eggs from the dog becomes the intermediate host because the eggs develop into larvae. The larvae in humans penetrate the bowel, and they enter the liver (most common) or other sites to produce the hydatid cyst. • May also be contracted by children eating grass contaminated with dog excreta containing the eggs • Rupture of cysts can produce anaphylaxis; therefore, care must be taken in removing the cysts at surgery.

CBD, Common bile duct; *CT,* computed tomography; *RUQ,* right upper quadrant.

2. Epidemiology
   a. Diagnosis of exclusion after viral other causes of hepatitis have been excluded
   b. Pathogenesis likely involves genetic susceptibility and a trigger (e.g., viral infection, medication).
   c. Mainly affects women (71%) at any age (but usually before the age of 40 years); however, it may also occur in patients older than 60 years of age who have concurrent autoimmune disorders (e.g., Hashimoto thyroiditis [HT], Graves disease [GD], rheumatoid arthritis).
   d. Two types of autoimmune hepatitis
      (1) Type 1 is the predominant form in the United States and worldwide (80% of cases).
      (2) Type 2 is uncommon in the United States.
   e. Range of presentations includes symptomatic hepatitis with increased transaminases, fulminant hepatitis, or cirrhosis.
   f. Associated with human leukocyte antigens (HLAs) DR3 and DR4 (see Chapter 4).
   g. Other autoimmune associations include HT and GD to name a few (see Chapter 23).
3. Clinical findings include fever, jaundice, and hepatosplenomegaly. Progression to cirrhosis is 36% in type 1 and 82% in type 1.
4. Laboratory findings for type 1 autoimmune hepatitis include:
   a. positive serum antinuclear antibody (ANA) test (>60% of cases).
   b. antibodies to soluble liver antigen (anti-SLA) have a high specificity (99%) but a low sensitivity (16%).

Dx of exclusion

Women; elderly with other diseases

Type 1 in U.S.
Type 2 uncommon in U.S.

Hepatitis, fulminant hepatitis, cirrhosis
HLA relationship
Other autoimmune associations: HT, GD
Fever, jaundice, hepatosplenomegaly

+Serum ANA

+Anti-SLA

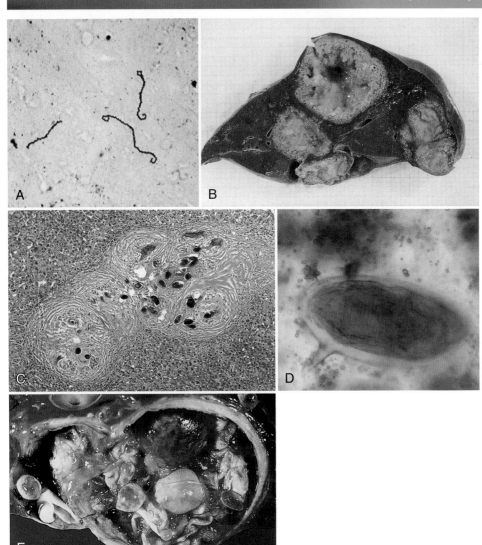

19-3: A, Silver staining of *Leptospira*, a spirochete. Notice the tightly coiled body with hooked ends. **B,** Amoebiasis with multiple amoebic abscesses, some of which show central areas of cavitation. **C,** Schistosomiasis chronic infection with pipestem cirrhosis and calcified Schistosoma eggs. **D,** *Schistosoma mansoni* egg. These eggs contain a miracidium and are enclosed in a thin shell with a prominent lateral spine. **E,** Hydatid cyst. A single cyst in the liver shows numerous daughter cysts containing larval forms (protoscoleces) in brood capsules. *(A and D from Murray PR, Rosenthal KS, Pfaller MA: Medical Microbiology, 6th ed, Philadelphia, Mosby Elsevier, 2009, pp 417, 877, respectively, Figs. 42.10, 84.9, respectively; B, C, and E from MacSween R, Burt A, Portmann B, et al: Pathology of the Liver, 4th ed, London, Churchill Livingstone, 2002, pp 383, 390, 388, respectively, Figs. 8.27, 8.41b, 8-35, respectively.)*

    c. anti–smooth muscle antibodies (>85% of cases).

    d. anti-actin, antisoluble liver antigen/liver pancreas.

    e. increased serum transaminases.

  5. Laboratory findings for type 2 autoimmune hepatitis include negative serum ANA, positive liver/kidney microsome (LKM) type 1 and 3 antibodies, and variable presence of liver cytosol (LC) type 1 antibodies.

C. Neonatal hepatitis

  1. **Definition:** Type of hepatitis of varied etiology that occurs soon after birth and is characterized by prolonged persistent jaundice that may progress to cirrhosis

  2. Epidemiology: may be idiopathic or associated with congenital infections (e.g., cytomegalovirus [CMV]) or inborn errors of metabolism (e.g., α_1-antitrypsin deficiency), cystic fibrosis, and bile duct obstruction, to name a few causes

  3. Liver biopsy shows multinucleated giant cells (MGCs; giant cell hepatitis; Link 19-32), cholestasis, giant cell change, extramedullary hematopoiesis (EMH; nucleated RBCs), inflammation, and fibrosis.

D. Reye syndrome

  1. **Definition:** Characterized by acute encephalopathy and a fatty liver that progresses to liver failure

  2. Epidemiology

    a. Postinfectious triad that defines Reye syndrome includes:

      (1) encephalopathy.

      (2) microvesicular fatty change (Fig. 19-4 A; Link 19-33).

      (3) serum transaminase elevation.

Margin notes:

+Anti-smooth muscle abs

Autoimmune hepatitis: + serum ANA, + anti–smooth muscle antibodies

+Serum ANA, +Anti LKM abs, Anti LC abs

Neonatal hepatitis

Persistent jaundice → cirrhosis

Idiopathic, congenital infections, inborn errors

MGCs, cholestasis, EMH, inflammation/fibrosis

Reye syndrome

Encephalopathy

Microvesicular fatty change

↑Transaminases

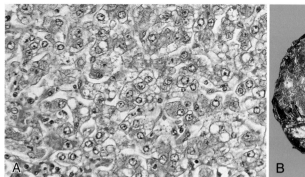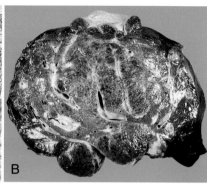

19-4: **A,** Reye syndrome showing microvesicular fatty change (clear spaces in cytosol). **B,** Fulminant liver failure. There is massive necrosis in the liver. The red zones represent necrosis with no hepatocytes, and the brown nodules are regenerative nodules. **(A** and **B** from MacSween R, Burt A, Portmann B, Ishak K, Scheuer P, Anthony P: Pathology of the Liver, 4th ed, London, Churchill Livingstone, 2002, pp 133, 315, respectively, Figs. 3.47, 7.1, respectively.)

Aspirin important role

Aspirin + infection (varicella, influenza)

mT damage
Disruption urea cycle
↑Serum ammonia

Defective β-oxidation FAs → fatty change

No inflammation

Hepatomegaly, liver dysfunction

Cerebral edema

Sleepy but respond → stuporous → obtundation → coma

↑Serum transaminases
N/↑serum bilirubin

↑Serum ammonia, PT
Hypoglycemia
Normal CSF analysis
High mortality rate
Acute fatty liver pregnancy

Abnormal β-oxidation FAs; microvesicular fatty change

Twin, 1st pregnancy
31 wks to 38 wks
Vomiting, pain, jaundice
Encephalopathy, renal failure

Deliver baby quickly

Preeclampsia

HTN, proteinuria, pitting edema, 3rd trimester

b. Uncommon since the role of aspirin was elucidated.
c. Usually develops in children <4 years old and often follows a varicella or influenza infection.
3. Pathogenesis includes:
  a. mitochondrial (mT; damage (? virus, salicylates).
  b. disruption of urea cycle (normally used to metabolize ammonia); causes an increase in serum ammonia.
  c. defective β-oxidation of fatty acids (FAs) in damaged mitochondria. More FAs are available to synthesize triglyceride (TG; fatty change; see Chapter 2).
4. Microvesicular fatty change is present in the liver.
  a. Small cytoplasmic globules are present in hepatocytes *without* nuclear displacement (Link 19-33).
  b. *No* inflammatory infiltrate
5. Clinical findings
  a. Initially, the neonate is afebrile, quiet, lethargic, sleepy, and vomiting. Hepatomegaly and liver dysfunction are present.
  b. Encephalopathy (cerebral edema with increased cerebral pressure) findings in progression include:
    (1) sleepy but responsive; vomiting.
    (2) stuporous, seizures, decorticate rigidity, intact papillary reflexes.
    (3) deepening coma, decerebrate rigidity, fixed pupils.
    (4) coma, loss of deep tendon reflexes, fixed dilated pupils, flaccidity or decerebrate.
    (5) death.
6. Laboratory findings include:
  a. increased serum transaminases (AST and ALT).
  b. normal to slight increase in TB.
  c. increased serum ammonia and prothrombin time (PT). Serum levels of ammonia and degree of prolongation of the PT predict the degree of severity.
  d. hypoglycemia caused by impaired glycogenesis and gluconeogenesis in the liver.
  e. cerebrospinal fluid (CSF) analysis is usually normal.
7. Mortality rate is ~ 25% to 50%.
E. **Acute fatty liver of pregnancy; epidemiology and clinical**
  1. **Definition:** Abnormality in the β-oxidation of FAs. Microvesicles of fat develop in the cytosol (microvesicular fatty change; Link 19-34).
  2. Epidemiology
    a. More common in twin and first pregnancies
    b. Presents between 31 weeks to 38 weeks with vomiting, abdominal pain, and jaundice. Severe cases may have encephalopathy, lactic acidosis, hyperuricemia, and renal failure.
  3. Must deliver baby quickly.
  4. Maternal and neonatal mortality rates are 1% and 7%, respectively.
F. **Preeclampsia** (see Chapter 22)
  1. **Definition:** Hypertension (HTN), proteinuria, and dependent pitting edema; usually occurs in the third trimester.

2. Liver cell necrosis is present around the portal triads (zone 1; see Fig. 2-6 B). Serum transaminases are increased.

3. Associated with the HELLP syndrome, which includes:
   a. <u>h</u>emolytic anemia with schistocytes (see Chapter 12).
   b. <u>e</u>levated serum transaminases.
   c. <u>l</u>ow platelets caused by disseminated intravascular coagulation (DIC; see Chapter 15).

G. **Fulminant hepatic failure (FHF)**
   1. **Definition:** Acute liver failure (ALF) with encephalopathy within 8 weeks of hepatic dysfunction in the absence of evidence of preexisting disease; does *not* represent a deterioration in liver function associated with chronic liver disease
   2. Epidemiology
      a. Occurs when there is insufficient synthetic and metabolic function to meet the needs of the patient
      b. Causes include:
         (1) drugs (e.g., acetaminophen [paracetamol] most common drug); account for most cases of ALF in the United States.
         (2) viral hepatitis (most common cause worldwide), hepatitis B.
         (3) viruses (e.g., herpes viruses, enteroviruses, parvovirus), hepatitis D. Reye syndrome, Wilson disease, and autoimmune hepatitis.
         (4) mushroom poisoning caused by *Amanita phalloides.*
   3. Gross and microscopic findings include (Fig. 19-4 B):
      a. wrinkled capsular surface caused by loss of the hepatic parenchyma (Link 19-35).
      b. dull red areas of necrotic parenchyma (Link 19-35 *interrupted circle*) with regenerative nodules (Link 19-35 *solid circle*) and blotches of green (bile).
      c. loss of hepatocytes and multinucleated giant cells (MCGs) (Link 19-36).
   4. Clinical findings include hepatic encephalopathy (see the following) and jaundice. Laboratory findings include:
      a. decrease in serum transaminases indicating that the liver parenchyma is destroyed.
      b. progressive increase in the PT (reduced synthesis of some coagulation factors) and serum ammonia (defective urea cycle).

V. **Circulatory Disorders of the Liver**
   A. **Prehepatic obstruction to blood flow**
      1. **Definition:** Obstruction of blood flow to the liver (i.e., hepatic artery, portal vein [PV])
      2. Hepatic artery thrombosis with infarction; epidemiology
         a. Liver infarction (usually pale infarction) is uncommon because of a dual blood supply (Fig. 19-5 A). Hepatic artery and portal vein (PV) tributaries normally empty blood into the sinusoids.
         b. Causes of hepatic artery thrombosis with infarction include:
            (1) liver transplant rejection.
            (2) vasculitis caused by polyarteritis nodosa (PAN; see Chapter 10).
      3. PV thrombosis; epidemiology
         a. Causes include:
            (1) pylephlebitis (inflammation of the PV).
               (a) Most often a complication of acute appendicitis (see Chapter 18)
               (b) Air is present in the PV from bacterial gas.

Zone 1 liver necrosis; ↑transaminases

Hemolytic anemia/schistocytes

Elevated transaminases

Low platelets

DIC

Fulminant hepatic failure

ALF/encephalopathy 8 wks; *no* preexisting disease

Insufficient synthetic/metabolic function

Drugs MCC

Acetaminophen MC drug

Viral hepatitis MCC worldwide

Wrinkled capsule

Necrosis, regenerative nodules

Loss hepatocytes; MGCs

Encephalopathy/jaundice

↓Transaminases, ↑PT, ammonia

Circulatory disorders

Prehepatic obstruction

Obstruction blood flow to liver

Hepatic artery thrombosis/infarction

Uncommon; dual blood supply

Hepatic artery/PV empty into sinusoids

Transplant rejection

PAN

Portal vein thrombosis

Pylephlebitis (inflammation PV)

Complication appendicitis

Air in PV

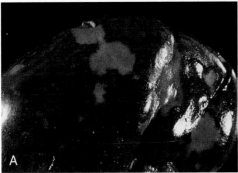
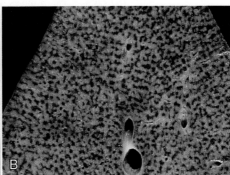

19-5: A, Liver infarctions showing multiple irregular pale areas of infarction. **B,** Centrilobular hemorrhagic necrosis ("nutmeg" liver). The liver has a mottled cut surface. Dark areas represent congested central venules and sinusoids. (***A** from my friend Ivan Damjanov, MD, PhD: Pathology for the Health-Related Professions, 2nd ed, Philadelphia, Saunders, 2000, p 134, Fig. 6-12; **B** from my friend Ivan Damjanov, MD, PhD, Linder J: Pathology: A Color Atlas, St. Louis, Mosby, 2000, p 146, Fig. 8-8.)*

(2) polycythemia vera (hyperviscosity of blood; see Chapter 13).

(3) hepatocellular carcinoma (HCC). Tumor invasion of the PV commonly occurs.

b. Clinical findings include portal hypertension, ascites, splenomegaly and no hepatomegaly.

B. **Intrahepatic obstruction to blood flow**

1. **Definition:** Intrahepatic obstruction of sinusoidal blood flow

2. Causes include:

a. cirrhosis (most common cause; see Section VIII).

b. centrilobular hemorrhagic necrosis (see later).

c. peliosis hepatis (see later).

d. sickle cell disease (see Chapter 12).

3. Centrilobular hemorrhagic necrosis

a. **Definition:** Hemorrhage and necrosis around the central venule caused by an increase in pressure in the vena cava from right-sided heart failure (RHF) or hypoperfusion in left-sided heart failure (LHF)

b. In LHF, the cardiac output is decreased, causing hypoperfusion of the liver. Hypoperfusion leads to ischemic necrosis of hepatocytes located around the central venules (zone III; Fig. 2-6 B). RHF causes a backup of systemic venous blood into the central venules and sinusoids and the PV.

c. The liver is enlarged and has a mottled red appearance ("nutmeg" liver; Fig. 19-5 B).

(1) Congestion of central venules and sinusoids is prominent.

(2) Necrosis of hepatocytes first occurs around the central venules in zone III. Other zones may be involved if central venous pressures remained increased.

d. Clinical findings include:

(1) painful hepatomegaly with or without jaundice.

(2) increased serum transaminases caused by ischemic necrosis of hepatocytes.

(3) possible progression to cirrhosis (known as "cardiac cirrhosis"). Fibrosis occurs around the central venules.

4. Peliosis hepatis

a. **Definition:** Sinusoidal dilation caused by blood

b. Causes include:

(1) anabolic steroids.

(2) *Bartonella henselae* causing bacillary angiomatosis (see Chapter 10); commonly occurs in AIDS

c. Potential for developing intraperitoneal hemorrhage

C. **Posthepatic obstruction to blood flow**

1. **Definition:** Obstruction of blood flow exiting the liver (e.g., hepatic vein obstruction)

2. Causes include hepatic vein thrombosis and venoocclusive disease.

3. Hepatic vein thrombosis (Budd-Chiari syndrome)

a. Causes include:

(1) polycythemia vera (caused by hyperviscosity; see Chapter 13); most common cause of hepatic vein thrombosis (up to 40% of cases).

(2) hypercoagulable state (20% of cases; see Chapter 15); for example:

(a) oral contraceptive pills (OCPs).

(b) proteins C and S deficiency.

(c) antiphospholipid syndrome (APLS).

(3) HCC <5% of cases. Cancer invades the hepatic vein.

b. Clinical findings include:

(1) painful hepatomegaly.

(2) Portal hypertension, ascites, and splenomegaly.

(3) high mortality rate.

c. Laboratory findings include increased serum transaminases and a prolonged PT.

d. Diagnostic tests include ultrasonography (US) with pulsed Doppler as a first-line test and magnetic resonance imaging (MRI).

e. Prognosis: mortality rate of 75% in the first year

4. Venoocclusive disease

a. **Definition:** A hepatic sinusoidal obstruction syndrome characterized by hepatomegaly with right upper quadrant (RUQ) pain, jaundice, and ascites

b. Complication of bone marrow (BM) transplantation

c. Fibrosis develops around the central venules.

D. **Hematobilia**

• **Definition:** Blood in the bile in patients with trauma to the liver

VI. Alcohol-Related and Drug- and Chemical-Induced Liver Disorders

A. Alcohol-related disorders; epidemiology

1. Risk factors for alcohol-related liver disease include the amount and duration of alcohol intake, female sex, and Asian descent (see Chapter 7).

2. Pathways for alcohol metabolism (see Chapters 2 and 7). Three enzyme systems in the liver are involved in the biotransformation of alcohol to acetaldehyde and include (1) alcohol dehydrogenase in the cytoplasm of hepatocytes; (2) the microsomal ethanol-oxidizing system (MEOS; see Chapter 2); and (3) peroxisomes, where catalase is the key enzyme.

3. Types of liver disease

   a. Fatty change is the most common type of disease (see Figs. 2-11, 2-12 A, B; Link 19-37).

      (1) **Definition:** Reversible disorder characterized by the presence of large vacuoles of TG in the cytoplasm of hepatocytes, which is called steatosis

      (2) Substrates of alcohol metabolism are used to synthesize liver TGs, which accumulate in the cytoplasm (see Chapter 2) and push the nuclei to the periphery of the liver cells.

      (3) Clinical and laboratory findings include painful hepatomegaly *without* fever and neutrophilic leukocytosis.

   b. Alcoholic hepatitis

      (1) **Definition:** Severe, progressive inflammatory disease of the liver characterized by fatty change, neutrophilic infiltration of the liver, and fibrosis

      (2) Epidemiology

         (a) Occurs in 15% to 20% of alcoholics

         (b) Majority are middle-aged men (40–50 years of age).

         (c) Women develop alcoholic hepatitis over a shorter time period than do men and with smaller amounts of alcohol because of decreased amounts of alcohol dehydrogenase (ALDH) in their gastric mucosa than in men's (see Chapter 7).

         (d) Increased incidence in minority groups (Hispanic ethnicity)

         (e) Pathophysiology relates to increased reactive oxygen species as well as inflammatory cytokines (e.g., tumor necrosis factor-α).

         (f) Stimulation of collagen synthesis around the central venules produces perivenular fibrosis (characteristic finding).

      (2) Microscopic findings include:

         (a) fatty change with neutrophil infiltration.

         (b) Mallory-Denk bodies in the cytoplasm, which represent damaged cytokeratin intermediate filaments (Fig. 2-11; Link 19-38). Mallory-Denk bodies are not a specific finding for alcoholic liver damage and can be seen in other diseases (Wilson's disease [25%], primary biliary cirrhosis [PBC; 24%], nonalcoholic cirrhosis [24%], HCC [23%], morbid obesity [8%], and intestinal bypass surgery [6%]).

         (c) perivenular fibrosis.

      (3) Clinical findings include:

         (a) fever, painful hepatomegaly.

         (b) ascites, hepatic encephalopathy.

         (c) possible progression to alcoholic cirrhosis.

      (4) Laboratory findings include (see Fig. 7-1 A, B):

         (a) absolute neutrophilic leukocytosis (12,000 to 14,000 cells/μL).

         (b) two times greater increase in serum AST than ALT because AST is located in the mitochondria (mT), and alcohol damages the mT in hepatocytes (see Chapter 7).

         (c) increase in serum alkaline phosphatase (ALP) and γ-glutamyltransferase (GGT), the latter enzyme a product of induction of the smooth endoplasmic reticulum by alcohol causing increased synthesis of the enzyme (see Chapter 7). Explains why serum GGT is disproportionately increased compared with ALP (see Table 19-2).

         (d) thrombocytopenia (<125,000 cells/μL; see Chapter 15) caused by sequestration in the enlarged spleen in portal hypertension, decreased production of thrombopoietin by the liver, and reduced synthesis of platelets from megakaryocytes in the bone marrow.

         (e) fasting hypoglycemia. Increased levels of nicotinamide adenine dinucleotide (NADH) convert pyruvate to lactate; hence, less pyruvate is available for gluconeogenesis (fasting state reaction). In addition, glycogen stores are decreased in alcoholics with severe liver disease.

↑AG metabolic acidosis

Lactic acidosis

↑β-OHB ketoacidosis; *not* detected with dipstick

Hyperuricemia

↑↑Serum TG (type IV)

↓Albumin, ↑γ-globulins

Polyclonal gammopathy

↑INR; ↓synthesis coagulation factors, ↓vitamin K

Macrocytic anemia; ↓folic acid, alcohol effect RBC membrane

Alcohol levels: blood, breath, urine tests

↑Urine ethyl glucuronide

↑Serum ferritin (APR)

NAFLD

Association with metabolic syndrome

Obese, diabetes mellitus (insulin resistance)

Hyperlipidemia, TPN

Bacterial overgrowth

Medications

Fatty change unrelated to alcohol; MC steatosis in U.S.

May progress to NASH, cirrhosis

MCC chronic ↑transaminases in children

Possible cirrhosis, portal hypertension, ascites, liver failure

Risk for HCC

Cirrhosis

Obstructive (cholestatic) liver disease

Mechanical block intra- or extrahepatic bile ducts

Intrahepatic cholestasis

Drugs MCC intrahepatic cholestasis

OCPs, anabolic steroids

Neonatal hepatitis

Pregnancy

Extrahepatic cholestasis

Gallstone block CBD

Stone from gallbladder

MCC extrahepatic cholestasis

PSC, EHBA

Carcinoma CBD, ampulla, head pancreas

Enlarged, green liver

Ducts distended, lakes, infarcts

(f) increased anion gap (AG) metabolic acidosis (see Chapter 5) caused by:
- lactic acidosis because NADH converts pyruvate to lactate.
- β-hydroxybutyric (β-OHB) ketoacidosis because excess acetyl CoA is converted to β-OHB acid in the liver. It is *not* detected with a urine dipstick or by the blood test for ketone bodies.

(g) hyperuricemia (potential for developing gout). Lactic acid and β-OHB excretion into the urine increases uric acid reabsorption in the proximal tubules, leading to hyperuricemia.

(h) hypertriglyceridemia. Caused by increased production of glycerol 3-phosphate, the key substrate that is required for TG synthesis in the liver. This is a type IV hyperlipoproteinemia (see Chapters 2 and 10).

(i) hypoalbuminemia, hypergammaglobulinemia (↑IgG and IgA; polyclonal gammopathy; see Chapter 3).

(j) increased international normalized ratio (INR) caused by decreased liver synthesis of coagulation factors and vitamin K deficiency (cannot activate vitamin K with epoxide reductase).

(k) macrocytic anemia caused by folic acid deficiency or alcohol's effect on RBC membrane.

(l) blood, breath, urine tests for alcohol (detection period, 8 hours or less).

(m) increased urine ethyl glucuronide (excellent indicator of recent alcohol ingestion; better than blood alcohol levels).

(n) increased serum ferritin (acute phase reactant [APR]; see Chapter 3). Levels may be as high as 5000 ng/mL (normal, 12–300 ng/mL).

c. Nonalcoholic fatty liver disease (NAFLD)

(1) Most commonly associated with metabolic syndrome in obese patients with diabetes mellitus (see Chapter 23). Insulin resistance is the hallmark of metabolic syndrome.

(2) Other risk factors include hyperlipidemia, prolonged total parenteral nutrition (TPN), bacterial overgrowth in small bowel, and certain medications (e.g., corticosteroids, calcium channel blockers, methotrexate).

(3) Fatty change (steatosis) occurs in the absence of alcohol intake. Most common liver disease in the United States causing fatty change of the liver (33% of population)

(4) May progress to nonalcoholic steatohepatitis (NASH), which involves inflammation of the liver and an increase in aminotransferases. May also progress to cirrhosis later in life (fifth to sixth decades of life).

(5) May occur in children and adolescents. Most frequent cause of chronic elevation of aminotransferases in children. Can lead to cirrhosis of the liver with concomitant portal hypertension, ascites, and liver failure. The increase of NASH in children is the growing epidemic of childhood obesity.

(6) Risk for HCC if fatty change is present for over 10 to 15 years

d. Cirrhosis (see later)

B. Chemical- and drug-induced liver diseases (Table 19-7; Link 19-39)

VII. Obstructive (Cholestatic) Liver Disease

A. Types of cholestatic liver disease

1. **Definition:** Mechanical blockage (cholestasis) of the intrahepatic or extrahepatic bile ducts (CBD) causing CB to enter the bloodstream, producing jaundice (Link 19-40)

2. Intrahepatic cholestasis; causes include:

a. drugs (e.g., OCPs, anabolic steroids). Drugs are the most common causes of intrahepatic cholestasis.

b. neonatal hepatitis (previously discussed).

c. pregnancy-induced cholestasis (estrogen).

3. Extrahepatic cholestasis; causes include (Link 19-41):

a. gallstone, blocking the CBD.

(1) Usually comes from the gallbladder

(2) Most common cause of extrahepatic cholestasis

b. primary sclerosing cholangitis (PSC), extrahepatic biliary atresia (EHBA).

c. carcinoma of the head of the CBD, ampulla of Vater, head of pancreas.

B. Gross and microscopic findings include:

1. enlarged, greenish colored liver.

2. bile ducts distended with bile (Fig. 19-6 A), bile lakes, and bile infarcts.

TABLE 19-7 Drug- and Chemical-Induced Liver Diseases

DISEASE	CAUSE
TUMORS	
Angiosarcoma (Link 19-71)	Vinyl chloride, arsenic, thorium dioxide (radioactive contrast material)
Cholangiocarcinoma (Link 19-74)	Thorium dioxide
Hepatocellular carcinoma (Links 19-69 and 19-70)	Vinyl chloride, aflatoxin (produced by *Aspergillus* mold)
Liver cell adenoma (Link 19-67)	OCPs, anabolic steroids
OTHER LIVER DISEASES	
Acute hepatitis	Isoniazid (caused by toxic metabolite), halothane, acetaminophen, methyldopa
Cholestasis (Link 19-39)	OCPs (estrogen interferes with intrahepatic bile secretion), anabolic steroids (same mechanism as OCPs)
Fatty change	Amiodarone (resembles alcoholic hepatitis; Mallory bodies and progression to cirrhosis), methotrexate
Fibrosis	Methotrexate, retinoic acid, amiodarone
HERBAL INJURIES	
	• Majority are idiosyncratic; others are dose dependent • Increase in serum transaminases most common • Peripheral blood eosinophilia with or without rash may be present • Cirrhosis or liver failure may occur • Germander (hepatitis), Chinese herbal tea (venoocclusive disease), Jin Bu Huan (hepatitis, fatty change), valerian (hepatitis), Gordo lobo yerba tea (venoocclusive disease), kava kava (hepatitis), Dai-saiko-to (hepatitis, fatty change, fibrosis), to name a few
Medication injuries	• Fatty change (steatosis): alcohol, tetracycline, amiodarone, prednisone • Cholestasis: estrogen, chlorpromazine, tricyclics, carbamazepine, clotrimazole, anabolic steroids • Granulomatous inflammation: quinidine, sulfonamides, allopurinol, sulfonylurea • Venoocclusive disease: azathioprine, pyrrolizidine, antineoplastics, alkaloids • Viral-like hepatitis: methyldopa, aspirin, phenytoin, isoniazid, amiodarone, propylthiouracil, sulfonamides

OCP, Oral contraceptive pill.

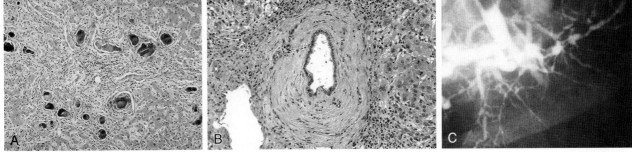

19-6: **A,** Cholestasis. Note the dilated bile ductules filled with yellowish-green bile. **B,** Liver biopsy in primary sclerosing cholangitis reveals prominent periductal fibrosis in the characteristic "onion-skin" pattern. **C,** Cholangiogram in primary sclerosing cholangitis reveals the characteristic beading pattern of bile ducts caused by multifocal strictures at those sites. (*A from Klatt E:* Robbins and Cotran Atlas of Pathology, *Philadelphia, Saunders, 2006, p 199, Fig. 8-11; **B** and **C** from McPherson R, Pincus M:* Henry's Clinical Diagnosis and Management by Laboratory Methods, *22nd ed, Philadelphia, Saunders, 2011, p 1014, Fig. 53.8B and A, respectively.)*

C. Clinical findings include:
1. jaundice with pruritus (severe itching of the skin). Pruritus is thought to be caused by bile salts deposited in the skin.
2. malabsorption of fat (see Chapter 18). Bile salts do *not* enter the small intestine, which causes malabsorption of fat.
3. cholesterol (CH) deposits in skin.
   a. Bile contains cholesterol.
   b. Example: xanthelasma (see Fig. 10-4 B).
4. light colored ("clay colored" stools) because of a lack of urobilin. CB does *not* enter the small intestine; therefore, intestinal bacteria *cannot* convert it into urobilinogen (UBG), which becomes urobilin (pigment responsible for stool color).

Jaundice, pruritus

Malabsorption of fat
CH deposits in skin
Bile contains CH
Xanthelasma

Light-colored stools; lack urobilin

↑TB with CB >50%

Bilirubinuria (CB in urine)

Absent UBG

↑ALP, ↑GGT, ↑5′ nucleotidase

Cholestasis: urine UBG 0, urine bilirubin ++

Benign intrahepatic cholestasis of pregnancy

Estrogen-induced cholestasis late pregnancy

MC pregnancy liver disorder

Estrogen inhibits intrahepatic bile secretion

↑Serum bile acids

Not dangerous to mother/fetus

Late second/early 3rd trimester

Pruritus palms/soles feet → generalized

Extrahepatic biliary atresia

EHBDs narrow/blocked/absent

3rd week of life → dark urine, acholic stools

No gender predilection

Not inherited

Inflammatory destruction all/part EH bile ducts

Bile duct proliferation portal triads

Hepatomegaly, +/− splenomegaly

Rectal exam: acholic stool

Immune response viral infection

Possible gene mutation

Common indication liver transplant

Primary sclerosing cholangitis

Cholestatic disorder; periductal fibrosis

Fibrosis intra/extrahepatic bile ducts

HLA association

Male dominant

Association ulcerative colitis > Crohn disease

Cirrhosis, cholangiocarcinoma

Jaundice

Pruritus

Hepatosplenomegaly

CB > 50%

Bilirubinuria

D. **Laboratory findings** (see Box 19-1 D) **include:**
1. increase in total bilirubin (TB) with CB representing >50% of the TB.
2. bilirubinuria (CB is soluble in urine). Urine is yellow because of CB.
3. absent urine UBG. Because CB in bile does not enter the bowel, intestinal bacteria cannot convert CB into UBG. Therefore, less UBG is reabsorbed (enterohepatic circulation), and less is excreted in the urine. Although the normal color of urine is caused by urobilin, the breakdown product of UBG, the yellow color of urine in cholestatic jaundice is caused by CB.
4. increase in serum ALP, GGT, and 5′ nucleotidase.
5. increase in serum cholesterol (present in bile).
6. urinalysis dipstick shows UBG 0, urine bilirubin++, signs of cholestasis.

E. **Benign intrahepatic cholestasis of pregnancy**
1. **Definition:** Reversible type of estrogen-induced cholestasis that occurs in genetically predisposed women in late pregnancy; characterized by intense pruritus with or without jaundice
2. Epidemiology
   a. Most common pregnancy-related liver disorders (1% of pregnancies)
   b. Caused by estrogen inhibition of intrahepatic bile secretion
   c. Serum bile acids are increased.
   d. *Not* dangerous to the mother or fetus
   e. Most commonly occurs in the late second or early third trimester
3. Clinical findings include generalized pruritus with pruritus beginning on the palms and soles of the feet.
4. Delivery is recommended at 37 weeks because of the intensity of the pruritus.

F. **Extrahepatic biliary atresia (EHBA)**
1. **Definition:** Fibro-obliterative destruction of the extrahepatic bile ducts (EHBDs) that occurs in the first 3 months of life
2. Epidemiology
   a. Causes jaundice in newborns that is first recognized in the third week of life. In addition, there is increasingly dark urine and acholic (light-colored) stools.
   b. *No* gender predilection; not inherited (80% of cases)
   c. Inflammatory destruction of all or part of the extrahepatic bile ducts
   d. Bile duct proliferation is present in the portal triads (Link 19-42).
   e. Hepatomegaly with or without splenomegaly
   f. Rectal exam reveals acholic stool.
   g. In 80% of cases, it is thought to be a pathological immune response to a viral infection (e.g., reovirus, rotavirus). Less commonly (20%), it may be a fetal malformation syndrome caused by mutation in a gene that is involved in regulating bile duct development.
   h. Common indication for liver transplantation in children

G. **Primary sclerosing cholangitis (PSC)**
1. **Definition:** Chronic progressive cholestatic disorder characterized by periductal fibrosis ("onion skinning") and chronic inflammation (CI) of both intrahepatic and extrahepatic bile ducts
2. Epidemiology
   a. Obliterative fibrosis of intrahepatic and extrahepatic bile ducts (see Fig. 19-6A, B; Link 19-43)
   b. Genetic predisposition for the disease and an association with HLA-DR52a (100%) and HLA-Cw7 (86%)
   c. Male dominant (70% of cases) and usually occurs in individuals <45 years old
   d. Associations with:
      (1) inflammatory bowel disease (IBD; 70% of cases; ulcerative colitis > Crohn disease).
      (2) other sclerosing disorders (retroperitoneal and mediastinal sclerosing fibrosis)
   e. Complications include cirrhosis and cholangiocarcinoma (cancer of the bile ducts). Other malignancy associations include gallbladder cancer and colorectal cancer.
3. Clinical findings in PSC include:
   a. jaundice.
   b. pruritus caused by deposition of bile salts/acids in skin.
   c. Hepatosplenomegaly (related to portal hypertension in cirrhosis).
4. Laboratory findings include:
   a. serum CB >50%.
   b. bilirubinuria.

      c. absent urine UBG and light-colored stools because CB does *not* enter the bowel for conversion to UBG.

      d. increase in serum ALP, GGT, and 5′ nucleotidase, the obstructive liver enzymes.

    5. Diagnosis is made with endoscopic retrograde cholangiopancreatography (ERCP), which shows narrowing and dilation of bile ducts ("beading"; Fig. 19-6 C; Links 19-43 and 19-44).

VIII. Cirrhosis

  A. Definition: Irreversible diffuse fibrosis of the liver with the formation of regenerative nodules (non-neoplastic nodules *without* sinusoids or portal triads)

  B. Regenerative nodules in cirrhosis

    1. Hepatocyte reaction to injury (Fig. 19-7)

    2. Lack portal triads and sinusoids (see Fig. 3-17)

    3. Nodules are surrounded by bands of fibrosis (Links 19-45, 19-46, 19-47, 19-48, and 19-49), which compress the sinusoids and central venules, leading to:

      a. intrasinusoidal HTN caused by an increase in hydrostatic pressure in the PV.

      b. reduction in the number of functional sinusoids.

      c. micronodular cirrhosis (nodule ~1 mm diameter; usually alcoholic cirrhosis; Link 19-47), macronodular cirrhosis (nodules >1 mm diameter and varying sizes; Link 19-46).

  C. Causes of cirrhosis include:

    1. alcoholic liver disease (ALD; most common cause of cirrhosis).

    2. postnecrotic cirrhosis caused by chronic hepatitis B or hepatitis C.

    3. autoimmune disease (PBC, autoimmune hepatitis).

    4. metabolic diseases, including hemochromatosis, Wilson's disease, α_1-antitrypsin (AAT) deficiency, and galactosemia (see Chapter 6).

  D. Complications associated with cirrhosis

    1. Hepatic failure

      a. **Definition:** End-point of progressive damage to the liver

      b. Numerous coagulation defects (see Chapter 15) caused by:

        (1) inability to synthesize coagulation factors, leading to a bleeding disorder.

        (2) decreased synthesis of protein C/S, causing the patient to be hypercoagulable.

      c. Hypoalbuminemia from decreased synthesis of albumin. Produces dependent pitting edema (see Fig. 5-3 C) and ascites (see Fig. 5-18 D) because of a decrease in plasma oncotic pressure (OP; see Chapter 5).

      d. Hepatic encephalopathy

        (1) **Definition:** Accumulation of toxic products that impair mental function in hepatic failure (Link 19-50)

        (2) Epidemiology

          (a) Reversible metabolic disorder

          (b) Increase in the blood of aromatic amino acids (e.g., phenylalanine, tyrosine, tryptophan) that are then converted into false neurotransmitters (e.g., γ-aminobutyric acid)

          (c) Increase in serum ammonia caused by a defective urea cycle in the liver that *cannot* metabolize ammonia

Ammonia derives from metabolism of amino acids and from the release of ammonia from amino acids by bacterial ureases in the bowel. Ammonia (NH_3) is diffusible and is reabsorbed into the portal vein for delivery to the urea cycle, where it is metabolized into urea. Ammonium (NH_4^+) is *not* reabsorbed in the bowel and is excreted in stool. Methods for reducing ammonia in the colon include restriction of protein intake (most cost-effective) and the use of oral neomycin, which destroys the colonic bacteria that synthesize ureases. Oral administration of lactulose results in the release of hydrogen ions, causing NH_3 to be converted to NH_4^+, which is excreted in the feces.

         (d) Factors precipitating encephalopathy include:

           • increased protein (most important factor) related to dietary sources or blood in the gastrointestinal tract, either of which leads to increased bacterial conversion of urea into ammonia.

           • metabolic alkalosis (e.g., from diuretics; see Chapter 5), which keeps ammonia in the NH_3 state (less H^+ ions in alkalosis; see earlier discussion of ammonia).

           • sedatives.

           • portosystemic shunts, which shunt ammonia away from the liver, the site that normally metabolizes ammonia in the urea cycle.

Margin notes:

Absent urine UBG

↑ALP/GGT/5′ nucleotidase

ERCP diagnostic; beading of bile ducts

Cirrhosis

Irreversible fibrosis; regenerative nodules

Regenerative nodules

Reaction to injury

Lack portal triads/sinusoids

Nodules surrounded by bands of fibrosis

Intrasinusoidal hypertension

↓Functional sinusoids

Micronodular/macronodular

ALD MCC cirrhosis

Postnecrotic: chronic HBV, HCV

Autoimmune: PBC, autoimmune hepatitis

Hemochromatosis, Wilson's disease

AAT deficiency, galactosemia

Complications of cirrhosis

Hepatic failure

End-point progressive liver damage

Coagulation defects

Bleeding: cannot synthesize factors

Hypercoagulable (↓protein C/S)

Hypoalbuminemia

Pitting edema, ascites (↓OP)

Hepatic encephalopathy

Toxic products impair mental function

Reversible metabolic disorder

Aromatic AAs → false neurotransmitters

↑Serum ammonia: defective urea cycle

Derives from amino acid metabolism and Urease-producing bacteria in bowel

↓Ammonia: ↓protein intake; antibiotics; lactulose

↑Protein

Metabolic alkalosis: NH_3 toxic

Sedatives

Portosystemic shunts

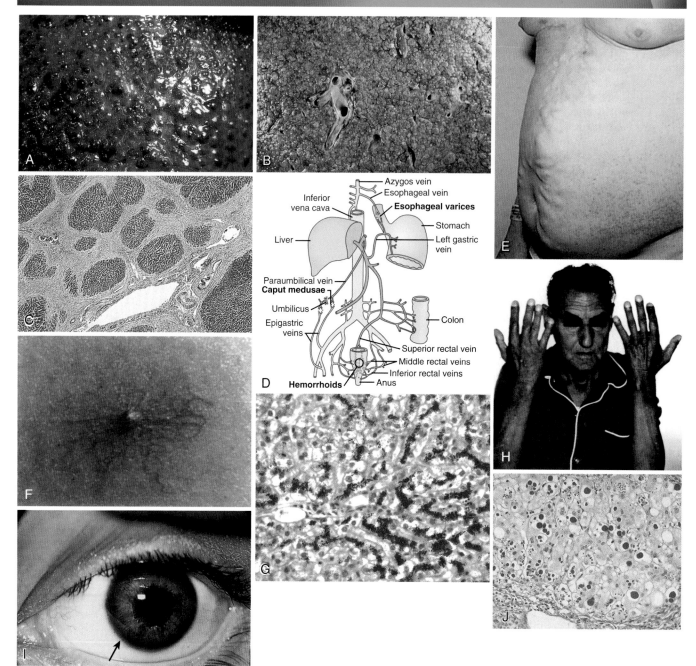

19-7: **A,** Surface of a liver with alcoholic cirrhosis showing a micronodular pattern. **B,** Cut section of a liver with alcoholic cirrhosis, showing micronodules representing regenerative nodules surrounded by collagen. **C,** Trichrome stain of a liver with alcoholic cirrhosis accentuating the regenerative nodules *(red)* and the fibrotic tissue *(blue).* **D,** Portal vein anatomy and anastomoses. Note that the portal vein derives from the splenic vein and the superior mesenteric veins. Portacaval anastomoses occur when there is reversed blood flow in portal hypertension. These lead to the development of esophageal varices (via anastomoses of the left gastric vein [portal] and the azygous vein [systemic]), caput medusae (via anastomoses of the paraumbilical vein [portal] with the superficial veins of the anterior abdominal wall [systemic]), and hemorrhoids (via anastomoses of the superior rectal vein [portal] and inferior rectal [systemic] veins). **E,** Patient with alcoholic cirrhosis showing ascites (abdominal distention), caput medusae (dilated superficial abdominal wall veins), and bilateral gyne-comastia. **F,** Spider angioma (telangiectasia) showing a single central arteriole and numerous radiating capillaries. **G,** Liver biopsy stained with Prussian blue in a patient with hereditary hemochromatosis. The hepatocytes are filled with blue iron granules. This is an early stage before parenchymal damage and fibrosis develop. **H,** Hemochromatosis in a male patient showing the characteristic bronze appearance of the skin. The hyperpigmentation results from the combination of iron deposited in skin plus and increase in melanin synthesis. Also note clubbing of the fingernails. **I,** Kayser-Fleischer ring *(arrow).* This shows deposition of a copper-colored pigment in the Descemet membrane in the cornea. **J,** α_1-Antitrypsin deficiency. The globules of α-1-antitrypsin accumulating in hepatocytes are periodic acid–Schiff positive. *(A, C, and J from MacSween R, Burt A, Portmann B, Ishak K, Scheuer P, Anthony P: Pathology of the Liver, 4th ed, London, Churchill Livingstone, 2002, pp 596, 280, 176, respectively, Figs. 13.13, 6.9, 4.21, respectively; B from my friend Ivan Damjanov, MD, PhD, Linder J: Pathology: A Color Atlas, St. Louis, Mosby, 2000, p 154, Fig. 8-42; D from Moore A, Roy W: Rapid Review Gross and Developmental Anatomy, 3rd ed, Philadelphia, Mosby Elsevier, 2010, p 95, Fig. 3.40; E from Swartz M: Textbook of Physical Diagnosis History and Examination, 5th ed, Philadelphia, Saunders Elsevier, 2006, p 497, Fig. 17.14; F from Gitlin M, Strauss R: Atlas of Clinical Hepatology, Philadelphia, Saunders, 1995, pp 3, 22, respectively; Fig. 1.4, 2.9 respectively; G from Kumar V, Fausto N, Abbas A: Robbins and Cotran Pathologic Basis of Disease, 7th ed, Philadelphia, Saunders, 2004, p 910, Fig. 18-28; I from Perkin GD: Mosby's Color Atlas and Text of Neurology, St. Louis, Mosby, 2002, p 151, Fig. 8-15.)*

(3) Clinical findings include:

    (a) alterations in the mental status.

    (b) somnolence and disordered sleep rhythms.

    (c) asterixis (i.e., inability to sustain posture, flapping tremor; Link 19-51).

    (d) coma and death in late stages.

2. Portal hypertension

  a. **Definition:** PV pressure that is greater than 10 mm Hg (normal pressure, 5–10 mm Hg)

  b. Epidemiology

    (1) PV anatomy is depicted in Fig. 19-7 D. The PV derives from the splenic vein and superior mesenteric vein (Link 19-52).

    (2) Pathogenesis involves:

      (a) prehepatic, hepatic, and posthepatic causes (Link 19-53).

      (b) intrahepatic is the most common cause and is due to resistance to intrahepatic blood flow due to intrasinusoidal HTN due to compression of sinusoids by regenerative nodules.

      (c) anastomoses between PV tributaries and the arterial system (Link 19-54).

  c. Complications include:

    (1) ascites (discussed later).

    (2) congestive splenomegaly.

      (a) Caused by increased hydrostatic pressure in the splenic vein, a branch of the PV

      (b) Congestive splenomegaly causes hypersplenism, producing various cytopenias (anemia, neutropenia, thrombocytopenia; see Chapter 14).

    (3) esophageal varices (see Chapter 18; see Fig. 18-15; see Links 18-41 and 18-42).

    (4) hemorrhoids (see Fig. 18-31 A).

    (5) periumbilical venous collaterals (caput medusae; Fig. 19-7 D, E).

  d. Shunts are used in treating portal hypertension to reduce pressure.

3. Ascites (Fig. 19-7 E)

  a. **Definition:** Accumulation of excess fluid (usually a transudate) in the peritoneal cavity (Link 19-55)

  b. Epidemiology; pathogenesis includes (see Chapter 3; Link 19-56):

    (1) Portal hypertension, which increases the portal vein hydrostatic pressure.

    (2) hypoalbuminemia, which decreases oncotic pressure (OP).

    (3) secondary hyperaldosteronism occurs because the:

      (a) cardiac output is decreased (see Chapter 5), resulting in decreased renal blood flow and activation of the renin-angiotensin-aldosterone (RAA) system, causing the retention of sodium (Na^+) and water.

      (b) diseased liver is unable to metabolize aldosterone (retains sodium and water).

  c. Clinical findings include:

    (1) abdominal distention with a prominent fluid wave, bulging flanks, flank dullness to percussion, and shifting dullness to percussion (turning patient on her or his left and right side) all have a low sensitivity (60%–80%) and specificity (47%–80%), *except* for detection of a prominent fluid wave, which has a specificity of 90%.

    (2) increased risk for developing spontaneous bacterial peritonitis (see Chapter 18 discussion).

Peritoneal fluid analysis is useful in distinguishing ascites of liver origin from ascites of peritoneal origin. The gradient between serum albumin and ascitic fluid albumin (serum albumin – ascitic fluid albumin) is very helpful in making this distinction. Whereas a difference >1.1 g/dL is ascites of liver origin, a difference <1.1 g/dL is of peritoneal origin (e.g., peritonitis). Recall that ascites of liver origin is a transudate, which is a protein-poor and cell-poor fluid; hence the expected difference between serum albumin and ascitic albumin is increased. However, ascitic fluid from peritonitis is an exudate, which is a protein- and cell-rich fluid; hence, the difference between serum and ascitic fluid is much less. Peritoneal fluid protein concentration and cell count are also useful. Whereas a total peritoneal fluid protein concentration <2.5 g/dL and white blood cell (WBC) count <300 cells/mm^3 + neutrophils <25% of the total count is consistent with a transudate, a concentration >2.5 g/dL and a WBC count >300 cells/mm^3 + neutrophils >25% of the total count indicates an exudate.

4. Hepatorenal syndrome

  a. **Definition:** A condition associated with advanced liver disease (e.g., cirrhosis) that causes a worsening of renal function with no other apparent cause (diagnosis of exclusion).

Margin notes:

Alterations mental status

Somnolence, disorder sleep

Asterixis: cannot sustain posture, flapping tremor

Coma → death

Portal hypertension

Portal vein pressure >10 mm Hg

PV: splenic vein + superior mesenteric vein

Intrasinusoidal hypertension, compression by nodules

PV: splenic vein + superior mesenteric vein

Ascites

Congestive splenomegaly

↑Hydrostatic pressure in splenic vein

Hypersplenism: cytopenias

Esophageal varices

Hemorrhoids

Caput medusae

Shunts to treat portal hypertension

Portal hypertension: ↑hydrostatic pressure

Hypoalbuminemia: ↓OP

Activation RAA: retain sodium/water

Liver cannot metabolize aldosterone

Abdominal distention; fluid wave

Risk for spontaneous peritonitis

Serum albumin – ascitic fluid albumin; >1.1 g/dL liver origin, <1.1 g/dL peritoneal origin

Hepatorenal syndrome

Advanced liver disease worsens renal function

Reversible renal failure without renal parenchymal disease

No shock, *no* volume depletion

No infection, *no* obstructive/parenchymal renal disease

Preservation renal tubular function

Random urine Na⁺ <20 mEq/L

Absence significant proteinuria; no hematuria

Dilation splanchnic vessels → pools blood → ↓renal blood flow

↑Serum BUN/creatinine

High mortality rate

Hyperestrinism in males

↑E in males

Liver *cannot* degrade estrogen and androstenedione

Androstenedione aromatized into E

Clinical findings hyperestrinism

Gynecomastia

Spider telangiectasia

Female hair distribution

Impotence, erectile dysfunction

SHBG binds FT → ↓FT

↓FT → ↓libido

Sialadenosis: bilateral parotid gland enlargement

Postnecrotic cirrhosis

Usually chronic HBV or HCV

↑Incidence HCC

Primary biliary cirrhosis

Granulomatous destruction bile ducts portal triads

Autoimmune disorder

IPF, SLE, DM, MCTD, RTA

CD8 T cells destroy bile duct epithelium in triads; granulomas

Antimitochondrial antibodies

b. Epidemiology
   (1) Reversible renal failure *without* renal parenchymal disease. Creatinine clearance is <40 mL/min (see Chapter 20).
   (2) Approximately 20% of people with hepatic failure die of this syndrome.
   (3) *Absence* of shock, volume depletion, infection, and obstructive or parenchymal renal disease

c. Preservation of renal tubular function
   (1) Random urine Na⁺ is <20 mEq/L (see Chapter 20).
   (2) Absence of significant proteinuria (protein in the urine; <500 mg/day) or hematuria (RBCs in the urine; see Chapter 20).

d. Dilation of the splanchnic vasculature pools blood, causing a drop in systemic vascular resistance and blood pressure that reduces renal blood flow. The serum blood urea nitrogen (BUN) and creatinine are both increased.

e. Mortality rate is >80%.

5. Hyperestrinism occurs in males.
   a. **Definition:** An increase in estrogen (E) in males that leads to the development of female external characteristics
   b. Pathogenesis
      (1) Diseased liver cannot degrade estrogen and 17-ketosteroids (e.g., androstenedione).
      (2) Androstenedione is then aromatized (converted by aromatase) into estrogen in adipose cells.
   c. Clinical findings of hyperestrinism in males include:
      (1) gynecomastia (Fig. 19-7 E).
      (2) spider telangiectasia (dilation of capillaries that causes them to have a spider-like appearance; see Chapter 10; Fig. 19-7 F).
      (3) female distribution of hair, in which the hair does *not* extend from the pubic area to the umbilicus (see Fig. 19-7 E).
      (4) impotence and erectile dysfunction (inability to have an erection during attempted intercourse).
         (a) Increased estrogen causes the synthesis of sex hormone–binding protein to increase. In turn, more free testosterone (FT) becomes bound to sex hormone–binding protein, resulting in less FT (see Chapter 21).
         (b) Decreased FT levels decreases libido (sexual desire), leading to erectile dysfunction

6. Protein-calorie deprivation is also present in cirrhosis. This may result in sialadenosis (sialosis) characterized by bilateral enlargement of the parotid glands.

7. Overview of clinical features of cirrhosis (Link 19-57)

E. **Postnecrotic cirrhosis**
   1. **Definition:** A type of cirrhosis that is most often caused by chronic hepatitis due to HBV or HCV
   2. Increased incidence of hepatocellular carcinoma (HCC; discussed later). The incidence of which virus is most commonly involved varies around the world.

F. **Primary biliary cirrhosis (PBC)**
   1. **Definition:** Type of cirrhosis associated with immune destruction of small bile ducts in the portal triads
   2. Epidemiology
      a. Autoimmune disorder often associated with other autoimmune disorders (80% of cases; e.g., Sjögren sicca syndrome most common, rheumatoid arthritis, progressive systemic sclerosis)
      b. Other associations: idiopathic pulmonary fibrosis (IPF), systemic lupus erythematosus (SLE), dermatomyositis (DM), mixed connective tissue disorder (MCTD), renal tubular acidosis (RTA)
      c. Pathogenesis
         (1) An environmental insult affecting mitochondrial proteins triggers CD8 T-cell destruction of intralobular bile duct epithelium (Link 19-58 A). Noncaseating granulomas are present in 25% of cases (Links 19-59 and 19-60).
         (2) Enzyme complex subunit in the mitochondrial membrane is the autoantigen that is recognized by the CD8 T cells.
         (3) IgM autoantibodies (antimitochondrial antibodies) develop against the mitochondria (97%). Presence of the autoantibody does *not* correlate with disease activity.

d. Primarily occurs in women (>90% of cases) between 40 and 50 years of age

e. Progresses from a chronic inflammatory reaction to cirrhosis with portal hypertension

f. Increased risk of ulcerative colitis in 70% to 80% of patients with PBC

g. Increased risk for developing HCC

3. Clinical findings include:

   a. pruritus (itchy skin; 20%–70% of cases).
      (1) Pruritus is of unknown etiology (it is *not* the deposition of bile salts in the skin).
      (2) Early finding that occurs well *before* jaundice appears

   b. painful hepatosplenomegaly.

   c. jaundice (60% of cases): late finding *after* most of the bile ducts have been destroyed.

   d. inflammatory arthropathy is commonly present (40%–70% of cases).

   e. xanthelasma (cholesterol deposited in the eyelids; 40% of cases; see Fig. 10-4 B); late finding caused by CH in bile backing up into the blood.

   f. Kayser-Fleischer ring in the cornea; caused by the retention of copper similar to that seen in Wilson's disease (discussed later).

   g. may develop lymphocytic or fibrosing alveolitis.

4. Laboratory findings include:

   a. antimitochondrial (mT) IgM antibodies (AMAs; 95%–98% of cases).

   b. positive serum ANA test (50% of cases; see Chapter 4).

   c. positive serum antibodies against antigens in the inner mitochondrial membrane (M2; 98%).

   d. increase in serum IgM (90%; characteristic finding).

   e. increased serum ALP and GGT.

   f. increased serum cholesterol (CH). Cholesterol is a component of bile.

5. Liver transplantation improves survival.

G. Secondary biliary cirrhosis

1. **Definition:** A complication of chronic extrahepatic bile duct obstruction from other causes. Example: Cystic fibrosis, in which bile is dehydrated (see Chapter 17)

2. Unlike PBC, there is *no* increase in serum antimitochondrial antibody or IgM.

H. Hereditary hemochromatosis (HHC)

1. **Definition:** An autosomal recessive (AR) disease in which there is unrestricted reabsorption of iron from the small intestine, leading to deposition of iron in various organs, causing dysfunction

2. Epidemiology

   a. An AR disorder with a 1/10 carrier rate; linked to the short arm of chromosome 6. HLA-A3 association

   b. Most common genetic disorder in people of North European ancestry

   c. Male-dominant disorder; the diagnosis is usually made in the fifth decade of life.

   d. In women, the diagnosis is usually made 10 to 20 years *after* menopause because the loss of iron during menses helps rid the body of excess iron during the reproductive period of life.

   e. Pathogenesis
      (1) Unrestricted reabsorption of iron in the small intestine
      (2) Mutations involving HHC gene (*HFE*). Two missense mutations (*C282Y* and *H63D*) occur on chromosome 6.
      (3) Iron stimulates the production of hydroxyl free radicals, which damage tissue and cause fibrosis (see Chapter 2).

The **normal function of the *HFE* gene protein product** (see Chapter 12 and Fig. 12-9) is to facilitate the binding of plasma transferrin (binding protein for iron) to the mucosal cell transferrin receptors in the duodenum. In general, if there is less transferrin-bound iron that binds to the receptor (indicating decreased iron stores), the synthesis and release of the hormone hepcidin by the liver is decreased, leading to increased duodenal reabsorption of iron. If there is more transferrin-bound iron that binds to the receptor (indicating increased iron stores), then there is increased liver synthesis and release of hepcidin, and less iron is reabsorbed by the duodenum. Because there is a mutated *HFE* gene in hemochromatosis, there is no binding of transferrin-bound iron to the transferrin receptor; therefore, *no* hepcidin is synthesized and released by the liver. This leads to unrestricted reabsorption of iron from the duodenum. Excess iron in the blood leads to excess iron in tissue. Iron in the tissue increases the formation of hydroxyl free radicals (see Chapter 2), causing tissue damage.

(4) Iron deposits in multiple organs, including the liver (target organ), pancreas, heart, joints, skin, pituitary, adrenals and testes.

Margin notes:

Female dominant

Cirrhosis/portal hypertension

↑Risk ulcerative colitis

↑Risk HCC

Pruritus

Pruritus *before* jaundice

Painful hepatosplenomegaly

Jaundice late finding

Inflammatory arthropathy

Xanthelasma

Kayser-Fleischer ring; retention copper

Lymphocytic or fibrosing alveolitis

Anti-mT IgM antibodies

+Serum ANA

Ab against antigens inner mitochondrial membrane (M2)

↑IgM

↑ALP/GGT

↑Serum CH

Liver transplantation

Secondary biliary cirrhosis

Chronic extrahepatic bile duce obstruction

Cystic fibrosis

No ↑IgM or anti-mT IgM abs

Hereditary hemochromatosis

AR; unrestricted iron reabsorption

AR disorder; 1/10 carrier rate

Short arm chromosome 6; HLA-A3

MC genetic disease people North European origin

Male dominant

Women *after* menopause become symptomatic

Unrestricted iron reabsorption

Missense mutations

Iron generates hydroxyl FRs

↓Hepcidin → unrestricted iron reabsorption by duodenum

Liver target organ; pancreas, heart, joints, pituitary, adrenals, testes

Hemosiderosis (secondary hemochromatosis) is caused by multiple blood transfusions (e.g., sickle cell anemia, thalassemia major), alcohol abuse (alcohol increases iron reabsorption), and well water (iron pipes). Iron deposits are more prevalent in macrophages than in parenchymal tissue.

Hemosiderosis: acquired
iron overload disease

Cirrhosis

Excess iron in hepatocytes

HCC risk

"Bronze diabetes"

Type I DM: destruction
β-islet cells

Skin hyperpigmentation

Malabsorption: loss
pancreatic exocrine function

Restrictive cardiomyopathy

Hypogonadism males/
female

2° Hypothyroidism

Amenorrhea: ↓E

Loss libido in men (↓T)

DJD

↑Serum iron, % saturation,
ferritin; ↓TIBC

% Transferrin saturation
best screen

TIBC >45%

↓TIBC (↓transferrin
synthesis)

↑↑Serum ferritin

Liver Bx for confirmation

Gene testing best for
screening relatives

Wilson disease

AR; inadequate biliary
excretion copper

Men = women

S/S late childhood

Acute hepatitis → cirrhosis
+ portal hypertension

Defect copper-transport
protein

↓Hepatocyte excretion
copper in bile

↓Incorporation copper into
ceruloplasmin

↑Unbound copper in blood

Copper loosely attached to
albumin

Copper toxic in tissue

3. Clinical findings include:
   a. cirrhosis (60% of cases).
      (1) Iron deposits primarily in hepatocytes (Fig. 19-7 G)
      (2) Increased risk for developing HCC
   b. "bronze diabetes."
      (1) Type I diabetes mellitus develops in 60% of cases and is caused by destruction of the β-islet cells in the pancreas.
      (2) Hyperpigmentation occurs in the skin in 75% of cases because excess iron in the skin increases melanin production (Fig. 19-7 H).
   c. malabsorption occurs because of destruction of the exocrine pancreas and the loss of pancreatic enzymes that are required for digestion (e.g., trypsin; see Chapter 18).
   d. restrictive cardiomyopathy occurs, leading to chronic heart failure (see Chapter 11).
   e. hypogonadism is caused by destruction of the pituitary gland, with associated loss of follicle-stimulating hormone (FSH) and luteinizing hormone (LH). Secondary hypothyroidism also occurs from lack of thyroid-stimulating hormone. Amenorrhea (absent menses) in women is caused by hypoestrinism (25% of cases). Loss of libido (desire for sex) in men is caused by decreased testosterone (T) levels (50% of cases).
   f. degenerative joint disease (DJD; chondrocalcinosis) occurs in >40% of cases (see Chapter 24; Link 19-61).
4. Laboratory findings include:
   a. increased serum iron, percent saturation, and ferritin (see Chapter 12).
      (1) Transferrin saturation is the best screening test.
      (2) Transferrin saturation (total iron binding capacity [TIBC]) values >45% indicate further evaluation is necessary to rule out hemochromatosis.
      (3) TIBC is decreased because transferrin synthesis is decreased when iron stores are increased (see Chapter 12).
      (4) Serum ferritin is elevated (>300 mg/L) and is used to follow therapy (phlebotomy, chelation).
   b. Liver biopsy is required to confirm the diagnosis (Link 19-62).
   c. Serum LH and FSH are decreased because of destruction of the anterior pituitary gland.
5. *HFE* gene testing for the *C282Y* mutation is used to screen relatives for hemochromatosis.
6. Link 19-63 summarizes clinical and laboratory findings in hemochromatosis.
7. Normal life expectancy if cirrhosis is *not* present.

I. **Wilson's disease (hepatolenticular degeneration)**
   1. **Definition:** An AR disorder of copper metabolism characterized by inadequate biliary excretion of copper that leads to copper accumulation and damage in multiple organs
   2. Epidemiology
      a. AR disorder that affects men and women equally
      b. Signs and symptoms of the disease are usually manifested in late childhood.
      c. Liver disease progresses from acute hepatitis to cirrhosis and portal hypertension.
      d. Pathogenesis
         (1) WD gene (*ATP7B*) codes for a P-type of adenosine triphosphatase (ATP), which is a copper-transport protein. A defect in this protein leads to:
            (a) defective hepatocyte transport of copper into bile for excretion.
            (b) defective incorporation of copper into ceruloplasmin (binding protein for copper in blood).
         (2) Unbound copper eventually accumulates in the blood.
            (a) Copper is loosely attached to albumin.
            (b) Copper that deposits in other tissues has a toxic effect.

Ceruloplasmin is a protein that is synthesized in the liver. It contains six copper atoms in its structure. Ceruloplasmin is secreted into the plasma, where it represents 90% to 95% of the total serum copper concentration. The remaining 5% to 10% of copper is free copper that is loosely bound to albumin. Ceruloplasmin is eventually taken up and degraded by the liver. The copper that was bound to ceruloplasmin is excreted into the bile. The gene defect in Wilson disease affects a copper transport system that produces a dual defect: decreased incorporation of copper into ceruloplasmin in the liver (ceruloplasmin is decreased) and decreased excretion of copper into bile (intrahepatic copper is increased). Accumulation of copper in the liver increases the formation of hydroxyl free radicals (Fenton reaction; see Chapter 2) that damage hepatocytes. Liver disease progresses from acute hepatitis to cirrhosis. In a few years, unbound copper is released from the liver into the circulation (increased in blood and urine), where it damages the brain, kidneys, cornea, and other tissues.

3. Clinical findings include:
   a. Kayser-Fleischer ring (~70% of cases).
      (1) Ring is caused by free copper deposits in Descemet membrane in the cornea (see Fig. 19-7 I).
      (2) *Not* pathognomonic of Wilson's disease because it is also seen in PBC
   b. central nervous system disease (>50% of cases; Fig. 26-21 A).
      (1) Copper deposits in the putamen; produces a movement disorder resembling parkinsonism
      (2) Copper deposits in the subthalamic nucleus; produces hemiballismus (violent movements of one lateral half of the body)
      (3) Copper is toxic to neurons in the cerebral cortex, producing dementia.
   c. cholestatic jaundice with hepatosplenomegaly (50% of cases).
      • Liver biopsy shows increased copper (gold standard for Dx), fibrosis, and cholestasis.
   d. Coombs-negative hemolytic anemia (see Chapter 12).
   e. renal disease.
      (1) Proximal tubule damage produces type II proximal renal tubular acidosis (see Chapter 5).
      (2) Nephrolithiasis (renal stones)
4. Laboratory findings include:
   a. decreased total serum copper caused by decreased ceruloplasmin.
   b. decreased serum ceruloplasmin (85%–95% sensitivity) with a normal serum copper level in its early stages; thus, normal serum copper levels do *not* exclude the diagnosis of Wilson's disease. If the ceruloplasmin is decreased or the 24-hour urine copper is increased, then a liver biopsy is performed for histology and quantitative copper determination in the tissue to secure the diagnosis. Usually the concentration is >250 mcg/g (dry weight) but may be as high as 3000 mcg/g.

J. **Alpha$_1$-antitrypsin (AAT) deficiency (PiZZ)**
   1. **Definition:** An AR disease associated with a deficiency in the protease inhibitor α_1-antitrypsin that results in a predisposition for developing emphysema in the lungs and cirrhosis in the liver
   2. Epidemiology
      a. AR disease
      b. Incidence is 1 in 1600 to 1 in 2000 live births. Prevalence in United States is 1 in 4800.
      c. By 15 years of age, more than 50% of patients have clinical manifestations of the disease.
         Pathogenesis
         (1) AAT is synthesized in the liver and is a protease inhibitor (Pi) that inhibits elastase, trypsin, collagenase, and proteases from neutrophils. If deficient in the lungs, emphysema may occur because of a progressive loss of elastic tissue within the airways. If deficient in the liver, aggregates of defective protein are found leading to cirrhosis.
         (2) Normal allele is M (95% frequency in the United States). PiMM is the normal genotype with a distribution of ~87%.
         (3) Deficient variant (decreased α_1-antitrypsin) has the Z allele (PiMZ; 1%–2% frequency) or the S allele (PiMS 8% frequency).
         (4) Severe deficiency most commonly occurs in the homozygous PiZZ variant.
            (a) Markedly decreased (<15% of normal) levels of α_1-antitrypsin in the serum. Incidence ranges from 1 in 2000 to 1 in 5000.
            (b) Associated with panacinar emphysema (all parts of the respiratory unit are destroyed; see Chapter 17).

Ceruloplasmin: protein synthesized in the liver that contains copper

Kayser-Fleischer ring

Excess copper Descemet membrane cornea

Kayser-Fleischer ring also in primary biliary cirrhosis

Parkinsonism (putamen deposition)

Hemiballismus (subthalamic nucleus deposits)

Dementia (cerebral cortex deposits)

Cholestatic jaundice, hepatosplenomegaly

↑Copper liver bx (gold standard)

Hemolytic anemia

Renal disease

Type II proximal renal tubular acidosis

Nephrolithiasis

↓Total serum copper (↓ceruloplasmin)

↓Serum ceruloplasmin, 24 hr urine copper increased. Quantitative copper in liver tissue >250 mcg/g (dry weight).

AAT deficiency

AR disease with ↓AAT; emphysema/cirrhosis

AR disease

Incidence 1/1600-2000 live births

AAT is Pi for elastase, trypsin, collagenase, proteases WBCs

↓AAT → emphysema, cirrhosis

M normal allele

PiMM normal genotype

Deficient variant has PiMZ or PiMS

Severe AAT deficiency usually PiZZ variant

Panacinar emphysema

(c) Associated with cirrhosis of the liver (see later). Clinically significant liver disease occurs in 10% to 15% of ZZ patients by 30 years of age.

(5) Risk of lung disease in heterozygotes (e.g., MZ) is uncertain.

(6) Other disorders that may occur in adults include membranoproliferative glomerulonephritis (GN) and systemic vasculitis.

3. Effect of increase AAT in hepatocytes
   a. In ~50% of homozygous ZZ patients, α_1-antitrypsin is *not* secreted properly from the hepatocytes.
   b. Pathologic accumulation of α_1-antitrypsin in hepatocytes causes liver damage.
   • Genetic mutation interferes with the folding of the AAT in the cisterns of rough endoplasmic reticulum (RER), inhibiting the transfer of proteins from the RER to the Golgi apparatus (Link 19-64). Periodic acid–Schiff stains and hematoxylin and eosin stains show red cytoplasmic granules (Fig. 19-7 J; Link 19-65).
   c. Presents as neonatal hepatitis with intrahepatic cholestasis (see previous discussion of neonatal hepatitis)
   d. Hepatitis progresses into cirrhosis. AAT deficiency is the most common cause of cirrhosis in children.
   e. Serum electrophoresis in AAT deficiency shows absence of the α_1 peak.
   f. Increased risk for developing HCC

K. Laboratory test abnormalities in cirrhosis include:
   1. decreased serum BUN and increased serum ammonia caused by disruption of the urea cycle.
   2. fasting hypoglycemia caused by defective gluconeogenesis and decreased glycogen stores.
   3. chronic respiratory alkalosis caused by overstimulation of the respiratory center by various toxic products originating from hepatic dysfunction (see Chapter 5).
   4. lactic acidosis caused by liver dysfunction (decreased conversion of lactic acid to pyruvate).
   5. hyponatremia occurs because of a decreased cardiac output in cirrhosis; the kidneys reabsorb a slightly hypotonic solution ($\uparrow$total body sodium [TBNa$^+$]/$\uparrow\uparrow$TBW), causing hyponatremia with clinical evidence of pitting edema caused by the excess in TBNa$^+$ (see Chapter 5).
   6. hypokalemia occurs because of secondary aldosteronism. This occurs when there is a decrease in cardiac output. This in turn causes a decrease in blood flow to the kidneys with activation of the RAA system. The elevated levels of aldosterone increase the renal exchange of Na$^+$ for K$^+$ in the aldosterone-enhanced Na$^+$ and K$^+$ epithelial channels in the late distal collecting tubules and the aldosterone-enhanced H$^+$/K$^+$-ATPase pump in the collecting ducts (see Chapter 5).
   7. Prothrombin time (PT) is increased because of decreased liver synthesis of the coagulation factors (see Chapter 15).
   8. hypoalbuminemia occurs because of decreased liver synthesis of albumin.
   9. hypocalcemia occurs because:
      a. hypoalbuminemia decreases the total serum calcium without affecting the ionized calcium level (see Chapter 23). Recall that approximately 40% of the total calcium is bound to albumin.
      b. vitamin D deficiency is present because of decreased liver 25-hydroxylation of vitamin D. Vitamin D normally acts to increase calcium absorption within the small bowel (SB) as well as reabsorption of calcium from the kidneys (see Chapters 8 and 23).
   10. mild increase in serum transaminase enzymes. Enzymes are *not* markedly increased because of the loss of liver parenchymal cells that normally synthesize the enzymes.

IX. Liver Tumors and Tumor-like Disorders
   A. Focal nodular hyperplasia (FNH)
      1. **Definition:** Localized non-neoplastic hyperplastic overgrowth of hepatocytes around a vascular anomaly, usually an arterial malformation
      2. Epidemiology
         a. Occurs in 0.4% of the population
         b. Tumor-like disorder of the liver (second most common "tumor")
         c. More common in women (80%–95% of cases) than men. OCP use has been implicated in the promotion of FNH but is generally *not* considered to be a causative factor.
         d. May occur in children with certain types of glycogen storage disease (GSD)
         e. May coexist with cavernous hemangiomas in 20% of cases

---

Liver cirrhosis

Membranoproliferative GN, systemic vasculitis

Homozygous ZZ: AAT not secreted properly from hepatocytes

Liver damage

Neonatal hepatitis with intrahepatic cholestasis

Hepatitis → cirrhosis in children

AAT deficiency MCC cirrhosis in children

SPE: absence of α_1 peak

$\uparrow$Risk HCC

Lab tests in cirrhosis

$\downarrow$Serum BUN, $\uparrow$serum ammonia

Fasting hypoglycemia: $\downarrow$gluconeogenesis/glycogen stores

Chronic respiratory alkalosis

Lactic acidosis

Hyponatremia

Hypokalemia (2° aldosteronism)

$\uparrow$PT: $\downarrow$synthesis coagulation factors

Hypoalbuminemia

Hypocalcemia: $\downarrow$total calcium, normal ionized calcium

$\downarrow$25(OH)-vitamin D

Vit D $\uparrow$ calcium absorption in SG/kidneys

Transaminases slightly increase

Tumors, tumor-like disorders

Focal nodular hyperplasia

Non-neoplastic overgrowth around vascular abnormality

Tumor-like disorder

Women > men

OCPs implicated in growth FNH, *not* causative

Children with GSD

Coexist with cavernous hemangiomas

f. In patients with multiple FNHs, one or more other lesions may occur, including hepatic hemangioma, berry aneurysms in the brain, and brain tumors (e.g., meningioma, astrocytoma).

3. Gross findings
   a. Poorly encapsulated nodule with a central depressed stellate scar that contains large blood vessels (Link 19-66)
   b. FNH: fibrous septae radiate to the periphery of the nodule

4. Diagnosis
   a. Computed tomography (CT) or magnetic resonance imaging (MRI) of the liver show a mass with a central scar.
   b. Angiography or Doppler US shows hypervascularity.
   c. Technetium 99 sulfur colloid scan shows normal or increased uptake in 60% to 70%.
   d. No surgery is required unless associated with pain.

B. **Cysts and abscesses**
   1. Benign cysts (single or multiple) occur in 1% of the adult population.
      a. Usually benign or congenital
      b. Usually recur after aspiration
   2. Hydatid cysts (see Table 19-7; Links 19-30 and 19-31)

C. **Benign tumors of the liver**
   1. Cavernous hemangioma
      a. **Definition:** Benign tumor of the liver composed of a proliferation of widely dilated blood vessels.
      b. Most common benign liver tumor (20% of the population)
      c. Most common in women as solitary (60%) or multiple asymptomatic masses
      d. Rare cause of intraperitoneal hemorrhage
      e. Best diagnosed with an enhanced CT scan
   2. Liver (hepatic) cell adenoma
      a. **Definition:** Benign hormone-induced liver tumor that has a predilection to hemorrhage into the peritoneal cavity
      b. Epidemiology of liver cell adenoma
         (1) More common in women than in men
         (2) Causes include:
            (a) OCPs (most common cause). Risk for adenoma correlates with duration of use and age older than 30 years.
            (b) anabolic steroids.
            (c) Von Gierke glycogenosis.
         (3) Highly vascular tumors that have a tendency to rupture during menstruation or pregnancy, causing intraperitoneal hemorrhage (30%) and possible death of the patient (Link 19-67)
         (4) Tend to regress if the patient stops taking OCPs or anabolic steroids
         (5) May transform into HCC; risk is greatest if they are >4 to 5 cm
      c. Surgical removal is usually recommended because of their risk for hemorrhage.

D. **Malignant tumors of the liver**
   1. Metastasis
      a. Most common liver cancer (Fig. 19-8 A; Link 19-68)
      b. Primary cancers of colon or rectum are the most common cancers, followed by the lung and breast cancer. Primary cancers that commonly extend into the liver include gallbladder, EHBD, pancreas, stomach cancers, and malignant melanoma. Other cancers include leukemia and lymphoma, particularly Hodgkin lymphoma (HL).
      c. Present as multiple nodular masses in the liver by physical exam or imaging studies
   2. Hepatocellular carcinoma (HCC)
      a. **Definition:** Malignancy originating from hepatocytes
      b. Epidemiology
         (1) Most common primary liver cancer. Third most common cancer worldwide caused by presence of hepatitis B and C. Hepatitis B can be associated with HCC *without* cirrhosis of the liver because chronic active hepatitis can progress to HCC.
         (2) Rapidly increasing in the United States because of an increase in HCV infections (80% of cases)
         (3) More common in males than females; peaks around the fifth and sixth decades of life

---

Multiple FNH: liver hemangioma, brain abnormalities

Poorly encapsulated nodule

Central stellate scar with large blood vessels

Fibrous septae radiate to periphery

CT/MRI

Angiography, Doppler US: hypervascularity

Technetium colloid scan: ↑uptake

Cysts/abscesses

Benign cysts (single, multiple)

Benign/congenital

Recur after aspiration

Hydatid cysts

Benign liver tumors

Cavernous hemangioma

Tumor with dilated vessels

MC benign liver tumor

Solitary (women) or multiple

Intraperitoneal hemorrhage rare

Enhanced CT scan

Liver cell adenoma

Benign hormone-induced liver tumor

May hemorrhage

Women > men

OCPs MCC

Anabolic steroids

Von Gierke glycogenosis

Tendency for rupture during menstruation/pregnancy

May regress with D/C OCPs/ anabolic steroids

HCC risk

Surgical removal

Metastasis

Metastasis MC liver cancer

Colorectal MC, breast

Gallbladder, EHBD, pancreas, stomach

Leukemia/lymphoma (HL)

Metastasis: MC liver cancer; colon/rectum MC primary site

Hepatocellular carcinoma

Arises from hepatocytes

MC 1° liver cancer

↑↑U.S. due to HCV

Males > females

5th – 6th decade

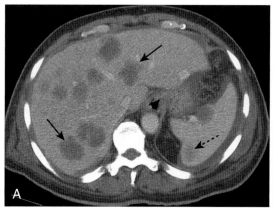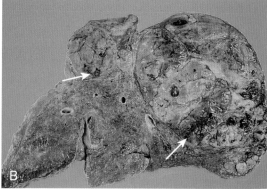

19-8: A, Computed tomography image showing metastases to the liver and spleen. Metastases usually appear as multiple, low-attenuation masses *(solid black arrows).* There are also low-attenuation lesions in the spleen *(dotted black arrow).* The patient had a primary adeno-carcinoma of the colon. **B,** Hepatocellular carcinoma. Multiple large, hemorrhagic tumor masses are present in the liver *(arrows).* There is also diffuse infiltration of tumor blending in with the remaining liver. *(**A** from Herring W: Learning Radiology Recognizing the Basics, 2nd ed, Philadelphia, Elsevier Saunders, 2012, p 187, Fig. 18.31; **B** from my friend Ivan Damjanov, MD, PhD, Linder J: Pathology: A Color Atlas, St. Louis, Mosby, 2000, p 161, Fig. 8-70.)*

Postnecrotic cirrhosis (HBV, HCV)	(4) Causes include:
	(a) postnecrotic cirrhosis, caused by chronic hepatitis B and chronic hepatitis C;
Malignant transformation regenerative nodules	malignant transformation of regenerative nodules.
Alcoholic cirrhosis	(b) alcoholic cirrhosis.
Aflatoxins	(c) aflatoxins (from *Aspergillus* mold in grains and peanuts).
HHC, Wilson's disease	(d) HHC and Wilson's disease.
PBC, AAT deficiency, tyrosinemia	(e) Primary biliary cirrhosis (PBC) AAT deficiency, tyrosinemia.
Anabolic steroids	(f) anabolic steroids.

(4) Causes include:
(a) postnecrotic cirrhosis, caused by chronic hepatitis B and chronic hepatitis C; malignant transformation of regenerative nodules.
(b) alcoholic cirrhosis.
(c) aflatoxins (from *Aspergillus* mold in grains and peanuts).
(d) HHC and Wilson's disease.
(e) Primary biliary cirrhosis (PBC) AAT deficiency, tyrosinemia.
(f) anabolic steroids.

Preexisting cirrhosis MC risk

Postnecrotic cirrhosis HBV/HCV MC risk factor

(5) Pathogenesis
(a) Most often associated with preexisting cirrhosis of the liver
(b) Postnecrotic cirrhosis caused by hepatitis B or C is the most common risk factor.

Focal, multifocal, diffuse

Vessel invader: portal/hepatic veins

Bile in neoplastic cells

c. Gross findings include:
(1) focal, multifocal, or diffusely infiltrating cancer with or without preexisting cirrhosis, the former being more common than the latter (Link 19-69).
(2) portal and hepatic vein invasion by the cancer is common.
d. Microscopic findings: Characteristic finding is the presence of bile in the cytoplasm of the cancer cells.

Pain MC

Fever (necrosis liver cells)

Hepatomegaly, arterial systolic hepatic bruit

Rapid liver enlargement in patient with cirrhosis

Bloody ascitic fluid

Lung MC site metastasis

e. Clinical findings include:
(1) abdominal pain, a common initial presentation.
(2) fever from necrosis of liver cells.
(3) hepatomegaly, arterial systolic hepatic bruit (caused by vascularity of tumor nodules; 25%).
(4) rapid enlargement of the liver occurs in patients with preexisting cirrhosis.
(5) development of bloody ascites is a very characteristic presentation.
(6) Lung is the most common site for metastasis.

↑AFP

Sudden ↑serum ALP, GGT

↑EPO: polycythemia

↑Insulin-like factor: hypoglycemia

PTH-related protein: hypercalcemia

Hypercholesterolemia: ↓expression LDL receptor

f. Laboratory findings include:
(1) increase in serum α-fetoprotein (AFP; 70% of cases). The sensitivity of this test ranges from 40% to 60%, and the specificity ranges from 80% to 94%.
(2) increased serum ALP and GGT. Sudden increase in these enzymes is a characteristic finding in HCC.
(3) production of ectopic hormones, which include:
(a) erythropoietin (EPO), producing secondary polycythemia (see Chapter 13).
(b) insulin-like factor, producing hypoglycemia (see Chapter 23).
(c) parathyroid hormone (PTH)–related protein, producing hypercalcemia (see Chapter 23).
(4) hypercholesterolemia, caused by reduced expression of low-density lipoprotein (LDL) receptor (decreased uptake of cholesterol from the blood).

Diagnosis

CT scan, US

Angiography

g. Diagnosis
(1) CT scan and US localize HCC.
(2) Angiography shows pooling and increased vascularity of the tumor.

h. Prognosis

(1) If unresectable, most patients die within 6 months.

(2) If resectable, the 5-year survival rate is 30% to 50%.

3. Fibrolamellar variant of HCC

a. **Definition:** Slow-growing variant of HCC that does *not* develop in a background of preexisting cirrhosis

b. Epidemiology

(1) Men and women are equally affected.

(2) *No* previous history of liver disease

(3) Develops in mid-20s

(4) Abdominal pain caused by a large, solitary, nodular hepatic mass in the left lobe of the liver (75%) (Link 19-70, *left*).

(5) Histologically, thin layers of fibrous tissue separate neoplastic cells, hence the term *fibrolamellar* (Link 19-70, *right*).

(6) Fibrous central scar is seen on imaging studies.

(7) Key finding is a normal serum AFP.

(8) Approximately 50% of patients have resectable tumors.

4. Angiosarcoma

a. **Definition:** Malignant neoplasm arising from the endothelial cells (ECs) lining blood vessels; may occur in any area of the body (Link 19-71). Recall that sarcomas arise from mesodermal cells.

b. Epidemiology

(1) Exposure to vinyl chloride is the most common cause.

(2) Other causes include arsenic and thorium dioxide.

X. Gallbladder and Biliary Tract Disease

A. Cystic diseases of the biliary tract include:

1. choledochal cyst.

a. **Definition:** Congenital cystic dilations of the extrahepatic biliary tract (Link 19-72)

b. Epidemiology

(1) Most common cyst in the biliary tract in children younger than 10 years old

(2) Occurs in 1 of 13,000 to 15,000 people

(3) Females outnumber males.

(4) Two-thirds present *before* 10 years of age.

(5) Increased incidence of cholelithiasis (gallstones), cholangiocarcinoma (cancer of bile ducts), and cirrhosis

c. Clinical findings include:

(1) epigastric or right-sided abdominal pain with persistent or intermittent jaundice.

(2) palpable mass in the RUQ of the abdomen in less than one-third of patients.

(3) classic triad of abdominal pain, jaundice, and palpable mass in <20% of patients.

(4) jaundice in infants, hepatomegaly.

d. Diagnosis

(1) US is the screening test of choice.

(2) ERCP or transhepatic cholangiography may be used.

(a) Useful in identifying intrahepatic and extrahepatic cysts

(b) Useful in identifying sites of obstruction

2. Caroli disease and Caroli syndrome

a. **Definition of Caroli disease:** Inherited disorder characterized by cystic dilation of the larger intrahepatic bile ducts (Fig. 19-9 A)

b. **Definition of Caroli syndrome:** Inherited disorder with dilation of large and small intrahepatic bile ducts

c. Both Caroli disease and syndrome are characterized by:

(1) congenital cystic dilations of the intrahepatic bile duct but *not* the extrahepatic bile ducts.

(2) diffuse or segmental dilation.

(3) increased risk for developing cholangiocarcinoma (carcinoma of the bile ducts).

d. Caroli disease

(1) Whereas the simple form is transmitted as an autosomal dominant trait, the complex form associated with polycystic kidney disease (PKD) is transmitted as an AR trait.

(2) Associated with cholestasis, which may lead to recurrent intrahepatic calculi and cholangitis (inflammation of the bile duct)

(3) Hepatic fibrosis is *not* present.

Poor prognosis

Fibrolamellar variant

Variant HCC *without* preexisting liver disease

Men = women

No preexisting liver disease

Mid-twenties

Abdominal pain; solitary mass; left lobe liver

Fibrous tissue separates neoplastic cells

Fibrous central scar (imaging)

Key: normal AFP

50% have resectable tumors

Angiosarcoma

Endothelial cell sarcoma

Vinyl chloride (plastic pipes), arsenic, thorium dioxide

Choledochal cyst

Congenital cystic dilations of extrahepatic biliary tract

MC biliary tract disease child <10 yrs old

Female > males

Majority present before 10 yrs of age

Cholelithiasis, cholangiocarcinoma, cirrhosis

Epigastric, right abdominal pain, intermittent jaundice

Palpable mass RUQ

Triad abdominal pain, jaundice, palpable mass

Jaundice in infants

Hepatomegaly

US screening test

ERCP, transhepatic cholangiography

Caroli disease/syndrome

Disease: inherited

Cystic dilation large intrahepatic bile ducts

Syndrome: dilation large/small intrahepatic bile ducts

Both: cystic dilations intrahepatic (*not* extrahepatic) bile ducts

Both: diffuse/segmental dilation

Both: ↑risk cholangiocarcinoma

Caroli disease

Simple form AD, complex form AR + PKD

Cholestasis, intrahepatic calculi, cholangitis

No hepatic fibrosis

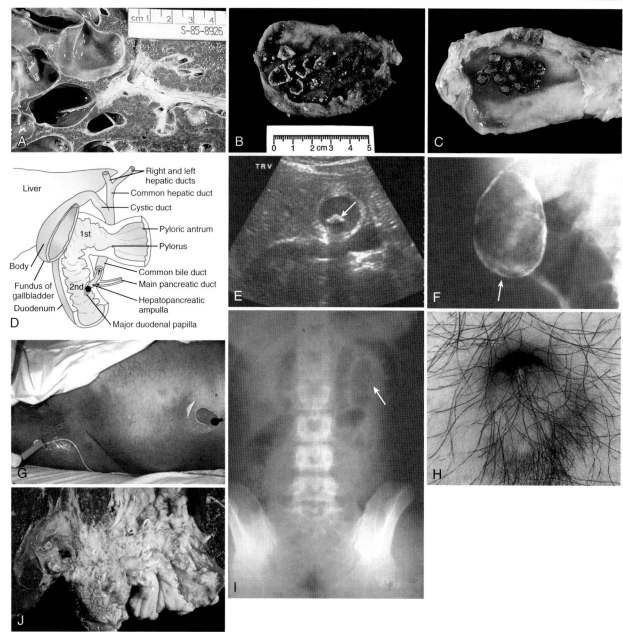

19-9: **A,** Caroli disease. Note the segmental dilation of the intrahepatic ducts. **B,** Yellow cholesterol stones with centers containing entrapped bile pigments. The wall of the gallbladder is scarred. **C,** Black pigmented stones. This type of stones is usually a sign of a chronic extravascular hemolytic anemia (e.g., hereditary spherocytosis, sickle cell disease), where there is an increase in unconjugated bilirubin (UCB) (macrophage destruction of spherocytes or sickle cells) and a corresponding increase in the uptake and conjugation of UCB to conjugated bilirubin (CB) in the liver. In the gallbladder, some of the CB is converted back to UCB, which combines with calcium to form calcium bilirubinate stones. **D,** Anatomy of gallbladder, common bile duct (CBD), pancreas, and main pancreatic duct. Note that a gallstone *(black circle)* that is lodged in the distal end of the CBD forces bile into the main pancreatic duct as well as the bile ducts in the liver *(arrows)*. This produces extrahepatic cholestasis with jaundice and acute pancreatitis. **E,** Ultrasound image showing gallstones *(arrow)*. **F,** Calcified gallbladder wall. The rimlike calcification *(solid white arrow)* identifies this as occurring in the wall of the gallbladder. This is a porcelain gallbladder, which occurs with chronic inflammation and stasis and is associated with gallstones and an increased incidence of carcinoma of the gallbladder. **G,** Grey-Turner sign. Note the purplish discoloration in the loins caused by tracking of hemorrhagic necrotic pancreatic material along the retroperitoneal planes. **H,** Cullen sign. Note the hemorrhagic discoloration around the umbilicus. It is caused by tracking of hemorrhagic necrotic pancreatic tissue around the falciform and umbilical ligaments. **I,** Sentinel loop from acute pancreatitis. A single, persistently dilated loop of small bowel is seen in the left upper quadrant *(solid white arrow)* in the prone radiograph of the abdomen. A sentinel loop or localized ileus often signals the presence of an adjacent irritative or inflammatory process. They are also seen in retrocecal acute pancreatitis. **J,** Pancreatic adenocarcinoma. Yellow tumor has extensively replaced the pancreas. *(A from MacSween R, Burt A, Portmann B, Ishak K, Scheuer P, Anthony P: Pathology of the Liver, 4th ed, London, Churchill Livingstone, 2002, p 125, Fig. 3.29; B and C from Kumar V, Fausto N, Abbas A: Robbins and Cotran Pathologic Basis of Disease, 7th ed, Philadelphia, Saunders, 2004, pp 930, 931, respectively, Figs. 18-50, 18-51, respectively; D from Moore A, Roy W: Rapid Review Gross and Developmental Anatomy, 3rd ed, Philadelphia, Mosby Elsevier, 2010, p 82, Fig. 3.27; E from Goldman L, Schafer AI: Cecil's Textbook of Medicine, 24th ed, Philadelphia, Saunders Elsevier, 2012, p 1017, Fig. 158-5; F and I from Herring W: Learning Radiology Recognizing the Basics, 2nd ed, Philadelphia, Elsevier Saunders, 2012, pp 157, 140, respectively; Figs. 16.3, 14-1B, respectively; G and H from Grieg JD: Color Atlas of Surgical Diagnosis, London, Mosby-Wolfe, 1996, p 162, Figs. 22-5, 22-4, respectively; J from Klatt F: Robbins and Cotran Atlas of Pathology, Philadelphia, Saunders, 2006, p 226, Fig. 9-14.)*

e. Caroli syndrome
(1) More common than Caroli disease and is transmitted as an AR trait
(2) Cystic dilation may occur in large or small intrahepatic bile ducts.
(3) Hepatic fibrosis is *always* present and may lead to portal hypertension.
(4) Polycystic liver disease (Link 19-73) can coexist with autosomal dominant PKD; associated with mutations in the *PKHD1* and *PKHD2* genes.
f. Clinical findings in Caroli disease and syndrome include:
(1) recurrent inflammation of the intrahepatic bile ducts.
(2) jaundice, rapid enlargement of liver.
(3) Portal hypertension in the type with congenital hepatic fibrosis (Caroli syndrome).

B. Cholangiocarcinoma
1. **Definition:** Malignancy of the bile ducts (may be intrahepatic or extrahepatic)
2. Epidemiology
   a. Most common malignancy of the bile ducts
   b. Causes of cholangiocarcinoma include disorders associated with chronic biliary inflammation, which include:
   (1) PSC (MCC; see earlier): most common cause of cholangiocarcinoma in the United States.
   (2) *Clonorchis sinensis* (Chinese liver fluke; particularly in northern Thailand).
   (3) choledochal cyst, Caroli disease or syndrome.
   (4) gallstones, chronic ulcerative colitis.
   c. Locations include:
   (1) intrahepatic bile ducts (20%–25% of cases; Link 19-74).
   (2) confluence of the right and left hepatic bile ducts at the liver hilum (50%–60% of cases; Klatskin tumor).
   (3) distal CBD (20% of cases).
3. Clinical and laboratory findings include:
   a. upper abdominal pain and weight loss in 50% of cases.
   b. obstructive jaundice.
   c. palpable gallbladder (Courvoisier sign). Only occurs if the cancer is located in the middle portion of the CBD or at the ampulla.
   d. hepatomegaly, increased levels of the tumor marker CA 19-9 in 80% of cases.
4. Diagnosis includes US, ERCP, combination of CT and MRI.
5. Mean survival time is less than 2 years.
6. Overview of cancers of the liver and biliary systems (Link 19-75)

C. Gallstones (cholelithiasis)
1. Anatomy of the gallbladder, duodenum, and biliary tract (Link 19-76)
   a. Fundus, body, and neck
   b. Cystic duct (CD) empties bile into CBD.
   c. Function: concentrates and stores bile between meals

Neural (cholinergic vagal stimulation), hormones (cholecystokinin, motilin) control filling and emptying of the gallbladder. Hormonal stimulation after meals causes the gallbladder to release concentrated bile (contraction) into the common bile duct and through the relaxed sphincter of Oddi into the duodenum for activation of digestive enzymes and further digestion of lipids (see Chapter 18).

2. Components of bile include:
   a. bile salts/acids (~67%).
   (1) Hepatic products of cholesterol (CH) metabolism
   (2) Water soluble
   (3) Detergent action renders cholesterol soluble in bile.
   b. phospholipid (PL; 22%): mainly composed of lecithin, hydrophobic, and solubilizes cholesterol in bile.
   c. protein (4.5%), free cholesterol (4%), and CB (0.3%).
   d. water, electrolytes, and bicarbonate.
3. Types of gallstones include:
   a. Mixed gallstones (80%)
   (1) Chronic cholecystitis is invariably present.
   (2) Various combinations of cholesterol, calcium bilirubinate, and calcium carbonate (Fig. 19-9 B; Links 19-77 and 19-78)

Marginal notes:

Caroli syndrome
Syndrome more common than disease; AR disease
Cysts large/small intrahepatic bile ducts
Hepatic fibrosis *always* present, portal hypertension
Polycystic liver disease + PKD
Caroli disease; clinical
Recurrent inflammation intrahepatic bile ducts
Jaundice
Rapid enlargement of liver
Portal hypertension in Caroli syndrome
Cholangiocarcinoma
Malignancy intrahepatic bile ducts
MC malignancy bile ducts
PSC MCC
Clonorchis sinensis
Chinese liver fluke (northern Thailand)
Choledochal cyst
Caroli disease/syndrome
Gallstones, chronic ulcerative colitis
Intrahepatic bile ducts
Confluence right/left hepatic bile ducts MC site; Klatskin tumor
Distal CBD
Upper abdominal pain, weight loss
Obstructive jaundice
Palpable gallbladder (Courvoisier sign)
Hepatomegaly
↑CA19-9
US, ERCP, CT/MRI
Poor survival
Gallstones (cholelithiasis)
Anatomy
Fundus, body, neck
Cystic duct → CBD
Concentrates/stores bile between meals

Components bile
Bile salts/acids
Product CH metabolism
Water soluble
CH soluble in bile
Phospholipid (lecithin)
Solubilized CH in bile
Protein, free CH, CB
Water, electrolytes, bicarbonate
Types gallstones
Mixed (MC)
Chronic cholecystitis
CH, calcium carbonate, bilirubin pigment

Multifaceted, laminated

Radiopaque (calcium carbonate)

Pure stones

Composed one substance

Pure CH stones *not* radiopaque

Pure CH stone; multiparous women

Calcium bilirubinate: jet black stone

Calcium bilirubinate: EHA, TPN

(3) Size and number may vary; usually multifaceted and laminated (layers on cut section). Radiopaque if they contain calcium carbonate (50% radiopaque).

b. Pure stones (10%)
   (1) Composed of only one substance
   (2) Pure cholesterol stones are usually single, spheroidal, and coarsely nodular and have a translucent bluish-white color. *Not* radiopaque. Majority are in multiparous women owing to alterations in cholesterol metabolism during pregnancy. There is *no* correlation of these stones with the cholesterol level in the blood during pregnancy.
   (3) Calcium bilirubinate stones are multiple, small, jet-black stones that have facets on their surface (see the following; Fig. 19-9 C, Link 19-79). They are most often associated with EHA (e.g., hereditary spherocytosis, sickle cell anemia, artificial cardiac valves) and TPN.

In extravascular hemolytic anemia (e.g., hereditary spherocytosis, sickle cell disease), there is an increase in unconjugated bilirubin (macrophage destruction of spherocytes or sickle cells) and a corresponding increase in the uptake and conjugation of unconjugated bilirubin to conjugated bilirubin in the liver. In the gallbladder, some of the conjugated bilirubin is converted back to unconjugated bilirubin, which combines with calcium to form calcium bilirubinate stones (Fig. 19-9 C; Link 19-79).

EHA: CB converted to UCB → UCB + calcium → calcium bilirubinate stones

Brown pigment stones

Sign CBD infection

Asians

Infection: CB → UCB → brown stone

Combined stones: large, single stones, chronic cholecystitis

Formation of gallstones

Enhanced intestinal absorption CH

Supersaturation bile with CH

Nucleation: CH crystals precipitate → CH stones

Bile stasis: hypomotility → enhances crystal nucleation

Biliary sludge: precipitates CH or calcium bilirubinate

Earliest stage gallstone formation

Risk factors

Female >40, pregnancy

Highest risk 5th/6th decades

Native/Mexican Americans, Scandinavians

OCPs, obesity

Rapid weight loss

Lipid-lowering drugs, octreotide, ceftriaxone

Diabetes mellitus, Crohn's disease

Symptomatic cholelithiasis: MC indication cholecystectomy

(4) Brown pigment stones
   (a) Sign of infection in the CBD; *not* seen in the gallbladder; commonly seen in Asians
   (b) Infection deconjugates CB, which increases UCB in the bile, leading to formation of brown pigment stones.

c. Combined stones (10%) are usually large, single stones that are associated with chronic cholecystitis (Link 19-78).

4. Major factors that are involved in the formation of most gallstones
   a. Enhanced intestinal cholesterol absorption: increased cholesterol absorption increases the total amount of cholesterol that is secreted into the bile by the liver
   b. Supersaturation of bile with cholesterol (CH): The amount of CH in bile exceeds the solubilizing capacity of bile acids and phospholipids.
   c. Nucleation: Cholesterol crystals precipitate from supersaturated bile, which enhances the formation of cholesterol stones (Fig. 19-9 B).
   d. Bile stasis: Hypomotility of the gallbladder from inflammation in the muscle wall accelerates crystal nucleation.
   e. Biliary sludge: composed of microscopic precipitates of cholesterol or calcium bilirubinate and represents the earliest stage of gallstone formation

5. Risk factors include:
   a. female >40 years old, pregnancy; two to three time more common than in men of the same age.
   b. Risk increases with age (highest incidence in fifth and sixth decades. In women and men 60 years of age, the prevalence of gallstones is 50% in women and 15% in men.
   c. Native Americans (e.g., endemic in Pima and Navajo Indians), Mexican Americans, Scandinavians
   d. use of OCPs, obesity (cholesterol is increased in bile in obese individuals).
   e. rapid weight loss, drugs (lipid-lowering, octreotide, ceftriaxone).
   f. diabetes mellitus , disease of terminal ileum causing decreased reabsorption of bile acids (Crohn's disease).

6. Symptomatic cholelithiasis is the most common indication for cholecystectomy.

Estrogen increases cholesterol stone formation by several mechanisms. Estrogen increases the synthesis of high-density lipoprotein, which transports cholesterol from peripheral tissue to the liver for excretion in bile. Estrogen upregulates low-density lipoprotein (LDL) receptor synthesis in hepatocytes, thus increasing the uptake of LDL, the primary vehicle for carrying cholesterol. Furthermore, estrogen increases 3-hydroxy-3-methyl-glutaryl-coenzyme A reductase (HMG-CoA) reductase activity (rate-limiting enzyme in cholesterol synthesis); therefore, more cholesterol is synthesized in the liver.

Estrogen: ↑HDL and delivery CH to liver; ↑synthesis LDL receptors; ↑HMG-CoA reductase activity → ↑CH synthesis

Cholecystitis MC

CBD obstruction

7. Acute symptoms related to cholelithiasis (Link 19-80)
8. Complications associated with stones include (Link 19-81):
   a. cholecystitis (most common).
   b. CBD obstruction (Fig. 19-9D; Link 19-82)

  c. Gallbladder cancer.

  d. acute pancreatitis.

 9. CT showing gallstones within the gallbladder (Link 19-83).

D. Acute cholecystitis

 1. **Definition:** Acute inflammation of the gallbladder; caused by gallstones in the majority of cases (Link 19-84)

 2. Epidemiology (see discussion on gallstones)

 3. Stages of development of acute cholecystitis

  a. Stage 1

   (1) Stone lodges in the CD.

    (a) Stimulus of food causes gallbladder contraction.

    (b) Stone is forced into the CD.

   (2) Midepigastric colicky pain (pain–pain-free interval–pain) occurs. Pain is caused by gallbladder contraction against the obstructed CD.

   (3) Fever, chills, nausea, and vomiting *without* pain relief

  b. Stage 2

   (1) Stone becomes impacted in the CD.

   (2) Mucus accumulates behind the obstruction.

   (3) Chemical irritation of the CBD mucosa. Mucosal damage releases phospholipase, which converts biliary lecithin to lysolecithin, a recognized mucosal toxin.

   (4) Bacterial overgrowth occurs with *no* invasion of the mucosa.

    (a) Most common pathogen is *Escherichia coli*, a gram-negative rod.

    (b) Less common pathogens include *Enterococcus, Bacteroides fragilis,* and *Clostridium perfringens* (gangrenous cholecystitis).

   (5) Pain shifts from the midepigastric area to the RUQ.

    (a) Dull, continuous aching pain

    (b) Pain radiation occurs to the right scapula or shoulder.

  c. Stage 3

   (1) Bacterial invasion through the mucosa into the gallbladder wall

   (2) Localized peritonitis with rebound tenderness

   (3) Positive Murphy sign (see later)

   (4) Absolute neutrophilic leukocytosis is present in a complete blood cell count.

   (5) Attack subsides if the stone passes through the CD.

    (a) Approximately 90% subside over the ensuing month.

    (b) If the attack does *not* subside, the gallbladder perforates (next stage).

  d. Stage 4 (perforation): Wall tension from gallbladder distention compresses lumens of intramural vessels, leading to gangrenous necrosis.

 4. Causes of cholecystitis *not* associated with stones include:

  a. AIDS, with infection caused by CMV or *Cryptosporidium.*

  b. severe volume depletion.

 5. Clinical findings include:

  a. fever (33% of cases).

  b. nausea and vomiting (>70% of cases).

  c. radiation of pain to the right scapula or shoulder.

  d. Murphy sign: the elicitation of pain on deep palpation of the RUQ as the inflamed gallbladder hits the examiner's finger as the patient inspires.

  e. jaundice (25%–50% of cases). Usually, this indicates a stone is present in the CBD. Jaundice is an indication for CBD exploration during surgery.

  f. palpable gallbladder (20% of cases).

  g. history of ingestion of a large fatty meal before the onset of pain.

  h. Acute pancreatitis with increased amylase: consider CBD stone and reflux of bile into pancreatic duct.

 6. Laboratory findings include:

  a. absolute neutrophilic leukocytosis with left shift (increased band neutrophils; see Chapter 3). WBC counts >12,000 cells/mm³ occur in >70% of cases.

  b. increased serum AST and ALT usually indicates a stone is present in the CBD.

  c. increased serum amylase suggests that acute pancreatitis is also present.

  d. increased serum bilirubin >4 mg/dL usually indicates a stone is present in the CBD.

 7. Tests to identify stones

  a. US is the preferred initial test (Fig. 19-9 E).

   (1) Gold standard test (>98% sensitivity)

   (2) Detects stones >12 mm in diameter

Detects sludge

Not effective in CBD stone detection

Plain film

ID stones CD

No HIDA in gallbladder

No HIDA in duodenum: stone CBD

MRI, ERCP, cholangiography

Complications acute cholecystitis

Gallstone ileus: bowel obstruction by stone

Gangrenous cholecystitis

Emphysematous cholecystitis: gas production

CBD exploration

Jaundice, dilated CBD

No stones gallbladder, acute pancreatitis

Chronic cholecystitis

Prolonged cholecystitis, repeated attacks

MC symptomatic gallbladder disease

Repeated attacks; cholelithiasis

Chemical inflammation

↑Wall thickness, fibrosis, CI

Persistent pain after eating in evening

Pain radiation right scapula

Recurrent epigastric distress, belching, bloating

Cholesterolosis

CH deposits in MPs in submucosa

Excess CH in bile

CH in MPs; speckled yellow mucosa

Usually asymptomatic; no clinical significance

US: small, fixed filling defects

Hydrops of gallbladder

GB dilation: chronic obstruction cystic duct

Chronic obstruction CD

Atrophy mucosa/muscle

Gallbladder cancer

Gallstones important role

Elderly women >70 years

Cholelithiasis 95% cases

Majority adenocarcinoma

      (3) Detects sludge and evaluates gallbladder wall thickness
      (4) *Not* effective in identifying CBD stones (<30% sensitivity)
  b. Plain film to detect radiopaque stones
  c. CT scan (see Link 19-83)
  d. Hepatobiliary iminodiacetic acid (HIDA) radionuclide scan
      (1) Identifies stone(s) in the CD; *no* visualization of the gallbladder
      (2) Tracer in the gallbladder but no tracer in the duodenum indicates that the stone is in the CBD.
  e. Magnetic resonance cholangiopancreatography, ERCP, and intraoperative cholangiography can detect CBD stones.

8. Complications of acute cholecystitis
  a. Gallstone ileus (see Chapter 18): bowel obstruction caused by a stone eroding into the duodenum from an inflamed gallbladder
  b. Gangrenous cholecystitis (Link 19-85): caused by ischemia of the gallbladder wall, usually in an older patient or a patient with CM
  c. Emphysematous cholecystitis: Often associated with gangrenous cholecystitis or infection caused by gas-producing bacteria (*E. coli,* 40%; *B. fragilis,* 30%; *C. perfringens,* 20%).

9. Indications for CBD exploration include jaundice, CBD dilation >12 mm, *no* stones in the gallbladder, and acute pancreatitis.

E. Chronic cholecystitis
1. **Definition:** Cholecystitis that has been present for a prolonged period of time (e.g., months) or is the result of repeated acute attacks of cholecystitis
2. Epidemiology
  a. Most common symptomatic disorder of the gallbladder
  b. Pathogenesis includes:
      (1) repeated attacks with a minor inflammatory reaction occur in a patient with cholelithiasis.
      (2) chemical inflammation of the mucosa (infection is uncommon).
3. Gross and histologic findings include thickening of the gallbladder wall. This is caused by muscular hypertrophy, submucosal fibrosis, and CI (Link 19-86).
4. Clinical findings
  a. Severe, persistent pain 12 hours after eating in the evening
  b. Pain radiates into the right scapular area.
  c. Recurrent epigastric distress, belching, and bloating.

F. Cholesterolosis
1. **Definition:** Condition in which cholesterol deposits in the macrophages (MP) in the submucosa of the gallbladder giving the mucosa a speckled yellow appearance ("strawberry gallbladder"; Link 19-87)
2. Pathogenesis
  a. An excess amount of cholesterol is present in the bile
  b. Cholesterol deposits in MPs in the submucosa produce a yellow, speckled mucosal surface.
3. Usually asymptomatic and has *no* clinical significance
4. US reveals small, fixed filling defects.

G. Hydrops of the gallbladder
1. **Definition:** Marked dilation of the gallbladder caused by chronic obstruction of the CD, resulting in the accumulation of a sterile mucoid or clear and watery fluid (Link 19-88)
2. Epidemiology
  a. Caused by chronic obstruction of the CD
  b. Long-standing distention of the gallbladder with fluid causes atrophy of the mucosa and muscle.
3. Treated with surgery

H. Gallbladder cancer
1. **Definition:** Rare cancer arising from the epithelial cells lining the gallbladder; usually associated with the presence of gallstones
2. Epidemiology
  a. Most commonly seen in women older than the age of 70 years
  b. Pathogenesis
      (1) Cholelithiasis is present in 95% of cases; believed to play a role in causing the cancer.
      (2) More than 90% of the cancers are adenocarcinomas (Link 19-89), with the remainder being anaplastic or squamous cancers.

(3) A porcelain gallbladder markedly increases one's risk for developing gallbladder cancer (Fig. 19-9 F).

Porcelain gallbladder important risk

(a) Refers to a gallbladder with extensive dystrophic calcification related to irritation of the mucosa by gallstones (see Chapter 2). Dystrophic calcification refers to the deposition of calcium phosphate in necrotic (damaged) tissue. Calcium enters the necrotic cells and binds to phosphate released from damaged membranes by phosphatase, producing calcium phosphate.

Gallbladder with dystrophic calcification

(b) When a porcelain gallbladder is diagnosed, it is mandatory to surgically remove the gallbladder because of a 50% risk for progression to cancer.

Porcelain gallbladder: immediate surgery

3. Five-year survival rate for gallbladder cancer is <2%.

XI. Pancreatic Disorders
A. Overview of anatomy and physiology of the pancreas (Links 19-90, 19-91, 19-92, 19-93, and 19-94)
B. Relative importance of most common pancreatic diseases (Link 19-95)
C. Embryologic abnormalities of the pancreas
1. Annular pancreas

Annular pancreas

a. **Definition:** Rare condition in which a ring of pancreatic tissue continuous with the head of the pancreas constricts the duodenum, causing bowel obstruction

Ring pancreatic tissue constricts duodenum

b. Epidemiology
(1) Embryologic anomaly in which the dorsal and ventral buds form a ring around the duodenum

Dorsal/ventral buds form ring

(2) Defect is associated with small bowel obstruction.

Small bowel obstruction

2. Aberrant pancreatic tissue (i.e., heterotopic rest, choristoma). Aberrant locations include the wall of stomach (most common), duodenum, jejunum, or Meckel diverticulum (Md).

Aberrant pancreatic tissue

Stomach wall MC, duodenum/jejunum, Md

3. Major pancreatic duct

Major pancreatic duct

a. Major pancreatic duct and CBD are confluent in their terminal part. Both empty their contents into the duodenum via the ampulla of Vater.

Major pancreatic duct/CBD confluent at terminal part

b. Major pancreatic duct is important in the pathogenesis of some causes of acute pancreatitis (Fig. 19-9 D).

Major pancreatic duct

(1) Gallstone(s) obstruct(s) the terminal part of the CBD.
(2) Increased backpressure causes bile to reflux into the major pancreatic duct.

Stone blocking CBD causes acute pancreatitis

(3) Bile activates the pancreatic proenzymes, causing acute pancreatitis.

Acute pancreatitis

D. Acute pancreatitis
1. **Definition:** Acute inflammation of the exocrine pancreas caused by activation of intrapancreatic enzymes causing autodigestion of the pancreatic tissue
2. Epidemiology, pathogenesis, and histology (Links 19-96, 19-97, and 19-98)
a. Alcohol abuse and gallstones are the major causes.

Alcohol, gallstones major causes

b. Must be activation of pancreatic proenzymes (inactive enzymes). Activation leads to autodigestion of the pancreas.

Activation pancreatic proenzymes

c. Mechanisms of activation of proenzymes include:
(1) obstruction of the main pancreatic duct (MPD) or terminal CBD, caused by:

Obstruction MPD or CBC

(a) gallstones (see Fig. 19-9 D; 40% of cases). This most often occurs in women with gallstones. Biliary sludge and microlithiasis are additional causes.

Stones (female dominant), sludge, microlithiasis

(b) thickened ductal secretions related to alcohol (40% of cases), which also increases duct permeability to the pancreatic enzymes. Alcohol-induced pancreatitis is most commonly seen in men.

Alcohol: thickened secretions

(c) pancreatic tumor.

Pancreatic tumor

(2) toxins: scorpion venom, methanol.

Scorpion venom, methanol, alcohol

(3) drugs (2% of causes): thiazides, estrogen, cimetidine, 6-mercaptopurine (6-MP).

Thiazides, estrogen

(4) metabolic: hypertriglyceridemia (>1000 mg/dL), hypercalcemia.

↑TG, hypercalcemia

(5) infectious: CMV, mumps, coxsackievirus, adenovirus, echovirus, EBV, HIV, parasites (*Ascaris lumbricoides, Clonorchis sinensis*).

CMV, mumps, parasites

(6) mechanical: Examples: seat belt trauma (MCC in children), bicycle handle bar, ERCP.

Seat belt trauma (MCC children), ERCP

(7) vascular: vasculitis, ischemia after cardiac surgery, malignant hypertension.

Vasculitis, ischemia

(8) hereditary: mutations in cationic trypsinogen gene (*PRSS1*), pancreatic secretory trypsin inhibitor (SPINK1), and cystic fibrosis transmembrane regulator (thick secretions block pancreatic ducts).

Hereditary (cystic fibrosis)

(9) miscellaneous: idiopathic (10% of cases), hypothermia, autoimmune pancreatitis, celiac disease, pregnancy, penetrating duodenal ulcer (DU).

Idiopathic, penetrating DU, autoimmune

d. Trypsin is important in the activation of proenzymes.

Trypsin activates proenzymes

(1) Proteases damage acinar cell structure.

Acinar damage

(2) Lipases and phospholipases produce enzymatic fat necrosis (see Chapter 2).

Fat necrosis

Vessel damage

Damage distant sites

Fever, N/V

Midepigastric pain, radiation ("knife-like") into back

Hypovolemic shock (3rd spacing)

(3) Elastases damage vessel walls and induce hemorrhage (see Fig. 2-16 I).
(4) Activated enzymes also circulate in the blood, causing damage in distant sites (e.g., phospholipase).
3. Clinical findings include:
   a. fever, nausea, and vomiting.
   b. severe, boring ("knife-like") midepigastric pain with radiation into the back. Radiation to the back is caused by the retroperitoneal location of the pancreas.
   c. hypovolemic shock caused by third space loss of fluids.

Third space fluid refers to fluid that is sequestered outside the vasculature (i.e., fluid that is unavailable for maintaining vascular volume). In acute pancreatitis, it refers to the peripancreatic collection of fluid that commonly occurs as the pancreas undergoes autodigestion. If conditions improve, the third-space fluid will reenter the vasculature, possibly causing fluid overload.

Fluid unavailable for volume maintenance in vascular compartment

Hypoxemia

Destruction surfactant pancreatic phospholipase

Atelectasis → intrapulmonary shunting

ARDS

Grey-Turner sign: flank hemorrhage

Cullen sign: periumbilical hemorrhage

DIC

Tetany

Hypocalcemia (enzymatic fat necrosis)

Tetany: calcium binds to FAs

Complications

Pancreatic necrosis

Systems signs occur earlier than usual

Fever higher than usual, tachycardia

↑↑Neutrophilic leukocytosis

Peripancreatic infections

Pancreatic fluid around pancreas

Abdominal mass; ↑amylase >14 days

Can produce pseudoaneurysms

Most resolve in 6 weeks

Pancreatic abscess

Late complication; pus within/around pancreas

Abdominal pain

High fever due to sepsis

E. coli, Pseudomonas spp.

Neutrophilic leukocytosis

Persistent hyperamylasemia

Diagnosis

CT scan shows bubbles

Pancreatic ascites: leaking pseudocyst

Pancreatic ascites

Fluid with ↑amylase/protein

Leaking pseudocyst/chronic pancreatitis

   d. hypoxemia.
   (1) Circulating pancreatic phospholipase destroys surfactant (alveoli, collapse).
   (2) Loss of surfactant induces atelectasis and intrapulmonary shunting.
   (3) Acute respiratory distress syndrome (ARDS) may occur (see Chapter 17).
   e. Grey-Turner sign (flank hemorrhage; Fig. 19-9 G).
   f. Cullen sign (periumbilical hemorrhage; Fig. 19-9 H).
   g. DIC (see Chapter 15) caused by activation of prothrombin by trypsin.
   h. tetany (spasms of the hands and feet caused by a decrease in serum ionized [unbound] calcium; see Chapter 23).
   (1) Hypocalcemia is caused by enzymatic fat necrosis.
   (2) Calcium binds to FAs, which decreases the serum level of ionized calcium.
4. Complications include:
   a. pancreatic necrosis.
   (1) Systemic signs occur earlier than usual.
   (2) Fever is higher than usual, and the patient has sinus tachycardia (rapid heartbeat).
   (3) Greater degree of neutrophilic leukocytosis in the peripheral blood than usual
   (4) Peripancreatic infections occur in 40% to 70% of cases.
   b. formation of a pancreatic pseudocyst (20% of cases).
   (1) **Definition:** A collection of digested pancreatic tissue encompassing the pancreas (example of third spacing) (Links 19-99 and 19-100)
   (2) Presents as an abdominal mass with persistence of serum amylase for >14 days. Amount of amylase in the fluid surpasses the renal clearance of amylase; hence, the increase in serum amylase persists for a longer period of time.
   (3) Can compress and erode surrounding structures, including blood vessels, producing pseudoaneurysms
   (4) Most resolve within 6 weeks.
   c. pancreatic abscess.
   Definition: Late complication of acute pancreatitis (>4 weeks after the initial attack) characterized by a collection of pus within and around the pancreas resulting from liquefactive necrosis (see Chapter 2) of pancreatic tissue and infection
   (1) Clinical and laboratory findings include:
       (a) abdominal pain.
       (b) high fever caused by sepsis. Usually secondary to gram-negative organisms such as *E. coli* or *Pseudomonas* spp.
       (c) neutrophilic leukocytosis.
       (d) persistent hyperamylasemia.
   (2) Diagnosis
       (a) CT scan shows multiple radiolucent bubbles in the retroperitoneum.
       (b) CT-guided aspiration of the abscess identifies the organisms producing the abscess.
   d. pancreatic ascites.
   (1) **Definition:** Increased amount of fluid in the peritoneal cavity; characterized by high levels of amylase and increased protein (>3 g/L)
   (2) Usually caused by leaking of a pancreatic pseudocyst or chronic pancreatitis (discussed in the following)
   (3) Usually resolves spontaneously

5. Laboratory findings in acute pancreatitis
   a. Level of enzymes does *not* correlate with severity of the disease.
   b. Increase in serum amylase (usually three times normal level).
      (1) *Not* specific for pancreatitis. Recall that amylase is also present in salivary glands and can be increased in mumps.
      (2) Sensitivity of 85% and specificity of 70% for diagnosing acute pancreatitis
      (3) Initial increase in amylase occurs after 2 to 12 hours; it peaks over 12 to 30 hours and returns to normal in 2 to 4 days because of increased renal clearance of the enzyme (Link 19-101).
      (4) Amylase is present in the urine for 1 to 14 days.
      (5) Persistent increase in serum amylase for >7 days suggests the presence of a pancreatic pseudocyst (see above discussion).
   c. Increase in urine amylase. Initial increase occurs over 4 to 8 hours; it peaks at 18 to 36 hours and returns to normal over 7 to 10 days.
   d. Increase in serum lipase.
      (1) More specific for acute pancreatitis than amylase; not excreted in the urine
      (2) Sensitivity of 80% and specificity of 75%
      (3) Initial increase in serum lipase occurs in 3 to 6 hours; it peaks in 12 to 30 hours and returns to normal over 7 to 14 days (Link 19-101).
   e. Serum ALT.
      (1) Elevation of ALT three times normal suggests a gallstone obstructing the CBD as the cause of pancreatitis.
      (2) Normal ALT does *not* rule out gallstone pancreatitis (test lacks sensitivity).
   f. Increase in serum immunoreactive trypsin (SIT)
      (1) Trypsin is specific for the pancreas.
      (2) Excellent newborn screen for cystic fibrosis
      (3) Sensitivity of 95% to 100% for diagnosing acute pancreatitis
      (4) Increases 5 to 10 times normal; remains increased for 4 to 5 days
   g. Decrease in fecal elastase; very sensitive and specific test for pancreatic exocrine dysfunction
   h. Absolute neutrophilic leukocytosis in the peripheral blood
   i. Hypocalcemia may occur because of binding of calcium to fatty acids (FAs).
   j. Hyperglycemia indicates destruction of β-islet cells.
6. Imaging studies in acute pancreatitis include:
   a. CT is the most informative test (Link 19-102). Shows pancreatic enlargement, peripancreatic fluid or debris, hemorrhage, necrosis, and abdominal fluid. Many physicians use CT as a predictor of severity. It is the gold standard for pancreatic imaging.
   b. Plain abdominal radiograph shows a sentinel loop in the subjacent duodenum or transverse colon (cut-off sign; Fig. 19-9 I); localized ileus, where the inflamed bowel lacks peristalsis
   c. Plain abdominal radiograph may also show a left-sided pleural effusion. Aspiration of the pleural fluid reveals an increase in amylase in 10% of cases.

Margin notes:
Level enzymes no correlation with severity

Amylase: *not* specific for pancreatitis; present in saliva

Normal in 2 to 4 days
↑Urine amylase; persists up to 14 days
↑Serum amylase >7 days → pseudocyst

↑Urine amylase
More specific than amylase
Not in urine

Normal 7–14 days
Serum ALT

↑↑↑Serum ALT: gallstone pancreatitis
↑SIT
Trypsin specific for pancreas
SIT excellent newborn screen for cystic fibrosis
↑↑Sensitivity for Dx acute pancreatitis
↓Fecal elastase: pancreatic exocrine dysfunction
Neutrophilic leukocytosis
Hypocalcemia: calcium binds to FAs
Hyperglycemia: destruction β-islet cells

CT gold standard

Sentinel loop: localized ileus

Left-sided pleural effusion
Fluid contains amylase

Ranson criteria are used to determine the patient prognosis in acute pancreatitis.

Admission (first 24 hours): age >55 years old, WBC count >16,000 cells/mm³, serum glucose >200 mg/dL, serum LDH >350 IU/L, and serum AST >250 U/L. Subsequent 48 hours: hematocrit drop >10% with hydration, serum BUN rise >5 mg/dL, PaO₂ <60 mm Hg (respiratory failure), base deficit >4 mEq/L (metabolic acidosis), calcium <8 mg/dL, and fluid sequestration >6 L. Those with three or four risk factors have a 15% mortality rate, but those with seven or more have a 100% mortality rate. Recent studies have begun to question whether the above criteria are an adequate indicator of severity. Other criteria assess severity by using vital signs, laboratory tests (WBC count, serum creatinine, hematocrit, arterial pH), age, and comorbidities as a predictor of mortality.

E. **Chronic pancreatitis**
   1. **Definition:** Recurrent or persistent chronic inflammatory disease characterized by fibrosis, chronic pain, and exocrine and endocrine insufficiency
   2. Epidemiology
      a. Occurs in men more often than women
      b. Majority of cases are idiopathic.
      c. Known causes of chronic pancreatitis

Margin notes:
Chronic pancreatitis

Fibrosis, pain, exocrine/endocrine dysfunction

Men > women
Majority idiopathic

(1) Alcohol abuse is the most common known cause (70%).

(2) Cystic fibrosis is the most common cause in children.

(3) Malnutrition is the most common cause in developing countries.

(4) Autoimmune disease may be the cause (15%).

    (a) Type 1 in United States (80%) and Japan (100%). Lymphoplasmacytic sclerosing pancreatitis; IgG4 relationship (increased in tissue); multiple organs involved

    (b) Type 2 in Europe: primarily centers around pancreatic ducts; no IgG4 relationship; no other organ involvement

(5) Hereditary pancreatitis (see previous discussion)

3. Pathogenesis/pathology

  a. Repeated attacks of acute pancreatitis eventually produce duct obstruction with dilation of the ducts and extensive fibrosis. Dilated ducts are frequently filled with stones (Link 19-103).

  b. Calcified concretions may also occur in the ducts. Radiographic dyes show a "chain of lakes" appearance in the major duct (Link 19-104).

  c. Additional findings in chronic pancreatitis are pseudocysts and nerve entrapment, producing the severe pain of chronic pancreatitis (Link 19-105).

4. Clinical findings include:

  a. severe pain radiating into the back.

  b. malabsorption (Link 19-106).

    (1) Indicates that >90% of the exocrine function of the pancreas is destroyed

    (2) Results in malabsorption with loss of protein in stool; ascites possible

  c. type 1 DM (70% of cases; Link 19-106) caused by loss of insulin.

5. Laboratory and radiographic findings include:

  a. variable levels of amylase and lipase. Serum amylase is less reliable than in acute disease. Values are either normal, borderline, or slightly increased. Serum lipase is *not* useful.

  b. decreased serum immunoreactive trypsin (SIT).

  c. 72-hour stool for fecal fat shows >7 g/24 hours while consuming a high-fat diet.

  d. decreased fecal elastase and chymotrypsin.

  e. tests for pancreatic insufficiency.

    (1) CT and plain films of the pancreas show dystrophic calcification (see Fig. 2-14 A), an excellent sign of chronic pancreatitis.

    (2) Functional tests include the:

      (a) secretin stimulation test (requires instrumentation): tests the ability of the pancreas to secrete fluids and electrolytes; abnormal in chronic pancreatitis

      (b) bentiromide test: tests the ability of pancreatic chymotrypsin to cleave orally administered bentiromide to *para*-aminobenzoic acid (measured in the urine); abnormal in chronic pancreatitis

  f. CT shows diffuse calcification in the pancreas (Link 19-107).

6. Approximately 50% 10-year mortality rate

F. **Exocrine pancreatic cancer**

1. **Definition:** An adenocarcinoma that is derived from the exocrine ductal epithelium

2. Epidemiology

  a. Second most common gastrointestinal malignancy after colorectal carcinoma

  b. Two times more common in men than women

  c. Usually occurs in the seventh and eighth decades of life

  d. Causes include:

    (1) smoking (most common cause); includes smokeless tobacco.

    (2) chronic pancreatitis.

    (3) hereditary pancreatitis.

    (4) DM, particularly in women.

    (5) obesity, high saturated fat diet, cirrhosis.

3. Pathogenesis

  a. High association with a *KRAS* gene mutation

  b. Mutations of suppressor genes (*p16* and *p53*)

4. Location of pancreatic cancer

  a. Most occur in the pancreatic head (60% of cases; Fig. 19-9 J), body (10%), tail (5%), and diffuse (25%) (Link 19-108).

  b. Often blocks the CBD, causing obstructive jaundice

5. Grossly, the cancers are infiltrative and firm (Link 19-109). Microscopically, they can be well, moderately, or poorly differentiated (Link 19-110).

6. Clinical findings
   a. Epigastric pain with weight loss (>90% of cases)
   b. Signs of CBD obstruction (carcinoma of head of pancreas)
      (1) Jaundice (>90% of cases; CB >50%)
      (2) Light-colored stools (absent UBG)
      (3) Palpable gallbladder (Courvoisier sign; 30% of cases)
   c. Superficial migratory thrombophlebitis (see Chapter 9)
   d. Metastasis to the left supraclavicular node (Virchow node); nonspecific; also occurs in stomach cancer
   e. Periumbilical metastasis (Sister Mary Joseph sign; Fig. 19-9 H). Also occurs in stomach cancer
   f. Additional signs that depend on location of the cancer are graphically summarized in Link 19-111.
7. Laboratory findings. Increase in CA19-9 is the gold standard tumor marker.
8. CT is used for imaging (Link 19-112) as well as for guiding percutaneous biopsy of the pancreatic mass to secure the diagnosis.
9. The overall survival rate is only 3% to 5%, with a median survival time of only 6 to 10 months if metastasis is *not* present and 3 to 5 months if metastasis is present.

Epigastric pain, weight loss

Signs CBD obstruction

Jaundice

Light-colored stools (absent UBG)

Palpable gallbladder

Superficial migratory thrombophlebitis

Metastasis to left supraclavicular node

CA19-9 gold standard tumor marker

Pancreatic carcinoma: CT scan best test

The **Whipple procedure** is an en bloc resection of the pancreatic head and neck (distal pancreas remains to prevent diabetes mellitus) and resection of part of the CBD. In some cases, there is resection of the antrum with vagotomy.

CHAPTER
20 Kidney Disorders

ABBREVIATIONS

MC most common   MCC most common cause   Rx treatment

I. Overview of the Kidney (Links 20-1, 20-2, 20-3, 20-4, 20-5, and 20-6)

Development of the kidney (Link 20-3). **A,** Lateral view of the early embryo showing mesonephros and metanephric primordia. **B,** Transverse section of the embryo from panel A. **C** and **D,** Successive stages of the metanephros. The metanephros is the last of the three embryonic kidneys (pronephros, mesonephros, metanephros). It appears early in week 5 and starts to function about week 9 as a permanent kidney. The kidney develops from metanephric mesoderm and the ureteric bud of the mesonephric duct. The ureteric bud repeatedly divides to form the ureter, renal pelvis, major and minor calyces, and collecting tubules. Metanephric mesoderm forms nephrons of the adult kidney, including the glomerulus, Bowman capsule, convoluted tubules, and loop of Henle. The developing kidney ascends from the pelvis to the adult position because of differential growth and decreased body curvature.

(Excerpt taken from Moore NA, Roy WA: Rapid Review Gross and Developmental Anatomy, 3rd ed, Philadelphia, Elsevier 2010, p 92.)

Excretes harmful waste products

Urea, Cr, uric acid

Maintain acid–base

HCO_3^-, H^+

Absorb essential substances

Na^+, glucose, amino acids

Water balance

Concentrate/dilute

Na^+ reabsorption

Vascular tone

ATII

VCs PVR arterioles, efferent arterioles

Synthesis/release aldosterone

↑Na^+ in PT

PGE_2: vasodilator afferent arteriole

EPO synthesis

2nd hydroxylation vit D

II. Renal Function Overview

   A. Excretes harmful waste products. Examples: urea, creatinine (Cr), uric acid

   B. Maintains acid–base homeostasis (see Chapter 5). Controls the synthesis and excretion of bicarbonate (HCO_3^-) and hydrogen (H^+) ions

   C. Reabsorbs essential substances. Examples: sodium (Na^+), glucose, amino acids

   D. Regulates water and sodium metabolism (see Chapter 5)
   - Controls water by concentrating and diluting urine and controls sodium reabsorption in the proximal and distal and collecting tubules

   E. Maintains vascular tone (see Chapter 5)
   1. Angiotensin II (ATII)
      a. Causes vasoconstriction of peripheral vascular resistance (PVC) arterioles and efferent arterioles
      b. Stimulates the synthesis and release of aldosterone from the zona glomerulosa of the adrenal cortex (via activation of 18-hydroxylase)
      c. Increases sodium reabsorption in the proximal tubule (PT)
   2. Renal-derived prostaglandin (PGE_2). Causes vasodilation of the afferent arterioles

   F. Produces erythropoietin (EPO; see Chapter 12)
   - Synthesized in the renal cortex by interstitial cells in the peritubular capillary bed

   G. Maintains calcium homeostasis (see Chapters 8 and 23)
   1. Second hydroxylation of vitamin D

a. 1-α-Hydroxylase (OHase) is synthesized in the proximal renal tubule cells (RTCs). Parathyroid hormone (PTH) is instrumental in the synthesis of the enzyme.

b. Enzyme converts 25-hydroxycholecalciferol (synthesized in the liver) to 1,25-dihydroxycholecalciferol.

2. Functions of vitamin D
   a. Increases small bowel reabsorption of calcium and phosphorus (P) and renal reabsorption of calcium in the distal tubules
   b. Promotes bone mineralization and maintains the serum calcium level

Vitamin D promotes bone mineralization by stimulating the release of alkaline phosphatase (ALP) from osteoblasts. ALP hydrolyzes pyrophosphate (removes the phosphate) and other inhibitors of calcium-phosphate crystallization.

   c. Increases monocytic stem cells to become osteoclasts

III. **Important Laboratory Findings in Renal Disease**
   A. **Hematuria**
      1. Upper urinary tract (UUT; kidneys, ureter) causes of hematuria include:
         a. Renal stone (most common cause)
         b. Glomerulonephritis (GN). Characterized by dysmorphic red blood cells (RBCs) (damaged RBCs with an irregular membrane)
         c. Renal cell carcinoma (RCC) and Wilms tumor
      2. Lower urinary tract (LUT; bladder, urethra, prostate) causes of hematuria include:
         a. Infection (most common)
         b. Urothelial carcinoma (old term, *transitional cell carcinoma*): most common noninfectious cause of hematuria
         c. Prostatic hyperplasia: most common cause of microscopic hematuria in men
      3. Drugs associated with hematuria
         a. Anticoagulants (warfarin, heparin)
         b. Cyclophosphamide
            (1) Hemorrhagic cystitis
            (2) Risk factor for urothelial carcinoma
   B. **Proteinuria**
      1. General
         a. **Definition:** Protein >150 mg/24 hours or >30 mg/dL (dipstick)
         b. Persistent proteinuria usually indicates renal disease.
         c. Qualitative tests include dipsticks and sulfosalicylic acid (SSA).
            (1) Dipsticks are specific for albumin.
            (2) SSA detects albumin and globulins.
         d. Quantitative test is a 24-hour urine collection.
      2. Types of proteinuria (Table 20-1; Link 20-7)

IV. **Renal Function Tests**
   A. **Serum blood urea nitrogen (BUN)**
      1. **Definition:** End-product of amino acids, pyrimidine, and ammonia metabolism
      2. Normal serum BUN is 7 to 18 mg/dL.
         a. Produced by the liver urea cycle
         b. Filtered in the kidneys
            (1) Urea is partly reabsorbed in the PT.
            (2) Amount reabsorbed is dependent on renal blood flow.
               (a) If glomerular filtration rate (GFR) is decreased, more is reabsorbed.
               (b) If GFR is increased, less is reabsorbed.
         c. Extrarenal loss (e.g., skin, bowel) may occur with very high serum concentration.
         d. Serum BUN levels depend on the following:
            (1) GFR.
            (2) protein content in the diet.
            (3) PT reabsorption.
            (4) functional status of the urea cycle in the liver. Example: In cirrhosis of the liver, the serum BUN is decreased.
      3. Causes of increased and decreased serum BUN (Table 20-2)

TABLE 20-1   Types of Proteinuria

TYPE	DEFINITION	CAUSES
Functional	• Protein <2 g/24 hr • *Not* associated with renal disease	• Fever, exercise, congestive heart failure • Orthostatic (postural): occurs with standing and is absent in the recumbent state. Urine protein is absent in the first morning void. *No* progression to renal disease.
Overflow	• Protein loss is variable • LMW proteinuria • Amount filtered > tubular reabsorption	• Multiple myeloma with BJ proteinuria • Hemoglobinuria: e.g., intravascular hemolysis (e.g., paroxysmal nocturnal hemoglobinuria) • Myoglobinuria: crush injuries, McArdle glycogenosis (deficient muscle phosphorylase). Increase in serum creatinine kinase.
Glomerular	• Nephritic syndrome: protein >150 mg/24 hr but <3.5 g/24 hr • Nephrotic syndrome: protein >3.5 g/24 hr	• Damage of GBM: nonselective proteinuria with loss of albumin and globulins. Example: poststreptococcal glomerulonephritis • Loss of negative charge on GBM: selective proteinuria with loss of albumin and *not* globulins. Example: minimal change disease (lipoid nephrosis)
Tubular	• Protein <2 g/24 hr • Defect in proximal tubule reabsorption of LMW proteins (e.g., amino acids at normal filtered loads)	• Heavy metal poisoning: e.g., lead and mercury poisoning • Fanconi syndrome: inability to reabsorb glucose, amino acids, uric acid, phosphate, and bicarbonate • Hartnup disease: defect in reabsorption of neutral amino acids (e.g., tryptophan) in the GI tract and kidneys

BJ, Bence Jones; *GBM,* glomerular basement membrane; *GI,* gastrointestinal; *LMW,* low molecular weight.

TABLE 20-2   Causes of Increased and Decreased Serum Blood Urea Nitrogen

CAUSE	COMMENTS
	INCREASED SERUM BUN
Decreased cardiac output	• CHF (MC overall cause), shock (e.g., hemorrhage) • ↓Cardiac output → ↓GFR → ↑proximal tubule reabsorption of urea → ↑serum BUN
Increased protein intake	• High-protein diet (athletes), blood in GI tract • ↑Amino acid degradation → ↑serum BUN (more synthesized)
Increased tissue catabolism	• Third-degree burns, postoperative state. • ↑Amino acid degradation → ↑serum BUN (more synthesized)
Acute glomerulonephritis	• Poststreptococcal glomerulonephritis • ↓GFR → ↑serum BUN (more reabsorbed in proximal tubules)
Acute or chronic renal failure	• ATN, diabetic glomerulopathy • ↓GFR → ↑serum BUN (backs up behind the failed kidneys)
Postrenal disease	• Urinary tract obstruction (e.g., urinary stone, prostatic hyperplasia) • ↓GFR backdiffusion of urea → ↑serum BUN
	DECREASED SERUM BUN
Increased plasma volume	• Normal pregnancy, SIADH (↑reabsorption pure water) • ↑↑Plasma volume → ↑↑ GFR → ↓serum BUN (less reabsorbed)
Decreased urea synthesis	• Cirrhosis, Reye syndrome, fulminant liver failure • Dysfunctional urea cycle → ↓serum BUN (less synthesized)
Decreased protein intake	• Kwashiorkor (↑CHO diet spares protein; see Chapter 8), starvation gluconeogenesis in kidneys • ↓Amino acid degradation → ↓serum BUN (less synthesized)

ATN, Acute tubular necrosis; *BUN,* blood urea nitrogen; *CHF,* congestive heart failure; *CHO,* carbohydrate; *GFR,* glomerular filtration rate; *GI,* gastrointestinal; *SIADH,* syndrome of inappropriate antidiuretic hormone.

Serum creatinine

End-product muscle creatinine

Cr: binds P for ATP synthesis

False ↑ with Cr supplements

Creatinine: filtered in kidney

Not reabsorbed/secreted

↑With age/muscle mass, ↓ with muscle wasting

Azotemia: ↑serum BUN + Cr

B. Serum creatinine (Cr)
1. **Definition:** Metabolic end-product of muscle creatine
2. Normal serum Cr is 0.6 to 1.2 mg/dL.
   a. Cr binds phosphate (P) in muscle for adenosine triphosphate (ATP) synthesis.
   b. Cr is falsely increased with Cr supplements used by body builders.
3. Cr is filtered in the kidneys but *not* reabsorbed or secreted. It is an excellent metabolite for renal clearance testing.
4. Serum concentration varies with age and muscle mass. It is increased with age and decreased with muscle wasting.
5. Increase in serum BUN and Cr is called azotemia.
6. Causes of increased and decreased serum Cr; similar to those for serum BUN

TABLE 20-3   Causes of Increased and Decreased Creatinine Clearance

CAUSE	COMMENTS
	INCREASED CCR
Normal pregnancy	• Normal increase in plasma volume causes an increase in the GFR, leading to an increase in CCr; highest at the end of the first trimester
Early diabetic glomerulopathy	• Efferent arteriole becomes constricted because of hyaline arteriolosclerosis, causing an increase in the GFR and CCr • Increased GFR damages the glomerulus (hyperfiltration injury)
	DECREASED CCR
Older adults	• GFR normally decreases with age causing a corresponding decrease in the CCr • Danger when using nephrotoxic drugs; therefore, the dose amount and interval must be adjusted accordingly for the person's age and CCr
Acute and chronic renal disease	• ARF caused by ATN • CRF caused by diabetic glomerulopathy, CPN, renal amyloidosis

ARF, Acute renal failure; *ATN,* acute tubular necrosis; *CPN,* chronic pyelonephritis; *CRF,* chronic renal failure; *GFR,* glomerular filtration rate.

C. **Creatinine clearance (CCr)**
  1. Correlates with GFR

Creatinine clearance
Correlates with GFR

Elderly patients normally have a decrease in creatinine clearance. Therefore, it is important to calculate the dose and dosing interval for nephrotoxic drugs (e.g., aminoglycosides) to prevent precipitating acute renal failure caused by nephrotoxic acute tubular necrosis.

  a. Annual decrease in CCr of 1 mL/min after age 50 years
  b. Useful in detecting renal dysfunction
  c. Relationship between serum Cr concentration and CCr (Link 20-8)
  2. CCr formula (Link 20-8)
   a. Measured CCr = UCr (mg/dL) × V (mL/min) ÷ PCr (mg/dL)
    (1) V = volume of a 24-hour urine collection in mL/minute, and UCr and PCr are the Cr concentration of urine and plasma, respectively.
    (2) CCr results are dependent on an accurate 24-hour urine collection.
   b. Normal adult CCr is 97 to 137 mL/min.
    (1) In general, CCr <100 mL/min is abnormal.
    (2) CCr <10 mL/min indicates renal failure.
    (3) ↑CCr is normal in pregnancy (because of a normal increase in plasma volume) and early diabetic glomerulopathy.
  3. Causes of increased and decreased CCr (Table 20-3)
D. **Serum BUN/Cr (Cr) ratio**
  1. Using normal values, the normal ratio is 15 (Fig. 20-1 A).
   a. Cr is filtered and is neither reabsorbed nor secreted.
   b. Urea is filtered and partly reabsorbed in the PT (earlier discussion).
   c. BUN/Cr ratio depends on changes in the following locations: before the kidneys (prerenal), within the kidney parenchyma (renal), and past the kidneys (postrenal).
  2. Prerenal, renal, and postrenal azotemia
   a. **Definition:** Azotemia is an increase in serum BUN and Cr.
   b. Prerenal azotemia (Link 20-9)
    (1) **Definition:** Azotemia caused by a decrease in cardiac output or volume depletion
     (a) Hypoperfusion of the kidneys decreases GFR.
     (b) *No* intrinsic renal parenchymal disease
    (2) Examples: volume loss (blood, sodium-containing fluid), congestive heart failure (CHF)
    (3) Serum BUN/Cr ratio >15 (Fig. 20-1 B, E)
     (a) Decreased GFR causes Cr and urea to accumulate in the blood. In prerenal azotemia, the ratio remains unchanged because of a proportionate increase in urea and Cr.
     (b) However, after filtration, proportionately more urea is reabsorbed back into the blood because of the decreased flow rate ($P_O > P_H$; see Chapter 5). Recall that urea reabsorption is flow dependent. All Cr is excreted in the urine.

Elderly normally have reduced CCr

Nephrotoxic drugs elderly: adjust dose/dose interval for CCr

CCr: normally ↓ with age
Detects renal dysfunction
CCr = UCr × V/PCr

CCr <100 mL/minute abnormal

CCr <10 mL/minute renal failure

↑CCr normal pregnancy, early diabetic glomerulopathy

Normal BUN/Cr ratio 15

Creatinine: filtered; *not* reabsorbed/secreted

Urea: filtered, partly reabsorbed

Prerenal, renal, postrenal

Azotemia: ↑BUN, Cr

Prerenal azotemia

↓Cardiac output, volume depletion

Hypoperfusion kidneys

No intrinsic disease

Volume loss, CHF

Prerenal azotemia: ↓cardiac output, ↓GFR; ratio >15

Ratio initially unchanged

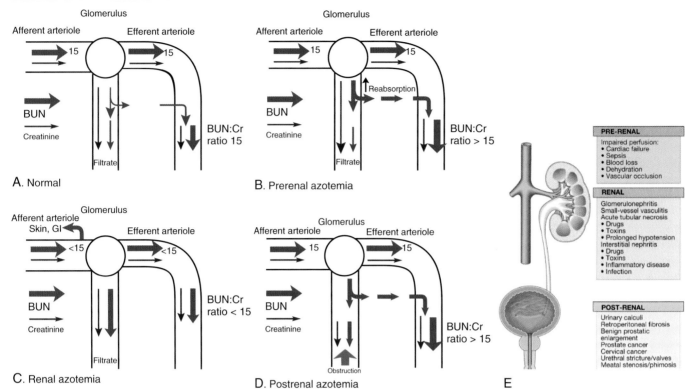

20-1: Blood urea nitrogen (BUN) and creatinine (Cr) ratios in normal persons (**A**) and in prerenal (**B**), renal (**C**), postrenal azotemia (**D**) and (**E**), causes of prerenal, renal, and postrenal azotemia. Thickness of *arrows* indicates degree of magnitude. Refer to the normal thickness of the arrows that is present in each schematic. See text for discussion. *GI*, Gastrointestinal. (*A to D from Goljan EF, Sloka KI: Rapid Review Laboratory Testing in Clinical Medicine, Philadelphia, Mosby Elsevier, 2008, p 102, Fig. 4-15. E from Walker BR, Colledge NR, Ralston SH, Penman ID: Davidson's Principles and Practice of Medicine, 22nd ed, St. Louis, Churchill Livingstone Elsevier, 2014, p 479, Fig. 17.10.*)

Ratio >15

Renal azotemia

Damage to kidneys

ATN, CRF

Ratio ≤15

Extrarenal loss urea (skin, bowel)

Serum BUN/Cr ratio remains ≤15

Postrenal azotemia

Post-kidney obstruction

No intrinsic kidney disease

Prostate hyperplasia, ureteral blockage

Serum BUN/Cr ratio >15

Obstructed urine flow ↓GFR

Initially, proportionate ↑BUN and Cr

↑↑Tubular pressure causes urea diffusion into blood

Initially ratio >15; ≤15 if obstruction persists

Urinalysis: gold standard test to evaluate renal disease

(c) Addition of proportionately more urea to blood increases the ratio to >15.
(d) Example: serum BUN 80 mg/dL, serum Cr 4 mg/dL. BUN/Cr ratio is 20 (80 ÷ 4).

c. Renal azotemia (uremia; Link 20-9)
   (1) **Definition:** Azotemia caused by parenchymal damage to the kidneys
   (2) Examples: acute tubular necrosis (ATN), chronic renal failure (CRF)
   (3) Serum BUN/Cr ratio ≤15 (Fig. 20-1 C, E)
      (a) Decreased GFR causes Cr and urea to accumulate in the blood, leading to increased extrarenal loss of urea (e.g., skin). BUN:Cr ratio is <15 because of extrarenal loss of urea (e.g., skin, bowel).
      (b) After filtration, both urea and Cr are lost in the urine. Proximal RTCs are sloughed off and are lost in the urine in renal failure.
      (c) Serum BUN/Cr ratio remains ≤15.
      (d) Example: serum BUN, 80 mg/dL; serum Cr, 8 mg/dL. BUN/Cr ratio is 10.

d. Postrenal azotemia (Link 20-9)
   (1) **Definition:** Azotemia caused by urinary tract obstruction distal to the kidneys; *no* intrinsic renal disease occurs unless obstruction persists
   (2) Examples: prostate hyperplasia, blockage of the ureters by stones or cancer
   (3) Serum BUN/Cr ratio >15 (Fig. 20-1 D, E)
      (a) Obstruction to urine flow decreases the GFR.
      (b) Both urea and Cr back up in the blood because of decreased GFR. Proportionate increase at this point. Ratio remains unchanged.
      (c) Increased tubular pressure related to the obstruction causes urea (*not* Cr) to diffuse back into the blood, causing a disproportionate increase in urea, leading to an increase in the ratio to >15.
   (4) Persistent obstruction damages tubular epithelium, causing renal azotemia (ratio ≤15).

E. Urinalysis (Table 20-4; Fig. 20-2; Links 20-10, 20-11, and 20-12)
   • Gold standard test in the initial workup of renal disease

TABLE 20-4   Urinalysis

COMPONENTS	COMMENTS
GENERAL EXAMINATION	
Color	• Dark yellow: concentrated urine, bilirubinuria, ↑UBG, vitamins • Red or pink: hematuria, hemoglobinuria, myoglobinuria, drugs (e.g., phenazopyridine, a urinary anesthetic), porphyria (see Chapters 25 and 26) • Pink diaper syndrome: benign condition in infants in which there is red-brown spotting caused by urate crystals, which turn pink on exposure to air. It can be scraped off the diaper, unlike blood. • Blue diaper syndrome: rare, autosomal recessive inborn error of amino acid metabolism caused primarily by defects in the intestinal reabsorption of tryptophan. Increased intestinal bacterial degradation of tryptophan leads to increased production and absorption of indican (a protein breakdown product). Increased loss of indican in the urine occurs, which on exposure to air oxidizes to an indigo blue color. Other manifestations of this syndrome include hypercalcemia, visual problems, and nephrocalcinosis. • Smoky-colored urine: acidic pH urine converts Hb to hematin; common finding in nephritic type of glomerulonephritis • Black urine after exposure to light: alkaptonuria (AR disease with deficiency of homogentisate oxidase; see Chapter 6) with an increase in homogentisic acid in the urine
Clarity	• Cloudy urine with alkaline pH: normal finding that is most often caused by phosphates • Cloudy urine with acid pH: normal finding that is most often caused by uric acid • Other causes: bacteria, WBCs, Hb, myoglobin also decrease clarity
Specific gravity	• Evaluates integrity of urine concentration and dilution • Specific gravity >1.023 (corresponds with a UOsm of 900 mOsm/kg). Indicates urine concentration and *excludes* intrinsic renal disease. • Hypotonic urine has a specific gravity <1.015 (corresponds with a UOsm of 220 mOsm/kg) • UOsm is the best indicator of urine concentration and dilution • Fixed specific gravity (1.008–1.010): correlates with lack of concentration and dilution (e.g., CRF)
CHEMICAL DIPSTICKS (LINK 20-10)	
pH	• Determined by diet and acid–base status of the patient • Pure vegan usually has alkaline pH (citrate converted into bicarbonate) • Those with high dietary meat ingestion usually have an acid pH (organic acids in meat) • Alkaline pH + smell of ammonia: urease-producing pathogen (e.g., *Proteus* spp.)
Protein	• Detects albumin (*not* globulins) • SSA: detects albumin and globulins (e.g., BJ protein) • Albuminuria: reagent strip and SSA have the *same* results • BJ protein: SSA *greater than* reagent strip result because SSA is detecting the light chains, but the reagent strip is not. Always confirm BJ protein with urine immunoelectrophoresis. • Microalbuminuria dipsticks: more sensitive than standard dipstick. Sensitive to 1.5–8 mg/dL. Microalbuminuria is the first sign of diabetic nephropathy.
Glucose	• Specific for glucose; does *not* detect fructose or other sugars • Detects urine glucose as low as 30 mg/dL • ↑Serum glucose + glucosuria: diabetes mellitus • Normal serum glucose + glucosuria: normal pregnancy (normally have a low renal threshold for glucose); benign glucosuria (low renal threshold for glucose)
Ketones	• Detects acetone, acetoacetic acid (*not* β-OHB). Nitroprusside in the test system only reacts with AcAc and acetone, *not* β-OHB. • Ketonuria: DKA, starvation, ketogenic diets, pregnancy (normal finding), isopropyl alcohol poisoning
Bilirubin (see Chapter 19)	• Detects conjugated (water-soluble) bilirubin. Unconjugated bilirubin (lipid-soluble) is never present in urine. • Bilirubinuria: viral hepatitis, obstructive jaundice
Urobilinogen (see Chapter 19)	• Normal to have trace amounts (normal urine color is due to urobilin) • Absent urine UBG, ↑urine bilirubin: obstructive jaundice • ↑Urine UBG, absent urine bilirubin: extravascular hemolytic anemia (e.g., hereditary spherocytosis) • ↑Urine UBG, ↑urine bilirubin: hepatitis
Blood	• Detects RBCs, Hb, and myoglobin • Hematuria: e.g., renal stone • Hemoglobinuria: e.g., intravascular hemolytic anemia • Myoglobinuria: e.g., crush injuries; ↑serum creatinine kinase
Nitrites	• Detects nitrites produced by nitrate reducing uropathogens (e.g., *Escherichia coli*). Test sensitivity and specificity are 30% and 90%, respectively. Requires ~4 hr for nitrate-reducing uropathogens to convert nitrates to nitrites, and those with UTIs commonly have increased frequency of urination, which explains the tests poor sensitivity.
Leukocyte esterase	• Detects esterase in neutrophils (pyuria; ~80% sensitivity) • Infections: urethritis, cystitis, pyelonephritis • Sterile pyuria (neutrophils present but *negative standard urine culture*): *Chlamydia trachomatis* urethritis, tuberculosis, drug-induced interstitial nephritis

Continued

TABLE 20-4 Urinalysis—cont'd

COMPONENTS	COMMENTS
	SEDIMENT
Cells	• Bacteria: usually a sign of a UTI • RBCs (hematuria; Link 20-11): renal stone, cancer (bladder, renal), glomerulonephritis (e.g., IgA nephropathy, Alport syndrome, thin basement membrane disease), urethritis, cystitis. Hematuria is >2–3 RBCs/HPF in centrifuged specimen. **Exercise-induced hematuria:** usually microscopic hematuria (RBC casts rare). ?Urinary bladder or glomerular origin. Seen in both contact and noncontact sports. Usually resolves 1–3 days after rest. • Dysmorphic RBCs: indicates hematuria of glomerular origin (see Fig. 20-2 A; Link 20-12). Damage occurs while passing through the glomerular basement membrane. More than 80% dysmorphic RBCs is diagnostic of glomerular hematuria. Sign of nephritic type of glomerulonephritis (inflammation damages RBCs). • Neutrophils (pyuria; see Fig. 20-2 B): UTI, sterile pyuria. Pyuria refers to ≥10 WBCs/HPF in a centrifuged specimen or ≥5 WBCs/HPF in an uncentrifuged specimen. • Oval fat bodies (see Fig. 20-2 C, D): renal tubular cells with lipid (nephrotic syndrome) • Renal tubular cells (see Fig. 20-2 E, F)
Casts	• Casts are formed in tubular lumens in the kidney and are composed of a protein matrix (Tamm-Horsfall protein) within which are entrapped cells, debris, or protein, which has leaked through the glomerulus. Their presence proves a renal origin of the disease. • Hyaline cast (see Fig. 20-2 G; Link 20-13): acellular, ghostlike cast containing protein. *No* clinical significance in the *absence* of proteinuria. Significant finding if proteinuria is present. • RBC cast (see Fig. 20-2 H; Link 20-13): nephritic type of glomerulonephritis (e.g., poststreptococcal glomerulonephritis) • WBC cast (see Fig. 20-2I; Link 20-13): acute pyelonephritis, acute tubulointerstitial nephritis • Renal tubular cell cast (see Fig. 20-2J; Link 20-13): ATN in acute renal failure • Fatty cast: contains lipid (e.g., cholesterol; Link 20-13): sign of nephrotic syndrome (e.g., lipoid nephrosis) • Waxy (broad) cast (see Fig. 20-2 K; Link 20-13): refractile, acellular cast; sign of CRF with tubular atrophy
Crystals	• Calcium oxalate: pure vegan diet, ethylene glycol poisoning, calcium oxalate stone • Uric acid: hyperuricemia associated with gout or massive destruction of cells after chemotherapy • Triple phosphate: may be a sign of UTI caused by urease-producing uropathogens (e.g., *Proteus* spp.) • Cystine: hexagonal crystal seen in cystinuria (inborn error of metabolism (see Fig. 20-2 L).

AcAc, Acetoacetic acid; *AR,* autosomal recessive; *ATN,* acute tubular necrosis; *β-OHB,* hydroxybutyric acid; *BJ,* Bence Jones; *CRF,* chronic renal failure; *DKA,* diabetic ketoacidosis; *Hb,* hemoglobin; *HPF,* high-powered field; *RBC,* red blood cell; *SSA,* sulfosalicylic acid; *UBG,* urobilinogen; *UOsm,* urine osmolality; *UTI,* urinary tract infection; *WBC,* white blood cell.

V. Clinical Anatomy of the Kidney

Clinical anatomy
Kidney blood supply
Cortex 90% blood supply
Medulla 10% blood supply (relatively ischemic)
Renal vessels end-arteries
No collateral circulation
Danger infarction
Afferent arterioles
JG apparatus: produce renin
Control blood flow: PGE₂
VD afferent arteriole
Direct blood into glomerular capillaries
Efferent arterioles
Drain glomerular capillaries
ATII (VC) controls efferent arteriole
Efferent arterioles become peritubular capillaries

A. Blood supply of the kidney

1. Renal cortex receives ~90% of the blood supply to the kidneys.
2. Renal medulla is relatively ischemic because of limited perfusion (10% of blood supply to the kidneys).
3. Renal vessels are end-arteries (see Chapter 2).
   a. *No* collateral circulation
   b. Occlusion of any branch of a renal artery produces infarction (see Chapter 2).
4. Afferent arterioles
   a. Contain the juxtaglomerular (JG) apparatus; produces the enzyme renin
   b. Blood flow controlled by renal-derived PGE_2 (vasodilator [VD])
   c. Direct blood into the glomerular capillaries
5. Efferent arterioles
   a. Drain the glomerular capillaries
   b. Blood flow controlled by ATII (vasoconstrictor [VC])
   c. Eventually become peritubular capillaries

Nonsteroidal antiinflammatory drugs (NSAIDs) inhibit production of PGE_2, therefore increasing the risk of renal medullary ischemia. This occurs because the intrarenal blood flow is controlled by the efferent arterioles, whose blood flow is maintained by ATII, a vasoconstrictor.

Terminology of the nephron. (1) *Filtration* is when a substance enters the nephron via the glomerulus through Bowman space. (2) *Secretion* is when a substance is pumped into the nephron at a site other than the glomerulus. (3) *Reabsorption* is when a substance is moved from the nephron back into the peritubular capillaries (and therefore back into the general circulation).

NSAIDS: inhibit production of PGE_2; risk medullary ischemia

Structure glomerulus

Fenestrated (holes) endothelium

B. Structure of the glomerulus (Fig. 20-3)

1. Glomerular capillaries contain fenestrated endothelium. Holes in the endothelial surface are important in the filtration process.

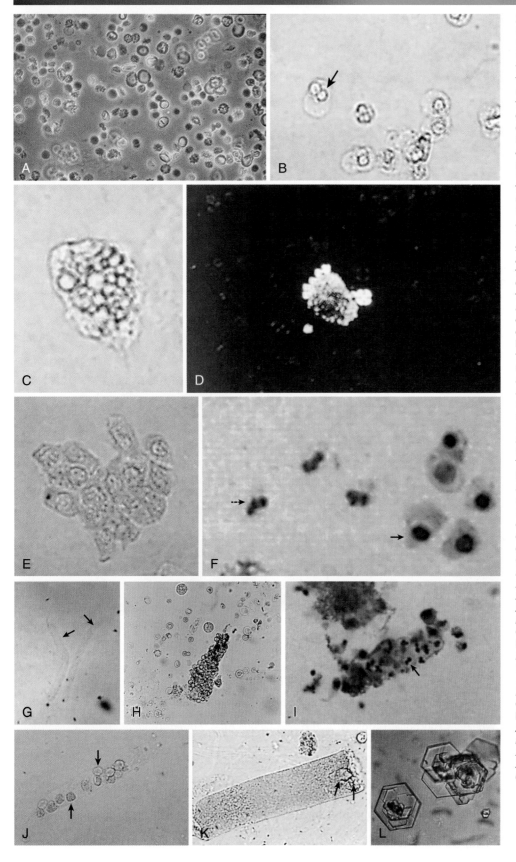

20-2: A, Dysmorphic red blood cells (RBCs). This phase contrast image of urine sediment shows dysmorphic RBCs *(arrows)* with protrusions from the RBC membrane related to damage from glomerular inflammation. They are a sign of hematuria of glomerular origin and are characteristic of the nephritic syndrome type of glomerulonephritis. **B,** Sediment with neutrophils. The *arrow* points to a bilobed neutrophil. **C,** Oval fat body with refractile lipid in the cytosol of the renal tubular cell (RTC). **D,** Oval fat body under polarization showing classic Maltese crosses. The Maltese crosses are caused by cholesterol, which is always increased in nephrotic syndrome. **E,** RTCs. **F,** RTCs *(solid arrow)* and neutrophils with multilobed nuclei *(interrupted arrow)*. **G,** Hyaline casts. The *arrows* show two hyaline casts that are acellular and have smooth borders. **H,** RBC cast in the urine. Note the cylindrical cast composed of red-staining cells. **I,** White blood cell cast. The cast is filled with multilobed cells *(arrow)* representing neutrophils. These casts are seen in acute pyelonephritis and acute drug-induced tubulointerstitial nephritis. **J,** RTC cast. The cast has numerous RTCs with round nuclei *(arrows)*. These casts are a sign of acute tubular necrosis. **K,** Waxy or broad cast in the urine sediment. The diameter of the cast is increased because of tubular atrophy. It has a refractile quality, with distinct margins. *Arrows* show degenerating RTCs. **L,** Hexagonal cystine crystals in a patient with hereditary cystinuria, an autosomal recessive disease affecting dibasic amino acids (cystine, arginine, and lysine). *(A and H from Forbes C, Jackson W:* Color Atlas and Text of Clinical Medicine, *3rd ed. London, Mosby, 2003, p 276, Figs. 6.10, 6.11, respectively; **B, D, G, I, J,** and **K** from Henry JB:* Clinical Diagnosis and Management by Laboratory Methods, *20th ed. Philadelphia, Saunders, 2001, Plates 18-4, 18-12, 18-13A, 18-17, 18-11, 18-14, respectively;* **C, E, F** *from McPherson RA, Pincus MR:* Henry's Clinical Diagnosis and Management by Laboratory Methods, *23rd ed, 2017, p 463, Figs. 28-12, 10, 11, respectively;* **L** *from Brown TA, Sonali SJ,* USMLE Step 1 Secrets, *ed 3, Philadelphia, 2013, Elsevier, pp 67-96.)*

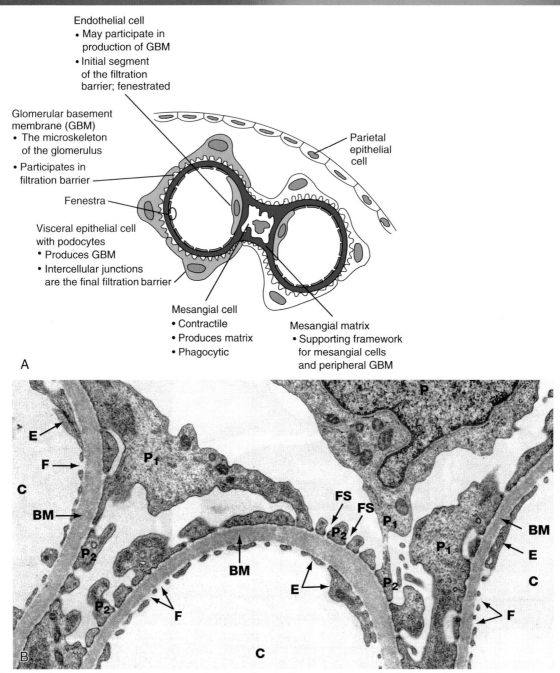

Endothelial cell
- May participate in production of GBM
- Initial segment of the filtration barrier; fenestrated

Glomerular basement membrane (GBM)
- The microskeleton of the glomerulus
- Participates in filtration barrier

Fenestra

Visceral epithelial cell with podocytes
- Produces GBM
- Intercellular junctions are the final filtration barrier

Parietal epithelial cell

Mesangial cell
- Contractile
- Produces matrix
- Phagocytic

Mesangial matrix
- Supporting framework for mesangial cells and peripheral GBM

20-3: **A,** Schematic of a normal glomerulus. See text for discussion. **B,** Electron micrograph of glomerular capillaries. *BC,* Bowman capsule; *BM,* basement membrane; *BS,* Bowman space; *C,* capillary loop; *E,* endothelial cell; *F,* fenestrations; *FS,* filtration slit; *GBM,* glomerular basement membrane; *M,* mesangial cell; *MM,* mesangial matrix; *P,* podocyte; *P₁,* podocyte primary process; *P₂,* podocyte secondary foot process. (**A** *Modified and reproduced with permission from Striker LJ, Olson JL, Striker GL: The Renal Biopsy, 2nd ed, Philadelphia, Saunders, 1990;* **B** *from Young B, Lowe J, et al: Wheater's Functional Histology: A Text and Colour Atlas, 5th ed, London, Churchill Livingstone Elsevier, 2006, p 313, Fig. 16-15b.)*

GBM
Type IV collagen
Size/charge determine protein filtration
Heparan sulfate – charge
GBM
Cationic proteins, LMW
Albumin – charge; *not* permeable
Loss – charge → albuminuria
Selective proteinuria (MCD)
GBM permeable: water, LMW proteins
GBM thickening

2. Glomerular basement membrane (GBM)
   a. Composed of type IV collagen
   b. Size and charge are the primary determinants of protein filtration.
      (1) Heparan sulfate produces the negative charge of the GBM.
      (2) Cationic proteins of low molecular weight (LMW) are permeable.
      (3) Albumin has a strong negative charge and is *not* permeable.
         (a) Loss of the negative charge causes loss of albumin in the urine.
         (b) Called selective proteinuria (e.g., minimal change disease [MCD])
      (4) GBM is permeable to water and LMW (<70,000 daltons) proteins (e.g., amino acids).
   c. Causes of GBM thickening

(1) Immunocomplex (IC) deposition. Example: membranous glomerulopathy

(2) Increased synthesis of type IV collagen. Example: diabetes mellitus (DM)

3. Visceral epithelial cells (VECs)

   a. Primarily responsible for production of the GBM

   b. Contain podocytes (footlike processes) and slit pores between the podocytes serve as a distal barrier for preventing protein loss in the urine.

   c. Fusion of the podocytes is present in any cause of the nephrotic syndrome.

4. Mesangial cells

   a. Support the glomerular capillaries

   b. Can release inflammatory mediators and proliferate in disease. Example: IgA glomerulopathy has mesangial IC deposits

5. Parietal epithelial cells

   a. Lining cells of Bowman capsule

   b. Proliferation causes "crescents" that encroach upon and destroy the glomerulus.

VI. Congenital Disorders and Cystic Diseases of the Kidneys

A. Horseshoe kidney

1. Most common congenital kidney disorder

2. Majority (90% of cases) are fused at the lower pole (Fig. 20-4). Kidney is trapped behind the root of the inferior mesenteric artery.

3. Clinical findings

   a. Increased incidence with Turner syndrome

   b. Increased risk of infection and stone formation

B. Cystic diseases of the kidney (Table 20-5)

VII. Glomerular Diseases

A. Terminology of glomerular disease (Table 20-6)

- Normal glomerulus (Fig. 20-5 A; Links 20-21, 20-22, 20-23, 20-24, 20-25, and 20-26)

B. Routine studies on biopsy specimens

1. H&E (hematoxylin and eosin stain) and other special stains: used to help classify the type of glomerular disease

2. Immunofluorescence (IF) stain

IC deposition

↑Synthesis type IV collagen

VECs

GBM synthesis

Podocytes (footlike)

Slit pores between podocytes

Prevent proteinuria

Fusion podocytes sign nephrotic syndrome

Mesangial cells

Support glomerular capillaries

Release inflammatory mediators

Parietal epithelial cells

Line Bowman capsule

Proliferation parietal epithelial cells → crescents

Congenital/cystic disorders

Horseshoe kidney

MC congenital kidney disorder

Fused at lower pole (90%)

Turner syndrome

Risk infection/stone formation

Cystic kidney diseases

H&E

IF stain

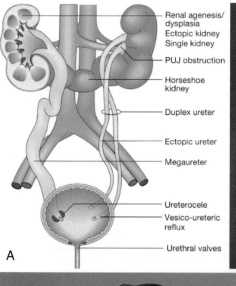

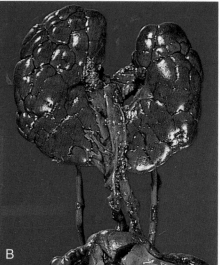

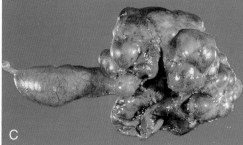

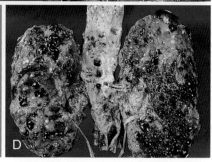

20-4: **A,** Congenital abnormalities of the urinary tract (upper and lower). **B,** Horseshoe kidney. Note that the lower poles of the kidneys are fused. **C,** Renal dysplasia. Note the multicystic deformed kidney and dilated ureter. **D,** Adult polycystic kidney disease. There is complete effacement of normal kidney architecture by cysts within the cortex and medulla of both kidneys. *(**A,** from Walker BR, Colledge NR, Ralston SH, Penman ID: Davidson's Principles and Practice of Medicine, Churchill Livingstone Elsevier, 22nd ed, 2014, p 510, Fig. 17.31; **B** to **D** from my friend Ivan Damjanov, MD, PhD, Linder J: Pathology: A Color Atlas, St. Louis, Mosby, 2000, pp 211, 213, 212, respectively; Fig. 11-3, 11-11, 11-7, respectively.)*

TABLE 20-5 Cystic Diseases of the Kidneys

CYSTIC DISEASE	COMMENTS
Renal dysplasia (see Fig. 20-4 C; Links 20-14 to 20-16)	• Most common cystic disease in children; accounts for 15%–20% of children with chronic renal insufficiency and ESRD • *No* inheritance pattern • Theories: mutations in renal development genes; altered interaction of the ureteric bud with extracellular matrix; abnormalities of renal growth factors; antenatal urinary tract obstruction • Abnormal development of one or both kidneys in utero. Abnormal structures persist in the kidneys (e.g., cartilage, immature collecting ductules) (Link 20-15). • Present as an enlarged, irregular, cystic, unilateral (bilateral) flank mass in a newborn; maternal history of polyhydramnios (excess amniotic fluid) • Bilateral dysplastic kidneys may lead to renal failure; accounts for ~20% of cases of CRF in children • Other urinary tract developmental anomalies that may be present: posterior urethral valves; prune-belly (Eagle-Barrett) syndrome; ureteropelvic junction obstruction; VACTERL; CHARGE, trisomy 13, 18, or 21 • Clinical course with bilateral involvement: progressive renal insufficiency in early childhood; nephrogenic diabetes insipidus, salt wasting, distal RTA • Multicystic renal dysplasia (Link 20-16): Kidneys are asymmetric with variably sized cysts. Small ureters lead to a hypoplastic bladder. Most severe form of renal dysplasia. Normal renal parenchyma replaced by cartilage and disorganized epithelial structures form primitive ducts. Multiple cysts of varying size and atresia of the renal pelvis and ureter.
Juvenile polycystic kidney disease	• AR inheritance; mutation of *PKHD1* gene, whose protein product codes for fibrocystin (modulates renal tubular formation by regulating polycystin-2 expression and function) • Enlarged kidneys at birth; most serious types are incompatible with life • Bilateral cystic disease; cysts in the cortex and medulla • Cysts also occur in the liver • Association with congenital hepatic fibrosis, leading to portal hypertension and esophageal variceal bleeding • Maternal oligohydramnios (decreased amniotic fluid). Newborns have Potter facies, a deformation caused by oligohydramnios. Physical findings include low-set ears, parrot-beak nose, and lung hypoplasia. • ESRD (>50% of cases) in first decade of life
Adult polycystic kidney disease (Fig. 20-4 D; Links 20-17 to 20-19)	• AD inheritance. Subtype 1 has a defect on chromosome 16 (85%–95%). Mutation in *PKD1* gene that encodes for polycystin (important in renal tubule development). Subtype 2 (5%–15%) has a gene on chromosome 4. • Family history of renal failure. Bilateral cystic disease develops by 20–25 years of age. Most express symptoms after the age of 30 years. Highest incidence of onset occurs between ages 45 and 65 years. Renal cysts are evident on CT or US by age 30 years in those with a positive family history • Bilaterally palpable kidneys • Cysts involve *all* parts of the nephron in the cortex and medulla • Cysts are also present in the liver (50% of cases), pancreas (10% of cases), and spleen (5% of cases) • Abdominal or flank pain caused by rupture of cysts, hemorrhage into cysts, passage of kidney stones (34%; urinary stasis), infection of cysts, recurrent UTIs major problem especially in women; hypertension (>80% of cases). • Associated with stroke (5%–10%) caused by rupture of intracranial berry aneurysms (aneurysms in <10% of cases), intracerebral hemorrhage, lacunar infarcts (see Chapter 26) • CRF begins at age 40–60 years because of destruction of kidneys by slowly expanding cysts; accounts for ~10% of cases of CRF; CRF is the most common cause of death • Other associations: sigmoid diverticulosis, hematuria, MVP, thoracic and abdominal aneurysms, ovarian cysts, hernias, and slight increased risk for developing RCC • AR disease: gene is located on chromosome 6. Can be diagnosed by US in utero when oligohydramnios (↓amniotic fluid) is present in the mother. Cysts develop from tubular ectasia of the collecting ducts. Liver abnormalities are always present and include liver fibrosis (most common), cholangitis, and portal hypertension with variceal bleeding. Death occurs in the perinatal period in 75% of cases. The remaining 25% of cases are milder and occur later in infancy, childhood, or early adulthood. The prognosis is much better in this latter group of patients.
Medullary sponge (cystic) kidney (Link 20-20)	• *No* inheritance pattern • Most commonly discovered with IVP. Striations present in the papillary ducts of the medulla ("Swiss cheese" appearance). Multiple cysts of the collecting ducts are present in the medulla (not present in the cortex). • Many patients are asymptomatic; recurrent UTIs, hematuria, and renal stones
Acquired polycystic kidney disease (Link 20-65)	• Most common cause is renal dialysis. Occurs in 80%–90% of patients on long-term dialysis for 5–10 years. Must be more than five cysts to secure the diagnosis. CT is more sensitive than US. • Tubules are obstructed by interstitial fibrosis or oxalate crystals • 50-fold increase in risk for developing RCC than the general population; predominates in males
Simple retention cysts	• Most common adult renal cyst (20% of adults); rare in children increase with age • Derived from tubular obstruction • May produce hematuria; may rupture if traumatized • Requires needle aspiration to distinguish it from RCC

AD, Autosomal dominant; *AR*, autosomal recessive; *CHARGE*, coloboma of the eye, heart anomaly, choanal atresia, retardation, and genital and ear anomalies; *CRF*, chronic renal failure; *CT*, computed tomography; *ESRD*, end-stage renal disease; *IVP*, intravenous pyelogram; *MVP*, mitral valve prolapse; *RCC*, renal cell carcinoma; *RTA*, renal tubular acidosis; *US*, ultrasonography; *UTI*, urinary tract infection; *VACTERL*, vertebral, anal, cardiac, tracheal, esophageal, renal, and limb.

TABLE 20-6   Nomenclature and Description of Glomerular Disorders

TERM	DESCRIPTION
Focal glomerulonephritis	Only a few glomeruli are abnormal
Diffuse glomerulonephritis	All glomeruli are abnormal
Proliferative glomerulonephritis	>100 nuclei in affected glomeruli
Membranous glomerulonephritis	Thick GBM; no proliferative change
Membranoproliferative glomerulonephritis	Thick GBM; hypercellular glomeruli
Focal segmental glomerulosclerosis	Fibrosis involving only a segment of the involved glomerulus
Crescentic glomerulonephritis	Proliferation of parietal epithelial cells around glomerulus
Primary glomerular disease	Involves only glomeruli and no other target organs (e.g., minimal change disease)
Secondary glomerular disease	Involves glomeruli and other target organs (e.g., SLE)

GBM, Glomerular basement membrane; *SLE,* systemic lupus erythematosus.

    a. IF identifies patterns and types of protein deposition
    b. Linear pattern (Fig. 20-5 B)
       (1) Characteristic finding in anti-GBM disease. Example: Goodpasture syndrome
       (2) Antibodies line up against evenly distributed antigens in the GBM. Antibodies are *not* detected by electron microscopy.
    c. Granular ("lumpy-bumpy") pattern (Fig. 20-5 C): usually indicates immunocomplex (IC) deposition in the glomerulus
  3. Electron microscopy (EM)
    a. ICs are electron dense.
    b. Detects submicroscopic defects in the glomerulus; examples include:
       (1) fusion of podocytes in the nephrotic syndrome (Fig. 20-5 D).
       (2) damage to visceral epithelial cells (VECs)
    c. Detects the site(s) of IC deposition
       (1) Deposits are electron dense (dark color).
       (2) Sites of deposition are designated as follows:
          (a) Subendothelial (Fig. 20-5 E). ICs are trapped between the endothelial cell (EC) and the GBM.
          (b) Subepithelial (Fig. 20-5 F). ICs pass through the GBM but are trapped beneath the podocytes.
          (c) Intramembranous. ICs deposit within the GBM.
          (d) Mesangial. ICs deposit in the mesangium.
  4. Patterns of glomerular involvement (Link 20-27)
C. Mechanisms producing glomerular disease
  1. ICs (example of type III hypersensitivity)
    a. ICs circulate and deposit in glomeruli or they develop in situ. Example: DNA–anti-DNA complexes in systemic lupus erythematosus (SLE).
    b. ICs activate the complement system.
       (1) Complement 5a (C5a) is produced, which is chemotactic to neutrophils.
       (2) Neutrophils damage the glomeruli. Damage to the glomeruli by neutrophils primarily occurs in nephritic types of GN (see later).
  2. Antibodies (abs) are directed against GBM antigens. Example: Goodpasture syndrome
  3. T-cell production of cytokines
    a. Cytokines cause the GBM to lose its negative charge.
    b. Cytokines damage podocytes, causing them to fuse.
    c. Example: MCD (lipoid nephrosis) in the nephrotic syndrome
D. Clinical manifestations of glomerular diseases
  1. Nephritic syndrome
  2. Nephrotic syndrome
  3. Chronic GN
E. Nephritic syndrome
  1. **Definition:** Glomerular injury is primarily due to neutrophils, causing hematuria, RBC casts, and proteinuria.
  2. Clinical and laboratory findings

Margin notes:

IF: patterns, types deposition

Linear IF: anti-GBM disease (e.g., Goodpasture syndrome)

Granular pattern: IC type glomerulonephritis

ICs electron dense
Submicroscopic defects
Fusion podocytes
Damaged VECs
Detects sites IC deposits
Deposits electron dense

Subendothelial

Subepithelial
Intramembranous
Mesangial
ICs: MC mechanism causing glomerulonephritis

ICs activate complement
C5a attracts neutrophils
Neutrophils damage glomeruli
Nephritic type GN
Goodpasture syndrome: abs against GBM
T cells produce cytokines
Cytokines cause GBM to lose negative charge
Cytokines damage podocytes (fuse)
Example: minimal change disease
Clinical manifestations
Nephritic syndrome
Nephrotic syndrome
Chronic glomerulonephritis
Nephritic syndrome
Hematuria, RBC casts, proteinuria
Clinical/lab findings

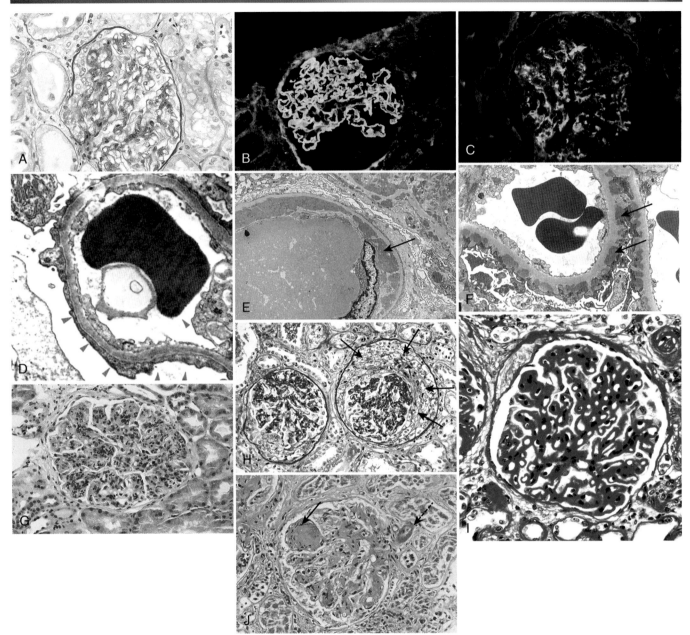

20-5: **A,** Normal glomerulus. **B,** Linear immunofluorescence. The uninterrupted smooth immunofluorescence along the glomerular basement membrane (GBM) is caused by deposition of IgG antibodies directed against the membrane (e.g., Goodpasture syndrome). **C,** Granular immunofluorescence. Granular irregular deposits in the capillaries are caused by immunocomplex deposition (e.g., poststreptococcal glomerulonephritis). **D,** Fusion of the podocytes. *Arrows* show fusion of the podocytes. The finding occurs in all glomerular diseases that present with the nephrotic syndrome (e.g., minimal change disease). **E,** Subendothelial immunocomplex deposits viewed with electron microscopy. The band of electron-dense material extends around the GBM and hugs the interface of the membrane with the capillary lumen. The *arrow* points to immune deposits directly beneath the nucleus of the endothelial cell. A thin rim of normal basement membrane *(light gray)* separates the deposits from the epithelial side of the membrane. The patient had diffuse proliferative glomerulonephritis caused by systemic lupus erythematosus. **F,** Subepithelial immunocomplex deposits viewed with electron microscopy. *Arrows* point to electron-dense deposits directly beneath the visceral epithelial cells in a patient with poststreptococcal glomerulonephritis. The normal basement membrane has a light gray appearance. **G,** Poststreptococcal diffuse proliferative glomerulonephritis. The glomerulus is hypercellular because of an increase in neutrophils and mesangial cells. **H,** Crescentic glomerulonephritis. *Arrows* point to a proliferation of parietal epithelial cells in Bowman capsule, occupying approximately 50% of the entire urinary space. The cells encase and compress the glomerular tuft. **I,** Diffuse membranous glomerulopathy. The hematoxylin and eosin)–stained biopsy shows glomerular basement membranes that are uniformly thickened. There is no proliferative component. **J,** Diabetic glomerulosclerosis. The *broken arrow* points to an afferent or efferent arteriole that has hyaline arteriolosclerosis, with an increase in proteinaceous material in the wall of the vessel. The *solid arrow* shows a mesangial nodule containing type IV collagen and trapped protein. *(A, F, and G from my friend Ivan Damjanov, MD, PhD: Pathology for the Health-Related Professions, 2nd ed, Philadelphia, Saunders, 2000, pp 329, 341, 329, Figs. 13-5A, 13-8C, 13-5B, respectively; B and H from Kumar V, Fausto N, Abbas A: Robbins and Cotran Pathologic Basis of Disease, 7th ed. Philadelphia, Saunders, 2004, pp 969, 977, Figs. 20-10E, 20-17, respectively; C, E, and J from my friend Ivan Damjanov MD, PhD, Linder J: Pathology: A Color Atlas, St. Louis, Mosby, 2000, pp 224, 229, Figs. 11-54, 11-64, respectively; D from Laszik ZG, Lajoie G, Nadasky T, Silva FG: Medical diseases of the kidney, in Silverberg SG, Delellis RA, Frable WJ [eds]: Principles and Practice of Surgical Pathology and Cytopathology, 3rd ed. New York, Churchill Livingstone, 1997, p 2079; I from Kern WF, Silva FG, Laszik ZG, et al [eds]: Atlas of Renal Pathology, Philadelphia, Saunders, 1999, p 53, Fig. 5-30.)*

a. Hypertension caused by salt retention
b. Periorbital puffiness caused by salt retention characteristic of that area
   (1) In some cases, edema is more generalized, resulting in pitting edema (see Chapter 5).
   (2) Sodium retention increases plasma hydrostatic (P_H) pressure.
c. Oliguria (~400 mL urine/day) caused by decreased GFR from inflamed glomeruli. Tubular function is intact.
d. Hematuria
   (1) Dysmorphic RBCs are present with irregular membranes (see Fig. 20-2 A).
   (2) Glomeruli become inflamed from IC deposition causing damage to RBC membranes (dysmorphic RBCs).
e. Neutrophils are present in the urine sediment (see Fig. 20-2 B), particularly in IC types of nephritic GN.
f. RBC casts are a key finding (50%–80%; see Fig. 20-2 H). Occasionally, white blood cell (WBC) casts are also present.
g. Proteinuria is >150 mg/day but <3.5 g/day.
h. Azotemia is present with a BUN/Cr ratio >15. Tubular function is intact in acute GN.
3. Primarily nephritic types of glomerular disease (Table 20-7)

F. Nephrotic syndrome
1. **Definition:** Proteinuria >3.5 g/24 hours caused by glomerular injury from cytokines rather than neutrophils.
   a. Cytokines damage podocytes, causing them to fuse.
   b. Cytokines destroy the negative charge of the GBM (massive loss of albumin).
2. Clinical and laboratory findings
   a. Key finding is proteinuria >3.5 g/24 hours.
   b. Hypoalbuminemia causes a decrease in plasma oncotic (P_O) pressure, resulting in generalized pitting edema and ascites.
      (1) Recall that pitting edema in *nephritic syndrome* is sodium retention causing an increase in P_H.
      (2) Increased risk for developing spontaneous peritonitis from *Streptococcus pneumoniae* or *Escherichia coli* (see Chapter 19)
   c. Hypertension in some types caused by sodium retention. Usually normal blood pressure in MCD and membranous nephropathy (MN). Blood pressure is frequently elevated in focal segmental glomerulosclerosis.
      • Hypercoagulable state caused by loss of antithrombin (AT, protein C/S in urine [see Chapter 15], increased platelet aggregation, and enhanced liver synthesis of procoagulant proteins). Potential for renal vein thrombosis (most common with membranous glomerulopathy).
   d. Hypercholesterolemia. Hypoalbuminemia increases synthesis of cholesterol. In response to a decrease in P_O, the liver increases the synthesis of lipoproteins.
   e. Hypogammaglobulinemia caused by the loss of γ-globulins in the urine
   f. Fatty/lipid casts with Maltese crosses (Link 20-13) and oval fat bodies (see Fig. 20-2 C, D): key finding of the nephrotic syndrome
3. Primarily nephrotic types of glomerular disease (Table 20-8)

G. Systemic diseases with nephrotic syndrome
1. Diabetic glomerulopathy (nephropathy)
   a. Sometimes called nodular glomerulosclerosis (Kimmelstiel-Wilson disease)
   b. Epidemiology
      (1) Nephropathy usually occurs after a several-year history of DM (≥10 years)
      (2) Glomerulopathy may occur in both type 1 and 2 DM. Occurs more often in type 1 (35%–45% of cases) than type 2 DM (20% of cases).
      (3) Most common cause of CRF in the United States; type 1 > type 2 DM
      (4) Risk factors
         (a) Poor glycemic control, hypertension
         (b) Diabetic retinopathy (type 1, 95; type 2, 50%–70%). High correlation with coexisting glomerulopathy in type 1 DM than type 2 DM. Patients with type 2 DM are less likely to have a coexisting retinopathy.
   c. Pathogenesis of renal disease
      (1) Nonenzymatic glycosylation (NEG) of the GBM and tubular basement membrane (BM; see Chapter 23)
         (a) Glycosylation refers to glucose attaching to amino acids.
         (b) Glycosylation increases the permeability of both vessel and tubular cell BM to proteins.

TABLE 20-7   Primarily Nephritic Types of Glomerular Disease

GLOMERULAR DISEASE	CLINICOPATHOLOGIC FINDINGS
IgA glomerulopathy (Berger disease) (Links 20-28 and 20-29)	• Most common nephropathy worldwide • Majority are nephritic (5% of cases are nephrotic) • Affects children and adults (young men); male:female ratio, 2:1; uncommon in blacks • Most common cause of chronic glomerulonephritis in children • Increased mucosal synthesis and decreased clearance of IgA • Increased serum IgA (50% of cases) • Focal proliferative glomerulopathy • Mesangial IgA IC deposits with granular IF; ICs activate the alternative complement pathway • Overlapping features with HSP may occur • Episodic bouts of hematuria (microscopic or gross) usually occur after a URI; HTN is common • Slow progression to CRF (20% of cases after 20 years) • Hematuria, RBCs casts (Link 20-13)
Poststreptococcal (see Fig. 20-5 C, F, and G; Links 20-30 B, 20-31, and 20-32)	• Most common type of postinfectious GN; other postinfectious causes include various viral infections (ECHO virus, HIV, adenovirus, influenza A, HBV, HCV), endocarditis-related glomerulonephritis, shunt-related endocarditis (usually *Staphylococcus aureus*), syphilis, and malaria • Usually follows group A streptococcal infection of skin (e.g., scarlet fever) or pharynx; *Streptococcus* types 12 and 49 are usually involved • Subepithelial IC deposits with granular IF; ICs activate the alternative complement pathway • Diffuse proliferative pattern with neutrophil infiltration • Hematuria 1–3 weeks after group A streptococcal infection by a nephritogenic strain (never produces acute rheumatic fever) • Clinical: presents 1–2 weeks after a sore throat with either grossly bloody or tea-colored urine. It may present after 2–3 weeks after impetigo. Periorbital edema occurs because of sodium retention. Edema can occasionally be more extensive and produce pitting in dependent areas (e.g., ankles). Hypertension is usually transient but may be severe in some cases. • Increased anti–DNase B titers. ASO titers increased in 70%. If the streptococcal infection causing GN is of skin origin, ASO is degraded by oil in the skin and is *not* increased. Streptozyme test is positive (90%) because it detects anti-DNAase B antibodies. Decreased serum C3 (90%). • Usually resolves. May recur within 1 year in 10% of patients. CRF is uncommon in children but common in adults. • Hematuria (Link 20-11), dysmorphic RBCs (Link 20-12), RBC casts (Link 20-13)
Diffuse proliferative glomerulonephritis (SLE) (see Fig. 20-5 C and E; Link 20-33 and 20-34)	• Diffuse proliferative GN is the most common subtype of glomerular disease in SLE. Approximately 40% of patients with SLE develop glomerulonephritis. Nearly 100% with major organ system involvement (cerebritis, pneumonitis, or vasculitis) will have renal involvement as well. • Subendothelial IC deposits with granular IF. DNA–anti-DNA ICs activate the classical complement pathway. "Wire looping" of capillaries corresponds with subendothelial ICs. • Neutrophil infiltration of the glomerulus with hyaline thrombi in capillary lumens is present. • Serum ANA test usually has rim pattern (see Chapter 4), corresponding with the presence of anti-dsDNA antibodies. • Evolves into RF in most cases; common cause of death in SLE. • Hematuria (Link 20-11), dysmorphic RBCs (Link 20-12), RBC casts (Link 20-13)
Rapidly progressive crescentic glomerulonephritis (see Fig. 20-5 B and H; Links 20-35 and 20-36)	• Clinical syndrome that may be a primary or secondary types of glomerular disease • Rapid loss of renal function progresses to ARF over days to weeks; very poor prognosis • May or may not be associated with crescent formation (crescentic GN; see Fig. 20-5 H) • Clinical associations: Goodpasture syndrome (kidney and pulmonary disease), Goodpasture disease (kidney disease only), microscopic polyarteritis (p-ANCA), Wegener granulomatosis (c-ANCA > p-ANCA), Churg-Strauss disease (p-ANCA > c-ANCA) • Goodpasture syndrome (Links 20-36 and 20-37): Male-dominant disease. 80% HLA-DR2 positive. Anti–basement membrane antibodies against collagen in glomerular and pulmonary capillaries. Linear IF (see Fig. 20-5 B, Link 20-37). EM has no electron-dense deposits. Anti-GBM antibodies are present in 90%–95% of patients. Crescentic GN (Goodpasture syndrome accounts for 5% of all cases). Begins with hemoptysis and ends with renal failure. • Hematuria (Link 20-11), dysmorphic RBCs (Link 20-12), RBC casts (Link 20-13)
Pauci-immune necrotizing crescentic glomerulonephritis (Link 20-38)	• Subtype of primary rapidly progressive crescentic GN; a crescentic glomerular disease in which immune deposits are *not* detected on immunofluorescence microscopy • 80%–90% have antineutrophil cytoplasmic antibodies • Causes of this subtype include Wegener granulomatosis (polyangiitis with granulomatosis), Churg-Strauss syndrome, and microscopic polyangiitis • Histologically, there is segmental necrosis with a break in the glomerular basement membrane. Fibrinoid necrosis and neutrophils accumulate in this area and initiate the formation of a cellular crescent in response to this break. The remainder of the glomerulus is normal. • Hematuria (Link 20-11), dysmorphic RBCs (Link 20-12), RBC casts (Link 20-13)

ANA, Antinuclear antibody; *ANCA,* antineutrophil cytoplasmic antibody; *ARF,* acute renal failure; *ASO,* anti–streptolysin O; *c-ANCA,* cytoplasmic antineutrophil cytoplasmic antibody; *CRF,* chronic renal failure; *ds,* double-stranded; *ECHO,* enteric cytopathic human orphan; *EM,* electron microscopy; *GBM,* glomerular basement membrane; *GN,* glomerulonephritis; *HSP,* Henoch-Schönlein purpura; *HTN,* hypertension; *IC,* immunocomplex; *IF,* immunofluorescence; *NAD,* nicotinamide adenine dinucleotidase; *p-ANCA,* perinuclear antineutrophil cytoplasmic antibodies; *RBC,* red blood cell; *SLE,* systemic lupus erythematosus; *URI,* upper respiratory infection.

TABLE 20-8 Primarily Nephrotic Types of Glomerular Disease

GLOMERULAR DISEASE	CLINICOPATHOLOGIC FINDINGS
Minimal change disease (MCD; lipoid nephrosis) (see Fig. 20-5 D; Links 20-39 and 20-40)	• Accounts for 80% of all cases of nephrotic syndrome; can be associated with NSAIDs • Most common cause of nephrotic syndrome in children <12 years old (girls>boys) and ~15% of adults (mid-60s) • T-cell cytokines cause the GBM to lose its negative charge, producing a selective proteinuria (albumin lost *not* globulins) • Secondary causes: Hodgkin lymphoma, NSAIDs, bee sting • Structurally normal glomeruli; positive fat stains in glomerulus and tubules • Often preceded by an URI or routine immunization • Usually normotensive (90% of cases), unlike other causes of nephrotic syndrome • Negative IF • EM shows fusion of podocytes and *no* electron-dense deposits • CRF is rare • Oval fat bodies (see Fig. 20-2C, D), fatty casts (Link 20-13)
Focal segmental glomerulosclerosis (FSG; Links 20-41 and Link 20-42)	• Primary or secondary disease; secondary causes: HIV (FSG most common glomerular disease in young black males), IV heroin abusers, and hyperfiltration associated with morbid obesity. Drugs: e.g., NSAIDs, captopril, gold therapy. Infections: HBV, *Plasmodium malariae*, syphilis. Malignancy: adenocarcinoma (breast, bowel, lung), Hodgkin lymphoma. Autoimmune disease: SLE (nephrotic presentation) • Second most common cause of nephrotic syndrome • Occurs in early teens to mid-30s • HTN early (20%) • Nonselective proteinuria, microscopic hematuria (60%–80%) • Microscopy shows focal and segmental glomerulosclerosis • IF shows nonspecific IgM deposition; *no* immunocomplexes are present • EM shows focal damage of VECs and fusion of the podocytes • Serum creatinine is normal. Elevation of creatinine is indicative of a poor prognosis. • Proteinuria is *not* massive (2–4 g/24 hr) • Poor prognosis particularly if associated with HIV, in which there is a rapid onset of renal failure with massive proteinuria; commonly progresses to CRF • Oval fat bodies (see Fig. 20-2 C, D), fatty casts (Link 20-13)
Diffuse membranous glomerulopathy (see Fig. 20-5 I; Links 20-43 to 20-45)	• Most common cause of nephrotic syndrome in adults • Highest incidence of renal vein thrombosis and DVT with PE most likely caused by loss of antithrombin in the urine • Associated with antiphospholipase A_2 (PLA_2) antibodies • Association with chronic HBV; less commonly associated with membranoproliferative glomerulonephritis • Can be associated with SLE • Can be associated with NSAIDs • Diffuse thickening of membranes; silver stains show "spike and dome" pattern beneath VECs • Subepithelial ICs with granular IF • Slow onset with a loss of the GFR usually over years • Proteinuria varies from subnephrotic range to massive (>20 g/24 hr) • Spontaneous remission in one third of patients • Serum creatinine is usually normal. If increased, it portends a poor prognosis and the possibility of renal vein thrombosis. • Oval fat bodies (see Fig. 20-2 C, D), fatty casts (Link 20-13)
Type I MPGN (Link 20-46, *left*)	• Most common type of MPGN. Nephrotic presentation (60% of cases). Some cases have a nephritic presentation. Presents most commonly between ages 7 and 30 years (70% present in second decade). Slight female predominance. Circulating ICs in 50% of cases. • Associations: chronic HBV, HCV (more common than HBV), IE, cryoglobulinemia (HCV is present in 80% to 90% of patients) • Subendothelial ICs with granular IF. ICs activate the classical and alternative complement pathways. IgG and C3 predominate. • EM shows tram tracks caused by splitting of the GBM by an ingrowth of mesangium. • Hypertension (35% of cases); majority have hematuria • Majority progress to CRF • Oval fat bodies (see Fig. 20-2 C, D), fatty casts (Link 20-13)
Type II MPGN (Links 20-46, *right*, and Link 20-47)	• Associated with the C_3 nephritic factor (C_3NeF), an autoantibody that binds to C_3 convertase (C_3bBb). Autoantibody prevents degradation of C_3 convertase, causing sustained activation of C_3 resulting in very low C_3 levels. • Diffuse intramembranous deposits ("dense deposit disease"). EM shows tram tracks. • HTN (35% of cases; poor prognostic sign); majority have hematuria • Majority progress to CRF • Oval fat bodies (see Fig. 20-2 C, D), fatty casts (Link 20-13)

CRF, Chronic renal failure; *DVT,* deep vein thrombosis; *EM,* electron microscopy; *GBM,* glomerular basement membrane; *GFR,* glomerular filtration rate; *HBV,* hepatitis B virus; *HCV,* hepatitis C virus; *HTN,* hypertension; *ICs,* immunocomplexes; *IE,* infective endocarditis; *IF,* immune-fluorescence; *IV,* intravenous; *MPGN,* membranoproliferative glomerulonephritis; *NSAID,* nonsteroidal antiinflammatory drug; *PE,* pulmonary embolism; *RBC,* red blood cell; *SLE,* systemic lupus erythematosus; *URI,* upper respiratory infection; *VEC,* visceral epithelial cell.

NEG afferent/efferent arterioles

Hyaline arteriolosclerosis

Efferent *before* afferent; ↑GFR

Osmotic damage ECs

Aldose reductase: glucose → sorbitol

Sorbitol osmotically active

Hyperfiltration damage to mesangium

Diabetic microangiopathy

DM microangiopathy: ↑type IV collagen GBM, TC BM, mesangium

Nonspecific IF

Fusion podocytes

Microangiopathy: ↑deposition of type IV collagen

Arteriolosclerosis afferent → GFR/CCr decrease

Nodules type IV collagen mesangial matrix

Microalbuminuria: sign diabetic glomerulopathy

Glomerulopathy: >10 yrs poor glycemic control

Microalbuminuria dipsticks

(2) NEG of the afferent and efferent arterioles.
    (a) Produces hyaline arteriolosclerosis (see Chapter 10)
    (b) NEG involves the efferent arterioles *before* the afferent arterioles. The increased pressure produces an increase in the GFR.
(3) Osmotic damage to glomerular capillary ECs (see Chapter 23)
    (a) Glucose is converted by aldose reductase into sorbitol.
    (b) Sorbitol is osmotically active, causing water to enter the ECs and damage them.
(4) Hyperfiltration damage to the mesangium caused by selective hyaline arteriolosclerosis of the efferent arterioles, which increases the GFR (CCr is increased) and damages the mesangial cells
(5) Diabetic microangiopathy
    • **Definition:** Increased deposition of type IV collagen in the GBM, tubular cell (TC) basement membranes, and mesangium
  d. Nonspecific IF.
  e. EM shows fusion of podocytes (Fig. 20-5 D).
  f. Microscopic findings (Fig. 20-5 J; Links 20-48 and 20-49)
    (1) Afferent and efferent hyaline arteriolosclerosis: When the afferent arteriole becomes hyalinized, the GFR and CCr decrease.
    (2) Nodular masses develop in the mesangial matrix. Nodules are caused by increased type IV collagen synthesis and trapped proteins.
  g. Clinical and laboratory findings
    (1) Microalbuminuria
      (a) Initial laboratory manifestation of diabetic glomerulopathy; usually begins after ~10 years of poor glycemic control
      (b) Microalbuminuria dipsticks detect albumin levels in the range of 1.5 to 8 mg/dL.

Because up to 20% of people with diabetes also have coexisting nondiabetic causes of proteinuria, all people with diabetes with proteinuria should be further evaluated to rule out coexisting systemic etiologies of proteinuria diseases such as monoclonal gammopathies, hepatitis B or C virus, and systemic lupus erythematosus. An **angiotensin-converting enzyme inhibitor** is prescribed when microalbuminuria is first detected because it slows the progression of diabetic glomerulopathy and retinopathy in both types of diabetes mellitus. One possible mechanism is by reducing pressure in the glomerular capillaries by decreasing angiotensin II vasoconstriction of the hyalinized efferent arterioles. Angiotensin receptor blockers are also useful, particularly in type 2 diabetes mellitus. These changes are independent of the abilities of both drugs to lower blood pressure.

ACE inhibitor/receptor blockers: slows progression nephropathy type 1/type 2 diabetes

DM: renal papillary necrosis, chronic pyelonephritis

Renal disease in primary/secondary amyloidosis

Hereditary glomerular diseases

Alport syndrome

XR MCC

Mutations α-chains type IV collagen in GBM

EM/MABs detect GBM defects

Hypertension, G/M hematuria men only, RBC casts, proteinuria

Sensorineural hearing loss

Cataracts, anterior lenticonus

ERSD by age 35

Thin BM disease: persistent hematuria

AD

Half normal thickness GBM

Normal renal function

Mild proteinuria, persistent microscopic hematuria

Chronic glomerulonephritis

RPGN and focal segmental glomerulosclerosis: MCCs chronic glomerulonephritis

    (2) Other renal diseases associated with DM include renal papillary necrosis (RPN) and acute and chronic pyelonephritis (CPN).
  2. Renal amyloidosis (see Chapter 4, Fig. 4-20 A to C): associated with primary and secondary amyloidosis

H. Hereditary glomerular diseases
  1. Alport syndrome
    a. X-linked recessive (XR most common; 80%) and autosomal dominant or recessive types; mutations in α-chains of type IV collagen in GBM
    b. EM or monoclonal antibody studies to detect GBM defects are useful in confirming the diagnosis.
    c. Hypertension, gross or microscopic hematuria, and RBC casts are common. Proteinuria occurs late in the disease. Family history of hematuria in men only.
    d. High-tone sensorineural hearing loss, cataracts, and anterior lenticonus (conical projection of the crystalline lens of the eye)
    e. End-stage renal disease (ESRD) is more common in men than in women. The majority have ESRD by age 35 years.
  2. Thin basement membrane disease ("benign familial hematuria")
    a. Autosomal dominant (AD) disorder
    b. Extremely thin GBMs (half normal thickness)
    c. Normal renal function
    d. Mild proteinuria with persistent microscopic hematuria

I. Chronic glomerulonephritis
  1. Causes in descending order of incidence include:
    a. rapidly progressive glomerulonephritis (RPGN).
    b. focal segmental glomerulosclerosis.

c. type I membranoproliferative glomerulonephritis (MPGN).

d. membranous glomerulopathy.

e. type IV diffuse proliferative GN in SLE.

f. IgA glomerulopathy.

2. Gross and microscopic findings in chronic GN include:

a. shrunken kidneys.

b. glomerular sclerosis and tubular atrophy.

VIII. Disorders Affecting Tubules and Interstitium

A. Acute renal failure (ARF)

1. **Definition:** Deterioration of renal function that develops in 24 hours that is manifested by an increase in serum Cr and BUN. ARF may be oliguric < 400 mL/day) or polyuric (>400 mL/day).

2. Epidemiology

a. Another term for acute renal failure is acute kidney injury.

b. Most common cause of ARF is ATN (see later). The second most common cause is prerenal azotemia caused by volume depletion (i.e., hypovolemic shock).

c. Greater than 10% of intensive care unit (ICU) patients develop ARF (see later).

d. More than 40% of hospital ARF is iatrogenic (doctor induced).

e. Hemolytic uremic syndrome (HUS) is the most common cause of intrinsic ARF in the United States (see Chapter 15).

f. ARF occurs in 20% of patients with sepsis.

g. ARF develops in >50% of patients with septic shock.

h. Can be subdivided into prerenal, renal, or postrenal causes (Link 20-50).

(1) Prerenal causes are from a decrease in effective arterial blood volume (EABV; see Chapter 5). Examples: vomiting, diarrhea, blood loss, CHF, shock (hypovolemic, septic, cardiogenic)

(2) Intrarenal causes are related to glomerular disease, tubular disorders, tubulointerstitial disorders, and vascular disorders.

(a) Examples: ATN, RPGN, HUS, thrombotic thrombocytopenic purpura (TTP), atheroembolic disease, contrast nephropathy (see later), vasculitis (e.g., polyarteritis nodosa), tubulointerstitial nephritis (TIN)

(b) Contrast nephropathy. Refers to an increase in serum Cr and BUN within 24 to 48 hours after administration of intravenous contrast (iodine). Cr and BUN usually peak within 7 days and return to normal within 10 days.

- Risk factors include renal insufficiency with a serum Cr >1.5 mg/dL (adults, 0.6–1.2 mg/dL); elderly (decrease in muscle mass may cause decreased values); diabetic nephropathy; CHF; cirrhosis; volume depletion; multiple myeloma with Bence Jones (BJ) protein.

- Usually reversible

(3) Postrenal causes related to obstruction of the urinary tract. Examples include bilateral renal vein thrombosis, RPN, prostate hyperplasia, urate nephropathy, ureteral obstruction (e.g., ureteral stones, invasive cervical cancer), bladder cancer, disseminated intravascular coagulation (DIC), and malignant hypertension.

B. Acute tubular necrosis (ATN)

1. **Definition:** ARF that is caused by necrosis of the renal tubular cells (RTCs); subdivided into ischemic and nephrotoxic types

2. Ischemic ATN

a. **Definition:** Caused by a decrease in renal blood flow to the kidney, resulting in the death of the RTCs

b. Epidemiology

(1) Most often caused by prerenal azotemia (decrease in cardiac output) due to hypovolemia

(2) Gross findings: The kidneys are swollen, and the renal cortex is pale (Link 20-51 A).

(3) Ischemia damages endothelial cells (EC).

(a) Causes a decrease in EC-derived vasodilators (VDs; nitric oxide [NO], PGI_2)

(b) Causes an increase in EC-derived vasoconstrictors (VC) (endothelin)

(c) Net effect is vasoconstriction of afferent arterioles, which decreases the GFR.

(4) Ischemia damages proximal RTCs (coagulation necrosis) and the basement membrane (BM).

(a) Proximal RTCs become detached into the lumen, causing obstruction of urine flow (Fig. 20-6 A; Links 20-51 B and 20-52). This produces pigmented proximal RTC casts (see Fig. 20-2 J; Link 20-13).

Type 1 MPGN

Membranous glomerulopathy

Type IV GN in SLE

IgA glomerulopathy

Shrunken kidneys

Glomerular sclerosis, tubular atrophy

Disorders tubules + interstitium

ARF

↓↓Renal function → ↑BUN, Cr → oliguric/polyruic

ARF = Acute kidney injury

MCC ATN, prerenal azotemia (2nd MCC)

ICU: >10% develop ARF

Hospital ARF: >40% iatrogenic

HUS: MCC intrinsic ARF in U.S.

ARF common in sepsis

ARF >50% in septic shock

Prerenal: ↓EABV

Blood loss, shock, CHF, vomiting/diarrhea

Intrarenal: glomerular, tubular, TIN, vascular

ATN, RPGN, HUS, TTP, TIN

↑Serum Cr/Bun 24–48 hrs post IV contrast

Serum Cr/BUN peak 7 days, normal within 10 days

Renal insufficiency; elderly; DM nephropathy; CHF; multiple myeloma; cirrhosis

Usually reversible

Obstruction urinary tract (postrenal)

Prostate hyperplasia, invasive cervical cancer. RPN, stones

Acute tubular necrosis (ATN)

ARF caused by necrosis RTCs

Ischemic, nephrotoxic ATN

Ischemic ATN

↓Renal blood flow → death RTCs

Prerenal azotemia MCC ischemic ATN

↓Cardiac output

Kidney swollen/pale

Ischemia damages ECs

↓EC-derived VDs (NO, PGI_2)

↑EC-derived VCs (endothelin)

Net effect → VC afferent arterioles → ↓GFR

Ischemia: damage proximal RTCs (coagulation necrosis) + BMs

Pigmented proximal RTC casts; key cast ATN

20-6: A, Acute tubular necrosis. Coagulation necrosis of proximal renal tubule cells *(arrows)* is evident with some detachment from the basement membrane. This detachment forms renal tubular cell casts. **B,** Normal and abnormal configuration of the ureteral orifices. The ureteral orifice on the left shows the normal angle of the intramural portion of the ureter in the bladder wall that prevents reflux during micturition. The intramural portion of the ureter on the right is incompetent and allows urine to reflux into the ureter, renal pelvis, and kidney to produce pyelonephritis. **C,** Acute pyelonephritis showing a neutrophil-dominant infiltrate in the tubular lumens *(arrow)* and interstitium. The neutrophils in the lumens are molded into white blood cell casts, which are passed in the urine along with free neutrophils and bacteria (pyuria). **D,** Chronic pyelonephritis. The renal cortex shows deep U-shaped scars. Sections through this scar would have revealed a blunt calyx directly beneath the base of the U. **E,** Analgesic nephropathy showing multiple brownish necrotic papillae *(arrows).* *(A, C, and D from Kern WF, Silva FG, Laszik ZG, et al [eds]:* Atlas of Renal Pathology, *Philadelphia, Saunders, 1999, pp 129, 149, respectively; Figs. 12-3, 13-15B, 13-16, respectively; B from Kliegman R:* Nelson Textbook of Pediatrics, *19th ed, Philadelphia, Elsevier Saunders, 2011, p 1834, Fig. 533.1A and D, respectively; E from Kumar V, Fausto N, Abbas A:* Robbins and Cotran Pathologic Basis of Disease, *7th ed, Philadelphia, Saunders, 2004, p 1003, Fig. 20-45.)*

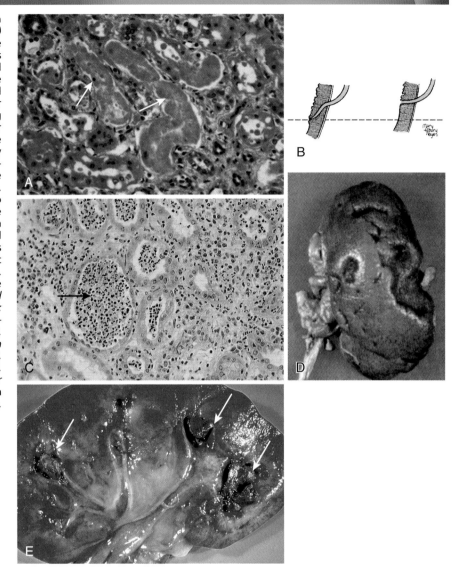

Casts ↓GFR

Fluid → interstitium

Oliguria

Sites of tubular damage

PT most susceptible to hypoxia

Medullary segment TAL

Location
Na⁺-K⁺-2Cl⁻ cotransporter

BM damaged → interferes with regeneration

Nephrotoxic acute tubular necrosis

Toxic agents damage RTCs

Aminoglycosides: MCC nephrotoxic ATN.

Radiocontrast agents

Lead, mercury

Myoglobin, Hgb

Microscopic findings

PTCs damaged

BM intact; good for regeneration

Regeneration may occur

Clinical/lab findings

Oliguria most cases

Pigmented RBCs

(b) Casts obstruct the lumen, causing an increase in the intratubular pressure. The increase in tubular pressure decreases the GFR by pushing fluid into the interstitium of the kidney. The net effect is oliguria (reduced urine flow).
  (5) Sites of tubular damage
      (a) Straight segment of PT. Most susceptible to hypoxia (see Chapter 2).
      (b) Medullary segment of the thick ascending limb (TAL; see Chapter 2); location of the Na^+-K^+-$2Cl^-$ cotransporter (see Chapter 5)
      (c) Tubular BMs are disrupted at these sites. This interferes with RTC regeneration.
  3. Nephrotoxic type of ATN
      a. **Definition:** Toxic agents delivered to the kidney cause the death of RTCs.
      b. Epidemiology
          (1) Causes
              (a) Aminoglycosides (e.g., gentamicin): most common cause
              (b) Radiocontrast agents
              (c) Heavy metals (e.g., lead, mercury)
              (d) Myoglobin or hemoglobin (Hgb)
          (2) Microscopic findings
              (a) Proximal tubule cells (PTCs) are primarily damaged.
              (b) Tubular BMs remain intact, allowing RTCs to regenerate properly.
  4. Clinical and laboratory findings
      a. Oliguria in most cases (~400 mL/24 hours), although some cases are polyuric (~800 mL/24 hours)
      b. Pigmented RTC casts in the urine (Fig. 20-2 F; Link 20-13)

BOX 20-1 Differential Diagnosis of Oliguria

Oliguria is defined as a urine output of less than 400 mL/day or less than 20 mL/hr. The major causes of oliguria include prerenal azotemia (most common cause), acute glomerulonephritis (nephritic type), acute tubular necrosis (renal azotemia), and postrenal azotemia. Laboratory tests that are commonly used in differentiating the types of oliguria include urine osmolality (UOsm), fractional excretion of sodium (FENa$^+$), random urine sodium (UNa$^+$), and the serum BUN/Cr (blood urea nitrogen/creatinine) ratio (see Section III). These tests evaluate tubular function. A UOsm greater than 500 mOsm/kg indicates good concentrating ability and intact tubular function, but a UOsm less than 350 mOsm/kg indicates poor concentrating ability and tubular dysfunction. The FENa$^+$ represents the amount of sodium excreted in the urine divided by the amount of sodium that is filtered by the kidneys. The calculation is as follows:

$$FENa^+ = [(UNa^+ \times PCr) \div (PNa^+ \times UCr)] \times 100$$

where UNa$^+$ is a random urine sodium, PNa$^+$ is plasma sodium, UCr is random urine creatinine, and PCr is plasma creatinine. Cr is used in the formula because the amount of sodium filtered is dependent on the glomerular filtration rate (GFR), which closely approximates the creatinine clearance (CCr). An FENa$^+$ below 1% indicates good tubular function and *excludes* acute tubular necrosis (ATN) as a cause of oliguria. An FENa$^+$ greater than 2% indicates tubular dysfunction and is highly predictive of ATN as the cause of oliguria. A random UNa$^+$ less than 20 mEq/L indicates intact tubular function, and a random UNa$^+$ greater than 40 mEq/L indicates tubular dysfunction. A serum BUN/Cr ratio greater than 15 indicates intact tubular function, but a serum BUN/Cr ratio of 15 or less indicates tubular dysfunction. In prerenal azotemia and acute glomerulonephritis (nephritic type), tubular function is preserved. To distinguish the two, the urine sediment examination is most useful. In prerenal azotemia, the urine sediment has *no* abnormal findings or may have a few hyaline casts. The sediment in acute glomerulonephritis (nephritic type) has hematuria and RBC casts. ATN and postrenal azotemia (long-standing obstruction) both have tubular dysfunction. Postrenal azotemia of short duration has normal tubular function with laboratory findings similar to prerenal azotemia. To distinguish ATN from postrenal azotemia as a cause of tubular dysfunction and oliguria, the urine sediment is most useful. In ATN, the sediment has pigmented renal tubular cell casts, but in postrenal azotemia, the sediment is usually normal. In addition, the patient will likely have a history of a renal stone, benign prostate hyperplasia, or cervical cancer, which commonly obstructs the ureters where they enter the urinary bladder.

Disorder	FENa$^+$ %	BUN/Cr	UNa$^+$	UOsm	Urinalysis
Prerenal azotemia	<1	>15	<20	>500	Normal sediment or hyaline casts
Acute glomerulonephritis	<1	>15	<20	>500	RBC casts, hematuria
Acute tubular necrosis	>2	≤15	>40	<350	Renal tubular cell casts
Postrenal azotemia (prolonged obstruction)	>2	≤15	>40	<350	Normal sediment

  c. Hyperkalemia (see Chapter 5)

  d. Increased anion gap (AG) metabolic acidosis (see Chapter 5)

  e. Azotemia (BUN/Cr ratio ≤15)

  f. Hypokalemia in the diuresis phase of ATN

  g. Increased susceptibility to infection

  5. Differential diagnosis of oliguria is discussed in Box 20-1.

C. **Tubular interstitial nephritis (TIN)**

  1. **Definition:** Primary injury to both the renal tubules and interstitial tissue that results in decreased renal function

  2. Epidemiology

   a. Acute pyelonephritis (APN; most common cause of TIN)

   b. Drugs (e.g., NSAIDS, rifampin)

   c. Infections. Examples: Legionnaires disease, leptospirosis

   d. SLE, lead poisoning (see Chapter 12), urate nephropathy, multiple myeloma (see Chapter 14)

  3. Acute pyelonephritis (APN)

   a. **Definition:** Acute bacterial infection of the kidney(s)

   b. Epidemiology

    (1) More common in women than men. Because women have short urethras, they are at increased risk of an infection spreading from the urethra, up to the bladder, and ultimately to the kidney(s), resulting in pyelonephritis.

    (2) *Escherichia coli* is the most common cause of APN. *Enterococcus* is second most common.

    (3) Risk factors

     (a) Indwelling urinary catheter (IUC), urinary tract (UT) obstruction

     (b) Medullary sponge kidney (MSK), DM

     (c) Pregnancy, sickle cell trait or disease

    (4) Pathogenesis

Hyperkalemia

↑AG metabolic acidosis

BUN/Cr ratio ≤15

Hypokalemia diuresis phase

Susceptibility to infection

FE$_{Na}$ very useful in distinguishing causes ARF

Tubulointerstitial nephritis

Injury tubules + interstitial tissue

Acute pyelonephritis

Drugs

Infections

SLE, Pb poisoning, urate nephropathy, myeloma

APN: MCC TIN

Acute kidney bacterial infection

Women > men

Women have short urethra

E. coli MCC

Enterococcus 2nd MCC

IUC, UT obstruction

MSK, DM

Pregnancy, sickle cell trait/disease

(a) Vesicoureteral reflux (VUR) with ascending infection (most common; Link 20-53 B, C). The intravesical portion of the ureter is normally compressed with micturition, preventing reflux of urine into the ureter(s) (Fig. 20-6 B, *left*). In VUR, the intravesical portion of the ureter is not compressed during micturition (Fig. 20-6 B, *right*). This allows infected urine to ascend up the ureter into the kidney. VUR is corrected by reimplantation of the ureter(s) or using stents.

(b) Ascending infection
- Most common cause of lower and upper urinary tract infections (UTIs) in females (Link 20-53 B)
- Distal urethra is normally colonized by *E. coli.*
- Organisms ascend into the urethra and bladder, causing urethritis and cystitis. If VUR is present, infected urine ascends to the renal pelvis and renal parenchyma (Link 20-53 C). This causes APN.

(c) hematogenous spread to the kidneys (Link 20-53 A). Uncommon cause of APN. Suspect hematogenous spread if *Staphylococcus aureus* is cultured in the urine.

c. Gross and microscopic findings
   (1) Grayish-white areas of microabscess formation in the cortex and medulla
   (2) Microabscess formation in the tubular lumens and interstitium (Fig. 20-6 C; Link 20-54)

d. Clinical findings include spiking fever, flank pain, increased frequency, and painful urination (dysuria).

e. Laboratory findings
   (1) WBC casts (key finding; Fig. 20-2 F; Link 20-13)
   (2) pyuria (pus in urine), bacteriuria (usually *E. coli*, gram-negative rod), and hematuria

f. Complications associated with APN
   (1) CPN (see later)
   (2) Perinephric abscess. **Definition:** Presence of purulent material (pus) around the kidney
   (3) RPN. Renal papillae are the apical end of the medullary pyramids and represent the dilated proximal part or the ureter for the outflow of urine from the collecting ducts.
   (4) septicemia (bacteria in the blood) with endotoxic shock (gram-negative shock; see Chapter 5).

4. Chronic pyelonephritis (CPN)
   a. **Definition:** Renal dysfunction secondary to fibrosis and tubular damage caused by chronic inflammation of the renal parenchyma
   b. Epidemiology
      (1) Most commonly preceded by APN that has *not* resolved
      (2) Commonly the result of VUR starting in young girls
      (3) Can be secondary to urinary tract obstruction and associated hydronephrosis (see later). Examples: prostate hyperplasia (see Chapter 21), renal stones (discussed later)
      (4) Reflux type of CPN is characterized U-shaped cortical scars (Fig. 20-6 D; Link 20-55 A) overlying a blunt calyx; visible with an intravenous pyelogram (IVP).
      (5) Obstructive type of CPN has uniform dilation of the calyces and diffuse thinning of cortical tissue.
      (6) Microscopic findings
         (a) Chronic inflammation (lymphocytes, plasma cells, and macrophages) and secondary scarring and obliteration of the glomeruli (Link 20-55 B)
         (b) Tubular atrophy manifested by the loss of tubules and tubules that contain eosinophilic material resembling thyroid tissue ("thyroidization"; Link 20-55 B)
   c. Clinical and laboratory findings
      (1) History of recurrent APN
      (2) Hypertension (retention of sodium). Reflux nephropathy is a cause of hypertension in children.
      (3) CRF (see later)
      (4) Laboratory findings (see laboratory finding in CRF)
      (5) Renal scan shows decreased uptake in the scarred kidneys (Link 20-55 C).

5. Acute drug-induced TIN

a. Common drug associations include:
 (1) penicillin, particularly methicillin.
 (2) rifampin, sulfonamides, NSAIDs, diuretics. NSAIDs can be associated with pure interstitial nephritis or glomerular diseases (MCD, membranous GN).
b. Epidemiology; pathogenesis
 (1) Combination of a type I and type IV hypersensitivity reaction (see Chapter 4)
 (2) Occurs ~2 weeks after beginning the drug
c. Clinical and laboratory findings
 (1) Abrupt onset of fever, oliguria (decreased urine volume), and rash. Withdrawal of the drug reverses the disease.
 (2) BUN/Cr ratio ≤15
 (3) Eosinophilia and eosinophiluria (eosinophils in the urine; highly predictive; 75% of cases)
 (4) Biopsy shows a marked mononuclear and eosinophil infiltrate in the interstitium (Link 20-56).
 (5) WBC casts, mild proteinuria
d. Rx: Withdraw the drug.
6. Contrast media nephropathy
 a. **Definition:** Impaired renal function within 48 to 72 hours of intravenous (IV) administration of contrast material
 b. Epidemiology
 (1) Impairment is manifested by a 25% increase in serum Cr from the previous baseline within 48 to 72 hours of administration of the IV contrast.
 (2) Pathogenesis
 (a) VC of renal vessels from the release of endothelin
 (b) High osmolality of the infused contrast material
 (c) Direct injury to the renal tubules
 (3) Risk factors include multiple myeloma with BJ proteinuria, underlying renal insufficiency, prerenal azotemia (e.g., congestive heart volume, volume depletion), diabetic nephropathy, chronic liver disease, and contrast material itself.
7. Analgesic nephropathy
 a. **Definition:** Renal papillary necrosis (RPN) and chronic interstitial nephritis (CIN) caused by the long-term consumption of analgesic agents (e.g., aspirin, acetaminophen, and other NSAIDs)
 b. Epidemiology
 (1) Common cause of chronic drug-induced TIN
 (2) More common in women than men
 (3) Usually occurs in persons with chronic pain
 (4) Initially recognized in patients who took phenacetin combined with caffeine and codeine
 (5) Pathogenesis of analgesic nephropathy caused by aspirin plus acetaminophen
 (a) History of chronic use of acetaminophen plus aspirin for 3 or more years
 (b) Acetaminophen free radicals damage renal tubules in the renal medulla (RPN; see Chapter 2).
 (c) Aspirin inhibits renal synthesis of PGE_2, leaving the VC effect of ATII unopposed. This decreases the blood flow to the renal medulla.
 c. Clinical complications
 (1) RPN (Fig. 20-6 E; Link 20-57)
 (a) **Definition:** Sloughing off of one or more renal papillae, producing gross hematuria, proteinuria, and flank pain
 (b) IVP shows a "ring defect" where one or more papillae used to reside.
 (c) Other causes of RPN include DM, sickle cell trait or disease, and APN.
 (2) Hypertension, CRF
 (3) Urothelial carcinoma (see later) of renal pelvis and urinary bladder (see Chapter 21)
8. Urate nephropathy
 a. **Definition:** Renal injury secondary to the deposition of urate crystals in the renal tubules and interstitium
 b. Epidemiology
 (1) Massive release of purines (the precursor of uric acid), usually after aggressive treatment of disseminated cancers (e.g., leukemia, malignant lymphoma)
 (2) Lead poisoning (see Chapter 12)
 (3) Gout (see Chapter 24)
 c. May lead to acute renal failure (ARF)

Methicillin

Rifampin, sulfonamides, NSAIDs

NSAIDs: pure interstitial nephritis, MCD, membranous GN

Type I/IV HSR

Two weeks after beginning drug

Acute drug-induced TIN: abrupt onset fever, oliguria, rash, eosinophilia

Abrupt onset fever, rash, oliguria

Withdrawal drug reverses disease

BUN/Cr ≤ 15

Eosinophilia, eosinophiluria

WBC casts, mild proteinuria

Withdraw drug

Contrast media nephropathy

Impaired renal function 2-3 days post-administration contrast material

Serum Cr ↑25% from baseline

Vasoconstriction (endothelin)

High osmolality infused contrast

Direct tubular injury

Multiple myeloma/BJ protein, renal insufficiency, CHF, DM, contrast material

Analgesic nephropathy

RPN, CIN long-term analgesics (aspirin, acetaminophen, NSAIDs)

Chronic drug-induced TIN

Women > men

Chronic pain syndromes

Chronic use acetaminophen + aspirin

Acetaminophen FRs; renal papillary necrosis

Aspirin inhibits renal synthesis PGE_2

Clinical complications

Renal papillary necrosis

Sloughing of renal papilla

IVP: ring defect

DM, sickle cell trait/disease, APN

Hypertension, CRF

Urothelial carcinoma renal pelvis/urinary bladder

Urate nephropathy

Urate crystals tubules/interstitium

Rx disseminated cancers

Lead poisoning

Gout

ARF

Patients with disseminated cancers should receive allopurinol, a xanthine oxidase inhibitor, *before* being treated with chemotherapy. This prevents urate nephropathy (tumor lysis syndrome) and acute renal failure.

9. Chronic lead (Pb) poisoning (see Chapters 7 and 12).
    a. Pathogenesis of lead poisoning causing TIN
        (1) Lead decreases the renal excretion of uric acid (urate nephropathy). Retention of uric acid can produce gout (see Chapter 24).
        (2) Lead also exhibits direct toxicity, resulting in TIN.
    b. PTCs contain characteristic nuclear acid-fast inclusions.
10. Multiple myeloma; mechanisms for renal disease include:
    a. BJ proteinuria (see Chapter 14).
        (1) BJ protein (light chains) produces tubular casts (Table 20-4). Light chains are toxic to renal tubular epithelium.
        (2) Casts obstruct the lumen and incite a foreign body giant cell reaction (FBGCR) involving tubules and interstitium, leading to renal failure (Link 20-58).
    b. nephrocalcinosis (see Chapter 2).
        (1) Hypercalcemia secondary to the lytic bone lesions produces metastatic calcification of the BM of collecting tubules (see Fig. 2-14 B).
        (2) Presenting symptoms of nephrocalcinosis are polyuria (nephrogenic diabetes insipidus [NDI]; see Chapter 23) and renal failure.
    c. Primary amyloidosis producing nephrotic syndrome (see Chapter 4). Light chains in multiple myeloma are converted to amyloid (see Fig. 4-20 B, C).

IX. **Chronic Renal Failure (CRF)**
    A. **Definition:** Progressive irreversible azotemia (abnormally high levels of BUN and other toxic substances) that develops over months to years and culminates in end-stage renal disease
    B. **Epidemiology**
        1. Kidneys no longer function well enough to sustain life.
        2. GFR is <10 mL/min.
        3. Causes
            a. DM (most common cause)
            b. Hypertension
            c. Chronic glomerulonephritis (CGN; Link 20-59), particularly when secondary to either RPGN or focal segmental glomerulopathy
            d. Cystic renal disease. Examples: renal dysplasia in children, adult polycystic kidney disease (APKD)
        4. Gross findings include bilateral, shrunken kidneys.
    C. **Clinical findings in CRF**
        1. Hematologic findings
            a. Normocytic anemia with a corrected reticulocyte count <3% (see Chapter 12). Primarily caused by decreased synthesis of erythropoietin (EPO) by the kidneys
            b. Qualitative (functional) platelet defects that are corrected by dialysis (see Chapter 15)
        2. Renal osteodystrophy (Links 20-60 and 20-61)
            a. **Definition:** Bone disease in secondary to CRF; characterized by softening of bone (osteomalacia), fibrous tissue replacement of bone, and formation of bone cysts
            b. Osteitis fibrosa cystica
                (1) **Definition:** Cystic bone lesions caused by an accelerated bone turnover as a result of hypovitaminosis D, causing hypocalcemia. The net effect of the chronic hypocalcemia is increased release of PTH (secondary hyperparathyroidism [2° HPTH]) causing chronic bone resorption.
                (2) Epidemiology
                    (a) Hypovitaminosis D is caused by the loss of 1-α-hydroxylase (OHase) in the PTs (see Chapter 8). Normally, kidney hydroxylation by 1-α-hydroxylase produces $1,25\text{-}(OH)_2\text{-}D$, which is the metabolically active form of vitamin D; calcitriol.
                    (b) Hypovitaminosis D produces hypocalcemia, which stimulates the production of PTH; called secondary HPTH (see Chapter 23). Elevated levels of serum phosphorous (P) also lower serum calcium through binding of phosphorous with calcium, causing tissue calcification (metastatic calcification; see Chapter 2).

(c) Increase in PTH increases bone resorption, causing cystic lesions in the bone (i.e., osteitis fibrosa cystica).

c. Osteomalacia
(1) **Definition:** Softening of bone secondary to decreased mineralization of the organic bone matrix (called osteoid; see Chapters 8 and 24)
(2) Hypovitaminosis D produces hypocalcemia, leading to decreased mineralization of osteoid (organic bone matrix).
(3) Impaired mineralization of the bone results in softening with associated pathologic fractures and bone pain.

d. Osteoporosis (see Chapter 24)
(1) **Definition:** The loss of *both* osteoid and mineralized bone, which causes an overall reduction in bone mass (density)
(2) In CRF, there is a chronic metabolic acidosis caused by retention of sulfuric acid, phosphoric acid, and uric acid (see Chapter 5).
(a) Bone is an important site for handling excess acid in the circulation.
(b) Net effect is increased uptake of excess H^+ ions by bone in exchange for surface Na^+ and K^+ and by dissolution of bone mineral, resulting in the release of buffer compounds, such as $NaHCO_3$, $CaHCO_3$, and $CaHPO_4$. Overall, this decreases mineralized bone.
(c) Loss of calcium in buffer compounds decreases mineralization of bone.
(3) Osteoblasts are also decreased in CRF; hence, the organic matrix of bone (osteoid) is decreased, called osteomalacia. Decrease in organic matrix and mineralized bone is called osteoporosis.
(4) Soft unmineralized bone causes fractures and bone pain.

3. Cardiovascular findings (see Chapters 10 and 11)
a. Hypertension from salt retention
b. Hemorrhagic fibrinous pericarditis; possible toxins include urea, Cr, PTH, uric acid, and others. BUN level is usually >60 mg/dL.
c. CHF: causes include volume overload (sodium retention), myocyte dysfunction, and increased interstitial fibrosis (IF) in the heart
d. Accelerated atherosclerosis. Due to endothelial damage from hypertension, toxins in uremia.

4. Miscellaneous clinical findings
a. Hemorrhagic gastritis
b. Uremic frost (urea crystals deposit on the skin; Link 20-62)

D. **Overview of clinical findings in chronic renal failure** (Links 20-63 and 20-64)
E. **Laboratory findings in CRF**
1. Acid–base and electrolyte findings
a. Hyperkalemia: caused by a transcellular shift in acidosis and decreased renal excretion (most common cause; see Chapter 5)
b. Increased anion gap (AG) metabolic acidosis from retention of phosphoric acid, sulfuric acid, and other acids (see Chapter 5)
2. Hypocalcemia; causes
a. Hypovitaminosis D: caused by decreased synthesis of 1-α-hydroxylase in PTCs, leading to decreased reabsorption of calcium from the small intestine
b. Hyperphosphatemia: caused by decreased renal excretion of phosphorus. Excess phosphorus binds with calcium and is deposited into bone and soft tissue (metastatic calcification; see Chapter 2).
3. Normocytic anemia: caused by decreased synthesis of erythropoietin (EPO) (see Chapter 12)
4. Prolonged bleeding time: caused by defects in platelet aggregation (see Chapter 15)
5. Increased serum cystatin C
a. Cysteine protease inhibitor that is produced by all nucleated cells
b. Filtered by the glomerulus but is *not* secreted
c. Level is less dependent on age, sex, race, and muscle mass than Cr.
d. Serum value >1.3 mg/L is consistent with renal dysfunction with an 88% sensitivity and 96% specificity.
6. Urinalysis findings in CRF
a. Fixed specific gravity
(1) Indicates a lack of both concentration and dilution related to tubular dysfunction
(2) Free water clearance is zero (see Chapter 5).
b. Waxy casts and broad casts (Fig. 20-2 K; Link 20-13)

Margin notes:

2° HPTH → ↑bone resorption → osteitis fibrosa cystica

Osteomalacia

↓Mineralization of osteoid

↓Vit D → ↓serum calcium →↓mineralization osteoid

Osteoid soft bone → pathologic fractures/pain

Osteoporosis

Loss osteoid/mineralized bone: ↓bone mass

CRF → chronic metabolic acidosis

Bone handles excess acid

Bone releases buffer compounds

Loss calcium in buffer compounds

↓Osteoblasts in CRF → ↓osteoid (organic matrix) in bone

CRF: osteomalacia/osteoporosis → pathologic bone fractures

Cardiovascular findings

Hypertension (salt retention)

Hemorrhagic fibrinous pericarditis

CHF

Volume overload, myocyte dysfunction, IF

Accelerated atherosclerosis (endothelial damage)

Hemorrhagic gastritis

Uremic frost

Lab findings CRF

Hyperkalemia

↑AG metabolic acidosis

Hypocalcemia

Hypovitaminosis D

Hyperphosphatemia → metastatic calcification

Normocytic anemia (↓EPO)

Prolonged bleeding time; aggregation defects

↑Serum cystatin C

Cysteine protease inhibitor

Filtered but *not* secreted

Marker renal dysfunction

Urinalysis findings CRF

Fixed specific gravity

No concentration/dilution

Free water clearance zero

Waxy/broad casts: signs of CRF

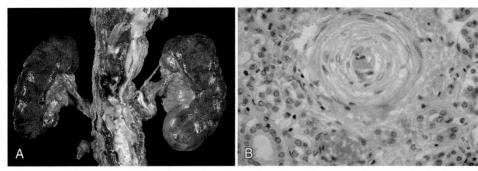

20-7: **A,** Nephrosclerosis. Kidneys have a scarred and granular external surface. The aorta shows marked atherosclerosis with fissuring and dystrophic calcification *(white areas).* **B,** Malignant hypertension. A feature of malignant hypertension is hyperplastic arteriolosclerosis caused by smooth muscle hyperplasia and basement membrane reduplication, giving the vessel an "onion skin" appearance. *(**A** from my friend Ivan Damjanov, MD, PhD, Linder J:* Pathology: A Color Atlas, *St. Louis, Mosby, 2000, p 216, Fig. 11-19;* **B** *from Klatt E:* Robbins and Cotran Atlas of Pathology, *Philadelphia, Saunders, 2006, p 7, Fig. 1-17.)*

E. **Dialysis kidney**
  • Patients that have been on long-term renal dialysis may develop cysts in the nonfunctional kidney (Link 20-65).

X. **Vascular Diseases of the Kidney**

  A. **Benign nephrosclerosis (BNS)**
    1. **Definition:** Renal changes that occur secondary to long-standing hypertension. These changes include a change in the size of the kidney, tubules, interstitium, and vasculature.
    2. Epidemiology
      a. Most common renal disease in primary hypertension
      b. Pathogenesis: Hyaline arteriolosclerosis of arterioles (see Chapter 10) in the renal cortex causes tubular atrophy, interstitial fibrosis, and glomerular sclerosis (Link 20-66; see Fig. 10-7 A).
      c. Grossly, both kidneys are small and have a finely granular cortical surface (Fig. 20-7 A; Link 20-67).
    3. Laboratory findings
      a. Mild proteinuria, hematuria (no RBC casts)
      b. Increase in serum BUN and Cr (renal azotemia)
  B. **Malignant hypertension**
    1. **Definition:** A sudden onset of accelerated hypertension
    2. Epidemiology
      a. Accelerated hypertension may occur in those with BNS (most common), normotensive individuals, or as a complication of various disorders (e.g., systemic sclerosis).
      b. Risk factors
        (1) Preexisting BNS (most common)
        (2) HUS (see Chapter 15)
        (3) Thrombotic thrombocytopenic purpura (TTP) (see Chapter 15), systemic sclerosis (see Chapter 4)
      c. Vascular damage to arterioles and small arteries
      d. Gross and microscopic changes
        (1) Fibrinoid necrosis, necrotizing arteriolitis, and glomerulitis manifested by pinpoint hemorrhages on the surface of both kidneys ("flea-bitten" kidneys)
        (2) Hyperplastic arteriolosclerosis ("onion skin" lesion; see Chapter 10; see Fig. 20-7 B and 10-7 B). Arterioles show smooth muscle cell (SMC) hyperplasia and reduplication of the BM.
    3. Clinical findings
      a. Rapid increase in blood pressure to ≥210/120 mm Hg
      b. Signs of hypertensive encephalopathy occur.
        (1) Cerebral edema: swelling of the brain and loss of the normal optic nerve disk margin (see Fig. 26-1 B).
        (2) Hypertensive retinopathy (see Box 10-1). Findings include flame hemorrhages, exudates, and changes in arterioles (arteriovenous nipping).
        (3) Potential for an intracerebral bleed (see Chapter 26)
      c. Oliguric ARF
    4. Laboratory findings
      a. Increase in serum BUN and Cr with BUN/Cr ratio ≤15
      b. Hematuria with RBC casts, proteinuria

C. **Renal infarction**
  1. **Definition:** Wedge-shaped pale areas of coagulation necrosis in the renal cortex of the kidney most commonly caused by embolization of thrombi from the left atrium in atrial fibrillation (AF) or cholesterol crystals from the proximal aorta (Ao) or renal arteries
  2. Epidemiology
    a. Causes
      (1) AF with embolization (most common). AF predisposes to left atrial thrombus formation and embolization into the systemic circulation. It is the most common cause of renal infarction.
      (2) Atheroembolic renal disease
        (a) Develops when atheromatous plaques within either the Ao or renal artery rupture, releasing cholesterol (CH) crystals into the renal arteries and their tributaries to produce pale, wedge-shaped infarctions in the renal cortex
        (b) Usually affect elderly individuals with diffuse erosive atherosclerosis in the renal arteries or the Ao proximal to the renal artery orifices
        (c) May also occur with catheter manipulation in the Ao or surgery
      (3) Vasculitis, particularly polyarteritis nodosa (PAN) (see Chapter 10)
    b. Gross and microscopic appearance
      (1) One or more irregular, wedge-shaped pale infarctions in the cortex (Links 20-68, 20-69, and 20-70)
      (2) Old infarctions have a V-shaped appearance caused by scar tissue (Link 20-71).
  3. Clinical finding: sudden onset of severe flank pain and hematuria
D. **Sickle cell nephropathy**
  1. **Definition:** Sickling of RBCs, causing occlusion of the small blood vessels in the kidneys
  2. Epidemiology: occurs with sickle cell trait (in hypoxic situations) or sickle cell disease
  3. Clinical presentation
    a. Asymptomatic hematuria (most common; see Chapter 12): caused by infarctions in the renal medulla
    b. Loss of concentrating ability in the kidney(s)
    c. Renal papillary necrosis (RPN), pyelonephritis
E. **Diffuse cortical necrosis**
  1. **Definition:** Uncommon cause of ARF that is secondary to ischemic necrosis of the renal cortex of both kidneys
  2. Epidemiology
    a. Complication of an obstetric emergency. Examples: preeclampsia, abruptio placentae (see Chapter 22)
    b. DIC *limited* to the renal cortex
      (1) Fibrin thrombi are present in arterioles and glomerular capillaries.
      (2) Bilateral, diffuse, pale infarctions of the renal cortex
    c. Anuria (*no* urine absence of urine production) in a pregnant woman caused by ARF
XI. **Obstructive Disorders of the Kidney**
  A. **Overview of causes of urinary tract obstruction (Link 20-72)**
  B. **Hydronephrosis**
    1. **Definition:** Dilation of the renal pelvis and calyces usually caused by obstruction of the ureter or less commonly the lower urinary tract (LUT) obstruction (e.g., prostate hyperplasia)
    2. Epidemiology
      a. Most common complication of an upper urinary tract (UUT) obstruction
      b. Children usually have congenital malformation. It is the most common renal abnormality detected on antenatal ultrasound (US).
        (1) Types of congenital malformations: bladder neck obstruction, posterior urethral valve (PUV), vesicoureteral reflux (VUR), ectopic ureter, megaureter (obstructive, nonobstructive), urethral atresia in prune belly syndrome
        (2) Idiopathic hypercalciuria is the most common cause of pediatric urinary calculi in the above abnormalities.
      c. Adults usually have acquired disease such as ureteral stone (most common cause) or prostate hyperplasia.
      d. Other causes of hydronephrosis include retroperitoneal fibrosis and invasive cervical cancer.
    3. Gross findings
      a. Dilated ureter and renal pelvis (Fig. 20-8 A; Links 20-73 and 20-74)
      b. Compression atrophy of the renal medulla and cortex from increased intraluminal pressure (see Chapter 2)
    4. May produce postrenal azotemia (increased in serum BUN and Cr)

Renal infarction

Pale wedge-shaped renal cortex

AF with embolization
Left atrial thrombus formation → systemic circulation
AF: MCC renal infarction
Atheroembolic renal disease
Rupture atheromatous plaques → embolization CH crystals
Elderly with erosive atherosclerosis proximal Ao, renal arteries
Catheter manipulation/surgery
Vasculitis (polyarteritis nodosa)
Wedge-shaped pale infarctions renal cortex
V-shaped appearance (scar tissue)
Sudden onset hematuria, flank pain
Sickle cell nephropathy
Sickling → vessel occlusion
Sickle cell trait/disease
Asymptomatic hematuria (medullary infarctions)
Loss urine concentration
Renal papillary necrosis
Pyelonephritis
Diffuse cortical necrosis
Ischemic necrosis renal cortex both kidneys
Preeclampsia, abruptio placenta
DIC
Fibrin thrombi arterioles/glomerular capillaries
Bilateral diffuse pale infarctions renal cortex
Pregnant woman: anuria → ARF
Obstructive disorders kidney
Hydronephrosis
Dilation renal pelvis/calyces from ureteral obstruction
MC complication UUT obstruction
Children: congenital malformations
Bladder neck obstruction, PUV, VUR
Ectopic ureter, megaureter
Urethral atresia (prune belly syndrome)
Idiopathic hypercalciuria MCC pediatric urinary calculi
Adults: ureteral stone MCC, prostate hyperplasia
Retroperitoneal fibrosis, invasive cervical cancer
Dilated ureter/renal pelvis
Compression atrophy renal medulla/cortex
Possible postrenal azotemia

20-8: A, Hydronephrosis of the kidney. There is marked dilation of the renal pelvis and calyces with thinning of the overlying cortex and medulla caused by compression atrophy. **B,** Staghorn calculi. Note the staghorn calculi in the renal calyces and the renal pelvis. (*A from Kumar V, Fausto N, Abbas A: Robbins and Cotran Pathologic Basis of Disease, 7th ed, Philadelphia, Saunders, 2004, p 1013, Fig. 20-56; B from Kern WF, Silva FG, Laszik ZG, et al [eds]: Atlas of Renal Pathology, Philadelphia, Saunders, 1999, p 155, Fig. 13-30.)*

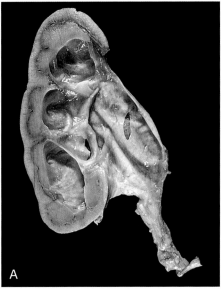
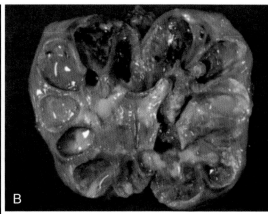

Renal stones

Mineral deposit in urinary tract

Males > females

Incidence greater in summer

↑Risk 2ⁿᵈ stone

↑Incidence children; ↑salt intake/↓fluid intake

Hypercalciuria (absence hypercalcemia)

MC metabolic abnormality

↑GI reabsorption calcium

Absorptive hypercalciuria

↓Urine volume concentrates urine

Hydration essential

↓Urine citrate

Urine pH alterations

Alkaline urine: calcium-phosphate stones

Acid urine: uric acid/cysteine stones

1° HPTH

↑Dietary phosphate, oxalates

Urinary infections urease producers

Types of renal stones

Calcium stones MC

Calcium oxalate stone MC (adults)

Hypercalciuria MC risk factor

Children stone composition: calcium, struvite, cysteine, uric acid, others

C. Renal stones (urolithiasis)
1. **Definition:** A small, hard mineral deposit that is formed within the urinary tract (kidney, ureter, urinary bladder, urethra)
2. Epidemiology
   a. More common in males than in females. In men, the lifetime prevalence of stones is 10%.
   b. Incidence is greater during the summer because of insufficient fluid intake.
   c. Fifty percent chance of a second stone occuring within 5 years of the first
   d. Fivefold increase in stones in children over the past 2 decades because of increased dietary salt and insufficient fluid intake
   e. Pathogenesis
      (1) Hypercalciuria (increased calcium in urine) in the absence of hypercalcemia
         (a) Most common metabolic abnormality producing stones
         (b) Caused by increased gastrointestinal reabsorption of calcium; called absorptive hypercalciuria
      (2) Decreased urine volume, which concentrates the urine. Hydration is essential in preventing stone formation.
      (3) Reduced urine citrate. Citrate normally chelates (binds to) calcium to form calcium citrate.
      (4) Urine pH alterations
         (a) Alkaline urine pH favors crystallization, which produces calcium- and phosphate-containing stones.
         (b) Acidic urine pH favors crystallization of uric acid and cysteine, which produces uric acid and cysteine stones.
      (5) Primary hyperparathyroidism (HPTH; 10% of cases) increases urine calcium concentration, producing calcium-containing stones.
      (6) Diets high in dairy products (contain phosphate) or oxalates form calcium phosphate and calcium oxalate stones.
      (7) Urinary infections caused by urease producers (e.g., *Proteus* spp.; ammonia smell of urine) increase the formation of stones containing ammonium (called struvite stones).
3. Types of renal stones
   a. Calcium stones (70%–80% of cases)
      (1) Calcium oxalate stones (~60%; most common type in adults), calcium phosphate stones (~10%), or calcium oxalate + phosphate stones (~10%). Risk factors for calcium oxalate stones include hypercalciuria (MC), hyperoxaluria (malabsorption states), decreased urine citrate (distal renal tubular acidosis [RTA], diarrhea), increased urinary uric acid.
      (2) Stone composition in children: calcium (58%), struvite (25%), cysteine (6%), uric acid or urate (9%), and others (2%)

(3) Risk factors for calcium phosphate stones include distal (type 1) renal tubular acidosis (RTA), primary hyperparathyroidism, and an alkaline urine pH.

  b. Magnesium ammonium phosphate (MAP) stone

  (1) Called a "staghorn calculus" or struvite stone, which occurs in 10% to 20% of cases; Fig. 20-8 B; Link 20-75)

  (2) Greatest risk factor is urine infections caused by urease producers (e.g., *Proteus* spp.).

  (3) Urine is alkaline and smells like ammonia.

  (4) Surgery is frequently necessary because of the large stone size.

  c. Uric acid stones occur in 10% to 12% of cases. Risk factors: hyperuricemia (e.g., gout, myeloproliferative disease [MPD] with a high cell turnover with increased release of purines, treatment of leukemia [increased release purines]).

  d. Cystine stones occur in (<1% of cases). Greatest risk factor is cystinosis, an autosomal recessive lysosomal storage disease with abnormal accumulation of the amino acid cystine.

4. Clinical findings

  a. Sudden onset of flank tenderness, nausea vomiting

  b. Colicky pain radiating into the ipsilateral groin; considered the worst pain in both men and women (other than childbirth)

  c. Gross hematuria may be evident.

5. Laboratory findings

  a. Hematuria, crystals in urine

  b. Hypercalcemia. If present, rule out primary HPTH.

  c. Straining the urine to collect stones

  (1) When stones are collected, they should always be sent for analysis.

  (2) More than 50% of patients pass the stone within 48 hours.

  (3) Recurrence of stone formation occurs in ~50% of patients.

6. Laboratory tests and diagnosis

  a. Noncontrast stone protocol computed tomography (CT) (Link 20-76)

  b. Standard studies include 24-hour urine collections for sodium, calcium, phosphate, Cr, urate, citrate, uric acid, oxalate, and cysteine. Studies also include urine pH (by meter not dipstick), urinalysis, urine culture (if leukocyte esterase and nitrites are present).

7. Treatment is tailored to the type of stone, which underscores why they should be collected and sent for analysis.

8. Hydration is the key to stone prevention.

XII. **Tumors of the Kidney and Renal Pelvis**

  A. **Overview of neoplasms of the urinary tract** (Link 20-77)

  B. **Angiomyolipoma**

  1. **Definition:** Hamartoma (see Chapter 9) composed of blood vessels, smooth muscle, and adipose cells

  2. Epidemiology: associated with tuberous sclerosis (see Chapter 26), manifestations of which include mental retardation, multisystem hamartomas, and hypopigmented skin lesions

  C. **Renal cell carcinoma (RCC)**

  1. **Definition:** Primary adenocarcinoma originating from the proximal RTCs

  2. Epidemiology

  a. Sporadic (most common) and hereditary types of RCCs

  b. Two times more common in men than women

  c. Most often occurs in the fourth to sixth decades of life

  d. Risk factors

  (1) Smoking (most common cause), obesity, renal dialysis

  (2) Von Hippel–Lindau disease (VHL; see Chapter 10)

  (a) Autosomal dominant disorder associated with hemangioblastomas located in the cerebellum and retina

  (b) Bilateral RCC occurs in 50% to 60% of cases.

  (3) Adult polycystic kidney disease (APKD)

  (4) Asbestos exposure, lead exposure, gasoline and petroleum product exposure

  e. Pathogenesis

  (1) Cytogenetic abnormalities occur in sporadic and hereditary cancers.

  (2) Translocations occur with a loss of the von Hippel–Lindau suppressor gene.

3. Gross and microscopic findings

  a. Clear cell adenocarcinoma is the most common type (70%–80% of cases).

  b. Present as an upper pole mass with cysts and hemorrhage; bright yellow mass often larger than 3 cm (75%–80% of cases; Fig. 20-9 A; Link 20-78 A)

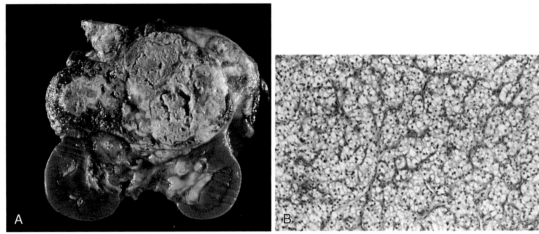

20-9: **A,** Renal cell carcinoma. The large, yellow upper pole mass with multifocal areas of hemorrhage extends into the renal pelvis. **B,** Renal cell carcinoma. This microscopic section of a renal cell carcinoma shows cells with a clear cytoplasm. *(**A** from my friend Ivan Damjanov, MD, PhD, Linder J:* Pathology: A Color Atlas, *St. Louis, Mosby, 2000, p 234, Fig. 11-79; **B** from Kern WF, Silva FG, Laszik ZG, et al [eds]:* Atlas of Renal Pathology, *Philadelphia, Saunders, 1999, p 281, Fig. 23-5.)*

Clear cells contain lipid/glycogen

Renal vein invasion → IVC

Metastatic sites

Lungs: MC site

Lungs MC metastatic site

Hemorrhagic nodules

X-ray: "cannonball" appearance

Bones: lytic lesions

RCC: invades renal vein; poor prognosis

Hemorrhagic skin nodules

Clinical findings

Often clinically occult; incidental finding

RCC triad: hematuria, flank pain, abdominal mass

Hematuria, abdominal mass

Flank pain, hypertension

Weight loss, fever

Left-sided varicocele

Hepatic dysfunction *without* metastasis

Laboratory findings

↑ESR

ACD

Ectopic hormones

EPO → 2° polycythemia

PTH-related peptide → hypercalcemia

US, CT, MRI

Late metastases

Renal vein invasion: poor prognosis

Renal pelvis cancer

Urothelial carcinoma

Cancer urothelial cells lining renal pelvis

c. Composed of clear cells that contain lipid and glycogen (Fig. 20-9 B; Link 20-78 B)
d. Tendency for renal vein invasion (15%–20% of cases) (Link 20-79); may invade inferior vena cava and extend to the right side of heart
e. Metastatic sites
  (1) Lungs: most common site for metastasis (50%–60% of cases). Metastatic nodules are hemorrhagic and have a "cannonball" appearance on radiographs.
  (2) Bones: lytic (radiolucent) lesions (30%–40% of cases)
  (3) Regional lymph nodes (15%–30% of cases)
  (4) Skin: Hemorrhagic nodules are present in the skin because of the increased vascularity of the tumor.
4. Clinical findings
  a. RCC may remain clinically occult for most of its course and is often an incidental finding on imaging.
  b. Triad (10% of cases): hematuria, abdominal mass, flank pain
  c. Hematuria (50%–60% of cases), abdominal mass (25%–45% of cases), flank pain (35%–40% of cases), hypertension (20%–40% of cases)
  d. Weight loss (30%–35% of cases), fever (5%–15% of cases)
  e. Left-sided varicocele (2%–3% of cases; see Chapter 21): relates to impaired drainage of the left spermatic vein secondary to tumor invasion of the left renal vein
  f. Hepatic dysfunction without the presence of metastasis (Stauffer syndrome)
5. Laboratory findings
  a. Elevated erythrocyte sedimentation (ESR) rate (nonspecific finding; 50%–60% of cases; see Chapter 3)
  b. Normocytic anemia (anemia of chronic disease [ACD]; 20%–40% of cases)
  c. Ectopic secretion of hormones (see Chapter 9)
    (1) EPO: produces secondary polycythemia (4% of cases; see Chapter 13)
    (2) PTH-related protein: produces hypercalcemia (3%–6% of cases)
6. Diagnosis includes US, abdominal CT (Link 20-80), and magnetic resonance imaging (MRI).
7. Prognosis
  a. Characteristically has late metastases; may recur 1 to 20 years after the tumor has been removed
  b. Average 5-year survival rate is 45% with metastasis. Up to 70% of cases do *not* have metastasis.
  c. Extension of the cancer into the renal vein or through the renal capsule conveys a poor prognosis (10%–15% 5-year survival rate).
D. Renal pelvis cancer
1. Urothelial carcinoma
  a. **Definition:** Cancer of the urothelial cells that line the renal pelvis; usually has a papillary appearance (Link 20-81)
  b. Epidemiology

(1) Most common type of renal pelvis cancer; grossly has a papillary pattern

(2) Approximately 50% have similar tumors elsewhere in the urinary tract (called "field effect").

c. Risk factors include smoking (most common), aromatic amines (aniline dyes), and cyclophosphamide.

2. Squamous cell carcinoma (SCC): Risk factors include renal stones and chronic infection, each of which produces chronic irritation, causing squamous metaplasia that progresses to SCC.

E. **Wilms tumor**

1. **Definition:** Malignant tumor of the kidney that is derived from the metanephric blastema, which are mesodermal cells (embryologic cells) that give rise to nephrons and the collecting ducts in the kidneys. Blastema is a mass of embryonic cells from which an organ or a body part develops.

2. Epidemiology

   a. Accounts for ~5% of childhood cancers; highest incidence is among blacks followed by whites and Asians

   b. Most common primary renal tumor in children

   c. Occurs between 2 and 5 years of age; slight female dominance, especially for bilateral disease; more than 75% diagnosed *before* 5 years of age

   d. Sporadic type is more common than the genetic type.

   e. Characteristics of the genetic type of Wilms tumor

      (1) Autosomal dominant inheritance (chromosome 11)

      (2) Association with WAGR syndrome: Wilms tumor, aniridia (absent iris), genitourinary abnormalities, retardation (mental)

      (3) Association with Beckwith-Wiedemann syndrome, trisomy 18

      • Beckwith-Wiedemann syndrome: Wilms tumor, macroglossia (enlarged tongue), enlarged body organs (liver, adrenal, pancreas), and hemihypertrophy of the extremities (one side or part of one side of the body is larger than the other)

3. Large, necrotic, gray-tan tumor that contains abortive glomeruli and tubules, primitive blastemal cells, and rhabdomyoblasts (immature skeletal muscle; mesoderm component). (Links 20-82 and 20-83)

4. Clinical findings

   a. Unilateral palpable mass in a child with hypertension. Hypertension is caused by ectopic renin secretion by the tumor which activates the renin-angiotensin-aldosterone system.

   b. Lungs are the most common site of metastasis.

5. Approximately 90% to 95% 5-year survival rate. Relapses beyond 5 years are rare.

Margin notes:

MC renal pelvis cancer; papillary

Similar cancer other sites urinary tract ("field effect")

Smoking MC risk factor, aniline dyes, cyclophosphamide

Squamous cell carcinoma

SCC risk factors: renal stones, chronic infection

Wilms tumor

Malignant tumor from metanephric blastema

Blastema: embryonic cells developing organ/body part

Incidence: blacks > whites.> Asians

MC 1° renal tumor in children

2 to 5 yrs of age

Sporadic > genetic type

Genetic type Wilms

AD inheritance

WAGR syndrome

Wilms, aniridia, GU abnormalities, retardation (mental)

Beckwith-Wiedemann syndrome, trisomy 18

Wilms, macroglossia, enlarged organs, hemihypertrophy extremities

Abortive glomeruli/tubules, blastemal cells, rhabdomyoblasts

Unilateral palpable mass with hypertension

Hypertension ectopic renin secretion

Lungs MC site metastasis

CHAPTER 21
Ureter, Lower Urinary Tract, and Male Reproductive Disorders

ABBREVIATIONS

MC most common
MCC most common cause

Dx diagnose

Hx history

I. **Overview** (Link 21-1)

- **The lower urinary tract (LUT) refer to the urinary bladder, prostate, and urethra.**

Bladder, prostate, urethra

II. **Common Ureteral Disorders**

A. **Primary obstructed nonrefluxing megaureter**

Megaureter

Dilated ureter

1. **Definition:** An abnormally dilated ureter (hydroureteronephrosis; Link 21-2)

2. Epidemiology

Aperistalsis distal ureter → dilation from retained urine

a. Aperistalsis of the distal ureter leads to urinary retention and thus increased intraluminal pressure, causing ureteral dilatation.

Males > females

b. More common in males than females; may be bilateral

May be bilateral

c. Often associated with other congenital anomalies (e.g., Hirschsprung disease)

Associated with Hirschsprung disease

B. **Ureteritis cystica**

Ureteritis cystica

1. **Definition:** Rare urothelial inflammatory response causing smooth cysts to project from the mucosa into the lumen (Link 21-3)

Cysts project into lumen

2. Epidemiology

Bladder may be involved

a. Similar findings may be present in the bladder.

Glandular metaplasia → adenocarcinoma

b. Cysts may undergo glandular metaplasia, which may progress to adenocarcinoma.

Ureteral stones

C. **Ureteral stones**

Ureters: MC site stones causing obstruction

- Ureters are the most common site for stones to cause obstruction.

Retroperitoneal fibrosis

D. **Retroperitoneal fibrosis**

Excessive fibrous tissue retroperitoneum

1. **Definition:** Excessive production of fibrous tissue in the retroperitoneum, causing entrapment of the ureters and other structures

Entraps ureters

2. Epidemiology

Idiopathic MCC

a. Most cases are idiopathic.

Causes/associations

b. Known causes and associations

Ergot derivatives; Rx migraines

(1) Ergot derivatives used in the treatment of migraines

Malignant lymphoma

(2) Malignant lymphoma within the retroperitoneum

Sclerosing conditions

(3) Other sclerosing conditions including:

PSC

(a) primary sclerosing cholangitis (PSC; see Chapter 19).

Sclerosing mediastinitis

(b) sclerosing mediastinitis (see Chapter 17).

Reidel thyroiditis

(c) Reidel thyroiditis (see Chapter 23).

Complications

3. Complications

Hydronephrosis MC complication

a. Hydronephrosis is the most common complication.

Right scrotal varicocele

b. Right scrotal varicocele (see section V). Fibrosis blocks the drainage of the right spermatic vein into the vena cava, unlike the left spermatic vein, which drains into the left renal vein.

Ureteral cancers

E. **Ureteral cancers**

UC MC ureteral cancer

- Urothelial carcinoma (UC) is the most common cancer (discussed under Urinary Bladder).

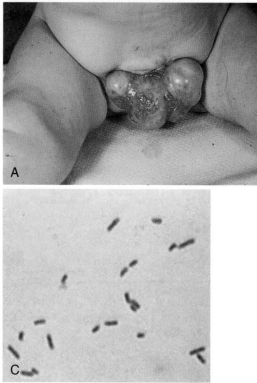

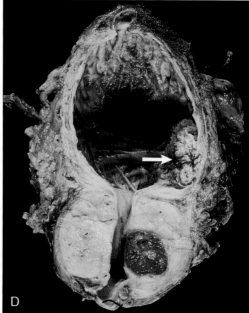

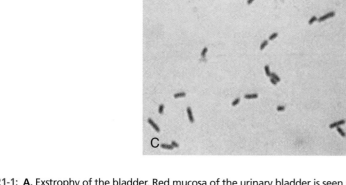

21-1: **A,** Exstrophy of the bladder. Red mucosa of the urinary bladder is seen protruding through the defect in the anterior abdominal wall. **B,** *Schistosoma haematobium* egg. These eggs are similar in size to those of *Schistosoma mansoni* but can be differentiated by the presence of a terminal rather than lateral spine. **C,** Gram stain of *Escherichia coli*. Note the gram-negative rods. **D,** Urothelial carcinoma (old term, *transitional cell carcinoma*) of the urinary bladder. The *arrow* shows a papillary exophytic mass arising from the mucosal surface of the bladder. The red lesion in the prostate gland is an infarction. *(A courtesy Dr. Roger D. Smith, Cincinnati, OH, and GRIPE; B from Murray PR, Rosenthal KS, Pfaller MA: Medical Microbiology, 6th ed, Philadelphia, Mosby Elsevier, 2009, p 878, Fig. 84.11; C from McPherson R, Pincus M: Henry's Clinical Diagnosis and Management by Laboratory Methods, 21st ed, Philadelphia, Saunders, 2006, Fig. 56-14; D from Rosai J, Ackerman LV: Surgical Pathology, 9th ed. St. Louis, Mosby, 2004, p 1328, Fig. 17-175.)*

III. Urinary Bladder Diseases
A. Congenital diseases of the urinary bladder
1. Exstrophy (Fig. 21-1 A)
   a. **Definition:** Developmental failure of the anterior abdominal wall and urinary bladder. The bladder mucosa is exposed to the body surface.
   b. Epidemiology
      (1) Often associated with epispadias (abnormal opening on the dorsal surface of the penis; see Section IV)
      (2) Complications
         (a) Inflammation predisposes to glandular metaplasia of the urinary bladder mucosa.
         (b) Increased risk for developing adenocarcinoma of the urinary bladder (see later)
2. Urachal cyst remnants
   a. **Definition:** A cyst development within the urachal remnants. In early embryologic development, it connects the umbilicus with the urinary bladder.
   b. Usually the embryonic allantois (part of the yolk sac) is obliterated to form the fibrous urachus that connects the apex of the bladder with the umbilicus; called the *median umbilical ligament* in adults.
      (1) If the lumen remains patent in a newborn (NB), a fistula (open connection) may develop between the urinary bladder and the umbilicus.
      (2) Midline cyst may persist that may drain urine to the opening on the umbilicus.

c. Cyst remnants predispose to adenocarcinoma of the urinary bladder; most common cause of a urinary bladder adenocarcinoma.
B. **Acute cystitis**
1. **Definition:** Acute inflammation (usually an infection) of the urinary bladder (Link 21-4)
2. Epidemiology; risk factors for LUT infections
   a. Female sex. Females have a short urethra, allowing pathogens a short passage into the urinary bladder (ascending infection; see Chapter 20).
   b. Indwelling urinary catheter (IUC)
      (1) Most common cause of sepsis in hospitalized patients
      (2) Accounts for 50% of nosocomial (hospital-acquired) urinary tract infections (UTIs)
   c. Sexual intercourse
      (1) "Honeymoon cystitis" occurs from trauma to the urethra from frequent sexual intercourse.
      (2) Voiding after intercourse reduces the risk for infection by flushing out urethral bacteria that would otherwise ascend into the urinary bladder.
   d. Diabetes mellitus (DM)
   e. Neurogenic bladder (stasis of urine)
   f. Cyclophosphamide
      (1) Produces hemorrhagic cystitis caused by liver metabolite acrolein that damages the urinary bladder mucosa (Link 21-5)
      (2) Prevented by taking mesna. Sulfhydryl compound given together with cyclophosphamide to inactivate damaging metabolites within the urinary bladder.
3. Epidemiology; pathogens causing acute cystitis
   a. *Escherichia coli*
      (1) Most common uropathogen (80%–90% of cases)
      (2) Gram-negative rod (Fig. 21-1 C)
      (3) UTIs account for 40% of hospital-acquired (nosocomial) infections.
      (4) Most common cause of sepsis in hospitalized patients
   b. Adenovirus causes hemorrhagic cystitis (Link 21-5). Other causes include *E. coli*, papovavirus, and influenza A.
   c. *Staphylococcus saprophyticus*
      (1) Causes acute cystitis in young, sexually active women; accounts for ~10% to 20% of LUT infections
      (2) Coagulase-negative gram-positive coccus
   d. Acute urethral syndrome in women
      (1) Female counterpart to nonspecific urethritis (NSU) in men (see later)
      (2) *Chlamydia trachomatis* is the most common cause of the acute urethral syndrome.
      (3) Identification of *Chlamydia* is made by using polymerase chain reaction (PCR) testing of voided urine.
   e. Schistosoma haematobium.
      (1) **Definition:** Trematode (fluke), whose first intermediate host is a snail and whose larvae enter veins in the urinary bladder wall, where they develop into adult worms (Link 21-6)
      (2) Transmission
         (a) Fork-tailed cercariae penetrate the skin.
         (b) Larvae enter veins in the urinary bladder wall.
         (c) Larvae develop into adult worms that deposit eggs.
         (d) Host develops an intense inflammatory response consisting of eosinophils (Eos) that surround the eggs. Eos release major basic protein (MBP), which kills helminths (see Chapter 3).
         (e) Inflammation causes squamous metaplasia of the bladder epithelium; may progress to dysplasia and squamous cancer.
      (3) Eggs have a large terminal spine (Fig. 21-1 B; Link 21-7).
   f. Other uropathogens: *Mycoplasma hominis, Ureaplasma urealyticum,* and *Neisseria gonorrhoeae*
4. Other types of cystitis
   a. Chronic cystitis: recurrent cystitis usually in women; leads to thickening of the urinary bladder wall and stone formation caused by stasis of urine (Link 21-8)
   b. Interstitial cystitis (Hunner cystitis)
      (1) Usually an adult or elderly woman who has cystitis with ulceration (Hunner ulcers) and marked submucosal edema of the urinary bladder, resulting in prominent lower

abdominal pain, suprapubic, or perineal pain and urinary frequency unresponsive to medical therapy

  (2) Edema, hemorrhage, and a mononuclear infiltrate with an increase in mast cells are present in the interstitial tissue.

  (3) Etiology remains obscure; however, autoimmune mechanisms may be involved.

 c. Eosinophilic cystitis

  (1) One clinical setting is seen in women and children who have allergic disorders and eosinophilia.

  (2) Another clinical setting is seen in older men with bladder injury related to other disorders of the urinary bladder or prostate. Rarely, it may be related to parasitic infestation.

  (3) In either setting, recurrent episodes of severe dysuria (painful urination) and hematuria may result in ureteral obstruction. Polypoid growths are present in the mucosa. Microscopically, there is a prominent infiltration of Eos, fibrosis, and myocyte necrosis with giant cells.

 d. Emphysematous cystitis.

  (1) Gas-filled vesicles in bladder wall caused by gas-forming bacteria (e.g., *Clostridium perfringens*)

  (2) May occur in patients with DM, neurogenic bladder, chronic urinary infections, or malignant hematologic disorders (leukemia, lymphoma)

5. Clinical findings in LUT infections

 a. Dysuria (painful urination)

 b. Increased frequency and urgency (feeling of having to urinate all the time)

 c. Nocturia (increased frequency of urination at night)

 d. Suprapubic discomfort caused by urinary bladder irritation; gross (visible) hematuria

6. Laboratory findings

 a. Pyuria (pus [white blood cells or WBCs] in the urine) with ≥10 WBCs per high-power field (HPF) in a centrifuged specimen; >2 WBCs/HPF in an uncentrifuged specimen

 b. Bacteriuria, hematuria

 c. Positive dipstick test for leukocyte esterase and nitrite (see Chapter 20)

 d. Urine culture showing ≥10^5 colony-forming units (CFUs)/mL. Urine culture is the gold standard criterion of infection.

7. Asymptomatic bacteriuria in women

 a. **Definition:** Two successive cultures with ≥10^5 CFUs/mL

 b. Epidemiology; causes

  (1) Pregnancy: Because acute pyelonephritis (APN) may occur in 1% to 2% of cases, asymptomatic bacteriuria is usually treated.

  (2) Older women in nursing homes; if asymptomatic and healthy, no treatment necessary

8. Sterile pyuria

 a. **Definition:** Neutrophils in the urine and lack of organisms in a standard culture after 24 hours; positive leukocyte esterase and a negative nitrite test

 b. Epidemiology; causes

  (1) *C. trachomatis:* cannot be detected with urine dipsticks; hence, the term "sterile"

  (2) Renal tuberculosis (TB): cannot be detected with urine dipsticks; hence, the term "sterile"

  (3) Acute tubulointerstitial nephritis (TIN; see Chapter 20)

9. Malakoplakia

 a. **Definition:** Rare infectious granulomatous disorder characterized by the presence erythematous papules, nodules, or ulcers involving the urinary bladder mucosa and other sites

 b. Epidemiology

  (1) Caused by defective phagolysosomal killing of bacteria by histiocytes, most commonly *E coli*; other pathogens include *Pseudomonas aeruginosa*

  (2) Usually a history of immunosuppression from renal transplantation, malignant lymphoma, long-term use of systemic corticosteroids, or DM, to name a few associations

  (3) Presents as erythematous papules, subcutaneous nodules, and ulcers

  (4) Foamy histiocytes are filled with laminated mineralized concretions called Michaelis-Gutmann bodies (calcium and iron), which are defective phagosomes that cannot degrade bacterial products (Link 21-9).

Mast cells prominent

?Autoimmune mechanisms

Eosinophilic cystitis

Women/children allergic disorders/eosinophilia

Old men bladder injury related to bladder or prostate problems

Severe dysuria, hematuria, ureteral obstruction

Polypoid growths; eosinophils, fibrosis

Myocyte necrosis/giant cells

Emphysematous cystitis

Gas-filled vesicles bladder wall

Clostridium perfringens

DM, neurogenic bladder, UTIs, leukemia/lymphoma

Clinical finding LUT infections

Dysuria

↑Frequency, urgency

Nocturia

Suprapubic pain

Gross hematuria

Laboratory findings

Pyuria

Bacteriuria, hematuria

+ Dipstick nitrite/leukocyte esterase

Urine culture ≥10^5 colony-forming units (CFUs)/mL

Urine culture: gold standard

Asymptomatic bacteriuria in women

Two successive cultures ≥10^5 CFUs/mL

Pregnancy

Usually treated (concern for APN)

Elderly women nursing homes

Sterile pyuria

Neutrophils in urine, lack of organisms *standard* culture

+Leukocyte esterase, −nitrite test

C. trachomatis (*not* detected with dipsticks)

Renal TB (*not* detected with dipsticks)

Acute TIN

Malakoplakia

Granulomatous infection; papules, nodules, ulcers

Defective histiocyte phagolysosomal killing *E. coli*

Immunosuppression, lymphoma, corticosteroids, DM

Papules, nodules, ulcers

Foamy histiocytes with Michaelis-Gutmann bodies (calcium/iron)

C. **Miscellaneous diseases of the urinary bladder**

1. Acquired diverticula
   a. **Definition:** Solitary or multiple outpouchings where mucosa herniates through areas of weakness in the urinary bladder wall
   b. Epidemiology
      (1) Most acquired diverticula are caused by benign prostate hyperplasia (BPH). BPH causes obstruction of urine outflow, which increases intravesical pressure, predisposing to diverticulum or diverticula formation through areas of weakness in the wall of the urinary bladder.
      (2) Diverticulitis and stone formation are common complications.

2. Cystocele
   a. **Definition:** Protrusion of the urinary bladder through the vaginal wall
   b. Epidemiology
      (1) Common in middle-aged to elderly women. Other causes include obesity, previous hysterectomy, and constipation (straining).
      (2) Mechanism
         (a) When the wall between bladder and vagina weakens, it allows the bladder to protrude into the vagina (Link 21-10).
         (b) Creates a pouch that collects residual urine
      (3) Urine leakage from incomplete emptying of the urinary bladder, particularly when laughing, coughing, sneezing

3. Cystitis cystica and glandularis
   a. **Definitions:** Cystitis cystica, the urinary bladder analog of ureteritis cystica, is characterized by mucosal cysts forming in the wall of the urinary bladder. Cysts are lined by urothelial cells. Cystitis glandularis refers to mucosal cysts that have undergone metaplastic transformation of urinary bladder urothelial cells to glandular cells (GCs).
   b. Epidemiology
      (1) Von Brunn (VB) nests are islands of benign-appearing transitional cell epithelium residing in the submucosa resulting from inward proliferation of the basal cell layer.
      (2) Cystitis cystica and cystitis glandularis are variants of VB nests with additional histologic changes.
         (a) In cystitis cystica, the center of the nests is filled with liquefied material as a result of chronic cystitis, bladder outlet obstruction (e.g., prostate hyperplasia [PH] or chronic irritation from bladder stones.
         (b) In cystitis glandularis, the urothelial epithelium has undergone glandular metaplasia, and the lining of the cysts is columnar with mucin-secretion.
            • Increased risk for developing adenocarcinoma from the mucus-secreting cells

---

Sidebar notes:

Acquired diverticula

Outpouchings in areas weakness bladder wall

Majority due to BPH

BPH obstruction → ↑intravesical pressure → diverticula thru areas weakness

Diverticulitis, stone formation

Cystocele

Protrusion bladder thru vaginal wall

Middle aged elderly women

Obesity, previous hysterectomy, constipation

Weakening between bladder and vaginal wall

Pouch with residual urine

Urine leakage (laugh, cough, sneeze), incomplete emptying bladder

Cystitis cystica

Cystitis glandularis

Mucosal cysts lined by urothelial cells (cystica)/GCs (glandularis)

VB nests submucosa: transitional epithelium

Cystitis cystica/glandularis variants VB nests

Cystitis cystica center liquefied material

Cystitis glandularis center lined by mucin-secreting cells

↑Risk adenocarcinoma

Retain urine: ↑sympathetic activity → relax detrusor muscle, contract internal sphincter muscle.

Void urine: ↑parasympathetic activity → contract detrusor muscle, relax internal sphincter muscle

---

Urinary bladder control and incontinence disorders (Link 21-11): Whereas relaxation of the detrusor muscle is involved in the storage of urine, contraction of the muscle is important in emptying the bladder. The sympathetic nervous system relaxes the detrusor muscle and contracts the internal sphincter; hence, it is important in the retention of urine in the bladder. In contradistinction, the parasympathetic nervous system is involved in emptying the bladder. It accomplishes this function by contracting the detrusor muscle and relaxing the internal sphincter muscle. There are four types of urinary incontinence: urge incontinence (40%–70% of cases), overflow incontinence, stress incontinence, and functional incontinence. **Urge incontinence** is caused by overactivity of the detrusor muscle, resulting in the production of low volumes of urine. Symptoms include increased urinary frequency, urgency, small volume voids, and nocturia. The most common causes are bladder irritation caused by benign prostate hyperplasia (BPH), atrophic urethritis, and infection. Treatment is with anticholinergics, which inhibit parasympathetic stimulation of detrusor contraction. The mechanisms for **overflow incontinence** are outflow obstruction (e.g., BPH) or detrusor underactivity related to autonomic neuropathy (e.g., diabetes mellitus). Symptoms include dribbling and low urine flow. Treatment involves the use of cholinergic drugs to enhance muscle tone (i.e., increase detrusor contraction) or, if obstruction is the cause (e.g., BPH), α-adrenergic blockers to relax smooth muscles in the bladder neck. The mechanism for **stress incontinence** is laxity of pelvic floor muscles with a concomitant lack of bladder support. This may be the result of not maintaining the posterior urethrovesical angle of 90 to 100 degrees or a lack of estrogen; hence, this type of incontinence primarily occurs in women. Symptoms relate to the loss of urine when there is an increase in intraabdominal pressure (e.g., laughing, coughing, sneezing). The mechanism for **functional incontinence** is inability to reach toilet facilities in time. Patients are normally continent; however, if they are taking diuretics or drinking too many caffeinated beverages, incontinence may occur.

D. Urinary bladder tumors
1. Bladder papilloma: very uncommon benign papillary tumor
2. UC (old term, *transitional cell carcinoma*; Links 21-12 to 21-15)
   a. **Definition:** Most common type of cancer that occurs in the renal pelvis, ureter, and urinary bladder. Urinary bladder cancer is more common than ureteral or renal pelvis cancer.
   b. Epidemiology
      (1) Most common urinary bladder cancer (93% of cases), renal pelvis (>95% of cases), and ureter cancer (>95% of cases). Sixth most common cancer in the United States. Seventh leading cause of cancer-related death. Squamous cancer accounts for 6% of urinary bladder cancer and adenocarcinoma for 1% of bladder cancers.
      (2) Incidence is decreasing in the United States; more common in men (3 : 1)
      (3) Increasing in women because of tobacco use; 10th most common cancer in women
      (4) Increased incidence with aging (seventh decade)
      (5) Most common sites for cancer are the lateral or posterior walls at the base of the urinary bladder. If UC is found in other sites, there is a high incidence of concurrent involvement (30%–50%) of the urinary bladder.
      (6) Causes
         (a) Smoking cigarettes (most common) leads to a four times greater risk; less risk for other tobacco products
         (b) Workers in dye, rubber, paint, and leather industries
         (c) Cyclophosphamide, arsenic exposure
         (d) Beer consumption (nitrosamines [carcinogens] are present in beer)
         (e) *Schistosoma haematobium* infections: Approximately 70% of the cancers are squamous cell carcinomas (SCCs), and 30% are UCs.
      (7) Pathogenesis
         (a) Genetic factors: Numerous chromosomes have been implicated (gains, losses, or rearrangements). Genes implicated include the *p53* and *RB* suppressor genes and *HRAS* proto-oncogene and alterations in the epidermal growth factor receptor (EGFR).
         (b) Environmental factors (see earlier discussion)
      (8) Multifocality ("field effect") and recurrence are the rule.
         • Common malignant stem cell abnormality that is present in all the urothelial epithelium; "diffuse genetic instability"
      (9) Reimplantation of the tumor from another site in the urinary system is a less common cause of recurrence.
      (10) Gross findings in UC correlate with the grade of the tumor; for example:
         (a) low-grade cancers (see Chapter 9) are usually papillary and typically are *not* invasive (Fig. 21-1 D).
         (b) high-grade cancers (see Chapter 9) are papillary or flat and are usually invasive.
   c. Clinical findings
      (1) Painless gross or microscopic hematuria occurs (70%–90% of cases); most common sign of UC of the urinary bladder
      (2) Dysuria (painful urination), increased frequency of urination
   d. Diagnosis
      (1) Excretory urography or intravenous pyelogram followed by cystoscopy with biopsy. Fluorescence cystoscopy is useful for flat lesions and carcinoma in situ.
      (2) Retrograde pyelography is the most useful test for upper urinary tract lesions (e.g., ureter).
   e. Prognosis
      (1) Improved prognosis when blood group antigens (A, B, or H; see Chapter 16) are present on the surface of the tumor
      (2) Five-year survival rate for all stages combined is 80%.
      (3) Potential for recurrence is greatest with high grade cancer, multifocal disease, and increasing size of the tumor.
3. Squamous cell carcinoma (SCC) of the urinary bladder
   a. **Definition:** Malignant neoplasm derived from bladder urothelium that has undergone squamous metaplasia as a reaction to chronic irritation; followed by progression to dysplasia and finally SCC
   b. Epidemiology
      (1) strong association with *Schistosoma haematobium* (Fig. 21-1 B). Eggs are located in the urinary bladder venous plexus.

Uncommon benign papillary tumor

UC MC cancer kidney, renal pelvis, bladder

UC MC bladder cancer

Incidence decreasing in U.S.

Men > women

Increasing in women: tobacco use

↑Incidence with aging

Lateral/posterior walls at base MC sites

Smoking cigarettes MCC

Workers dye/rubber/paint/leather industries

Cyclophosphamide, arsenic

Beer consumption (nitrosamines)

SCC/UCs bladder: *S. haematobium* infection

Genetic factors

Chromosomal (gains, losses, rearrangements)

p53 and *RB* suppressor genes, *HRAS* proto-oncogene

Alterations EGFR

Environmental factors

Multifocality, recurrence

"Field effect"

"Diffuse genetic instability" of urothelium

Reimplantation

Gross findings

Low-grade papillary; *not* invasive

High-grade papillary/flat; usually invasive

Clinical findings

Painless gross/ microscopic hematuria MC sign

Dysuria

↑Frequency urination

Diagnosis

Excretory urography/IV pyelogram

Fluorescence cystoscopy

Retrograde pyelography: upper urinary tract lesions

Better prognosis blood group A, B, or H

Recurrence: high grade, multifocal, ↑tumor size

Squamous cell carcinoma bladder

Chronic irritation → squamous metaplasia → dysplasia → SCC

S. haematobium; eggs urinary bladder venous plexus

Common cancer in Egypt
Eos around eggs
IgE abs attached to eggs
Eos have Fc receptors for IgE
Eos attach to receptors → release MBP → destroy egg
Type II HSR involving Eos + antibodies
Chronic irritation → metaplasia → dysplasia → SCC
Adenocarcinoma urinary bladder
Rare cancer of bladder
Most from urachal remnants
Others from cystitis glandularis, exstrophy
Embryonal rhabdomyosarcoma
Derived from rhabdomyoblasts (striated muscle)
MC sarcoma in children; boys > girls
Bladder MC site for boys; vagina for girls
"Grape-like" mass urethral orifice boys; cervical polyp in girls
Cancers invading bladder: cervical/prostate cancer
Cause obstruction → hydronephrosis → postrenal azotemia → death
Urethral diseases
4 Components
Male urethra
Longer than female urethra
Common outlet for urinary/genital systems
Female urethra: short
Thru UVSM (controls urine outflow), perineal membrane
USVM ends as external urethral orifice vestibule vagina
Urethra fused to anterior wall vagina
Urethral infections
STD urethritis: *C. trachomatis, N. gonorrhoeae*
Urethra MC site STDs
Reactive arthritis: chlamydial urethritis, conjunctivitis, HLA-B27 arthritis
E. coli MC non-STD urethritis
Urethral caruncle
Female: friable, red, painful urethral mass
Chronically inflamed granulation tissue → bleeding
Urethral diverticulum females
Outpouching female urethra
Defect periurethral fascia
0.5%–5% normal females, rare in males
Variable size, single/multiple
Congenital or acquired
Vaginal aspect of urethra
Distal 2/3rd urethra, periurethral glands opening

(2) Common cancer in Egypt, where approximately 70% of the cancers are SCC and 30% are UCs

(3) Pathogenesis of SCC of the urinary bladder caused by *S. hematobium*. Eggs are surrounded by Eos. IgE antibodies (abs) are attached to the eggs. Eos have Fc receptors for IgE. Eos attach to receptors and release MBP, which destroys the egg (type II hypersensitivity reaction [HSR]).

(4) Chronic bladder irritation or infection causes squamous metaplasia → squamous metaplasia progresses to dysplasia → squamous dysplasia progresses to SCC

4. Adenocarcinoma of urinary bladder
   a. **Definition:** Rare cancer characterized by the formation of glands that infiltrate the wall of the urinary bladder
   b. Epidemiology
      (1) Most arise from urachal remnants (see previous discussion).
      (2) Other cancers arise from cystitis glandularis or exstrophy of the urinary bladder.

5. Embryonal rhabdomyosarcoma (sarcoma botryoides)
   a. **Definition:** Malignant soft tissue tumor that is derived from rhabdomyoblasts, the embryonic derivative of skeletal muscle tissue
   b. Epidemiology
      (1) Most common sarcoma in children; slightly more common in boys than girls Accounts for ~3% of childhood cancers
      (2) Most common site for boys is the urinary system (urinary bladder). Most common site in girls is the vagina. Presents as "grape-like" mass protruding from the urethral orifice (Link 21-16) or a cervical polyp in girls.

6. Cancers that invade the bladder include cervical cancer and prostate cancer. They obstruct the urethra and the ureters, producing hydronephrosis, postrenal azotemia, and death by renal failure.

IV. Urethral Diseases

A. Segments of the urethra in the male
- Prostate urethra, membranous urethra, bulbous urethra, and penile urethra

B. Comparison between male and female urethras
1. Male urethra is 20 cm to 30 cm long and serves as a common outlet for both the urinary and genital systems.
2. Female urethra is ~5 cm in length and passes through the urethrovaginal sphincter muscle (UVSM; controls outflow of urine) and the perineal membrane and ends as the external urethral orifice in the vestibule of the vagina. The urethra is fused to the anterior wall of the vagina.

C. Infections of the urethra
1. Chlamydial and gonococcal infections occur in men and women (see Chapter 22).
   a. The urethra is the most common site for these sexually transmitted diseases (STDs; Link 21-17).
   b. Chlamydial urethritis is a common component of reactive arthritis in men. Manifestations of reactive arthritis include urethritis, sterile conjunctivitis, and human leukocyte antigen (HLA)-B27–associated arthritis (see Chapter 24).
2. Nonvenereal diseases causing urethritis are most commonly due to *E.coli*, a gram-negative rod.

D. Urethral caruncle
1. **Definition:** Female-dominant disease characterized by a friable, red, painful mass at the urethral orifice
2. Composed of chronically inflamed granulation tissue that causes bleeding

E. Urethral diverticulum in females
1. **Definition**: Outpouching caused by a defect in the periurethral fascia the leaves of which form the outer portion of the envelope from which the diverticulum develops
2. Epidemiology and clinical findings (Excerpted from Resnick, MI, Novick, AC: Urology Secrets, 3rd ed, Hanley & Belfus, Philadelphia, 2003, An imprint of Elsevier, pp 185–187.)
   a. May occur in 0.5% to 5% of the normal female population. They may be small or large, single or multiple, or completely surround the urethra. They are rare in males and if present are usually congenital. They are not discussed here.
   b. May be congenital or acquired from surgery, trauma, or infection; acquired is the most common cause
   c. Always located on the vaginal aspect of the urethra (anterior vaginal wall) on the distal two-thirds of the urethra where the periurethral glands open

d. Infection or obstruction of the periurethral glands (PUGs) produce retention cysts, which rupture into the lumen, resulting in the formation of a diverticulum.

e. Cysts may enlarge and cause partial obstruction or complete obstruction of urine flow. Inflammation may also occur in the cysts. The most common pathogens are *N. gonorrhoeae* (GC), *C. trachomatis*, and *E. coli*.

f. Stasis of urine within the cyst and infection may lead to stone formation.

g. Classic "three D" triad is dribbling, dysuria, and dyspareunia (painful intercourse).

h. Symptoms include urinary urgency, hematuria, recurrent UTIs, urinary retention, and urinary incontinence.

i. Signs include a palpable suburethral mass or expression of purulent material.

j. Diagnosis: Magnetic resonance imaging (MRI) is the gold standard; voiding cystourethrography and positive-pressure retrograde urethrography may be used to confirm the diagnosis.

F. **Posterior urethral valve (PUV) and anterior urethral valve (AUV)**

1. PUV in males

a. **Definition:** Abnormal congenital mucosal folds in the prostate urethra (similar to a thin membrane); impairs urinary bladder drainage. Females do *not* get PUVs.

b. Epidemiology and clinical

(1) Incidence 1:8000 males

(2) Prenatal: oligohydramnios (decreased amniotic fluid; see Chapter 22), ultrasound (US) shows hydronephrosis (often first sign) and ascites (filtration of urine secondary to increased intraluminal pressure; *not* a perforation.)

(3) NBs: delayed voiding, leakage of urine, distended bladder, bilateral hydronephrosis

(4) Older children: urinary incontinence, dysuria, UTIs, gross or microscopic hematuria

(5) Vesicoureteral reflux (VUR) 50% of boys

c. Potential for postrenal failure (see Chapter 20)

d. Diagnose with voiding cystourethrogram

2. AUV and diverticulum in males

a. **Definition:** A wide-mouthed anterior urethral diverticulum; distal lip of the diverticulum fills during voiding, causing compression of the distal urethra

b. All occur in the bulbous urethra. Valve mechanism is usually formed by an associated diverticulum. The diverticulum may arise from incomplete formation of the ventral corpus spongiosum, an incomplete urethral duplication, or a congenital cystic dilation of a periurethral gland.

c. Cystic mass is present on the ventral aspect of the penoscrotal junction. The mass increases in size during voiding.

d. Diagnosed with voiding cystourethrogram

G. **SCC of the urethra; epidemiology**

1. Most common cancer of the urethra in both males and females

2. Most common cause is chronic irritation associated with urethral stricture in men and urethral diverticula in women.

3. Females present with hematuria or urethral bleeding. Dysuria or obstructive difficulties in urination indicate advanced disease.

4. Men present with similar signs and symptoms. In addition, a persistent urethral stricture or a fistula between the urethra and skin indicates advanced disease.

5. Common metastatic sites for both men and women are regional lymph nodes (pelvic lymph nodes [deep inguinal lymph nodes])

V. **Penis Diseases**

A. **Link 21-17 is an overview of infections of the male reproductive tract.**

B. **Table 21-1**

C. **Malformations of the urethral groove of the penis**

1. Hypospadias

a. **Definition:** Abnormal opening on the ventral (underside) surface of the penis rather than the tip of the penis (Fig. 21-2 A; Link 21-18, *left*)

b. Epidemiology

(1) Most common malformation of the urethral groove

(2) Risk factors

(a) Father or male sibling with the defect

(b) Monozygotic twins (see Chapter 22): insufficient production of human chorionic gonadotropin (hCG) by a single placenta

---

Margin notes:

Infection/obstruction PUGs → cysts → rupture → diverticulum

GC, *C. trachomatis*, *E. coli*

Stone formation

3 D's: dribbling, dysuria, dyspareunia

Urgency, hematuria, UTIs, urine retention, urine incontinence

Suburethral mass

MRI gold standard

PUV only in males

Mucosal folds prostate urethra → obstruction bladder drainage

Do *not* occur in females

Prenatal oligohydramnios, hydronephrosis, ascites

NBs: delayed voiding, bladder distention, urine leakage, bilateral hydronephrosis

Older child: urinary incontinence, dysuria, UTIs, hematuria

VUR 50% boys

Potential postrenal failure

Dx: voiding cystourethrogram

AUV/diverticulum males

Wide-mouth anterior urethral diverticulum

All in bulbous urethra

Usually formed in association with diverticulum

Cystic mass ventral aspect penoscrotal junction

Increased size with voiding

Dx: voiding cystourethrogram

SCC urethra

SCC MCC urethral cancer males/females

Chronic irritation urethral stricture men

Urethral diverticula women

Females: hematuria or urethral bleeding; dysuria/obstructive urination

Men: similar to female + fistula between urethra and skin

Metastasis pelvic lymph nodes men/women

Pelvic nodes: deep inguinal modes

Penis diseases

Hypospadias

Abnormal opening ventral surface penis

MC malformation urethral groove

Hx father, previous male sibling

Monozygotic twins

Insufficiency production hCG

TABLE 21-1 Homologues in Urogenital Development

INDIFFERENT STRUCTURE	MALE DERIVATIVE	FEMALE DERIVATIVE
Genital ridge	Testis	Ovary
Mesonephric duct	• Epididymis • Ductus deferens • Ejaculatory duct	• Appendix of ovary* • Gartner duct*
Paramesonephric duct	• Appendix of testis* • Prostate utricle*	• Uterine tubes • Uterus • Upper vagina
Upper urogenital sinus	• Urinary bladder • Prostate urethra	• Urinary bladder • Urethra
Lower urogenital sinus	Spongy urethra	• Lower vagina • Vaginal vestibule
Genital tubercle	Penis	Clitoris
Urogenital folds	Spongy urethra (base)	Labia minora
Labioscrotal swellings	Scrotum	Labia majora

*Vestigial structures of potential medical significance.
From Moore NA, Roy WA: *Rapid Review Gross and Developmental Anatomy,* 3rd ed, Philadelphia, Elsevier, 2010, p 134, Table 4-8.

21-2: **A,** Hypospadias. The *arrow* shows the urethral opening on the ventral surface of the penis. **B,** Phimosis. Note the long foreskin with nonretractile prepuce. *(A from Kliegman, R:* Nelson Textbook of Pediatrics, *19th ed, Philadelphia, Elsevier Saunders, 2011, p 1853, Fig. 538.1B; B from Taylor S, Raffles A:* Diagnosis in Color Pediatrics, *London, Mosby-Wolfe, 1997, p 182, Fig. 6.18.)*

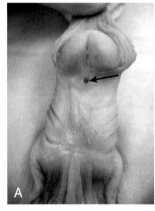
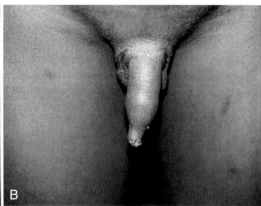

If downward curvature (chordee)

Painful intercourse

Faulty closure urethral folds

Opening in distal penis

?Abnormal androgen production

Epispadias

Abnormal dorsal opening on penis

Defect genital tubercle

Dorsal curvature; incomplete dorsal foreskin

Phimosis

Prepuce cannot retract over head of penis; infections

NBs commonly have adhesions that resolve

Paraphimosis: incarceration retracted foreskin behind glans

Balanoposthitis

Infection of glans/prepuce

(3) Frequently associated with downward curvature of the penis (called chordee; Link 21-18 right); painful intercourse
(4) Pathogenesis
  (a) Caused by faulty closure of the urethral folds
  (b) Ventral opening is usually in the distal penis rather than the penoscrotal junction.
  (c) May be related to abnormal androgen production
2. Epispadias
  a. **Definition:** Abnormal opening on the dorsal (topside) surface of the penis (Link 21-19)
  b. Caused by a defect in the genital tubercle
  c. Dorsal curvature of the penis and an incomplete foreskin dorsally are also characteristic.
D. Phimosis
  1. **Definition:** A condition in uncircumcised males characterized by narrowing of the distal foreskin, preventing its retraction over the glans penis (Fig. 21-2 B); commonly associated with infections
  2. In NBs, retraction of the foreskin may be difficult because of normal adhesions; normally resolves spontaneously.
  3. Paraphimosis occurs when the foreskin left in the retracted position becomes swollen, and then is unable to be returned to its normal position (Link 21-20).
E. Balanoposthitis
  1. **Definition:** Infection of the glans and prepuce, the fold of skin that covers the head of the penis (Link 21-21)

a. Usually occurs in uncircumcised males with poor hygiene.

b. Accumulation of smegma, a cheese-like, sebaceous secretion that collects beneath the foreskin, leads to infection. Infectious agents include *Candida*, pyogenic bacteria, and anaerobes.

2. Inflammatory scarring may produce an acquired phimosis.

F. **Miscellaneous disorders of the penis**

1. Peyronie disease

   a. **Definition:** Type of fibromatosis (see Chapter 24) that causes lateral curvature of the penis and pain on erection

   b. Epidemiology: estimated to affect 5% of men; increasing incidence with age

   c. Clinical findings: In addition to pain on erection, there are painful intercourse (both partners) and erectile dysfunction (ED); may cause infertility.

2. Priapism

   a. **Definition:** Persistent and painful erection

   b. Causes include sickle cell disease and penile trauma.

3. Balanitis xerotica obliterans (BXO)

   a. **Definition:** Patchy white lesion (leukoplakia) involving the glans and prepuce; may undergo malignant transformation to a SCC. Xerosis refers to abnormally dry skin.

   b. Patchy white lesions predispose to the development of painful erosions and fissures and SCC.

   c. Urethra meatus stenosis causes obstruction.

G. **Carcinoma in situ (CIS) of the penis**

1. Bowen disease

   a. **Definition:** Leukoplakia (white plaque-like lesion) involving the mucus membrane of the glans penis (Link 21-22)

   b. Epidemiology

      (1) Usually occurs in those >35 years of age

      (2) Association with human papillomavirus (HPV) type 16

      (3) Precursor for invasive SCC (~10% of cases)

      (4) Association with other types of visceral cancer

2. Erythroplasia of Queyrat

   a. **Definition:** A red patch of squamous CIS that mainly occurs on the mucosal surface of the glans penis, the prepuce, or the urethral meatus of older men

   b. Epidemiology

      (1) HPV type 16 association

      (2) Some pathologists consider it to be Bowen disease.

      (3) Presents as a shiny, moist, raised erythematous plaque that appears exclusively under the foreskin of the uncircumcised penis (Link 21-23).

3. Bowenoid papulosis

   a. **Definition:** Brown verrucous (wartlike) lesions of the external genitalia with pathologic features of carcinoma in situ (CIS)

   b. Epidemiology

      (1) Association with HPV type 16

      (2) Does *not* develop into invasive SCC; only CIS with *no* predisposition for invasion

   c. Clinical findings: multiple pigmented reddish brown papules that are located on the external genitalia (Link 21-24)

H. **Squamous cell carcinoma (SCC) of the penis**

1. Epidemiology

   a. Erythroplasia of Queyrat (EoQ), Bowen disease, and BXO may progress to invasive SCC.

   b. Circumcision protects against developing SCC of the penis.

      (1) Most common cancer of the penis; usually affects men 40 to 70 years old

      (2) Most common sites are the glans or the mucosal surface of the prepuce (Links 21-25 and 21-26).

   c. Two-thirds of the cases are associated with HPV types 16 and 18. Products from smoking tobacco may act as cocarcinogens with HPV.

   d. Risk factors

      (1) Lack of circumcision is the greatest risk factor.

      (2) Bowen disease, EoQ, BXO, and genital herpes infections

2. Metastasize to the inguinal and iliac nodes

VI. Testis, Scrotal Sac, and Epididymis Diseases
A. Overview of testis (see Fig. 6-26 A; Links 21-27, 21-28, 21-29, and 21-30)

Development of the male reproductive system: The mesonephric tubules differentiate into the different parts of the male duct system (see the following figure). The caudal end of the mesonephric tubules becomes the epididymis. The next portion acquires a smooth muscle coat and becomes the ductus deferens. In the 10th week of gestation, the seminal vesicles bud from a region where the mesonephric tubule joins the pelvic urethra. The portion of the mesonephric tubule that is distal to the seminal vesicle bud is then called the ejaculatory duct. The prostate gland develops in the 10th week as an endodermal outgrowth of the pelvic urethra. Its development is dependent on the presence of dihydrotestosterone, an androgenic hormone whose precursor is testosterone. The testis cords remain solid until puberty, when there is an increase in the circulating levels of testosterone. This increase brings about canalization of the testis cords, which then becomes the seminiferous tubules.

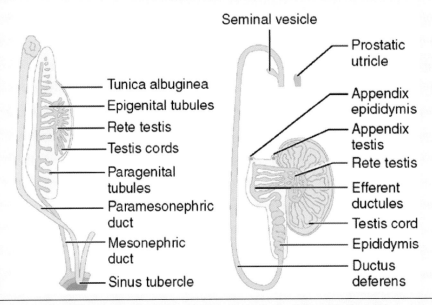

(From Bogart BI, Ort FH: *Elsevier's Integrated Anatomy and Embryology*, St. Louis, Mosby Elsevier, 2007, p 170, Fig. 7-20.)

Cryptorchidism
Descent of testes
Transabdominal phase
Testes descend to lower abdomen or pelvic brim
MIS responsible transabdominal phase
Inguinoscrotal phase
Descent thru inguinal canal → scrotum
Androgen and hCG-dependent
Cryptorchidism
Incomplete/improper descent testis into scrotal sac
MC GU disorder in boys
Premature males, full-term males
Cryptorchid testis association
AIS, KS, CF
Locations
High scrotal area MCC site
Palpable mass; majority unilateral
Many spontaneously descend 3 mths age
Combination androgens/hCG
Descent uncommon after 3 mths
Potential for infertility
Arrest germ cell maturation
Testicular atrophy
~ Changes normal descended contralateral testis

B. Cryptorchidism of the testes
1. Normal descent of testes (Link 21-31)
   a. Transabdominal phase
      (1) Testes descend to the lower abdomen or pelvic brim.
      (2) Müllerian inhibitory substance (MIS) is responsible for this phase.
   b. Inguinoscrotal phase
      (1) Descent through the inguinal canal into the scrotum
      (2) Androgen and hCG dependent
2. Cryptorchidism
   a. **Definition:** Incomplete or improper descent of the testis into the scrotal sac
   b. Epidemiology
      (1) Most common genitourinary (GU) disorder in boys
      (2) Occurs in 30% of premature boys and 5% of full-term boys
      (3) Associations include androgen insensitivity syndrome (AIS), Kallmann syndrome (KS), and cystic fibrosis (CF).
      (4) Locations
         (a) High scrotal area is the most common site (60%), followed by the inguinal canal (25%) and abdomen (15%; Link 21-32).
         (b) Palpable mass; majority are unilateral (90% of cases).
      (5) Many spontaneously descend by 3 months of age.
         (a) Combination of androgens and hCG
         (b) Spontaneous descent is uncommon after 3 months.
   c. Complications if uncorrected
      (1) Potential for infertility
         (a) Arrest in germ cell maturation
         (b) Testicular atrophy
         (c) Similar changes may occur in the normally descended contralateral testis.

       (2) Increased risk for developing a seminoma (see later)

          (a) Risk for cancer in the cryptorchid testis increases by 5- to 10-fold.

          (b) Increased risk also applies to the normally descended testicle.

       (3) Increased risk of torsion in the undescended testis (see later)

C. Orchitis

   1. **Definition:** Acute or chronic inflammation of one or both testicles

   2. Epidemiology; causes

     • Mumps

       (1) Contracted by inhalation of respiratory droplets → replicates in lymphoid tissue in lymph nodes → spreads to the salivary glands and other sites (testicles)

       (2) Infertility is uncommon. Most cases are unilateral.

       (3) Orchitis is more likely to occur in an older child or adult.

       (4) Congenital or acquired syphilis

       (5) Human immunodeficiency virus (HIV), extension of acute epididymitis

       (6) Extension of acute epididymitis

D. Epididymitis

   1. **Definition:** Acute or chronic inflammation of the epididymis caused by infection or trauma

   2. Epidemiology and pathogens (Link 21-17)

     a. Common pathogens in those <35 years old include sexually transmitted *N. gonorrhoeae* (30%) and *C. trachomatis* (70%).

     b. Common pathogens in persons >35 years old include *E. coli* and *Pseudomonas aeruginosa*.

     c. *Mycobacterium tuberculosis* begins in the epididymis and then spreads to the seminal vesicles, prostate, and testicles. It is a caseating granulomatous inflammation (see Chapter 2).

     d. HIV in AIDS

   3. Clinical and laboratory findings

     a. Unilateral scrotal pain with radiation of the pain into the spermatic cord or flank

     b. Scrotal swelling and epididymal tenderness. Urethral discharge is commonly present if sexually transmitted.

     c. Prehn sign is present: Elevation of the scrotum decreases the pain.

     d. Urinalysis reveals pyuria (increased neutrophils). Doppler US shows normal or increased blood flow.

   4. Torsion of the appendix testis or epididymis

     a. Embryologic remnants; normally undetectable on routine examination

     b. Torsion of the appendix may occur early in early puberty. It may be difficult to differentiate from torsion of the spermatic cord.

     c. Torsion of appendix or epididymis presents with acute scrotal pain and the presence of a tender mass on the upper anterior surface of the testis or epididymis (Link 21-33)

E. Varicocele

   1. **Definition:** Dilated veins of the pampiniform plexus of the spermatic cord; commonly located on the left (Link 21-34)

   2. Epidemiology

     a. Occurs in 15% to 20% of all males; usually presents between 15 and 25 years of age; rare after 40 years of age; occurs in 40% of infertile males

     b. Most common cause of left-sided scrotal enlargement in adults

     c. Pathogenesis

       (1) Left spermatic vein drains into the left renal vein at a 90-degree angle, where there is an increased resistance to blood flow because of the small caliber of the vessel. Drainage of a varicocele is into the deferential vein, saphenous vein, and inferior epigastric vein.

       (2) Therefore, blockage of the left renal vein causes backup of blood into the left spermatic vein, leading to incompetency of the valves (similar in concept to varicose veins in the legs; see Chapter 10) and development of a varicocele in the left scrotal sac.

         (a) Examples of disorders that can block the left renal vein include renal cell carcinoma (RCC), which commonly invades the renal vein (see later), and compression of the left renal vein between the superior mesenteric artery (SMA) and the aorta (Ao; nutcracker phenomenon).

         (b) Smoker with sudden onset of left-sided varicocele consider RCC with invasion of left renal vein

---

Margin notes:

Cryptorchid testis: ↑risk for seminoma

Fivefold to tenfold increase

↑Risk seminoma normal descended testicle

↑Risk torsion

Orchitis

Inflammation testicle(s)

Mumps

Inhalation respiratory droplets

Replicates in lymph nodes

Salivary glands, testicles

Infertility uncommon

Usually unilateral

Orchitis more likely older child/adult

Congenital/acquired syphilis

HIV

Extension epididymitis

Epididymitis

Acute/chronic inflammation infection/trauma

<35: *N. gonorrhoeae*, *C. trachomatis*

>35: *E. coli*, *P. aeruginosa*

TB begins epididymis → seminal vesicles, prostate, testes

Caseating granulomatous inflammation

HIV

Unilateral scrotal pain radiating into cord/flank

Swelling, tenderness

Urethral discharge if STD

Prehn sign: elevation scrotum ↓pain

Urinalysis: pyuria

Doppler US

Torsion appendix testis/epididymis

Embryologic remnants

Difficult to differentiate from torsion spermatic cord

Torsion appendix/epididymis: acute scrotal pain; tender mass

Varicocele

Dilated veins pampiniform plexus in spermatic cord

15–25 yrs of age, rare after 40

40% infertile males

MCC left-sided scrotal enlargement in adult

Left spermatic vein drains into left renal vein (90° angle; ↑resistance)

RCC, compression left renal vein between SMA and Ao

Smoker sudden onset varicocele consider RCC with L renal vein invasion

(3) Right spermatic vein drains into the vena cava; therefore, there is *no* increased resistance to blood flow in the large caliber vena cava. However, in retroperitoneal fibrosis (see earlier), thrombosis of right renal vein or inferior vena cava, or increased pressure within the right spermatic vein pressure will cause a right-sided varicocele.

3. Clinical findings
   a. Heaviness or dull ache in scrotum with prolonged standing
   b. Dragging sensation in the affected testicle
   c. Visible "bag of worms" that disappears when the patient is supine and increases in size with a Valsalva maneuver (Fig. 21-3 A)
   d. Infertility (33% of adults): heat from the increased vascularity may decrease spermatogenesis (controversial) and increase reactive oxygen species (peroxide, superoxide free radicals) damage sperm; increase in sperm antibodies
   e. Failure of left testicular growth
4. Diagnosed by US

F. Testicular torsion
1. **Definition:** Twisting of the spermatic cord leading to a decrease in testicular blood flow and severe pain in the scrotal sac
2. Epidemiology
   a. Majority occur between 12 and 18 years old
   b. Most common urologic emergency in males
   c. Predisposing factors
      (1) Violent movement and physical trauma are the most common causes of torsion.
      (2) Other causes include a cryptorchid testis or atrophy of the testis.
   d. Twisting of the spermatic cord cuts off the venous and arterial blood supply to the testis, which may cause a hemorrhagic infarction of the testicle (Fig. 21-3 B; Link 21-35).
   e. One-third spontaneously remit.
3. Clinical findings
   a. Sudden onset of severe testicular pain
   b. Absence of the cremasteric reflex (key diagnostic finding). Normal cremasteric reflex is retraction of the scrotum after stroking the inner thigh with a tongue blade.
   c. Visible evidence of the testicle drawn up into the inguinal canal (Fig. 21-3 C)
4. Testicular torsion is diagnosed with US.

G. Hydrocele
1. **Definition:** Collection of serous fluid between the two layers of the tunica vaginalis (Link 21-36)
2. Epidemiology
   a. Most common cause of scrotal enlargement in boys (Fig. 21-3 D)
   b. Often associated with testicular tumors (20%)
   c. Pathogenesis
      (1) Tunica vaginalis fails to close.
      (2) Fluid accumulates in the serous space between the layers of the tunica vaginalis.
   d. Invariably associated with an indirect inguinal hernia (see Chapter 18)
3. Diagnosis: US distinguishes fluid versus a testicular mass causing scrotal enlargement.
4. Other fluid accumulations
   a. Hematocele (contains blood)
   b. Spermatocele (contains sperm): common in adolescents; located in the upper pole of the epididymis

H. Testicular tumors
1. Epidemiology
   a. Most common male malignancy between ages 15 and 35 years
   b. Occurs more often in whites than blacks (rare)
   c. Risk factors
      (1) Three age peaks: boys from birth to age 10 years, between ages 20 and 40, men >60 years
      (2) Cryptorchid testicle (20- to 40-fold increase)
         (a) Overall most common risk factor for testicular cancer
         (b) Greatest risk is an intraabdominal cryptorchid testis
      (3) Androgen insensitivity syndrome (AIS; see Chapter 6), Klinefelter syndrome (XXY) (see Chapter 6), Peutz-Jeghers syndrome (Sertoli-Leydig cell tumor), possibly Marfan syndrome, inguinal hernia, mumps, orchitis, others (prior testicular cancer,

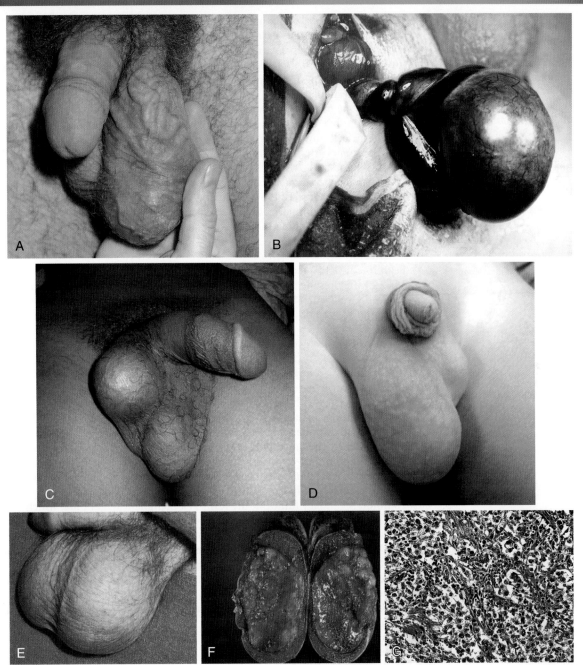

21-3: A, Varicocele in the left scrotal sac. Note the "bag of worms" appearance. **B,** Left testicular torsion in an adolescent. The testis is enlarged, discolored, and necrotic (hemorrhagic infarction). **C,** "Late phase torsion" in an adolescent with severe testicular pain 1 month previously. Note the absence of inflammation and the high position of the testis in the scrotum. **D,** Hydrocele in the right scrotal sac. **E,** Seminoma of the testicle showing the scrotal mass. **F,** Seminoma that has been surgically removed. Note that the tumor replaces most of the testicle. **G,** Microscopic section of a seminoma. Note the large tumor cells with fibrous septa infiltrated by numerous lymphocytes. (*A from Swartz MH:* Textbook of Physical Diagnosis, *5th ed, Philadelphia, Saunders Elsevier, 2006, p 545, Fig. 18-27; **B, C,** and **D** from Kliegman R:* Nelson Textbook of Pediatrics, *19th ed, Philadelphia, Elsevier Saunders, 2011, pp 1861, 1863, respectively, Fig. 539.2A and B, 539.6 respectively; **E** and **F** from Grieg JD:* Color Atlas of Surgical Diagnosis, *London, Mosby-Wolfe, 1996, p 307, Fig. 38-8; **G** from Rosai J, Ackerman LV:* Surgical Pathology, *9th ed, St. Louis, Mosby, 2004, p 1421, Fig. 18-57.)*

testicular microlithiasis [calcification]), electric blankets, briefs rather than boxer underwear, prior testicle trauma, elevated scrotal temperature)

   d. Types of testicular tumors

     (1) Malignant testicular tumors most often have a germ cell origin (95% of cases).

     (2) Benign testicular tumors are usually sex cord–stromal tumors (5% of cases).

     (3) Classification of germ cell tumors

        (a) 40% are of one cell type. Seminoma is the most common type (30% of cases).

Microlithiasis, ↑heat, briefs, prior trauma
Types testicular tumors
Malignant testicular tumors: most have germ cell origin
Benign tumors usually sex cord–stromal tumors
Classification
40% One cell type: seminoma MC

(b) 60% of cases are mixtures of two or more patterns (i.e., seminomas or nonseminomatous germ cell tumors). Nonseminomatous germ cell tumors include embryonal carcinoma, teratoma, choriocarcinoma, and yolk sac tumor.

(c) The majority (90%) arise in the testicles, and 10% occur in the pineal gland, mediastinum, or retroperitoneum.

(4) Types of testicular tumors and age

(a) Yolk sac tumors and pure teratomas <4 years old

(b) Seminoma, embryonal carcinoma, choriocarcinoma (chorio), and mixed germ-cell tumors postpubertal men up to age 40 years

(c) Spermatocytic seminoma, malignant lymphoma, or secondary tumors in men >50 years old

(d) Cytogenetic characteristic of germ cell tumors is a duplication of the short arm of chromosome 12 (90% of cases).

(e) Table 21-2 summarizes all the testicular tumors.

2. Most common clinical finding in testicular cancer is a unilateral, painless enlargement of the testis

3. Tumor markers

a. α-Fetoprotein (AFP) for yolk sac (endodermal sinus) tumor

b. β-hCG for the presence of a choriocarcinoma, a malignant tumor containing syncytiotrophoblast and cytotrophoblast (see Chapter 22)

c. Elevation of β-hCG or AFP is present in 80% to 90% of nonseminomatous germ cell tumors.

d. Elevated AFP indicates the presence of nonseminomatous elements.

e. False positive (FP) for β-hCG is seen with marijuana use and hypogonadism.

f. FP for AFP may occur in liver disease (e.g., hepatocellular carcinoma [HCC]).

g. Lactate dehydrogenase (LDH): nonspecific marker of cell breakdown; degree of elevation correlates with size of the tumor mass

4. Most frequent sites of metastasis for seminomas and nonseminomatous germ cell tumors are paraaortic lymph nodes at the level of the renal vessels (MC; Link 21-41) followed in descending order by the lung, liver, brain, bone, and kidney. They do *not* metastasize to the inguinal lymph nodes. Involvement of paraaortic lymph nodes produces low back pain. Presence of chest pain, dyspnea, cough, or hemoptysis indicates lung metastasis or anterior mediastinal lymphadenopathy.

5. Most common secondary tumor of the testis is a malignant lymphoma, which causes diffuse enlargement of both testes. Primary malignant lymphoma of the testis occurs as well. If cancer cells spread from a primary cancer to another part of the body, they may continue to divide and form a secondary tumor (metastasis) in the new location.

6. The most common metastatic tumors to the testis are prostate, lung, gastrointestinal tract, kidney, and malignant melanoma.

7. The most common mesenchymal tumors (derive from mesoderm) are fibromas, angiomas, leiomyomas, and neurofibromas.

8. Diagnosis: US, computed tomography (CT) scan, or MRI of the pelvis and abdomen

VII. Prostate Diseases

A. Clinical anatomy of the prostate

1. Dihydrotestosterone (DHT) is responsible for developing the prostate.

2. Zones of the prostate (Link 21-42)

a. Peripheral zone: palpated during a digital rectal examination (DRE); primary site for prostate cancer

b. Transitional zone: primary site for the glandular component of PH

c. Periurethral zone: primary site for the fibromuscular (stromal) component of PH

B. Acute and chronic prostatitis

1. **Definition:** Acute or chronic inflammation of the prostate gland

2. Epidemiology

a. Approximately 50% of men develop prostatitis in their lifetime. Chronic prostatitis is more common the acute prostatitis.

b. Characterized as bacterial or nonbacterial

c. Acute prostatitis

(1) Caused by intraprostate reflux of urine from the posterior urethra or urinary bladder

(2) Often associated with acute cystitis; occurs in young to middle-aged men

(3) Postulated pathways of infection (Link 21-43)

TABLE 21-2   Testicular Tumors*

TUMOR	AGE (YR)	MORPHOLOGIC OR CLINICAL FINDINGS	TUMOR MARKER(S)	PROGNOSIS
Seminoma (see Fig. 21-3 E and G); Link 21-37	30–35, >65; mean age, 40	• Most common germ cell tumor (50% of cases); may be mixed with other germ cell tumors. • Yellow tumor usually *without* significant hemorrhage or necrosis • Neoplastic cells are large and have a centrally located nucleus containing prominent nucleoli • Stroma has a prominent lymphocytic infiltrate; granulomas frequent; *not* complicated by sarcoma • Metastasis: lymphatic (paraaortic lymph nodes) metastasis *before* hematogenous (lungs)	↑hCG in 10% of cases	• Excellent • Extremely radiosensitive
Spermatocytic seminoma		• *Not* a variant of seminoma; occurs in 1% of males • Age at diagnosis ranges from 19–92 yr (mean, 53.5 yr) • *Not* linked to cryptorchidism • *Not* a primary cancer in extragonadal sites • Bilaterality in <5% of cases; may be complicated by sarcoma • *No* serum marker associations • Multinodular • Lymphocytic infiltrate *not* as prominent as in a seminoma; cell size variation is uncommon, unlike a seminoma • Nuclear pleomorphism • Cytoplasmic borders indistinct • Mitosis rate is high • Benign clinical course • Metastasis uncommon		
Embryonal carcinoma (Link 21-38)	20–25	• Bulky tumor with hemorrhage and necrosis • Contains embryoid bodies • Other tumor types are often present • Metastasis: hematogenous *before* lymphatic	↑AFP or hCG in 90% of cases	• Intermediate • Less radiosensitive than seminomas
Yolk sac (endodermal sinus) tumor (Link 21-39)	MC testicular tumor children <4 yr old	Characteristic perivascular Schiller-Duval bodies (attempt at formation of an embryonic yolk sac)	↑AFP in all cases	Good
Choriocarcinoma	20–30	• Most commonly mixed with other tumor types • Contains trophoblastic tissue (syncytiotrophoblast and cytotrophoblast (see Chapter 22) • May produce gynecomastia (hCG is an LH analogue)	↑hCG in all cases	• Poor • Most aggressive testicular tumor • Hematogenous spread to lungs.
Teratoma (Link 21-40)	Affects males of all ages	• Contains derivatives from ectoderm, endoderm, mesoderm • If mixed with embryonal carcinoma, it is called a teratocarcinoma	↑AFP or hCG in 50% of cases	• Good • Usually benign in children and malignant in adults (usually SCC)
Malignant lymphoma	MC testicular cancer in men >60 yr of age	Secondary involvement of both testes by diffuse large cell lymphoma	None	Poor

*Listed in order of prognosis (good to poor).
AFP, α-Fetoprotein; *hCG*, human chorionic gonadotropin; *LH*, luteinizing hormone; *MC*, most common; *SCC*, squamous cell carcinoma.

(4) Pathogens that are likely in those <35 years of age include *C. trachomatis* and *N. gonorrhoeae.*

(5) Pathogens that are more likely in those >35 years old include *E. coli, P. aeruginosa,* and *Klebsiella pneumoniae.*

  d. Prostadynia: symptoms consistent with prostatitis, but cultures of prostate secretions after rectal exam are negative and neutrophils are absent; most likely related to bladder neck dysfunction (spasms) leading to reflux of urine into the prostate and ejaculatory ducts

Acute prostatitis <35 years old: consider *Chlamydia, Neisseria*

E. coli, P. aeruginosa, K. pneumoniae

Prostadynia

Symptoms prostatitis: negative cultures/no WBCs

Bladder neck dysfunction (spasms) → reflux into prostate/ejaculatory ducts

Chronic prostatitis

Persistent bacterial infection

MCC *E. coli*

Gonococcal, tuberculous, parasitic, mycotic, nonspecific

Common in cyclists

Clinical findings

Dysuria, urgency, ↑frequency

Fever acute *not* chronic

Low back, perineal, suprapubic pain

Painful/swollen gland rectal exam

Hematuria some cases

>20 WBCs/HPF and/or bacteria in urine taken at end of micturition

Prostate hyperplasia

Hyperplasia, *not* hypertrophy

Age-dependent change

MCC enlarged prostate in men >50 yrs old

Blacks > whites

Transitional/periurethral zones

DRE sensitivity 50% (coin toss)

30% with PH have occult cancer

↑DHT sensitivity

DHT → hyperplasia glandular/stromal cells

Stromal cells → 5α-reductase → DHT synthesis

Hyperplasia glandular/stromal cells → nodules

Glandular hyperplasia transitional zone

Stromal hyperplasia periurethral zone → urethral obstruction

Signs obstruction MC finding

Problem initiation + completely stopping (dribbling)

Incomplete emptying bladder

Nocturia

↑Frequency urination

Intermittency (starting/stopping until feels empty)

↑Urgency

Weak urinary stream

Having to strain to begin urination

Microscopic hematuria

Prostate specific antigen

Proteolytic enzyme, ↑sperm motility

Normal or slightly increased

Rarely >10 ng/mL

e. Chronic prostatitis
 (1) Chronic bacterial infection caused by persistent bacterial infections with inflammatory cells in prostate secretions despite antibiotic treatment. May form prostate calculi.
 (2) Usually caused by *E. coli* (most common). Other bacteria include *Enterobacter, Proteus, Klebsiella,* and *Pseudomonas* spp.
 (3) Other forms of prostatitis include gonococcal prostatitis, tuberculous prostatitis, parasitic prostatitis, mycotic prostatitis, and nonspecific granulomatous prostatitis.
 (4) Prostatitis is common in cyclists, caused by prolonged seat compression on the prostate gland.
3. Clinical findings
 a. Dysuria, urgency, and increased frequency of urination
 b. Fever in acute prostatitis (*not* chronic prostatitis)
 c. Lower back, perineal, or suprapubic pain or combinations of these symptoms
 d. Painful or swollen gland on rectal examination; hematuria in some cases
 e. Diagnosis of prostatitis: >20 WBCs/HPF taken at the end of micturition (prostate component). Increased bacterial in urine taken at the end of micturition is confirmatory.

C. **Prostate hyperplasia (PH) (old term, *benign prostate hyperplasia*)**
 1. **Definition:** An enlarged prostate gland caused by hyperplasia of both the glandular and stromal tissue. Many books and clinicians use the term *benign prostate hypertrophy,* which is incorrect. Hyperplasia is an increase in cell number, and hypertrophy is an increase in cell size.
 2. Epidemiology
 a. Age-dependent change (see Chapter 6); majority of men develop PH as they age; approximately 80% have PH at 80 years of age; more common in blacks than whites
 b. Develops in the transitional (glands) and periurethral (stroma) zones of the prostate gland
 c. DRE has a sensitivity of 50% for detection of PH. Approximately 30% of men with PH have occult prostate cancer.
 3. Pathogenesis
 a. Primary cause is increased sensitivity of prostate tissue to dihydroxytestosterone (DHT), which is involved in the embryonic development of the gland.
 b. DHT causes hyperplasia of the glandular and stromal cells in the prostate (see Fig. 2-15 E).
 c. Stromal cells contain 5α-reductase and are the site of DHT synthesis.
 4. Gross and microscopic findings
 a. Hyperplasia of both the GCs and stromal cells.
 (1) Leads to nodule formation (Fig. 21-4; Links 21-44 and 21-45)
 (2) Nodules are yellow-pink and are soft on digital palpation.
 b. Glandular hyperplasia develops nodules in the transitional zone.
 c. Stromal hyperplasia develops nodules in the periurethral zone, which is most responsible for obstruction of the urethra.
 5. Clinical and laboratory findings
 a. Signs of obstruction are the most common findings.
 (1) Trouble in initiating and completely stopping the urinary stream (dribbling)
 (2) Incomplete emptying of the urinary bladder (sensation of feeling that the bladder is *not* completely empty after voiding)
 (3) Nocturia (frequent nighttime urination)
 (4) Increased frequency of urination (have to urinate again in less than two hours after urinating)
 (5) Intermittency while urinating (stopping and starting again until the bladder feels empty)
 (6) Increased urgency (difficult to postpone urination), weak urinary stream, and having to strain to begin urination
 b. Hematuria may occur; however, it is usually microscopic and is *not* evident while urinating.
 c. Prostate-specific antigen (PSA)
 (1) Proteolytic enzyme that increases sperm motility and maintains seminal secretions in the liquid state
 (2) Usually normal (0–4 ng/mL) or between 4 and 10 ng/mL in 30% to 50% of cases of PH
 (3) Rarely >10 ng/mL in PH

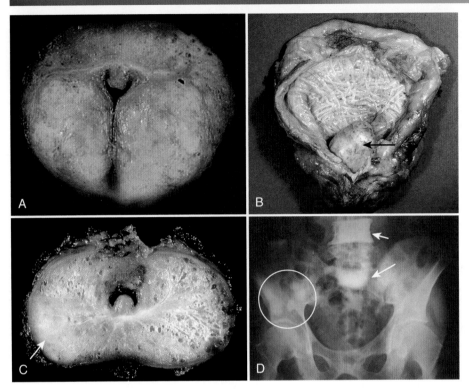

21-4: **A,** Prostate hyperplasia (PH). The gross section of prostate shows yellow periurethral nodular masses, causing narrowing of the lumen of the urethra. **B,** PH *(arrow)* causing obstructive uropathy and dilation of the urinary bladder. The trabeculated appearance of the wall of the bladder results from hyperplasia and hypertrophy of the smooth muscle. **C,** Prostate cancer. The *arrow* points to a triangular area of prostate cancer located at the periphery of the gland. The remainder of the gland has a normal, spongy appearance. **D,** Osteoblastic metastases from carcinoma of the prostate. There are osteoblastic (sclerotic) lesions seen in the L4 and S1 vertebral bodies *(solid white arrows).* Also present are multiple lesions in the right ilium *(white circle)* and other areas throughout the pelvis. (**A** from my friend Ivan Damjanov, MD, PhD, Linder J: Pathology: A Color Atlas, St. Louis, Mosby, 2000, p 249, Fig. 12-31; **B** from my friend Ivan Damjanov, MD, PhD: Pathology for the Health-Related Professions, 2nd ed, Philadelphia, Saunders, 2000, p 15, Fig. 1-17; **C** from Kumar V, Fausto N, Abbas A: Robbins and Cotran Pathologic Basis of Disease, 7th ed, Philadelphia, Saunders, 2004, p 1052, Fig. 21-34; **D** from Herring W: Learning Radiology Recognizing the Basics, 2nd ed, Philadelphia, Elsevier Saunders, 2012, p 221, Fig. 21.6.)

6. Complications (Link 21-46)
   a. Obstructive uropathy
      (1) Most common complication
      (2) Postrenal azotemia may occur (increase in serum blood urea nitrogen and serum creatinine (see Chapter 20). There is the potential for postrenal azotemia to progress into acute renal failure if left untreated.
      (3) Bilateral hydronephrosis may occur (see Chapter 20).
      (4) Bladder diverticula may develop in the urinary bladder wall caused by increased intravesical pressure (see previous discussion).
      (5) Bladder wall smooth muscle cell hypertrophy and hyperplasia may occur (Fig. 21-4 B).
   b. bladder infections (cystitis), caused by residual urine remaining after urination.
   c. prostate infarctions are pale infarctions (Fig. 21-1D; Link 21-47). There is pain on DRE of the prostate. PSA values are increased because of infarction.
   d. *No* risk for hyperplasia to progress into carcinoma
7. Diagnosis
   a. DRE is an insensitive test. It has a minimal effect on increasing serum PSA levels.
   b. Transrectal US with biopsy is usually performed if nodules are palpated or if there is an increased serum PSA level (see later discussion).

D. Prostate cancer
   1. **Definition:** Cancer of the prostate gland; most commonly an adenocarcinoma arising from the periphery of the gland
   2. Epidemiology
      a. Most common cancer in men (1 in 6 lifetime risk); second most common cancer-related death in men (lung or bronchus most common cause cancer-related death)
      b. Approximately 65% of all prostate cancers are diagnosed in men ≥65 years old. Average age of diagnosis is 72 years old.
      c. More common in blacks (~10% lifetime risk) than whites. Rare in Asians. Japanese and mainland Chinese have the lowest rates of prostate cancer.
      d. Adenocarcinomas are the most common types of cancer in the prostate. Less common types are small cell neuroendocrine cancers.
      e. Usually asymptomatic until advanced; peripheral location in the majority of cases
      f. Risk factors
         (1) Advancing age is the most important risk factor.
         (2) Prostate cancer in first-degree relatives (father and brothers)
         (3) Black race, smoking cigarettes, diet high in saturated fat

Complications PH
Obstructive uropathy MC
Possible postrenal azotemia
Renal failure
Bilateral hydronephrosis
Bladder diverticula
↑Intravesical pressure
Thickening bladder wall (SMC hypertrophy/hyperplasia)
Bladder infections (residual urine)
Prostate infarctions (pale)
Prostate pain DRE
↑PSA
No risk for BPH → prostate cancer
DRE insensitive test; minimal effect PSA levels
Transrectal US with biopsy: nodules palpated, ↑PSA
Prostate cancer
Usually adenocarcinoma, periphery
MC cancer men
2nd MC cancer-related death in men
Majority diagnosed in men ≥65 years old
Blacks > whites; rare in Asians
Adenocarcinoma MC cancer type
Asymptomatic until advanced
Peripheral location
Advancing age (most important)
Prostate cancer first-degree relative
Black race
Smoking cigarettes
High-saturated fat diet

3. Pathogenesis: DHT-dependent cancer
4. Prostate intraepithelial neoplasia (PIN)
   a. **Definition:** Foci of atypia or dysplasia in the prostate gland
   b. May be a precursor lesion for prostate cancer
5. Gross and microscopic of prostate cancer
   a. Invasive cancer has a firm, gritty, yellow appearance (Fig. 21-4 C; Link 21-48). Glands vary in morphology depending on the grade of the cancer (Link 21-49).
   b. Hallmarks of malignancy
      (1) Invasion of the capsule around the prostate
      (2) Blood vessel or lymphatic invasion, perineural invasion
      (3) Extension into the seminal vesicles or base of the urinary bladder
6. Clinical findings in symptomatic prostate cancer
   a. Positive predictive value (PV⁺) of DRE for detecting prostate cancer is 15% to 30%.
   b. Obstructive uropathy implies extension of the cancer into the bladder base.
   c. Low back and pelvic pain
      (1) Portends that bony metastases may have occurred to the vertebrae and pelvic bones; caused by spread of the cancer via the Batson venous plexus (Fig. 9-7 E).
      (2) Alkaline phosphatase (ALP) is increased.
         (a) Caused by osteoblastic metastases (cytokines from the cancer initiate reactive bone formation; Fig. 21-4 D). Density of bone is increased on radiographs.
         (b) Osteoblasts contain the enzyme ALP.
   d. Compression of the spinal cord may occur.
7. Diagnosis of prostate cancer
   a. Screening tests for prostate cancer
      (1) DRE and PSA are recommended annually beginning at 40 years of age. A new guideline recommends against screening men older than age 75 years because harm outweighs the benefits.
      (2) Normal value for a serum PSA is 0 to 4 ng/mL.
         (a) PSA >10 ng/mL is highly predictive of cancer (PV⁺) of 70%.
         (b) PSA between 4 and 10 ng/mL is a gray zone; may be an early prostate cancer or BPH
      (3) A normal serum PSA does *not* exclude the possibility of having prostate cancer. Studies have shown that 16% of men with prostate cancer have PSA values below 1 ng/mL (false-negative test result).
8. Spread of prostate cancer (Link 21-50)
   a. Perineural invasion
   b. Lymphatic spread is to the regional lymph nodes (internal iliac nodes).
   c. Hematogenous spread
      (1) Bone is the most common extranodal site of metastasis (Fig. 21-4 D). Bones involved in descending order include the lumbar spine, proximal femur, and pelvis.
      (2) Lungs and liver are additional sites for hematogenous spread.
9. Diagnosis using transrectal needle core biopsies of prostate; indications include abnormal PSA value (see earlier), abnormal DRE results, and previous diagnosis of atypia or CIS.
10. Histologic grade uses the Gleason score. It is based on the degree of glandular differentiation (well differentiated, moderately differentiated, or poorly differentiated) and growth pattern of the tumor in two regions of the prostate gland under low-power magnification.
11. Imaging tests for prostate cancer
    a. Radionuclide bone scan (Link 21-51): evaluates for presence of bone metastasis
    b. CT and MRI
    c. Transrectal US evaluates the extent of disease.
12. Prognosis of prostate cancer: The dramatic increase in survival from prostate cancer is caused by early detection and improved therapy. The 5-year survival rate for all stages is almost 99%.

VIII. **Male Hypogonadism**
   A. **Normal male reproductive physiology** (Link 21-52)
      1. Follicle-stimulating hormone (FSH)
         a. Stimulates spermatogenesis in the seminiferous tubules of the testes
         b. Negative feedback relationship with the hormone inhibin
            (1) Decreased inhibin causes an increase in FSH
            (2) Inhibin is synthesized by the Sertoli cells in the seminiferous tubules of the testes.
      2. Luteinizing hormone (LH)

    a. LH stimulates testosterone (T) synthesis in the Leydig cells in the testes.

    b. Testosterone has a negative feedback with LH. A decreased testosterone level causes an increase in LH.

3. Testosterone

    a. Maintains male secondary sex characteristics, increases libido (sexual desire)

    b. Enhances spermatogenesis in the seminiferous tubules

    c. Decreased testosterone causes hypogonadism, infertility, and decreased libido (impotence).

4. Sex hormone–binding globulin (SHBG or androgen-binding globulin)

    a. Binding protein for testosterone and estrogen (E)

       (1) In both men and women, SHBG is mainly synthesized in the liver.

       (2) In men, the Sertoli cells also synthesize SHBG.

       (3) Estrogen increases the synthesis of SHBG in the liver.

       (4) Androgens, insulin, obesity, and hypothyroidism all cause decreased synthesis of SHBG.

    b. SHBG has a higher binding affinity for testosterone than estrogen.

       (1) Increased serum SHBG decreases free serum testosterone levels.

       (2) Decreased SHBG increases free serum testosterone levels.

B. Pathogenesis of male hypogonadism

1. **Definition:** A condition in which a man is *not* producing enough testosterone or has a resistance to testosterone caused by androgen receptor deficiency

2. Decreased production of testosterone occurs in hypopituitarism and Leydig cell dysfunction.

3. Resistance to testosterone occurs in androgen receptor deficiency in the androgen insensitivity (AIS; testicular feminization; see Chapter 6).

C. Causes of male hypogonadism

1. Primary hypogonadism caused by Leydig cell dysfunction

    a. Causes

       (1) Chronic alcoholic liver disease: There is inhibition of the binding of LH to Leydig cells (caused by toxins that are increased in chronic liver disease).

       (2) Chronic renal failure (CRF), in which toxins are known to have a direct toxic effect on the Leydig cells

       (3) Irradiation, orchitis, testicular trauma

    b. Laboratory findings in Leydig cell dysfunction

       (1) Decreased serum testosterone, caused by destruction of Leydig cells or the lack of binding of LH to Leydig cells

       (2) Increased serum LH caused by a decrease in serum testosterone via negative feedback. This type of primary hypogonadism is called <u>hyper</u>gonadotropic hypogonadism because serum LH is increased.

       (3) Decreased sperm count caused by decreased serum testosterone, which normally enhances spermatogenesis

       (4) Normal levels of serum FSH. Inhibin is present in Sertoli cells (*not* Leydig cells); therefore, serum FSH levels are *not* altered by Leydig cell dysfunction.

2. Primary hypogonadism caused by Leydig cell and seminiferous tubule dysfunction

    a. Causes are the same as listed for Leydig cell dysfunction

    b. Laboratory findings in primary hypogonadism caused by Leydig cell and seminiferous tubule dysfunction

       (1) Decreased serum testosterone caused by destruction of Leydig cells or lack of binding of luteinizing hormone to Leydig cells

       (2) Increased serum LH caused by decreased serum testosterone

       (3) Decreased sperm count caused by testosterone deficiency and seminiferous tubule dysfunction

       (4) Increased serum FSH caused by a decrease in serum inhibin related to Sertoli cell dysfunction. Note that in Leydig cell dysfunction alone, FSH is normal because inhibin is normal (see 1.b earlier).

3. Secondary hypogonadism caused by hypothalamic or pituitary dysfunction; causes include:

    a. constitutional delay in puberty (most common cause): normal laboratory test findings.

    b. hypopituitarism (see Chapter 23).

       (1) Causes of hypopituitarism

         (a) Craniopharyngioma in children and a nonfunctioning pituitary adenoma in adults

         (b) Prolactinoma: Prolactin inhibits gonadotropin-releasing hormone (GnRH) production in the hypothalamus); therefore, both serum FSH and serum LH are decreased.

LH stimulates T synthesis in Leydig cells

T negative feedback with LH

↓T, ↑LH

Testosterone

Maintains male 2° sex characteristics

Increases libido

Enhances spermatogenesis

↓T: hypogonadism, infertility, ↓libido (impotence)

SHBG: binding protein T and E

Men/women: SHBG synthesized liver

Sertoli cells synthesize SHBG

E ↑SHBG in liver

↓Synthesis SHBG: androgens, insulin, obesity, hypothyroidism

SHBG greater affinity for T than E

↑SHBG causes ↓free testosterone

↓SHBG causes ↑free testosterone

Pathogenesis male hypogonadism

Male *not* producing enough T; androgen receptor deficiency

↓T: hypopituitarism, Leydig cell dysfunction

T resistance: androgen receptor deficiency in AIS

Causes male hypogonadism

1° Hypogonadism: Leydig cell dysfunction

Chronic alcoholic liver disease

LH inhibition of binding to Leydig cells

CRF: toxic effect on Leydig cells

Irradiation, orchitis, testicular trauma

Laboratory findings in Leydig cell dysfunction

↓T: destruction Leydig cells/binding to Leydig cells

↑LH: due to ↓serum T

Hypergonadotropic (↑LH) hypogonadism

↓Sperm count

Normal FSH

Inhibin present in Sertoli cells *not* Leydig cells

Primary hypogonadism: Leydig cell + seminiferous tubule dysfunction

↓Serum T

↑LH due to ↓serum T

↓Sperm count

↑FSH due to ↓inhibin in Sertoli cell dysfunction

2° Hypogonadism: hypothalamic/pituitary dysfunction

Constitutional delay MCC, lab studies normal

Hypopituitarism

Causes hypopituitarism

Craniopharyngioma

Prolactinoma

Prolactin inhibits GnRH (↓FSH + ↓LH)

Lab findings in
hypopituitarism
↓FSH, ↓LH, ↓T, ↓sperm
count
Hypogonadotropic (↓LH)
hypogonadism
Hypothalamic dysfunction:
Kallmann syndrome
AD disorder
Maldevelopment olfactory
bulbs (anosmia) + GnRH
Clinical findings male
hypogonadism
Impotence
Failure to sustain erection:
attempted intercourse or
during
Impotence MC
manifestation male
hypogonadism

(2) Laboratory findings in hypopituitarism

    (a) Decrease in FSH, serum LH, serum testosterone, and sperm count

    (b) Because LH is decreased, this type of hypogonadism is called <u>hypogonadotropic</u> hypogonadism

  c. hypothalamic dysfunction: KS.

    (1) Autosomal dominant disorder

    (2) Maldevelopment of the olfactory bulbs (anosmia [lack of smell] and GnRH-producing cells in the hypothalamus. GnRH normally stimulates the release of LH and FSH from the anterior pituitary; hence, laboratory findings are the same as those listed earlier for hypopituitarism.

D. Clinical findings for male hypogonadism

  1. Impotence

    a. **Definition:** Failure to sustain an erection during attempted intercourse or during intercourse

    b. Most common manifestation of impotence

Testosterone, per se, does *not* have any role in producing an erection (parasympathetic response) or ejaculation (sympathetic response). However, decreased testosterone decreases libido, which decreases psychic desire and leads to impotence.

↓Testosterone → ↓Libido
→ impotence
Loss 2° male sex
characteristics
E activity unopposed
Female hair distribution,
gynecomastia, soft skin
Osteoporosis
T normally ↓osteoclastic
activity, ↑osteoblastic
activity
↓T → ↑osteoclastic activity,
↓osteoblastic activity
Infertility: ↓spermatogenesis
Male infertility
Inability to cause pregnancy
fertile female for at least
1 yr
Epidemiology/pathogenesis
↓Sperm count: from—
1° Testicular dysfunction
Leydig cell dysfunction
Seminiferous tubule
dysfunction (90% male
infertility)
Varicocele, Klinefelter,
orchitis
T, LH normal
↓Sperm count
↑FSH, ↓inhibin
2° Hypogonadism caused by
pituitary and/or
hypothalamic dysfunction
End-organ dysfunction
Obstruction vas deferens
Disorders accessory sex
organs or ejaculation

  2. Loss of male secondary sex characteristics

    a. Estrogen activity is unopposed if testosterone is decreased or unable to bind to receptors.

    b. Findings include a female hair distribution (hair does *not* extend to the umbilicus; Link 21-53), gynecomastia (subareolar gland proliferation; Link 21-53), and soft skin.

  3. Osteoporosis

    a. Testosterone normally inhibits osteoclastic activity and increases osteoblastic activity.

    b. Decreased testosterone increases osteoclastic activity and decreases osteoblastic activity.

  4. Infertility caused by decreased spermatogenesis

E. Summary of causes of male hypogonadism (Table 21-3)

IX. Male Infertility

  A. Definition: Inability to cause pregnancy in a fertile woman for a least 1 year

  B. Epidemiology and pathogenesis

    1. Decreased sperm count

      a. Primary testicular dysfunction

        (1) Leydig cell dysfunction (see VIIIC)

        (2) Seminiferous tubule dysfunction (~90% of cases of male infertility; see IX.A)

          (a) Causes of seminiferous tubule dysfunction include varicocele (see VIE), Klinefelter syndrome (see Chapter 6), and orchitis (see Section VI)

          (b) Serum testosterone and serum LH are normal because Leydig cells are intact.

          (c) Sperm count is decreased caused by dysfunction of the seminiferous tubules.

          (d) Serum FSH is increased because inhibin is decreased caused by Sertoli cell dysfunction.

      b. Secondary hypogonadism caused by pituitary or hypothalamic dysfunction (see section VII)

    2. End-organ dysfunction

      a. Causes

        (1) Obstruction of the vas deferens

        (2) Disorders involving the accessory sex organs or ejaculation

      b. Laboratory findings

TABLE 21-3 Summary of Causes of Male Hypogonadism

DYSFUNCTION	TESTOSTERONE	SPERM COUNT	LH	FSH
PRIMARY				
Leydig dysfunction	↓	↓	↑	N
Seminiferous tubule dysfunction	N	↓	N	↑
Leydig cell and seminiferous tubule dysfunction	↓	↓	↑	↑
SECONDARY				
Hypopituitarism	↓	↓	↓	↓

FSH, Follicle-stimulating hormone; *LH*, luteinizing hormone; *N*, normal.

(1) Variable sperm count

(2) Normal serum testosterone, FSH, LH, and prolactin

C. **Laboratory tests for infertility**

1. Semen analysis

   a. Gold standard test for infertility

   b. Components of semen

      (1) Spermatozoa derive from the seminiferous tubules.

      (2) Coagulant derives from the seminal vesicles.

      (3) Enzymes to liquefy semen derive from the prostate gland

   c. Components evaluated in a standard semen analysis

      (1) Volume is *not* positively correlated with the number of sperm.

         • Normal volume is 2 to 5 mL.

      (2) Sperm count. Normal count is 20 to 150 million sperm/mL.

      (3) Sperm morphology: Morphology is very abnormal in reconnections of a vasectomy.

      (4) Sperm motility

2. Serum gonadotropins, testosterone, and prolactin

X. **Erectile Dysfunction (Impotence)**

A. **Definition:** Persistent inability to obtain or maintain a penile erection adequate for coitus

B. **Causes**

1. Psychogenic

   a. Most common cause of impotence in young men

   b. Causes include work stress, marital conflicts, and performance anxiety.

   c. Nocturnal penile tumescence (NPT; erection)

      (1) **Definition:** Erections that occur at night

      (2) Average male has ~5 erections while asleep.

      (3) Nocturnal penile tumescence is preserved in impotence secondary to psychogenic causes.

      (4) All other causes of impotence have a loss of nocturnal penile tumescence.

2. Decreased testosterone. Decreased libido (sexual desire; see Section VII).

3. Vascular insufficiency

   a. Most common cause of impotence in men >50 years of age

   b. Clinical findings

      (1) Impotence caused by vascular insufficiency related to aortoiliac atherosclerosis with decreased penal blood flow

      (2) Claudication (cramping pain when walking); muscle atrophy (see Chapter 10)

      (3) Diminished femoral artery pulse with bruits (see Chapter 10)

4. Neurologic disease

   a. Parasympathetic system (S2–S4) is necessary for erection.

   b. Sympathetic system (T12–L1) is necessary for ejaculation.

   c. Neurogenic causes of impotence

      (1) Multiple sclerosis (MS; see Chapter 26)

      (2) Autonomic neuropathy caused by DM (see Chapter 23)

      (3) Radical prostatectomy

5. Drug effects; examples:

   a. Leuprolide (gonadotropin-releasing hormone agonist [stimulates an action])

   b. Methyldopa, psychotropics

6. Endocrine disease; examples

   a. DM: autonomic neuropathy and vascular insufficiency

   b. Primary hypothyroidism: decreased thyroxine, increased thyrotropin-releasing hormone [TRH]), which increases prolactin, which, in turn inhibits GnRH release, causing a decrease in LH and FSH

   c. Prolactinoma: Prolactin inhibits GnRH release (↓serum FSH/LH).

7. Penis disorders (see Section V): Peyronie disease (fibromatosis), priapism (permanent erection)

8. Pneumonic: IMPOTENCE

I = inflammatory (prostatitis), M = mechanical (Peyronie disease), P = postsurgical (radical prostatectomy), O = occlusive vascular (atherosclerosis), T = traumatic (pelvic fracture), E = endurance factors (chronic renal failure), N = neurogenic, C = chemicals (antihypertensive drugs), E = endocrine (diabetes)

(Taken from Resnick MI, Novick AC: What are the organic causes of erectile dysfunction in *Urology Secrets*, 3rd ed, Philadelphia, Hanley & Belfus, 2003, An Imprint of Elsevier, p 43, 5.)

Variable cell count
Normal T, FSH, LH, and prolactin
Gold standard test for infertility
Spermatozoa (seminiferous tubules)
Coagulant (seminal vesicles)
Enzymes liquefy semen (prostate gland)
Volume
Normal volume 2–5 mL
Sperm count
Normal count 20 to 150 million sperm/mL
Sperm morphology
Morphology abnormal reconnection after vasectomy
Sperm motility
Lab tests: serum gonadotropins, T, prolactin
Erectile dysfunction
Cannot obtain/maintain erection for coitus
Psychogenic MCC ED young men
Work stress, marital conflicts, performance anxiety
NPT: erections at night
Average male 5 erections while asleep
NPT preserved in psychogenic causes impotence
All other causes impotence: loss of NPT
ED from ↓T due to ↓libido
Vascular insufficiency
MCC impotence men >50
Aortoiliac atherosclerosis → ↓penal blood flow
Claudication, muscle atrophy
Diminished femoral artery pulse/bruits
Neurologic disease
Parasympathetic for erection: S2–S4
Sympathetic for ejaculation: T12–L1
Neurogenic causes impotence
MS
Autonomic neuropathy DM
Radical prostatectomy
Drugs causing ED: leuprolide, methyldopa, psychotropics
DM → autonomic neuropathy, vascular insufficiency (enhance atherosclerosis)
1° Hypothyroidism
1° Hypothyroidism ↓LH, FSH
Prolactinoma: prolactin inhibits GnRH release
Penis disorders
Peyronie disease (fibromatosis)
Priapism
Impotence

ABBREVIATIONS

MC most common	Dx diagnosis	S/S signs/symptoms
MCC most common cause	Hx history	

I. **Overview of Female Reproductive Organs** (Links 22-1 to 22-3)

II. **Sexually Transmitted Diseases (STDs) and Other Genital Infections**
   A. A summary of infections is listed in Table 22-1 and Figure 22-1. Link 22-4 shows examples of each of the STDs.
   B. STDs are declining in the United States.

III. **Vulva Disorders**
   A. **Vulva anatomy**
   - Composed of the labia majora, labia minora, mons pubis, clitoris, vestibule, urinary meatus, vaginal orifice, hymen, Bartholin glands, Skene ducts, and vestibulovaginal bulbs (Link 22-1 B)
   B. **Bartholin gland cyst**
      1. **Definition:** Swelling of the Bartholin gland usually secondary to obstruction of Bartholin gland duct by mucus and edema; may become secondarily infected, forming an abscess
      2. Bartholin glands are located on each side of the opening of the vagina (Link 22-1 B).
   C. **Bartholin gland abscess** (Link 22-40)
      1. **Definition:** A collection of pus in the Bartholin gland(s)
      2. Common causes include *Neisseria gonorrhoeae* (MCC), *Staphylococcus* spp, *Escherichia coli*, and *Streptococcus* spp.
   D. **Non-neoplastic dermatoses**
      1. Lichen sclerosus (Fig. 22-2 A; Links 22-41 and 22-42)
         a. **Definition:** Benign, chronic disorder characterized by thinning of the epidermis with edema and hyalinization of the dermis; shrinkage of the labia and stenosis of the introitus (entrance into the vaginal canal) are noted as well
         b. Epidemiology
            (1) Usually occurs in prepubertal girls and postmenopausal women
            (2) Strong association with autoimmune disorders and a link to human leukocyte antigen (HLA)-DQ7
            (3) White parchment-like appearance of the skin (leukoplakia); usually symmetrical; labia minora lost
            (4) Clinical findings include pruritus and painful intercourse (dyspareunia).
            (5) May be associated with squamous cell carcinoma (SCC) in a small percentage (~5%) of women
      2. Psoriasis (see Chapter 25)

Margin notes (left column):

STDs declining in U.S.
Vulva disorders

Bartholin gland cyst

Duct obstruction by mucus/edema

May become infected

Glands each side vaginal opening

Bartholin gland abscess

Collection pus in gland

N. gonorrhoeae MCC

Nonneoplastic dermatoses

Lichen sclerosis

Thin epidermis, hyalinization dermis

Prepubertal girls, postmenopausal women

HLA association

Leukoplakia

Labia minora lost

Pruritus, dyspareunia

Small SCC risk

Psoriasis

TABLE 22-1 Sexually Transmitted Diseases and Other Genital Infections

PATHOGEN	DESCRIPTION AND TREATMENT
Candida albicans (see Fig. 22-1 A; Links 22-5 to 22-8)	• Other Candida species include Candida glabrata and Candida tropicalis • Saline microscopy of the vaginal fluid shows yeasts and pseudohyphae (elongated yeasts; indicate infection; Link 22-8) • Part of the normal vaginal flora • Bubbles are not present in the discharge • Second most common cause of vaginitis in the United States. Accounts for 20% to 25% of cases of vaginitis. Allergic responses to Candida spp. may involve the penis immediately after coitus; characterized by erythema, edema, severe pruritus, and irritation of the penis. • Risk factors: diabetes mellitus, antibiotics, pregnancy, OCPs • Recurrent yeast infections are thought to be caused by colonization of the GI tract, which becomes a repository of the pathogen • Pruritic vaginitis with a white or thick ("cottage cheese") discharge and fiery red vaginal mucosa. Women may also have bladder symptoms and be misdiagnosed as having cystitis rather than vaginitis. • Diagnosis: Vaginal pH <4.5 (normal). Amine test (smell of vaginal fluid caused by release of amines) after mixing a sample of vaginal discharge with a few drops of KOH is negative (not malodorous). Saline microscopy shows yeasts and pseudohyphae (40%–50% sensitivity). 10% KOH microscopy is positive in 60%–90% of cases.
Chlamydia trachomatis (see Fig. 22-1 B; Link 22-9)	• Second most common STD • Often coexists with Neisseria gonorrhoeae (45% of cases) • Incubation period, 7–12 days after exposure. Noninfective intracellular inclusions (reticulate bodies) are present in phagosomes of metaplastic endocervical squamous cells in the cervix. Reticulate bodies divide to form extracellular elementary bodies, which are the infective bodies producing infection. Elementary bodies enter metaplastic endocervical squamous cells and become noninfective reticulate bodies. • Infections in males: NSU (sterile pyuria), epididymitis, proctitis • Infections in females: urethritis (sterile pyuria [negative standard culture], neutrophils present), cervicitis, PID, perihepatitis (FHC syndrome: scar tissue between the peritoneum and surface of the liver caused by pus from previous PID; movement produces pain), proctitis, Bartholin gland abscess • Eye infections in newborns: conjunctivitis (ophthalmia neonatorum). Erythromycin eye drops are normally used in all neonates to prevent infection by Chlamydia trachomatis or N. gonorrhoeae. Silver nitrate eye drops are no longer used. • Newborn pneumonia (see Chapter 17) • Nucleic acid amplification test has the highest sensitivity and specificity
C. trachomatis subspecies (see Fig. 22-1 C; Link 22-10)	• STD, called lymphogranuloma venereum • Incubation period, 3 days–3 weeks • Papules or ulcerations • Inguinal lymphadenitis with granulomatous microabscesses and draining sinuses • Lymphedema of scrotum or vulva. Women may also develop rectal strictures.
Gardnerella vaginalis and other bacteria (see Fig. 22-1 D; Links 22-11 to Link 22-13)	• Gram-negative rod that causes bacterial vaginosis. It is not caused by a single organism, but is the result of a massive overgrowth of anaerobic bacteria, including Gardnerella vaginalis, Bacteroides spp., peptostreptococci, and genital mycoplasma. The organisms are found in the urethras of men who are partners of women with bacterial vaginosis. • Most common vaginitis. Accounts for 40% to 50% of infectious vaginitis. Bubbles are present in the white- or gray-colored vaginal discharge. No inflammation is present. • Douching alters the microenvironment by decreasing lactobacilli (gram-positive rods that produce lactic acid and the normal vaginal pH of 3.8–4.5). IUDs are also a risk factor. • Increases susceptibility to STDs and preterm birth. • Diagnosed in 17–19% of women seeking gynecologic care. • New or multiple sex partners also predispose to this vaginitis. Organisms are located in the urethras of infected men. • pH of semen is >4.7 (often alkaline with pH 7.2–7.8). At this pH, the bacteria proliferate and produce decarboxylases that release amines, causing a malodorous vaginal discharge. The result of the amine test (adding a drop of KOH to discharge material) is positive (release of amines). Neutrophils are not present within the discharge. • Organisms adhere to (not invasive) squamous cells, producing "clue cells." These are squamous cells that have the bacteria adherent to their surface. They are best seen with a Pap smear but can also be identified using saline microscopy. • Increased incidence of preterm delivery and low-birth-weight newborns • Treatment of sexual partners is reserved for women who have recurrent infections. • Obstetric complications include chorioamnionitis, preterm labor, prematurity, and postpartum fever. • Gynecologic complications include postabortion and posthysterectomy fever, chronic mast cell endometritis, cervicitis, and low-grade cervical dysplasia. • Mobiluncus curtisii is a common bacterium in women with bacterial vaginosis. The bacterial cells are curved and have pointed ends (Link 22-13).
Haemophilus ducreyi (Links 22-14, 22-15, and 22-16)	• STD. Bacterium is a gram-negative rod. Produces a disease called chancroid. • Incubation period, 3–10 days • Male-dominant disease (10:1) • High incidence of HIV is present in affected patients. • Painful genital and perianal papules that break down to form painful ulcers. Suppurative inguinal nodes are frequently present. • Diagnosed with Gram stain ("school of fish" appearance) and culture

Continued

TABLE 22-1   Sexually Transmitted Diseases and Other Genital Infections—cont'd

PATHOGEN	DESCRIPTION AND TREATMENT
HSV-2 (see Fig. 22-1 E, F; Links 22-17, 22-18, 22-19, and 22-20)	• Fifth most common STD. Virus remains latent in the sensory ganglia, hence the propensity for recurrences of the infection. • Incubation period, 2–10 days • Characterized by recurrent vesicles that ulcerate. Locations: penis, vulva, cervix, and perianal area • Tzanck preparation: Scrapings removed from the base of an ulcer show multinucleated squamous cells with eosinophilic intranuclear inclusions. • Pregnancy: If lesions are present, the baby is delivered by cesarean section.
HPV (see Fig. 22-1 G; Links 22-21, 22-22, 22-23, and 22-24)	• Most common overall STD. Types 6 and 11 (90% of cases; low-risk types) produce condyloma acuminata (venereal [genital] warts). • Incubation period, 3 weeks–8 months • Warts are fernlike or flat lesions located in the genital area (e.g., penis, vulva, cervix, perianal). Approximately 80% of sexually active women will have acquired HPV by age 50 yr. • Virus produces koilocytic change in the squamous epithelium (Fig. 22-4 B). Cells have wrinkled pyknotic nuclei surrounded by a clear halo (Link 22-24; see Fig. 22-4 C). • Approximately 90% of the warts spontaneously clear within 2 yr (most within 8 mo). Older women more often have persistent disease because of a decrease in cellular immunity associated with aging. • HPV vaccine decreases the risk for developing venereal warts.
Klebsiella granulomatis (Links 22-25 and 22-26)	• STD; gram-negative coccobacillus that causes granuloma inguinale • Organism is phagocytized by macrophages (Donovan bodies). • Creeping, raised sore that heals by scarring; no lymphadenopathy • Diagnosis: detection of Donovan bodies. No FDA-cleared molecular tests are available for the detection of *K. granulomatis* DNA.
Neisseria gonorrhoeae (see Fig. 22-1 H and I; Links 22-27, 22-28, and 22-29)	• Fourth most common STD. Gram-negative diplococcus that infects glandular or urothelial epithelium. Other sites of infection include the rectum, oropharynx, and conjunctiva. Gonococci attach to the epithelium via pili. • Virulence factors include lipopolysaccharide, pili, outer membrane proteins, iron-binding proteins (iron required for growth), IgA protease (destroys mucosal IgA, which is part of the local immune system), and β-lactamase (destroys the β-lactam ring of penicillin). • Major reservoir for continued spread of gonorrhea is the asymptomatic patient. Among infected women, 30%–50% are asymptomatic and show no symptoms. Among infected men, only 5%–10% are asymptomatic. • Risk for acquiring the infection in men is ~20% after a single vaginal exposure to an infected woman and rises to 60%–80% after four or more exposures. • Transmission rate from male to female is ~50% per contact and rises to 90% after three exposures. This is caused by the greater exposed mucosal surface in the vagina. Gonococci can also be transmitted via oral–genital contact or rectal intercourse. • Symptoms appear 2–7 days after sexual exposure. • Infection sites are similar to those for *C. trachomatis*. • Complications: ectopic pregnancy, male sterility, disseminated gonococcemia (C6–C9 deficiency is a risk factor). Disseminated gonococcemia is associated with septic arthritis (knee MC site), FHC syndrome, tenosynovitis (hands, feet), pustules (hands, feet); more common in women than men. • Nucleic acid amplification test has the highest sensitivity and specificity. Other tests: urethral swab in symptomatic males with Gram stain or endocervical swab for culture in women
Treponema pallidum (see Fig. 22-1 J, K, and L; Links 22-30, 22-31, 22-32, 22-33, 22-34, and 22-35)	• Sixth most common STD; gram-negative spirochete that causes syphilis • Incubation period, ~2 weeks • Primary syphilis: solitary painless, indurated chancre; chancre locations: penis, labia, anus, mouth • Secondary syphilis: maculopapular rash on trunk, palms, soles; generalized painful lymphadenopathy; condylomata lata, which are flat lesions in the same area as condylomata acuminata caused by HPV; alopecia (hair loss) • Tertiary syphilis: neurosyphilis, aortitis, gummas • Congenital syphilis (see Chapter 6) • Nonspecific screening tests: RPR or VDRL. Titers decrease after treatment. • Confirmatory treponemal test: FTA-ABS; positive with or without treatment • Jarisch-Herxheimer reaction: Intensification of the rash in secondary syphilis may occur because of proteins released from dead organisms after treatment with penicillin.
Trichomonas vaginalis (see Fig. 22-1 M; Links 22-36, 22-37, 22-38, and 22-39)	• Third most common STD; flagellated protozoan with jerky motility in a wet saline preparation of the discharge (80%–90% sensitivity) • Most women are asymptomatic or have a profuse, purulent, pruritic, and malodorous vaginal discharge. The discharge is yellow. Painful intercourse is common (dyspareunia). Men are asymptomatic carriers (present in prostatic urethra) and serve as a reservoir for infection in women. Increased susceptibility for HIV (breaks in vaginal mucosa from inflammation) and increased HIV shedding. • Produces vaginitis (15%–20% of cases), cervicitis, urethritis, PID, preterm delivery, and low-birth-weight babies. Present in 13%–25% of women attending gynecology clinics. Present in 50%–75% of prostitutes and 7%–35% of women in STD clinics. • Strawberry-colored cervix and fiery red vaginal mucosa. Discharge is yellow and has bubbles. Vaginal fluid pH is 5.0–6.0. • Diagnosis: nucleic acid amplification test has the highest sensitivity and specificity. Other tests: culture, monoclonal fluorescent antibody staining, saline microscopy shows organisms and numerous neutrophils. Oral and rectal tests are not recommended. • Must treat both partners

FDA, Food and Drug Administration; *FHC,* Fitz-Hugh–Curtis; *FTA-ABS,* fluorescent treponeme antibody-absorption test; *GI,* gastrointestinal; *HPV,* human papillomavirus; *HSV,* herpes simplex virus; *IFN,* interferon; *IUD,* intrauterine device; *NSU,* nonspecific urethritis; *OCP,* oral contraceptive pill; *PCR,* polymerase chain reaction; *PID,* pelvic inflammatory disease; *RPR,* rapid plasma reagin; *STD,* sexually transmitted disease; *VDRL,* Venereal Disease Research Laboratory.

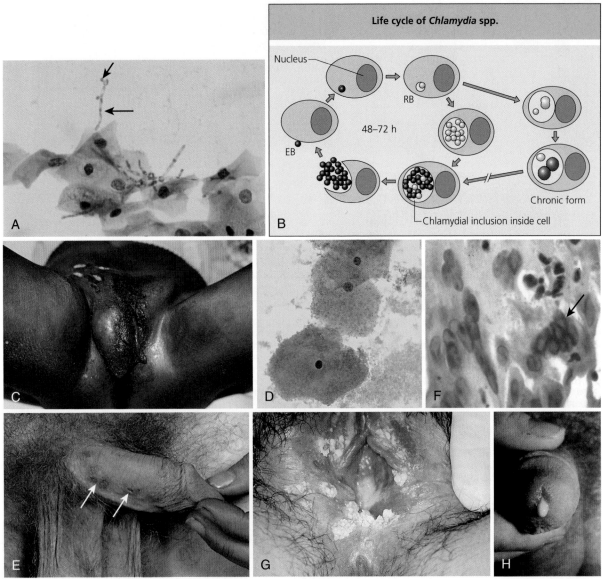

22-1: Genital infections. **A,** *Candida* spp. *Bottom arrow* shows elongated yeasts (pseudohyphae); *top arrow* shows yeasts. **B,** *Chlamydia trachomatis* life cycle. See Table 22-1 for discussion. **C,** Lymphogranuloma venereum (*Chlamydia trachomatis* subspecies). The patient has unilateral vulvar lymphedema and inguinal ulcerations (four white areas). **D,** *Gardnerella vaginalis.* Superficial squamous cells (SCs) are covered by granular material representing bacterial organisms attached to (not invading) the surface. **E,** Herpes type 2. *Arrows* show ulcerated, red lesions on the shaft of the penis. **F,** Herpes type 2. Biopsy showing a multinucleated SC with smudged, "ground-glass" nuclei with intranuclear inclusions *(arrow).* **G,** Human papillomavirus. Numerous keratotic papillary (fernlike) processes are present on the surface of the labia. These are called venereal warts or condylomata acuminata. **H,** *Neisseria gonorrhoeae* purulent penile discharge.

Continued

E. **Benign and malignant tumors**
1. Papillary hidradenoma (hidradenoma papilliferum)
   a. **Definition:** Benign tumor of the apocrine sweat gland in the vulva
   b. Epidemiology: painful nodule located on the labia majora of the vulva
2. Vulvar intraepithelial neoplasia (VIN)
   a. **Definition:** Dysplasia of the vulvar squamous epithelium; ranges from mild to carcinoma in situ (CIS) (Link 22-43)
   b. Epidemiology
      (1) Accounts for 4% of gynecologic cancers
      (2) Strong association with human papillomavirus (HPV) type 16 (70% of cases). The virus integrates into the host cell's genome and causes loss of transcriptional regulation and overexpression of oncoproteins E6 and E7 and ultimately uncontrolled promotion of cell cycle progression. HPV E6 protein binds to p53 protein, and HPV E7 binds to retinoblastoma protein (Rb), thereby disabling these tumor suppressor genes.

Benign/malignant tumors

Papillary hidradenoma

Benign apocrine sweat gland tumor

Painful nodule labia majora

Vulvar intraepithelial neoplasia

HPV type 16 MCC

E6 protein binds p53 protein

E7 protein to Rb suppressor protein

Suppressor genes disabled

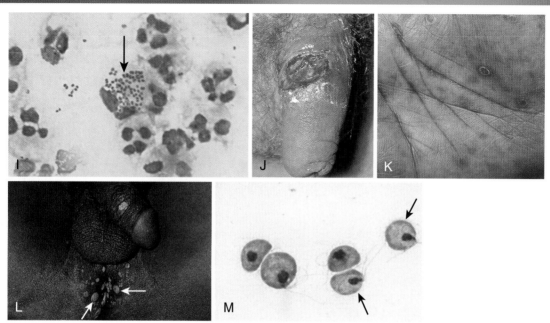

22-1 cont'd: **I,** *N. gonorrhoeae.* Neutrophils *(arrow)* show numerous, phagocytosed gram-negative diplococci. **J,** *T. pallidum.* Note the well-demarcated primary chancre just distal to the glans penis. **K,** *Treponema pallidum.* Note the characteristic palmar papules and plaques of secondary syphilis. **L,** *Treponema pallidum.* Note the flat, plaque-like lesions *(arrows)* of condyloma latum. **M,** *Trichomonas vaginalis.* Note the numerous pear-shaped, flagellated organisms *(arrows).* *(A and F from Atkinson BF: Atlas of Diagnostic Cytopathology, Philadelphia, Saunders, 1992, pp 76, 78, 80, respectively, Figs. 2-49B, 2-55, and 2-63, respectively; B from Cohen J, Opal SM, Powderly WG: Infectious Diseases, 3rd ed, St. Louis, Mosby Elsevier, 2010, p 1817, Fig. 177.1; C from Cohen J, Powderly W: Infectious Diseases, 2nd ed. St. Louis, Mosby, 2004; D and G from my friend Ivan Damjanov, MD, PhD, Linder J: Pathology: A Color Atlas, St. Louis, Mosby, 2000, pp 261, 260, respectively, Figs. 13-10B, 13-8, respectively; E from Bouloux P-M: Self-Assessment Picture Tests: Medicine, Vol 1. London, Mosby-Wolfe, 1996, p 17, Fig. 33; H from Marx J: Rosen's Emergency Medicine Concepts and Clinical Practice, 7th ed, Philadelphia, Mosby Elsevier, 2010, p 1291, Fig. 96.10; I from Greer I, Cameron IT, Kitchener HC, Prentice A: Mosby's Color Atlas and Text of Obstetrics and Gynecology, St. Louis, Mosby, 2000, p 274, Fig. 10-50; J and L from Swartz MH: Textbook of Physical Diagnosis, 5th ed, Philadelphia, Saunders Elsevier, 2006, p 537, 553, respectively, Fig. 18-13, 18-39, respectively; K from Lookingbill D, Marks J: Principles of Dermatology, 3rd ed, Philadelphia, Saunders, 2000, p 124, Fig. 10-17; M from Kumar V, Fausto N, Abbas A: Robbins and Cotran Pathologic Basis of Disease, 7th ed. Philadelphia, Saunders, 2004, p 1064, Fig. 22-4.)*

Younger than age 40 years; ?role smoking

VIN: precursor SCC

Squamous cell carcinoma vulva

MC cancer vulva

6th decade; with/without inflammatory dermatitis

Risk factors

HPV type 16

Smoking cigarettes

AIDS, lichen sclerosus, obesity, hypertension, DM

Inguinal/pelvic node metastasis

Extramammary Paget disease

Intraepithelial adenocarcinoma

Red/white crusted vulvar lesion

Intraepithelial adenocarcinoma

Contain mucin

Spread along epithelium; rarely invade dermis

Most are curable

Malignant melanoma

(3) Mean age for VIN has recently decreased from older than 50 years to younger than age 40 years. May be attributed to increased cigarette smoking in young women.
(4) VIN is a precursor for the development of SCC.
3. Squamous cell carcinoma (SCC) of the vulva; epidemiology (Fig. 22-2 B, C)
   a. Most common cancer of the vulva (Links 22-44 and 22-45)
   b. Most common in women in the sixth decade; may or may not be associated with an inflammatory dermatitis.
   c. Risk factors
      (1) HPV type 16, the most common risk factor; smoking cigarettes
      (2) Immunodeficiency disorders (e.g., AIDS), lichen sclerosus, obesity, hypertension, and diabetes mellitus (DM)
   d. Metastasis to inguinal nodes or pelvic nodes depending on location of the tumor
4. Extramammary Paget disease
   a. **Definition:** Intraepithelial adenocarcinoma limited to the vulva
   b. Epidemiology
      (1) Red intermixed with white (leukoplakia), crusted vulvar lesion ("cake-icing effect"; Fig. 22-2 D; Link 22-46 A)
      (2) It is an intraepithelial adenocarcinoma that derives from primitive epithelial progenitor cells.
      (3) Malignant Paget cells contain mucin (Fig. 22-2 E), a characteristic finding of an adenocarcinoma. Mucin is positive with the periodic acid–Schiff (PAS) stain.
      (4) Malignant cells spread along the epithelium but rarely invade the dermis (Link 22-46 B).
      (5) Most cases are curable.
5. Malignant melanoma (see Chapter 25)
   a. **Definition:** Malignancy of melanocytes in the epidermis (Link 22-47)
   b. Epidemiology

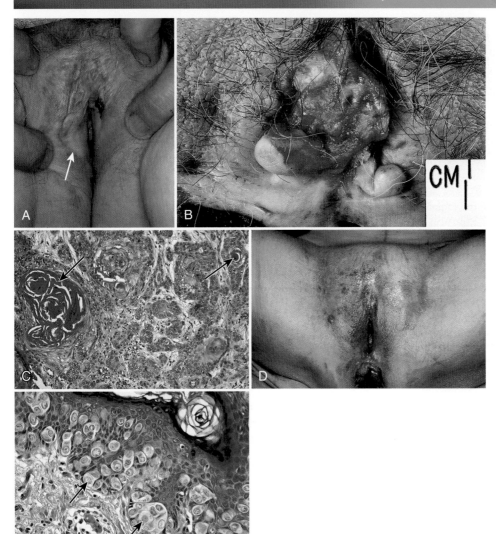

22-2: **A,** Lichen sclerosis. The vulva shows a parchment-like appearance *(arrow).* **B,** Gross appearance of invasive squamous cell carcinoma (SCC) of the vulva. Note the huge tumor mass involving all vulvar structures. **C,** Microscopic appearance of invasive SCC of the vulva. It is a well-differentiated tumor. Note the keratin squamous pearls *(arrows),* a very characteristic finding in SCCs. **D,** Clinical and gross appearance of vulvar Paget disease. Note the extensive red, crusted lesion. **E,** Extramammary Paget disease. Large, pink-staining, malignant Paget cells *(arrows)* are disposed singly and in clusters within the epidermis. In Paget disease of the nipple, the same kinds of cells are present in the epidermis. (*A from Savin JAA, Hunter JAA, Hepburn NC:* Diagnosis in Color: Skin Signs in Clinical Medicine, *London, Mosby-Wolfe, 1997, p 124, Fig. 4.81; **B** to **E** from Rosai J:* Rosai and Ackerman's Surgical Pathology, *9th ed, St. Louis, Mosby, 2004, pp 1489, 1490, 1492, respectively, Figs. 19.11D, 19.12A, 19.16A, 19.17B, respectively.*)

(1) Majority develop on the labia majora, labia minor, or the clitoris

(2) Second most common vulvar malignancy

(3) White women are at greater risk than African American women for developing vulvar melanoma.

(4) Five-year survival rate ranges from 15% to 54%; survival is worse for African American women than white women.

IV. Vagina Disorders

A. Imperforate hymen

1. **Definition:** Canalization abnormality at the site where the vaginal plate contacts the urogenital sinus (UGS)

2. Epidemiology/clinical

   a. After birth, it presents as a bulging, membrane-like structure in the vestibule of the vagina behind which is blood (neonatal hematocolpos [vagina fills with menstrual blood]). It is caused by exposure to estrogen (E) in utero. Glands in the endometrial mucosa undergo hyperplasia. When the baby is delivered, the E source is lost, and the endometrial tissue is sloughed off, causing a small amount of vaginal bleeding.

   b. Most common and most distal form of vaginal outflow obstruction (Link 22-48)

   c. Anatomic cause of primary amenorrhea

B. Rokitansky-Küster-Hauser (RKH) syndrome

1. **Definition:** Congenital disorder associated with an absence or underdevelopment of the vagina and uterus. The ovaries are usually present and functional.

2. Epidemiology

Labia majora/minor, clitoris

2nd MC vulvar malignancy

Risk: white > African American women

Poor survival

Vagina disorders

Imperforate hymen

Canalization abnormality (vaginal plate contacts UGS)

Bulging membrane vaginal vestibule

MC/most distal vaginal outflow obstruction

Anatomic cause 1° amenorrhea

RKH syndrome

Vagina/uterus underdeveloped or absent

Ovaries present/functional

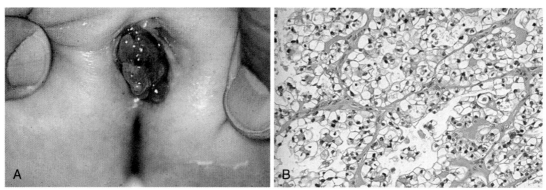

22-3: A, Embryonal rhabdomyosarcoma of the vagina. Note the bloody, necrotic mass protruding out of the vagina. **B,** Clear cell carcinoma of the vagina. Note the clear, vacuolated cells with ill-defined glandular spaces. *(A from my friend Ivan Damjanov, MD, PhD, Linder J: Pathology: A Color Atlas, St. Louis, Mosby, 2000, p 266, Fig. 13-29; B from Klatt E: Robbins and Cotran Atlas of Pathology, Philadelphia, Saunders, 2006, p 295, Fig. 13-12.)*

Genetic/environmental factors

Some AD inheritance

Anatomic cause 1° amenorrhea

Gartner duct cyst vagina

Wolffian duct remnant

Cyst lateral wall vagina

Rhabdomyoma

Benign tumor skeletal muscle

Tongue, heart (tuberous sclerosis)

Embryonal rhabdomyosarcoma

Skeletal muscle malignancy

MC sarcoma girls <5yrs of age

Grapelike mass vagina

Clear cell adeno

Intrauterine exposure to DES

DES: was used to prevent spontaneous abortion

Inhibits Müllerian differentiation

Vaginal adenosis

Benign remnants vaginal Mullerian glands

Red ulcerations upper vagina

Precursor clear cell adeno in vagina

Cancer involves upper vagina/cervix

Abnormal shaped uterus: impaired implantation

Cervical incompetence; recurrent abortions

Vaginal SCC

HPV type 16

Extension cervical SCC into vagina

Inguinal lymph node metastasis

Cervix disorders

Cervix = endocervix + exocervix

Exocervix non-keratinizing squamous cells

a. Most likely results from a combination of genetic and environmental factors
b. Some cases appear to have an autosomal dominant (AD) inheritance pattern.
c. Anatomic cause of primary amenorrhea (failure of menses to occur by age 16 years)

C. Gartner duct cyst of the vagina
1. **Definition:** Remnant of the wolffian (mesonephric) duct
2. Epidemiology: presents as a cyst on the lateral wall of the vagina

D. Benign and malignant tumors of the vagina
1. Rhabdomyoma
   a. **Definition:** Benign tumor (? hamartoma) of skeletal muscle
   b. Other locations for a rhabdomyoma include the tongue and the heart, the latter site associated with tuberous sclerosis (see Chapter 26).
2. Embryonal rhabdomyosarcoma
   a. **Definition:** Malignancy of skeletal muscle composed of rhabdomyoblasts with cross-striations
   b. Epidemiology
      (1) Most common sarcoma (mesodermal origin) in girls younger than 5 years of age
      (2) Presents as a necrotic, grapelike mass that protrudes from the vagina (Fig. 22-3 A; Link 22-49)
3. Clear cell adenocarcinoma of the vagina (Fig. 22-3 B)
   a. **Definition:** Rare adenocarcinoma linked to diethylstilbestrol (DES), a drug that was used prevent a threatened abortion (see Chapter 6)
   b. Epidemiology
      (1) Occurs in women with intrauterine exposure to DES. DES was used to prevent spontaneous abortion.
      (2) DES inhibits müllerian differentiation. Müllerian structures include fallopian tubes, uterus, cervix, and upper one-third of the vagina.
      (3) Vaginal adenosis
         (a) **Definition:** Benign remnants of Müllerian glands in the vagina (Link 22-50)
         (b) Epidemiology: presents as red, superficial ulcerations in the upper portion of the vagina. Precursor lesion for clear cell adenocarcinoma. Risk for developing the cancer is small (1:1000). Cancer involves the upper vagina or cervix.
   c. Other DES abnormalities
      (1) Abnormally shaped uterus with impaired implantation
      (2) Cervical incompetence, a common cause of recurrent abortions
4. Vaginal squamous cell carcinoma (SCC)
   a. Primary SCC of the vagina is associated with HPV type 16.
   b. Most cancers are an extension of a cervical SCC into the vagina rather than arising from the vaginal epithelium.
   c. Primary cancers metastasize to the inguinal lymph nodes.

V. Cervix Disorders
A. Clinical anatomy and histology
1. The cervix includes the exocervix and endocervix. The exocervix begins at the cervical os (opening of the cervix).
2. The exocervix is normally lined by nonkeratinizing squamous epithelium.

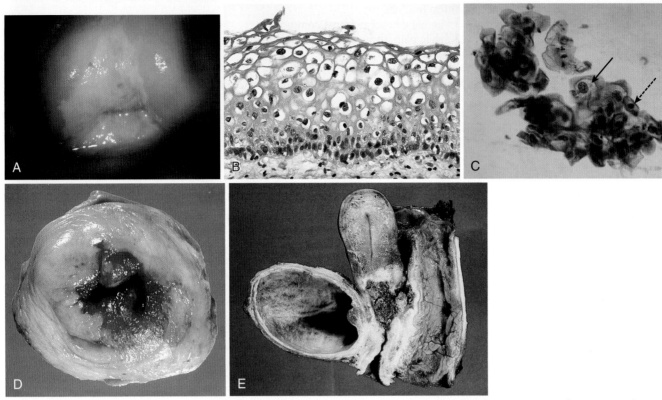

22-4: A, Appearance of the cervix after application of 3% to 5% acetic acid. Note the well-defined, opaque acetowhite area, with regular margins, involving a large part of the visible squamocolumnar junction. **B,** Koilocytosis caused by human papillomavirus (HPV). The squamous cells have wrinkled pyknotic nuclei surrounded by a clear halo. **C,** Papanicolaou stain of the exfoliated cervicovaginal squamous epithelial cells, showing the perinuclear cytoplasmic vacuolization termed koilocytosis (vacuolated cytoplasm; solid arrow) and nuclear pyknosis *(interrupted arrow)*, which are characteristic of HPV infection. **D,** Squamous cell carcinoma (SCC) of the cervix. Note the bleeding and ulceration in the cervical os. **E,** SCC of cervix with extension down into the vagina, wall of the urinary bladder *(solid arrow)*, and wall of the rectum *(interrupted arrow)*. (*A from Cohen J, Opal SM, Powderly WG: Infectious Diseases, 3rd ed, St. Louis, Mosby Elsevier, 2010, p 653, Fig. 59.2; B from Rosai J, Ackerman LV: Surgical Pathology, 9th ed, St. Louis, Mosby, 2004, p 1530, Fig. 19-74; C from Murray PR, Rosenthal KS, Pfaller MA: Medical Microbiology, 6th ed, Philadelphia, Mosby Elsevier, 2009, p 504, Fig. 51.7; D and E courtesy of Dr. Hector Rodriguez-Martinez, Mexico City, Mexico.)*

3. The endocervical glands are normally lined by mucus-secreting columnar cells.
4. The endocervical epithelium (ETM) normally migrates down to the exocervix (Fig. 22-4 A).
   a. Exposure to the acid pH of the vagina causes the endocervix to develop benign squamous metaplasia. *Lactobacilli* (gram-positive rods) produce lactic acid, maintaining an acid pH in the vagina.
   b. Area undergoing metaplasia is called the transformation zone (TZ; Links 22-51 and 22-52). TZ is where squamous dysplasia and cancer develop. TZ must be sampled when performing a cervical Papanicolaou (Pap) smear (Links 22-53 and 22-54 A).
   c. Metaplastic squamous cells (SCs) block endocervical (EC) gland orifices. Obstruction of outflow of mucus produces nabothian cysts. Nabothian cysts are a normal finding in women.

B. Acute and chronic cervicitis
   1. **Definition:** Acute or chronic inflammation of the cervix
   2. Epidemiology
      a. Accounts for 20% to 25% of women presenting with vaginal discharge
      b. Can be found in any sexually active woman
      c. Subdivided into acute and chronic cervicitis
   3. Acute cervicitis
      a. **Definition:** Refers to acute inflammation in the TZ
      b. Epidemiology; causative agents:
         (1) *Chlamydia trachomatis, N. gonorrhoeae* (GC), *Trichomonas vaginalis, Candida* spp., human herpesvirus 2 (HSV-2), and HPV
         (2) Note: HPV vaccine is directed against HPV 16 and 18 serotypes (subtypes associated with cervical cancer) and HPV 6 and 11.

Endocervix mucus-secreting columnar cells
Endocervical ETM → exocervical ETM
Acid pH → squamous metaplasia
Lactobacilli: gram + rod; produce lactic acid
TZ site squamous metaplasia
TZ: site for squamous dysplasia/cancer
Must sample TZ when performing cervical Pap
Cervical Pap: sample TZ
Metaplastic squamous cells block EC gland orifices
Nabothian cysts: obstruction EC gland orifices
Nabothian cysts normal finding
Acute/chronic inflammation cervix
Vaginal discharge
Sexually active women
Cervicitis: common cause of vaginal discharge
Acute cervicitis
Acute inflammation in TZ
Chlamydia, GC, Trichomonas, *Candida*, HSV-2, HPV
HPV vaccine against HPV 16/18 subtypes

c. Clinical findings
   (1) Vaginal discharge (most common)
   (2) Pelvic pain, dyspareunia (painful intercourse), pain on palpation of cervix during pelvic exam
   (3) Easy bleeding when obtaining cultures from the cervical os
   (4) Erythematous cervical os that may be covered by an exudate
d. Diagnosis
   (1) DNA probe to detect *C. trachomatis* and *N. gonorrhoeae*
   (2) These organisms account for >50% of cases of acute cervicitis.
   (3) Wet mount for visualizing *T. vaginalis* (jerky movements caused by the flagella). Examination of a cervical Pap smear shows numerous neutrophils.
4. Chronic cervicitis
   a. **Definition:** Condition that occurs when acute cervicitis persists
5. Follicular cervicitis
   a. **Definition:** Type of cervicitis that is caused by *C. trachomatis* characterized by pronounced lymphoid follicles with germinal centers present in a cervical biopsy
   b. Epidemiology
      (1) *C. trachomatis* infects metaplastic squamous cells (SCs)
         (a) Metaplastic cells contain vacuoles (phagosomes) with inclusions called reticulate bodies (Fig. 22-1 B).
         (b) Reticulate bodies divide into elementary bodies, which are the infective particles of *C. trachomatis*.
      (2) Cervicitis is the primary source for *C. trachomatis*, *N. gonorrhoeae* conjunctivitis (ophthalmia neonatorum), and pneumonia in newborns. Newborn contact with an infected cervix during delivery is an example of vertical transmission of an infection to a newborn.

C. Cervical Pap smear
1. Purpose of a cervical Pap smear
   a. Screening test to rule out (R/O) squamous dysplasia and cancer
   b. Used to evaluate the hormone status of a woman
2. Sample sites include the vagina, exocervix, and the TZ.

Because the transformation zone is the site for squamous dysplasia and squamous cancer, it must be adequately sampled. The presence of metaplastic squamous cells or mucus-secreting columnar cells indicates proper sampling. Absence of these cells means that the Pap smear must be repeated.

---

3. Interpretation of a cervical Pap smear (Link 22-54 B; Fig. 22-5)
   a. Presence of superficial SCs indicates that E levels are adequate.
   b. Intermediate SCs indicate progesterone (P) levels are adequate.
   c. Parabasal cells indicate that there is a lack of E and P stimulation.
   d. Normal nonpregnant women should have approximately 70% superficial SCs and 30% intermediate SCs.
      (1) Superficial SCs have small, contracted nuclei, and the cytoplasm is stained red because of cytoplasmic keratin.
      (2) Intermediate SCs are deeper cells with plump nuclei and blue-green cytoplasm on Pap stain.
   e. Pregnant woman should have 100% intermediate SCs (from P, the primary hormone of pregnancy).

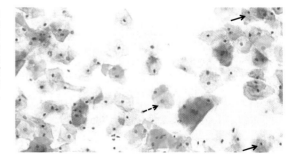

22-5: Normal cervical Pap smear in a young woman. Normal nonpregnant women should have approximately 70% superficial squamous cells and 30% intermediate squamous cells. Superficial squamous cells have a small, contracted nuclei and the cytoplasm is stained red because of the cytoplasmic keratin (two *dark black arrows*). Intermediate squamous cells are deeper cells, and the cells have plump nuclei of normal appearance, and the cytoplasm is stained blue-green (*interrupted black arrow*). (From Young B, O'Dowd G, Woodford P: *Wheater's Functional Histology: A Colour Text and Atlas,* 6th ed, Churchill Livingstone Elsevier, 2014, p 369, Fig. 18.25.)

f. Elderly woman usually lack E and P and have an atrophic smear with predominantly parabasal cells (small, round cells that are normally located along the basement membrane) and inflammatory cells.

g. Women with continuous exposure to E *without* P should have 100% superficial SCs. This indicates that the woman may be taking E *without* P or she has a tumor that is secreting E (e.g., granulosa cell tumor of the ovary).

D. Endocervical (EC) polyp

1. **Definition:** Non-neoplastic polyp that protrudes from the cervical os
2. Epidemiology
   a. Arises from the endocervix, *not* the exocervix
   b. Most commonly seen in perimenopausal women and multigravida women between 30 and 50 years of age; *not* a precancerous polyp
   c. Pathogenesis: inflammation, trauma, and pregnancy have been implicated in their development
3. Clinical findings of an EC polyp include postcoital bleeding and vaginal discharge.

E. Cervical intraepithelial neoplasia (CIN)

1. **Definition:** Dysplasia of squamous cells that normally line the surface epithelium of the cervix
2. Epidemiology
   a. Majority of cases are associated with HPV.
      (1) Types 6 and 11 carry a low risk for developing SCC.
      (2) Types 16 and 18 carry a high risk for developing SCC. HPV genotyping is available to identify these subtypes of HPV.
      (3) HPV produces koilocytosis in SCs (Fig. 22-4 B and C; Link 22-24). Koilocytic SCs have a clear halo containing wrinkled, pyknotic nuclei.
   b. Peak incidence for CIN is 25 to 29 years of age.
   c. The false-negative rate for detecting dysplasia on a cervical Pap smear is ~40%, indicating that it has a low sensitivity for detecting cervical dysplasia.
   d. Risk factors for CIN
      (1) Early age of onset of sexual intercourse; multiple, high-risk partners
      (2) High-risk types of HPV in a biopsy
      (3) Cigarette smoking, oral contraceptive pills (OCPs)
      (4) Immunodeficiency (e.g., human immunodeficiency [HIV] virus infection)
3. Classification of CIN (Links 22-55 and 22-56)
   a. CIN I: mild dysplasia involving the lower one-third of the epithelium
   b. CIN II: moderate dysplasia involving the lower two-thirds of the epithelium
   c. CIN III: severe dysplasia to CIS involving the full thickness of the epithelium (Fig. 2-15 H)
   d. Microinvasion is identified by a greater degree of squamous differentiation and location below the basement membrane (Links 22-56 D and 22-57).
4. Progression from CIN I to CIN III is *not* inevitable. Reversal to normal is more likely in CIN I. Requires ~10 years for progression from CIN I to CIN III. Requires ~10 years for progression from CIN III to invasive cancer. The average age for developing cervical cancer is ~45 years.
5. Clinical findings in CIN
   a. CIN is *not* usually visible to the naked eye and requires colposcopy of a 3% acetic acid prepared cervix (Link 22-58 right). Colposcopy refers to direct visualization of the cervix with a scope.
   b. Colposcopy findings of CIN, after application of 3% acetic acid include blood vessel loops reaching the surface epithelium (called punctation) and networks of fine-caliber vessels that are in close proximity to each other (called mosaics).

F. Cervical cancer

1. **Definition:** Penetration of the basement membrane of the cervix by malignant cells
2. Epidemiology
   a. Cervical cancer is the third most common gynecologic cancer and the third most common gynecologic cancer leading to death in the United States. Overall, cervical cancer is the eighth most common cancer in women. The median age at diagnosis is 48 years.
   b. Higher incidence of cervical cancer in developing countries because of a lack of easily accessible health care. In the U.S. population, the incidence of cervical cancer in descending order is Hispanic, black, and white.
   c. Majority of cervical cancers are SCC (75%–80% of cases). Small cell cancer and adenocarcinoma are less common types of cervical cancer.

Elderly: 100% parabasal (atrophic); inflammatory cells

Woman taking E alone, granulosa cell tumor: 100% superficial

Endocervical polyp

Non-neoplastic

Arises from endocervix

Perimenopausal/ multigravida women

Not precancerous

Inflammation, trauma, pregnancy

Postcoital bleeding; vaginal discharge

Cervical intraepithelial neoplasia

Dysplasia surface squamous cells

Majority due to HPV

HPV 6,11 low risk

HPV 16, 18 high risk

HPV effect → koilocytosis

Clear halo/pyknotic nucleus

Peak incidence 25 to 29

Pap smear low sensitivity for detecting cervical dysplasia

Early onset of sex

Multiple, high-risk partners

HPV 16/18

Cigarette smoking

OCPs

Immunodeficiency

Cervical dysplasia: precursor for SCC

CIN I mild dysplasia

CIN II moderate dysplasia

CIN III severe dysplasia/CIN

Microinvasion: below basement membrane; ↑squamous differentiation

Progression *not* inevitable

Average age cervical SCC ~45 years

Colposcopy required to visualize CIN

Punctation, mosaics signs of CIN

Cervical cancer

Penetration basement membrane by malignant cells

Least common gynecologic cancer; cancer with lowest mortality

Incidence higher in developing countries

U.S. incidence: Hispanic→black→white

Majority SCCs

Small cell cancer/ adenocarcinoma less common

d. Cause and risk factors are the same as those listed for CIN. Cervical Pap smears have markedly reduced the incidence and mortality from cervical cancer. However, the incidence of cervical cancer has recently reached a plateau because of the number of women who fail to be screened.

Pap smear most responsible for ↓incidence/mortality

(1) Pap smear detection of low-grade cervical dysplasia has a sensitivity of ~70% and a specificity of 75%.

(2) Pap smear detection of high-grade cervical dysplasia has a sensitivity of 75% and a specificity of 95%.

Abnormal vaginal bleeding postcoital MC sign

Malodorous discharge

Cancer characteristics

Down into vagina

Out into lateral wall cervix, vagina

Cervical cancer: renal failure common COD

Para-aortic lymph nodes

Lungs, liver, bones

3. Clinical findings in cervical cancer (Fig. 22-4 D; Link 22-59 A, B): abnormal vaginal bleeding (most common), usually postcoital; malodorous discharge

4. Cervical cancer characteristics (Fig. 22-4 E)
   a. Extension *down* into the vagina; extension *out* into the lateral wall of the cervix and vagina
   b. Infiltration into the bladder wall causing obstruction of the ureters. Postrenal azotemia leading to renal failure is a common cause of death (COD).
   c. Spreads to paraaortic lymph nodes; distant hematogenous metastasis particularly to lungs, liver, and bones

5. As expected, survival rates depend on the stage of disease (Link 22-60).

VI. **Reproductive Physiology and Selected Hormone Disorders**
   A. **Sequence to menarche** (Link 22-61)

Breast budding

Growth spurt, pubic hair

Axillary hair, menarche

Menarche (mean 12.8 yrs)

Anovulatory cycles 1 to 1.5 yrs

1. Breast budding (thelarche) → growth spurt → pubic hair → axillary hair → menarche
2. Menarche: Mean age of menarche is 12.8 years. Anovulatory cycles (lack of ovulation) last for 1 to 1.5 years.

   B. **Synthesis of sex hormones in thecal cells of the ovary** (Fig. 22-6)
   C. **Development of the dominant follicle (oocyte) in the ovary in the menstrual cycle**

Ovarian follicles are fluid-filled sacs containing immature oocytes called primordial follicles (PFs). They are encompassed by a layer of granulosa cells that aid in the growth of the follicles. The oocyte in a PF is arrested in the diplotene* phase of meiosis I. The PFs go through various stages of development and eventually become antral follicles. During each menstrual cycle, a cohort of antral follicles is recruited for development out of which usually one is selected. During the sixth to ninth day of the menstrual cycle, one of the recruited antral follicles is selected and becomes the **dominant follicle** (?greater sensitivity to follicle-stimulating hormone [FSH] than the other antral follicles), and all the other antral follicles undergo atresia. FSH provides a further signal for growth of the dominant follicle and rescues it from atresia. When the dominant follicle (oocyte) is released into the fallopian tube, it is signaled to continue meiosis. It progresses from the diplotene stage of meiosis I to arrest at the metaphase stage of meiosis II. At this point, the first polar body can be seen (Link 22-64). The metaphase stage of meiosis II is only completed if fertilization occurs. If fertilization by a sperm does occur, a mature ovum is formed that has a second polar body. Without fertilization, the egg remains in metaphase stage of meiosis II. The area in the ovary from which the dominant follicle ruptured has residual cell layers left behind. They form a new structure called the corpus luteum, which produces P for the secretory phase of the menstrual cycle.

---

*Diplotene stage of meiosis I is the fourth stage of the prophase of meiosis, during which the paired homologous chromosomes separate except at the places where genetic exchange has occurred.
(Taken from Mularz A, Dalati S, Pedigo R: *OB/GYN Secrets*, 4th ed, St. Louis, Elsevier, 2017, pp 8–9.)

   D. **Phases of the menstrual cycle** (Taken from Mularz A, Dalati S, Pedigo R: OB/GYN Secrets, 4th ed, St. Louis, Elsevier, 2017, pp 7–13.)

Menarche: 10–12 years old

1. Menarche (first menstrual period) begins at ages 10–12 years old.
2. Overview of the menstrual cycle

The endocrine changes in the menstrual cycle affect both the **ovary** and the **endometrium**. In the **ovary**, the proliferative phase *(follicular phase)* of the menstrual cycle matures the ovum in preparation for ovulation. The secretory phase *(luteal phase)* occurs after ovulation, and its function is to maintain the corpus luteum. During this phase, the ovum moves through the fallopian tubes and prepares for fertilization and implantation. The **endometrium** matches the proliferative phase by causing endometrial gland proliferation via a rise in estrogen (E). After ovulation, the secretory phase of the endometrium is characterized by preparation of the endometrium for possible implantation. Under the influence of progesterone (P), there is increased endometrial gland tortuosity and secretion and edema of stromal cells. If implantation does *not* occur, the sudden drop-off in serum E and P initiates menses by causing apoptosis of endometrial cells.

E-mediated gland proliferation phase

Most variable phase

3. Proliferative (follicular) phase of the menstrual cycle (Fig. 22-7; Links 22-62 and 22-63 A)
   a. **Definition:** E-mediated proliferation of the endometrial glands; *most* variable phase of the menstrual cycle

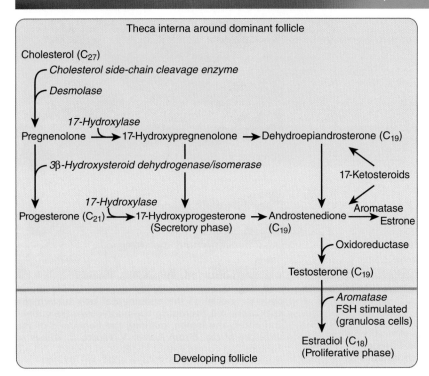

Theca interna around dominant follicle

Cholesterol (C_{27})
  Cholesterol side-chain cleavage enzyme
  Desmolase

17-Hydroxylase
Pregnenolone → 17-Hydroxypregnenolone → Dehydroepiandrosterone (C_{19})

3β-Hydroxysteroid dehydrogenase/isomerase

17-Ketosteroids

17-Hydroxylase
Progesterone (C_{21}) → 17-Hydroxyprogesterone → Androstenedione — Aromatase
(Secretory phase)   (C_{19})   → Estrone

Oxidoreductase

Testosterone (C_{19})

Aromatase
FSH stimulated
(granulosa cells)

Estradiol (C_{18})
(Proliferative phase)

Developing follicle

22-6: Synthesis of sex hormones in the ovaries. Luteinizing hormone is responsible for stimulation of hormone synthesis in the theca interna surrounding the developing follicle. Follicle-stimulating hormone increases the synthesis of aromatase in granulosa cells. Aromatase converts testosterone to estradiol. *(Modified from Goljan EF: Star Series: Pathology, Philadelphia, Saunders, 1998, Fig. 18-1.)*

  b. E surge occurs 24 to 36 hours *before* ovulation.
    (1) E surge stimulates a marked increase in luteinizing hormone (LH) from the anterior pituitary gland (called the LH surge).
    (2) Example of a positive feedback function of E
    (3) E also stimulates the release of follicle-stimulating hormone (FSH) from the anterior pituitary gland. It has positive feedback on both FSH and LH; however, E has a greater positive feedback on LH than FSH. Note the greater increase in LH than FSH in Figure 22-7.
    (4) The LH surge initiates ovulation. It is primarily driven by rising E production from the dominant follicle in the ovary, which peaks approximately 24 to 36 hours before ovulation. The LH surge induces an inflammatory-like response that allows prostaglandins and proteases to break down the cell layers of the dominant follicle, causing the release of the oocyte.
    (5) Testosterone (T) normally increases *before* ovulation in the normal menstrual cycle. It is responsible for the libido (sexual desire) that normally occurs *before* ovulation.
  4. Ovulation (also see previous discussion)
    a. **Definition:** Release of a dominant follicle from the ovary that enters the fallopian tube between days 14 and 16
    b. Ovulation indicators
      (1) Increase in body temperature, an effect of progesterone (P)
      (2) Subnuclear vacuoles in endometrial cells (Fig. 22-8)
        (a) Best sign of ovulation in a biopsy specimen of endometrium
        (b) Vacuoles contain glycogen and glycoproteins. Glycogen is important for nutrition for the fertilized ovum.
      (3) Mittelschmerz (midcycle pain). Blood from the ruptured follicle locally irritates the peritoneum.
  5. Secretory phase (luteal phase) of the menstrual cycle (see Fig. 22-7; Links 22-62 and 22-63 A)
    a. P-mediated phase of the menstrual cycle. P is produced by the corpus luteum. This is the *least* variable phase of the menstrual cycle.
    b. P increases gland tortuosity and secretion.
    c. P increases the number of subnuclear vacuoles in the endometrial glands.
    d. P increases edema of stromal cells.
    e. Other functions of P.

E surge 24–36 hrs before ovulation

E stimulates increase in LH → LH surge

+Feedback function of E

E stimulates release FSH; LH > FSH

Ovulation: E surge → LH surge → ovulation

LH surge → ovulation

↑T *before* ovulation

↑T responsible for libido

Ovulation

Release dominant follicle

Between days 14 and 16

Ovulation indicators

↑Body temperature (P)

Subnuclear vacuoles

Best sign ovulation

Glycogen nutrition for fertilized ovum

Mittelschmerz: mid-cycle pain

Localized peritoneal irritation

P-mediated; produced by corpus luteum

Least variable phase

↑Gland tortuosity/secretion

↑Number subnuclear vacuoles

Edema of stromal cells

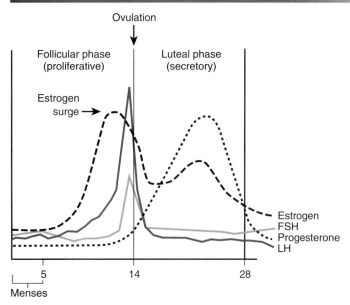

22-7: Menstrual cycle. Estrogen is most important in the proliferative phase and progesterone in the secretory phase of the cycle. Estrogen surge causes the luteinizing hormone (LH) surge, which initiates ovulation. Note the positive feedback of estrogen on LH is greater than follicle-stimulating hormone (FSH). *(From Brown TA: Rapid Review Physiology, Philadelphia, Mosby, 2007, p 99, Fig. 3-15.)*

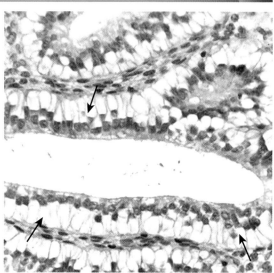

22-8: Subnuclear vacuoles *(arrows)* containing mucin push the nuclei of the endometrial cells toward the apex of the cell. Eventually, the mucin passes the nucleus and enters the lumen, marking the beginning of the secretory phase. *(From Kumar V, Fausto N, Abbas A: Robbins and Cotran Pathologic Basis of Disease, 7th ed. Philadelphia, Saunders, 2004, p 1081, Fig. 21-5B.)*

↓GnRH → ↓secretion FSH/LH

Causes hypothalamus to ↑basal body T

(1) Negative feedback at the level of the hypothalamus decreases gonadotropin-releasing hormone (GnRH), which reduces secretion of FSH and LH secretion.

(2) Causes the hypothalamus to increase the basal body temperature (T)

  f. Summary of ovarian changes in menses (Link 22-63 B)

In **fertility workups**, endometrial biopsies are commonly performed on day 21 to determine if ovulation has occurred. The presence of a secretory endometrium on day 21 confirms that ovulation has occurred.

Secretory endometrium day 21 confirms ovulation

Menses
Monthly flow blood/ endometrial tissue
Basal layer (overlies myometrium), functional layer (overlies basal layer)
Blastocyst implantation, hormone sensitive, shed during menses
Sudden drop E and P

6. Menses
    a. **Definition:** The monthly flow of blood and endometrial tissue from the uterus
        (1) The two layers of the endometrium are the *basal layer*, which overlies the myometrium and the *functional layer*, which overlies the basal layer.
        (2) The functional layer is the site for blastocyst implantation (see later). It is sensitive to hormones and is shed during menses.
    b. Menses initiated by the sudden drop-off in serum levels of E and P (see Fig. 22-7); signal for apoptosis of endometrial cells

Mother's increased E levels causes hyperplasia of endometrial glands in a female fetus. Newborn baby girls may have vaginal bleeding because of the sudden drop of maternal hormones with delivery.

Maternal E causes fetal endometrial gland hyperplasia; NB vaginal bleeding.
Plasmin prevents menstrual blood from clotting
Excess clotting indicates menorrhagia
Fertilization
Fertilization in ampullary portion of fallopian tube
Takes 6 days for fertilized egg to implant
Blastocyst forms day 4

Blastocyst implants day 6

    c. Plasmin prevents menstrual blood from clotting. Excess clotting is a sign of menorrhagia (excessive bleeding) because it implies that plasmin did *not* have enough time to lyse fibrinogen in the clot material.
7. Fertilization
    a. Fertilization (sperm penetrating the egg) usually takes place in the ampullary portion of the fallopian tube (Link 22-64).
    b. The fertilized egg spends 4 days in the fallopian tube and approximately 2 days in the uterine cavity *before* implantation.
        (1) While in the fallopian tube, the fertilized egg becomes a blastocyst (fourth day).
        (2) The blastocyst implants in the endometrial mucosa by the sixth day, which corresponds to day 21 in the menstrual cycle.

    c. An exaggerated secretory phase (greater gland tortuosity and secretion) occurs in pregnancy. It is called the Arias-Stella phenomenon (Link 22-65).

8. Summary of functions of FSH in the menstrual cycle
   a. Prepares the dominant follicle of the month
      (1) Unstimulated follicles in the ovary are arrested in the meiosis I prophase.
      (2) FSH causes the follicle to enlarge.
   b. FSH increases aromatase synthesis in the granulosa cells in the follicle.
   c. FSH increases the synthesis of LH receptors. LH is important in stimulating estradiol synthesis in the theca interna around the dominant follicle. It does this by first synthesizing androstenedione, which in a few steps produces estradiol (see Fig. 22-6). Estradiol is the key hormone of the proliferative phase of the menstrual cycle.

9. Summary of functions of luteinizing hormone (LH) in the menstrual cycle
   a. LH in the **proliferative phase** of the menstrual cycle
      (1) LH increases the synthesis of 17-ketosteroids (17-KS) in the theca interna surrounding the developing follicle (see Fig. 22-6). Dehydroepiandrosterone (DHEA) and androstenedione are 17-ketosteroids (17-KS).
      (2) DHEA is converted to androstenedione.
      (3) Oxidoreductase converts androstenedione to T.
      (4) After entering the granulosa cells within the developing follicle, T is converted by an aromatase enzyme to estradiol. This reaction is known as aromatization. Estradiol is the key hormone in the proliferative phase of the menstrual cycle.
   b. LH surge is induced by a sudden increase in E (see earlier discussion).
      (1) Ovulation occurs when LH is *greater* than FSH.
      (2) LH-stimulated follicle moves from meiosis I prophase into meiosis II metaphase.
      (3) Fertilization of the stimulated follicle by the spermatozoa causes the follicle to develop into a mature oocyte with 23 chromosomes.
   c. LH in the secretory phase of the menstrual cycle. In the secretory phase of the cell cycle, the theca interna primarily synthesizes 17-hydroxyprogesterone (17-OH-progesterone; see Fig. 22-6).

10. Hormone changes in pregnancy
    a. Human chorionic gonadotropin (hCG)
       (1) Synthesized in the syncytiotrophoblast lining the chorionic villus in the placenta. Levels of hCG can be detected 7 days after fertilization, which is 4 to 5 days after implantation. It should rise by at least 66% every 48 hours during early pregnancy. When levels reach 3000 mIU/mL, a gestational sac can usually be seen.
       (2) Acts as a LH analogue by maintaining the corpus luteum of pregnancy
       (3) The corpus luteum synthesizes P for ~8 to 10 weeks.
    b. The corpus luteum involutes after ~8 to 10 weeks.
       (1) Placenta synthesizes P for the remainder of the pregnancy (Link 22-66 A). P is important in maintaining pregnancy.
       (2) Spontaneous abortion may occur at this time of the pregnancy if the placental production of P is inadequate.
    c. Estriol is the primary E of pregnancy (see later).

E. **Oral contraceptive pills (OCPs)**
   1. Mixture of E + progestins (P)
      a. Baseline levels of E in the OCPs prevent the midcycle E surge, which prevents the LH surge, which prevents ovulation.
      b. Progestins arrest the proliferative phase and cause gland atrophy (Links 22-67 and 22-68).
      c. Progestins cause stromal cells to become plump ("decidualized"; Links 22-67 and 22-68).
      d. Progestins inhibit LH, which also prevents the LH surge.
   2. OCPs alter fallopian tube motility

F. **Sources and types of E**
   1. Estradiol
      a. Primary E in nonpregnant women
      b. Principally derived from the ovaries by the conversion of T to estradiol by aromatase (see Fig. 22-6)
      c. Primary hormone that is responsible for the proliferative (follicular) phase of the menstrual cycle (see earlier discussion).
      d. Stimulates the growth of the stroma (connective tissue) in the endometrium
      e. Stimulates elongation of the spiral arteries, which supply the endometrium.

Exaggerated secretory phase that occurs in pregnancy

FSH prepares follicle of month

Unstimulated follicles in meiosis I prophase

Follicle gets larger

FSH ↑aromatase synthesis granulosa cells

FSH ↑synthesis LH receptors

LH functions menstrual cycle

LH ↑synthesis 17-KS

17-KS: DHEA, androstenedione

DHEA → androstenedione

Androstenedione → T

T converted to estradiol by aromatase in granulosa cells

LH surge due to ↑E

LH > FSH initiates ovulation

LH: follicles progress to meiosis II metaphase

Fertilized follicle → mature oocyte with 23 chromosomes

LH secretory phase: synthesizes 17-OH-progesterone

Hormone changes in pregnancy

hCG

hCG synthesized in syncytiotrophoblast

hCG: LH analogue; maintains corpus luteum

Corpus luteum synthesizes P

Corpus luteum involutes ~8 to 10 wks

Placenta synthesizes P for remainder of pregnancy

P maintains the pregnancy

Spontaneous abortion if P inadequate

Estriol primary E of pregnancy

OCPs

Estrogen + progestins

OCP: low E prevents LH surge and ovulation

Progestins cause gland atrophy

Stromal cells "decidualized"

Progestins inhibit LH

Alter fallopian tube motility

Sources estrogen

Estradiol

1° estrogen nonpregnant woman

Derived from ovaries

Proliferative phase hormone

Stimulates stromal growth

Elongates spiral arteries

Cervical mucus watery
Sperm now able to move thru cervix
"Ferning" cervical mucus in proliferative phase
Growth/development female reproductive system
Breast development, prolactin secretion, maintaining pregnancy
Estrone
Weak estrogen of menopause
Adipose cell aromatization androstenedione → estrone
Androstenedione derived from adrenal cortex *not* ovaries
Estriol
Estrogen of pregnancy
Fetal adrenal/liver → placenta → maternal liver
Sources/types androgens
Androstenedione = derivation ovaries/adrenal cortex
Most DHEA from adrenal cortex
Remainder DHEA ovaries
DHEA-S: adrenal cortex
Testosterone
T synthesized ovaries/adrenal glands
Androstenedione → T
Peripheral conversion to DHT by 5-α-reductase
SHBG
Binding protein T/E
Synthesized in liver
E ↑synthesis in liver
Androgens, obesity, hypothyroidism ↓synthesis
Greater binding affinity for T than E
↑SHBG, ↓FT
↓SHBG; ↑FT
↑FT → hirsutism
Menopause
Permanent cessation menses without pathologic cause
51.4 years of age
Before 40 years of age 1° ovarian failure
Perimenopause: hot flashes, sleep problems, vaginal dryness
Perimenopause 2 to 8 yrs
Physiologic menopause
Waxing/waning E levels
↓Ovarian function
Depletion granulosa/thecal cells
Lack ovarian response to gonadotropins
↑LH → ↑androgens (ovarian stromal cells)

f. Causes increased secretion of watery cervical mucus
  (1) Watery mucous allows sperm to move through the cervix.
  (2) In the proliferative phase, estradiol is responsible for "ferning" when a sample of cervical mucus is spread out on a glass slide and allowed to dry.
g. Stimulates growth and development of the female reproductive system
h. Important in normal breast development, prolactin secretion, and maintaining pregnancy

2. Estrone
  a. Weak E that is produced during menopause.
  b. Derived from adipose cell aromatization of androstenedione into estrone (see Fig. 22-6). Because the ovaries are atrophic after menopause, androstenedione is synthesized in the adrenal cortex.

3. Estriol
  a. Primary E of pregnancy
  b. Derives from the fetal adrenal gland and liver, placenta, and maternal liver (Link 22-66 B; see Section X)

G. Sources and types of androgens
1. Androstenedione has equal derivation from the ovaries (see Fig. 22-6) and the adrenal cortex.
2. Dehydroepiandrosterone (DHEA)
  a. Most DHEA is synthesized in the adrenal cortex (80%).
  b. The remainder is synthesized in the ovaries (see Fig. 22-6).
3. DHEA-sulfate (DHEA-S) is almost exclusively synthesized in the adrenal cortex.
4. Testosterone (T)
  a. T is synthesized in the ovaries and adrenal glands.
  b. Derived from conversion of androstenedione to T by oxidoreductase (see Fig. 22-6)
  c. Peripherally converted to 5-α-dihydrotestosterone (DHT) by 5-α-reductase, located in the ovaries, adrenal glands, and liver.

H. Sex hormone–binding globulin (SHBG) (Fig. 22-9)
1. **Definition:** Binding protein for T and E (also see Chapter 21)
  a. In both men and women, SHBG is synthesized in the liver.
  b. E increases synthesis of SHBG in the liver.
  c. Androgens, obesity, and hypothyroidism all decrease the synthesis of SHBG.
2. SHBG has a greater binding affinity for T than for E.
  a. Increased levels of SHBG decrease the level of free testosterone (FT) level.
  b. Decreased levels of SHBG increase the level of FT; common cause of hirsutism in obese women (see later discussion).

I. Menopause
1. **Definition:** Permanent cessation of menses (amenorrhea) for 12 months *without* a pathologic cause
  a. Average age of menopause is 51.4 years of age; earlier in smokers and nulliparous women (no pregnancies)
  b. Menopause *before* 40 years of age is called primary ovarian failure.
  c. Perimenopause (before menopauses) refers to the time period of menstrual irregularities (hot flashes [>75%], insomnia, vaginal dryness) until 1 year after menopause; averages 2 to 8 years
2. Epidemiology
  a. Causes
    (1) Physiologic menopause
    (2) Waxing and waning of the E levels caused by decreased ovarian function
      (a) Depletion of granulosa cells and thecal cells
      (b) Lack of an ovarian response to gonadotropins
      (c) Increased LH stimulates androgen production in the stromal cells of the ovaries.

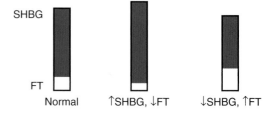

22-9: Schematic of sex hormone–binding globulin (SHBG). See text for discussion. *FT,* Free testosterone. *(From Goljan EF, Sloka KI: Rapid Review Laboratory Testing in Clinical Medicine, Philadelphia, Mosby Elsevier, 2008, p 366, Fig. 10-11.)*

(3) Surgical removal or radiation of the ovaries

(4) Turner syndrome (see Chapter 6), family history of early menopause, left-handedness

b. Average age of menopause is 51 years old.

(1) Age at which menopause occurs is genetically determined.

(2) Smokers reach menopause earlier than nonsmokers.

3. Clinical findings in menopause

a. Secondary amenorrhea. **Definition:** When a woman who has been having normal menstrual cycles stops having menses for 6 months or longer

b. Hot flashes

(1) **Definition:** Sudden sensation of warmth that lasts 1 to 5 minutes

(2) Warmth occurs in the upper body and face and then becomes more generalized. Palpitations and anxiety may also occur.

(3) Result from alterations in the hypothalamic thermoregulatory center (HTRC) caused by fluctuations in steroid and peptide hormone levels

c. Atrophic vaginitis

(1) **Definition:** Vaginal inflammation caused by thinning and shrinking of the vaginal mucosa as well as decreased lubrication caused by the lack of E

(2) Clinical findings include pruritus, burning, bleeding, and dyspareunia (painful intercourse) caused by the dry vaginal mucosa.

d. Mood swings, anxiety, depression, and insomnia

e. Some women may have increased libido (sexual desire); others have decreased libido.

(1) Free testosterone (FT) is thought to be the key hormone that determines libido in a woman.

(2) Because estradiol (E) decreases in menopause, a decrease in SHBG synthesis leads to higher FT levels and increased libido.

f. ↓High-density lipoprotein (HDL), ↑low-density lipoprotein (LDL; ↑cholesterol [CH]).

g. Urinary incontinence (see Chapter 21)

h. Headaches, tiredness, and lethargy

i. Osteoporosis (see Chapter 24): increased risk for vertebral fractures and Colles fractures (fracture of the distal radius with or without fracture of the ulnar styloid (see Chapter 24)

4. Laboratory findings in menopause

a. Increase in serum FSH and serum LH caused by the drop in E and P, respectively

b. Increased serum FSH is the best marker of menopause.

c. Decrease in serum estradiol (E)

J. Hirsutism and virilization in females

1. **Definition of hirsutism:** Excess hair in normal hair-bearing areas (Fig. 22-10 A). It occurs in 5% to 10% of reproductive-age women.

2. **Definition of virilization:** Hirsutism plus the development of male secondary sex characteristics (see later)

3. Epidemiology of hirsutism and virilization

a. Androgens produced in the ovary include T (25%), androstenedione (50%), and DHEA (20%).

b. Androgens produced by the adrenal gland cortex include T (25%), androstenedione (50%), DHEA (50%), and DHEA-S (100%).

c. Peripheral tissue conversion (adipose and skin) includes T from androstenedione (50%), DHEA from DHEA-S (30%), and dihydrotestosterone (DHT) from T.

d. Modulators of androgen action (only free hormone is active, *not* hormones bound to binding proteins)

(1) Sex hormone–binding protein (80%) and albumin (20%) bind to circulating androgens, thereby decreasing the amount of free androgens. Only free hormones can act on target tissues.

(2) 5-α-reductase converts T to DHT (more potent and active than T) at the level of the skin.

e. Male secondary sex characteristics

(1) Increased muscle mass

(2) Male hair distribution from the mons pubis to the umbilicus (Fig. 22-10 B); acne (see Chapter 25)

(3) An enlarged clitoris (clitoromegaly; Fig. 22-10 C) is the most important clinical finding in the diagnosis of virilization.

f. Both hirsutism (H) and virilization (V) are caused by increased androgens of ovarian or adrenal origin.

22-10: A, Hirsutism. This woman has excess hair above the lip and on the chin. **B,** Virilization. This woman has a male distribution of hair from the mons pubis to the umbilicus. **C,** Clitoromegaly. Note the elongation of the clitoris, which is the gold standard sign of virilization. **D,** Polycystic ovary syndrome (PCOS) showing an enlarged ovary with multiple subcortical cysts. **E,** PCOS shown on an ultrasound image with an enlarged ovary demonstrating multiple subcortical cysts *(arrows).* (**A** *from Goljan EF, Sloka KI: Rapid Review Laboratory Testing in Clinical Medicine, Philadelphia, Mosby Elsevier, 2008, p 369, Fig. 10-12;* **B** *and* **C** *from Bouloux P: Self-Assessment Picture Tests: Medicine, Vol. 1. London, Mosby-Wolfe, 1997, pp 47, 4, respectively, Figs. 93, 7, respectively;* **D** *from my friend Ivan Damjanov, MD, PhD, Linder J: Pathology: A Color Atlas, St. Louis, Mosby, 2000, p 262, Fig. 13-17A;* **E** *from Pretorius ES, Solomon JA: Radiology Secrets, 2nd ed, Philadelphia, Mosby, 2006, p 204, Fig. 24-7.)*

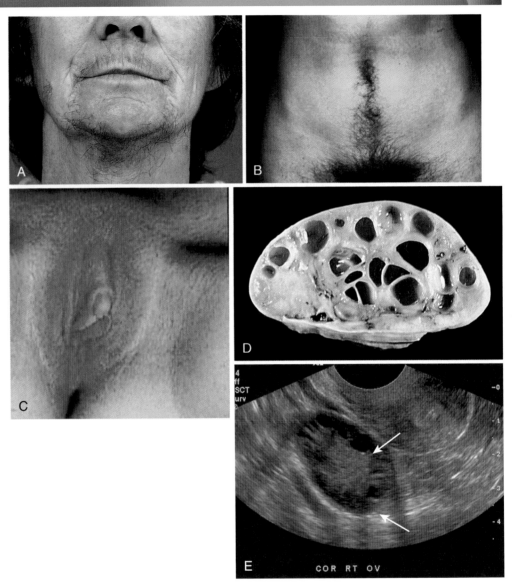

Ovaries only ↑T

Adrenals: ↑DHEA-S + T

Causes H/V

MCC PCOS

Irregular menses, insulin resistance, obesity

Idiopathic: normal menses, ↑androgens

Idiopathic: ↑5-α-reductase activity skin; normal menses/androgens

Classic, nonclassic CAH

Insulin resistance syndrome

Drugs

Ovarian tumors: LC, SL cell tumors

Adrenal tumors

Obesity (↓SHBG → ↑FT)

Hypothyroidism (↓SHBG → ↑FT)

PCOS

Incompletely developed ovarian follicles anovulation; ↑androgens

    (1) Ovarian origin: T is primarily increased.
    (2) Adrenal origin: Both DHEA-S and T are increased. Both are androgenic hormones.
  g. Causes of hirsutism and virilization
    (1) Polycystic ovary syndrome (PCOS; 75% of cases): associated with irregular menses, insulin resistance, and obesity
    (2) Idiopathic hyperandrogenemia: associated with normal menses and increased androgens
    (3) Idiopathic hirsutism: normal menses, normal androgen levels; most likely caused by increased 5-α-reductase activity in the skin
    (4) Nonclassic and classic adrenogenital syndrome (congenital adrenal hyperplasia [CAH]; see Chapter 23)
    (5) Insulin resistance syndrome (see Chapter 23)
    (6) Drugs: androgenic progestins, phenytoin, cyclosporin, minoxidil
    (7) Ovarian tumor: Leydig cell (LC) tumor, Sertoli-Leydig (SL) cell tumor
    (8) Adrenal tumor: adenoma or carcinoma producing Cushing syndrome (see Chapter 23)
    (9) Obesity (see Chapter 8): Decreased SHBG causes an increase in FT.
    (10) Hypothyroidism (↓SHBG, ↑FT; see Chapter 23)
 4. Polycystic ovarian syndrome (PCOS)
  a. **Definition:** Characterized by the presence of incompletely developed ovarian follicles in the ovaries ("cysts") caused by anovulation and an increase in androgens, causing hirsutism (virilization less common)

b. Epidemiology
   (1) Occurs in 6% to 25% of reproductive-age women
   (2) Signs and symptoms begin around menarche.
   (3) Associated with an increase in the incidence of obesity (40%–50% of cases), insulin resistance (metabolic syndrome; see Chapter 23), and acanthosis nigricans (AN; see Chapter 25)
   (4) Key to the pathogenesis of PCOS is increased secretion of LH by the anterior pituitary gland relative to the secretion of FSH (LH/FSH ratio >3).
      (a) May result from either increased hypothalamic secretion of gonadotropin releasing hormone (GnRH) or, less likely, from a primary anterior pituitary abnormality
      (b) Increased LH produces hyperplasia of the ovarian theca cells around the ovarian follicles (called follicular hyperthecosis) and an increase in the production of T (T) and androstenedione (hyperandrogenicity; see earlier discussion).
   (5) Pituitary secretion of FSH is decreased relative to LH secretion.
      (a) The effect of this imbalance leads to decreased ovarian granulosa cell aromatization of androgens (As) to estrogens (Es; normally a function of FSH]. Clinical problems related to this imbalance are hyperandrogenicity and chronic anovulation (caused by decreased E).
      (b) Another clinical effect is follicular arrest (lack of further maturation of the follicle) leading to the formation of subcortical cysts that enlarge the ovaries (Fig. 22-10 D and E).
   (6) Excess androstenedione is converted to estrone. Although a weak E, increased levels of estrone can lead to endometrial gland hyperplasia or cancer and breast cancer (see later).
c. Clinical findings
   (1) Oligomenorrhea (infrequent menses), anovulatory infertility
   (2) Hirsutism (more common than virilization), acne, infertility, obesity, and impaired glucose intolerance (IGT; caused by insulin resistance)
   (3) Endometrial gland hyperplasia or cancer (e.g., vaginal bleeding)
d. Laboratory findings
   (1) LH/FSH ratio >3
   (2) Increase in serum FT and androstenedione
   (3) Decrease in serum sex hormone binding globulin (SHBG)
   (4) Normal to decreased serum FSH

K. Menstrual dysfunction
1. Two most common times for irregular menstrual cycles is 2 years after puberty and 3 years before menopause (called perimenopause).
2. Menorrhagia
   a. **Definition:** Blood loss >80 mL per period
   b. Menorrhagia characteristics
      (1) Staining of sheets at night with heavy protection
      (2) Excessive passage of clots: indicates that plasmin, an enzyme that normally lyses fibrin clots in the uterine cavity, does *not have* enough time to dissolve the clot because of the rapidity of blood flow (see Chapter 15)
3. Premenstrual syndrome (PMS)
   a. **Definition:** Cyclic and behavioral symptoms in the days preceding menses, causing interference with work or lifestyle. Symptoms are followed by a symptom-free interval.
   b. Epidemiology and clinical
      (1) Symptoms occur the same time each cycle. Usually correspond with the luteal phase of the cycle, and abate by day 4 of menstruation. PMS affects 20% to 40% of women, mostly with mild to moderate symptoms. A minority (5%–8%) are severely affected.
      (2) Common symptoms include bloating or abdominal discomfort, irritability, anxiety, depression, mood swings, weight gain, acne, breast fullness or pain, headache, fatigue, and food cravings (particularly for sweets).
      (3) Multifactorial: estrogen (E)/P, fluids and electrolytes (activation of renin-angiotensin-aldosterone [RAA] system), neurotransmitters (NTs; serotonin, γ-aminobenzoic acid [GABA]), and other hormones (endorphins, androgens, glucocorticoids)
      (4) Clinical diagnosis (i.e., presence of the previous clinical findings); no specific laboratory tests required

---

6% to 25% reproductive-age women

S/S begin around menarche

↑Incidence obesity, metabolic syndrome, AN

PCOS: LH/FSH ratio >3

↑Hypothalamic secretion GnRH or 1° pituitary abnormality

↑LH → follicular hyperthecosis → ↑T, androstenedione → hyperandrogenicity

↓FSH relative to LH

↓Ovarian granulosa cell aromatization As to Es (normally FSH function)

Chronic anovulation, hyperandrogenicity

Follicular arrest → subcortical cysts

↑androstenedione → estrone → endometrial hyperplasia/cancer, breast cancer

Oligomenorrhea

Hirsutism, obesity, infertility, IGT

Endometrial hyperplasia/cancer (vaginal bleeding)

LH/FSH ratio >3

↑Serum FT, androstenedione

↓Serum SHBG

Serum FSH N/↓

Menstrual dysfunction

Irregular cycles 2 yrs after puberty, perimenopause

Menorrhagia

Blood loss >80 mL per period

Staining sheets at night

Excess clots

Premenstrual syndrome

Cyclic/behavioral symptoms preceding menses

Symptoms during luteal phase → day 4 menses

Bloating/discomfort, craving for sweets

E/P, RAA, NTs

History sufficient for Dx

Dysmenorrhea

Painful menses

50% women
Primary types
1° only in ovulatory cycles

↑PGF$_{2\alpha}$ → ↑uterine contractions, cervical stenosis
2° Dysmenorrhea

Endometriosis MCC
Adenomyosis: functioning glands/stroma in myometrium
Leiomyomas: smooth muscle tumor
Cervical stenosis
Dysfunctional uterine bleeding
Abnormal bleeding in absence of pregnancy

Hormone imbalance common
DUB: menorrhagia MC abnormal bleeding
Regular normal intervals with ↓ blood flow
Irregular intervals with excessive flow/duration
Irregular/excessive bleeding menses + between periods
Menses at intervals >35 days apart
Menses at intervals <21 days apart
Postmenarchal, perimenopausal (MC)
Perimenopausal *before* menopause
Average age 47.5 years
Majority DUB anovulatory, remainder ovulatory
DUB reproductive age ovulatory
Anovulatory DUB: ↑↑E stimulation, ↑P stimulation
Absent secretory phase
↑↑E stimulation → EGH → ↑bleeding

4. Dysmenorrhea
   a. **Definition:** Painful menses with crampy, midline pain primarily in the lower abdomen
   b. Epidemiology
      (1) Approximately 50% of women have dysmenorrhea. Approximately 10% of women are incapacitated for 1 to 3 days.
      (2) Primary type of dysmenorrhea
         (a) Only occurs in ovulatory cycles
         (b) Caused by increased prostaglandin F 2α (PGF 2α). Prostaglandins cause uterine contractions leading to increased uterine pressure. When uterine pressure exceeds the pressure within uterine blood vessels, uterine ischemia develops. The net effect is pain (dysmenorrhea) caused by the accumulation of anaerobic metabolites.
      (3) Secondary dysmenorrhea is associated with other disorders.
         (a) Endometriosis (most common; functioning endometrial glands and stroma outside the uterus; see later)
         (b) Adenomyosis (functioning endometrial glands and stroma within the myometrium; see later)
         (c) Leiomyomas (benign smooth muscle tumors [SMTs] in the uterine wall; see later)
         (d) Cervical stenosis (blood cannot exit the cervical os properly)
5. Dysfunctional uterine bleeding (DUB)
   a. **Definition:** Abnormal uterine bleeding in regards to volume, regularity, frequency, or duration in the absence of pregnancy
   b. Epidemiology
      (1) Hormonal imbalances are frequently present. Accounts for 33% of gynecologist office visits. Up to 70% of gynecology consultations in those perimenopausal or postmenopause are for DUB.
      (2) Types of abnormal bleeding (Table 22-2)
         (a) Menorrhagia (most common): regular normal intervals between periods that have excessive blood flow and duration of blood flow but with normal intervals between periods
         (b) Hypomenorrhea: decreased bleeding at regular normal intervals
         (c) Metrorrhagia: irregular intervals between periods of excessive blood flow and duration
         (d) Menometrorrhagia: irregular or excessive bleeding during both menstruation as wells between periods
         (e) Oligomenorrhea: menses at intervals that are > days apart
         (f) Polymenorrhea: menses at intervals that are <21 days apart
      (3) Most cases of DUB are postmenarchal (after the first menses) and perimenopausal (most common).
         (a) Perimenopause is the period of time *before* menopause occurs.
         (b) Average age of perimenopause is 47.5 years.
      (4) Overall, ~90% of cases of DUB are anovulatory (no ovulation); the remaining 10% are ovulatory types of DUB.
      (5) During the reproductive ages, 80% are ovulatory types of DUB.
   c. Pathogenesis of anovulatory DUB
      (1) Excessive E stimulation relative to P stimulation of the endometrial mucosa.
      (2) Absent secretory phase of the menstrual cycle
      (3) Excessive E stimulation produces hyperplasia and excessive bleeding.

TABLE 22-2 Categorization of Abnormal Uterine Bleeding and the PALM-COIEN Mnemonic System

TYPE OF BLEEDING	STRUCTURAL CAUSES (PALM)	NONSTRUCTURAL CAUSES (COEIN)
Abnormal uterine bleeding	Polyp	Coagulopathy
Heavy menstrual bleeding	Adenomyosis	Ovulatory dysfunction
Intermenstrual bleeding	Leiomyoma	Endometrial
Postmenopausal bleeding	Malignancy or hyperplasia	Iatrogenic Not yet classified

Structural causes (mnemonic PALM) taken from Mularz A, Dalati S, Pedigo R: *OB/GYN Secrets,* 4th ed, St. Louis, Elsevier, 2017, p 15.

TABLE 22-3   Causes of Abnormal Bleeding by Age

AGE BRACKET	CAUSES OF BLEEDING
Prepubertal	• Vulvovaginitis: poor hygiene, infection (e.g., gonorrhea), sexual abuse, foreign bodies • Embryonal rhabdomyosarcoma
Menarche to 20 yr	• Anovulatory DUB (most common cause) • von Willebrand disease (see Chapter 15)
20–40 yr	• Pregnancy and its complications (most common cause) • Ovulatory types of DUB • PID, hypothyroidism, submucosal leiomyomas, adenomyosis, endometrial polyp, endometriosis
≥40 yr	• Anovulatory DUB (most common cause in perimenopausal period) • Endometrial hyperplasia or cancer (most common cause in menopause)

DUB, Dysfunctional uterine bleeding; *PID,* pelvic inflammatory disease.

    d. Ovulatory types of DUB include inadequate luteal phase (ILP) and irregular shedding of the endometrium (ISE).
      (1) Inadequate luteal phase is caused by inadequate maturation of the corpus luteum, which leads to reduced synthesis of P.
        (a) Delay in the development of the secretory phase
        (b) Inadequate luteal phase has been implicated in infertility, recurrent pregnancy loss, and irregular cycles (<26 days).
        (c) Inadequate luteal phase is documented by decreased serum 17-hydroxyprogesterone (OHP) levels after ovulation.
      (2) ISE is caused by a persistent luteal phase with continued secretion of P. It is characterized by a mixture of proliferative and secretory glands in the menstrual effluent.
    e. Breakthrough bleeding
      (1) **Definition:** Bleeding that occurs between menstrual periods
      (2) Occurs in DUB caused by ISE of the endometrium, women taking OCPs, and uterine leiomyomas (see later)
  6. Causes of abnormal bleeding by age are listed in Table 22-3.
L. Amenorrhea
  1. **Definition:** The absence of menses in a woman of reproductive age
    • Definition of reproductive age varies from 12 to 49 years of age or 15 to 49 years of age (World Health Organization).
  2. Epidemiology
    a. Primary amenorrhea
      (1) **Definition:** Absence of menses by 16 years of age in the presence of normal secondary sexual characteristics (breast development, pubic hair, growth acceleration). However, in the absence of these secondary sexual features by the age of 14 years, the clinician should begin a workup for primary amenorrhea.
      (From Ferri FF: 2017 Ferri's Clinical Advisor, Philadelphia, Elsevier, 2017, p 63.)
      (2) Incidence of primary amenorrhea is <1%.
      (3) Most cases are caused by constitutional; usually a family history of delayed onset of menses.
    b. Secondary amenorrhea
      (1) **Definition:** The absence of menses for >6 months in a patient who has had normal previous P withdrawal cycles
      (From Ferri FF: 2017 Ferri's Clinical Advisor, Philadelphia, Elsevier, 2017, p 63.)
      (2) Incidence of secondary amenorrhea is 5% to 7%.
      (3) Most cases of secondary amenorrhea are caused by pregnancy.
  3. Pathogenesis of amenorrhea
    a. Hypothalamic or pituitary disorder
      (1) Decreased synthesis of FSH and LH
        (a) Results in a decreased synthesis of E and P, respectively
        (b) Called hypogonadotropic (↓FSH and ↓LH) hypogonadism
      (2) *No* withdrawal bleeding after receiving P because the endometrial mucosa is *not* E stimulated
      (3) Examples

Margin notes:

Ovulatory DUB: ILP; ISE

ILP: inadequate maturation corpus luteum → ↓P

ILP: delay development secretory phase

ILP: infertility, recurrent pregnancy loss, irregular cycles

ILP Dx: ↓serum 17-OHP after ovulation

ISE: persistent luteal phase, continued P secretion

Mixture proliferative/secretory glands

Breakthrough bleeding

Bleeding between menstrual periods

DUB due to ISE, OCPs, uterine leiomyomas

Amenorrhea

Absence menses reproductive age

Primary amenorrhea

Absence menses by 16 (normal 2° sex characteristics)

Incidence <1%

MCC 1° amenorrhea constitutional delay

Usually family Hx delayed menses

Secondary amenorrhea

Absence menses >6 mths; Hx normal P withdrawal cycles

Incidence 5% to 7%

MCC pregnancy

Pathogenesis

Hypothalamic or pituitary disorder

↓Synthesis FSH + LH

↓Synthesis E + P, respectively

Called hypogonadotropic hypogonadism

No bleeding *after* receiving P

Hypothalamic/pituitary cause: ↓FSH, LH, E

TABLE 22-4 Differential Diagnosis of Amenorrhea

DISORDER	FSH AND LH	ESTROGEN	EXAMPLES
Hypothalamic or pituitary disorder	↓	↓	Hypopituitarism Anorexia nervosa, prolactinoma
Ovarian disorder	↑	↓	Turner syndrome
End-organ defect	N	N	Imperforate hymen, Asherman syndrome
Constitutional delay	N	N	Family history of delayed onset of menses

FSH, Follicle-stimulating hormone; *LH*, luteinizing hormone; *N*, normal.

Hypopituitarism (no FSH/LH), prolactinoma (↓GnRH)

Anorexia nervosa (↓GnRH)

Ovarian disorder

↓Ovarian synthesis E and P

Corresponding ↑FSH and LH

Hypergonadotropic hypogonadism

No bleeding *after* receiving P

Turner syndrome

Surgical removal ovaries

End-organ defect

Defect prevents egress of blood

Usually a 1° amenorrhea

Normal FSH, LH, E, P

No bleeding after receiving P

Imperforate hymen, RKH syndrome

Removal stratum basalis by excessive curettage

Uterine disorders

Uterine prolapse

Descent uterus into vagina and beyond

Uterosacral/cardinal ligaments relaxed

Cervix sags downwards into vagina

Asymptomatic, vaginal bulge

Entire uterus prolapses

May occur any age

Pregnancies, vaginal birth, myopathy/neuropathy

Endometritis

Infection following delivery/abortion

(a) Hypopituitarism (no synthesis of FSH and LH) and prolactinoma (prolactin inhibits GnRH; see Chapter 23)

(b) Anorexia nervosa (excessive weight loss inhibits the secretion of GnRH; see Chapter 8). Kallmann syndrome (lack of GnRH)

b. Ovarian disorder

  (1) Decreased synthesis of E and P

    (a) Corresponding increase in serum FSH and LH, respectively, because of negative feedback

    (b) Called hypergonadotropic (↑FSH and ↑LH) hypogonadism

  (2) *No* withdrawal bleeding after receiving P because the endometrial mucosa is *not* E-stimulated

  (3) Examples

    (a) Turner syndrome (see Chapter 6)

    (b) Surgical removal of ovaries

c. End-organ (target organ) defect

  (1) Defect that prevents the normal egress of blood in menses; more likely to be a cause of primary amenorrhea

  (2) Normal levels of FSH, LH, E, and P

  (3) *No* withdrawal bleeding after receiving P

  (4) Examples

    (a) Imperforate hymen, Rokitansky-Küster-Hauser (RKH) syndrome (see previous discussion)

    (b) Asherman syndrome is the development of intrauterine adhesions because of trauma (e.g., repeated endometrial curettage).

d. A summary of the differential diagnosis of amenorrhea is listed in Table 22-4 and Link 22-69.

VII. Uterine Disorders

  A. Uterine (pelvic organ) prolapse

    1. **Definition:** Descent of the uterus into the vagina and beyond (Link 22-70).
(From Mularz A, Dalati S, Pedigo R: OB/GYN Secrets, 4th ed, St. Louis, Elsevier, 2017, p 79, #4.)

    2. Epidemiology and clinical

      a. Descent of the uterus occurs when the supporting structures (e.g., uterosacral ligaments and the cardinal ligaments) relax and allow the relationship between the uterus and the vaginal axis to be altered. This allows the cervix to sag downward into the vagina.

      b. Some women are asymptomatic, but others complain of feeling a vaginal "bulge" or pelvic pressure. Symptoms worsen with the length of time the woman is standing. Heavy lifting and straining also exacerbate symptoms.

      c. In some cases, the entire uterus prolapses (called *procidentia*).

      d. May occur at any age

      e. Predisposing causes include congenital defects, trauma during childbirth, and multiple deliveries.

      f. Classified as first, second, and third degree according to the level to which the uterus has descended. It is one of the most common reasons for hysterectomy.

  B. Endometritis

    1. **Definition**: An infection of the endometrial mucosa; usually follows delivery or abortion

    2. Epidemiology

a. Rate of postpartum endometritis is 1% to 8%.
b. Most common genital tract infection after delivery
c. More common in preterm deliveries than in term deliveries
3. Acute endometritis
   a. **Definition:** Acute inflammation (AI) of the endometrial mucosa
   b. Epidemiology
      (1) Most often caused by a bacterial infection after a delivery, miscarriage, prolonged labor, or cesarean section (greatest risk factor for the development of postpartum endometritis)

Clostridium perfringens is isolated from the genital tracts of 1% to 10% of healthy women. Before legalization of elective abortion in the United States, *C. perfringens* was isolated in ~25% after abortion in whom uterine infection was suspected and cultures were taken.

      (2) Multiple pathogens are usually involved in the infection.
         (a) Group B streptococcus *(Streptococcus agalactiae)* is a common pathogen.
         (b) Other pathogens include group A streptococcus, *Staphylococcus aureus, Bacteroides fragilis, C. trachomatis, N. gonorrhoeae,* and *E. coli.*
   c. Clinical findings include fever, abdominal pain with uterine tenderness to palpation, and the presence of a purulent or foul vaginal discharge (called *lochia*).
4. Chronic endometritis
   a. **Definition:** Chronic inflammation of the endometrial mucosa (plasma cells are the key finding)
   b. Causes chronic endometritis
      (1) Retained placenta
      (2) *N. gonorrhoeae*
      (3) Intrauterine device (IUD) associated with an *Actinomyces israelii* infection with the classic sulfur granules (Link 22-71)
   c. A key histologic finding is the presence of plasma cells in a biopsy (Link 22-72).
C. **Adenomyosis**
   1. **Definition:** Chronic condition characterized by invagination of the stratum basalis of the endometrial mucosa into the underlying myometrium, causing abnormal uterine bleeding and dysmenorrhea
   2. Epidemiology
      a. Glands and stroma thicken the myometrial tissue (Fig. 22-11 A; Link 22-73)
      b. Enlarged globular uterus
      c. Highest incidence occurs in women in the mid to late 40s.
      d. Common finding in hysterectomy specimens.
   3. Clinical findings in adenomyosis include menorrhagia, dysmenorrhea, and pelvic pain.
   4. Definitive diagnosis is secured with a myometrial biopsy. Magnetic resonance imaging (MRI) shows a thickened junctional zone (interface between the endometrium and myometrium). High-resolution ultrasonography can also identify this junction.
D. **Endometriosis**
   1. **Definition:** Chronic inflammatory condition in which functioning glands and stroma are located *outside* the confines of the uterus (Link 22-74)
   2. Epidemiology
      a. Cyclic bleeding of gland and stromal implants wherever they are located
      b. Prevalence is highest in women with dysmenorrhea (40%–60% of cases).
      c. Average age at the time of diagnosis is 25 to 29 years old.
      d. Multifactorial inheritance has been implicated (see Chapter 6). There is a 7% occurrence rate in first-degree female relatives.
      e. Pathogenesis
         (1) Reverse menses theory, whereby endometrial tissue enters the fallopian tubes (most common), with implantation of viable endometrial cells in fallopian tube and various locations in the abdominal cavity (e.g., intestines) and pelvic cavity (e.g., ovaries)
         (2) Coelomic metaplasia theory, in which serosal cells in the peritoneal cavity develop into functioning endometrial tissue

MC genital infection following delivery

Acute endometritis: uterine infection following delivery or abortion

Acute endometritis

AI endometrial mucosa

Bacterial infection p. delivery/miscarriage/prolonged labor/C-section

Group B streptococcus (*S. agalactiae*) is common pathogen

Acute endometritis: fever, uterine pain, discharge

Chronic endometritis

Chronic inflammation endometrial mucosa (plasma cells)

Retained placenta

N. gonorrhoeae

IUD; Actinomyces israelii

Chronic endometritis: plasma cells in biopsy

Adenomyosis

Functioning endometrial mucosa in myometrium

Glands/stroma thicken myometrium

Enlarged globular uterus

Women mid to late 40s

Menorrhagia, dysmenorrhea, pelvic pain

Myometrial biopsy; MRI junctional zone

Endometriosis

Functioning glands/stroma outside uterus

Endometriosis: functioning glands/stroma outside confines of uterus

↑Prevalence women with dysmenorrhea

25 to 29 yrs old

Multifactorial inheritance

Reverse menses theory

Coelomic metaplasia theory

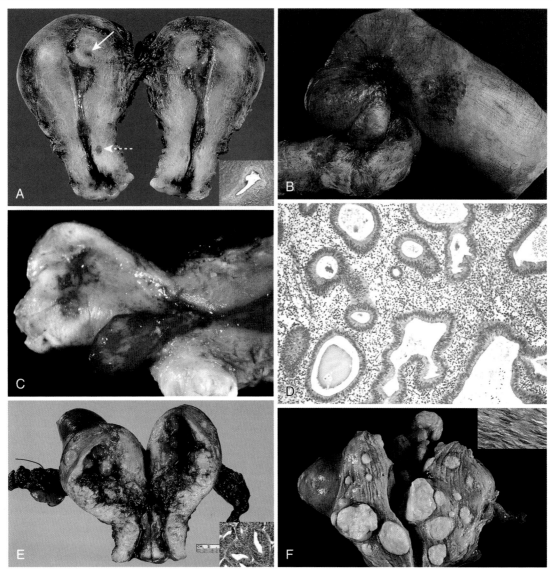

22-11: **A,** Adenomyosis. The *solid arrow* shows an area of hemorrhage surrounded by irregularly thickened endometrial stroma. The *interrupted arrow* shows a nabothian cyst in the endocervical canal. The microscopic section shows an endometrial gland and stroma in the myometrium. **B,** Endometriosis implants on a loop of intestine. Note that the serosal surface has multiple areas of hemorrhage with a "powder burn" appearance. **C,** Endometrial polyp. Note the hemorrhagic polyp arising from the endometrial mucosa. It is a common cause of uterine bleeding. **D,** Simple hyperplasia of endometrial glands showing cystic dilation and focal areas of glandular outpouching. There is no gland crowding or stratification of the epithelial lining. **E,** Endometrial carcinoma showing necrotic tumor filling the uterine cavity and extending completely through the uterine wall and into the endocervical canal. Snippet in right lower quadrant is a well-differentiated adenocarcinoma with crowding of the glands and hyperchromatic nuclei. **F,** Leiomyomas. In sagittal section, multiple well-circumscribed, gray-white nodules (leiomyomas) are dispersed throughout the myometrium. Submucosal leiomyomas are a common cause of uterine bleeding. Snippet in the *right upper corner* shows elongated spindle-shaped smooth muscle cells. *(A and E from Rosai J, Ackerman LV:* Surgical Pathology, *9th ed, St. Louis, Mosby, 2004, pp 1578, 1586, respectively, Figs. 19-123, 19-136B, respectively.* **Snippet in corner of A and E** *from Rosai J, Ackerman LV:* Surgical Pathology, *10th ed, St. Louis, Mosby, 2011, p 1485, Fig. 19.124, 137A, respectively;* **B** *and* **F** *from my friend Ivan Damjanov, MD, PhD, Linder J:* Pathology: A Color Atlas, *St. Louis, Mosby, 2000, pp 126, 277, respectively, Figs. 7-77, 13-49, respectively.* **Snippet in right upper corner of F** *from Rosai J:* Rosai and Ackerman's Surgical Pathology, *10th ed, St. Louis, Mosby Elsevier, 2011, p 1509, Fig. 19.169;* **C** *and* **D** *from Kumar V, Fausto N, Abbas A:* Robbins and Cotran Pathologic Basis of Disease, *7th ed, Philadelphia, Saunders, 2004, pp 1082, 1086, respectively, Figs. 22-27C, 22-31A, respectively.)*

Vascular/lymphatic spread theory

Induction theory

Hormonal/immunologic/inflammatory factors stimulate differentiation into endometrial tissue

Ovaries MC site of implantation

(3) Vascular or lymphatic spread theory
(4) Induction theory in which certain hormonal, immunologic, or inflammatory factors stimulate differentiation into endometrial tissue or allow ectopic endometrial cells to implant and proliferate; caused by activated macrophages (MPs) releasing proinflammatory cytokines (interleukins 6 and 8 and tumor necrosis factor-α)

3. Common sites of endometriosis include the ovaries (most common site; Link 22-75), rectal pouch, fallopian tubes, and intestine.

The **rectal pouch of Douglas** is anterior to the rectum and posterior to the uterus. It is the most dependent portion of the female pelvis and can be palpated by digital rectal examination. It is a common site to collect blood (e.g., ruptured tubal pregnancy), malignant cells (e.g., seeding by ovarian cancer), endometrial implants, and pus (e.g., pelvic inflammatory disease [PID]).

4. Clinical findings
   a. Dysmenorrhea (most common finding)
   b. Abnormal bleeding, including premenstrual spotting and menorrhagia
   c. Painful stooling during menses. Bleeding implants on the rectal serosa in the pouch of Douglas are stretched with stooling.
   d. Intestinal obstruction and intestinal bleeding during menses
   e. Increased risk for an ectopic pregnancy because of scarring of fallopian tubes by implants
   f. Infertility caused by implants on the ovaries or fallopian tubes; dyspareunia (painful intercourse)
   g. Enlargement of the ovaries caused by blood-filled cysts
   h. Endometriosis triad: dysmenorrhea, dyspareunia, and infertility
5. Diagnosis
   a. Laparoscopy is useful for both diagnosis and treatment. Implants have a "powder burn" appearance (Fig. 22-11 B).
   b. Increase in serum cancer antigen 125 (CA125)
      (1) Excellent sensitivity but poor specificity (increased false-positive results)
      (2) CA125 is also a cancer antigen that is increased in surface-derived ovarian cancers and other gynecologic disorders, hence the increase in false positives
      (3) More useful in excluding endometriosis when negative

E. **Endometrial polyp** (Fig. 22-11 C)
   1. **Definition:** Benign polyp in the uterine cavity that enlarges with E stimulation
   2. Epidemiology
      a. Does *not* develop into an endometrial carcinoma
      b. Can protrude through the cervix into the vagina
   3. Clinical findings
      a. Common cause of menorrhagia in the 20- to 40-year-old age bracket
      b. Spotting occurs between menstrual periods or after menopause.
      c. Malignancy in 3.6%
   4. Diagnosis: vaginal ultrasound or MRI, dilation and curettage (D&C)

F. **Endometrial hyperplasia**
   1. **Definition:** Abnormal proliferation of E-stimulated endometrial glands and stroma from exogenous or endogenous sources (Link 22-76)
   2. Epidemiology
      a. Risk factors
         (1) Early menarche or late menopause (both increase the amount of time available for E stimulation)
         (2) Nulliparity
         (3) Obesity, DM. Adipose cells contain aromatase, which converts androgens to E.
         (4) PCOS
         (5) Taking E *without* P
         (6) Anovulatory menstrual cycles.
         (7) Tamoxifen use
         (8) Hereditary nonpolyposis colorectal cancer (HNPCC, Lynch syndrome; see Chapter 9)
      b. Classification
         (1) Simple hyperplasia (Fig. 22-11 D; Link 22-77 A)
            (a) Increased number of cystically dilated glands
            (b) Absence of glandular crowding
         (2) Complex hyperplasia
            (a) Increased number of dilated glands with branching
            (b) Glandular crowding is present with less intervening stromal tissue.
         (3) Atypical complex hyperplasia (Link 22-77 B)
            (a) Glandular crowding and dysplastic epithelial cells line the glands.
            (b) Greatest risk for progressing into endometrial cancer (42% of cases)

Rectal pouch of Douglas: site for collection of blood, malignant cells, pus, endometrial implants

Dysmenorrhea MC

Premenstrual spotting, menorrhagia

Painful stooling during menses

Intestinal obstruction during menses

Ectopic pregnancy

Infertility

Dyspareunia

Enlarged ovaries (cysts)

Triad: dysmenorrhea, dyspareunia, infertility

Laparoscopy useful for Dx/Rx

↑CA125

Endometrial polyp

Benign polyp enlarges with E stimulation

No transformation to cancer

Protrude thru cervix into vagina

Common cause menorrhagia 20 to 40

Spotting between periods, after menopause

Malignancy 3.6%

Vaginal ultrasound/MRI

D&C

Endometrial hyperplasia

Abnormal E stimulated gland/stroma

Early menarche/late menopause

Nulliparity

Obesity, DM

Adipose contains aromatase (androgens → E

PCOS

Taking E without P

Anovulatory cycles

Tamoxifen use

HNPCC

Simple hyperplasia

Cystically dilated glands

No glandular crowding

Complex hyperplasia

Dilated glands/branching

Glandular crowding

Atypical hyperplasia

Glandular crowding, dysplastic epithelium

↑↑Risk endometrial carcinoma

Meno-, metro-, menometrorrhagia

Postmenopausal bleeding

Endometrial biopsy

Malignancy glands (MC) and/or stroma

2ⁿᵈ MC gynecologic cancer

2ⁿᵈ MC gynecologic cancer causing death

Median age 60 years

Prolonged E stimulation

OCPs ↓risk (progestins)

Types endometrial cancer

Well-differentiated adeno MC type

Adenoacanthoma: adenocarcinoma with foci benign squamous tissue

Adeno + SCC

Papillary adenocarcinoma is aggressive

Cancer characteristics

Down into endocervix

Out into uterine wall

Lungs MC site for metastasis

Postmenopausal bleeding MC

Dx endometrial Bx

Uterine leiomyoma

Benign monoclonal SMT

Leiomyoma: MC benign connective tissue tumor in women; blacks > whites

Somatic mutation monoclonal myometrial cell line

More sensitive to E than P

MC overall benign tumor; regress menopause

Women >30 yrs old

Blacks > whites

E sensitive; enlarge in pregnancy

Commonly degenerate, calcify, hyalinize

Single/multiple

Submucosal, intramural, subserosal

Menorrhagia

Obstructive delivery

Menstrual cramping

Pressure on colon (constipation)

Pressure on bladder

Dx ultrasound/MRI

3. Clinical findings
   a. Menorrhagia, metrorrhagia, and menometrorrhagia
   b. Postmenopausal bleeding
4. Diagnosis secured by endometrial biopsy

G. **Endometrial carcinoma**
   1. **Definition:** A malignancy arising from endometrial glands (MC), stroma (adenocarcinoma), or both (Link 22-78)
   2. Epidemiology and pathogenesis
      a. Most common gynecologic cancer in the United States (ovarian cancer is second) and second most common gynecologic cancer causing death
      b. Median age at onset is 60 years old
      c. Pathogenesis is prolonged E stimulation; same risk factors as endometrial hyperplasia
      d. OCPs decrease risk because of to the anti-E effect of progestins. **Note:** There is a slightly increased risk for developing breast cancer with OCPs because E also has a role in the stimulating ductal epithelial cells.
      e. Types of endometrial cancer
         (1) Well-differentiated endometrial adenocarcinoma (adeno; Link 22-79).
            (a) Most common type of endometrial carcinoma
            (b) Adenoacanthoma: cancer that contains foci of benign squamous tissue, the latter having *no* prognostic significance
            (c) Adenosquamous carcinoma: cancer that contains foci of malignant SCC and has a worse prognosis than endometrial adenocarcinoma alone
         (2) Papillary adenocarcinoma is a highly aggressive endometrial cancer. Papillary means that the cancer has a branching pattern.
      f. Cancer characteristics (Link 22-78)
         (1) Spreads down into the endocervix
         (2) Spreads out into the uterine wall (Fig. 22-11 E)
         (3) Lungs are the most common site of metastasis.
   3. Clinical findings: postmenopausal bleeding occurs in 90% of cases
   4. Diagnosis secured by endometrial biopsy

H. **Uterine leiomyoma (fibroids)**
   1. **Definition:** Benign monoclonal smooth muscle tumor (SMT; Fig. 22-11 F; Link 22-80).
   2. Epidemiology
      a. Pathogenesis: somatic mutation of a monoclonal myometrial cell line. Factors initiating mutation include intrinsic abnormalities of myometrium, congenital increase in E receptors in myometrium, hormonal changes, and ischemic injury at the time of menses. Leiomyomas contain E and P receptors and are most sensitive to E. Factors increasing overall lifetime exposure to E (e.g., obesity, early menarche) increase their incidence.
      b. Most common overall benign tumor in women of reproductive age. They regress after menopause because of a reduction in E.
      c. Occurs in 20% to 50% of women >30 years old; more common in blacks than whites
      d. E-sensitive tumor and may become larger during pregnancy
      e. Commonly undergo degeneration, dystrophic calcification (calcification of damaged tissue), and hyalinization (resembling glass); may be single or multiple
      f. Locations: submucosal (may prolapse into cervix), intramural, and subserosal (Links 22-81 and 22-82)
   3. Clinical findings
      a. When they are located in the submucosa, they can ulcerate and bleed very severely, leading to menorrhagia (excessive bleeding).
      b. *Not* a major cause of infertility (2%–3%)
      c. Pregnancy: Cause of an obstructive delivery. Increased risk preterm delivery, placenta previa (see later), postpartum hemorrhage, and C-section. Unpredictable effect on growth of leiomyomas. Degeneration of leiomyomas during pregnancy may cause acute pain.
      d. Cramping during menses; pressure on colon may produce constipation
      e. Pressure on the bladder may increase frequency (frequent urination), urgency (sense of having to urinate), and incontinence (see Chapter 21).
   4. Diagnosis is made using transabdominal or transvaginal ultrasound or MRI.

I. **Uterine leiomyosarcoma**
   1. **Definition:** Malignancy (sarcoma) of smooth muscle in the myometrium. Recall that sarcomas are malignancies of connective tissue, which is derived from the mesoderm (see Chapter 9).
   2. Epidemiology
      a. Most common sarcoma of the uterus
      b. Unlike leiomyomas, which are benign SMTs, leiomyosarcomas have numerous atypical mitoses and foci of necrosis, key features that differentiate them from leiomyomas.
J. **Carcinosarcoma (malignant müllerian tumors)**
   1. **Definition:** Combination of an adenocarcinoma and a malignant mesenchymal (stromal) tumor
   2. Epidemiology
      a. Primarily occur in postmenopausal women
      b. Bulky, necrotic tumors that often protrude through the cervical os
      c. Mesenchymal component in stroma may include muscle, cartilage, and bone.
      d. Strong association with previous irradiation; poor prognosis
VIII. **Fallopian Tube Disorders**
   A. **Hydatid cysts of Morgagni**
      1. **Definition:** Benign cystic müllerian remnants most often located around the fimbriated end of the fallopian tube
      2. Epidemiology: may undergo torsion (>25% of cases), causing abdominal pain that could be misdiagnosed as acute appendicitis if located on the right side or acute diverticulitis if located on the left side
   B. **Pelvic inflammatory disease (PID)**
      1. **Definition:** Polymicrobial infection that involves the upper genital tract, including the endometrial mucosa (endometritis), fallopian tub (salpingitis), ovary (oophoritis, tuboovarian abscess), and peritoneum (peritonitis) if pus spills into the peritoneal cavity
      2. Epidemiology
         a. Diagnosed in 2% to 5% of women in STD clinics
         b. Most common cause of female infertility and ectopic pregnancy because of scar tissue formation
         c. Risk factors
            (1) Young age; multiple sexual partners; high-risk sexual partners (men with gonorrhea or *Chlamydia* infections); bacterial vaginosis
            (2) Previous episodes of PID; damaged fallopian tubes increase the risk; unprotected sex
         d. Most but *not* all cases of PID are STDs.
         e. Causes
            (1) Most often caused by *N. gonorrhoeae* or *C. trachomatis*
            (2) Coexisting infection in 45% of cases (both pathogens), which is why antibiotic therapy is given to treat both organisms
            (3) Other nonsexually transmitted pathogens: *B. fragilis*, streptococci, *C. perfringens*, *Mycobacterium tuberculosis*, and cytomegalovirus (CMV)
         f. Spread of PID (Link 22-83)
      3. Gross findings
         g. Fallopian tubes are filled with pus (Fig. 22-12 A)
         h. Resolution of the infection commonly leads to hydrosalpinx (Link 22-84). As pus resorbs, clear fluid is left behind, causing distention of the fallopian tubes.
      4. Clinical findings
         a. May be asymptomatic
         b. Fever usually >38.3°C (101°F)
         c. Lower abdominal pain, pain with cervical motion ("chandelier sign") and palpation of the adnexa and uterus during pelvic examination, and pain in the right upper quadrant (RUQ; 5% of cases). RUQ pain is a perihepatitis. Perihepatitis is caused by pus from the fallopian tube collecting underneath the diaphragm of the liver, which later develops fibrous tissue strands between the surface of the liver and diaphragm, causing pain with movement (called the Fitz-Hughes–Curtis syndrome; see Table 22-1; Link 22-85).
         d. Abnormal uterine bleeding; vaginal discharge and mucopurulent discharge in the cervical os
      5. Diagnosis
         a. Cervical motion tenderness and adnexal tenderness on pelvic examination
         b. Culture or polymerase chain reaction (PCR) of cervical discharge for *N. gonorrhoeae* and *C. trachomatis*
         c. Laparoscopy, transvaginal ultrasound, MRI (best sensitivity and specificity)

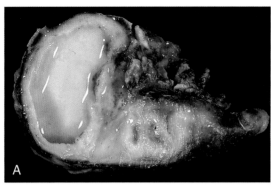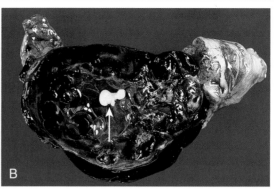

22-12: A, Pelvic inflammatory disease. Note the pus filling the lumen of the fallopian tube. **B,** Ruptured ectopic tubal pregnancy showing marked hemorrhage (hematosalpinx) and an embryo *(arrow)* in the center of the clot material. *(A and B from Rosai J, Ackerman LV:* Surgical Pathology, *9th ed, St. Louis, Mosby, 2004, pp 1638, 1639, respectively, Figs. 19-192B, 19-198, respectively.)*

↑ESR/CRP
WBCs saline microscopy
Gram stain WBCs with G– diplococci
Salpingitis isthmica nodosa
SIN: tubal diverticulosis
Nodules narrow lumen
?Postinfectious reaction to previous STD
Infertility, ectopic pregnancy
Hysterosalpingography shows "beading appearance"
Ectopic pregnancy
Embryo implants outside uterine cavity (usually fallopian tube)
1% to 2% pregnancies
MCC pregnancy-related maternal death 1st trimester
Ectopic pregnancy: MCC is previous PID
MCC scarring previous PID
Endometriosis → scarring of fallopian tube
Altered tubal motility (OCPs)
Previous SIN
IUD, smoking (ciliary dysmotility [fallopian tubes])
Previous tubal ligation
Majority ectopic pregnancies implant in fallopian tube
MC site ampullary portion below fimbriae
Interstitial part fallopian tube, abdominal cavity
Heterotopic pregnancy: coexistence IUP + ectopic pregnancy
Abdominal pain and/or vaginal bleeding
Immediately order pregnancy test
Negative test excludes ectopic pregnancy
Positive test: further studies
Adnexal tenderness
Peritoneal signs rebound tenderness
Hypovolemic shock
Classic triad: vaginal bleeding, adnexal pain, adnexal mass
Complications of ectopic pregnancy
Rupture FP → IAD → shock
MC COD early pregnancy

d. Increased erythrocyte sedimentation rate (ESR) and C-reactive protein (CRP)
e. White blood cells (WBCs) on saline microscopy of exudate (absence eliminates PID); gram stain showing WBCs with gram-negative diplococci (Link 22-83 inset)

C. **Salpingitis isthmica nodosa (SIN)**
1. **Definition:** Invagination of the fallopian tube mucosa into the muscle ("tubal diverticulosis")
2. Epidemiology
   a. Produces nodules in the tube that narrow the lumen
   b. Probably a postinfectious reaction to a previous infection (e.g., *C. trachomatis* or *N. gonorrhoeae* infection)
3. Complications include infertility and ectopic pregnancy.
4. Diagnosis is made by hysterosalpingography, which shows a "beading appearance" in the areas of constriction.

D. **Ectopic pregnancy**
1. **Definition:** Embryo implants outside the uterine cavity, usually in the fallopian tube or rarely in other sites (e.g., abdominal cavity)
2. Epidemiology
   a. Occurs in 1% to 2% of pregnancies
   b. MCC of pregnancy-related maternal death in the first trimester; accounts for 13% of maternal deaths
   c. Risk factors
      (1) Scarring from previous PID (most common cause)
      (2) Endometriosis with scarring of the fallopian tube
      (3) Altered tubal motility (OCPs)
      (4) SIN
      (5) IUD, smoking (causes ciliary dysmotility in fallopian tubes); previous tubal ligation
   d. Sites of implantation of an ectopic pregnancy
      (1) Majority (97.7%) occur within the fallopian tube (Fig. 22-12 B; Link 22-86). Most ectopic pregnancies are located in the broad ampullary portion below the fimbriae (>80%), isthmus of tube (12%), and fimbrial region (5%).
      (2) Less common sites include the interstitial part of the fallopian tube (2.3% pregnancies [part of the fallopian tube that penetrates the muscular layer of the uterus]) and abdominal cavity.
      (3) Heterotopic pregnancy: coexistence of an intrauterine pregnancy (IUP) and ectopic pregnancy; occurs in 1 in 4000 pregnancies
3. Clinical findings
   a. Two key findings: abdominal pain or tenderness (95% cases) or vaginal bleeding (75% of cases) that occurs ~6 weeks after a previous normal menstrual period
   b. Always order a pregnancy test (detects levels of hCG as low as 20 mIU/mL). Negative pregnancy test excludes an ectopic pregnancy. A positive test requires additional evaluation.
   c. Adnexal tenderness (87%–99% of cases); peritoneal signs of rebound tenderness (>70% of cases)
   d. Hypovolemic shock from intraperitoneal bleeding (2%–17% of cases)
   e. Classic triad for an ectopic pregnancy is vaginal bleeding, adnexal pain, and adnexal mass.
4. Complications of ectopic pregnancy
   a. Rupture of fallopian tube with intraabdominal bleed (IAD), leading to hypovolemic shock; most common cause of death in early pregnancy

TABLE 22-5   Differential Diagnosis of Adnexal Masses

BENIGN	MALIGNANT
Physiologic (Functional) Ovarian Cysts • Follicular cyst • Corpus luteum cyst • Theca lutein cyst	**Ovarian Malignancies** • Epithelial cell • Sex cord stromal cell • Germ cell
Nonfunctional Ovarian Cysts • Endometrioma (endometriosis implant) • Polycystic ovaries	**Fallopian Tube Cancer** • Nongynecologic cancers • Gastrointestinal tumors • Lymphoma • Other metastases
Benign Ovarian Neoplasms • Mature cystic teratoma • Fibroma, adenofibroma, cystadenofibroma • Serous cystadenoma, mucinous cystadenoma • Brenner tumor	
Fallopian Tube Origin • Ectopic pregnancy • Paratubal cyst • Hydrosalpinx, hematosalpinx • Tubo-ovarian abscess	
Nonadnexal • Diverticulitis • Appendiceal abscess • Pelvic kidney • Leiomyomas	

Taken from Mularz A, Dalati S, Pedigo R: *OB/GYN Secrets,* 4th ed, St. Louis, Elsevier, 2017, p 65, Table 15-1.

b. Hematosalpinx (blood in the fallopian tube). Ectopic pregnancy is the most common cause of this complication.

5. Diagnosis

c. Urine screen for β-human chorionic gonadotropin (β-hCG) test is the best screening test. Usually sensitive enough to detect an ectopic pregnancy. The serum test is used if the urine screen result is negative. A positive test result does not prove that an ectopic pregnancy is present, only that the patient is pregnant.

d. Vaginal ultrasound is the confirmatory test. Yolk sac or fetal pole has a 100% predictive value for ectopic pregnancy.

e. Laparoscopy is used in equivocal cases.

IX. Differential Diagnosis of Adnexal Masses (Table 22-5)

The patient's age and menstrual status are most important when evaluating adnexal structures (fallopian tubes, ovaries). If a woman is menstruating regularly, adnexal structures are usually physiologic findings in the ovaries (follicular cysts, corpus luteum, theca lutein cysts). Malignant adnexal masses are usually found in women >45 years old. Exceptions to this rule are germ cell and sex-cord stromal tumors (discussed later), which occur in both younger women and postmenopausal women.

X. Ovarian Disorders

A. Follicular cyst

1. **Definition:** Accumulation of fluid in a follicle or a previously ruptured follicle
2. Epidemiology
   a. Most common ovarian mass
   b. Non-neoplastic cyst (e.g., follicular cyst; Link 22-87)
   c. Rupture of the cyst produces a sterile peritonitis with pain.
   d. Most follicular cysts spontaneously regress.
3. Ultrasound is the best screening test.

B. Corpus luteum cyst

1. **Definition:** An accumulation of fluid in the corpus luteum during pregnancy
2. Epidemiology
   a. Most common ovarian mass in pregnancy
   b. Non-neoplastic cyst (Link 22-88)
   c. May be confused with an amniotic sac on ultrasound
   d. Most corpus luteum cysts regress spontaneously.

C. Oophoritis

1. **Definition:** Inflammation of one or both ovaries
2. Epidemiology: may be a complication of mumps or PID

Marginal notes:

Ectopic pregnancy MCC hematosalpinx (blood in tube)

Urine hCG best screen

Vaginal ultrasound confirmatory test; detects yolk sac or fetal pole

Laparoscopy equivocal cases

Ovarian disorders
Follicular cyst
Fluid in follicle/previously ruptured follicle
MC ovarian mass
Non-neoplastic cyst
Rupture → sterile peritonitis/pain
Most regress spontaneously
Ultrasound best screening test
Corpus luteum cyst: MC ovarian mass in pregnancy; nonneoplastic
Accumulation fluid in corpus luteum during pregnancy
MC ovarian mass in pregnancy
Non-neoplastic cyst
Often confused with amniotic sac on ultrasound
Most regress spontaneously
Oophoritis: complication of mumps or PID
Inflammation one/both ovaries
Complication mumps, PID

D. **Stromal hyperthecosis**
  1. **Definition:** A hypercellular ovarian stroma
  2. Epidemiology
     a. Primarily occurs in obese postmenopausal women (sixth or seventh decades of life)
     b. Causes bilateral ovarian enlargement
     c. Within the hypercellular ovarian stroma are vacuolated (luteinized) stromal hilar cells that synthesize excess androgens; may cause hirsutism or virilization
  3. Clinical findings
     a. Hirsutism or virilization
     b. Association with acanthosis nigricans (see Chapter 25), insulin resistance (see Chapter 23), and PCOS
     c. Hypertension (?cause)

E. **Ovarian torsion**
  1. **Definition:** A rotation of the adnexa on its fibrovascular pedicle, compromising the blood flow and leading, in some cases, to infarction of the tube or ovary
  2. Epidemiology and clinical
     a. Fifth most common surgical gynecologic emergency
     b. Two clinical settings
        (1) In infants and children, the twisted ovary is usually normal (no cysts or tumor).
        (2) In adults, the ovary usually has a cyst or a tumor (benign or malignant).
     c. In adults, it presents as acute abdominal pain simulating acute appendicitis along with nausea and vomiting. Pelvic mass may be palpable. Right adnexa is more frequently involved than the left. Intermittent pain occurs in chronic torsions.
     d. Grossly, the ovary is usually enlarged dark red (Link 22-89). The cut surface shows blood and edema fluid. Hemorrhagic coagulation necrosis is present on histologic exam.

F. **Ovarian tumors**
  1. **Definition:** An ovarian mass that may be benign or malignant, unilateral or bilateral, and may secrete androgens or estrogen (E)
  2. Epidemiology
     a. Tumors are more likely benign in women <45 years of age. Risk for developing ovarian tumors increases with age.
     b. Median age of presentation is 61 years. Incidence peaks in women in their late 70s.
     c. Ranks first for cancer-deaths related to gynecologic disease; ranks fifth for all cancer deaths in women
     d. Risk factors
        (1) Nulliparity (a woman has never given birth to a child or has never been pregnant)
        (2) Greater the number of ovulatory cycles, the greater the risk for developing a surface-derived ovarian tumors (see later)
        (3) Hereditary factors (Link 22-90)
           (a) Inactivation of the BRCA1 and BRCA2 suppressor genes (serous carcinomas; see Chapter 9)
           (b) Li-Fraumeni syndrome (teratoma; see Chapter 9)
           (c) Turner syndrome (see Chapter 6): increased risk for developing a dysgerminoma
           (d) Peutz-Jeghers syndrome (PJS; see Chapter 18): increased incidence of ovarian sex cord tumors
        (4) History of breast cancer or postmenopause E therapy
        (5) Obesity (increased E)
     e. OCPs and pregnancy decrease the risk for surface-derived ovarian cancers (see later) because the patient has experienced a decreased number of ovulatory cycles.
     f. Typical stage of presentation of ovarian cancer. Approximately 60% of malignant ovarian tumors present with distant disease (cancer has metastasized), 15% are localized (confined to the primary site), 19% are regional (spread to the regional lymph nodes), and 6% are unknown.
  3. Classification of ovarian tumors (Table 22-6; Fig. 22-13)
     a. Surface-derived tumors (epithelial; Links 22-91, 22-92, 22-93, 22-94, and 22-95)
        (1) Account for 70% of all ovarian tumors
        (2) Derive from the coelomic epithelium. The coelomic epithelium is the outermost layer of the male and female gonads; as such, it is important in forming the germinal epithelium in males and females.
        (3) Account for the greatest number of malignant ovarian tumors

TABLE 22-6   Classification of Ovarian Tumors

TUMOR	CHARACTERISTICS
SURFACE (COELOMIC EPITHELIUM)-DERIVED TUMORS (70% OF ALL OVARIAN TUMORS)	
Serous tumors (see Fig. 22-14; Links 22-91 and 22-92)	• Most common group of primary benign and malignant tumors (40% of surface-derived tumors) • Most common group of tumors that can be bilateral • Cysts are lined by ciliated cells (similar to the fallopian tube) • Serous cystadenoma: most common benign ovarian tumor. Some are classified as borderline malignancy. • Serous cystadenocarcinoma: malignant; has psammoma bodies (dystrophically calcified tumor cells); most common malignant tumor that is bilateral
Mucinous tumors (Links 22-93 and 22-94)	• Cysts are lined by mucus-secreting cells (similar to the endocervix); account for 10%–15% of surface-derived ovarian tumors • Large, multiloculated tumors • Seeding may produce pseudomyxoma peritonei (Link 22-94); most common primary site for pseudomyxoma peritonei is not mucinous tumors of the ovary but mucinous tumors of the appendix • Mucinous cystadenoma: benign; may be associated with Brenner tumor • Mucinous cystadenocarcinoma: malignant
Endometrioid	• Accounts for 15% of ovarian tumors; commonly associated with endometrial carcinoma (15%–30% of surface-derived cancers); histology of the cancer resembles endometrial carcinoma • Commonly bilateral
Brenner tumor (Link 22-95)	• Accounts for 1% of ovarian tumors • Usually benign • Contain Walthard cell rests (urothelial-like epithelium)
Other surface-derived tumors	• Clear cell carcinoma (6% of surface-derived ovarian tumors) • Undifferentiated (1% of surface-derived ovarian tumors)
GERM CELL TUMORS (15% OF ALL OVARIAN TUMORS)	
Cystic teratoma (see Figs. 9-1 C and 22-14C; Links 22-96, 22-97, and 22-98)	• Account for 20% of germ cell tumors; most are benign; rarely bilateral (<5% of cases); <1% become malignant (usually cell carcinoma) • Most common benign germ cell tumor; arise from three germ cell layers: ectodermal (e.g., hair), mesodermal (e.g., muscle), and endodermal tissues (e.g., thyroid) • Ectodermal differentiation (hair, sebaceous glands, teeth) is the most prominent component. • Most of the above derivatives are found in a nipple-like structure in the cyst wall called a Rokitansky tubercle. • Immature malignant types contain mature and immature components (e.g., muscle, neuroepithelium). Histologic grade is determined by the quantity of immature neural tissue. • Struma ovarii type has functioning thyroid tissue and will take up radioactive iodine-123 (Link 22-98). • Struma carcinoid of the ovary is an unusual form of ovarian teratoma composed of an intimate mixture of thyroid and carcinoid tissues. A small number of patients exhibit clinical signs of androgen production with virilism. *No* patients have carcinoid syndrome. When confined to the ovary, struma carcinoid is almost always benign.
Dysgerminoma	• Most common malignant germ cell tumor (~50%) • Same histologic appearance as a seminoma of the testis (see Fig. 21-3 G) • Associated with the streak gonads of Turner syndrome • Characteristic increase in serum LDH
Yolk sac tumor (endodermal sinus tumor) (Link 22-99)	• Second most common germ cell tumor (25%) • Malignant tumor (similar to yolk sac tumor in males) • Only 5% are bilateral • Most common ovarian cancer in girls <4 yr old. However, the average age of occurrence of the tumor is 23 yr old. • Contain Schiller-Duval bodies (resemble yolk sac)
Mixed germ cell tumors	• Increased serum AFP in the majority of cases • Mixed germ cell tumors account for 8% of germ cell tumors. • Mixed germ cell tumors include at least two different malignant germ cell tumors. Most common combination is a dysgerminoma with an endodermal sinus tumor.
Embryonal carcinoma	• Embryonal carcinoma is usually a component of a mixed germ cell tumor. • Rare and aggressive when present • May secrete estrogen and be associated with precocious puberty or irregular bleeding • Secretes hCG and AFP
Choriocarcinoma	• Choriocarcinoma is a very rare ovarian tumor. • Children present with precocious puberty. • Tumors secrete hCG primary amenorrhea. • Patient karyotype 45,X or mosaicism with 45,X/46, XY. • Majority are phenotypic women (80%); the remainder are phenotypic men with hypospadias, cryptorchidism, and internal female sex organs. Among phenotypic women, half are normal in appearance, and the other half are virilized with primary amenorrhea or external genitalia.

Continued

TABLE 22-6   Classification of Ovarian Tumors—cont'd

TUMOR	CHARACTERISTICS
SEX CORD–STROMAL TUMORS (10% OF ALL OVARIAN TUMORS)	
Thecomas (Link 22-100) and fibroma (Link 22-101)	• Rarely malignant • Rare before puberty; usually seen in perimenopausal or postmenopausal women • Thecomas (Link 22-100) may produce estrogen. • Fibromas (Link 22-101) are benign tumors associated with Meigs syndrome (ascites, right-sided pleural effusion). Regression of effusions follows removal of the tumor. Commonly have dystrophic calcification that is visible on radiography
Granulosa cell tumors (Links 22-102 and 22-103)	• Yellow tumor that primarily secretes estrogen and progesterone, in some cases • Low-grade malignant tumor with juvenile or adult variants • Juvenile variants occur in women <30 yr of age. Children may show signs of precocious puberty because of secretion of estrogen by the tumor. • Older women may have amenorrhea or irregular bleeding. • Tumor contains Call-Exner bodies (microfollicles).
Sertoli-Leydig cell tumor (androblastoma)	• Rare, benign masculinizing tumor that produces androgens • Average presenting age is 25 yr old • Majority are masculinizing, some are estrogenic, and others do not secrete any hormones. • Pure Leydig cell tumors contain cells with crystals of Reinke. • Association with Peutz-Jeghers syndrome
Gonadoblastoma (Link 22-104)	• Rare malignant tumor with mixture of a germ cell tumor (dysgerminoma) and sex cord–stromal tumor • Associated with abnormal sexual development in 80% of cases • Commonly have dystrophic calcification that is visible on radiography
TUMORS METASTATIC TO OVARY (<3% OF ALL OVARIAN TUMORS)	
Metastasis	• May effect one or both ovaries; usually hematogenous spread and less commonly caused by seeding • Müllerian origin: uterus, fallopian tubes, contralateral ovary • Extramüllerian origin: breast, GI tract
Krukenberg tumor (see Figs. 18-19 C and 22-14 D; Link 22-105)	• May affect one or both ovaries • Contains signet-ring cells most commonly from hematogenous spread of a gastric cancer (diffuse carcinoma [linitis plastica]). Less commonly, a variant of breast cancer with signet ring cells can also metastasize to the ovaries.

AFP, α-Fetoprotein; *GI,* gastrointestinal; *hCG,* human chorionic gonadotropin; *LDH,* Lactate dehydrogenase.

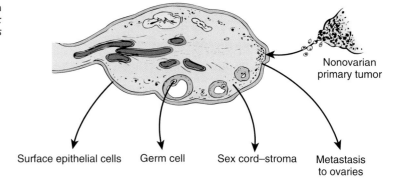

22-13: Schematic showing the derivation of primary ovarian tumors. *(From Kumar V, Abbas AK, Fausto N, Mitchell RN: Robbins Basic Pathology, 8th ed. Philadelphia, Saunders Elsevier, 2007, p 729, Fig. 19-16.)*

Nonovarian primary tumor

Surface epithelial cells   Germ cell   Sex cord–stroma   Metastasis to ovaries

Malignant surface-derived commonly seed omentum

Germ cell tumors

Germ cell: 15%

Similar to testicular cancers

Late teens and 20s

Abdominal pain, ↑abdominal girth, uterine bleeding

Germ cell tumors: most benign, few malignant

Sex cord-stromal tumors

Sex cord-stromal tumors: 10%

Derive from stromal cells

(4) Because they are on the ovarian surface, malignant surface-derived tumors commonly detach and seed the omentum (see Chapter 9). Recall that cancer cells lose their cell-to-cell attachments (cadherins; see Chapter 9).

b. Germ cell tumors (Links 22-96, 22-97, 22-98, and 22-99)

(1) Account for 15% of all ovarian tumors

(2) Cancers are similar to those seen in the testicle (see Chapter 21).

(3) Usually manifest in women in their late teens and 20s

(4) Present with abdominal pain, increase in abdominal girth, abnormal uterine bleeding

(5) Derive from primitive germ cells of the embryonic gonad

(6) Most are benign.

c. Sex cord–stromal tumors (Links 22-100, 22-101, 22-102, 22-103, and 22-104)

(1) Account for 10% of all ovarian tumors

(2) Derive from stromal cells (structural tissue cells analogous to fibroblasts)

(3) Some are hormone producing (e.g., granulosa cell tumor produces E and T).

(4) The majority are benign.

d. Metastasis to the ovaries

(1) Accounts for <3% of all ovarian tumors

(2) The majority are hematogenous metastasis.

(3) Seeding is a less common type of metastasis (e.g., primary colon cancer seeds the ovaries).

(4) Common primary cancers that metastasize to the ovaries

(a) Malignant tumors of müllerian origin from the cervix, uterus, and fallopian tubes. Recall that the müllerian ducts in females develop into the fallopian tubes, uterus, cervix, and upper portion of the vagina.

(b) Primary ovarian cancer in the contralateral ovary

(c) Breast cancer and cancer in the gastrointestinal tract

(d) Krukenberg tumor, which is unique in that signet ring cells are present; suggests either and implicate diffuse cancer of the stomach or breast cancer as the primary site (Fig. 22-14 D; Link 22-105; see Chapter 18)

4. Clinical findings

a. Abdominal enlargement caused by fluid (the most common sign)

(1) Malignant ascites is most often caused by seeding.

(2) Signs of malignant ascites caused by seeding

(a) Induration in the rectal pouch on digital rectal examination (see Chapter 9)

(b) Intestinal obstruction with colicky pain (pain alternating with pain free intervals; see Chapter 18)

b. Palpable ovarian mass in a postmenopausal woman. The ovaries should *not* be palpable in menopausal women because they normally undergo atrophy.

c. Malignant pleural effusion: The pleural cavity is a common site for ovarian cancer metastasis.

d. Torsion (twisting around its vascular pedicle and ligamentous supports) leading to infarction. Most often occurs with cystic teratomas of the ovary. Radiographs may show calcification from bone or teeth (see Fig. 9-1 C).

Some stromal cells produce hormones (E, T)

Majority benign

Metastasis <3%

Majority hematogenous metastasis

Seeding less common

Malignant tumors of Mullerian origin (e.g., uterus)

Primary cancer in contralateral ovary

Breast, GI cancers

Krukenberg tumors: signet ring cells (stomach/breast cancer)

Ovarian cancer: abdominal enlargement due to fluid MC sign

Malignant ascites: seeding MCC

Malignant ascites: induration in rectal pouch; intestinal obstruction

Palpable ovarian mass

Ovaries should not be palpable in menopause

Pleural cavity: common site for ovarian metastasis

Torsion of ovary

Cystic teratoma MC

Radiograph shows calcification (bone/teeth)

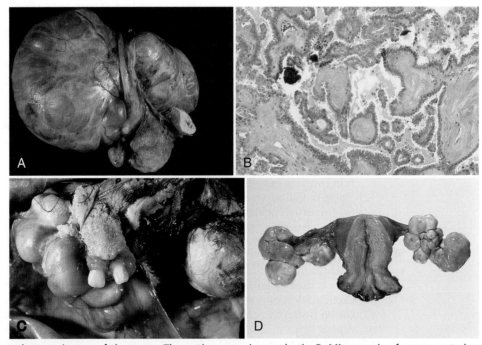

22-14: A, Serous cystadenocarcinoma of the ovary. The entire ovary is neoplastic. **B,** Microscopic of serous cystadenocarcinoma showing papillary fronds and red-blue concretions called psammoma bodies (example of dystrophic calcification). **C,** Well-developed teeth in ovarian cystic teratoma. Also note the hair and sebum. **D,** Typical gross appearance of Krukenberg tumors of the ovary. The involvement is bilateral, and the tumors are characterized by a multinodular outer appearance. Most cases are caused by hematogenous metastasis from a diffuse gastric carcinoma (linitis plastica) with signet ring cells. (*A and B from my friend Ivan Damjanov, MD, PhD:* Pathology for the Health-Related Professions, *2nd ed, Philadelphia, Saunders, 2000, Figs. 15-15A, 15-15B, respectively; C and D from Rosai J:* Rosai and Ackerman's Surgical Pathology, *9th ed, St. Louis, Mosby, 2004, pp 1687, 1708, respectively, Figs. 19.290, 19.340, respectively; D courtesy of Dr. R. A. Cooke, Brisbane, Australia; from Cooke RA, Stewart B:* Colour Atlas of Anatomical Pathology, *Edinburgh, Churchill Livingstone, 2004.*)

e. Signs of hyperestrinism from E-secreting tumors (e.g., granulosa cell tumor)
   (1) Vaginal bleeding occurs from endometrial hyperplasia or cancer.
   (2) 100% superficial squamous cells present in a cervical Pap smear.
f. Signs of hirsutism or virilization are associated with androgen-secreting tumors (e.g., Sertoli-Leydig cell tumors).

5. Tumor markers
   a. Surface-derived serous ovarian cancers release CA125 in 80% of cases. CA125 is *not* released by other epithelial-derived cancers (e.g., mucinous, endometrioid cancers). CA125 has a low sensitivity and specificity in predicting malignancy. It is most useful in monitoring women who have been treated for an ovarian serous carcinoma. Low sensitivity and specificity preclude its use as a screening test of ovarian cancer.
   b. Other tumor markers include human epididymis protein 4 (HE4) and OVA1 (combines 5 ovarian CA biomarkers). HE4 is primarily used to monitor women who have been treated for epithelial ovarian cancer.

6. The prognosis in ovarian cancer is better in those <65 years of age.

XI. **Gestational Disorders**
A. **Placental anatomy**
   1. Overview of placenta (Links 22-106 and 22-107)
   2. Fetal surface (Fig. 22-15 A; Link 22-108)
      a. Surface is entirely covered by the chorionic plate.
      b. Chorionic villus vessels converge with the umbilical cord.
      c. Chorion is covered by the amnion.
      d. Meconium-stained (fetal stool) fetal surface (Link 22-109). This may occur in term or postterm placentas; often a sign of fetal distress from hypoxia. Meconium also increases the risk for infection.
   3. Maternal surface (Fig. 22-15 B; Link 22-110)
      a. Maternal surface contains cotyledons covered by a layer of decidua basalis.
      b. Cotyledons contain fetal vessels, chorionic villi, and the intervillous space (IVS).
      c. Chorionic villi project into the IVS.
         (1) IVS contains maternal blood from which O₂ is extracted.
         (2) Spiral arteries from the uterus empty into the IVS.
      d. Chorionic villi are lined by trophoblastic tissue (Fig. 22-15 C; Link 22-107 B).
         (1) The outside layer of chorionic villi is composed of syncytiotrophoblast (Link 22-107 B).
            (a) Synthesizes hCG (see earlier discussion)
            (b) Synthesizes human placental lactogen (HPL). Amount of human placental lactogen directly correlates with the placental mass. Human placental lactogen has anti-insulin activity and is similar to human growth hormone (GH).
         (2) Inside layer of the chorionic villi is composed of cytotrophoblast (Link 22-107 B). Cytotrophoblastic cells play an important role in the implantation of a newly fertilized egg in the uterus.
      e. Vessels within chorionic villi coalesce to form the umbilical vein (contains fetal blood with O₂ attached to hemoglobin F [HbF]).
      f. Umbilical cord
         (1) Contains one umbilical vein and two umbilical arteries (Link 22-111). The umbilical vein contains oxygenated blood (an exception to the rule for a vein).
         (2) Single umbilical artery (UA) has clinical significance.
            (a) Increased incidence of congenital anomalies (20% of cases)
            (b) Congenital anomalies include cardiovascular defects, trisomy 18, and esophageal atresia.
B. **Placental infections**
   1. Epidemiology
      a. Most are caused by an ascending bacterial infection from the vagina.
         (1) Complication of premature rupture of membranes (PROM)
         (2) Group B streptococcus (*Streptococcus agalactiae*) is a common pathogen in the vagina.
         (3) Other pathogens: *B. fragilis*, *Prevotella bivia*, group A streptococcus
      b. Congenital infections (e.g., CMV, syphilis).
   2. Funisitis and placentitis
      • **Definition:** Infections of the umbilical cord and placenta, respectively
   3. Chorioamnionitis (Link 22-112)
      a. **Definition:** Infection of the fetal membranes (amnion and chorion)
      b. Increases risk for neonatal sepsis and meningitis

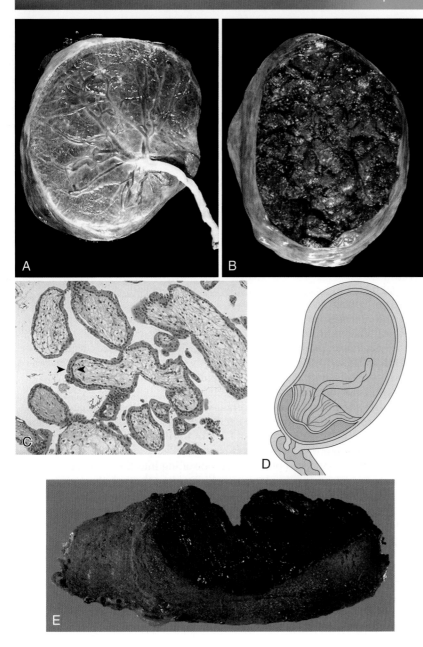

22-15: A, Normal placenta showing the fetal side. Covered by the chorionic plate. Chorionic villi vessels converge with the umbilical cord. The chorion is covered by the amnion. **B,** Normal placenta showing the maternal side. Note the cotyledons covered by a layer of decidua basalis. **C,** Chorionic villi. The outer layer of the villus is covered by two layers of cells called the trophoblast *(arrowheads).* The outer layer of the trophoblast is lined by syncytiotrophoblast, and the inner layer is lined by cytotrophoblast. The vessels in the chorionic villi converge to become the umbilical vein, which is the vessel with the highest O₂ content. **D,** Schematic of placenta previa. Note how the placenta is implanted over the cervical os. **E,** Abruptio placentae. Note the retroplacental blood clot that separated the placenta from its implantation site. *(A, B, C, and E from Klatt F: Robbins and Cotran Atlas of Pathology, Philadelphia, Saunders, 2006, p 326 for A, B, and C, p 327 for E, respectively, Figs. 13-108A, B, 13-109, 13-112. respectively; D from Greer I, Cameron IT, Kitchener HC, Prentice A: Mosby's Color Atlas and Text of Obstetrics and Gynecology, St. Louis, Mosby, 2000, p 184, Fig. 7-28.)*

Maternal-to-fetal infections (vertical transmission) are transmitted from the mother to the fetus, either across the placenta during fetal development (prenatal) or during labor and delivery as the baby passes through the birth canal (perinatal). Pathogens include cytomegalovirus, toxoplasmosis, HIV, rubella, and syphilis, to name a few. See Chapter 6.

C. **Selected placental abnormalities**
1. Placenta previa (Fig. 22-15 D; Link 22-113)
   a. **Definition:** Implantation of the placenta over the internal cervical os (opening of the cervix)
   b. Epidemiology: A previous cesarean section (C-section) increases a woman's risk for developing placenta previa in a future pregnancy.
   c. Clinical findings
      (1) Usually presents with *painless* vaginal bleeding in the second or third trimester
      (2) Uterus is soft and nontender.
      (3) Fetal distress is *not* usually present.
   d. Placenta previa recurs in 4% to 8% of subsequent pregnancies.
   e. Diagnosis: Transabdominal ultrasound localizes the placenta over the opening to the cervical os. Digital pelvic exam is contraindicated!!! Danger of vaginal hemorrhage.

Placenta implants over internal cervical os

Previous C-section ↑risk

Clinical findings

Painless vaginal bleeding 2nd or 3rd trimester

Uterus soft/nontender

No fetal distress

4% to 8% recurrence subsequent pregnancies

Dx transabdominal ultrasound

2. Abruptio placenta
   a. **Definition:** Premature separation of the placenta caused by formation of a retroplacental clot (Fig. 22-15 E; Link 22-114)
   b. Epidemiology
      (1) Most common cause of late pregnancy bleeding
      (2) Occurs in 1:830 pregnancies. Incidence ranges between 0.4% and 1% of pregnancies.
      (3) Three locations are subchorionic (between placenta and membranes), retroplacental (between placenta and myometrium; worse prognosis for fetal survival), and preplacental (between the placenta and amniotic sac).
      (4) Fetal mortality rate is 20% to 40%.
      (5) Risk factors for developing an abruptio placenta
         (a) Maternal hypertension (greatest risk factor; 40%–50% of cases)
         (b) Smoking cigarettes, cocaine use
         (c) Advanced maternal age, trauma
         (d) Chorioamnionitis, PROM
         (e) History of a previous abruptio placentae
   c. Clinical findings
      (1) Painful vaginal bleeding (originates from uterus); presents with vaginal bleeding (80% of cases) or concealed bleeding (20%)
      (2) Forceful uterine contractions (~15% of cases) or signs of preterm labor
      (3) Evidence of fetal distress is usually present.
      (4) Abruptio placentae triad: painful vaginal bleeding, abdominal or back pain, and fetal compromise
   d. Diagnosis is made by ultrasound. Pelvic exam is contraindicated.
3. Placenta accreta, increta, and percreta
   a. **Definition:** Placenta accreta is when the placental villi adhere to the myometrium as a result of a partial or complete absence of the decidua basalis and faulty development of Nitabuch's layer. Nitabuch's layer is normally a layer of fibrinoid degeneration between the invading trophoblasts and the decidua basalis.
   b. **Definition:** Placenta increta refers to placental villi invading into the myometrium.
   c. **Definition:** Placenta percreta refers to placental villi invading through the uterine serosa.
   d. Epidemiology
      (1) Great risk for hemorrhage during delivery
      (2) Commonly requires surgery to control bleeding
      (3) Risk factors for the development of placenta accreta
         (a) Placenta previa in patients with a previous history of a cesarean section (most important risk factor)
         (b) Advanced maternal age, multiparity, previous endometrial curettage
      (4) Hysterectomy is often necessary.
      (5) Risk of recurrence 5% to 15%. After two consecutive abruptions, the risk for the third increases to 20% to 25%.
4. Velamentous insertion
   a. **Definition:** Insertion of the umbilical cord away from the placental edge resulting in vessels coursing unprotected through the membranes (Links 22-115 and 22-116).
   b. Epidemiology
      (1) Increased risk for hemorrhage if vessels are torn. Vessels are *not* protected by Wharton jelly (WJ). WJ is a gelatinous substance within the umbilical cord that is largely comprised of mucopolysaccharides (hyaluronic acid and chondroitin sulfate).
      (2) Can be diagnosed by ultrasound
      (3) Baby may require cesarean delivery to prevent a vessel tear.
      (4) Congenital anomalies occur in 30% of cases, an increase of premature delivery in ~17% of cases, and small newborn size for dates in ~35% of cases.
5. Succenturiate placenta
   a. **Definition:** Placenta in which one or more lobes of the placenta are located separately from the main placenta (Link 22-117)
   b. Epidemiology
      (1) Usually a vascular connection is between the main lobe and the extra lobe
      (2) Increased risk for hemorrhage if the lobe is detached
      (3) Increased risk for infection if it is *not* recognized at delivery because extra lobe may be retained in the uterus

6. Marginal cord insertion (battledore placenta)
   a. **Definition:** Insertion of the cord at the margin of the placenta
   b. Epidemiology
      (1) Present in 7% of pregnant women; incidence higher in multiple gestations
      (2) *No* known clinical significance
7. Placentomegaly (large placenta): Causes include DM (see Chapter 23), Rh hemolytic disease of newborn (Rh HDN; see Chapter 16), and congenital syphilis (see Chapter 6).
8. Twin placentas (Fig. 22-16)
   a. Monochorionic types (monoamniotic or diamniotic) are associated with identical twins (see Fig. 22-16).
      (1) Identical twins derive from a single zygote (diploid cell resulting from the fusion of two haploid gametes; a fertilized ovum).
      (2) Most identical twins have a monochorionic diamniotic placenta (65%–70%) (see Fig. 22-16 B). Monochorionic monoamniotic placenta for identical twins is the type of placenta for conjoined twins and has the potential for tangling of umbilical cords.
      (3) Diamniotic with separate amniotic sacs (see Fig. 22-16 B)
      (4) Fetal-to-fetal transfusion can occur in either type (A or B; Link 22-118).
   b. Dichorionic placentas
      (1) May be associated with either monozygotic ("identical") or dizygotic ("fraternal") twins (Link 22-119). Dizygotic ("fraternal") twins occur when separate eggs are fertilized.
      (2) Placentas can be dichorionic diamniotic fused (40%; Fig. 22-16 C) or dichorionic diamniotic separated (most common type [60%]; Fig. 22-16 D).
D. **Preeclampsia and eclampsia (toxemia of pregnancy)**
   1. **Definition of preeclampsia:** A pregnant woman with new-onset hypertension (≥140 mm Hg systolic or ≥90 mm Hg diastolic) accompanied by proteinuria (>300 mg in 24-hr urine collection or 30 mg/dL [1+ dipstick])
   2. **Definition of eclampsia:** Preeclampsia plus generalized seizures
   3. Epidemiology of preeclampsia
      a. Usually occurs after the 20th week of pregnancy
      b. Occurs in 0% to 14% of primigravidas and 5.7% to 7.3% of multigravidas
      c. Risk factors for preeclampsia
         (1) Extremes of age: <15 years of age and >35 years of age
         (2) Nulliparity, blacks > whites
         (3) Hx previous preeclampsia or positive family history, multiple gestations
         (4) DM, obesity
         (5) Thrombocytosis, renal or collagen vascular diseases, antiphospholipid syndrome (APLS)
      d. May be associated with hydatidiform moles (see later discussion); complete mole in 1% of cases; partial mole in 5% of cases

e. Pathogenesis of preeclampsia
  (1) Abnormal placentation
    (a) Incomplete trophoblastic invasion into the maternal spiral arteries leads to poor placental perfusion and hypoxia, which in turn leads to the production of free radicals and oxidative stress.
    (b) Mechanical or functional obstruction of the spiral arteries
  (2) Imbalance favoring vasoconstrictors (VCs) over vasodilators (VDs)
    (a) Normal VDs are decreased. Example: prostaglandin E$_2$ (PGE$_2$)
    (b) VCs are increased. Example: thromboxane A$_2$. Increased sensitivity to angiotensin II (ATII) by the muscular walls of the arteries
    (c) Increase in various growth factors (e.g., vascular endothelial growth factor [VEGF], placental growth factor [PGF]). PGF is a member of the VEGF subfamily.
  (3) Net effect in preeclampsia is placental hypoperfusion
f. Pathologic findings in preeclampsia
  (1) Premature aging of the placenta
  (2) Multiple placental infarctions with pale coagulation necrosis (see Chapter 2; Links 22-120 and 22-121)
  (3) Spiral arteries show intimal atherosclerosis (reduces blood flow to placenta).
4. Clinical and laboratory findings in preeclampsia
  a. Hypertension caused by increased vasoconstrictors. Blood pressure ranges from just below 140/90 mm Hg (mild) to >160/110 mm Hg (severe).
  b. Proteinuria in the nephrotic range (>3.5 g/24 hours). Total protein is usually >5 g in a 24-hour urine collection.
  c. Dependent pitting edema caused by loss of albumin in the urine causing a decrease in plasma oncotic pressure (P$_O$; see Chapter 5).
  d. Weight gain >4 lb/week caused by retention of sodium
  e. Generalized seizures
    (1) Preeclampsia + seizures is called eclampsia.
    (2) About 1% of patients with preeclampsia develop eclampsia. Magnesium sulfate is used for treatment of eclampsia.
  f. Renal disease; swollen endothelial cells (ETCs) in the glomerular capillaries, which produces oliguria (<400 mL/24 hr)
  g. Liver disease
    (1) RUQ pain and hepatomegaly
    (2) Periportal necrosis with increased transaminases (serum alanine [ALT] and aspartate aminotransferase [AST])
  h. HELLP syndrome (see Chapter 19)
    (1) **H**emolytic anemia with schistocytes (see Chapter 12)
    (2) **EL**evated serum transaminases
    (3) **L**ow **p**latelets caused by disseminated intravascular coagulation
E. Gestational trophoblastic neoplasms
  1. Hydatidiform mole
    a. **Definition:** Benign tumor of the chorionic villi in the placenta.
    b. Epidemiology
      (1) Complete mole; all the chorionic villi are neoplastic and look like "grapes" (Link 22-122)
      (2) Partial mole: only some of the chorionic villi are neoplastic; other chorionic villi are normal
      (3) More common at the extremes of age
      (4) In United States, it occurs in 1:1200 pregnancies. In Indonesia, it occurs in 1:200 pregnancies.
      (5) Complete mole is the most common type
        (a) **Definition:** All of the chorionic villi are neoplastic.
        (b) Chorionic villi are dilated and swollen because of the influx of water, and they do *not* contain fetal blood vessels or fetal parts (Fig. 22-17 A).
        (c) Ovum is 46,XX in 90% of cases. Ovum lacks maternal chromosomes (called an empty ovum). Chromosomes are paternally derived (Link 22-123 A). There is duplication of a 23X sperm in the ovum (46XX; most common ovum) or two separate 23X or Y sperm enter the ovum (called dispermy; 46XX or 46XY ovum).
        (d) Increased risk for developing a choriocarcinoma (a malignancy composed of syncytiotrophoblast and cytotrophoblast; see later) in (15%–20%) of cases.

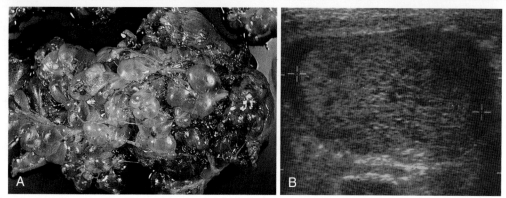

22-17: A, Complete hydatidiform mole. The enlarged and edematous villi are interconnected by thin cordlike structures. No fetus is present. **B,** Ultrasound image of a complete hydatidiform mole showing the classic "snowstorm" appearance. **(A** from my friend Ivan Damjanov, MD, PhD, Linder J: Pathology: A Color Atlas, St. Louis, Mosby, 2000, p 290, Fig. 13-111A; **B** from Greer I, Cameron IT, Kitchener HC, Prentice A: Mosby's Color Atlas and Text of Obstetrics and Gynecology, St. Louis, Mosby, 2000, p 94, Fig. 4-22.)

(e) Clinical findings
- Vaginal bleeding at 6 to 16th week gestational age (80%–90% of cases).
- Severe vomiting (hyperemesis gravidarum; 8% of cases); risk for developing metabolic alkalosis (see Chapter 5)
- Preeclampsia in 1% of cases
- Uterus that is too large for gestational age (~30% of cases)
- Increased β-hCG for gestational age (>100,000 mIU/mL; 15% of cases)
- Bilateral theca lutein cysts, which develop in response to high levels of β-hCG (15% of cases)
- "Snowstorm appearance" on ultrasound (Fig. 22-17 B)

(f) In treating a complete mole by D&C, all of the complete mole must be removed because of a danger of developing a choriocarcinoma (see later). Serial measurements of β-hCG levels after the D&C should go down to zero!!!

c. Partial mole
(1) **Definition:** Normal villi are intermixed with neoplastic villi.
(2) Fetal parts are intermixed with neoplastic villi.
   (a) Amnion and fetal vessels with fetal erythrocytes are present within the mesenchyme of the neoplastic villi.
   (b) Ovum is triploid (69 XXY in 70% of cases; XXX in 27% of cases).
   (c) Most commonly caused by fertilization of a maternally derived 23X ovum by two sperm that are either 23X or Y, producing an ovum with 69XXY (most common; Link 22-123 B) or, less commonly, XXX
(3) Preeclampsia is present in 5% of patients.
(4) *No* risk for developing a choriocarcinoma. Recall that it is a risk with a complete mole.
(5) Clinical findings
   (a) Incomplete or missed abortion (90% of cases; Link 22-124)
   (b) Vaginal bleeding (75% of cases), uterine enlargement (5% of cases)
   (c) Theca lutein cysts and hyperemesis gravidarum (extremely rare)
   (d) β-hCG elevated for gestational age (<100,000 mIU/mL) in the majority of cases. Recall that it is >100,000 mIU/mL in a complete mole.
(6) Treatment of a partial mole is the same as that for a complete mole.

2. Choriocarcinoma
a. Malignant tumor composed of syncytiotrophoblast and cytotrophoblast (Links 22-125 and 22-126). Chorionic villi are *not* present.
b. Risk factors
(1) Complete mole (50% of cases), spontaneous abortion (25% of cases)
(2) Full term pregnancy (22% of cases), ectopic pregnancy (3% of cases)
c. Common sites of metastasis include the lungs, vagina, liver, and brain. Metastatic lesions are hemorrhagic (recall that renal cell carcinoma also has hemorrhagic metastases).
d. Excellent response to chemotherapy (methotrexate) in gestationally derived choriocarcinomas; hence, low mortality rate

F. **Amniotic fluid (AF)**
  1. **Definition:** The yellowish-colored fluid that surrounds a fetus within the amniotic sac
  2. Composition
     a. Predominantly fetal urine.
     b. High salt content that causes "ferning" when dried on a slide
        (1) Excellent sign of premature rupture of the amniotic sac
        (2) Do *not* confuse this "ferning" with the type that is seen in watery cervical mucus.
     c. Amniotic fluid is swallowed and recycled by the fetus.
     d. Polyhydramnios
        (1) **Definition:** An excessive amount of amniotic fluid in the amniotic sac
        (2) Causes
            (a) Tracheoesophageal (TE) fistula, which prevents amniotic fluid from being reabsorbed in the intestine for excretion in the urine (see Chapter 18)
            (b) Duodenal atresia, which prevents amniotic fluid from being reabsorbed in the intestine for excretion in the urine (see Chapter 18)
            (c) Maternal DM (20% of cases)
                • Maternal hyperglycemia → fetal hyperglycemia → fetal polyuria (caused by the osmotic effect of glucose in the urine)
            (d) Anencephaly caused by craniospinal defects that allow cerebrospinal fluid (CSF) to empty into the amniotic fluid
     e. Oligohydramnios
        (1) **Definition:** A decreased amount of amniotic fluid in the amniotic sac
        (2) Causes
            (a) Juvenile polycystic kidney disease (JPKD; see Chapter 20)
            (b) Fetal genitourinary (GU) obstruction, uteroplacental insufficiency
            (c) Premature rupture of membranes (PROM)
G. **α-Fetoprotein (AFP) in pregnancy**
  1. Increased maternal AFP is present in an open neural tube defect.
     a. Related to folic acid deficiency in the pregnant woman

---

Folic acid acts as a coenzyme and is important in an unborn child for the normal growth of cells, tissues, and organs. The enzyme methionine synthase (see Fig. 6-8) is an important enzyme that converts homocysteine into methionine. This biochemical reaction requires a methyl group, which is provided by folic acid. Therefore, if folic acid is decreased, the methyl group is unavailable, which causes an increase in homocysteine. An increase in homocysteine prevents the closure of the neural tube, hence increasing the risk for developing an open neural tube defect as well as other manifestations.

---

  b. Folic acid stores should be adequate *before* pregnancy because the neural tube is already developed by the end of the first month of gestation.
  2. Decreased AFP is seen in trisomy 21 (Down syndrome; see Chapter 6).
H. **Urine estriol in pregnancy**
  1. Multiple sites for synthesis
  2. Estriol is derived from the fetal adrenal gland, placenta, and maternal liver.
     a. Fetal zone of the adrenal cortex
        (1) Converts pregnenolone synthesized in the placenta to dehydroepiandrosterone sulfate (DHEA-S)
        (2) Fetal zone adrenal cortex is absent in anencephaly, a type of neural tube defect associated with an absence of the brain (see Chapter 26).
     b. Fetal liver. In the fetal liver, DHEA-S is 16-hydroxylated to 16-OH-DHEA-S.
     c. Placenta
        (1) Placental sulfatase cleaves off the sulfate from 16-OH-DHEA-S.
        (2) 16-OH-DHEA is converted by aromatase to free unbound estriol.
     d. Maternal liver
        (1) Free estriol is conjugated to estriol sulfate and estriol glucosiduronate.
        (2) Both compounds are excreted in maternal urine and bile.
  3. Decreased levels of estriol are a sign of fetal–maternal–placental dysfunction.
  4. Down syndrome triad
     a. Decreased urine estriol
     b. Decreased AFP (see earlier)
     c. Increased serum β-hCG
  5. Lamellar body count is the MC test used to assess fetal lung maturity. Test is performed on blood analyzer (lamellar bodies same size as platelets). Lamellar bodies contain surfactant.

Nipple/areola complex	Lactiferous sinus	Major duct	Terminal duct	Lobule	Stroma

22-18: Locations for breast lesions. See text for discussion. (*Redrawn from Goljan EF: Star Series: Pathology, Philadelphia, Saunders, 1998, Fig. 18-3.*)

Paget's disease	Intraductal papilloma	Fibrocystic change	Tubular carcinoma	Lobular carcinoma	Fibroadenoma
Breast abscess	Breast abscess	Ductal cancer		Sclerosing adenosis	Phyllodes tumor
	Plasma cell mastitis				

XII. Breast Disorders

A. Clinical anatomy
1. Overview of anatomy (Links 22-127 and 22-128)
   High-density locations of breast tissue are located in the
   a. Upper outer quadrant (UOQ): underscores why breast cancer is most commonly located in this quadrant.
   b. Area beneath the nipple.
2. Hormone effects during menstrual cycle
   a. E stimulates ductal and alveolar cell growth, fat, and stroma.
   b. P stimulates alveolar cell proliferation and lobule differentiation for milk production (it does *not* stimulate secretion) and breast swelling in the secretory phase.
3. Hormone effects in lactation
   a. Prolactin stimulates and maintains lactogenesis (production of milk) and secretion.
   b. Oxytocin stimulates the expulsion of milk into the ducts; released by the suckling reflex
4. Lymph nodes
   a. Outer quadrant cancers drain to the axillary lymph nodes.
   b. Inner quadrant cancers drain to the internal mammary nodes.

B. Locations of breast lesions (Fig. 22-18)

C. Nipple discharges
1. Galactorrhea (excessive production of milk); causes other than lactation
   a. Physiologic causes include prolonged sucking of nipple and sexual intercourse.
   b. Prolactinoma (see Chapter 23): most common pathologic cause of galactorrhea (Fig. 22-19 A)
   c. Primary hypothyroidism (see Chapter 23).
      (1) Most common nonpituitary endocrine disease causing galactorrhea
      (2) Decreased serum thyroxine increases thyrotropin-releasing factor (TRF), which stimulates the release of prolactin.
   d. Drugs. Examples– OCPs, phenothiazines, methyldopa, H_2-receptor blockers, anxiolytics, and tricyclic antidepressants (TCAs)
2. Bloody nipple discharge: Causes include intraductal papilloma and ductal cancer.
3. Purulent nipple discharge.
   a. Acute mastitis caused by *S. aureus* infection (Link 22-129)
   b. Acute mastitis usually occurs during lactation or breastfeeding (2%–3%). Treat with antibiotics, and the patient should continue breastfeeding.
4. Greenish brown nipple discharge occurs in mammary duct ectasia (plasma cell mastitis; see later).

D. Breast pain (mastalgia)
1. Occurs in two-thirds of menstruating women
2. Cyclic pain is usually diffuse, bilateral, and most often associated with fibrocystic change (FCC; see later)
3. Noncyclic breast pain is localized and is most often caused by a cyst or mass.
4. Pain alone is rarely a presenting symptom of a malignancy.
5. Mondor disease
   a. Superficial thrombophlebitis of veins overlying the breast
   b. Presents as a palpable, painful cord

E. Examples of benign types of microcalcifications in mammograms
- Popcorn calcifications (Fig. 22-19 B) and round calcifications (Fig. 22-19 C)

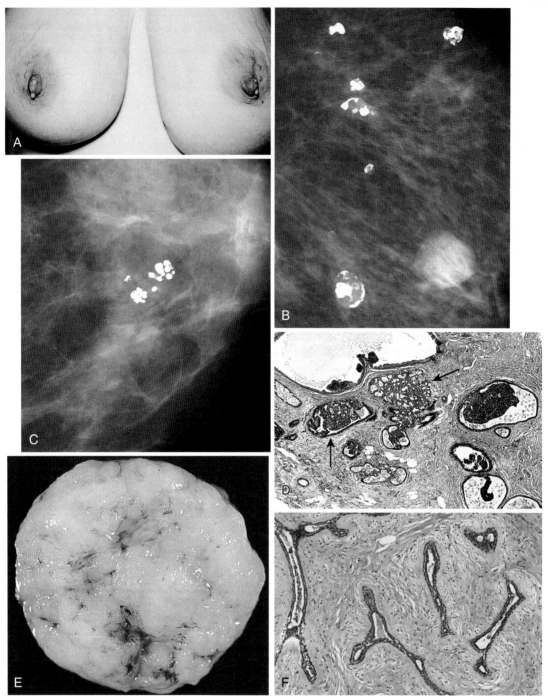

22-19: **A,** Galactorrhea in a patient with a prolactinoma. **B,** Mammogram with benign "popcorn" calcifications. **C,** Mammogram with benign round calcifications. **D,** Fibrocystic change. The microscopic section shows cystic spaces surrounded by a dense fibrous stroma. The large cyst at the top has eosinophilic staining cells exhibiting apocrine metaplasia. The smaller cysts *(arrows)* show extensive ductal hyperplasia with a sieve-like pattern. **E,** Fibroadenoma. Note the bulging gray-white surface of this benign stromal tumor. **F,** Fibroadenoma. A microscopic section shows compressed, elongated benign ducts surrounded by neoplastic stromal tissue. *(**A** from Mansel R, Bundred N: Color Atlas of Breast Disease, St. Louis, Mosby, 1995; **B** and **C** from Pretorius ES, Solomon JA: Radiology Secrets Plus, 3rd ed, Philadelphia, Mosby Elsevier, 2011, p 40, Figs. 6.8, 6.7, respectively; **D** from Rosai J, Ackerman LV: Surgical Pathology, 9th ed. St. Louis, Mosby, 2004, p 1780, Fig. 20-30; **E** from my friend Ivan Damjanov, MD, PhD, Linder J: Pathology: A Color Atlas, St. Louis, Mosby, 2000, p 298, Fig. 14-3; **F** from my friend Ivan Damjanov, MD, PhD: Pathology for the Health-Related Professions, 2nd ed, Philadelphia, Saunders, 2000, p 405, Fig. 16-5B.)*

F. Fibrocystic change (FCC)
  1. **Definition:** It is *not* a disease and is characterized the presence of cysts, fibrosis, and hyperplasia in the ducts and stroma of the normal female breast.
  2. Epidemiology
    a. Most common painful breast mass in women <50 years old
    b. Occurs in >50% of women in the reproductive period of life
    c. Distortion of normal cyclic breast changes
  3. Small and large cysts (Fig. 22-19 D; Links 22-130 to 22-132)
    a. "Lumpy bumpy" feeling on breast exam
    b. Some cysts hemorrhage into the cyst fluid; called "blue-domed" cysts
    c. Cysts vary in size with the menstrual cycle; *no* malignant potential
    d. May have to be surgically removed if recurrent
  4. Ductal hyperplasia
    a. **Definition:** Excess proliferation of ductal cells (DCs)
    b. Epidemiology
      (1) Duct epithelium is E sensitive and responds to hormone hormonal changes that occur normally in the proliferative phase of the menstrual cycle. Recall that the proliferative phase of the cell cycle is predominantly controlled by E.
      (2) Histologic changes
        (a) Papillary proliferation, which is called papillomatosis
        (b) Apocrine metaplasia refers to the presence of large, pink-staining cells.
        (c) Atypical ductal hyperplasia (similar to atypical endometrial hyperplasia) is a cause of concern because there is an increased risk for developing cancer because of excess E stimulation that may progress to breast cancer.
  5. Fibrosis in the stroma has *no* malignant potential.
G. Sclerosing adenosis
  1. **Definition:** A proliferation of small ductules or acini in the lobule (Link 22-133)
  2. Epidemiology
    a. Histologic pattern is often confused with infiltrating ductal cancer
    b. Often contains microcalcifications
H. Inflammation
  1. Acute mastitis (see earlier discussion)
  2. Mammary duct ectasia (plasma cell mastitis)
    a. **Definition:** An excess buildup of debris that fills the main duct(s), causing them to dilate and become inflamed with a prominent plasma cell infiltration (Link 22-134)
    b. Epidemiology
      (1) Affects 25% of postmenopausal women
      (2) Main ducts fill up with debris.
        (a) This causes dilation, rupture, and inflammation that is characterized by a heavy plasma cell infiltration around the main ducts.
        (b) Ductal debris produces a greenish brown nipple discharge.
      (3) May produce skin and nipple retraction that simulates breast cancer.
      (4) *No* increased risk for developing breast cancer
  3. Traumatic fat necrosis.
    a. **Definition:** Necrosis that occurs in fatty tissue as a result of blunt trauma or surgery (see Chapter 2)
    b. Microscopic findings
      (1) Lipid-laden macrophages with foreign body giant cells (FBGCs; Link 22-135)
      (2) Fibrosis and dystrophic calcification.
    c. Clinical findings: initial painful mass in the acute stage after trauma followed by the presence of a painless, indurated mass that may produce skin retraction simulating breast cancer
  4. Silicone breast implant
    a. **Definition:** A polymer of silica, oxygen, and hydrogen
    b. Epidemiology
      (1) May have leakage or rupture
      (2) Silicone produces a foreign body (FB) inflammatory reaction composed of multinucleated giant cells and chronic inflammatory cells
      (3) An association with initiating an autoimmune disease (AD) has *not* been proven.
I. Benign breast tumors
  1. Fibroadenoma
    a. **Definition:** Benign tumor derived from the stroma of the breast

MC breast tumor <35 yrs old

Cyclosporine (renal transplantation)

Discrete, moveable, painless/painful mass

Single or multiple lesion

Proliferating stroma compresses ducts

↑Size during pregnancy (E sensitive)

May disappear/involute during menopause

Not progress to cancer

Dx FNA

Phyllodes tumor

Rare bulky tumor derived from stromal cells

Most commonly benign

Hypercellular stroma + mitoses signs malignancy

Lobulated tumor with cystic spaces

Often reaches massive size

Intraductal papilloma

Benign papillary tumor lactiferous duct/sinuses

MCC nipple discharge <50 yrs old

No risk for developing cancer

Breast cancer

Invasive cancer ducts or lobules

Breast cancer: MC cancer in women

Second MCC cancer death in women

Mean age 64 yrs old

Risk ↑ with age

Japan, Asia lowest death rates

MC breast mass women >50 years old

Prevalence decreasing: early detection

Risk factors

Family Hx and genetics

Genetic basis <10% of cases

AD BRCA1/BRCA2

Li-Fraumeni multicancer syndrome (inactivation *p53*)

RAS, ERBB2, RB1 suppressor gene, *PTEN, CDH1*

Early menarche, late menopause

Nulliparity

Postmenopausal obesity

E hormone replacement *without* progestins

DCIS, LCIS

b. Epidemiology
(1) Most common breast tumor in women <35 years old
(2) Fibroadenomas develop in 50% of women who receive cyclosporine after renal transplantation.
(3) Present as a discrete movable, painless or painful mass (Fig. 22-19 E). Multiple fibroadenomas may be present in 10%–15% of cases.
(4) Stroma proliferation compresses the surrounding ducts (Fig. 22-19 F). The duct epithelium is *not* neoplastic only the stroma.
(5) Because they are sensitive to the effects of E, fibroadenomas may increase in size during pregnancy.
(6) May spontaneously disappear or involute during menopause because of a decrease in E
(7) Does *not* progress into cancer; however, breast cancer may secondarily develop within duct epithelial cells as a separate event in 3% of cases.
  • Diagnosis is secured with a fine-needle aspiration (FNA; small-needle diameter) or core needle (larger needle diameter) biopsy.
2. Phyllodes tumor
  a. **Definition:** Rare, benign, borderline, or malignant bulky tumor that is derived from stromal cells
  b. Epidemiology
  (1) Most often a benign tumor; however, it can be malignant in some cases. A hypercellular stroma with mitoses is a sign of malignancy.
  (2) Lobulated tumor with cystic spaces that contain leaf-like extensions
  (3) Often reaches a massive size
3. Intraductal papilloma
  a. **Definition:** Benign papillary tumor that arises within the lactiferous ducts or sinuses (Link 22-136)
  b. Epidemiology
  (1) Most common cause of a bloody nipple discharge in women <50 years old
  (2) *No* increased risk for developing into cancer

J. Breast cancer
1. **Definition:** Invasive cancer of the breast that arises from the ducts or lobules that can develop in women or rarely in men (1%)
2. Epidemiology
  a. Most common cancer in adult women (1:8 lifetime risk; 12%) and the second most common cancer producing death in women
  (1) Mean age for breast cancer is 64 years old. Risk increases with age.
  (2) Japan and Asia have the lowest death rates. England and Wales have the highest.
  b. Most common breast mass in women >50 years old
  c. Currently a decrease in prevalence in breast cancer because of early detection and treatment
  d. Risk factors
  (1) Family history and genetics
    (a) Increased risk if breast cancer involves first-generation relatives (mother, sister)
    (b) Genetic basis is involved in <10% of cases (see Chapter 9).
      • Autosomal dominant *BRCA1* and *BRCA2* mutation association (the breasts or ovaries are frequently prophylactically removed). High penetrance. Lifetime risk is breast cancer risk is 40% to 85%.
      • Li-Fraumeni multicancer syndrome (inactivation of *p53* suppressor gene [see Chapter 9])
    (c) Other gene relationships: *RAS* oncogene, *ERBB2*, *RB1* suppressor gene, *PTEN* (phosphatase and tensin homolog) and *CDH1* (cadherin-1 gene)
  (2) Prolonged E stimulation; causes include:
    (a) early menarche or late menopause, nulliparity (never been pregnant).
    (b) Postmenopause obesity caused by increased aromatization of androstenedione to estrone.
    (c) E hormone replacement therapy without the use of progestins.
  (3) Ductal carcinoma in situ (DCIS) and lobular carcinoma in situ (LCIS), both of which can become invasive cancers
  (4) Other risk factors include atypical ductal hyperplasia, endometrial or ovarian cancer, ionizing radiation, smoking cigarettes, high breast density (determined by mammogram), combined E and P hormone therapy, two first-degree relatives with breast cancer, menopause after the age of 55 years (longer E exposure), and a history of cancer in the opposite breast

3. Factors that *decrease* the risk for breast cancer include breastfeeding, moderate or vigorous physical activity, and healthy body weight. Prophylactic oophorectomy decreases breast cancer risk by 50%, and prophylactic mastectomy decreases breast cancer risk by 90%.

4. Clinical findings
   a. Painless breast mass; usually (*not* always) in the upper outer quadrant
   b. Other potential findings include skin or nipple retraction, painless axillary adenopathy, hepatomegaly, bone pain if metastasis has occurred

5. Mammography
   a. Breast cancer screening recommendations are controversial.
   b. Some studies show that breast cancer screening is associated with an overall 19% reduction of breast cancer mortality (~15% for women in their 40s and ~32% for women in their 60s).
   c. Purpose of mammography is to detect nonpalpable masses.
   d. Diagnostic mammography is the first imaging study performed in a newly discovered breast mass.
   e. Mammography screening has a sensitivity of 67.8% and a specificity of 75%.
   f. Mammography does *not* distinguish benign from malignant, although some findings are highly suggestive of malignancy.
   g. Screening usually starts annually at age 40 years (recommendations vary) but earlier if the patient is high risk.
   h. It identifies microcalcifications and spiculated masses with or without microcalcifications (30%–50% of cases).
      (1) Microcalcifications most often occur in DCIS and sclerosing adenosis in fibrocystic change (false positive).
      (2) Microcalcification patterns that suggest malignancy include five or more tightly clustered microcalcifications that are punctate (Fig. 22-19 B, C), microlinear (Fig. 22-20), or branching (see Fig. 22-20).
   i. MRI screening is reserved for high-risk (>20%) women such as *BRCA* carriers.
   j. FNA (cannot detect if in situ or invasive) or core or excisional biopsy (can differentiate in situ from invasive)

6. Types of breast cancer are listed in Table 22-7 and depicted in Figure 22-21.

7. Natural history and prognosis of breast cancer (Link 22-147)
   a. First spreads by lymphatics (local spread) and then progresses to the hematogenous route (more widespread; see Chapter 9)
      (1) Outer quadrant cancer spreads to the axillary nodes.
      (2) Inner quadrant cancers spread to the internal mammary nodes.
   b. Extranodal metastasis
      (1) Common sites of metastasis include the lungs (MCC breast cancer), bone (MCC breast cancer), liver, brain, and ovaries.
      (2) May metastasize 10 to 15 years after treatment
      (3) Pain in a bone metastasis is relieved with local radiation.
   c. Staging of breast cancer
      (1) Extranodal metastasis has greater significance than nodal metastasis (see Chapter 9).
      (2) Sentinel lymph node biopsy

Margin notes:
Painless mass
Usually UOQ
Skin/nipple retraction
Painless axillary adenopathy
Screening recommendations controversial
Reduction in breast cancer mortality
Detects non-palpable masses
Breast mass detected → 1st step mammography
Specificity > sensitivity
Not distinguish benign from malignant

IDs microcalcifications and speculated masses with/without calcification

DCIS, sclerosing adenosis

Punctate, microlinear, branching
MRI high risk BRCA carriers

FNA, core/excisional biopsy

Lymphatics → hematogenous
Outer quadrant → axillary nodes
Inner quadrant internal mammary nodes
MC cancer metastatic to lungs/bone
Delayed metastasis not uncommon
Bone pain from metastasis relieved by radiation
Extranodal spread has greater significance than nodal metastasis alone

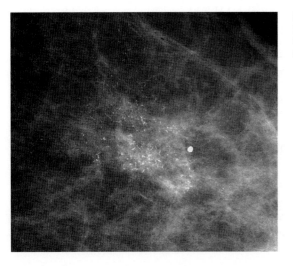

22-20: Mammogram showing breast cancer with microlinear, branching malignant microcalcifications. *(From Pretorius ES, Solomon JA: Radiology Secrets Plus, 3rd ed, Philadelphia, Mosby Elsevier, 2011, p 39, Fig. 6-5.)*

TABLE 22-7 Types of Breast Cancer

TYPE	COMMENTS
NONINVASIVE	
Ductal carcinoma in situ (DCIS) (see Fig. 22-21 A; Link 22-137 C, D)	• Nonpalpable • Patterns: cribriform (sieve-like), comedo (necrotic center) • Commonly contain microcalcifications • Cannot be detected by mammogram unless microcalcifications are present • One-third eventually invade
Lobular carcinoma in situ (LCIS; see Fig. 22-21 B)	• Nonpalpable • Virtually always an incidental finding in a breast biopsy for other reasons • *Cannot* be identified by mammography (*no* calcifications) • Lobules are distended with bland neoplastic cells • One-third eventually invade • Usually positive for estrogen and progesterone receptors • Increased incidence of cancer in the opposite breast (20%–40% of cases)
INVASIVE	
Infiltrating ductal carcinoma (see Fig. 22-21 C and D; Links 22-137 A, B, 22-138, 22-139, and 22-140)	• Stellate morphology (noted in the gross specimen and mammogram), indurated, gray-white tumor • One-third have amplification of the *ERBB2* oncogene • Gritty on cut section • Induration is caused by reactive fibroplasia (desmoplasia) of the stroma to the tumor
Paget disease of nipple (Fig. 22-21 E; Link 22-141)	• Extension of DCIS into the lactiferous ducts and skin of the nipple producing a rash, with or without nipple retraction • Paget cells are present (see Fig. 22-2 E; extramammary Paget disease). Paget disease of the breast is an adenocarcinoma of the breast that is invading the epithelium. This is different than vulvar Paget disease, which is an adenocarcinoma limited to the epithelium. • Palpable mass is present in 50%–60% of cases.
Medullary carcinoma (Link 22-142)	• Associated with *BRCA1* mutations • Bulky, soft tumor with large cells and a lymphoid infiltrate • Majority are negative for estrogen and progesterone receptors
Inflammatory carcinoma (see Fig. 22-21 F; Link 22-143)	• Erythematous breast with dimpling like an orange (peau d'orange) caused by fixed opening of the sweat glands, which cannot expand with lymphedema • Not a specific type of cancer but is rather a clinical manifestation caused by plugs of tumor blocking the lumen of dermal lymphatics causing localized lymphedema • Very poor prognosis
Invasive lobular carcinoma (Link 22-144)	• Neoplastic cells are arranged linearly ("called Indian filing") or in concentric circles (bull's-eye appearance) in the stroma • Invasive carcinoma develops in the contralateral breast in 5%–10% of cases.
Tubular carcinoma (Link 22-145)	• Develops in terminal ductules • Increased incidence of cancer in opposite breast (10% of cases)
Colloid (mucinous) carcinoma (Link 22-146)	• Usually occurs in elderly women • Neoplastic cells are surrounded by extracellular mucin.

Lymph nodes first metastasize to:

Bx determines if cancer spread into lymphatics

Negative Bx: other nodes okay

Positive Bx: chance others involved

Most often positive postmenopausal women

Better prognosis if positive

Candidate for antiestrogen Rx

Poor prognosis if amplification/overexpression *ERBB2*

(a) **Definition:** Lymph node (s) that the cancer would initially drain into (and thus first metastasize to)

(b) Sentinel node biopsy is used to determine if breast cancer has spread beyond the primary site into the lymphatics.

(c) If the biopsy is negative for metastasis, the other nodes in that group are usually negative.

(d) If the biopsy is positive for metastasis, there is a chance that other nodes in that group have metastases.

d. E and P receptor assays (ERA and PRA, respectively)

(1) Assays are most often positive in postmenopausal women.

(2) Clinical significance of a positive ERA and PRA

(a) Confers an overall better prognosis; however, this improvement decreases as the follow-up interval increases

(b) Indicates that the patient is a candidate for antiestrogen therapy (e.g., tamoxifen, oophorectomy)

e. Another test that is performed on breast cancer tissue is the *ERBB2 (HER-2)* oncogene test.

(1) Poor prognosis if amplification or overexpression are present in the malignant cells (see Chapter 9)

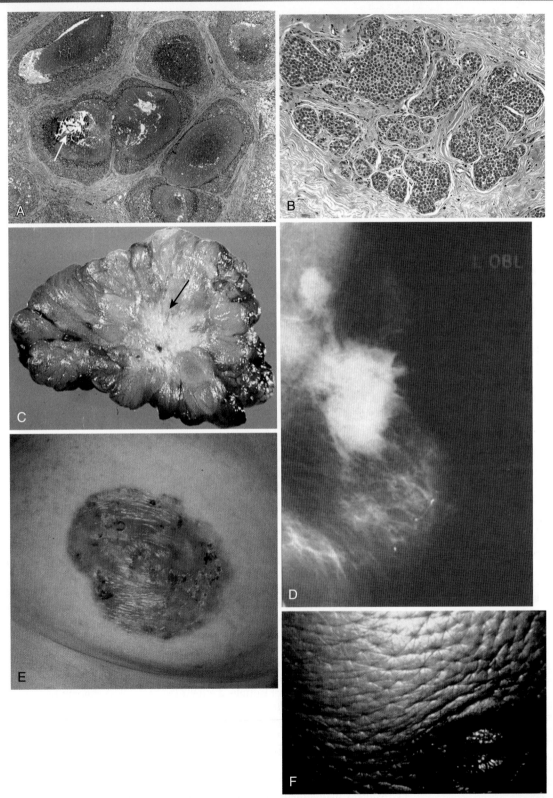

22-21: A, Ductal carcinoma in situ showing dilated ducts lined by layers of neoplastic cells. Central areas of necrosis (comedo pattern) are present, some of which contain microcalcifications *(white arrow).* **B,** Lobular carcinoma in situ showing complete replacement and expansion of a lobule by a monomorphic population of cells. **C,** Infiltrating ductal carcinoma showing a stellate-shaped scar *(arrow)* in the fat tissue of the breast. **D,** Mammogram showing a large irregular spicular mass lesion, which on biopsy showed an infiltrating ductal carcinoma. **E,** Paget disease of the breast showing an erythematous rash around the nipple. **F,** Inflammatory carcinoma of the right breast. Note the dimpled appearance of the breast (peau d'orange). *(A and B from Kumar V, Fausto N, Abbas A:* Robbins and Cotran Pathologic Basis of Disease, *7th ed, Philadelphia, Saunders, 2004, pp 1139, 1142, Figs. 23-16B, 23-20, respectively; **C** from my friend Ivan Damjanov, MD, PhD, Linder J:* Pathology: A Color Atlas, *St. Louis, Mosby, 2000, p 304, Fig. 14-14A; **D** and **F** from Grieg JD:* Color Atlas of Surgical Diagnosis, *London, Mosby-Wolfe, 1996, p 33, Figs. 6-22, 6-23, respectively; **E** from Swartz MH:* Textbook of Physical Diagnosis, *5th ed. Philadelphia, Saunders Elsevier, 2006, p 464, Fig. 16-7.)*

(2) In gene amplification in a cancer cell, multiple copies of the gene are made; in overexpression in a cancer cell, there is increased gene transcription, resulting in the production of certain proteins or other substances that may play a role in cancer development.

f. Surgical procedures in breast cancer.
- Modified radical mastectomy includes the nipple–areolar complex, all the breast tissue, and an axillary lymph node dissection.

A **winged scapula** may occur from damage to the long thoracic nerve (Link 22-148). There is also a risk of developing lymphedema.

Winged scapula: damage long thoracic nerve. Lymphedema risk.

Subareolar gland proliferation male breast due to E

Unilateral > bilateral

↑E

↓Androgens (E unopposed)

Defect androgen receptors (E unopposed)

Peripheral tissue aromatization

T → estradiol

Androstenedione → estrone

Leydig cells in testis

Physiologic gynecomastia

Newborns (common)

Puberty

Elderly persons

Cirrhosis MCC

Cannot metabolize E

Cannot metabolize 17-KS

17-KS aromatized to estrone

Genetic diseases

Klinefelter syndrome

Androgens → E in Leydig cells

AIS

↓Androgen receptor synthesis

E displaced from SHBG

Examples: spironolactone, ketoconazole

↑E activity

Examples: DES, digoxin

Block androgen receptors

Examples: spironolactone, flutamide

↓Androgen production

Example: leuprolide

Choriocarcinoma synthesizes hCG (LH analogue)

↓Androgen production

1° hypogonadism

Example: Leydig cell dysfunction

2° hypogonadism

Example: pituitary/hypothalamic dysfunction

Rare

Inactivation *BRCA2* suppressor gene

Klinefelter syndrome

Same prognosis as women

(1) Breast conservation therapy
  (a) Lumpectomy with microscopically free margins
  (b) Sentinel node biopsy
(2) Breast irradiation

K. **Gynecomastia**
1. **Definition:** Benign subareolar glandular proliferation in the male breast caused by E (Link 22-149)
  a. More often unilateral than bilateral
  b. Caused by increased E stimulation related to
    (1) Increase in E
    (2) Decrease in androgens (leaves E unopposed)
    (3) Defect in androgen receptors (leaves E unopposed)
  c. Sources of E
    (1) Peripheral tissue aromatization (85% of cases)
      (a) T is converted to estradiol by aromatase.
      (b) Androstenedione is converted to estrone by aromatase.
    (2) Leydig cells in testis (15% of cases).
2. Physiologic gynecomastia
  a. Gynecomastia is normal in:
    (1) newborns (present in 60%–90% of cases).
    (2) puberty (peaks at ages 13–14 years).
    (3) older adults (occurs between 50 and 80 years of age).
  b. In general, surgery is *not* indicated.
3. Pathologic gynecomastia
  a. Cirrhosis (most common pathologic cause)
    (1) The liver cannot metabolize E.
    (2) The liver *cannot* metabolize 17-KS. 17-KS is peripherally aromatized to estrone.
  b. Genetic diseases
    (1) Klinefelter syndrome (see Chapter 6): increased aromatization of androgens to estrogens in Leydig cells and decreased responsiveness of T to androgen receptors
    (2) Androgen insensitivity syndrome (AIS; testicular feminization; see Chapter 6); decreased androgen receptor synthesis
  c. Drugs
    (1) Drug displacement of E from SHBG leading to increased free E fraction. Examples: spironolactone, ketoconazole
    (2) Drugs with E activity. Example: diethylstilbestrol (DES), digoxin (activates E receptors)
    (3) Drugs that block androgen receptors. Examples: spironolactone, flutamide
    (4) Drugs that decrease androgen production. Example: leuprolide
  d. Cancer
    - Choriocarcinoma of the testis produces hCG, which is a LH analogue (hCG acts like LH).
  e. Disorders with decreased androgen production
    (1) Primary hypogonadism. Example: Leydig cell dysfunction (see Chapter 21)
    (2) Secondary hypogonadism. Example: pituitary or hypothalamic dysfunction (see Chapter 21)

L. **Breast cancer in men; epidemiology**
1. Breast cancer in men is extremely rare.
2. Risk factors
  a. Inactivation of the *BRCA2* suppressor gene (normally regulates DNA repair)
  b. Klinefelter syndrome (see Chapter 6)
3. Stage for stage, breast cancer in men has the same prognosis as in women.

ABBREVIATIONS

MC most common
MCC most common cause

COD cause of death

Rx treatment

I. **Overview of Endocrine Disease**
   A. **Clinical significance of various endocrine diseases** (Link 23-1)
   B. **Location of endocrine glands** (Link 23-2)
   C. **Hormones in the endocrine system** (Link 23-3)
   D. **Examples of cell-to-cell signaling** (Link 23-4)
      • Neurocrine, endocrine, paracrine, autocrine
   E. **Endocrine axis and feedback mechanisms** (Link 23-5)
   F. **Negative feedback loops** (Link 23-6)
      1. **Definition:** Inverse relationship between the concentration of a hormone and the concentration of the stimulant that controls an increase or a decrease in hormone production; attempt to maintain a target level of a hormone
      2. Example of a negative feedback loop: Increase in serum ionizing calcium (Ca) level leads to a decrease in the synthesis and release of parathyroid hormone (PTH) by the parathyroid glands.
      3. Example of a negative feedback loop: Increased serum cortisol level leads to a decrease in adrenocorticotropic hormone (ACTH) release by the anterior pituitary gland.
   G. **Positive feedback loops**
      1. **Definition:** Amplification of a hormone away from a target level
      2. Example of a positive feedback loop: In the proliferative phase of the menstrual cycle, a surge in estradiol causes luteinizing hormone (LH) to increase to a greater degree than follicle-stimulating hormone (FSH). This "LH surge" stimulates ovulation (see Fig. 22-7).
   H. **Stimulation tests evaluate hypofunctioning disorders**
      1. Example: ACTH stimulation test is used in the workup of hypocortisolism to determine whether hypocortisolism is caused by adrenal hypofunction or pituitary or hypothalamic hypofunction.
         a. If ACTH does *not* cause an increase in serum cortisol, the problem is adrenal hypofunction.
         b. If ACTH causes an increase in serum cortisol, the problem is either hypopituitarism or hypothalamic hypofunction.
      2. Causes of endocrine hypofunction (Links 23-7 and 23-8)
         a. Autoimmune destruction (MCC of hypofunction). Examples: Addison disease, Hashimoto thyroiditis
         b. Infarction (see Chapter 2). Examples: Sheehan postpartum necrosis, Waterhouse-Friderichsen syndrome (WFS) in meningococcemia (sepsis from *Neisseria meningitidis*)

Negative feedback loops

Inverse relation controls ↑/↓ in hormone production

↑Serum ionized calcium: ↓serum PTH

↑Plasma cortisol, ↓serum ACTH

Positive feedback loops

Hormone amplification away from target level

+ Feedback: ↑estradiol → ↑LH > FSH→ ovulation

Stimulation tests: hypofunction disorders

ACTH stimulation test in hypocortisolism

No ↑cortisol: adrenal hypofunction

↑Cortisol: hypopituitarism/ hypothalamic hypofunction

Endocrine hypofunction

MCC autoimmune disease

Addison disease, Hashimoto thyroiditis

Infarction

WFS: meningococcemia

c. Decreased gland stimulation. Example: Decreased thyroid-stimulating hormone (TSH) in hypopituitarism causes a decrease in thyroid production of thyroxine (T_4).

d. Other causes of endocrine hypofunction include enzyme deficiency, infection, metastasis, or a congenital disorder.

I. **Suppression tests**

1. Suppression tests evaluate hyperfunctioning endocrine disorders.
   a. Example: The low-dose dexamethasone (DXM; cortisol analogue) suppression test evaluates hypercortisolism caused by pituitary, adrenal, or the ectopic Cushing syndrome.
   b. Cortisol is *not* suppressed in Cushing syndrome with a low dose of DXM.
2. Most hyperfunctioning endocrine disorders *cannot* be suppressed.
   a. Notable *exceptions* are prolactinoma and pituitary Cushing syndrome.
   b. Dopamine analogues (e.g., cabergoline) can suppress prolactin secretion from a prolactinoma.
   c. High-dose of DXM (cortisol analogue) can suppress ACTH production in pituitary Cushing syndrome causing a decrease in cortisol.
3. Causes of endocrine hyperfunction (Links 23-7 and 23-8) include benign (MCC) and malignant tumors, hyperplasia, and acute inflammation. Examples of each:
   a. Benign adenoma of the adrenal cortex can synthesize excess cortisol producing Cushing disease.
   b. Small cell carcinoma (SCC) of the lung releases antidiuretic hormone (ADH), causing hyponatremia (syndrome of inappropriate antidiuretic hormone secretion [SIADH]).
   c. Parathyroid gland hyperplasia produces hypercalcemia.
   d. Acute thyroiditis (acute inflammation) causes release of stored thyroid hormone, producing hyperthyroidism.

II. **Hypothalamus Disorders**

A. **Tumors or tumor-like conditions altering hypothalamic function**
   1. Pituitary adenoma (see section IV): most common tumor affecting hypothalamic function
   2. Craniopharyngioma (see Section IV)
   3. Midline hamartoma: *not* a neoplasm and produces precocious puberty in boys
   4. Langerhans histiocytosis (see Chapter 14). Metastasis of malignant histiocytes to the hypothalamus leads to decreased production of ADH (diabetes insipidus). This results in an excessive loss of water in the kidneys.

B. **Inflammatory disorders altering hypothalamic function**
   1. Sarcoidosis (see Chapter 17): produces granulomatous inflammation in the hypothalamus, leading to decreased ADH and diabetes insipidus with a loss of excessive amounts of water in the urine.
   2. Infectious diseases involving the hypothalamus (e.g., meningitis, brain abscesses, encephalitis; see Chapter 26) may alter hypothalamic function.

C. **Clinical findings of hypothalamic dysfunction**
   1. Secondary hypopituitarism
      a. **Definition:** Occurs when hypothalamic dysfunction decreases the synthesis and release of various releasing factors that normally stimulate the anterior or posterior pituitary gland to synthesize and release their hormones
      b. Example: deficiency of gonadotropin-releasing hormone (GnRH) in the hypothalamus causes a decrease in FSH and LH synthesis by the anterior pituitary gland
      c. Example: deficiency of corticotropin-releasing hormone (CRH) in the hypothalamus causes a decrease in ACTH produced by the anterior pituitary gland, which in turn leads to a decrease in the synthesis of cortisol in the adrenal cortex
   2. Central diabetes insipidus (CDI; discussed fully in Chapter 5)
   3. Hyperprolactinemia: Loss of dopamine from the hypothalamus removes the inhibition of prolactin synthesis in the anterior pituitary, leading to an increase in prolactin and a corresponding increase in milk production in females (galactorrhea).
   4. Precocious puberty: A midline hamartoma (see later) in the hypothalamus in a boy causes precocious puberty.

"True" precocious puberty implies a central nervous system (CNS) origin for the disorder. Alternatively, pseudoprecocious puberty implies a peripheral cause (e.g., adrenogenital syndrome). True precocious puberty in boys is the onset of puberty *before* 9 years of age. A common cause is a midline hamartoma in the hypothalamus. True precocious puberty in girls is the onset of puberty *before* 8 years of age. Usually idiopathic, it is less likely to be caused by a midline hamartoma (non-neoplastic overgrowth of disorganized nerve tissue).

5. Visual field disturbances: usually bitemporal hemianopia caused by compression of the optic chiasm by a suprasellar mass (e.g., craniopharyngioma) or a large pituitary adenoma

6. Mass effects
   a. Mass lesion in the brain causes an obstructive (noncommunicating) hydrocephalus (see Chapter 26).
   b. Example: A large pituitary adenoma may compress the third ventricle, producing a noncommunicating hydrocephalus.

7. Growth disorders: Dwarfism may occur in children because of to a lack of growth hormone-releasing hormone (GHRH) from the hypothalamus.

8. Primary amenorrhea caused by Kallmann syndrome. In this syndrome, there is decreased synthesis of GnRH by the hypothalamus, which in turn decreases the synthesis and release of FSH and LH in the anterior pituitary gland, leading to primary amenorrhea.

III. Pineal Gland Disorders
A. Clinical anatomy of the pineal gland
1. Pineal gland is located in the midline location above the quadrigeminal plate in the midbrain.
2. Site for melatonin production
   a. Superior cervical sympathetic ganglia stimulates receptors on pinealocytes, causing the release of melatonin into the spinal fluid and blood.
   b. Melatonin functions
      (1) Important in sleep, mood, and circadian rhythms
      (2) Released at night; used in the treatment of sleep and mood disorders

B. Pineal gland disorders
1. Dystrophic calcification of the pineal gland begins in childhood.
   a. Calcification is useful in radiology to show shifts caused by mass lesions in the brain.
   b. Approximately 80% of pineal glands are calcified by 70 to 80 years of age.
2. Pineal gland tumors
   a. The majority are germ cell tumors resembling seminomas in the testis (see Chapter 21).
   b. A minority of tumors are teratomas with ectodermal, endodermal, and mesodermal components (see Chapter 9).

C. Clinical findings in pineal gland tumors
1. Visual disturbances causing paralysis of upward conjugate gaze (Parinaud syndrome; see Fig. 26-3 B)
2. Obstructive hydrocephalus caused by compression of the cerebral aqueduct draining the third ventricle (see Chapter 26)

IV. Pituitary Gland Disorders
A. Pituitary gland hormones (Link 23-9)
B. Overview of signs and symptoms of pituitary sella disorders
1. Clinical syndromes of excess hormone production (hyperfunction; e.g., acromegaly, pituitary Cushing disease, galactorrhea or secondary amenorrhea from prolactinoma)
2. Clinical syndromes caused by hypofunction of the pituitary (e.g., secondary hypothyroidism, hypocortisolism, infertility)
3. Compression syndromes (hydrocephalus, frontal headaches, visual disturbances [bitemporal hemianopsia]).

C. Anterior pituitary hypofunction
1. **Definition:** Partial or complete loss of secretion of one or more hormones synthesized in the anterior pituitary gland
2. Epidemiology
   a. Pituitary gland includes anterior and posterior parts.
   b. Infarctions of the pituitary gland invariably lead to panhypopituitarism (all hormones are decreased).
   c. Types of pituitary gland dysfunction
      (1) Primary hypopituitarism (pituitary dysfunction): At least 75% of the gland must be destroyed.
      (2) Secondary hypopituitarism (hypothalamic dysfunction): decreased synthesis and release of hypothalamic releasing factors
3. Causes of hypopituitarism

Dysfunction: visual field defects

Mass effects

Large pituitary adenoma → obstructive hydrocephalus

Growth disorders

Dwarfism in children

1° Amenorrhea: Kallmann syndrome

↓GnRH → ↓FSH/LH → 1° amenorrhea

Pineal gland disorders

Midline above quadrigeminal plate

Melatonin synthesis

Superior cervical sympathetic ganglia

Melatonin functions

Sleep, mood, circadian rhythms

Released at night

Rx sleep, mood disorders

Pineal gland disorders

Dystrophic calcification

Shows shifts in mass lesions

Pineal gland tumors

Majority germ cell tumors

Minority teratomas

Paralysis upward gaze ("setting sun" sign)

Obstructive hydrocephalus (compression cerebral aqueduct)

Pituitary gland disorders

Hyperfunction

Hypofunction

Compression syndromes

Anterior pituitary hypofunction

Loss one/more anterior pituitary hormones

Anterior/posterior pituitary

Infarction: panhypopituitarism

1° Hypopituitarism

>75% Gland destroyed

2o Hypopituitarism (hypothalamic dysfunction)

Causes hypopituitarism

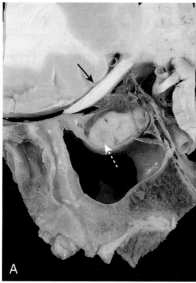
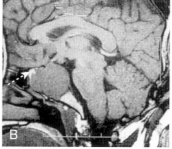
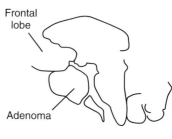

23-1: **A,** Pituitary adenoma. The *interrupted arrow* shows a well-circumscribed mass that has almost completely replaced the pituitary gland. A thin rim of sella turcica is present at the base of the tumor. The *solid arrow* shows the optic nerve and its proximity to the sella turcica. **B,** Magnetic resonance images of the pituitary gland. Sagittal view of a large pituitary adenoma lifting and distorting the optic chiasm *(white arrow)* and impinging on the frontal lobe. *(A from Burger PC, Scheithauer BW, Vogel KS:* Surgical Pathology of the Nervous System, *4th ed, London, Churchill Livingstone, 2002, p 444, Fig. 9-20. B from Melmed S, Polonsky KS, Larsen PR, Kronenberg HM:* Williams Textbook of Endocrinology, *13th ed, Philadelphia, Elsevier Saunders, 2016, p 233, Fig. 9-1B.)*

Nonfunctioning pituitary adenoma

MCC hypopituitarism in adults

Microadenoma <10 mm; macroadenoma ≥10 mm

MEN I: pituitary adenoma, HPTH, pancreatic tumor

Craniopharyngioma

Benign tumor Rathke pouch remnants

MCC hypopituitarism in children

a. Nonfunctioning (null) pituitary adenoma (Fig. 23-1; Links 23-10 and 23-11)
   (1) MCC of hypopituitarism in adults; accounts for 45% of overall sellar masses
   (2) Called a microadenoma if <10 mm or a macroadenoma if ≥10 mm; called a pituitary incidentaloma if discovered in a patient without symptoms in brain imaging for other disorders
   (3) Association with multiple endocrine neoplasia (MEN) I syndrome, which includes pituitary adenoma, hyperparathyroidism (HPTH), and pancreatic tumor (e.g., Zollinger-Ellison syndrome or insulinoma).
b. Craniopharyngioma
   (1) **Definition:** Benign pituitary tumor derived from Rathke pouch remnants
   (2) Epidemiology
      (a) MCC of hypopituitarism in children

Rathke pouch is derived from the oral ectoderm. It develops into the anterior lobe of the pituitary gland.

Rathke pouch derived from oral ectoderm. Develops anterior lobe.
Above sella turcica
Destroys pituitary gland
Cystic tumor, hemorrhage, calcification
Bitemporal hemianopia
CDI
Sheehan postpartum necrosis
Hypovolemic shock blood loss → pituitary infarction
Pale infarction
Sudden loss lactation (loss prolactin)
Eventual hypopituitarism
Pituitary enlargement pregnancy: ↑synthesis prolactin; progesterone inhibits secretion

      (b) Located *above* the sella turcica (contains the pituitary gland). Extends into the sella turcica and destroys the pituitary gland.
      (c) Cystic tumor with hemorrhage and dystrophic calcification (Links 23-12 and 23-13)
   (3) Clinical findings
      (a) Bitemporal hemianopia (compresses the optic chiasm)
      (b) CDI by destroying the posterior pituitary gland, which stores ADH (see Chapter 5)
c. Sheehan postpartum necrosis
   (1) **Definition:** An infarction of the pituitary gland caused by hypovolemic shock secondary to blood loss during parturition
   (2) Epidemiology
      (a) Pale infarction (see Chapter 2)
      (b) Classic presentation of Sheehan postpartum necrosis is the sudden cessation of lactation caused by a sudden loss of prolactin.
      (c) Eventual development of hypopituitarism

The **pituitary gland** doubles in size during pregnancy because of increase synthesis of prolactin. During pregnancy, prolactin release is inhibited by high levels of progesterone.

d. Pituitary apoplexy
   (1) **Definition:** "Apoplexy" refers to a sudden onset of pituitary dysfunction
   (2) Epidemiology
      (a) Most often caused by hemorrhage or infarction within a preexisting pituitary adenoma
      (b) Predisposing factors include trauma, pregnancy (Sheehan postpartum necrosis, a nontumorous cause), and treatment of a prolactinoma with bromocriptine.
   (3) Clinical findings in pituitary apoplexy include a sudden onset of headache, mental status dysfunction, visual disturbances, and hormone dysfunction.
e. Sickle cell anemia (HbSS; see Chapter 12). Pituitary infarction occurs from vascular occlusion of the blood vessels by sickled red blood cells (RBCs).
f. Lymphocytic hypophysitis
   (1) **Definition:** Female-dominant autoimmune destruction of the pituitary gland
   (2) Epidemiology: occurs during or after pregnancy
g. Empty sella syndrome
   (1) **Definition:** Brain imaging shows an empty sella in the sphenoid bone (Link 23-14).
   (2) Epidemiology
      (a) Primary type of empty sella syndrome
         • Often seen in obese hypertensive women
         • Anatomic defect is present above the pituitary gland.
         • Subarachnoid space extends into the sella turcica and fills up with cerebrospinal fluid (CSF).
         • Increase in pressure on the pituitary gland causes it to flatten out and undergo atrophy (compression atrophy).
      (b) Secondary type of empty sella syndrome caused by regression in size of the pituitary gland caused by radiation, trauma, or surgery
4. Clinical and laboratory findings in anterior pituitary hypofunction (Table 23-1; Fig. 23-2). The metyrapone test distinguishes hypocortisolism caused by pituitary dysfunction or adrenal dysfunction.
5. Diagnosis of anterior pituitary hypofunction
   a. A computed tomography (CT) scan or magnetic resonance imaging (MRI; preferred) of the sella turcica, which is located in the sphenoid bone. MRI visualizes the pituitary fossa, sella turcica with the anterior and posterior clinoid processes, optic chiasm, pituitary stalk, and the cavernous sinuses.
   b. Stimulation tests are performed to identify the various pituitary hormone deficiencies (e.g., arginine stimulation shows a decrease in growth hormone [GH] and insulinlike growth factor-1 [IGF-1]).
   c. Hypothalamic dysfunction (see section II)

Margin notes:
Pituitary apoplexy
Sudden loss pituitary function
Hemorrhage/infarction preexisting pituitary adenoma
Trauma, pregnancy, Rx prolactinoma with bromocriptine
Sudden onset headache, mental/visual/hormone dysfunction
Sickle cell anemia
Infarction from vascular occlusion by sickled cells
Lymphocytic hypophysitis
Female dominant autoimmune destruction
Occurs during/after pregnancy
Empty sella syndrome
Brain imaging shows empty sella in sphenoid bone
Primary type
Obese hypertensive women
Anatomic defect above pituitary gland
Subarachnoid space extends in sella turcica (↑CSF)
Compression atrophy pituitary gland
2° Type: ↓size due to radiation, trauma, surgery
Metyrapone test: pituitary vs adrenal dysfunction
Dx anterior pituitary hypofunction
MRI/CT sella turcica
Stimulation test for hormone deficiencies
Hypothalamic dysfunction

TABLE 23-1 Clinical Findings in Hypopituitarism

TROPHIC HORMONE DEFICIENCY	DISCUSSION
Gonadotropins (FSH, LH)	• Children have delayed puberty. • Women have secondary amenorrhea. Produces osteoporosis, hot flashes (lack of estrogen), and decreased libido (sexual desire). • Men have impotence caused by decreased libido from decreased testosterone (see Chapter 21). • GnRH stimulation test: *no* significant increase of FSH and LH in hypopituitarism; eventual increase of FSH and LH in hypothalamic disease as the pituitary gland regains function
Growth hormone (GH)	• Decreased GH decreases synthesis and release of IGF-1. • Children have growth delay: delayed fusion of epiphyses. Bone growth does *not* match the age of the child. • Adults have hypoglycemia: decreased gluconeogenesis, loss of muscle mass, and increased adipose around the waist. • Arginine and sleep stimulation tests: *no* increase in GH or IGF-1
Thyroid-stimulating hormone (TSH)	• Secondary hypothyroidism: decreased serum T_4 and TSH • Cold intolerance, constipation, weakness • *No* increase in TSH after TRF stimulation
Adrenocorticotropic hormone (ACTH) (see Fig. 23-2)	• Metyrapone test: stimulation test of pituitary ACTH and adrenal gland reserve. The inhibition of adrenal 11-hydroxylase by metyrapone causes a decrease in cortisol and a corresponding increase in plasma ACTH (pituitary) and 11-deoxycortisol (adrenal) proximal to the enzyme block. In hypopituitarism, neither ACTH nor 11-deoxycortisol is increased. In adrenal disease, ACTH is increased, but 11-deoxycortisol is decreased.

ADH, Antidiuretic hormone; *FSH,* follicle-stimulating hormone; *GnRH,* gonadotropin-releasing hormone; *IGF,* insulin-like growth factor; *LH,* luteinizing hormone; *SIADH,* syndrome of inappropriate antidiuretic hormone; *T_4,* thyroxine; *TRF,* thyrotropin-releasing factor.

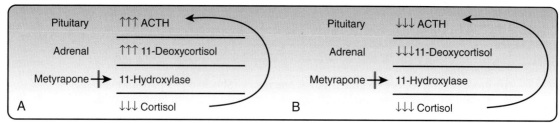

23-2: Schematic of the metyrapone test: a normal response (**A**) and the response expected in hypopituitarism (**B**). **A,** Metyrapone blocks 11-hydroxylase in the adrenal cortex. This decreases cortisol, leading to an increase in adrenocorticotropic hormone (ACTH) and 11-deoxy-cortisol. **B,** A decrease in cortisol does *not* increase pituitary ACTH, indicating hypopituitarism as the cause of hypocortisolism. Because ACTH is *not* increased, there is *no* increase in 11-deoxycortisol proximal to the enzyme block.

Posterior pituitary hypofunction

Function posterior pituitary

Stores ADH

Controls TBW

↑ADH concentrate urine

↓ADH dilute urine: loss free water

CDI: deficiency ADH

SIADH: increased ADH

Release oxytocin after suckling

Paraventricular nucleus hypothalamus

Causes milk ejection/uterine contractions

Pituitary hyperfunction disorders

30% Adenomas non-functioning

Prolactinoma

Benign tumor secretes prolactin

Benign adenoma

MC pituitary tumor

Dopaminergic pathways inhibit

May secrete GH

2° amenorrhea + galactorrhea

↑Prolactin→ ↓GnRH → ↓FSH/LH

Promotes lactation in nonpregnant women

Excess prolactin men

Men: impotence

Loss libido: ↓T from ↓LH

Headache

Pituitary tumor larger men>women

Galactorrhea rare in men

Serum prolactin >200 ng/mL

↓Serum FSH/LH

↑Prolactin→ ↓GnRH

↓FSH → ↓E; ↓LH → ↓P

↓E + ↓P → 2° amenorrhea

D. Posterior pituitary hypofunction
1. Normal function of the posterior pituitary
   a. Stores antidiuretic hormone (ADH)
      (1) ADH controls total body water (TBW).
      (2) The presence of ADH induces the concentration of urine by allowing free water to be reabsorbed from the collecting ducts (see Chapter 5).
      (3) Absence of ADH produces dilution of urine by allowing free water to be lost in the urine (see Chapter 5).
      (4) CDI caused by a deficiency of ADH and SIADH (increased ADH) are discussed in Chapter 5.
   b. Releases oxytocin after suckling
      (1) Oxytocin is primarily produced in the paraventricular nucleus in the hypothalamus.
      (2) Causes milk ejection and uterine contractions
2. See Chapter 5 for a complete discussion of diabetes insipidus.

E. Pituitary hyperfunction disorders
1. Thirty percent of pituitary adenomas are nonfunctioning.
2. Prolactinoma
   a. **Definition:** Benign tumor prolactin secreting tumor of the anterior pituitary gland
   b. Epidemiology
      (1) Benign adenoma
      (2) Overall MC pituitary tumor (35% of all tumors)
      (3) Dopaminergic pathways normally inhibit prolactin.
      (4) Also secretes GH in 7% of cases
   c. Clinical and laboratory findings (Link 23-15)
      (1) In women, it produces secondary amenorrhea (loss of menses), galactorrhea (lactation; see Fig. 22-19 A), oligomenorrhea without ovulation, infertility, and osteoporosis (caused by estrogen [E] deficiency). Women can be premenopausal or postmenopausal and still develop galactorrhea.
         (a) Prolactin inhibits GnRH, which decreases FSH and LH, resulting in a decrease in E synthesis in the ovaries.
         (b) Prolactin promotes lactation even though the woman is *not* pregnant.
      (2) Excess prolactin in men
         (a) Impotence (inability to sustain and erection and/or ejaculate during sexual intercourse) and loss of libido. Loss of libido (sexual desire) is caused by a decrease in testosterone (T) from decrease in serum LH.
         (b) LH related to increased prolactin
         (c) Headache from the tumor: Pituitary tumors tend to be larger in men than in women.
         (d) Galactorrhea is rare in men because of their lack of estrogenic stimulation of glandular tissue.
      (3) Serum prolactin level is usually >200 ng/mL.
      (4) Decrease in serum FSH and LH
         (a) Increased prolactin levels suppress release of GnRH.
         (b) A decrease in FSH and LH causes a decrease in serum E and serum progesterone (P), respectively.
         (c) Responsible for secondary amenorrhea in women
   d. Other causes of galactorrhea are discussed in Chapter 22.

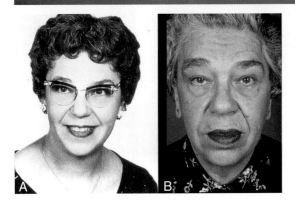

23-3: Acromegaly showing the patient before development of the tumor (**A**) and after development of the tumor (**B**). Note the coarse facial features and enlargement of the jaw and lips. Looking at previous photographs is very useful in suspecting acromegaly. *(From my friend Ivan Damjanov, MD, PhD: Pathology for the Health-Related Professions, 2nd ed, Philadelphia, Saunders, 2000, p 407.)*

3. Growth hormone adenoma
   a. **Definition:** Benign pituitary tumor that secretes excess GH, resulting in gigantism in children and acromegaly in adults
   b. Epidemiology
      (1) Accounts for 20% of all pituitary adenomas. Adenomas secreting GH and prolactin account for 7% of all adenomas.
      (2) Functions of GH
         (a) GH stimulates liver synthesis and release of IGF-1.
         (b) GH stimulates gluconeogenesis and amino acid uptake in muscle.
         (c) GH has a negative feedback relationship with glucose and IGF-1. Where hyperglycemia inhibits GH, hypoglycemia stimulates GH.
         (d) GH has an antinatriuretic action (causes the retention of sodium).
      (3) Functions of IGF-1: stimulates the growth of bone (linear and lateral), cartilage, and soft tissue. It is synthesized in the liver.
   c. Clinical and laboratory findings
      (1) Children develop gigantism.
         (a) Gigantism is caused by an increase linear bone growth because the epiphyses have not fused yet.
         (b) Lateral bone growth is also increased.
      (2) Adults develop acromegaly (Fig. 23-3; Links 23-16, 23-17, 23-18, 23-19, and 23-20).
         (a) Increased lateral bone growth (e.g., hands, feet, jaw); no linear bone growth because the epiphyses in adults are fused
         (b) Prominent jaw and spacing between the teeth
         (c) Frontal bossing caused by an enlarged frontal sinus. This increases hat size.
         (d) Macroglossia (large tongue) is present, which makes it difficult to chew.
         (e) Dilated cardiomyopathy is present (see Fig. 11-23; Link 11-56 B, Chapter 11). MCC of death.
         (f) Increased risk for developing colon polyps and tumors
         (g) Hypertension occurs because of sodium retention, which is related to an increase in GH and insulin. Hyperglycemia increases the release of insulin, which has a mineralocorticoid activity, leading to retention of sodium and hypertension (see Chapter 10).
         (h) Visceral organomegaly with dysfunction in the heart, liver, kidneys, and thyroid gland (Links 23-17 and 23-18)
         (i) Muscle weakness caused by myopathy
         (j) Headache and visual field defects occur because of an enlarged sella turcica.
         (k) Serum GH and IGF-1 are both increased, the latter test being the more sensitive test. Bone hormones are *not* suppressed by glucose administration.
         (l) Hyperglycemia is a secondary cause of diabetes mellitus (DM). It is caused by an increase in gluconeogenesis (GH is gluconeogenic).
   d. Diagnosis of excess GH conditions
      (1) Imaging with CT and MRI (best test)
      (2) Suppression tests
4. Pituitary adenoma secreting ACTH 7% of adenomas (see section VII). Pituitary adenomas secreting TSH, LH, FSH account for 1% of tumors.
5. Syndrome of inappropriate antidiuretic hormone (SIADH; see Chapter 5)

GH adenoma

Excess GH → gigantism child, acromegaly adult

Functions GH

GH → ↑liver synthesis IGF-1

GH ↑gluconeogenesis + amino acid uptake muscle

GH −feedback with glucose and IGF-1

Hyperglycemia: ↓GH; hypoglycemia:↑GH

GH antinatriuretic (retention sodium)

Insulin-like growth factor-1

IGF-1: stimulates bone, cartilage, soft tissue

Clinical/lab findings

Gigantism (children)

↑Linear/lateral bone growth in children

↑Lateral bone growth

Acromegaly (adults)

↑Lateral bone growth; no linear bone growth

Prominent jaw; spacing between teeth

Frontal bossing; ↑hat size

Macroglossia

Dilated cardiomyopathy; MC COD

↑Risk colon polyps/tumors

Hypertension: salt retention (GH + insulin effect)

Hyperglycemia → ↑insulin (retains sodium)

Organomegaly

Myopathy

Headache, visual field defects

↑IGF-1 greater sensitivity than ↑GH

Hormones *not* suppressed by ↑glucose

Secondary DM

↑Gluconeogenesis from GH

Dx excess GH conditions

MRI best test; CT

Suppression tests

ACTH, TSH, LH, FSH

V. Thyroid Gland Disorders

A. Overview of thyroid gland (Links 23-21 and 23-22)

B. Steps in thyroid hormone synthesis (Link 23-23)

Trapping I TSH-mediated

1. Trapping of iodide (I–) is mediated by TSH
   - If TSH is *not* stimulating the thyroid gland (e.g., hypopituitarism or a person is taking excess thyroid hormone that suppresses TSH release), the thyroid gland undergoes atrophy.

↓TSH → gland atrophy

Iodides → iodine peroxidase mediated

I + T → MIT, DIT

Organification TSH mediated

MIT + DIT = T_3

DIT + DIT = T_4

Stored as colloid

Proteolysis TSH mediated

T4/T3 bind to TBG

1/3rd TBG sites occupied

FT_4 → FT_3: outer ring deiodinase

FT_3 active hormone

FT_4 prohormone

FT_3: – feedback with TSH/TRH

↑FT_3→ ↓TSH, ↓TRH

↓FT_3→↑TSH, ↑TRH

2. Oxidation of iodides to iodine (I) is peroxidase mediated.
3. Organification
   a. Iodine is incorporated into tyrosine (T) to form MIT (monoiodotyrosine) and DIT (diiodotyrosine).
   b. Organification is TSH mediated.
4. Coupling of MIT with DIT produces triiodothyronine (T_3).
5. Coupling of DIT with DIT produces T_4.
6. Hormones are stored as colloid.
7. Proteolysis of colloid by lysosomal proteases is TSH mediated.
8. T_4 and T_3 bind to thyroid-binding globulin (TBG). One-third of TBG binding sites are normally occupied.
9. Free T_4 (FT_4) is peripherally converted to free T_3 (FT_3) by an outer ring deiodinase.
   a. FT_3 is the metabolically active hormone.
   b. FT_4 is considered a prohormone (not metabolically active).
   c. FT_3 has a negative feedback relationship with TSH.
      (1) Increase in FT_3 should decrease serum TSH and decrease thyrotropin-releasing hormone (TRH).
      (2) Decrease in FT_3 should increase TSH and increase TRH.

Thyroid-stimulating hormone (TSH) secretion is regulated by two reciprocal factors: (1) thyrotropin-releasing hormone (TRH) from the hypothalamus stimulates the secretion of TSH from the anterior pituitary gland, and (2) thyroid hormones inhibit the secretion of TSH by downregulating the TRH receptor on the thyrotrophs, thus decreasing their sensitivity to stimulation by TRH. This negative feedback effect of thyroid hormones is mediated by free triiodothyronine (FT_3), which is possible because the anterior lobe contains thyroid deiodinase (converting thyroxine (T_4) to triiodothyronine [T_3]). The reciprocal regulation of TSH secretion by TRH and negative feedback by FT_3 results in a relatively steady rate of TSH secretion, which in turn produces a steady rate of secretion of thyroid hormones (in contrast to growth hormone secretion, whose secretion is pulsatile).

(Excerpt taken from Costanzo LS: *Physiology*, 5th ed, Philadelphia, Saunders Elsevier, 2014, p 411.)

Functions thyroid hormone

BMR

Growth/maturation tissue

Turnover hormones/vitamins

Cell regeneration

Synthesis LDL receptors

Synthesis β-adrenergic receptors for catecholamines

Thyroid function tests

Total serum T_4

Total serum T_4: T4 bound to TBG + FT_4

C. Functions of thyroid hormone

1. Controls the basal metabolic rate (BMR; see Chapter 8)
2. Controls the growth and maturation of tissue (e.g., brain)
3. Controls the turnover of hormones and vitamins; involved in cell regeneration
4. Controls the synthesis of low-density lipoprotein (LDL) receptors for LDL, the main vehicle for transporting cholesterol (CH) in the blood
5. Controls the synthesis of β-adrenergic receptors for catecholamines

D. Thyroid function tests

1. Total serum T_4 (Fig. 23-4 A)
   a. Represents T_4 that is bound to TBG and free (unbound) T_4 (FT_4)
      (1) **Note:** The values used in the schematic do *not* represent true values for each of the components.
      (2) Figure 23-4 A shows one-third of TBG binding sites on two TBGs occupied by T_4. Six molecules of T_4 are bound to TBG.
      (3) Serum FT_4 is 4.
      (4) Total serum T_4 is 10 (6 bound to TBG and 4 to FT_4 = 10).
      (5) TSH is normal because the serum FT_4 is normal.
   b. Increase in TBG synthesis by the liver will result in an increased total serum T_4 (Fig. 23-4 B).

E: ↑TBG → ↑total serum T4 but not FT_4

↑E: pregnancy, OCPs, hormone replacement

      (1) Estrogen (E) increases the synthesis of TBG.
      (2) Causes of increased E include pregnancy, taking oral contraceptive pills (OCPs), and hormone replacement in menopause.
      (3) Extra TBG in the schematic has one-third of its binding sites occupied by T_4. This increases the total amount of T_4 bound to TBG from 6 to 9.

       (4) The 3 FT_4s used to bind to the extra TBG are immediately replaced by 3 T_4 released from the thyroid gland; therefore, the serum FT_4 remains normal (4).

       (5) Total serum T_4 is increased (9 + 4 = 13) because of T_4 bound to the extra TBGs.

       (6) TSH is normal because the serum FT_4 is normal.

       (7) *No* signs of thyrotoxicosis are present because the serum FT_4 is normal.

  c. A decrease in TBG synthesis results in a decreased total serum T_4.

       (1) Causes of a decrease in TBG include anabolic steroids and the nephrotic syndrome (urinary loss of TBG).

       (2) Total serum T_4 is decreased because the amount of TBG is decreased.

       (3) Serum FT_4 and the serum TSH remain normal.

       (4) *No* signs of hypothyroidism because the serum FT_4 is normal

  d. Clinical situations involving TBG

       (1) TBG is normal, and the serum FT_4/FT_3 is increased in Graves disease (increased synthesis of FT_4) and thyroiditis (release of FT_4 from colloid in the inflamed thyroid).

       (2) TBG is normal and serum FT_4/FT_3 is decreased in hypothyroidism.

       (3) TBG is decreased and serum FT_4/FT_3 is normal in a person taking anabolic steroids and in the nephrotic syndrome, in which TBG is lost in the urine along with other proteins.

       (4) TBG is increased and serum FT_4/FT_3 is normal in a woman taking E or during pregnancy because E increases the synthesis of TBG.

2. Serum thyroid stimulating hormone (TSH)

  a. Excellent screening test for evaluating thyroid dysfunction

  b. Examples of serum TSH alterations

       (1) Increased serum TSH is present in primary hypothyroidism, because a decrease in the synthesis of FT_4/FT_3 by the thyroid gland results in an increase in serum TSH by negative feedback.

       (2) Decreased serum TSH

          (a) Thyrotoxicosis (e.g., Graves disease). Increased synthesis of FT_4/FT_3 decreases the serum TSH by negative feedback.

          (b) Hypopituitarism: A decrease in the synthesis of TSH causes a decrease in the synthesis of FT_4/FT_3 by the thyroid gland (called secondary hypothyroidism).

          (c) Hypothalamic dysfunction: A decrease in the synthesis of TRH decreases the synthesis and release of TSH from the anterior pituitary, which in turn decreases the synthesis of FT_4/FT_3 by the thyroid gland (called tertiary hypothyroidism).

3. ^{123}I (radioactive) uptake

  a. ^{123}I uptake is used to evaluate the synthetic activity of the thyroid gland. Recall that iodide (I) is used to synthesize thyroid hormone.

  b. Increased ^{123}I uptake indicates increased thyroid synthesis of T_4. Examples include Graves disease and toxic nodular goiter (Link 23-24).

  c. Decreased ^{123}I uptake

       (1) Inactivity of the thyroid gland

          (a) Example: If a patient is taking thyroid hormone, this decreases TSH, which in turn decreases ^{123}I uptake.

          (b) Because TSH is decreased, the thyroid gland undergoes atrophy (see Chapter 2).

       (2) Inflammation of the thyroid gland. Example: In acute, subacute, and chronic thyroiditis, inflammation of the gland interferes with the normal functions of the gland.

  d. ^{123}I uptake evaluates the functional status of thyroid nodules (see later).

       (1) Decreased ^{123}I uptake in a nodule is called a "cold" nodule. Examples of "cold nodules" in the thyroid include a cyst, an adenoma (e.g., follicular adenoma), and thyroid cancer (e.g., follicular cancer; see Fig. 23-5).

       (2) Increased ^{123}I uptake in a thyroid nodule is called a "hot" nodule and is seen in a toxic nodular goiter (see later).

4. Serum thyroglobulin is used as a marker for thyroid cancer.

E. Thyroiditis

1. Acute thyroiditis

  a. **Definition:** Acute inflammatory disease of the thyroid that leads to thyroid gland destruction and release of hormones

  b. Epidemiology; causes

Margin notes:

↓TBG: ↓total serum T_4 but not FT_4

↓TBG: anabolic steroids, nephrotic syndrome

Changes in TBG: alter total serum T_4; no effect on FT_4 and TSH

Clinical situations involving TBG

Graves/thyroiditis: TBG normal, ↑serum FT_4/FT_3

Hypothyroidism: TBG normal, ↓serum FT_4/FT_3

Steroids/anabolics: ↓TBG, normal serum FT_4/FT_3

Pregnancy, taking E: ↑TBG, normal serum FT_4/FT_3

Serum TSH

Excellent screening test thyroid dysfunction

Serum TSH alterations

↑Serum TSH: primary hypothyroidism

↓Serum TSH: thyrotoxicosis

Hypopituitarism

↓Serum TSH: hypopituitarism

↓Serum FT_4/FT_3: secondary hypothyroidism

Hypothalamic dysfunction

↓Serum TSH: hypothalamic dysfunction

↓TRH → ↓TSH → ↓serum FT_4/FT_3

Tertiary hypothyroidism

^{123}I uptake

Evaluates synthetic activity thyroid gland

I: synthesis thyroid hormone

↑^{123}I uptake: ↑synthesis thyroid hormone

Graves disease, toxic nodular goiter

↓^{123}I uptake

↓^{123}I uptake: inactive thyroid gland

↓^{123}I uptake: patient taking thyroid hormone

↓TSH → thyroid gland atrophy

↓^{123}I uptake: thyroiditis

^{123}I uptake: evaluates functional status thyroid nodules

↓^{123}I uptake: cold nodule (non-functioning)

Cyst, follicular adenoma, thyroid cancer

Hot nodule: ↑^{123}I uptake, toxic nodular goiter

↑Serum thyroglobulin: marker thyroid cancer

Thyroiditis

Acute thyroiditis

Inflammation releases hormones

A Normal B Additional TBG

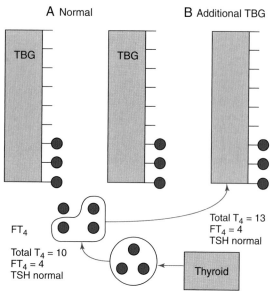

23-4: Schematic of total serum thyroxine (T_4) in a normal individual (**A**) and an individual with an increase in thyroid-binding globulin (TBG) (**B**). The actual numbers do not represent the true concentration of T_4 and free T_4 (FT_4). The *bars* represent TBG, and the *circles* are T_4 bound to TBG and T_4 that is free (FT_4). FT_4 normally has a negative feedback with thyroid-stimulating hormone (TSH). Refer to the text for a complete discussion. *(From Goljan EF: Star Series: Pathology, Philadelphia, Saunders, 1998, Fig. 19-1.)*

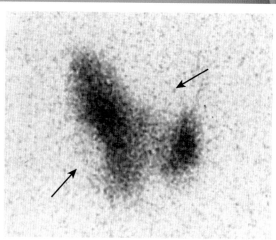

23-5: Nuclear scan of thyroid showing "cold" nodules (lack of uptake or radioactive iodine) in both lobes of the thyroid *(arrows)*. *(From Katz D, Math K, Groskin S: Radiology Secrets, Philadelphia, Hanley & Belfus, 1998, p 531, Fig. 2.)*

Bacterial infections: *S. aureus* MCC
Fungi, parasites
Direct trauma
Fever
Tender gland, cervical adenopathy
Initial thyrotoxicosis
↑Serum T_4, ↓serum TSH
Permanent hypothyroidism uncommon
↓^{123}I uptake
Subacute granulomatous thyroiditis
Subacute thyroiditis: granulomatous inflammation, MGCs
MCC painful thyroid
Virus MCC (coxsackievirus, mumps)
Women 40 to 50 yrs old
Clinical findings
Often preceded by viral URI
No cervical adenopathy
Initial thyrotoxicosis (gland destruction)
↑Serum T_4, ↓serum TSH
Permanent hypothyroidism uncommon
↓^{123}I uptake
Self-limited disease
Hashimoto thyroiditis
Chronic lymphocytic autoimmune disease → 1° hypothyroidism
MCC 1° hypothyroidism
↑Incidence with age
Women > men
HLA associations
Turner, Down, Klinefelter syndromes
↑Incidence PA

(1) Bacterial infections (e.g., *Staphylococcus aureus* is the MCC).
(2) Less common pathogens (e.g., fungi and parasites in immunocompromised patients)
(3) Direct trauma to the thyroid gland
   c. Clinical findings
(1) Fever, tender gland with painful cervical adenopathy
(2) Initial thyrotoxicosis from gland destruction. Increase in serum T_4 and a decrease in serum TSH.
(3) Permanent hypothyroidism is uncommon.
   d. ^{123}I uptake is decreased.
2. Subacute granulomatous thyroiditis
   a. **Definition:** Type of thyroiditis associated with granulomatous inflammation and multinucleated giant cells (MGCs)
   b. Epidemiology
(1) MCC of a painful thyroid gland
(2) Most commonly caused by a viral infection (e.g., coxsackievirus, mumps)
(3) Most often occurs in women 40 to 50 years old
   c. Clinical findings
(1) Often preceded by an upper respiratory infection (URI)
(2) Cervical adenopathy is not prominent.
(3) Initial thyrotoxicosis occurs from gland destruction. Serum T_4 is increased, and serum TSH is decreased.
(4) Permanent hypothyroidism is uncommon.
   d. ^{123}I uptake is decreased.
   e. Disease is self-limited and does *not* require treatment.
3. Hashimoto thyroiditis
   a. **Definition:** Chronic lymphocytic autoimmune disease that produces primary hypothyroidism
   b. Epidemiology
(1) MCC of primary hypothyroidism
(2) Incidence increases with age; more common in women than men
(3) Human leukocyte antigen (HLA)-DR3 and HLA-DR5 associations; increased incidence in Turner syndrome, Down syndrome, and Klinefelter syndrome and increased incidence of other autoimmune diseases (e.g., pernicious anemia [PA])

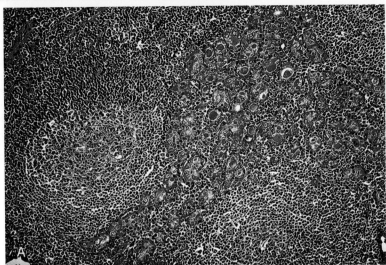
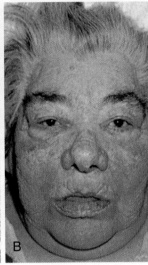

23-6: **A,** Microscopic section of Hashimoto thyroiditis. Note the prominent germinal follicle and heavy infiltrate of lymphocytes throughout the gland with destruction of the thyroid follicles. **B,** Primary hypothyroidism in a patient with Hashimoto thyroiditis. The patient has a puffy face, particularly around the eyes (localized myxedema), and coarse hair. (**A** *from Rosai J, Ackerman LV: Surgical Pathology, 9th ed, St. Louis, Mosby, 2004, p 522, Fig. 9-10;* **B** *from Forbes C, Jackson W: Color Atlas and Text of Clinical Medicine, 2nd ed, London, Mosby, 2002, p 325, Fig. 7-72.)*

(4) Risk factor for developing a primary B-cell malignant lymphoma of the thyroid gland (see later)

(5) Pathogenesis is multifactorial.

    (a) Cytotoxic T cells destroy the parenchyma (type IV hypersensitivity reaction [HSR]); initial thyrotoxicosis and eventual primary hypothyroidism

    (b) Blocking antibodies are present against the TSH receptor (type II HSR); decrease in hormone synthesis

    (c) Helper (CD_4) T cells release cytokines, attracting macrophages that damage thyroid tissue (type IV HSR).

    (d) Antimicrosomal and antithyroglobulin antibodies destroy thyroid parenchyma (type II HSR).

(6) Gross and microscopic findings

    (a) Gland is enlarged and has a fleshy white appearance with numerous rounded protuberances projecting from the surface (Links 23-25 and 23-26).

    (b) Gland has a prominent lymphocytic infiltrate with numerous lymphoid follicles with germinal centers (Fig. 23-6 A).

  c. Clinical findings

    (1) Initial thyrotoxicosis from gland destruction. This phase is known as hashitoxicosis.

    (2) Signs of hypothyroidism eventually occur (see later discussion).

4. Riedel thyroiditis

  a. **Definition:** Rare chronic inflammatory disease characterized by fibrous tissue replacement (sclerosis) of the gland with extension of fibrosis into surrounding tissues

  b. Epidemiology

    (1) Extension of fibrosis into the surrounding tissue can obstruct the trachea.

    (2) Associated with other sclerosing conditions (e.g., sclerosing mediastinitis; see Chapter 17)

    (3) Primary hypothyroidism may occur.

5. Subacute painless lymphocytic thyroiditis (SPLT)

  a. **Definition:** Autoimmune disease that develops postpartum

  b. Epidemiology: Unlike Hashimoto thyroiditis, the thyroid gland *lacks* the lymphoid follicles with germinal centers.

  c. Clinical findings

    (1) Abrupt onset of thyrotoxicosis caused by gland destruction

    (2) Thyroid gland is slightly enlarged and *painless.*

    (3) Progresses to primary hypothyroidism in 40% to 50% of cases

    (4) Antimicrosomal antibodies are present in 50% to 80% of cases.

Risk factor 1° B-cell malignant lymphoma thyroid

Multifactorial pathogenesis

Type IV HSR: cytotoxic T cells

Initial thyrotoxicosis → 1° hypothyroidism

Blocking abs against TSH receptor (type II HSR).

↓Hormone synthesis

CD_4 T cell release cytokines → damage (type IV)

Antimicrosomal/ antithyroglobulin abs (type II HSR)

Gray appearance; lymphoid infiltrate

Prominent lymphoid infiltrate/follicles

Initial thyrotoxicosis from gland destruction

Hashitoxicosis

Eventual signs hypothyroidism

Riedel thyroiditis

Chronic disease with fibrosis

Fibrous tissue into surrounding tissue

Tracheal obstruction

Association with sclerosing mediastinitis

Hypothyroidism may occur

Subacute painless lymphocytic thyroiditis

Autoimmune disease postpartum

Thyroid lacks lymphoid follicles

Abrupt onset thyrotoxicosis (gland destruction)

Enlarged and painless

Hypothyroidism 50%

Antimicrosomal abs

F. **Hypothyroidism**
   1. **Definition:** Reduced secretion of thyroid hormone
   2. Epidemiology
      a. Incidence increases with age and is more common in women than men.
      b. Types of hypothyroidism
         (1) Primary hypothyroidism MCC (>90%): thyroid gland dysfunction; see earlier discussions
         (2) Secondary hypothyroidism (pituitary hypofunction). See earlier discussion.
         (3) Tertiary hypothyroidism (hypothalamic hypofunction). See earlier discussion.
         (4) Tissue resistance to thyroid hormone
      c. Patients are hypometabolic. Basal metabolic rate (BMR) is decreased (see Chapter 8).
      d. β-receptor and low density lipoprotein (LDL) receptor synthesis is decreased.
      e. Causes of hypothyroidism
         (1) Hashimoto thyroiditis (90% of cases; see earlier)
         (2) Subacute painless lymphocytic thyroiditis (see earlier); Reidel thyroiditis (see earlier)
         (3) Hypopituitarism, hypothalamic dysfunction (see earlier)
         (4) Iodine deficiency, enzyme deficiency, congenital
         (5) Drugs, including amiodarone, lithium, sulfonamides, and phenylbutazone
   3. Congenital hypothyroidism
      a. **Definition:** Hypothyroidism that occurs in infancy or early childhood
      b. Epidemiology
         (1) Fetal thyroid starts developing during the seventh week of pregnancy and produces hormone by the 12th week of gestation.
         (2) Brain requires T_4 for its maturation during the first year of life.
         (3) Causes
            (a) Congenital disease; approximately 85% associated with abnormal thyroid gland development (dysgenesis) or with an ectopic gland (migration problem). Hormonogenesis defect (10%–15%; synthesis defect); pituitary or hypothalamic defect (5% of cases)
            (b) Maternal hypothyroidism: must be present *before* the fetal thyroid is developed
            (c) Acquired disorders. Hashimoto thyroiditis, low iodide intake (countries that do not iodize their salt), exposure to neck radiation
      c. Clinical findings
         (1) Severe mental impairment
         (2) Increased weight and short stature. In contrast, pituitary dwarfism is characterized by decreased weight and short stature.
         (3) Newborns (NBs) and infants: delayed development and poor growth, prolonged hyperbilirubinemia, feeding difficulties, delayed stooling, bradycardia, large anterior and posterior fontanelles, macroglossia (enlarged tongue), hoarse cry, umbilical hernia, facial puffiness, unconjugated hyperbilirubinemia (Link 23-27).
   4. Clinical findings in adult hypothyroidism
      a. Proximal muscle myopathy: very common finding in hypothyroidism. Serum creatine kinase (CK) is increased.
      b. Weight gain caused by a hypometabolic state with retention of water and sodium
      c. Dry and brittle hair (Link 23-28); loss of the outer one-third of the eyebrow (Link 23-29)
      d. Bradycardia (slow heart rate) because there are fewer β-adrenergic receptors
      e. Coarse yellow skin: Decreased conversion of β-carotenes into retinoic acid results in carotenemia, giving the skin a yellow discoloration that can be confused with jaundice.
      f. Periorbital puffiness (edema) and a hoarse voice (only present in Hashimoto thyroiditis)
         (1) Caused by myxedema (Fig. 23-6 B; Links 23-28 and 23-30)
         (2) Myxedema is caused by an increased amount of hyaluronic acid in the interstitial tissue; nonpitting edema because hyaluronic acid gives increased viscosity to the interstitial tissue.
      g. Fatigue, cold intolerance, and constipation
      h. Menstrual irregularities (most often menorrhagia)
      i. Diastolic hypertension caused by retention of sodium and water; dilated cardimyopathy with biventricular congestive heart failure (CHF) (see Chapter 11)
      j. Atherosclerotic coronary artery disease (CAD)
      k. Delayed recovery of Achilles deep tendon reflex (DTR), mental slowness, and dementia
   5. Overview of clinical findings in hypothyroidism (Link 23-31)

6. Laboratory findings in hypothyroidism
   a. Decreased serum T$_3$/T$_4$ and increased serum TSH
   b. Increased antimicrosomal, antiperoxidase, and antithyroglobulin antibodies
   c. Occurs in Hashimoto thyroiditis and subacute painless lymphocytic thyroiditis (SPLT)
   d. Hypercholesterolemia caused by decreased synthesis of LDL receptors (type II hyperlipoproteinemia [HLP]; see Chapter 10)
6. Myxedema coma
   a. Definition: A loss of brain function as a result of severe, long-standing hypothyroidism
   b. Epidemiology
      (1) Most commonly occurs in elderly patients with untreated or inadequately treated hypothyroidism
      (2) Superimposed events that can precipitate myxedema coma include prolonged cold exposure, infection, surgery, trauma, acute myocardial infarction (AMI), CHF, pulmonary embolism, stroke, gastrointestinal bleeding, and various drugs (sedatives, opiates). (*Excerpt from McDermott MT: Endocrine Secrets, 6th ed, Philadelphia, Elsevier Saunders, 2013, p 311, # 14.*)
   c. Clinical findings in myxedema coma
      (1) Progressive stupor, hypothermia
      (2) Bradycardia, hypoventilation
      (3) Hypoglycemia, hypocortisolism, syndrome of inappropriate antidiuretic hormone (SIADH)
   d. Mortality rate ranges from 0% to 45%.
G. **Thyroid hormone excess**
   1. Classification
      a. Thyrotoxicosis. **Definition:** Thyroid hormone excess regardless of cause (e.g., Graves disease, thyroiditis, increased intake of thyroid hormone)
      b. Hyperthyroidism: **Definition:** Thyroid hormone excess caused by increased synthesis of the hormone. Examples: Graves disease and toxic nodular goiter
   2. Patients are hypermetabolic because there is an increase in the BMR (see Chapter 8).
   3. Graves disease
      a. **Definition:** Female-dominant hypermetabolic state caused by B-cell production of IgG antibodies that stimulate the TSH receptors
      b. Epidemiology
         (1) MCC of hyperthyroidism and thyrotoxicosis (80% of cases)
         (2) Female-dominant autoimmune disease
         (3) HLA-B8 and HLA-DR3 association with Graves disease in the white population
         (4) Pathogenesis
            (a) T cells induce specific B cells to produce IgG antibodies against the TSH receptor; stimulating type of antibody as opposed to a blocking antibody; type II HSR (see Chapter 4)
            (b) Antimicrosomal and antithyroglobulin antibodies are present.
            (c) Inciting events that may initiate onset of the disease include infection, withdrawal of steroids, iodide excess, and the postpartum state.
         (5) On physical exam, there is symmetrical, nontender thyromegaly.
         (6) Histologic exam reveals scant colloid and papillary infolding of the glands (Links 23-32 and 23-33).
         (7) Increased incidence of type 1 DM, rheumatoid arthritis (RA), immune thrombocytopenia (IT), and vitiligo (autoimmune destruction of melanocytes causes patchy skin depigmentation)
      c. Clinical and laboratory features unique to Graves disease and *not* found in other causes of thyrotoxicosis
         (1) Infiltrative ophthalmopathy (exophthalmos) occurs in 50% of cases.
            (a) Proptosis (protrusion) and muscle weakness of the eye (Figs. 23-7 A and B; Links 23-34 and 23-35)
            (b) Caused by increased swelling of the orbital tissue (adipose and muscle caused by water retention from hydrophilic mucopolysaccharides and a lymphocytic infiltrate)
            (c) Increased fibroblast growth in the orbital tissue may cause fibrosis of the orbital muscles.
         (2) IgG-TSH receptor antibodies cross the placenta, producing transient hyperthyroidism in the fetus.
         (3) Pretibial myxedema occurs in 1% to 2% of cases (Fig. 23-7 C; Links 23-36 and 23-37) caused by excess glycosaminoglycans (hyaluronic acid) in the dermis.

23-7: A, Graves disease. The patient has exophthalmos and a diffuse enlargement of the thyroid gland (goiter). **B,** Severe exophthalmos in Graves disease. Note the proptosis of the eye, increased vascularity of the conjunctiva, and enlarged lacrimal gland. **C,** Pretibial myxedema in Graves disease. Note the thickened area of erythema involving the pretibial area and dorsum of the foot. **D,** Schematic of euthyroid sick syndrome (ESS). In ESS, the outer ring deiodinase is blocked, and the inner ring deiodinase converts T₄ to reverse T₃, which is inactive. (*A from Forbes C, Jackson W:* Color Atlas and Text of Clinical Medicine, *2nd ed, London, Mosby, 2002, p 323, Fig. 7-61; B from Swartz MH:* Textbook of Physical Diagnosis, *5th ed, Philadelphia, Saunders Elsevier, 2006, p 232, Fig. 10-35;* **C** *courtesy of R. A. Marsden, MD, St. George's Hospital, London;* **D** *courtesy of Edward Goljan, MD.*)

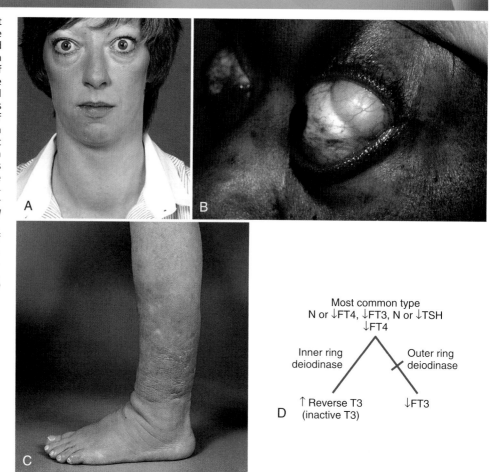

Most common type
N or ↓FT4, ↓FT3, N or ↓TSH
↓FT4

Inner ring deiodinase   Outer ring deiodinase

↑ Reverse T3 (inactive T3)   ↓FT3

D

(4) Thyroid acropachy may be present.
   (a) **Definition:** Digital swelling and clubbing of the fingers (Link 23-38). Periosteal reaction of the metacarpals and phalanges is present on radiographs (Link 23-39).
   (b) Nails separate from the nail bed (lifted up).
   (c) Exophthalmos and pretibial myxedema are usually present.
(5) Hematologic changes unique to Graves disease include a normal to slightly low white blood cell (WBC) count; neutropenia; a relative lymphocytosis (the percentage is increased, but the absolute number of lymphocytes is normal); an absolute increase in monocytes; and in severe cases of Graves disease, a normocytic anemia.
(6) Clinical findings in Graves disease (Link 23-40)
4. Clinical findings in Graves disease in the elderly (also called apathetic hyperthyroidism)
   a. Cardiac abnormalities include atrial fibrillation (AF; key finding) and congestive heart failure (CHF).
   b. Muscle weakness and apathy (lack of affect); thyromegaly
5. Toxic multinodular goiter (Plummer disease)
   a. **Definition:** A multinodular goiter that becomes TSH-independent and produces hyperthyroidism
   b. ¹²³I scan shows "hot" nodules (increased uptake of ¹²³I), and the remainder of the thyroid gland undergoes atrophy because of the lack of stimulation of the gland by TSH.
   c. Distinctions from Graves disease include a *lack* of exophthalmos, pretibial myxedema, and associations with other autoimmune diseases.
6. Clinical signs in *all* causes of thyrotoxicosis
   a. Signs in thyrotoxicosis
   (1) Weight loss in the presence of a good appetite
   (2) Fine tremor of the hands
   (3) Heat intolerance, diarrhea, and anxiety

Thyroid acropachy: digital swelling/clubbing

Nails lifted up

Exophthalmos/pretibial myxedema usually present

Neutropenia

Monocytosis, normocytic anemia

Apathetic hyperthyroidism in elderly

AF key finding; CHF

Muscle weakness, apathy

Thyromegaly

Toxic multinodular goiter

TSH-independent → hyperthyroidism

"Hot" nodules (↑uptake ¹²³I)

No exophthalmos/pretibial myxedema; *no* autoimmune disease associations

Clinical signs all causes thyrotoxicosis

Weight loss (good appetite)

Fine hand tremor

Heat intolerance, diarrhea, anxiety

(4) Menstrual irregularities (usually oligomenorrhea; see Chapter 22)

(5) Lid stare (Links 23-34 and 23-35): caused by increased sympathetic stimulation of the levator palpebrae superioris in the eyelid

  b. Cardiac findings in thyrotoxicosis

    (1) Sinus tachycardia (>90 beats/min)

    (2) Increased risk for developing AF (a key clinical finding)

    (3) Systolic hypertension (see Chapter 10)

    (4) High-output congestive heart failure (high output-CHF; see Chapter 11)

      (a) Thyroid hormone increases β-receptor synthesis in the heart.

      (b) Excess hormone has an inotropic effect on the heart (increases the strength of the muscle contraction) and a chronotropic effect on the heart (increases the heart rate).

  c. Brisk DTRs

  d. Osteoporosis may occur because of increased bone turnover (see Chapter 24).

7. Laboratory findings in thyrotoxicosis

  a. Increased serum T_3/T_4 and decreased serum TSH

  b. Increased ^{123}I uptake: occurs in Graves disease (diffuse uptake of ^{123}I) and toxic multinodular goiter (uptake of ^{123}I is limited to the "hot," overactive nodules)

  c. Decreased ^{123}I uptake: occurs in thyroiditis (inflamed thyroid glands) in its early stages and in those taking excess thyroid hormone (TSH is suppressed, and the glands cannot take up the ^{123}I)

  d. Hyperglycemia: caused by increased glycogenolysis (breakdown of glycogen) and an increased incidence of type I DM in Graves disease only

  e. Hypocholesterolemia caused by increased metabolism of cholesterol

  f. Hypercalcemia caused by increased bone turnover

8. Comparison of hyperthyroidism with hypothyroidism (Link 23-41)

9. Thyroid storm

  a. **Definition:** Life-threatening condition characterized by and exaggeration of the manifestations of thyrotoxicosis

    (*From McDermott MT*: Endocrine Secrets, *6th ed, Philadelphia, Elsevier Saunders, 2013, p 309, #1.*)

  b. Epidemiology: most often occurs in patients who have unrecognized or inadequately treated thyrotoxicosis and a precipitating event such as thyroid or nonthyroid surgery, infection, or trauma

  c. Clinical findings

    (1) Tachyarrhythmia (arrhythmia with increased heart rate)

    (2) Hyperpyrexia (dangerously high temperatures)

    (3) Tachypnea (rapid, shallow breathing)

    (4) Volume depletion from vomiting and diarrhea

    (5) Uncontrollable activity or muscle movement; coma

10. Euthyroid sick syndrome (ESS)

  a. **Definition:** Serum levels of T_3 and T_4 are abnormal, but thyroid gland function appears to be normal.

  b. Epidemiology

    (1) Associated with malignancy, CHF, anorexia nervosa (AN), chronic renal failure (CRF), sepsis, acute myocardial infarction (AMI), and other disorders

    (2) Laboratory test alterations usually return to normal with resolution of the illness.

    (3) Pathogenesis (Fig. 23-7 D)

      (a) In the normal condition, a peripheral tissue outer ring deiodinase converts FT_4 into metabolically active FT_3.

      (b) In ESS, the outer ring deiodinase is blocked, and the inner ring deiodinase converts FT_4 into inactive reverse T_3.

      (c) There are also abnormalities in TBG.

    (4) Laboratory findings in the MC variant of ESS

      (a) Normal to decreased serum FT_4; decreased serum FT_3

      (b) Normal to decreased serum TSH

      (c) Increased serum reverse T_3: Converting T_4 to RT_3 is a way to remove any unneeded T_4. It is metabolically inactive.

H. Summary of laboratory findings in thyroid disorders (Table 23-2)

I. Nontoxic goiter

1. **Definition:** Thyroid enlargement caused by an excess of colloid (fluid that contains the prohormone thyroglobulin; Fig. 23-8 A; Link 23-42)

Margin notes:

Oligomenorrhea

Lid stare

Stimulation levator palpebrae superioris

Cardiac findings

Sinus tachycardia

AF

Systolic hypertension

HO-CHF

$\uparrow\beta$-receptor synthesis in heart

Thyroid hormone: inotropic/chronotropic effect

Brisk DTRs

Osteoporosis

Lab findings thyrotoxicosis

$\uparrow$Serum T_3/T_4, $\downarrow$TSH (negative feedback)

$\uparrow^{123}$I uptake

Graves diffuse uptake, TMG limited to "hot" nodules

$\downarrow^{123}$I uptake: thyroiditis (early stage), taking excess hormone

Hyperglycemia: $\uparrow$glycogenolysis; $\uparrow$ type 1 DM

$\downarrow$Serum CH

Hypercalcemia ($\uparrow$bone turnover)

Thyroid storm

Life-threatening thyrotoxicosis

Unrecognized/inadequately Rx thyrotoxicosis + precipitating event

Tachyarrhythmia

Hyperpyrexia

Tachypnea

Volume depletion (vomiting/diarrhea)

Uncontrollable activity/muscle movement

Coma

Euthyroid sick syndrome

Serum T_3/T_4 abnormal; normal gland function

Malignancy, CHF, AN, CRF, sepsis, AMI

Lab tests return normal post resolution illness

Normal: outer ring deiodinase converts FT_4 to FT_3

Block of iodinase; FT_4 converted to inactive reverse T_3

Lab MC variant

N to $\downarrow$serum FT4

$\downarrow$Serum FT3

N to $\downarrow$serum TSH

$\uparrow RT_3$ (reverse T_3): metabolically inactive

Nontoxic goiter

Goiter: thyroid enlargement from excess colloid

Thyroid enlargement; excess colloid (thyroglobulin)

TABLE 23-2 Laboratory Findings in Thyroid Disease

DISORDER	SERUM T_4	FREE T_4	SERUM TSH	^{123}I UPTAKE
Graves disease	↑	↑	↓	↑
Patient taking excess hormone	↑	↑	↓	↓
Initial phase of thyroiditis	↑	↑	↓	↓
Primary hypothyroidism	↓	↓	↑	↔
Secondary hypothyroidism (hypopituitarism)	↓	↓	↓	↔
Increased TBG (e.g., excess estrogen)	↑	N	N	↔
Decreased TBG (e.g., anabolic steroids)	↓	N	N	↔

N, Normal; *T_4,* thyroxine; *TBG,* thyroid-binding globulin; *TSH,* thyroid-stimulating hormone; *↔, not* indicated.

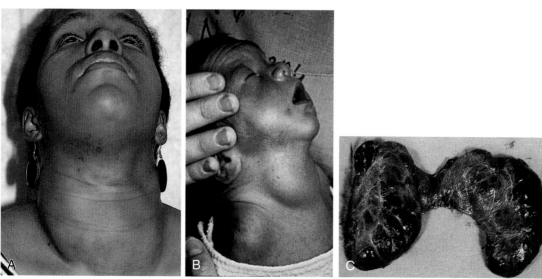

23-8: **A,** Patient with a multinodular goiter. Note the diffuse enlargement of the lower anterior neck. **B,** Newborn infant with iodide-induced goiter caused by Lugol's solution treatment of the mother during the third trimester. This illustrates the danger of chronic excess iodide administration during pregnancy. **C,** Thyroid gland with multinodular goiter. Note the diffusely enlarged gland with numerous cystic nodules filled with excess colloid. Hemorrhage has occurred into many of the cysts. *(**A** from Swartz MH: Textbook of Physical Diagnosis, 5th ed, Philadelphia, Saunders Elsevier, 2006, p 799, Fig. 9-7; **B,** from Melmed S, Polonsky KS, Larsen PR, Kronenberg HM: Williams Textbook of Endocrinology, 13th ed, Philadelphia, Elsevier Saunders, 2016, p 352, Fig. 11-11; **C** from Grieg JD: Color Atlas of Surgical Diagnosis, London, Mosby-Wolfe, 1996, p 268, Fig. 33-3.)*

Endemic MC goiter; iodide deficiency

Sporadic: goitrogens, enzyme deficiency, puberty, pregnancy

Absolute/relative ↓thyroid hormone

Combination hyperplasia/hypertrophy

Bouts hyperplasia/hypertrophy → gland involution

Initially diffuse enlargement → nodular

Goiter complications

Sudden enlargement: hemorrhage into cysts

Compression JV: neck congestion

1° hypothyroidism

Toxic nodular goiter

One/more nodules TSH independent ("hot") → thyrotoxicosis

2. Epidemiology
   a. Types of goiter
      (1) Endemic type is caused by iodide deficiency (MC type)
      (2) Sporadic type is caused by goitrogens (e.g., cabbage), enzyme deficiency, puberty, or pregnancy
   b. Pathogenesis
      (1) Absolute or relative deficiency of thyroid hormone
      (2) Combination of two growth alterations, hyperplasia and hypertrophy (work hypertrophy). The thyroid gland attempts to increase hormone synthesis.
      (3) Bouts of hyperplasia and hypertrophy are followed by gland involution. Involution is caused by failure of the gland to sustain hormone synthesis.
      (4) Initially, the thyroid is diffusely enlarged; with time, it becomes multinodular (Fig. 23-8 B, C; Link 23-43).
   c. Complications associated with goiters
      (1) Hemorrhage into cysts: produces a sudden, painful, thyroid gland enlargement
      (2) Compression of the jugular vein (JV) causing neck congestion; called the Pemberton sign
      (3) Primary hypothyroidism
      (4) Toxic nodular goiter: One or more nodules become TSH independent and develop into "hot" nodules, producing excess thyroid hormone (thyrotoxicosis; sometimes called Plummer disease).

(5) Hoarseness (caused by compression of the recurrent laryngeal nerve, a branch of the vagus nerve)

(6) Dyspnea (difficulty with breathing caused by compression of the trachea)

J. Overview of palpable thyroid nodules

1. Palpable nodules occur in ~6% of the population.
2. Malignancy is present in ~10% of all thyroid nodules and in ~8% of palpable thyroid nodules.
3. Incidence increases with age and are more frequently present in women than men.

K. Solitary thyroid nodule

1. **Definition:** Palpation of a distinct mass in an otherwise normal thyroid gland
2. Epidemiology
   a. Majority are "cold" (nonfunctioning) nodules (95% of cases).
   b. Causes of a solitary thyroid nodule in adult women
      (1) Majority are cysts in a goiter (60% of cases) or a follicular adenoma (25% of cases; Link 23-44).
      (2) Approximately 15% are malignant.
      (3) Approximately 85% to 90% of solitary nodules are euthyroid (normal thyroid function).
   c. Causes of a solitary thyroid nodule in adult men and children: Causes are similar to those in women, but there is an increased risk of malignancy.
   d. History of radiation to the head and neck increases risk of the nodule being malignant (40% of cases).
3. Diagnosis: Fine-needle aspiration (FNA) is the most important initial step. Thyroid hormone studies are used to rule out a functioning nodule.

L. Benign and malignant tumors of the thyroid

1. Comparison of a benign versus a malignant tumor of the thyroid (Link 23-45)
   a. Benign tumors are usually surrounded by a complete capsule and have a homogeneous cut surface (no cysts or hemorrhage).
   b. Malignant tumors have a nonhomogeneous cut surface (necrosis, hemorrhage) and invasive growth into adjacent tissue and may have evidence of metastasis to local lymph nodes.
2. Follicular adenoma
   a. **Definition:** MC benign tumor of the thyroid; presents as a solitary "cold" nodule
   b. Epidemiology
      (1) Surrounded by a complete capsule (Link 23-44)
      (2) Approximately 10% progress to a follicular carcinoma.
3. Papillary adenocarcinoma
   a. **Definition:** MC primary cancer of the thyroid; composed of papillary fronds intermixed with follicles and calcified concretions called psammoma bodies
   b. Epidemiology
      (1) MC endocrine cancer as well as the MC primary thyroid cancer (88% of cases)
      (2) More common in women than in men (3:1); usually occurs between ages 40 to 80 years
      (3) Associated with radiation exposure
      (4) Cancer is TSH dependent.
   c. Gross and microscopic findings (Links 23-46, *left* and 23-47)
      (1) Usually multifocal
      (2) Papillary fronds are intermixed with follicles.
      (3) Psammoma bodies are present in 35% to 45% of cases; these represent dystrophically calcified cancer cells (Fig. 23-9).
   d. Lymphatic invasion is common; metastasize to the cervical nodes and lung.
   e. Diagnose is made with FNA.
   f. Five-year survival rate is >95%.
4. Follicular carcinoma
   a. **Definition:** Primary cancer of the thyroid gland that arises from follicular cells
   b. Epidemiology
      (1) Accounts for 10% of the primary thyroid cancers
      (2) MC thyroid cancer that presents as a solitary cold nodule
      (3) Female-dominant cancer; occurs between the ages of 45 and 80 years
   c. Gross and microscopic findings
      (1) Cancer can be encapsulated or invasive through capsule or into vessels.
      (2) Neoplastic follicles invade blood vessels (Links 23-46, *second from left* and 23-48).
      (3) Lymph node metastasis is uncommon; hematogenous rather than lymphatic spread
   d. Metastasize to the lung and bone. The 5-year survival rate is ~80%.

Hoarseness: compression recurrent laryngeal nerve

Dyspnea: tracheal compression

Palpable thyroid nodules

Occur in ~6% of population

Malignancy ~10% thyroid nodules

Incidence ↑with age; women > men

Solitary thyroid nodule

Mass in otherwise normal thyroid

Majority cold nodules (nonfunctioning)

Causes adult women

Women: majority cysts in goiter; follicular adenoma

Small number malignant

Majority euthyroid

Causes men, children

Men/children: greater chance malignancy

Prior Hx radiation: greater risk for malignancy

FNA

Thyroid hormone studies

Benign/malignant tumors

Benign: complete capsule, homogeneous surface

Malignant: necrosis, hemorrhage, invasive growth, metastasis

Follicular adenoma

MC benign thyroid tumor; "cold" nodule

Complete capsule

Small risk progression → follicular carcinoma

Papillary adenocarcinoma

MC thyroid cancer; psammoma bodies

MC endocrine cancer; MC primary cancer thyroid

Women > men

Ages 40 to 80

Associated with radiation exposure

TSH-dependent

Gross/microscopic

Multifocal

Papillary fronds + follicles

Psammoma bodies

Lymphatic invasion common

Cervical nodes/lung

Dx FNA

Follicular carcinoma

Arises from follicular cells

10% thyroid cancers

Presents as solitary cold nodule

Female dominant

45 to 80 yrs old

Gross/microscopic

Encapsulated and/or invasive

Blood vessel invasion

Nodal metastasis uncommon

Hematogenous spread

Lung/bone metastasis

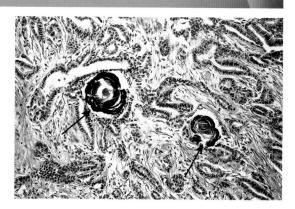

23-9: Papillary carcinoma of thyroid showing branching papillae and blue concretions *(arrows)* representing psammoma bodies. *(From Rosai J, Ackerman LV: Surgical Pathology, 9th ed, St. Louis, Mosby, 2004, p 534, Fig. 9-37A.)*

Medullary carcinoma

Derives from parafollicular C cells (calcitonin)

3 to 4% thyroid cancers

Sporadic > familial

Familial type

AD MEN IIa/IIb

IIa: MC, 1° HPTH, pheochromocytoma

IIb: MC, neuromas lips/tongue, pheo, Marfan-like

Familial better prognosis than sporadic

Ectopic ACTH (Cushing syndrome)

C cells: synthesize calcitonin

Calcitonin: ↓serum calcium (suppresses osteoclasts)

Calcitonin tumor marker

Possible hypocalcemia

Calcitonin converted into amyloid (Acal)

C-cell hyperplasia → medullary carcinoma

Diagnosis

FNA

↑Serum calcitonin

Pentagastrin infusion → ↑serum calcitonin

Primary B-cell lymphoma

Most often derives from Hashimoto thyroiditis

25 to 70 yrs old

<1% Thyroid cancers

Fair prognosis

Anaplastic thyroid cancer

Undifferentiated, rapidly aggressive

1% Thyroid cancers

Elderly women

Multinodular goiter; Hx follicular cancer

Rapidly aggressive; uniformly fatal

Parathyroid gland disorders

Superior (4th), inferior (3rd) pharyngeal pouches

Thymus 3rd pharyngeal pouch

3rd/4th pharyngeal pouches undeveloped; hypoparathyroidism + no thymic shadow

5. Medullary carcinoma
   a. **Definition:** Malignant tumor that derives from parafollicular C cells that normally synthesize calcitonin
   b. Epidemiology
      (1) Accounts for 3% to 4% of thyroid cancers
      (2) Types of medullary carcinoma: sporadic (80% of cases), familial (20% of cases)
      (3) Familial type of medullary carcinoma
         (a) Associated with autosomal-dominant (AD) MEN syndromes IIa and IIb
         (b) MEN IIa syndrome includes medullary carcinoma, primary hyperparathyroidism, and pheochromocytoma (usually a benign tumor that secretes catecholamines (Link 23-49).
         (c) MEN IIb (III) syndrome includes medullary carcinoma, mucosal neuromas (lips and tongue; Link 23-50), pheochromocytoma (pheo), and a Marfanoid body habitus.
      (4) Familial type has a better prognosis than the sporadic type.
      (5) Ectopic ACTH can also be secreted by the tumor, resulting in Cushing syndrome.
   c. Pathogenesis and histology
      (1) Tumor derives from the parafollicular C cells (Links 23-46, *third from left* and 23-51).
      (2) C cells normally synthesize calcitonin, whose function is to lower blood calcium levels by suppressing osteoclast activity in the bones and by increasing calcium excretion in the urine.
         (a) Calcitonin is a tumor marker for medullary carcinoma of the thyroid (see Chapter 9).
         (b) Increased levels of calcitonin may produce hypocalcemia; however, this is an uncommon finding.
         (c) Calcitonin can be converted into amyloid (A cal; see Chapter 4).
      (3) C-cell hyperplasia is a precursor lesion for medullary carcinoma.
   d. Diagnosis
      (1) FNA: measurement of serum calcitonin levels (increased)
      (2) Infusion of pentagastrin increases the calcitonin levels.
6. Primary B-cell malignant lymphoma
   a. Most often develop from Hashimoto thyroiditis
   b. Age of onset is 25 to 70 years old.
   c. Accounts for <1% of thyroid cancers; fair prognosis
7. Anaplastic thyroid cancer
   a. **Definition:** Undifferentiated, rapidly aggressive thyroid cancer that is uniformly fatal
   b. Epidemiology
      (1) Accounts for 1% of thyroid cancers; most often occurs in elderly women
      (2) Risk factors for anaplastic cancer include multinodular goiter and a history of follicular cancer.
      (3) Rapidly aggressive and uniformly fatal; 5-year survival rate is 5%

VI. Parathyroid Gland Disorders
   A. Clinical anatomy and physiology
   1. Superior and inferior parathyroid gland (Fig. 23-10)
      a. Glands derive from the fourth pharyngeal pouch and the third pharyngeal pouch, respectively.
      b. Thymus also develops from the third pharyngeal pouch.
      c. In DiGeorge syndrome, the third and fourth pharyngeal pouches fail to develop; hence, patients have hypoparathyroidism and a pure T-cell deficiency with no thymic shadow (absent thymus; see Chapter 4).

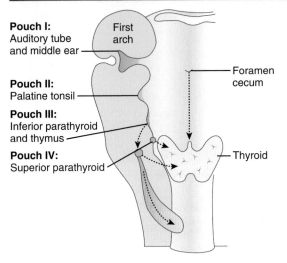

Pouch I:
Auditory tube
and middle ear

Pouch II:
Palatine tonsil

Pouch III:
Inferior parathyroid
and thymus

Pouch IV:
Superior parathyroid

First
arch

Foramen
cecum

Thyroid

23-10: Developmental origins of thyroid, parathyroid, and thymus glands. *Arrows* show pathways of migration. Note how pouch III develops into the inferior parathyroid gland and the thymus (synthesizes T cells), and pouch IV develops into the superior parathyroid glands. *(From Moore A, Roy W: Rapid Review Gross and Developmental Anatomy, 3rd ed, Philadelphia, Mosby.)*

2. PTH functions (Link 23-52)
   a. Increases Ca reabsorption in the early distal tubule (DT)
   b. Decreases phosphorus (Ph) reabsorption in the proximal tubule
   c. Increases intestinal reabsorption of Ca and Ph
   d. Decreases bicarbonate reclamation in the proximal tubule (see Chapter 5)
   e. Maintains the ionized Ca level in the blood by increasing bone resorption and renal reabsorption of Ca. Ionized Ca, *not* bound Ca, is functionally active.
   f. Increases the number and activity of osteoclasts, which increase bone resorption
   g. Increases the synthesis of 1-α-hydroxylase in the proximal renal tubule, which increases the synthesis of 1,25-$(OH)_2$D (dihydroxycholecalciferol; calcitriol)
   h. PTH is stimulated by hypocalcemia and hyperphosphatemia.
   i. PTH is suppressed by hypercalcemia and hypophosphatemia.
3. Role of vitamin D (D) in Ca metabolism (see Fig. 8-6; see Chapter 8)
   a. Preformed vitamin D in the diet consists of cholecalciferol (in fish) and ergocalciferol (in plants).
   b. Endogenous synthesis of vitamin D in the skin occurs by solar photoconversion of 7-dehydrocholesterol to vitamin D_3 (cholecalciferol).
   c. Reabsorption of vitamin D occurs in the small intestine.
   d. Hydroxylation of precursor vitamin D to 25-hydroxyvitamin D (25-[OH]D; calcidiol) occurs in the liver cytochrome P-450 system.
   e. 25-(OH)D is secreted into the blood and bound to a protein for delivery to the proximal tubules of the kidneys.
   f. Kidney hydroxylation of 25-(OH)D by 1-α-hydroxylase (1-α-OHase) produces 1,25-$(OH)_2$-D, the active form of vitamin D, called calcitriol. If PTH is decreased, 1-α-hydroxylase is decreased, and calcitriol is also decreased.
   g. Calcitriol attaches to nuclear receptors in target tissues.
   h. Functions of calcitriol (see Chapter 8)
      (1) Increases Ca reabsorption in the duodenum
      (2) Increases Ph reabsorption in the jejunum and ileum
      (3) Increases Ca reabsorption in the distal tubule (DT) of the kidney
      (4) Increases bone resorption to help maintain serum ionized Ca level (minor role of calcitriol). Calcitriol induces monocytic stem cells to become osteoclasts that increase bone resorption.
      (5) Increases bone mineralization (major role)
   i. Feedback control of calcitriol is Ca mediated.
      (1) Decreased serum Ca: ↑PTH → ↑synthesis 1-α-hydroxylase → ↑synthesis l,25-$(OH)_2$D
      (2) Increased serum Ca: ↓PTH → ↓synthesis of 1-α-hydroxylase → ↓synthesis 1,25-(OH)2D
4. Total serum Ca
   a. Components of the total serum Ca (Fig. 23-11 A)
      (1) Ca bound to albumin (40%) and Ph and citrate (13%)
         (a) Albumin has the most acidic amino acids (e.g., aspartate, glutamate) that have carboxyl groups (COOH, COO⁻).

↑Ca reabsorption early DT
↓Ph reabsorption proximal tubules
↑Intestinal reabsorption Ca + Ph
↓Bicarbonate reclamation Proximal tubule
Maintains ionized Ca levels (functional Ca)
↑Number osteoclasts → ↑bone resorption
↑Synthesizes 1-α-hydroxylase in proximal tubules
↑Synthesis 1,25-(OH)2D
PTH stimulation: ↓Ca, ↑Ph
PTH suppression: ↑Ca, ↓Ph
Role of vitamin D
Preformed D diet: cholecalciferol, ergocalciferol
Endogenous synthesis
Sunlight synthesis skin: major source D

7-Dehydrocholesterol → cholecalciferol
D reabsorbed small intestine
Liver 25-hydroxylase: cholecalciferol → 25-(OH)D (calcidiol)
25-(OH)D → proximal tubules
25-(OH)D → 1,25-(OH)2-D by 1-α-OHase
↓PTH → ↓1-α-OHase→ ↓calcitriol
Calcitriol attaches to nuclear receptors in tissue
Functions calcitriol
↑Ca reabsorption duodenum
↑Ph reabsorption jejunum/ duodenum
↑Ca reabsorption DT kidney
↑Bone resorption → maintain serum ionized C (minor role)
Calcitriol: ↑osteoclast production: bone resorption
↑Bone mineralization (major role)
Feedback control calcitriol
↓Ca: ↑PTH → ↑1-α-OHase → ↑synthesis l,25-(OH)2D
↑Ca: ↓PTH → ↓1-α-OHase → ↓synthesis l,25-(OH)2D
Total serum calcium
Ca bound to albumin, Ph, citrate
Albumin most COO–
Acid amino acids: aspartate, glutamate

23-11: Total serum calcium in a normal individual with a normal pH (**A**), an individual with hypoalbuminemia and normal pH (**B**), and an individual with respiratory alkalosis and alkaline pH (**C**). Refer to the text for discussion. *PTH*, Parathyroid hormone.

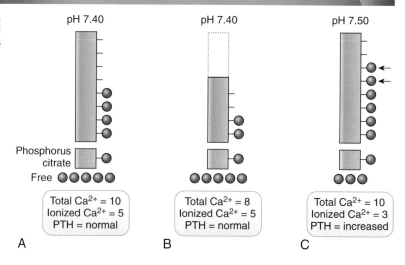

Normal PH: ~40% Ca²⁺ binds to COO−

Free ionized Ca²⁺ 47%

Metabolically active

Hypoalbuminemia

↓Total serum Ca (↓Ca bound to albumin)

Ca²⁺, PTH normal

Normal Ca²⁺ → no tetany

Correction formula for hypoalbuminemia

RAlk

RAlk: ↑↑negative charges

Less H+ → more COO−

↑COO− on albumin→ ↑binding Ca²⁺

Total serum Ca normal

↓Serum Ca²⁺ (ionized Ca)

↑Serum PTH

Signs of tetany

RAlk: normal total serum Ca; ↓ionized C, ↑PTH; tetany

Tetany: ↓serum ionized Ca (Ca²⁺)

Eₜ comes close to Eₘ; initiates action potential

Clinical findings tetany

Carpopedal spasm: thumb adducts into palm

Chvostek sign: facial twitching after tapping CN VII

Hypoparathyroidism

Hypofunction parathyroid glands

Causes

MCC autoimmune

Previous thyroid surgery

(b) At a normal pH of 7.4, ~40% of the acidic groups are COO⁻ and bind to positively charged Ca (Ca²⁺).

(2) Free, ionized Ca (Ca²⁺; 47%); metabolically active

b. Hypoalbuminemia (Fig. 23-11 B).

(1) Total serum Ca is decreased, caused by a decrease in Ca bound to albumin.

(2) Free ionized level of Ca and serum PTH levels remain normal.

(3) *No* evidence of tetany because the free ionized Ca level is normal

(4) Formula that corrects total serum Ca when hypoalbuminemia is present is as follows: corrected serum Ca when hypoalbuminemia is present = serum Ca − serum albumin + 4

c. Respiratory alkalosis (RAlk; Fig. 23-11 C)

(1) RAlk increases the number of negative charges on albumin.

(a) This is because there are fewer H⁺ ions on the COOH groups of acidic amino acids in an alkalotic state where there are less H⁺ ions. COOH groups change to COO⁻ because there are less H⁺ ions in RAlk.

(b) Extra negative charges on albumin are now available to bind some of the ionized Ca (two *black arrow*s in Fig. 23-11 C).

(2) Total serum Ca remains normal.

(3) Because some Ca ions are bound to albumin, serum ionized Ca is decreased.

(4) Because the ionized serum Ca is decreased, serum PTH is increased (normal negative feedback relationship).

(5) Because the serum ionized Ca is decreased, the patient will develop signs of tetany (see later). Although serum PTH is in equilibrium with ionized Ca, it cannot keep pace with the binding of ionized Ca to the additional negative charges on albumin in RAlk; hence, tetany occurs. Breathing into a paper bag will correct the alkalosis, and tetany will disappear (rebreathing CO₂).

d. Tetany is caused by a decreased serum ionized Ca concentration.

(1) Decrease in the serum ionized Ca level causes partial depolarization of nerves and muscle (Link 23-53).

(a) This lowers the threshold potential (Eₜ), which allows it to come closer to the resting membrane potential (Eₘ).

(b) This allows the action potential to be initiated with a smaller stimulus.

(2) Clinical findings of tetany

(a) Carpopedal spasm in which the thumb flexes into the palm (Fig. 23-12 A)

(b) Chvostek sign, which refers to increased facial twitching after tapping the facial nerve (cranial nerve [CN] VII)

B. **Hypoparathyroidism**

1. **Definition:** Hypofunction of the parathyroid glands leading to hypocalcemia

2. Epidemiology; causes

a. Autoimmune hypoparathyroidism (MCC)

b. Previous thyroid surgery; *not* a common complication in current day thyroid surgery

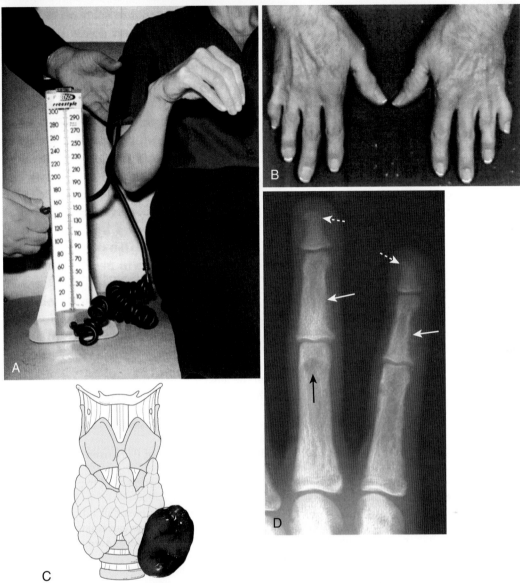

23-12: **A,** Carpal spasm (Trousseau sign; thumb adducts into the palm) is a manifestation of tetany, which is caused by a decrease in the ionized calcium level in blood. Its onset can be provoked by inflating a sphygmomanometer cuff to just above the systolic pressure for at least 2 minutes. **B,** Pseudohypoparathyroidism. Note the short fourth and fifth digits, producing the classic "knuckle-knuckle-dimple-dimple" sign. **C,** Parathyroid adenoma in primary hyperparathyroidism. **D,** Subperiosteal resorption in primary hyperparathyroidism. The radiologic hallmark of hyperparathyroidism is subperiosteal bone resorption, seen especially well on the radial aspect of the middle phalanges of the index and middle fingers *(solid white arrows)*. Here the cortex appears shaggy and irregular, compared with the cortex on the opposite side of the same bone, which is well defined. This patient also displays two other findings of hyperparathyroidism: a small brown tumor *(solid black arrow)* and resorption of the terminal phalanges (acroosteolysis) *(dotted white arrows)*. **(A** from Forbes C, Jackson W: Color Atlas and Text of Clinical Medicine, 3rd ed, London, Mosby, 2004, p 314, Fig. 7.73; **B** from Bouloux P: Self-Assessment Picture Tests: Medicine, Vol. 3, London, Mosby-Wolfe, 1997, p 14, Fig. 27; **C** from Rosai J, Ackerman LV: Surgical Pathology, 9th ed, St. Louis, Mosby, 2004, p 597, Fig. 10-2; **D** from Herring W: Learning Radiology Recognizing the Basics, 2nd ed, Philadelphia, Elsevier Saunders, 2012, p 225, Fig. 21-14.)

   c. DiGeorge syndrome (failure of development of the third and fourth pharyngeal pouch, which results in an absent thymus and parathyroid glands; see Chapter 4).

   d. Hypomagnesemia

      (1) MCC hypocalcemia in a hospital setting

      (2) Magnesium (Mg) is a cofactor for adenylate cyclase. Cyclic adenosine monophosphate (cAMP) is required for PTH activation and secretion → hypoparathyroidism.

      (3) Causes of hypomagnesemia include diarrhea, aminoglycosides, diuretics, and alcoholism.

DiGeorge syndrome: absent thymus/PTH glands

Hypomagnesemia MC pathologic cause of hypocalcemia in hospital

Mg cofactor adenylate cyclase

cAMP required for PTH activation/secretion

Hypoparathyroidism

Diarrhea, aminoglycosides, diuretics, alcoholism

TABLE 23-3 Other Causes of Hypocalcemia

DISORDER	COMMENTS
Acute pancreatitis	• Calcium is bound to fatty acids in enzymatic fat necrosis. • Poor prognostic sign
Hypovitaminosis D	• Lack of sunlight: decreased photoconversion of cholesterol to (nonrenal) vitamin D_3 (cholecalciferol) in the skin • Malabsorption (e.g., celiac disease): ↓reabsorption of fat-soluble vitamin D; ↓25-(OH)D → 1,25-(OH)$_2$D. ↓Serum calcium, ↓serum phosphorus, ↑serum PTH (2° HPTH) • Cirrhosis: decreased synthesis of 25-(OH)D → ↓1,25-(OH)$_2$D; ↓serum calcium, ↓serum phosphorus, ↑serum PTH • Drugs that stimulated the cytochrome system (e.g., alcohol, phenytoin): increased metabolism of 25-(OH)D into an inactive metabolite; decreased 25-(OH)D → ↓1,25-(OH)$_2$D; ↓serum calcium, ↓serum phosphorus, ↑serum PTH (2° HPTH) • Chronic renal failure (most common cause): ↓synthesis of 1,25-(OH)$_2$D (↓1-α-hydroxylation); ↓serum calcium, ↑serum phosphorus (retained by failed kidney), ↑serum PTH (2° HPTH),
Pseudohypoparathyroidism (see Fig. 23-12 B; Links 23-54 and 23-55)	• Autosomal dominant disease • End-organ resistance to PTH (includes its ability to synthesize 1-α-hydroxylase in the proximal tubule) • Mental retardation, basal ganglia calcification, short fourth and fifth metacarpals ("knuckle-knuckle-dimple-dimple" sign) • Hypocalcemia, normal to ↑PTH, normal 25-(OH)D, ↓1,25-(OH)$_2$D; ↓serum calcium, ↓serum phosphorus.

2° HPTH, Secondary hypoparathyroidism; *25-(OH)D*, calcidiol; *1,25-(OH)$_2$D*, calcitriol; *PTH*, parathyroid hormone.

Clinical findings
Tetany
Dystrophic calcification basal ganglia
Metastatic calcification
↑Serum Ph hypoparathyroidism → drives Ca into tissue
Cataracts
Candida infections
Hypoparathyroidism: ↓serum PTH, ↓serum Ca, ↑serum Ph
Other causes hypocalcemia
Primary hyperparathyroidism
Excessive production/secretion PTH
MCC non-malignant/outpatient hypercalcemia
Malignancy MCC hypercalcemia in hospital
Postmenopausal women; women > men
Often asymptomatic
1° HPTH: MEN I, IIa association
MCC 1° HPTH: benign adenoma
Single adenoma
Chief cells, no adipose
Other glands atrophic
Right inferior parathyroid gland MC site
Primary hyperplasia
Primary hyperplasia: all 4 glands involved
Chief cell hyperplasia
Clear cell hyperplasia: ↑↑serum Ca
Carcinoma uncommon
Renal findings
Renal stones MC presentation
Nephrocalcinosis
Metastatic calcification basement membrane CDT
NDI, renal failure
Gastrointestinal findings

3. Clinical findings in hypoparathyroidism
   a. Tetany (hypocalcemia)
   b. Calcification of the basal ganglia: caused by metastatic calcification (see Chapter 2). Increased serum Ph in primary hypoparathyroidism drives Ca into the brain tissue.
   c. Cataracts (opacification of the lens); *Candida* infection (? cause)
4. Laboratory findings in hypoparathyroidism include hypocalcemia, hyperphosphatemia, and a decrease in serum PTH.
5. Other causes of hypocalcemia are listed and discussed in Table 23-3.

C. **Primary Hyperparathyroidism (HPTH)**
   1. **Definition:** Excessive production and secretion of PTH from the parathyroid glands
   2. Epidemiology
      a. MC nonmalignant cause of hypercalcemia and cause of hypercalcemia in an outpatient setting
      b. Malignancy is the MCC of hypercalcemia in a hospitalized patient. Primary HPTH and malignancy account for 90% of all causes of hypercalcemia.
      c. Occurs most frequently in postmenopausal women; more common in women than men; asymptomatic in >50% of people
      d. Association with MEN I and IIa (Link 23-49)
      e. Causes of HPTH (Link 23-56)
         (1) Adenoma (~80% of cases; Fig. 23-12 C)
             (a) Usually a single adenoma
             (b) Histologic findings include sheets of chief cells with *no* intervening adipose (Link 23-57).
             (c) The remainder of that parathyroid gland, as well as the other parathyroid glands, becomes atrophic. Hypercalcemia suppresses PTH produced by normal parathyroid gland tissue.
             (d) Right inferior parathyroid gland is the MC site for a parathyroid adenoma.
         (2) Primary hyperplasia (~20% of cases)
             (a) All four glands are involved in primary hyperplasia (Link 23-56, *left*).
             (b) Usually a chief cell hyperplasia
             (c) Clear cell hyperplasia (called wasserhelle cell hyperplasia) is associated with a greater increase in serum Ca levels than parathyroid adenoma.
         (3) Carcinoma (uncommon)
   3. Clinical findings
      a. Renal findings
         (1) Ca stones, the MC presentation
         (2) Nephrocalcinosis (see Chapters 2 and 20): caused by metastatic calcification of the basement membrane of the collecting duct tubules (CDT) causing refractoriness to ADH and polyuria (increased frequency of urination); causes nephrogenic diabetes insipidus (NDI) and renal failure
      b. Gastrointestinal finding

(1) Peptic ulcer disease (PUD; see Chapter 18). Ca stimulates gastrin, which increases gastric acid, leading to peptic ulcers in the stomach and proximal duodenum.

(2) Acute pancreatitis (see Chapter 19): Ca activates phospholipase, which hydrolyzes the fatty tissue within and around the pancreas.

(3) Constipation: Hypercalcemia decreases the neuron membrane permeability to sodium ions, thus decreasing the excitability, leading to hypotonicity of smooth muscle cell (SMC) in the bowel.

  c. Bone and joints

(1) Osteitis fibrosa cystica

(a) Characterized by cystic and hemorrhagic bone cysts caused by increased osteoclastic activity mediated by excess PTH

(b) Commonly involves the jaw

(2) Radiographic findings

(a) Subperiosteal bone resorption of the phalanges (Fig. 23-12 D; Links 23-58, 23-59, and Link 23-60, *right*) and tooth sockets

(b) "Salt and pepper" appearance of the skull (Link 23-60 left)

(c) Resorption of the distal phalanges, called acroosteolysis (Fig. 23-12 D; Links 23-59 and 23-60, right)

(3) Osteoporosis (loss of both organic bone matrix [called osteoid] and mineralized bone; see Chapter 24)

(4) Chondrocalcinosis (pseudogout): Ca pyrophosphate is deposited in cartilage (see Chapter 24).

  d. Diastolic hypertension is caused by hypercalcemia-induced increase in smooth muscle contraction of the peripheral resistance arterioles, thus increasing the diastolic pressure (see Chapter 10).

  e. Eyes: Band keratopathy, caused by metastatic calcification, refers to the presence of a band across the central cornea.

  f. Central nervous system findings include psychosis, confusion, anxiety, and coma.

  g. An excellent mnemonic is "stones, bones, abdominal groans, and psychic moans."

4. Laboratory findings and metabolic consequences in primary HPTH (Link 23-61)

  a. Increased serum PTH, increased serum Ca, and decreased serum Ph. Intact serum parathyroid hormone (iPTH) is the best initial screening test.

  b. Normal anion gap metabolic acidosis (NAGMA) (see Chapter 5)

(1) Caused by decreased proximal tubule reclamation of bicarbonate

(2) Example of type II renal tubular acidosis (RTA; see Chapter 5)

  c. Chloride/Ph ratio is >33.

(1) Recall that in a NAGMA, an increase in serum chloride counterbalances the loss of negative charges related to the decrease in bicarbonate. Therefore, in primary HPTH, the increase in serum chloride from the NAGMA plus the decrease in serum Ph leads to an increase in the chloride/Ph ratio.

(2) Chloride/Ph ratio <29 *excludes* primary HPTH.

  d. Decreased serum 1,25-$(OH)_2$D (hypovitaminosis D)

(1) Hypercalcemia decreases the synthesis of 1-α-hydroxylase in the proximal renal tubule, which decreases the synthesis of 1,25-(OH)2D.

(2) Protective effect so that serum Ca is not too high

  e. Electrocardiogram (ECG) shows shortening of the QT interval

5. Localization of a parathyroid adenoma is made using a technetium-99m-sestamibi radionuclide scan (Link 23-62).

6. Other causes of hypercalcemia are listed and discussed in Table 23-4.

  a. Primary HPTH and the hypercalcemia of malignancy (see Chapter 9) together account for ~80% of all cases of hypercalcemia; malignancy MCC hypercalcemia in hospital setting

  b. Primary differentiating feature between these two diagnoses is serum PTH.

(1) Serum PTH is increased in primary HPTH.

(2) Serum PTH is decreased in hypercalcemia of malignancy, whether it is caused by lytic lesions (MC) or PTH-related peptide.

  c. Hypercalcemia in pregnancy can produce hypocalcemia in fetus caused by suppression of PTH in the fetus. Tetany may occur in the fetus.

D. Secondary Hyperparathyroidism (HPTH)

1. **Definition:** Excessive parathyroid secretion of the PTH occurring as a compensatory response to hyperphosphatemia, hypocalcemia, or decreased serum calcitriol levels

PUD

↑Gastrin → ↑acid → PUD (prox stomach, duod)

Acute pancreatitis

Ca activates pancreatic phospholipase

Constipation

↑C → ↓neuron membrane permeability to Na → SMC hypotonicity

Bone and joints

Osteitis fibrosa cystica

Cystic/hemorrhagic bone cysts

↑Osteoclastic activity (↑PTH)

Jaw common site

Radiographic findings

Subperiosteal bone resorption phalanges/tooth sockets

Salt/pepper skull

Resorption distal phalanges

Osteoporosis

Chondrocalcinosis (pseudogout)

Ca pyrophosphate deposition in cartilage

1° HPTH: diastolic hypertension

Eyes: band keratopathy

Psychosis, confusion, anxiety, coma

"Stones, bones, abdominal groans, and psychic moans"

Intact serum PTH (iPTH): best initial screen

NAGMA

↓Proximal tubule reclamation bicarbonate

Type II RTA

Chloride/Ph ratio >33

Chloride/Ph ratio <29 excludes 1° HPTH

↓Serum 1,25-(OH)2D (hypovitaminosis D)

↑Serum Ca → ↓ synthesis 1-α-OHase → ↓1,25-(OH)2D

Protective effect

ECG shortening QT interval

Sestamibi scan: localize parathyroid adenoma

1o HPTH, malignancy 80% all hypercalcemias

Malignancy: MCC of hypercalcemia in the hospital

↑PTH in 1° HPTH

↓PTH in malignancy (lytic lesions, PTH-related peptide)

1° HPTH vs. malignancy: ↑PTH in former, ↓PTH in latter

↑Ca pregnancy → ↓fetal PTH → ↓fetal Ca → fetal tetany

Secondary HPTH

2° HPTH: compensation for hypocalcemia

2° HPTH: hyperphosphatemia, ↓serum calcitriol/calcium

TABLE 23-4   Other Causes of Hypercalcemia

DISORDER	COMMENTS
Hypervitaminosis D	Increased calcium reabsorption in the jejunum and kidneys
Malignancy induced	Mechanisms: • Bone metastasis with local activation of osteoclasts (most common): produces lytic lesions in bone; ↑serum calcium → ↓serum PTH • Ectopic secretion of a PTHrP (e.g., SCC of lung, RCC): generalized activation of osteoclasts *without* producing lytic lesions in bone; uses the same receptor site as PTH to perform its functions; ↑serum calcium → ↓serum PTH; ↑PTHrP (measured in special laboratories) • Multiple myeloma: localized increased secretion of osteoclast-activating factor (IL-1) by malignant plasma cells; produces lytic lesions in bone; ↑serum calcium → ↓serum PTH
Familial hypocalciuric hypercalcemia	• Autosomal dominant with 100% penetrance • Mutation causing altered set point for calcium-sensing receptor on renal tubule and parathyroid gland; normal to slightly increased serum PTH but very low urinary calcium levels (increased in primary hyperparathyroidism)
Sarcoidosis	Mechanism: macrophages in granulomas synthesize 1-α-hydroxylase, causing hypervitaminosis D
Thiazides	Mechanism: increases early distal tubule reabsorption of calcium (PTH-mediated channel); always consider a possible underlying parathyroid adenoma if hypercalcemia develops in a patient taking thiazides (order serum intact PTH)

IL, Interleukin; *PTH,* parathyroid hormone; *PTHrP,* parathyroid hormone–related protein; *RCC,* renal cell carcinoma; *SCC,* squamous cell carcinoma.

23-13: Schematic showing serum calcium and serum parathyroid hormone (PTH) in different disorders. The *center square with the shaded areas* represents the normal serum calcium and PTH. *Area A* describes primary hypoparathyroidism (↓serum calcium, ↓serum PTH); *area B* represents hypoalbuminemia (↓serum calcium, normal serum PTH); *area C* represents secondary hyperparathyroidism (↓serum calcium, ↑serum PTH); *area D* represents respiratory alkalosis (normal serum calcium, ↑serum PTH from ↓ionized calcium level); *area E* represents primary hyperparathyroidism (↑serum calcium, ↑serum PTH); and *area F* represents hypercalcemia associated with malignancy (↑serum calcium, ↓serum PTH).

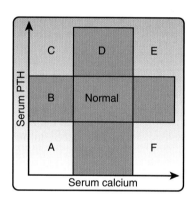

2. Epidemiology
   a. Hyperplasia of all four parathyroid glands
      (1) Physiologic compensation for hypocalcemia
      (2) Example: hypovitaminosis D caused by renal failure or malabsorption produces hypocalcemia and secondary HPTH
   b. In secondary HPTH, the serum Ca is decreased, and the serum PTH is increased.
   c. May develop tertiary HPTH
      (1) Glands become autonomous regardless of the Ca level; *not* a physiologic response.
      (2) May bring the serum Ca into a normal or increased range
   d. A Rugger-jersey spine in secondary HPTH. It is characterized by a bandlike osteosclerosis of the superior and inferior margins of the vertebral bodies. It is *only* seen in secondary, *not* primary HPTH (Link 23-63).
   e. Mechanism of how CRF produces secondary HPTH (Link 23-64)

E. Schematic summarizing serum PTH and Ca relationships (Fig. 23-13)

F. Phosphorous (Ph) disorders
   1. The causes of hypophosphatemia are listed and discussed in Table 23-5.
   2. Clinical findings in hypophosphatemia
      a. Muscle weakness (lack of adenosine triphosphate [ATP])
      b. Decreased synthesis of ATP causes muscle weakness.
      c. Muscle paralysis and rhabdomyolysis (rupture of muscle) may occur.
         (a) Rupture of muscle produces myoglobinuria.
         (b) Urine has a red color, the dipstick for blood is positive (does *not* distinguish hemoglobin [Hb] from myoglobin), and the serum CK is markedly increased (see Chapter 20).
      d. RBC hemolysis: RBCs require ATP to maintain ion pumps and membrane integrity.
      e. Osteomalacia (soft bones). Ph is required to mineralize bone (see Chapter 8).

Margin notes (left column):

Hyperplasia all 4 glands

Physiologic compensation for hypocalcemia

Renal failure, malabsorption

2° HPTH: ↓serum Ca, ↑serum PTH

May develop tertiary HPTH

Tertiary HPTH: glands become autonomous

Serum Ca normal or increased

Rugger-jersey spine

Muscle weakness

↓ATP synthesis

Muscle paralysis/rhabdomyolysis

Myoglobinuria

Urine red; +urine dipstick for blood; ↑↑serum CK

RBC hemolysis

RBC hemolysis: ↓ATP

Osteomalacia

Ph required for bone mineralization

TABLE 23-5   Causes of Hypophosphatemia

DISORDER	COMMENTS
Hypovitaminosis D (extrarenal causes)	Decreased reabsorption of phosphorus from the small intestine
Insulin Rx in DKA	Increased uptake of glucose into cells requires phosphorus for phosphorylation (traps glucose in the cell).
Primary HPTH	Increased PTH decreases phosphorus reabsorption in the proximal tubules.
PTH-related peptide	Uses the same receptor as PTH; decreases phosphorus reabsorption in the proximal tubules
Respiratory or metabolic alkalosis	Alkalosis activates phosphofructokinase, the rate-limiting reaction of glycolysis, causing increased phosphorylation of glucose; most common cause of hypophosphatemia in hospitalized patients

DKA, Diabetic ketoacidosis; *HPTH,* hyperparathyroidism; *PTH,* parathyroid hormone; *Rx,* treatment.

TABLE 23-6   Causes of Hyperphosphatemia

DISORDER OR CONDITION	COMMENTS
Chronic renal failure (most common cause)	Decreased excretion of phosphorus as titratable acid (see Chapter 5)
Normal child	Children require increased serum phosphorus to drive calcium into bone for mineralization (see Chapter 1).
Primary hypoparathyroidism	Decreased excretion of phosphorus as titratable acid
Pseudohypoparathyroidism	• Autosomal dominant disease (see Table 23-3) • End-organ resistance to PTH (includes its ability to synthesize 1-α-hydroxylase in the proximal tubule)

PTH, Parathyroid hormone.

TABLE 23-7   Summary of Calcium and Phosphorus Disorders

DISORDER	SERUM CALCIUM	SERUM PHOSPHORUS	SERUM PTH
Primary hypoparathyroidism	↓	↑	↓
Vitamin D deficiency (renal)	↓	↑	↑
Vitamin D deficiency (nonrenal)	↓	↓	↑
Primary HPTH	↑	↓	↑
Malignancy-induced hypercalcemia (lytic)	↑	–	↓
Malignancy-induced hypercalcemia (PTHrP)	↑	–	↓

PTH, Parathyroid hormone; *PTHrP,* parathyroid hormone–related peptide.

3. Causes of hyperphosphatemia are listed and discussed in Table 23-6.
4. Clinical findings in hyperphosphatemia include metastatic calcification because excess Ph drives Ca into normal tissue (see Chapter 2).
   G. **Summary table integrating Ca, Ph, and PTH in Ca and Ph disorders** (Table 23-7)
VII. **Adrenal Gland Disorders**
   A. **Regulation of cortisol secretion** (Link 23-65)
   B. **Overview of adrenal cortex hormones** (Fig. 23-14; Link 23-66)
      1. Zona glomerulosa produces mineralocorticoids (e.g., aldosterone). Angiotensin II activates 18-hydroxylase, which converts corticosterone to aldosterone.
      2. Zona fasciculata produces glucocorticoids.
         a. 11-Deoxycortisol and cortisol are called 17-hydroxycorticoids (17-OH).
         b. Cortisol and ACTH have a diurnal variation; both are higher in the morning and lower in the evening (see Chapter 1).
      3. Zona reticularis produces sex hormones, which are called 17-ketosteroids (17-KSs).
         a. Dehydroepiandrosterone (DHEA) and androstenedione are 17-KSs.
         b. Testosterone (T)
            (1) Androstenedione is converted by oxidoreductase into T.
            (2) T is converted to dihydrotestosterone (DHT) by 5α-reductase in peripheral tissues.
            (3) Peripheral tissue sites that produce DHT include the skin, testes, prostate, seminal vesicles (SVs), epididymis, liver, and ovaries.

Causes hyperphosphatemia

Hyperphosphatemia: metastatic calcification

Glomerulosa: mineralocorticoids (e.g., aldosterone)

ATII activates 18-OHase → corticosterone to aldosterone

Fasciculata: glucocorticoids

11-Deoxycortisol, cortisol: 17-hydroxycorticoids (17-OH)

Cortisol/ACTH diurnal

Reticularis: sex hormones

DHEA, androstenedione: 17-KS

Testosterone (T)

Androstenedione → T

T → DHT by 5α-reductase peripheral tissue

DHT: skin, testes, prostate, SV, epididymis, liver, ovaries

23-14: Adrenocortical hormone synthesis. The zona glomerulosa produces mineralocorticoids (e.g., aldosterone), the zona fasciculata produces glucocorticoids (e.g., cortisol), and the zona reticularis produces sex hormones (e.g., testosterone). The 17-hydroxycorticoids (17-OH) are 11-deoxycortisol and cortisol. The 17-ketosteroids (17-KSs; weak androgens) are dehydroepiandrosterone and androstenedione. Testosterone is converted to dihydrotestosterone (DHT) by 5α-reductase in extraadrenal tissue. *17OHP*, 17-hydroxyprogesterone.

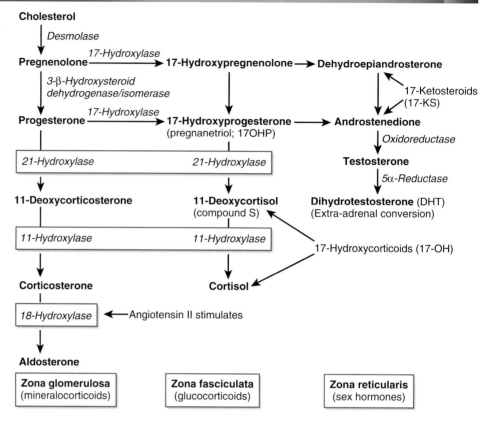

C. **Overview of adrenal medulla hormones** (Fig. 23-19 A)
  1. Adrenal medulla is of neural crest origin.
  2. Produces catecholamines (epinephrine [EPI] and norepinephrine [NOR])
  3. Metabolic products of EPI and NOR include metanephrine and vanillylmandelic acid (VMA).
  4. Metabolic product of dopamine is homovanillic acid (HVA).
D. **Adrenocortical hypofunction (primary hypocortisolism)**
  1. Acute adrenocortical insufficiency
    a. **Definition:** A sudden lack of production of glucocorticoids or mineralocorticoids by the adrenal cortex
    b. Epidemiology and causes
      (1) Causes of acute adrenocortical insufficiency
        (a) Abrupt withdrawal of corticosteroids (MCC). If a person is on long-term corticosteroid therapy, the plasma ACTH is suppressed, and the adrenal cortex undergoes atrophy.
        (b) WFS (see later), anticoagulation therapy (hemorrhage into adrenals)
      (2) Waterhous-Friderichsen syndrome (WFS)
        (a) **Definition:** Acute adrenal failure caused by disseminated intravascular coagulation (DIC) caused by septicemia, which results in acute bilateral hemorrhagic infarctions of the adrenal glands (Link 23-67)
        (b) Epidemiology
          • Septicemia (pathogens in the blood) is usually caused by *Neisseria meningitides*, a gram-negative diplococcus.
          • Patients develop endotoxic shock (see Chapter 5).
          • In endotoxic shock, the release of tissue thromboplastin activates the extrinsic coagulation system and damages the endothelial cells, causing DIC (see Chapter 15).
          • Fibrin clots in small vessels in DIC cause hemorrhagic infarction in the loose-textured adrenal cortex in both adrenal glands.
  2. Chronic adrenal insufficiency (Addison disease)
    a. **Definition:** Chronic adrenal insufficiency characterized by decreased production of glucocorticoids and mineralocorticoids, with a corresponding increase in ACTH

Adrenal medulla hormones

Neural crest origin

Produces catecholamines (EPI, NOR)

Metabolic end-products EPI/NOR: metanephrines, VMA

Dopamine → HVA

Adrenocortical hypofunction (primary hypocortisolism)

Acute adrenocortical insufficiency

Sudden lack hormone production in cortex

Abrupt withdrawal long-term corticosteroids MCC

Plasma ACTH suppressed

Adrenal cortex atrophic

WFS

Anticoagulation Rx

WFS

Sepsis → DIC → bilateral adrenal hemorrhage (infarction)

N. meningitides MCC

Endotoxic shock

DIC

Fibrin clots vessels → hemorrhagic infarction

Chronic adrenal insufficiency (Addison disease)

↓Production glucocorticoids/mineralocorticoids → ↑ACTH

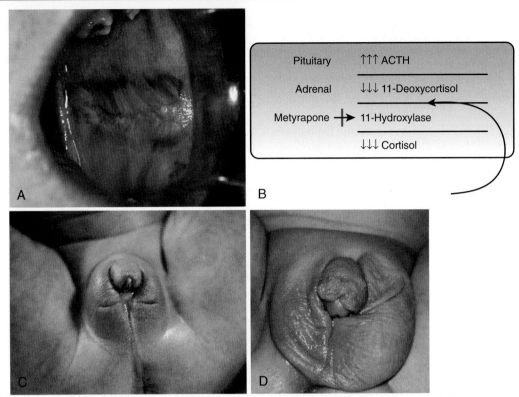

23-15: A, Addison disease. Note the increased melanin pigmentation of the buccal mucosa. **B,** Schematic of the metyrapone test in Addison disease. Metyrapone blocks 11-hydroxylase in the adrenal cortex. This further decreases cortisol, leading to a marked increase in adreno-corticotropic hormone (ACTH) caused by a loss of negative feedback. However, the increase in ACTH does *not* increase the synthesis of 11-deoxycortisol in the adrenal cortex, which is destroyed in Addison disease. **C,** Newborn girl with ambiguous genitalia. Note the enlarged clitoris and the partially fused labia majora, suggesting the presence of a scrotum. **D,** Virilized external genitalia in a female infant with adrenogenital syndrome caused by 21-hydroxylase deficiency. *(A from Savin JAA, Hunter JAA, Hepburn NC: Diagnosis in Color: Skin Signs in Clinical Medicine, London, Mosby-Wolfe, 1997, p 1105, Fig. 4.44; B courtesy of Edward Goljan, MD; C courtesy of Patrick C. Walsh, MD, Johns Hopkins School of Medicine; D from Goldman L, Schafer AI: Cecil's Medicine, 24th ed, Philadelphia, Saunders Elsevier, 2012, p 1514, Fig. 241-4.)*

   b. Epidemiology and causes
      (1) Autoimmune destruction; MCC and accounts for 80% of cases
      (2) Miliary tuberculosis (7%–20%): MCC in developing countries. Disseminated histoplasmosis can also produce adrenal insufficiency.
      (3) Adrenogenital syndrome is the MCC in children (see later discussion).
      (4) Metastasis, most often from a primary lung cancer; AIDS (30% develop Addison disease)
   c. Clinical findings in Addison disease (Links 23-68 and 23-69)
      (1) Weakness, tiredness, fatigue, and anorexia (100%)
      (2) Hypotension (<110 mm Hg) caused by sodium loss from mineralocorticoid and glucocorticoid deficiency (88%–94%)
      (3) Diffuse hyperpigmentation (94% of cases; Fig. 23-15 A)
         (a) Increased plasma ACTH stimulates melanocytes.
         (b) Pigmentation is prominent in the buccal mucosa (Link 23-70), skin, and skin creases.
      (4) Electrolyte disturbances (see later; 92% of cases)
   d. Laboratory findings in Addison disease
      (1) Short and prolonged ACTH stimulation test: *no* increase in serum cortisol or 17-OH in both tests
      (2) Metyrapone test shows an increase in plasma ACTH and *no* increase in serum cortisol (Fig. 23-15 B).
      (3) Increased plasma ACTH
      (4) Electrolyte findings include hyponatremia (88%), hyperkalemia (64%), and normal anion gap metabolic acidosis (NAGMA) (see Chapter 5).
      (5) Anemia (55%): sometimes macrocytic caused by pernicious anemia (PA)
      (6) Increased serum blood urea nitrogen (BUN) and creatinine (azotemia) caused by volume loss fluid and electrolytes in urine (55%)

Autoimmune destruction MCC

Miliary TB MCC developing countries; histoplasmosis

Adrenogenital syndrome MCC children

Metastasis: lung cancer MCC

AIDS

Weakness, tiredness, fatigue, anorexia

Addison disease: diffuse hyperpigmentation; hypotension, weakness

Electrolyte disturbances

Short/prolonged ACTH: *no* ↑serum cortisol, 17-OH

Metyrapone test: ↓cortisol → ↑ACTH → ↓11-deoxycortisol

↑Plasma ACTH

↓Serum sodium, cortisol, bicarbonate; ↑serum potassium; NAGMA

Anemia; sometimes PA

Azotemia: volume loss fluid/electrolytes

Aldosterone enhances the exchange of sodium for potassium in the kidneys (see Fig. 5-9 A). Hence, its deficiency leads to a hypertonic loss of sodium in the urine (hyponatremia), retention of potassium (hyperkalemia), and retention of hydrogen ions (metabolic acidosis). Aldosterone also enhances the proton pump (see Fig. 5-10). Deficiency of aldosterone leads to retention of protons and metabolic acidosis (normal anion gap type).

Fasting hypoglycemia: loss gluconeogenesis

Eosinophilia, lymphocytosis, neutropenia

Adrenogenital syndrome

Cortex enzyme deficiency(ies) → ↓cortisol → ↑ACTH

AR disorder

Enzyme deficiency → ↓cortisol, ↑ACTH

↑ACTH → cortex hyperplasia → diffuse skin pigmentation

Ambiguous genitalia: 1st step determine genetic sex with chromosome analysis

Male infants: enlarged penis only

Precocious puberty males/females

Girls: irregular menses; infertility

Rapid childhood growth; fusion epiphyses (short stature)

↑Androgens → acne

↓17-KS, T, DHT: hypogonadism male/females

Females: delayed menarche/2° sex characteristics

Males: pseudohermaphroditism; external genitalia requires DHT

↑M: Na⁺ retention → hypertension

↓Mineralocorticoids

↓M: hyponatremia, hyperkalemia

↓M: hypotension (possible shock)

↑Ss proximal to enzyme block

↓Ss distal to enzyme block

Classic 21-OHase deficiency

MC enzyme deficiency

Mutation CYP21A2 gene

↑17-KS, ↑T, ↑DHT

Ambiguous genitalia female only

Enlarged penis in male infants

Postnatal virilization males/females

↓Mineralocorticoids: salt losers

Mineralocorticoids distal to enzyme block

Danger hypovolemic shock

↓17-OH (11-deoxycortisol, cortisol)

↑17-Hydroxyprogesterone

Nonclassical 21-OHase deficiency

Cortisol, M activity normal (no sodium loss)

(7) Because cortisol is a gluconeogenic hormone, the loss of gluconeogenesis leads to fasting hypoglycemia.

(8) Hematologic findings caused by a loss of cortisol include eosinophilia (17%), lymphocytosis, and neutropenia (see Chapter 13).

3. Adrenogenital syndrome (congenital adrenal hyperplasia)
   a. **Definition:** Group of genetic diseases characterized by one or more adrenal cortex enzyme deficiencies involved in the synthesis of cortisol, resulting in overstimulation of the adrenal cortex by ACTH
   b. Epidemiology/clinical
      (1) Autosomal-recessive (AR) disorder
      (2) Enzyme deficiency causes hypocortisolism and a corresponding increase in ACTH.
      (3) Increase in ACTH causes adrenocortical hyperplasia and diffuse skin pigmentation caused by stimulation of melanocytes.
      (4) An increase in 17-KS, T, and DHT results in ambiguous genitalia in female infants (Fig. 23-15 C, D; Link 23-71). This is primarily caused by the increase in DHT and its effect on the external genitalia. Key point: The first step when identifying ambiguous genitalia in a newborn (NB) child is to check the genetic sex of the NB with a chromosome analysis.
         (a) Male infants have enlarged penises but do *not* develop ambiguous genitalia.
         (b) Precocious puberty may develop in males and females. In girls, the excess androgens are aromatized in peripheral tissue to produce estrogen (E).
         (c) Girls experience irregular menses and infertility as adults.
         (d) Both sexes have rapid growth in childhood and early fusion of the epiphyses and thus most are short in stature as adults.
         (e) Increase in androgens predisposes both sexes to acne.
      (5) Decreases in 17-KS, T, and DHT cause hypogonadism in both sexes.
         (a) Menarche and development of secondary sex characteristics are delayed in females. Recall that female hormones are derived from androgens.
         (b) Males develop pseudohermaphroditism. Male external genitalia development requires DHT (see Chapter 6).
      (6) Increase in mineralocorticoids (M) causes sodium retention, leading to hypertension.
      (7) Decrease in mineralocorticoids
         (a) Sodium loss (hyponatremia) and hyperkalemia
         (b) Hypotension and possible hypovolemic shock
      (8) Increased substrates (Ss) proximal to an enzyme block
      (9) Decreased Ss distal to an enzyme block
   c. Classic 21-hydroxylase (21-OHase) deficiency (Fig. 23-16); epidemiology
      (1) MC enzyme deficiency (90%–95% of cases)
      (2) Mutation of the *CYP21A2* gene, which encodes the adrenal steroid 21-OH enzyme
      (3) Increase in 17-KS, T, and DHT
         (a) All of these hormones are proximal to the enzyme block.
         (b) Ambiguous genitalia is present in female infants but *not* in male infants.
         (c) External genitalia in male infants show enlarged penises.
         (d) Postnatal virilization occurs in males and female infants.
      (4) Decrease in mineralocorticoids; therefore, affected patients lose salt.
         (a) Mineralocorticoids are distal to the enzyme block; therefore, they are salt losers.
         (b) Similar to Addison disease, in which mineralocorticoids are also decreased, there is a risk of developing hypovolemic shock from loss of excess sodium in the urine.
      (5) Decrease in 17-OH (decrease in 11-deoxycortisol and cortisol). All the 17-OH (17-hydroxycorticoids) are distal to the enzyme block (Fig. 23-14).
      (6) Increase in 17-hydroxyprogesterone because it is proximal to the enzyme block
   d. Nonclassical 21-OHase deficiency; epidemiology
      (1) *Unlike* classic 21-OHase deficiency, cortisol and mineralocorticoid (M) activity are normal, and there is *no* loss of sodium in the urine.

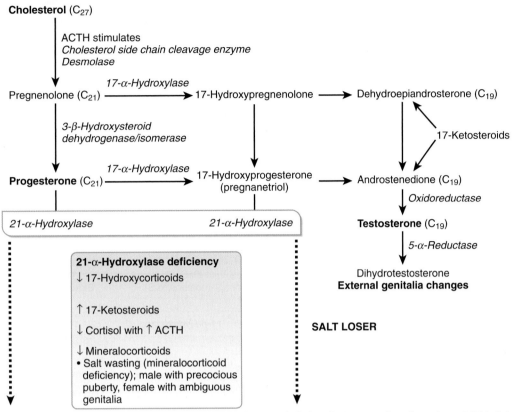

Cholesterol (C_{27})

ACTH stimulates
Cholesterol side chain cleavage enzyme
Desmolase

Pregnenolone (C_{21}) $\xrightarrow{\text{17-}\alpha\text{-Hydroxylase}}$ 17-Hydroxypregnenolone $\longrightarrow$ Dehydroepiandrosterone (C_{19})

3-β-Hydroxysteroid
dehydrogenase/isomerase

17-Ketosteroids

Progesterone (C_{21}) $\xrightarrow{\text{17-}\alpha\text{-Hydroxylase}}$ 17-Hydroxyprogesterone (pregnanetriol) $\longrightarrow$ Androstenedione (C_{19})

Oxidoreductase

21-α-Hydroxylase   *21-α-Hydroxylase*

Testosterone (C_{19})

5-α-Reductase

21-α-Hydroxylase deficiency
↓ 17-Hydroxycorticoids

↑ 17-Ketosteroids

↓ Cortisol with ↑ ACTH

↓ Mineralocorticoids
• Salt wasting (mineralocorticoid deficiency); male with precocious puberty, female with ambiguous genitalia

Dihydrotestosterone
External genitalia changes

SALT LOSER

23-16: Schematic for adrenogenital syndrome: 21-hydoxylase deficiency (salt loser). See text for discussion. *ACTH,* Adrenocorticotropic hormone.

(2) Increased prevalence in Ashkenazi Jewish, Mediterranean, Middle Eastern, and Indian populations

(3) Asymptomatic at birth; develops in late childhood, adolescence, or adulthood with symptoms of excessive androgen secretion

(4) In adolescent and adult females, the symptoms of increased androgens include hirsutism (excess hair in normal hair-bearing areas), acne, menstrual irregularity, increased risk for spontaneous miscarriages, and impaired fertility.

(5) In both sexes, there is tall stature caused by accelerated linear growth of bone, and advanced skeletal maturation for age.

(6) Examination of the external genitalia in females may reveal clitoral enlargement in some girls *without* genital ambiguity.

(7) Enlargement of the penis with prepubertal testes may be noted in boys.

e. 11-Hydroxylase deficiency (11-OHase; Fig. 23-17)

(1) Decrease in the synthesis of cortisol because it is distal to the enzyme block

(2) Decrease in cortisol results in increased plasma levels of ACTH; causes adrenocortical hyperplasia.

(3) Increase in 17-KS, T, and DHT because they are all proximal to the enzyme block

(a) In severe forms of 11-hydroxylase deficiency, female infants exhibit ambiguous genitalia and virilization, and males develop enlarged penises.

(b) In mild forms of 11-OHase deficiency, the increased androgen effects in both sexes appear in mid-childhood as early development of pubic hair, an increase in linear bone growth, and an accelerated bone age.

(4) Increase in the weak mineralocorticoid 11-deoxycorticosterone (proximal to the enzyme block) to a level that causes salt retention and hypertension

(5) Increase in 17-OH because 11-deoxycortisol is proximal to the enzyme block. Cortisol is decreased.

(6) Increase in 17-hydroxyprogesterone because it is proximal to the enzyme block

f. Diagnosis of adrenogenital syndrome (congenital adrenal hyperplasia)

(1) Serum 17-hydroxyprogesterone (17-OHP) is an excellent screening test because it is proximal to the enzyme block in both 21- and 11-OHase deficiency.

Ashkenazi Jews, Mediterranean

Middle-Eastern, Indian

Asymptomatic at birth; late childhood→

Excessive androgen secretion

Adolescent/adult females: signs ↑androgens

Both sexes: tall stature, accelerated linear bone growth

Both sexes: advanced skeletal maturation for age

Clitoral enlargement without genital ambiguity

Enlargement penis; prepubertal testes in boys

11-Hydroxylase deficiency

↓Serum cortisol

↑Plasma ACTH → adrenocortical hyperplasia

↑17-KS, T, DHT: proximal to block

Severe: infant females ambiguous genitalia, males enlarged penis

Mild: late childhood; pubic hair, ↑bone growth

↑11-deoxycorticosterone (weak); hypertension

↑17-OH (11-deoxycortisol); ↓cortisol

↑17-Hydroxyprogesterone

Serum 17-OHP screen: ↑in 21/11-OHase deficiency

23-17: Schematic for adrenogenital syndrome: 11-hydoxylase deficiency (salt retainer). See text for discussion. *ACTH*, Adrenocorticotropic hormone.

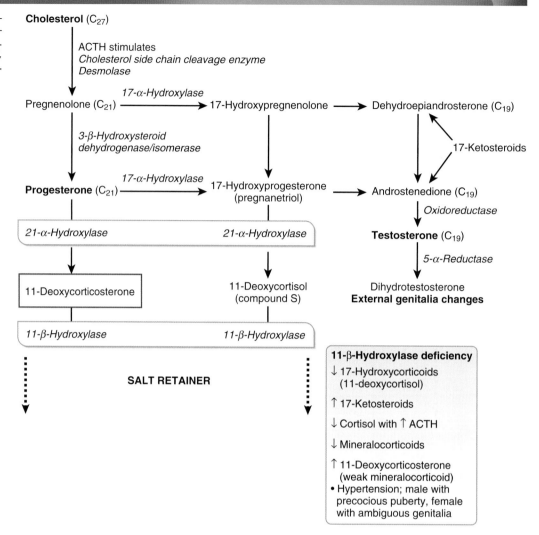

11-β-Hydroxylase deficiency

↓ 17-Hydroxycorticoids (11-deoxycortisol)

↑ 17-Ketosteroids

↓ Cortisol with ↑ ACTH

↓ Mineralocorticoids

↑ 11-Deoxycorticosterone (weak mineralocorticoid)
• Hypertension; male with precocious puberty, female with ambiguous genitalia

TABLE 23-8 Summary of Adrenogenital Syndromes

LABORATORY MEASUREMENT	21-OHASE DEFICIENCY	11-OHASE DEFICIENCY
17-Ketosteroids	↑	↑
17-Hydroxyprogesterone	↑	↑
17-Hydroxycorticoids	↓	↑
Mineralocorticoids	↓	↑

OHase, Hydroxylase.

Chorionic villous sampling

Confirmation: ↑urine 17-OH/17-KS

   (a) Measured prenatally with chorionic villous sampling
   (b) Newborn (NB) screening test for serum 17-OHP is performed in most but *not* all states.
  (2) Confirmation of the diagnosis is made by measuring the urine 17-hydroxycorticoids and 17-KS, both of which are increased in adrenogenital syndrome.
 g. Summary of adrenogenital syndrome is presented in Table 23-8.

Cushing syndrome

Excess cortisol

MCC corticosteroid Rx (iatrogenic)

Pituitary Cushing MC pathologic cause

Pituitary adenoma; ↑ACTH → ↑cortisol

 E. **Adrenocortical hyperfunction** (Link 23-72)
  1. Cushing syndrome
   a. **Definition:** Clinical abnormalities that occur caused by excess production of cortisol
   b. Epidemiology; causes
    (1) Prolonged corticosteroid therapy is the MCC.
    (2) Pituitary Cushing syndrome (Cushing disease; Links 23-73 and 23-74 C)
     (a) Accounts for 60% of cases of Cushing syndrome
     (b) Caused by a pituitary adenoma producing increased amounts of ACTH, leading to excess production of cortisol by the adrenal cortex

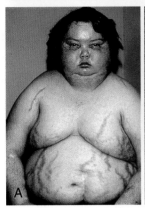
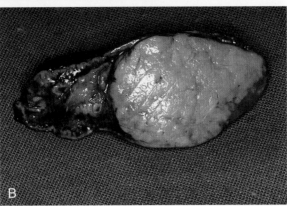

23-18: A, Patient with Cushing syndrome showing moon facies, truncal obesity, and purple abdominal striae. **B,** Benign adenoma in the adrenal cortex from a person with primary aldosteronism. Benign adenomas producing adrenal Cushing syndrome would look the same, but they would be producing excessive amounts of cortisol. *(A from my friend Ivan Damjanov, MD, PhD:* Pathology for the Health-Related Professions, *2nd ed, Philadelphia, Saunders, 2000, p 426; **B** from Bouloux, P:* Self-Assessment Picture Tests Medicine, *Vol. 1, London, Mosby-Wolfe, 1997, p 56, Fig. 112.)*

(3) Adrenal Cushing syndrome
    (a) Accounts for 25% of cases of cases of Cushing syndrome
    (b) Most often caused by an adenoma arising in the adrenal cortex (Links 23-74 B and 23-75)
    (c) Increase in serum cortisol causes a decreased synthesis and release of ACTH by negative feedback.
(4) Ectopic Cushing syndrome
    (a) Accounts for 15% of cases of cases of Cushing syndrome (Link 23-73 and 23-74 D)
    (b) Most commonly caused by a small cell carcinoma (SCC) of the lung secreting excess amounts of ACTH, leading to excess synthesis and release of cortisol by the adrenal cortex
    (c) Less common causes include excess ectopic ACTH production by the thymus (thymoma) and thyroid (MC of the thyroid).
    (d) Both plasma ACTH and serum cortisol are increased.
c. Clinical findings in Cushing syndrome (Links 23-76, 23-77, and 23-78)
    (1) Weight gain caused by hyperinsulinism from hyperglycemia
        (a) Insulin increases the storage of fat (triglyceride) in adipose tissue (see later discussion). Fat deposition occurs in the face (moon facies), upper back ("buffalo hump"), and trunk (truncal obesity; Fig. 23-18 A).
        (b) Insulin also exhibits mineralocorticoid effects, leading to sodium (and thus water) retention.
    (2) Muscle weakness.
        (a) Cortisol breaks down muscles in the extremities (thin extremities).
        (b) Degrading muscles supply amino acids (e.g., alanine) for gluconeogenesis, which produces hyperglycemia (DM).
    (3) Diastolic hypertension
        (a) Caused by the increased production of weak mineralocorticoids (e.g., corticosterone, 11-deoxycorticosterone), glucocorticoids, and insulin, each of which has increased mineralocorticoid activity
        (b) Aldosterone is *not* increased because it requires angiotensin II to be present.
    (4) Hirsutism and virilization are caused by increased androgens (17-KS, T) and insulin (increases androgen synthesis in the ovaries).
    (5) Purple abdominal stria (stretch marks): Excess cortisol weakens collagen, causing rupture of blood vessels in the stretch marks (Link 23-78).
    (6) Osteoporosis: Hypercortisolism causes increased breakdown of bone.
d. Laboratory findings
    (1) Increased free (unbound) cortisol levels in a 24-hour collection of urine: very high positive and negative predictive value for diagnosing Cushing syndrome (see Chapter 1)
    (2) Low-dose dexamethasone (DXM; cortisol analogue) suppression test: A low dose of DXM cannot suppress cortisol in all types of Cushing syndrome (see previous discussion).
    (3) High-dose DXM suppression test: A high dose of DXM can suppress cortisol in pituitary Cushing syndrome but *not* in the other types (ectopic Cushing and adrenal Cushing syndromes).

Margin notes:

Adrenal Cushing syndrome

2nd MCC

Adrenal adenoma MCC

Adrenal Cushing: ↑cortisol → ↓ACTH

SCC lung MCC

Less common: thymoma, medullary carcinoma

Ectopic Cushing: ↑↑ACTH, ↑cortisol

Weight gain: hyperglycemia → ↑insulin

Insulin ↑TG in adipose

Moon facies, buffalo hump, truncal obesity

Insulin mineralocorticoid effect

Muscle weakness

Cortisol degrades muscle

Degrading muscles → amino acid (alanine) → hyperglycemia

Diastolic hypertension

↑Weak mineralocorticoids

Aldosterone *not* increased

Hirsutism/virilization: androgens, insulin

Osteoporosis

Breakdown of bone

↑Urine free cortisol (excellent screen)

Low-dose DXM: no suppression cortisol all types

High-dose DXM; only suppresses pituitary Cushing

Hyperglycemia

Cortisol enhances gluconeogenesis

Hyperglycemia→ ↑insulin → central obesity; hypertension

Hypokalemia; metabolic alkalosis

Nelson syndrome

Bilateral adrenalectomy → uncovers ACTH pituitary adenoma

Prior: ↑cortisol suppresses CRH (hypothalamus)

After adrenalectomy: ↑CRH → ↑size pituitary adenoma

Headache

Diffuse hyperpigmentation (ACTH effect)

Hyperaldosteronism

Primary aldosteronism

Hypernatremia, hypokalemia, metabolic alkalosis

Benign adenoma zona glomerulosa

Clinical findings

Diastolic hypertension (excess Na⁺)

Muscle weakness (↓K⁺)

Tetany (metabolic alkalosis)

Laboratory findings

N/↑Na⁺, ↓K⁺, metabolic alkalosis

↓PRA

↑PV → ↑RBF → ↓activation JG apparatus → PRA

↑Plasma aldosterone

Secondary aldosteronism

Compensatory reaction from ↓ECF volume

(4) Hyperglycemia (DM)
  (a) Cortisol enhances gluconeogenesis.
  (b) Hyperglycemia stimulates the release of insulin, which increases centrally located adipose tissue deposits. In addition, hyperinsulinemia also contributes to producing hypertension because of its mineralocorticoid effect of increasing sodium retention.
(5) Hypokalemic metabolic alkalosis: caused by increased production of weak mineralocorticoids in Cushing syndrome (see Table 5-8)

e. Nelson syndrome
  (1) **Definition:** Bilateral adrenalectomy causes enlargement of a preexisting undiagnosed ACTH-secreting pituitary adenoma.
  (2) Epidemiology
    (a) Before adrenalectomy, an undiagnosed pituitary adenoma secreting ACTH stimulates the adrenal cortex to increase the synthesis and release of serum cortisol. An increase in serum cortisol suppresses the release of corticotropin-releasing hormone (CRH) by the hypothalamus (Link 23-23 A, B).
    (b) After bilateral adrenalectomy, normalization of the serum cortisol levels removes the suppressive effect on CRH release by the hypothalamus. The net effect is an increase in the release of CRH by the hypothalamus and an increase in the size of the pituitary adenoma as well as an increase in the production and release of ACTH.
  (3) Clinical findings
    (a) Headache caused by enlargement of the preexisting pituitary adenoma
    (b) Diffuse hyperpigmentation caused by an increase in production of the pituitary adenoma of ACTH by the pituitary adenoma

f. A summary of laboratory findings in pituitary, adrenal, and ectopic Cushing syndrome is presented in Table 23-9.

g. Comparison of findings in Addison disease and Cushing syndrome (Link 23-79)

2. Hyperaldosteronism
  a. Primary aldosteronism (Conn syndrome; see Chapter 5 for full discussion)
    (1) **Definition:** Clinical syndrome characterized by hypernatremia, hypokalemia, and metabolic alkalosis caused by excessive aldosterone secretion
    (2) Epidemiology: most often caused by a benign adenoma in the zona glomerulosa of the adrenal cortex secreting excess aldosterone (Fig. 23-18 B; Links 23-80 and 23-81)
    (3) Clinical findings
      (a) Diastolic hypertension caused by excess sodium
      (b) Muscle weakness caused by hypokalemia
      (c) Tetany caused by metabolic alkalosis (see previous discussion)
    (4) Laboratory findings (see Chapter 5; see Fig. 5-9)
      (a) High normal or mild hypernatremia, hypokalemia, and metabolic alkalosis
      (b) Decreased plasma renin activity (PRA). In primary aldosteronism, plasma volume (PV) is increased from sodium retention, which increases the renal blood flow (RBF) and decreases activation of the juxtaglomerular (JG) apparatus and the release of renin (↓PRA).
      (c) Increase in plasma aldosterone levels in the blood
  b. Secondary aldosteronism (see Chapter 5)
    (1) **Definition:** Compensatory reaction related to a decrease in extracellular fluid (ECF) volume
    (2) Epidemiology

TABLE 23-9 Summary of Pituitary, Adrenal, and Ectopic Cushing Syndrome (CS)

LABORATORY TEST	PITUITARY CS	ADRENAL CS	ECTOPIC CS
Serum cortisol	↑	↑	↑
Urine free cortisol	↑	↑	↑
Low-dose dexamethasone	Cortisol *not* suppressed	Cortisol *not* suppressed	Cortisol *not* suppressed
High-dose dexamethasone	Cortisol suppressed	Cortisol *not* suppressed	Cortisol *not* suppressed
Plasma ACTH	"Normal"* to ↑	↓	Markedly ↑

*"Normal": a plasma adrenocorticotropic hormone (ACTH) in the normal range is *not* normal in the presence of an increase in serum cortisol.

A decrease in extracellular fluid volume (e.g., hemorrhage or Na$^+$ depletion [hypertonic loss of Na$^+$]) causes a decrease in renal blood flow, which increases renin secretion by the juxtaglomerular cells of the kidney. Renin, an enzyme, catalyzes the conversion of angiotensinogen to angiotensin I. Angiotensin-converting enzyme catalyzes the conversion of angiotensin I to angiotensin II, which then acts on the zona glomerulosa to stimulate aldosterone synthesis. This increase in aldosterone is called secondary aldosteronism. Aldosterone increases sodium reabsorption in the late distal tubule Na$^+$–K$^+$ channels.

(Modified excerpt from Costanzo LS: *Physiology*, 5th ed, Philadelphia, Saunders Elsevier, 2014, p 421.)

F. **Adrenal medulla hyperfunction**
1. **Definition:** Increased production of catecholamines resulting in hypertension
2. Pheochromocytoma
   a. **Definition:** Tumor arising from the adrenal medulla that releases excessive amounts of catecholamines, usually norepinephrine (NOR) (MC) and epinephrine (EPI)
   b. Epidemiology
      (1) Unilateral in ~90% of cases
      (2) Benign adenoma in ~90% of cases
      (3) Arises in the adrenal medulla in ~90% of cases. Other sites of origin include the wall of the urinary bladder, organ of Zuckerkandl near the bifurcation of the aorta, and posterior mediastinum.
      (4) N-Methyltransferase converts NOR to EPI (see Fig. 23-19 A).
         (a) Adrenal medulla and the organ of Zuckerkandl (Z) contain the N-methyltransferase. Produce NOR and EPI.
         (b) Other sites lack N-methyltransferase; therefore, tumors arising in these sites (e.g., posterior mediastinum) only produce NOR, not EPI.
      (5) Associations of pheochromocytoma
         (a) Neurofibromatosis (5% in type 1; see Chapter 26)
         (b) Multiple endocrine neoplasia (MEN) IIa and IIb (MEN III). MEN is caused by a mutation in the *RET* proto-oncogene.
         (c) Von Hippel–Lindau disease (VHL; often bilateral pheochromocytomas)
            • Caused by a mutation in the *VHL* gene.
   c. Tumor characteristics: brown, hemorrhagic, and often necrotic (Links 23-82 to 23-84)
   d. Clinical findings of a pheochromocytoma
      (1) Diastolic hypertension
         (a) MC manifestation; sustained in 55% of cases
         (b) Paroxysmal bursts occur in 45% of cases. These bursts are *not* present in primary hypertension.

↓ECF → ↓RBF → activates JG cells → renin converts ATG to ATI → ACE converts ATI to ATII → ATII acts on zona glomerulosa to synthesize aldosterone
Adrenal medulla hyperfunction
↑Production catecholamines
Pheochromocytoma
Tumor adrenal medulla releasing excess NOR, EPI
Unilateral ~90%
Benign adenoma 90%
Arises adrenal medulla ~90%
Bladder, organ Zuckerkandl
Posterior mediastinum
N-methyltransferase → NOR to EPI
N-methyltransferase: adrenal medulla, organ of Z
Lack N-methyltransferase: e.g., posterior mediastinum, secrete NOR only
Associations pheochromocytoma
Neurofibromatosis
MEN IIa, MEN IIb
MEN: mutation RET protooncogene
VHL: often bilateral pheo
Mutation *VHL* gene
Brown, hemorrhagic, necrotic
Clinical findings
Diastolic hypertension
Hypertension MC finding
Sustained 55%
Paroxysmal bursts hypertension 45%
No paroxysmal bursts in 1° hypertension

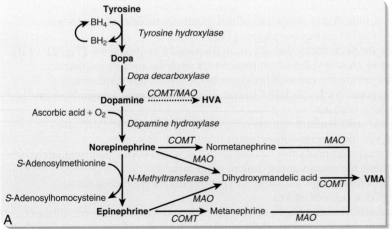

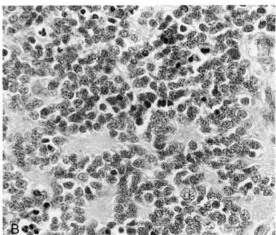

23-19: A, Schematic of catecholamine synthesis and degradation in adrenal medulla. Note the role of tyrosine in the synthesis of catecholamines. Catecholamines are important neurotransmitters and are involved in cardiac contraction, vasoconstriction, and gastrointestinal motility. **B,** Neuroblastoma of the adrenal medulla with Homer-Wright rosettes (neuroblasts are located around a central space). *BH$_2$,* Dihydrobiopterin; *BH$_4$,* tetrahydrobiopterin; *COMT,* catechol-O-methyltransferase; *HVA,* homovanillic acid; *MAO,* monoamine oxidase; *VMA,* vanillylmandelic acid. (*A* from Pelley J, Goljan E: *Rapid Review Biochemistry, 2nd ed, Philadelphia, Mosby, 2007, p 144, Fig. 8-6; B from my friend Ivan Damjanov, MD, PhD:* Pathology for the Health-Related Professions, *2nd ed, Philadelphia, Saunders, 2000, Fig. 17-16.*)

Pounding headache
Palpitations
Palpitations with/without tachycardia
Palpitations *not* in 1° hypertension
Drenching sweats
Correlates with paroxysms hypertension
Hyperhidrosis *not* present in 1° hypertension
Anxiety correlates with paroxysms hypertension
Anxiety *not* present in 1° hypertension
Chest pain: subendocardial ischemia
Postural hypotension
Drop BP standing up from sitting/lying down
Reduced PV
Ileus: lack bowel peristalsis
Plasma free metanephrines best screen/confirm
↑Plasma normetanephrine
↑24-Hour urine metanephrine (best screening test)
↑24-Hour urine for VMA
Lack NOR suppression with clonidine
Hyperglycemia: glycogenolysis, gluconeogenesis
Neutrophilic leukocytosis: marginating pool now circulating
Neuroblastoma
Malignant tumor postganglionic sympathetic neurons
Secretes excess catecholamines
MC children <5 yrs old
3rd MC cancer children
Mean age 18 mths
Adrenal medulla MC site; posterior mediastinum
Amplification N-MYC oncogene
Malignant neuroblasts
Homer-Wright rosettes
Neuroblasts around central space
EM secretory granules
Opsoclonus-myoclonus syndrome
Paraneoplastic syndrome
20% to 50%
Myoclonic jerks extremities
Chaotic eye movements
Skin, bone metastasis common
Majority patients have metastasis
Prognosis age dependent
Palpable abdominal mass (do *not* palpate)
Bluish lesions on skin infants (metastasis)
Diastolic hypertension
Neck nodules, bone pain, proptosis, "raccoon eyes," fever/weight loss

(2) Pounding headache in 80% of cases; heart palpitations in 70% of cases
   (a) Palpitations may occur with or without tachycardia (increased heart rate).
   (b) Palpitations are *not* present in primary hypertension.
(3) Drenching sweats (hyperhidrosis) is present in 70% of cases. Correlates with the paroxysms of hypertension. Hyperhidrosis is *not* present in primary hypertension. Sweat glands receive sympathetic innervation but have muscarinic acetylcholine receptors, which are normally stimulated by the parasympathetic nervous system.
(4) Anxiety. Correlates with the paroxysms of hypertension. Anxiety is *not* present in primary hypertension.
(5) Chest pain from subendocardial ischemia arises as a result of vasoconstriction of the coronary arteries.
(6) Orthostatic (postural) hypotension.
   (a) **Definition:** Low blood pressure that occurs when standing up from sitting or lying down
   (b) Plasma volume (PV) is reduced owing to vasoconstriction of arterioles and venules by catecholamines.
(7) Ileus (lack of bowel peristalsis) caused by inhibition of peristalsis by catecholamines
  e. Laboratory findings (Fig. 23-19 A; Link 23-85)
   (1) Increase in plasma free metanephrines, which is the best test to screen and to confirm the presence of a pheochromocytoma
   (2) Increase in plasma normetanephrine
   (3) Increase in a 24-hour urine level of metanephrine (100% sensitivity for diagnosing a pheochromocytoma)
   (4) Increased in a 24-hour urine level of vanillymandelic acid (VMA)
   (5) Lack of suppression of plasma norepinephrine (NOR) with clonidine (antihypertensive drug)
   (6) Hyperglycemia caused by catecholamine enhanced increase in glycogenolysis and gluconeogenesis
   (7) Neutrophilic leukocytosis caused by inhibition of neutrophil adhesion molecules that allow the marginating pool of neutrophils to become part of the circulating pool, thus increasing the neutrophil count in the peripheral blood (see Chapter 3)
3. Neuroblastoma
  a. **Definition:** Malignant tumor arising from postganglionic sympathetic neurons that originates in the adrenal medulla or the sympathetic chain of ganglion cells that secrete excess amounts of catecholamines
  b. Epidemiology
   (1) Most often occurs in children <5 years old. Third MC cancer in children. Mean age of onset is 18 months.
   (2) Primarily located in the adrenal medulla; less commonly located in the posterior mediastinum (paraspinal location)
   (3) Caused by an amplification of the *N-MYC* oncogene, a nuclear transcriber (see Chapter 9)
   (4) "Small cell" tumor that is composed of malignant neuroblasts (Link 23-86)
     (a) Homer-Wright rosettes are present (Link 23-87).
     (b) Rosettes are neuroblasts that are located around a central space (Fig. 23-19 B). Electron microscopy shows neurosecretory granules in the cytoplasm.
   (5) Neuroblastomas are the cause of the opsoclonus-myoclonus syndrome.
     (a) Paraneoplastic syndrome (see Chapter 9): associated with a neuroblastoma in 20% to 50% of cases
     (b) Myoclonic jerks (sudden muscle contractions) occur in the extremities.
     (c) Chaotic eye movements (opsoclonus) occur in all directions.
   (6) Neuroblastomas commonly metastasize to the skin and bones. Approximately 70% of patients have metastases at the time of diagnosis.
   (7) Prognosis depends on age. Children <1 year old have a good prognosis.
  c. Clinical findings of a neuroblastoma
   (1) Palpable abdominal mass, which upon palpation may cause increased release of catecholamines. For this reason, abdominal palpation should *not* be performed on future physical examinations.
   (2) Infants show bluish, bruise-like nodules on the skin (metastasis).
   (3) Diastolic hypertension
   (4) Signs of metastatic disease: firm, nontender lesions on the neck, bone pain, proptosis of the eyes, "raccoon eyes," fever, weight loss

TABLE 23-10 Summary of Islet Cell Tumors

TUMOR	DESCRIPTION
Glucagonoma	• Malignant tumor of α-islet cells • Clinical: hyperglycemia, rash (necrolytic migratory erythema)
Insulinoma	• Benign tumor of β-islet cells; most common islet cell tumor • Approximately 80% have MEN I syndrome • Clinical: fasting hypoglycemia causing mental status abnormalities • Laboratory: fasting hypoglycemia; increase in serum insulin and C-peptide (proteases split proinsulin into insulin + C-peptide); C-peptide is a marker of endogenous insulin production by β-islet cells • Surreptitious injection of insulin: fasting hypoglycemia, increased insulin, *decreased* C-peptide (hypoglycemia suppresses β-islet cells)
Somatostatinoma	• Malignant tumor of δ-islet cells; somatostatin is an inhibitory hormone • Inhibition of gastrin causes achlorhydria • Inhibition of cholecystokinin causes cholelithiasis and steatorrhea • Inhibition of gastric inhibitory peptide causes diabetes mellitus • Inhibition of secretin causes steatorrhea
VIPoma (pancreatic cholera)	• Malignant tumor with excessive secretion of VIP • Clinical: secretory diarrhea, achlorhydria • Laboratory: hypokalemia, NAGMA (loss of bicarbonate in stool)
Zollinger-Ellison (see Chapter 18)	• Malignant tumor (60%–90% of cases) that secretes excess gastrin and causes hyperacidity • Majority are located in the duodenum (60% of cases) and less commonly in the pancreatic islet cells (30% of cases); radiolabeled octreotide is used to localize the tumor • Sporadic in two-thirds of cases; associated with MEN type I in one-third of cases • Ulcers are single and in the usual locations, or there may be multiple ulcers • Clinical: peptic ulceration, diarrhea, maldigestion of food • Laboratory: serum gastrin >1000 pg/mL

MEN, Multiple endocrine neoplasia; *NAGMA*, normal anion gap metabolic acidosis; *VIP*, vasoactive intestinal peptide.

d. Diagnosis
    (1) Increased urine VMA and HVA (derived from dopamine; 90%–95% sensitivity); increased in 90% of cases
    (2) Imaging studies
        (a) Body scan with ^{131}I-MIBG (<u>m</u>eta<u>i</u>odo<u>b</u>enzylguanidine). Malignant cells pick up the radioactive material.
        (b) Bone scans to detect lytic lesions
e. Prognosis
    (1) Neuroblastomas in infants can spontaneously regress!
    (2) Overall survival rate is 40%. Children <1 year old have a 90% cure rate.

VIII. Islet Cell Tumors (Table 23-10)

In the β-islet cells, proinsulin is cleaved into insulin and C-peptide (Link 23-88 A, B). In a patient with an insulinoma arising from the islet cells, both the serum insulin and C-peptide are increased. However, if a person is self-injecting insulin, the serum insulin is increased, but the C-peptide is decreased. The excess insulin injected will produce hypoglycemia; however, the hypoglycemia will have a negative feedback on the person's islet cells, causing suppression of endogenous synthesis of insulin and a decrease in the serum C-peptide level. All of the islet cell tumors are summarized in Links 23-89 and 23-90.

IX. Diabetes Mellitus
  A. Definition: Syndrome of hyperglycemia that involves many systems and has many causes and is broadly classified into type 1 and type II DM
  B. Functions of insulin (*Excerpted from Herschel R: Physiology Secrets, 2nd ed, Philadelphia, Hanley & Belfus, 2003, p 224, #112 table.*)
    1. Anabolic functions of insulin
      a. Liver
        (1) Increases glycogen storage (glycogenesis)
        (2) Increases the synthesis of very-low-density lipoprotein (VLDL)
        (3) Increases glycolysis (breakdown of glucose to pyruvic acid)
      b. Muscle
        (1) Increases amino acid uptake and protein synthesis
        (2) Increases glucose transport and glycogen synthesis
      c. Adipose increases glucose uptake and triglyceride storage.

Margin notes:

Diagnosis

↑Urine VMA, HVA

Imaging studies

^{131}I-MIBG: neuroblasts take up material

Bone scans: detect lytic lesions

Can spontaneously regress in infants

Insulinoma: ↑serum insulin, ↑C-peptide. Patient injecting excess insulin: ↑serum insulin, ↓C-peptide (suppressed)

Diabetes mellitus

Hyperglycemia syndrome

Type I/II DM

Anabolic functions insulin

Liver

↑Glycogen storage

↑Synthesis VLDL

↑Glycolysis

Muscle

↑Amino acid uptake/protein synthesis

↑Glucose transport, ↑glycogen synthesis

Adipose: ↑glucose uptake, ↑TG storage

Anticatabolic functions insulin
Liver inhibits glycogenolysis, ketogenesis, gluconeogenesis
Muscle: inhibits glycogen phosphorylase
Adipose inhibits glycolysis

2. Anticatabolic functions of insulin
   a. Liver inhibits glycogenolysis, ketogenesis, and gluconeogenesis.
   b. Muscle inhibits glycogen phosphorylase.
   c. Adipose inhibits lipolysis.

Insulin action: Insulin is **synthesized** by pancreatic β cells as an inactive precursor, proinsulin. Proteolytic cleavage of proinsulin yields C-peptide and active insulin, consisting of disulfide-linked A and B chains (Link 23-88). **Secretion** of insulin is regulated by circulating substrates and hormones. Insulin secretion is **stimulated** by increased blood glucose (most important), increased individual amino acids (e.g., arginine, leucine), and gastrointestinal hormones (e.g., secretin), which are released after ingestion of food. Insulin is **inhibited** by somatostatin, low glucose levels, and hypokalemia. **Metabolic actions** of insulin are most pronounced in the liver, muscle, and adipose tissue. The overall effect is to promote storage of excess glucose as glycogen in the liver and muscle and as triacylglycerols in adipose tissue. The **insulin receptor** (Link 23-91) is a tetramer whose cytosolic domain has tyrosine kinase activity for generating second messengers. Insulin binding triggers signaling pathways that produce several cellular responses (i.e., postreceptor functions). Increased adipose tissue mass downregulates insulin receptor synthesis, and loss of adipose upregulates receptor synthesis. Increased glucose uptake by muscle and adipose tissue is prompted by translocation of insulin-sensitive glucose transporter 4 (GLUT4) receptors to the cell surface. Dephosphorylation from insulin action activates energy-storage enzymes (e.g., glycogen synthase) and inactivates energy-mobilizing enzymes (e.g., glycogen phosphorylase). Increased enzyme synthesis from insulin action (e.g., glucokinase, phosphofructokinase) is caused by activation of gene transcription.

(Excerpt taken from Pelley JW, Goljan EF: *Rapid Review Biochemistry*, 3rd ed, St. Louis, Mosby Elsevier 2011, p 113.)

Incidence 9% to 10%
↑Incidence Native Americans
Legal blindness
Peripheral neuropathy
CRF
Below-the-knee amputation
↑Incidence rate with age
Classification DM
Types 1 and 2 DM
Secondary causes
Pancreas: CF, chronic pancreatitis
Drugs
Glucocorticoids, pentamidine, thiazide, α-interferon
Endocrine disease
Pheochromocytoma, Cushing, glucagonoma
Genetic disease
Hemochromatosis, metabolic syndrome, MODY
Insulin receptor deficiency
Acanthosis nigricans
Infections
Infections: mumps, CMV
IGT
GDM
MODY
Mutations AD gene: interferes with insulin production
AD disorder
HNF1-α gene (70%)
Gene ↓amount insulin produced
Usually <25; *not* obese
Mild to severe hyperglycemia
Reduced amount insulin in β-cells
No ketoacidosis
May progress to type 2 DM
Metabolic syndrome
Insulin resistance syndrome
Hyperglycemia, dyslipidemia
Abdominal obesity, hypertension

3. Figure 23-20 A summarizes the functions of insulin in the fed state and the fasting state. Figure 23-20 B summarizes the actions of insulin on target tissues.

C. Epidemiology
1. Affects 9% to 10% of the population in the United States; increased incidence in Native Americans (e.g., 35% of Pima Indians have DM)
2. Leading cause in the United States of legal blindness, peripheral neuropathy, chronic renal failure (CRF), and below-the-knee amputation
3. Incidence rate increases with age.

D. Classification of diabetes mellitus
1. Types 1 and type 2 DM (Table 23-11)
2. Secondary causes of DM
   a. Pancreatic disease. Examples: cystic fibrosis (CF), chronic pancreatitis
   b. Drugs. Examples: glucocorticoids, pentamidine, thiazides, α-interferon
   c. Endocrine disease. Examples: pheochromocytoma, glucagonoma, Cushing syndrome
   d. Genetic disease. Examples: hemochromatosis, metabolic syndrome, maturity onset diabetes of the young (MODY)
   e. Insulin-receptor deficiency: Acanthosis nigricans is a phenotypic marker for this secondary cause of DM (Link 23-92).
   f. Infections. Examples: mumps and cytomegalovirus (CMV; AIDS patients)
3. Impaired glucose tolerance (IGT)
4. Gestational diabetes mellitus (GDM)
5. MODY
   a. **Definition:** Any of several hereditary different forms of diabetes caused by mutations in an autosomal dominant (AD) gene that interfere with insulin production in the β-cells of the pancreas
   b. Epidemiology
      (1) Accounts for 2% to 5% cases of DM
      (2) AD disease
         (a) Hepatocyte nuclear factor 1-α (HNF1-α) gene causes about 70% of cases of MODY.
         (b) Gene causes DM by reducing the amount of insulin that is produced by the pancreas.
      (3) Patients are usually <25 years old and are *not* obese.
      (4) Present with mild to severe hyperglycemia caused by reduced amounts of insulin in the β-cells
      (5) Diabetic ketosis is *not* present.
      (6) May progress into type 2 DM
6. Metabolic syndrome
   a. **Definition:** Insulin resistance syndrome characterized by hyperglycemia, dyslipidemia, abdominal obesity, and hypertension

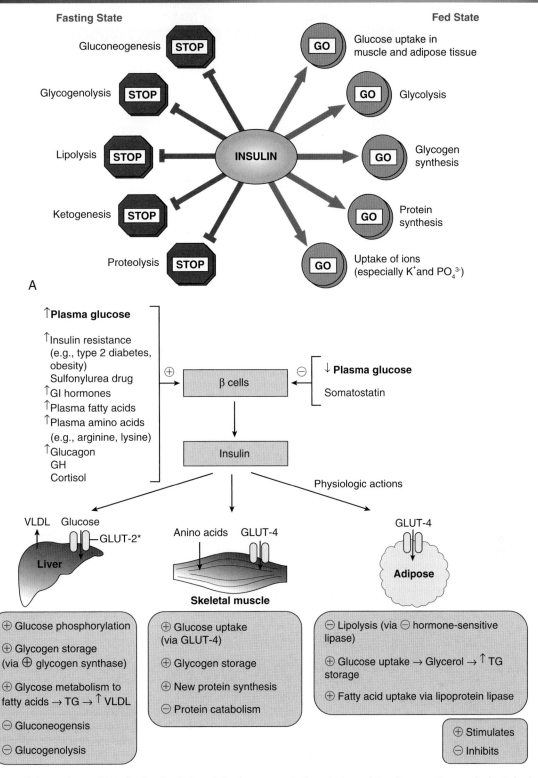

23-20: A, Overview of the actions of insulin in the fed and fasting state. **B,** Regulation of insulin secretion and physiologic actions of insulin. *GH,* Growth hormone; *GI,* gastrointestinal; *GLUT,* glucose transporter; *K+,* potassium; *PO₄³⁻,* phosphate; *TG,* triglyceride; *VLDL,* very-low-density lipoprotein. (*A From Gaw A, Murphy MJ, Srivastava R, Cowan RA, O'Reilly Denis St J:* Clinical Biochemistry: An Illustrated Colour Text, *5th ed, Churchill Livingstone Elsevier, 2013, p 62, Fig. 31.2; B from Brown TA:* Rapid Review Physiology, *2nd ed, St. Louis, Mosby Elsevier, 2012, p 93, Fig. 3-19.*)

TABLE 23-11   Comparison Between Type 1 and Type 2 Diabetes Mellitus

CHARACTERISTIC	TYPE 1	TYPE 2
Prevalence (%)	• 5–10	• 90–95
Age at onset	• <30 yr	• Usually >40 yr but any age
Speed of onset	• Rapid	• Insidious
Body habitus	• Usually thin • History of weight loss *before* presentation	• Usually obese (80% of cases) or overweight • History of weight gain *before* diagnosis
Genetics	• Family history uncommon (<20% first degree relatives with diabetes) • 35%–50% concordance in monozygotic twins • Environmental factors required for expression • HLA-DR3 and HLA-DR4	• Strong family history of first-degree relatives with diabetes • 60%–90% concordance in monozygotic twins • *No* HLA association • Increased in Native Americans and blacks
Associations	Other autoimmune diseases: Graves disease, Hashimoto thyroiditis, pernicious anemia, Addison disease, vitiligo	• *No* other autoimmune associations
Pathogenesis (Links 23-93 and 23-94)	• Precipitating factors largely unknown • Risk factors: microbial, chemical, dietary • Endogenous insulin levels low or absent • Pancreas devoid of β-islet cells • Insulitis: T-cell cytokine destruction (type IV HSR) and autoantibodies against β-islet cells (>80%) and insulin (>50%) (type II HSR); glutamic acid decarboxylase antibodies • Triggers for destruction—e.g., viruses	• Relative deficiency of insulin (Link 23-95) • Early stages have hyperinsulinemia • Insulin resistance related to receptor and postreceptor problems • Decreased insulin receptors: downregulation by increased adipose • Postreceptor defects: most important factor. Examples: tyrosine kinase defects (normally is activated when insulin attaches to its receptor [muscle, adipose]); GLUT-4 abnormalities (normally moves from the cytoplasm to the cell membrane to attach to glucose and transport glucose into the cytoplasm) • Fibrotic β-islet cells contain amyloid • *No* autoantibodies
Clinical findings	• Polyuria (osmotic diuresis from glucosuria), polydipsia (↑POSM), polyphagia, weight loss	• Insidious onset of symptoms • Recurrent blurry vision: alteration in lens refraction from sorbitol • Recurrent infections: bacterial, *Candida* • Target organ disease: nephropathy, retinopathy, neuropathy, coronary artery disease • Reactive hypoglycemia: too much insulin released in response to a glucose load (early finding) • Increased risk for Alzheimer disease (see Chapter 26)
	• Ketoacidosis (hyperglycemia, coma, production of ketone bodies) • Lactic acidosis from shock (losing sodium by osmotic diuresis from glucosuria) • Greater daily variability in glucose values • Exaggerated hyperglycemic response to stressors and meals • Normal insulin sensitivity • C-peptide: very low or undetectable	• HHS: enough insulin to prevent ketoacidosis but *not* enough to prevent hyperglycemia • Lactic acidosis may occur from shock (losing sodium by osmotic diuresis from glucosuria) • Blood sugars stable throughout the day • Very reduced insulin sensitivity • C-peptide levels: detectable or elevated

GLUT, Glucose transport unit; *HLA,* human leukocyte antigen; *HHS,* hyperglycemic hyperosmolar state; *HSR,* hypersensitivity reaction.

Insulin resistance syndrome
Genetic defect exacerbated by obesity
Women: African American, Mexican American
↑With weight
Commonly associated with POS
Associated with acanthosis nigricans
↑Alzheimer disease risk
Clinical/lab findings
Hyperinsulinemia
↑Synthesis VLDL; ↑TG
Hypertension ≥130/85 mm Hg
Insulin causes sodium retention
CAD
↑ Insulin damages endothelial cells
Obesity exacerbates insulin resistance

b. Epidemiology
   (1) Affects ~25% of the United States adult population
   (2) Insulin resistance syndrome
       (a) A genetic defect causes insulin resistance that is exacerbated by obesity
       (b) Increased prevalence in women, with an increased prevalence in African Americans and Mexican Americans. Prevalence increases with weight.
       (c) Commonly associated with polycystic ovary syndrome (PCOS) in women (see Chapter 22).
       (d) Associated with acanthosis nigricans (see Chapters 22 and 25)
       (e) Associated with an increased risk for developing Alzheimer disease (see Chapter 26)
c. Clinical and laboratory findings in metabolic syndrome
   (1) Hyperinsulinemia, which leads to:
       (a) increased synthesis of VLDL (hypertriglyceridemia). Serum triglyceride (TG) is ≥150 mg/dL.
       (b) Hypertension (≥130/85 mm Hg); increased insulin increases sodium retention by the renal tubules
       (c) Coronary artery disease (CAD). Increased insulin damages endothelial cells.
   (2) Obesity exacerbates insulin resistance.

TABLE 23-12   Complications of Diabetes Mellitus

COMPLICATION CATEGORY	DISCUSSION
Atherosclerotic disease (see Figs. 2-16 D and 10-5; Links 23-11 and 23-14; see Chapter 10)	• Increased incidence of strokes, CAD, and peripheral vascular disease • Acute MI is the most common cause of death • Gangrene of the lower extremities. Diabetes is the most common cause of nontraumatic amputation of the lower extremity.
Renal disorders (see Fig. 20-5 J, Links 23-100, 23-101; see Chapter 20)	• Renal failure caused by nodular glomerulosclerosis (see Chapter 20) • Renal papillary necrosis

Ocular disorders (see Fig. 23-21B) (Links 23-96 and 23-97)	• Increased risk for cataracts and glaucoma
	• Retinopathy (15%):
	  • *Nonproliferative:* microaneurysm formation, flame hemorrhages, exudates.
	  • *Proliferative:* formation of new vessels (neovascularization), increased risk for retinal detachment and blindness, annual ophthalmologic examination is mandatory (photocoagulate microaneurysms)

Peripheral nerve disorders (Fig. 23-21A)	• Diabetes mellitus is the most common cause of peripheral neuropathy in the United States; occurs in 70%–80% of cases. • Sensory: paresthesias, patients complain of burning feet, ↓pinprick sensation, ↓proprioception (ataxia) • Motor dysfunction: muscle weakness, ↓deep tendon reflexes • Neuropathy is the most important risk factor for neuropathic ulcers on the bottom of the feet (patient cannot feel pain).
Autonomic nervous system disorders	• Autonomic neuropathy: gastroparesis (delayed emptying of stomach), impotence, neurogenic bladder, orthostatic hypotension
CN disorders	• Diabetes is the most common cause of multiple cranial nerve palsies. • CNs most often involved: CN III, IV, and VI
Infectious disorders	• Urinary tract infections • *Candida* infections: e.g., vulvovaginitis (see Links 22-5 to 22-8; Chapter 22). • Malignant external otitis caused by *Pseudomonas aeruginosa* • Rhinocerebral mucormycosis: *Mucor* extends from the frontal sinuses to the frontal lobes, producing infarction (invades vessels) and abscesses (see Fig. 26-16 B) • Cutaneous infections: usually *Staphylococcus aureus* abscesses
Skin disorders	• Necrobiosis lipoidica diabeticorum: well-demarcated yellow plaques over the anterior surface of the legs or dorsum of the ankles (Links 23-98 and 23-99) • Lipoatrophy: atrophy at insulin injection sites caused by impure insulin • Lipohypertrophy: increased fat synthesis at insulin injection sites
Joint disorders	• Neuropathic joint: related to lack of sensation; bone or joint deformity from repeated trauma (see Chapter 24)

CAD, Coronary artery disease; *CN*, cranial nerve; *MI*, myocardial infarction.

(a) Increased adipose downregulates insulin receptor synthesis (type 2 DM).
(b) Definition for obesity in the metabolic syndrome is as follows:
  • abdominal waistline girth in men >40 inches.
  • abdominal waistline girth in women >35 inches.
(3) Serum high-density lipoprotein cholesterol (HDL-CH) <40 mg/dL in men and <50 mg/dL in women.
(4) Fasting serum glucose >100 mg/dL or taking insulin or glucose-lowering medications; type 2 DM
E. **Pathologic processes and complications in DM** (Table 23-12)
  1. Poor glycemic control
    a. Hyperglycemia is the key factor that produces organ damage.
    b. Glucose (G) control reduces onset and severity of complications. Complications are related to retinopathy, neuropathy, and nephropathy, in descending order.
  2. Nonenzymatic glycosylation (NEG)
    a. **Definition:** Glucose combines with amino groups in proteins.
    b. Advanced glycosylation products (AGPs) are produced.
      (1) Products increase blood vessel (BV) permeability to protein.
      (2) Products increase atherogenesis (formation of lipid plaques) on the endothelium of vessels.
    c. Role of nonenzymatic glycosylation in the pathology of DM
      (1) Production of glycosylated hemoglobin A1c (Hb_{A1c})
      (2) Hyaline arteriolosclerosis (HALS; see Chapter 10), diabetic glomerulopathy (DG; see Chapter 20)
      (3) Ischemic heart disease (IHD see Chapter 11), strokes (small vessel strokes; see Chapter 26), peripheral vascular disease (PVD; see Chapter 10)

↑Adipose: downregulates insulin receptor synthesis (type 2 DM)

Definition obesity: abdominal waistline girth

↓Serum HDL men/women

↑Fasting glucose; taking insulin or glucose lowering meds

Type 2 DM

Pathologic processes/complications

Poor glycemic control

Hyperglycemia key in organ damage

G control reduces complications

Good G control prevents complications

Nonenzymatic glycosylation (NEG)

Glucose combines with amino groups in proteins

AGPs produced

AGPs ↑BV permeability to proteins

AGPs ↑atherogenesis

NEG and pathology

↑Hb_{A1c}

HALS, DG

IHD, strokes, PVD

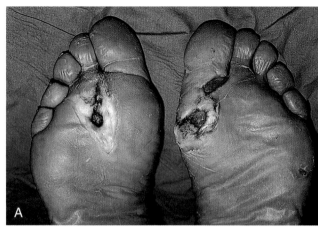 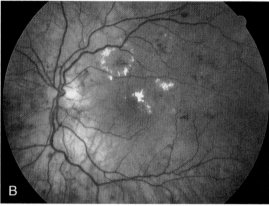

23-21: A, Neuropathic ulcers. Note the areas of ulcerations over the pressure points on the plantar surfaces of both feet. The patient had no sensation for pain in these areas because of a peripheral neuropathy. This emphasizes the importance for checking pain sensation of the feet in all diabetic patients. **B,** Background diabetic retinopathy (right eye). Exudates are the sharp white areas, and microaneurysms are the areas with small hemorrhages. (*A from Swartz MH:* Textbook of Physical Diagnosis, *5th ed, Philadelphia, Saunders Elsevier, 2006, p 641, Fig. 20-72; B from Goldman L, Schafer AI:* Cecil's Medicine, *24th ed, Philadelphia, Saunders Elsevier, 2012, p 2438, Fig. 431-24.*)

Osmotic damage
Aldose reductase: converts G to sorbitol; osmotic damage
Osmotic damage in DM
Cataracts
Peripheral neuropathy
Osmotic damage Schwann cells
Neuropathic ulcers
Cannot feel pain
Retinopathy; microaneurysms
Diabetic microangiopathy
↑Type IV collagen synthesis
Basement membrane/mesangium
Diabetic glomerulopathy: nephrotic syndrome
Clinical findings DM
Insulin-induced hypoglycemia
Hypoglycemia MC complication
Destruction of neurons
Clinical hypoglycemia
SNS signs
Sweating, tachycardia
Palpitations, shaking
PNS signs
Nausea, hunger
Focal neurologic deficits, mental confusion, coma
Diabetic ketoacidosis
DKA: complication type 1 DM
Hyperglycemia, ketoacidosis
Only type 1DM
Medical illness, omission insulin
Severe volume depletion → shock, coma
Osmotic diuresis
Mechanisms hyperglycemia
↑Gluconeogenesis
↑Glucagon, EPI
Gluconeogenesis: key mechanism for hyperglycemia

3. Osmotic damage
   a. Aldose reductase converts glucose (G) to sorbitol. Sorbitol, like glucose, is osmotically active and draws water into tissue, causing damage.
   b. Role of osmotic damage in DM
      (1) Formation of cataracts (opacifications in the lens of the eye; see Chapter 26)
      (2) Peripheral neuropathy (see Chapter 26)
         (a) Osmotic damage of Schwann cells causes demyelination and sensorimotor peripheral neuropathy (see Chapter 26).
         (b) Peripheral neuropathy leads to neuropathic ulcers on the bottom of the feet (Fig. 23-21 A). Patient cannot feel pain.
      (3) Retinopathy (see Chapter 26): Osmotic damage to pericytes produces microaneurysms of the retinal vessels (Fig. 23-21 B).
4. Diabetic microangiopathy
   a. Increased synthesis of type IV collagen in the basement membranes and mesangium of the renal glomeruli (see Fig. 20-5 J).
   b. Important in diabetic glomerulopathy and development of the nephrotic syndrome (excess urinary loss of albumin; see Chapter 20)
F. **Clinical findings in DM**
   1. Insulin-induced hypoglycemia
      a. MC complication of DM
      b. Produces irreversible brain damage by destroying neurons
      c. Clinical findings in hypoglycemia
         (1) Sympathetic nervous system (SNS) signs: sweating, tachycardia (rapid heart rate), palpitations (feeling of have a rapid, pounding heart), and tremulousness (shaking)
         (2) Parasympathetic nervous system (PNS) signs: nausea and hunger
         (3) Focal neurologic deficits, mental confusion, coma
   2. Diabetic ketoacidosis (DKA; Fig. 23-22)
      a. **Definition:** Life-threatening complication of poorly controlled type 1 DM that is characterized by an increased anion gap type of metabolic acidosis, ketonemia, and severe hyperglycemia
      b. Epidemiology
         (1) Complication of type 1 DM
         (2) Precipitated by medical illness or omission of insulin
         (3) Produces severe volume depletion, causing hypovolemic shock and coma (see Chapter 5). Volume depletion is caused by the loss of sodium and water caused by osmotic diuresis (excess glucose in urine; see Chapter 5).
         (4) Mechanisms for hyperglycemia in DKA
            (a) Increased gluconeogenesis caused by an increase in glucagon and epinephrine (EPI) (counterregulatory hormones that normally oppose insulin); most important mechanism of hyperglycemia in DKA

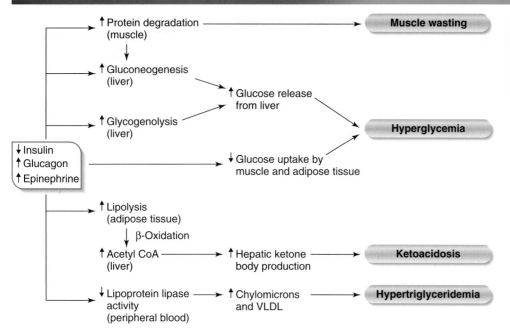

23-22: Metabolic changes in diabetic ketoacidosis (DKA). Refer to the text for discussion. *VLDL,* Very-low-density lipoprotein. *(From Pelley J, Goljan FF:* Rapid Review: Biochemistry, *Philadelphia, Mosby, 2004, p 176, Fig. 9-5.)*

(b) Increased glycogenolysis in the liver is caused by the release of glucagon and EPI and is short-lived as glycogen stores are rapidly depleted.

(c) Decreased uptake of glucose by muscle and adipose tissue (minor role)

(5) Mechanism for ketone bodies in DKA

(a) Increased lipolysis of adipose tissue by increased levels of EPI and cortisol causes the release of fatty acids (FAs) into the blood. Occurs because there is *no* inhibition of hormone-sensitive lipase (HSL, an enzyme that is normally inhibited by insulin to prevent lipolysis of the adipose tissue).

(b) With the increase in fatty acids (FAs) from lipolysis, the FAs undergo β-oxidation, which increases the production of acetyl CoA.

(c) Acetyl CoA is then converted by the liver into ketone bodies, which include acetone (fruity odor to the breath), acetoacetic acid, and β-hydroxybutyric acid (β-OHBA). The latter two ketoacids are responsible for the increased anion gap metabolic acidosis that is called DKA.

(6) Mechanism for hypertriglyceridemia in DKA

(a) Lack of insulin decreases the synthesis of capillary lipoprotein lipase (CLL) in the peripheral blood. Insulin normally increases the synthesis of CLL (see Chapter 10).

(b) Because CLL is decreased, chylomicrons (CMs) and VLDL accumulate in the blood and can no longer be converted into FAs and glycerol. This produces a type V hyperlipoproteinemia (HLP), which is characterized by an increase in both chylomicrons and VLDL (see Chapter 10; Table 10-1). Plasma is turbid (see Fig. 10-3).

(c) Hypertriglyceridemia may precipitate acute pancreatitis and eruptive xanthomas in the skin (see Fig. 10-4 D), called the hyperchylomicronemia syndrome (see Chapter 10; Table 10-1).

c. Laboratory findings in DKA

(1) Hyperglycemia: Glucose ranges from 250 to 1000 mg/dL.

(2) Increased Hb_{A1c} (≥6%)

(3) Dilutional hyponatremia (see Chapter 5)

(a) Glucose overrides sodium in controlling the osmotic gradient.

(b) Water shifts out of the intracellular fluid (ICF) compartment into the ECF compartment and dilutes the serum sodium.

(4) Hyperkalemia (see Chapter 5): In metabolic acidosis, there is a transcellular shift as excess H^+ ions enter cells in exchange for potassium (see Fig. 5-12).

(5) Increased anion gap metabolic acidosis (see Chapter 5) caused by ketoacidosis (KA) and lactic acidosis (LA), the latter caused by decreased tissue perfusion from hypovolemia related to the loss of sodium and glucose in the urine (osmotic diuresis)

(6) Prerenal azotemia (see Chapter 20)

↑Glycogenolysis (liver): glucagon, EPI

↓Uptake G by muscle/ adipose

Ketone bodies in DKA

↑Lipolysis → release FAs in blood

No inhibition HSL

↑β-oxidation FAs → ↑acetyl CoA

Acetyl CoA → acetone, acetoacetic acid, β-OHBA

Ketoacids: acetoacetic acid/β-OHBA

↑TG in DKA

↓Synthesis CLL

↑↑CM, VLDL

Type V HLP; turbid plasma

Acute pancreatitis, eruptive xanthomas

Hyperchylomicronemia syndrome

Hyperglycemia

↑HbA1c (glycosylated Hb)

Dilutional hyponatremia

Water ICF → ECF

Hyperkalemia: transcellular shift H^+ for K^+

↑AG metabolic acidosis

↑KA + LA (hypovolemic shock)

Prerenal azotemia

TABLE 23-13 Diagnostic Categories: Diabetes Mellitus and At-Risk States

FASTING PLASMA GLUCOSE LEVEL	2-HOUR (75-G) OGTT RESULT		
	<140 MG/DL	140–199 MG/DL	≥200 MG/DL
<100 mg/dL	Normal	IGT*	DM
100-125 mg/dL	IFG *	IGT*	DM
≥126 mg/dL	DM	DM	DM
Hb$_{A1c}$ level (%)	<5.7 Normal	5.7–6.4 High risk*	≥6.5 DM

*May be referred to as prediabetes.
DM, Diabetes mellitus; *IFG,* impaired fasting glucose; *IGT,* impaired glucose tolerance, *OGTT,* oral glucose tolerance test.
Modified from Ferri FF: *2017 Ferri's Clinical Advisor,* St. Louis, Elsevier, 2017, p 365, Table 1D-9. Taken from Goldman L, Schafer AI: *Goldman's Cecil Medicine,* 24th ed, Philadelphia, Saunders, 2012.

Prerenal azotemia

Volume depletion from osmotic diuresis

Mortality rate 5% to 10%

Hyperosmolar hyperglycemic state

Complication of type 2 DM

Lab Dx DM

Glycosylated hemoglobin (Hb$_{A1c}$)

Glucose attached to Hb

Marker long-term glycemic control

Mean glucose previous 8-12 wks

Normal Hb$_{A1c}$: <5.7%

Prediabetes: Hb$_{A1c}$ 5.7% to 6.4%

Diabetes: Hb$_{A1c}$ 6.5% or higher

Impaired glucose tolerance

Hyperglycemia nondiagnostic for DM

Prediabetic state; insulin resistance

Risk for type 2 DM

Macrovascular disease, peripheral nephropathy

Dx IGT

FPG 100 mg/dL to 126 mg/dL

2-hr glucose: >140 mg/dL to 199 mg/dL

Gestational diabetes mellitus

Glucose intolerance developed during pregnancy

Anti-insulin effect HPL, cortisol, P

↑Risk GDM future pregnancies

Macrosomia

Hyperglycemia fetus → release insulin

Insulin ↑fetal fat stores in adipose

Insulin↑muscle mass

RDS

Insulin inhibits fetal surfactant production

Risk open neural tube defects

(a) **Definition:** An increase in the serum blood urea nitrogen and serum creatinine caused by renal hypoperfusion secondary to a decrease in cardiac output. The decreased renal perfusion leads to a proportionately greater increase in urea from the kidneys than creatinine, causing the serum BUN to creatinine level to be >15 (see Fig. 20-1 B).

(b) In DKA, the volume depletion is from osmotic diuresis, which decreases the cardiac output and the renal blood flow to the kidneys.

d. Mortality rate in DKA is 5% to 10%.

3. Hyperosmolar hyperglycemic state (HHS; see Table 23-11)

a. **Definition:** Complication of type 2 DM in which there is enough insulin to prevent ketoacidosis but *not* enough to prevent hyperglycemia

b. Epidemiology: increased mortality rate (20%–50%) because patients tend to be older and usually have underlying cardiac and renal problems

G. **Overview of complications of DM** (Links 23-100 and 23-101)

H. **Laboratory diagnosis of DM**

1. Criteria for the diagnosis of DM (Table 23-13)

2. Hemoglobin (Hb)$_{AIC}$

a. **Definition:** Hb to which glucose is attached

b. Epidemiology

(1) Evaluates long-term glycemic control

(2) Represents the mean glucose value for the preceding 8 to 12 weeks. Normal range in a nondiabetic adult is <5.7%.

(3) Prediabetes (IGT) is 5.7% to 6.4%. Increased risk for type 2 DM. DM is 6.5% or higher.

I. **Impaired glucose tolerance (IGT)**

1. **Definition:** A patient who has hyperglycemia that is nondiagnostic for DM

2. Epidemiology

a. Represents a prediabetic state with insulin resistance

b. Approximately 30% develop type 2 DM within 10 years.

c. Increased risk for macrovascular (large vessel) disease and peripheral neuropathy

3. Diagnosis of IGT

a. Fasting plasma glucose (FPG) is 100 to 126 mg/dL.

b. Two-hour glucose is 140 mg/dL to 199 mg/dL after 75-g oral glucose.

J. **Gestational diabetes mellitus (GBS)**

1. **Definition:** Glucose intolerance that develops during pregnancy

2. Epidemiology

a. Caused by the anti-insulin effect of human placental lactogen (HPL), cortisol, and progesterone (P) in pregnancy

b. Increased risk for GDM in future pregnancies

c. Newborn (NB) risks in mothers with GDM

(1) Macrosomia (Fig. 23-23)

(a) Hyperglycemia in the fetus causes release of insulin.

(b) Insulin increases fat stores in the adipose tissue.

(c) Insulin increases muscle mass by increasing amino acid uptake in muscle (growth hormone effect of insulin).

(2) Respiratory distress syndrome (RDS; see Chapter 17, Fig. 17-4). Insulin inhibits the fetal production of surfactant.

(3) Increased risk for developing open neural tube defects

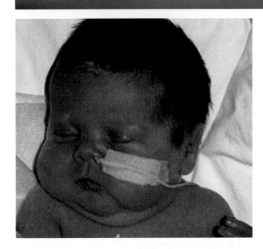

23-23: Hyperglycemia in a fetus causes release of insulin. Insulin increases fat stored in adipose tissue. Insulin increases muscle mass by increasing amino acid uptake in muscle (growth hormone effect of insulin). *(From Taylor S, Raffles A:* Diagnosis in Color Pediatrics, *London, Mosby-Wolfe, 1997, p 36, Fig. 1-71.)*

       (4) Increased risk for developing neonatal hypoglycemia (Link 23-102)

          (a) If the mother is *not* in good glycemic control, the fetus islet cells produce insulin in response to the hyperglycemia.

          (b) High insulin level at birth drives the NBs glucose into the hypoglycemic range, which may cause serious damage, such as neurologic damage resulting in mental impairment, recurrent seizures activity, developmental delay, and personality disorders.

          (c) To reduce the possibility of severe damage to the NB, it is important to give the newborn glucose after birth to prevent the above complications.

          (d) If women with GDM *cannot* control their blood by diet alone, then insulin is recommended to maintain their glucose levels within the normal range.

     d. Women who have had GDM in a previous pregnancy are at risk for developing type 2 DM.

  3. Screening for GDM

     a. Pregnant women are screened between 24 and 28 weeks' gestation.

     b. Criteria vary among different associations.

X. Polyglandular Deficiency Syndromes

  A. Type I polyglandular syndrome

    1. **Definition:** Rare autosomal recessive (AR) disease with immune-cell dysfunction leading to multiple endocrine diseases

    2. Epidemiology

     a. Mean age of onset is 12 years old; *no* HLA relationship

     b. Endocrine disorders associated with the syndrome: Addison disease, primary hypoparathyroidism

     c. Mucocutaneous candidiasis is also commonly present.

  B. Type II polyglandular syndrome

    1. **Definition:** Rare autosomal dominant disease with immune-cell dysfunction (ICD) leading to multiple endocrine diseases

    2. Epidemiology

     a. Mean age of onset is 24 years old; association with HLA-DR3 and HLA-DR4

     b. Endocrine disorders associated with the syndrome: Addison disease, Hashimoto thyroiditis, type 1 DM

XI. Hypoglycemia

  A. Definition

    • Ranges have been anywhere from 40 to 70 mg/dL (normal fasting, 70–110 mg/dL). Reasonable cutoff point is <50 mg/dL.

  B. Fed state hypoglycemia

    1. **Definition:** Hypoglycemia that develops ~1 to 5 hours after eating

    2. Epidemiology

     a. Reactive type of hypoglycemia in that it is associated with food intake

     b. Causes

      (1) Insulin treatment in type 1 DM

       (a) MCC of fed state hypoglycemia

       (b) Sulfonylurea-related hypoglycemia is less common.

      (2) IGT or type 2 DM. An excessive amount of insulin is released for the amount of glucose that is absorbed.

Risk fetal hypoglycemia

↑G mother → ↑G fetus → ↑fetal insulin

↑Fetal insulin at birth → fetal hypoglycemia

Neurologic damage

Give NB glucose at birth

Women with GDM risk type 2 DM

Screening for GDM

Polyglandular deficiency syndromes

Type I polyglandular syndrome

AR disease, multiple endocrine diseases

Mean age 12 yrs old

No HLA association

Addison disease

1° Hypoparathyroidism

Mucocutaneous candidiasis

Type II polyglandular syndrome

Autoimmune disease, ICD, multiple endocrine diseases

Mean age 24 yrs old

HLA-DR3/DR4 association

Addison disease

Hashimoto thyroiditis

Type 1 DM

Hypoglycemia

Fasting glucose <50 mg/dL

Fed state hypoglycemia

Hypoglycemia ~1 to 5 hours after eating

Reactive type associated with food intake

Insulin Rx in type 1 DM MCC

IGT or type 2 DM

More insulin released than required

3. Clinical findings are adrenergic type signs
   a. Sweating, trembling, anxiety, palpitations, tachycardia, mydriasis (dilated pupils caused by contraction of the radial muscle in the iris)
   b. Numbness and tingling, most likely related to anxiety and rapid breathing producing respiratory alkalosis and signs of tetany (see previous discussion)

Idiopathic postprandial syndrome (IPS): This syndrome is characterized by the presence of adrenergic symptoms *without* demonstrable evidence of hypoglycemia. Patients also complain of lack of energy, mental dullness, and inability to concentrate. Symptoms usually disappear if mixed carbohydrate–protein meals are eaten at frequent intervals.

4. Diagnosis: Measure blood glucose when the person is symptomatic.
C. **Fasting type of hypoglycemia**
   1. **Definition:** Hypoglycemia that develops 4 to 6 hours after a meal
   2. Epidemiology; causes (Link 23-103; Whipple triad)
      a. Alcohol (MCC; see Chapter 7)
         (1) Increased nicotinamide adenine dinucleotide (NADH) from alcohol metabolism converts pyruvate to lactate. Less pyruvate is available for gluconeogenesis; therefore, there is less glucose being synthesized during fasting.
         (2) Decreased glycogen stores in hepatocytes in severe liver disease (e.g., cirrhosis) caused by excess alcohol
      b. Renal failure: Kidney is a site for gluconeogenesis; therefore, severe kidney disease interferes with normal functions such as gluconeogenesis.
      c. Malnutrition: extreme muscle wasting from breakdown of muscle protein for energy, leading to less amino acids available for gluconeogenesis
      d. Chronic liver disease: Decreased liver gluconeogenesis and glycogen stores are depleted.
      e. Insulinoma
         (1) Increased insulin leads to increased uptake of glucose (into liver and muscle and adipose cells) from the blood, leading to hypoglycemia.
         (2) Serum insulin and serum C-peptide are both increased (see previous discussion).
      f. Hypopituitarism: Decreased growth hormone (GH) and cortisol decrease gluconeogenesis.
      g. Ketotic hypoglycemia in childhood
         (1) **Definition:** MCC of hypoglycemia in childhood that typically occurs when illness limits food intake
         (2) Epidemiology
            (a) MCC of hypoglycemia from 18 months to mid-childhood
            (b) Children with ketotic hypoglycemia have markedly reduced levels of alanine in the basal state and even lower with prolonged fasting. Recall that alanine is a key amino acid for gluconeogenesis. Alanine aminotransferase (ALT) transaminates alanine to pyruvate, an important substrate for gluconeogenesis in the fasting state.
            (c) Other causes of ketogenic hypoglycemia
               • Inborn errors of metabolism: maple syrup urine disease, galactosemia, hereditary fructose intolerance, and von Gierke glycogen storage disease (see Chapter 6)
               • Carnitine deficiency

Carnitine is required for the synthesis of carnitine acyltransferase (CAT). CAT is the rate-limiting reaction of β-oxidation of fatty acids, which are an important source of energy in the fasting and starvation states for muscle tissue. Any excess of acetyl CoA, the end-product of β-oxidation, is used by the liver to synthesize ketone bodies. Ketone bodies are used for energy by muscle in the fasting state and by the brain in starvation. Therefore, in carnitine deficiency, a decrease in CAT significantly reduces the amount of ketone bodies as a source of energy. This leaves glucose as the only fuel available for all tissues to use for energy, which results in hypoglycemia.

   h. Beckwith-Wiedemann syndrome: characterized by hypoglycemia (hyperinsulinemia from islet cell hyperplasia), macroglossia, omphalocele, gigantism, visceromegaly, and hemihypertrophy (Link 23-104)
   3. Neuroglycopenic symptoms of hypoglycemia predominantly occur in the fasting state.
      a. Dizziness, confusion, headache, inability to concentrate
      b. Motor disturbances, seizures, visual disturbances, and coma
   4. Diagnosis of a fasting state hypoglycemia: supervised 24-hour fast to provoke hypoglycemia

ABBREVIATIONS

MC most common   MCC most common cause

I. Bone Disorders

A. Osteogenesis imperfecta (brittle bone disease)

1. **Definition:** Inherited generalized disorder of connective tissue characterized by defective synthesis of type I collagen
2. Epidemiology
   a. MC type is autosomal dominant (AD) disease
   b. Increase in perinatal death. Families with severe postmenopausal osteoporosis should be evaluated for possible osteogenesis imperfecta.
3. Clinical findings
   a. Pathologic fractures occur at birth with minimal trauma (Link 24-1).
   b. Patients have blue sclera (Fig. 24-1 A). Reflection of the underlying choroidal veins through the thin sclera. Sclera is thin because of the lack of type I collagen.
   c. Presenile deafness occurs in patients in their 20s and 30s.
   d. Other findings: short stature, scoliosis, brittle teeth, short limbs

B. Achondroplasia

1. **Definition:** Hereditary condition associated with impaired proliferation of cartilage at the growth plate; results in very short limbs and sometimes a face that is small in relation to the (normal-sized) skull
2. Epidemiology
   a. AD disease
   b. Mutation in the fibroblast growth factor receptor 3 (*FGFR3*) gene. Gene mutations increase with paternal age.
3. Clinical and laboratory findings (Fig. 24-1 B; Link 24-2)
   a. Macrocephaly, depressed nasal bridge
   b. Shortened arms and legs, redundant skin folds in arms and legs
   c. Normal serum growth hormone (GH) and insulin-like growth factor 1 (IGF-1) levels

C. Osteopetrosis (marble bone disease)

1. **Definition:** Rare inherited disease caused by a failure of the osteoclasts to reabsorb bone; net result is the formation of dense but disorganized bone, resulting in bone fractures
2. Epidemiology
   a. The three distinct clinical forms of the disease are infantile (autosomal recessive [AR]), intermediate (AR), and adult onset (AD).
   b. Adult form has a good prognosis; the other types have a poor prognosis.
   c. Overgrowth and sclerosis of the cortical bone ("too much bone")
3. Clinical findings
   a. Pathologic fractures
   b. Anemia caused by replacement of marrow cavity by bone
   c. Cranial nerve compression causing visual and hearing loss

---

Bone disorders

Osteogenesis imperfecta

Inherited: defective type I collagen

AD MC type
↑Perinatal death
Adult women severe osteoporosis

Pathologic fractures at birth

Blue sclera

Reflection underlying choroidal veins

Sclera lacks type I collagen

Presenile deafness

Short stature, scoliosis, brittle teeth, short limbs

Achondroplasia

Impaired cartilage at growth plate

AD

Mutation *FGFR3* gene

Gene mutations ↑ with paternal age

Macrocephaly, depressed nasal bridge

Short legs, redundant skin folds

Normal GH, IGF-1 levels

Osteopetrosis

Failure osteoclasts to resorb bone; fractures

Three types

Adult good prognosis, other type poor prognosis

Overgrowth/sclerosis cortical bone; "too much bone"

Pathologic fractures

Anemia

Visual/hearing loss

24-1: A, Osteogenesis imperfecta. Note the faint blue tint of the sclera representing the reflection of the underlying choroidal veins. **B,** Child with achondroplasia. The head is a normal size; however, the lower extremities show tibial bowing. *(A from Forbes CD, Jackson WF:* Color Atlas and Text of Clinical Medicine, *3rd ed, St. Louis, Mosby, 2003 p 135, Fig. 3.118. B from Mir MA:* Atlas of Clinical Diagnosis, *London, Saunders, 1995; B from Kliegman R:* Nelson Textbook of Pediatrics, *19th ed, Philadelphia, Elsevier Saunders, 2011, p 2429, Fig. 687-3C.)*

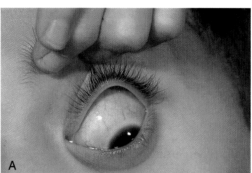
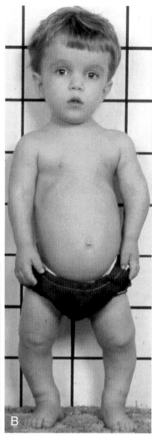

Osteomyelitis

Bacterial bone infection

Acute osteomyelitis

S. aureus MCC acute osteomyelitis

Contiguous, hematogenous, direct implantation

Contiguous source

MCC osteomyelitis

Diabetic foot ulcers

Polymicrobial

Sepsis → hematogenous spread to bone

Metaphysis MC site (hematogenous)

Nutrient artery metaphysis

Tibia/fibula MC sites child

Calcaneus bone foot

Vertebrae common site adults

S. aureus: MC pathogen

Viral infections uncommon

D. Osteomyelitis
1. **Definition:** Acute or chronic infection of bone; most commonly caused by a bacterium and less commonly by fungi and viruses
2. Acute osteomyelitis
   a. *Staphylococcus aureus* is the overall MC pathogen causing acute osteomyelitis (70% to 89%) followed by *Streptococcus* (*Streptococcus pyogenes*, viridans *Streptococcus*, *Streptococcus pneumoniae*).
   b. Sources of infection include contiguous, hematogenous, and direct implantation (trauma or surgery).
   c. Contiguous source
      (1) MCC of osteomyelitis
      (2) Refers to extension of infection into bone from adjacent soft tissue (diabetic foot ulcers, decubitus ulcers), injury, or surgery
      (3) Most of these infections are polymicrobial, with *S. aureus* commonly present as well.
   d. Hematogenous source (bloodstream infection) is a common cause of osteomyelitis in both children and adults; commonly monomicrobial.
      (1) Metaphysis in bone is a common site of infection (Link 24-3 A). Vascular supply is best in the metaphysis (nutrient artery), which favors hematogenous spread of the infection to that area of the bone.
      (2) Tibia and fibula are the MC sites for osteomyelitis in children. These are rapidly growing tubular bones that receive a lot of blood, hence the predisposition to osteomyelitis
      (3) Calcaneus bone in the foot is a nontubular bone that develops osteomyelitis.
      (4) Vertebrae are a common site for osteomyelitis in adults. Pathogens include *Mycobacterium* spp., *S. aureus*, gram-negative bacteria (e.g., *Pseudomonas aeruginosa*, *Serratia* spp.), and *Candida* spp.
      (5) Infection is most often caused by *S. aureus* in adults (90% of cases). Other pathogens include *S. pyogenes*, *Klebsiella kingae* (children <3 years old; 32% of cases), *S. pneumoniae* (children <3 years old; 18%), *P. aeruginosa* (intravenous drug abusers [IVDAs]; second MCC in adults), *Serratia* spp. (IV drug abusers), *Eikenella* (IVDAs),

Enterobacteriaceae (third MCC in adults), *Salmonella paratyphi* (sickle cell disease [SCD]), *Mycobacteria* spp., and fungi.

    (6) Osteomyelitis in SCD (see Chapter 12)

        (a) *S. paratyphi* is the usual causative agent (50%–70% of cases). *S. aureus* is the next MCC.

        (b) Sickling of blood vessels in the spleen results in repeated infarctions, rendering it dysfunctional, small, and fibrotic. Net result is impaired removal of opsonized encapsulated organisms (e.g., *Salmonella* spp.).

    (7) Tuberculous osteomyelitis

        (a) Hematogenous spread of tuberculosis from a primary lung focus.

        (b) Targets vertebral column (Pott disease)

    (8) IVDAs

        (a) Bones involved include the vertebrae and sternoclavicular and pelvic bones.

        (b) Common organisms include *P. aeruginosa* and *Serratia marcescens*. Other pathogens include *S. aureus* and *Eikenella* spp.

  e. Direct implantation

    (1) Direct implantation of *P. aeruginosa* caused by puncture of a foot through rubber footwear produces a localized osteomyelitis.

    (2) Prosthetic joints: microorganisms typically grow in biofilm, which protects bacteria from antimicrobial treatment and the host immune response.

3. Chronic osteomyelitis; epidemiology

  a. Treatment of refractory acute osteomyelitis (osteo) is the most frequent cause.

  b. Approximately 10% to 30% of acute osteomyelitis progresses into chronic osteomyelitis.

  c. In elective trauma surgery, chronic osteomyelitis occurs in 1% to 5% after closed fractures and, depending on severity, 3% to 50% after open fractures.

  d. Neutrophils enzymatically destroy the bone in chronic osteomyelitis (Fig. 24-2).

    (1) Devitalized bone is called sequestra.

    (2) Reactive bone formation occurs in the periosteum (called involucrum).

  e. Draining sinus tracts to the skin surface often occur; increased risk of squamous cell carcinoma (SCC) developing at the orifice of the sinus tracts.

4. Clinical findings of osteomyelitis include abrupt fever, bone pain (usually back in 86% of cases), and swelling. If chronic, a draining sinus tract(s) may also be present.

5. Diagnosis

  a. Increased erythrocyte sedimentation rate (ESR; ~90% of cases) and C-reactive protein (CRP; ~98% of cases; see Chapter 5).

  b. Peripheral white blood cell (WBC) count is increased in 20% of cases.

  c. Bone aspiration and blood for culture: Together, they are diagnostic in 50% to 80% of cases.

  d. Imaging studies: plain radiography (Link 24-3 B, *left*), magnetic resonance imaging (MRI; Link 24-3 B, *right*) is the most accurate (test of choice for vertebral osteomyelitis), technetium bone scan (detects early lesions), gallium scintigraphy with single-photon emission computed tomography (SPECT)

E. Osteoporosis

1. **Definition:** The progressive loss of both organic bone matrix (osteoid) and mineralized bone

---

Margin notes:

Osteomyelitis sickle cell disease

S. paratyphi: MC osteomyelitis

Spleen dysfunctional (infarctions) for bacteria removal

Tuberculous osteomyelitis

Hematogenous spread 1° lung focus

Vertebral column (Pott disease)

IVDA

Vertebrae, sternoclavicular, pelvic

IVDA: *P. aeruginosa, S. marcescens*

Direct implantation

P. aeruginosa: puncture foot through rubber footwear

Prosthetic joints: bacteria grow in biofilm

Chronic osteomyelitis

Rx-refractory acute osteo MCC chronic osteo

Acute → chronic 10% to 30%

Elective trauma surgery closed/open fractures

Sequestra devitalized bone

Involucrum reactive bone formation in periosteum

Draining sinuses: danger SCC at sinus drainage orifice

Bone pain, abrupt fever, erythema, swelling, possible sinus tract (chronic)

Dx osteomyelitis

↑ESR/CRP

↑Peripheral WBC count

Bone aspiration/biopsy culture

MRI most accurate; SPECT

Osteoporosis

Loss organic/mineralized bone

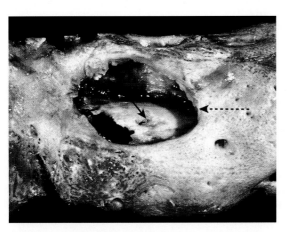

24-2: Chronic osteomyelitis. The *solid arrow* points to necrotic bone in the center of a draining abscess (sequestrum). The *interrupted arrow* is a rim of new bone formation (involucrum). *(From Kumar V, Abbas AK, Fausto N, Mitchell RN: Robbins Basic Pathology, 8th ed, Philadelphia, Saunders Elsevier, 2007, p 810, Fig. 21-7.)*

2. Epidemiology
   a. MC metabolic abnormality of bone
   b. Risk factors
      (1) Family history of osteoporosis; currently smoking cigarettes
      (2) Thin body habitus; current use of corticosteroids (MC secondary cause)
      (3) Sedentary life tyle, premature menopause, heavy alcohol intake
   c. Bone mass peaks at age 30 years and is slightly greater in men than women.
   d. During the fourth and fifth decades of life, both sexes start losing bone.
   e. Loss of both organic bone matrix (osteoid) and mineralized bone produces decreased bone mass and density.
      (1) Decreased thickness of the cortical and trabecular bone (Link 24-4)
      (2) Radiographs of osteoporotic bone show osteopenia (a washed-out appearance).
   f. Osteoporosis is more common in women than men. Men have greater bone mass to begin with; therefore, it takes longer for them to develop osteoporosis.
   g. Primary osteoporosis
      (1) Affects 80% of women and 60% of men
      (2) Subdivided into idiopathic (not discussed), type I (postmenopausal women), and type II (involutional involving men and women)
   h. Secondary osteoporosis
      (1) Accounts for 20% to 40% of osteoporosis in both men and women
      (2) Refers to osteoporosis that exists in other disease processes, inherited disease, or as a result of a medication side effect
3. Type I osteoporosis
   a. **Definition:** Type of osteoporosis typically seen in postmenopausal women caused by a deficiency of estrogen (E); commonly results in vertebral and distal forearm fractures
   b. Role of E in maintaining bone mass
      (1) E normally enhances osteoblastic activity and inhibits osteoclastic activity in bone.
      (2) Effect on bone mass is mediated through the inhibition of cytokines (cks; e.g., interleukin [IL]-1, IL-6, tumor necrosis factor [TNF]) that modulate osteoclastogenesis (osteoclast differentiation, activation, life span, and function).
   c. In E deficiency, there is an increase in secretion of the previously mentioned cks by monocytes and cells in the bone marrow.
      (1) These cks have the following *normal* effects.
         (a) Enhance expression of *RANKL* (receptor activator of nuclear factor κB ligand) and RANK genes (receptor activator of nuclear factor κB), which increase osteoclastogenesis (increase in recruitment and activity of osteoclasts)
         (b) Inhibit the expression of osteoprotegerin (OPG), a receptor produced by osteoblasts that inhibits *RANKL/RANK* interaction
      (2) In postmenopausal osteoporosis, osteoclastic activity is greater than osteoblastic activity, so there is a loss of bone mass.
   d. Clinical findings (Link 24-5)
      (1) Compression fractures of the vertebral bodies (Fig. 24-3 A, C)
         (a) MC fracture in postmenopausal osteoporosis
         (b) Patients lose stature (height).
      (2) Dowager's hump (Fig. 24-3 B, C)
         (a) Kyphosis (forward bending of the spine) is caused by advanced osteoporosis.
         (b) Interferes with respiration, if severe
      (3) Increased risk for Colles fracture of the distal radius
   e. Diagnosis of osteoporosis
      (1) Dual-energy x-ray absorptiometry (DEXA) is a noninvasive test that evaluates bone marrow density (BMD).
      (2) World Health Organization uses a T-score to define osteoporosis (Link 24-6).
         (a) Calculated by subtracting the mean BMD (in g/cm^2) of a young adult reference population from the patient's BMD and dividing this by the standard deviation (SD) of the young adult reference population.
         (b) Using the T-score, osteoporosis is defined as −2.5 SD and below.
4. Type II osteoporosis
   a. **Definition:** Senile type of osteoporosis that is caused by defective differentiation of bone marrow stromal cells into adipocytes rather than osteoblasts. This type of osteoporosis is especially associated with fractures of the wrist, proximal humerus, vertebrae, pelvis, femoral neck, and tibia.

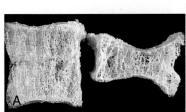 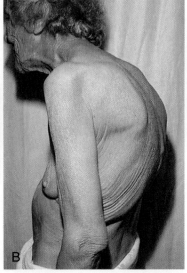 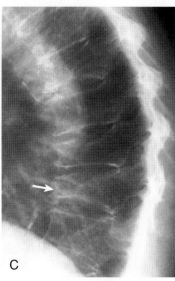

24-3: **A,** Osteoporosis of the vertebral column. The vertebral body on the right shows decreased bone mass caused by compression fractures compared with a normal vertebral body on the left. **B,** Older woman with osteoporosis showing the classic dowager's hump. **C,** Radiograph of the spine showing radiolucency (loss of bone mass), compression fractures *(white arrow),* and kyphosis of the spine in a patient with osteoporosis. *(A from Kumar V, Fausto N, Abbas A: Robbins and Cotran Pathologic Basis of Disease, 7th ed, Philadelphia, Saunders, 2004, p 1284, Fig. 26-12; B from Seidel HM, Ball JW, Danis JE, Benedict GW: Mosby's Guide to Physical Examination, 6th ed, St. Louis, Mosby Elsevier, 2006, p 756, Fig. 21-78. C, From Ashar BH, Miller RG, Sisso SD: The Johns Hopkins Internal Medicine Board Review, 4th ed, Elsevier, 2012, p 316, Fig. 39-6. Taken from Goldman L, Bennett JC, Ausiello D: Cecil Medicine, 22nd ed, Philadelphia, Elsevier Saunders, 2004, Fig. 258.4).*

   b. Epidemiology
     (1) Occurs in women and men who are >70 years old
     (2) Progressive decline in osteoblasts and increased activity of osteoclasts (bone resorption exceeds bone formation). Decreased physical activity puts less stress on bone, resulting in decreased bone formation (decreased osteoblastic activity).
     (3) In addition, there is decreased production of $1,25(OH)_2D_3$, the active form of vitamin D that is derived from the kidneys. Results in decreased calcium absorption and increased secretion of parathyroid hormone (PTH; increases bone resorption).
     (4) Fractures commonly occur in the wrist, hip, and vertebrae.
  5. Secondary osteoporosis
    a. **Definition:** Osteoporosis that is caused by medical conditions or treatments that interfere with the formation of the organic bone matrix (osteoid) or mineralized bone
    b. Epidemiology and causes
     (1) Underlying disease: endocrine (hypercortisolism), bone marrow (multiple myeloma, leukemia), connective tissue (Ehlers-Danlos syndrome, Marfan syndrome), or gastrointestinal (GI; malabsorption syndromes)
     (2) Drugs (e.g., prolonged heparin use, corticosteroids, cyclosporine)
     (3) Hypogonadism (e.g., in hypopituitarism, there is a decrease in GH and IGF-1; decrease in E in women and testosterone in men)
     (4) Malnutrition (e.g., anorexia nervosa is associated with hypoestrinism)
     (5) Space travel (lack of gravity reduces bone stress)
F. Avascular necrosis (AVN)
  1. **Definition:** Cellular death of bone components caused by interruption of the blood supply
  2. Epidemiology
    a. Sites
     (1) Femoral head and condyle (MC site; Legg-Calvé-Perthes [LCP] disease)
     (2) Capitellum of distal humerus (Panner disease)
     (3) Scaphoid (navicular) and lunate bones (Burns disease) in the wrist
     (4) Tarsal navicular bone in the foot (Kohler disease)
    b. Causes
     (1) Corticosteroids (35% of cases): produce the death of osteocytes, especially in association with excessive alcohol ingestion
     (2) Alcohol (22% of cases)

Margin notes:
Women/men >70 yrs old

Decline osteoblasts, ↑osteoclast activity

↓Activity → less stress on bones

↓Production $1,25(OH)_2D_3$

↓Ca absorption, ↑PTH: ↑bone resorption

Fractures wrist, hips, vertebrae

Secondary osteoporosis

Medical conditions

Interference with osteoid and/or mineralized bone formation

Underlying disease: e.g., hypercortisolism

Heparin, corticosteroids, cyclosporine

Hypogonadism

Malnutrition

Space travel (lack of gravity)

Avascular necrosis

Cellular death bone components

Femoral head MC site

Distal humerus

Scaphoid (navicular)/lunate bones

Tarsal navicular bone foot

Corticosteroids MCC

Death osteocytes

Alcohol

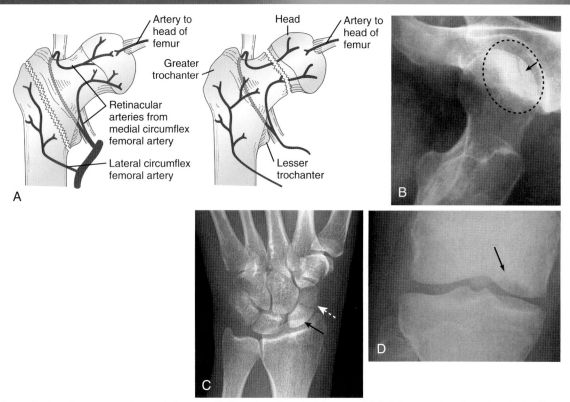

24-4: A, Schematic showing a pertrochanteric fracture *(left)* and a subcapital fracture *(right)*. See text for discussion. **B,** Radiograph showing avascular necrosis (AVN) of the femoral head from a subcapital fracture. The *interrupted circle* highlights an area of increased bone density, within which is a fracture site *(arrow)*. **C,** AVN of the scaphoid bone in the wrist. The *interrupted white arrow* shows the area of fracture, and the *black arrow* shows sclerotic bone, representing reactive bone formation. **D,** Osteochondritis dissecans. The *arrow* indicates a subcortical radiolucency in the knee of an adolescent female patient with chronic medial knee pain. *(A from Moore NA, Roy WA: Rapid Review Gross and Developmental Anatomy, 2nd ed, Philadelphia, Mosby Elsevier, 2007, p 147, Fig. 5-4; B from Rosai J, Ackerman LV: Surgical Pathology, 9th ed, St. Louis, Mosby, 2004, p 2144, Fig. 24-8A; C from Herring W: Learning Radiology Recognizing the Basics, 2nd ed, Philadelphia, Elsevier Saunders, 2012, p 244, Fig. 22-26; D from Marx J: Rosen's Emergency Medicine Concepts and Clinical Practice, 7th ed, Philadelphia, Mosby Elsevier, 2010, p 657, Fig. 54.8.)*

Idiopathic	(3) Other causes (43% of cases)
Fractures	(a) Idiopathic, fractures
Altered lipid metabolism: femoral head	(b) Altered lipid metabolism. Lipids enter the femoral head, causing ischemia.
Femoral head aseptic necrosis	c. Femoral head aseptic necrosis (Link 24-7)
	(1) About 20% to 50% of AVN is bilateral.
20% to 50% bilateral	(2) Common site for fracture older adults, often in association with falling
Elderly who fall	(a) Peritrochanteric fracture is extracapsular and does *not* compromise the
Peritrochanteric fracture no AVN	blood supply to the femoral head; therefore, no aseptic necrosis occurs
	(Fig. 24-4 A left).
	(b) A subcapsular fracture disrupts the blood supply (retinacular arteries from medial
AVN subcapsular fracture disrupts retinacular arteries	circumflex femoral artery); therefore, aseptic necrosis occurs (see Figs. 24-4 A, *right* and 24-4 B).
SCD AVN femoral head	(3) In SCD, sickle cells occlude blood vessels in the femoral head (vasoocclusive disease; see Chapter 12).
Corticosteroids long-term	(4) Long-term use of corticosteroids (see earlier)
AVN scaphoid bone	d. Scaphoid bone aseptic necrosis (Fig. 24-4 C)
Thumb side of wrist	(1) Located on the thumb side of the wrist
	(2) MC bone in the wrist that is fractured. Bone is perfused from distal to proximal, so a
MC wrist bone fractured; poor blood supply	fracture can lead to disruption of perfusion to the proximal aspect of the scaphoid bone.
	e. Digits in SCD: Dactylitis (painful swelling in the hands) occurs in sickle cell anemia caused by vascular occlusion and subsequent infarction of the metacarpal bones (see Fig.
Dactylitis metacarpal bones	12-24 B; see Chapter 12).
Imaging studies	3. Imaging studies for aseptic necrosis
MRI most sensitive early test	a. MRI: most sensitive test (sensitivity, 75%–100%) for early detection of aseptic (avascular) necrosis; classic "double line" sign

b. Computed tomography (CT) scan: shows central necrosis and areas of collapse *before* it is visible with a standard radiography

c. Bone scan (Tc^{99}m-methylene diphosphonate)

(1) Early signs show *no* uptake (cold area; sensitivity, 70%).

(2) Late signs show increased uptake caused by bone remodeling.

d. X-ray study

(1) Most insensitive test in the early phases

(2) In later phases, radiographs show radiolucency (resorption of dead bone) with a sclerotic (increased density) border caused by reactive bone formation.

4. Osteochondrosis

a. **Definition:** AVN of ossification centers (epiphyses) in children with subsequent fragmentation and repair

b. Legg-Calvé-Perthes (LCP) disease

(1) **Definition:** AVN involving the femoral head ossification center (Link 24-8)

(2) Epidemiology

(a) Occurs most often in boys 4 to 8 years of age; male:female ratio is 4:1

(b) Presents with pain in the knee (referred pain) or a painful limp

(c) Delayed bone age; more common in whites and Asians; rare in blacks

(d) Secondary osteoarthritis (OA) is common.

G. Osteochondritis dissecans

1. **Definition:** Variant of osteochondrosis that is limited to the articular epiphysis characterized by separation between a portion of articular cartilage and underlying subchondral bone from the surrounding tissue (Fig. 24-4 D)

2. Epidemiology

a. Causes

(1) Trauma is the primary insult. Ischemia is a secondary injury.

(2) Portion of articular cartilage and underlying subchondral bone becomes detached.

b. Occurs between 9 and 18 years of age; four times more common in males than females

c. Knee is the MC joint involved.

(1) Lateral portion of the medial femoral condyle is the most frequent site (85% of cases).

(2) Piece of cartilage along with a thin layer of bone becomes detached.

3. Clinical findings

a. Localized pain in the knee; morning stiffness

b. Locking of the knee joint by a loose body

c. Tenderness at the site of lesion in the knee; limp with stiffness

d. Osteoarthritis (OA) is a common complication (see the following).

4. Diagnosis of osteochondritis dissecans

• Anteroposterior, lateral, and tunnel view radiographs. MRI is the gold standard test.

H. Osgood-Schlatter disease (OSD)

1. **Definition:** A developmental condition of adolescence characterized by painful swelling of the tibial tuberosity caused by inflammation of the patellar tendon at its insertion site (apophysitis)

2. Epidemiology

a. Occurs in physically active boys (ages 11–15 years) and girls (ages 8–13 years); male:female ratio is 3:1

b. Prevalence is estimated to be ~20% of adolescent athletes and 4.5% in nonatheletes; particularly associated with sports involving repetitive quadriceps contraction (e.g., football, track).

c. *No* adverse effect on bone growth

3. Clinical findings

a. Pain is aggravated by squatting, climbing stairs, or extending the knee with resistance.

b. Thick patellar ligament and tenderness of the tibial tubercle (Link 24-9)

c. Bilateral symptoms are present in 30% of patients.

d. End result is permanent knobby-appearing knees as a result of callous formation.

I. Paget disease (osteitis deformans)

1. **Definition:** Focal disorder of chaotic bone remodeling (both formation and resorption) that results in thick, weak bone at risk for pathologic fractures

2. Epidemiology

a. Primarily occurs in men >50 years of age. Family history positive in 40% of cases.

b. Sites of involvement in descending order: pelvis, lumbar spine, sacrum or femur, skull, tibia, humerus, scapula; uncommon in hand, foot, and fibula

---

CT scan shows AVN before radiograph

Bone scan

No uptake early

Uptake later

X-ray

Insensitive early phase

Radiolucency later phase

Osteochondrosis

AVN of ossification centers children

Legg-Calvé-Perthes

AVN femoral head ossification center

Boys 4 to 8 years

Knee pain (referred)/painful limp

Delayed bone age

Whites, Asians; rare in blacks

2° arthritis common

Osteochondritis dissecans

Osteochondrosis limited to articular epiphysis

Trauma primary insult

Ischemia secondary injury

Portion articular cartilage + subchondral bone separates

Ages 9 to 18

Males > females

Knee MC joint

Lateral portion medial femoral condyle MC site

Piece cartilage + thin layer bone detached

Clinical findings

Localized pain in knee; morning stiffness

Locking of knee joint by loose body

Tenderness at site of lesion

Limp with stiffness

OA late complication

Diagnosis

Radiographs of knee

MRI gold standard

Osgood-Schlatter disease

Painful swelling tibial tuberosity

Inflammation patellar tendon

Active boys/girls

Adolescent athletes > nonathletes

Repetitive quadriceps contraction (football, track)

No adverse effect on bone growth

Pain squatting

Pain climbing stairs

Pain extending knee with resistance

Thick patellar ligament; tender tibial tubercle

Bilateral symptoms 30%

Permanent knobby-appearing knees

Paget disease

Chaotic bone remodeling

Pathologic fractures

Men >50 years of age

Family history some cases

Pelvis, lumbar spine, skull

Uncommon hand, foot, fibula

Paramyxovirus infection osteoclasts

Early phase osteoclastic resorption

Late phase osteoblastic bone formation

↑↑Serum ALP

Thick/weak bone (mosaic pattern)

Clinical findings

Bone pain MC

Headaches/hearing loss

↑Hat size

Pathologic bone fractures

Pain/swelling overlying bone

Risk osteosarcoma

Risk of high-output heart failure

AV connections in bone

Bx: woven bone, weak bone

Haphazard deposition osteoid

Bone scan shows "hot spots"; best test

Radiographs show thickened bone, radiolucencies

↑↑Serum ALP, normal calcium/phosphorus

Fibrous dysplasia

Replacement medullary bone with fibrous tissue

Defect in osteoblast differentiation/maturation

Monostotic, polyostotic

No sex predilection

10 to 30 yrs of ag

Medullary bone replaced by fibrous tissue with cyst formation

c. Pathogenesis
  (1) Possible association with paramyxovirus infection of osteoclasts; possible genetic factors
  (2) Early phase of osteoclastic resorption of bone; produces shaggy-appearing lytic lesions in the bone
  (3) Late phase of increased osteoblastic bone formation
    (a) Produces a markedly increased level of serum alkaline phosphatase (ALP)
    (b) Produces thick, weak bone in a mosaic pattern (Link 24-10 A)
3. Clinical findings in Paget disease
  a. Bone pain is the MC complaint.
  b. Headaches and hearing loss occur if the skull is affected.
  c. Hat size is increased with skull involvement. As an integration point, recall that acromegaly caused by GH excess also increases hat size.
  d. Clinical findings and complications
    (1) Pathologic bone fractures
    (2) Pain and swelling overlying the bone
    (3) Increased risk for developing osteosarcoma or fibrosarcoma, malignancies of bone (<1%)
    (4) Increased risk for developing high-output heart failure (see Chapter 11); caused by numerous arteriovenous (AV) connections in the vascular bone
4. Diagnosis of Paget disease
  a. Bone biopsy shows woven bone (weak bone; "mosaic bone") with haphazard deposition of osteoid. Osteoclasts are also present, causing bone resorption (Link 24-10 A).
  b. Bone scans show "hot spots" (Fig. 24-5 B; Link 24-10 B); best test for showing the extent of Paget disease in the skeleton.
  c. Radiographs show thickened bone with shaggy areas of radiolucency (Fig. 24-5 A; Links 24-10 C and 24-10 D).
  d. Serum ALP is markedly increased; however, serum calcium and phosphorus are normal.
5. Overview of clinical findings in Paget disease (Link 24-11)

J. Fibrous dysplasia
1. **Definition:** Defect in bone-forming cells causing medullary bone to be replaced by fibrous tissue
2. Epidemiology
  a. Skeletal developmental anomaly with a defect in osteoblast differentiation and maturation
  b. May involve a single bone (monostotic; 70%–80% of cases) or multiple bones (polyostotic; McCune-Albright syndrome; see later)
  c. *No* sex predilection; occurs between 10 and 30 years of age
  d. Cysts may develop in the fibrous tissue matrix (Link 24-12).

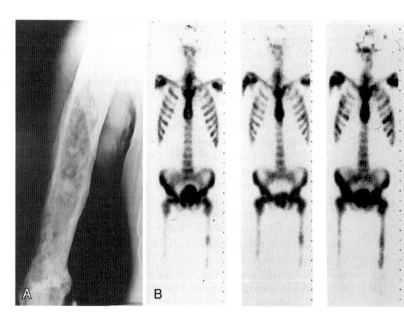

24-5: **A,** Radiograph of the humerus in Paget disease. Note the cortical thickening of the bone and the ragged appearing lytic areas throughout the bone matrix. **B,** Bone scan showing "hot spots" in Paget disease. (***A** from Katz D, Math K, Groskin S:* Radiology Secrets, *Philadelphia, Hanley & Belfus, 1998, p 311, Fig. 1;* ***B** from Bouloux P:* Self-Assessment Picture Tests Medicine, *Vol. 4, London, Mosby-Wolfe, 1997, p 82, Fig. 163.)*

e. MC locations for fibrous dysplasia
   (1) Ribs (28% of cases), femur (24% of cases)
   (2) Tibia or fibula (Link 24-12) or craniofacial bones (10%–25% of cases)
       (a) In the craniofacial bone, it produces cherubism.
       (b) Cherubism refers to bilateral swelling at the angle of the mandible, sometimes involving the entire jaw, imparting a cherubic look to the face, similar to the cherubs in Renaissance paintings.
   (3) Other bones that may be involved include the humerus and vertebrae.
f. McCune Albright syndrome.
   (1) **Definition:** Syndrome characterized by polyostotic fibrous dysplasia and other clinical signs
   (2) Clinical findings
       (a) Patches of pigmented skin called "café-au-lait" spots (ovoid, flat, coffee-colored lesions)
       (b) Precocious puberty
       (c) Hyperthyroidism, excess GH (gigantism [child] or acromegaly [adult]), hypercortisolism (Cushing syndrome), and other uncommon conditions

K. Neoplastic disorders of bone; epidemiology
1. Metastasis is the MC malignancy of bone (see Fig. 9-7 E, F, G). Breast cancer is the MC primary tumor that metastasizes to bone.
2. Primary malignant tumors of bone, in descending order of frequency
   • Multiple myeloma (see Chapter 14), osteosarcoma, chondrosarcoma, and Ewing sarcoma
3. Summary of bone tumors is found in Table 24-1; MC sites for bone tumors (Link 24-13).

II. Joint Disorders
A. Synovial fluid analysis
1. Routine studies performed on synovial fluid include WBC count and differential, crystal analysis, culture, and Gram stain.
2. Crystal identification
   a. Monosodium urate (MSU)
      (1) **Definition:** Needle-shaped (monoclinic) crystal
      (2) Special polarization of the crystals shows negative birefringence.
          • **Definition:** A crystal that is yellow when parallel to the slow ray of the compensator (Fig. 24-6 A)
   b. Calcium pyrophosphate
      (1) **Definition:** Monoclinic-like or triclinic (rhomboid) crystal
      (2) Special polarization of the crystals shows positive birefringence (Fig. 24-6 B).
          • **Definition:** A crystal that is blue when parallel to the slow ray of the compensator

B. Classification of joint disorders
1. Group I
   a. Noninflammatory joint disease
   b. Examples: OA, neuropathic joint
2. Group II
   a. Inflammatory joint disease
   b. Examples: rheumatoid arthritis (RA), gout
3. Group III
   a. Septic joint disease
   b. Examples: Lyme disease (LD), disseminated gonococcemia (GC)
4. Group IV
   a. Hemorrhagic joint disease
   b. Examples: trauma, hemophilia A and B (see Chapter 15)

C. Signs and symptoms of joint disease
1. *Arthralgia* is a general term for joint pain.
2. Arthritis connotes inflammation of the joint associated with pain, swelling, tenderness, and warmth.
3. Morning stiffness
   a. **Definition:** Pain or stiffness in the joints that lasts >30 minutes
   b. Examples: RA, systemic lupus erythematosus (SLE), polymyalgia rheumatica
4. Abnormal joint mobility
   a. Caused by damage to ligaments and the joint capsule
   b. Example: a tear of the anterior cruciate ligament (ACL) in the joint

TABLE 24-1   Tumors of Bone

TUMOR TYPE	EPIDEMIOLOGY	PRIMARY LOCATION	CHARACTERISTICS
BENIGN			
Osteochondroma (Link 24-14)	• Males, 10–30 yr • Solitary or multiple • May be pedunculated	Metaphysis of distal femur (70%) and tibia	• Outgrowth of bone (exostosis) capped by benign cartilage • Bone marrow of the lesion is often in continuity with the bone marrow of the femur or tibia • Most common benign tumor of bone; rarely symptomatic
Enchondroma (Link 24-15)	• Equal distribution in males and females 20–50 yr of age • Solitary or multiple • Most common nonaggressive lesions of the hands • Maffucci syndrome: a rare congenital disorder of mesodermal dysplasia characterized by enchondromatosis and soft tissue hemangiomas (benign vascular tumors); malignant transformation to a chondrosarcoma is common	• Medullary location in the diaphysis • Located in small tubular bones in the hands and feet	• Multiple enchondromas (Ollier disease) are at risk for chondrosarcoma • Malignant transformation occurs in 1% of solitary enchondromas
Nonossifying fibroma (fibrous cortical defect) (Link 24-16)	Common finding in children and adolescents (30%–40%)	• Distal radius • Cortical and metaphyseal based	With skeletal maturation, these lesions typically fill in with bone
Unicameral (simple) bone cyst (Link 24-17)	<20 yrs of age	Long tubular bones, especially the proximal ends of the humerus and femur (90% of cases)	• Usually asymptomatic unless traumatized • Pathologic fracture can lead to in-filling of the lesion with healing of bone
Aneurysmal bone cyst (Link 24-18)	• Second decade of life (50%–70%) • Posttraumatic or reactive response to a preexisting bony lesions, possibly related to hemodynamic alterations (e.g., venous obstruction and arteriovenous fistulas) • Slightly increased incidence in females	• Expansile cystic lesion • May occur in any bone in the body • ~60%–70% arise in long tubular bones, usually originating from the metaphysis; also may arise from posterior elements of the vertebrae	• May affect any bone • Benign but locally aggressive and may weaken bone, leading to pathologic fractures • Recurrence is common after intralesional curettage • "Soap bubble" appearance • Blood-filled spaces in the lesion; ?vascular malformation • May accompany other bone lesions (e.g., fibrous dysplasia, osteosarcoma, chondrosarcoma)
Osteoma	• Male-to-female ratio, 2:1 • 40–50 yr	Skull and facial bones	Associated with Gardner polyposis syndrome (see Chapter 18)
Osteoid osteoma (Link 24-19)	• Male-to-female ratio, 2:1 • 10–30 yr	• Cortex of metaphysis • Proximal femur, tibia, humerus, hands and feet, vertebrae, fibula	• Radiographic finding: radiolucent focus surrounded by sclerotic bone • Nocturnal pain relieved by aspirin
Osteoblastoma (Link 24-20)	• Male-to-female ratio, 2:1 • 10–30 yr	• Medulla of metaphysis • Vertebrae, tibia, femur, humerus, pelvis, ribs	• Similar to osteoid osteoma • Sometimes called a giant osteoid osteoma
Giant cell tumor (Link 24-21)	• Male-to-female ratio, 5:4 • Females 20–40 yr	Epiphysis and metaphysis of distal femur or proximal tibia, radius	• Reactive multinucleated giant cells resemble osteoclasts • Neoplastic mononuclear cells
MALIGNANT			
Chondrosarcoma (Link 24-22)	• Male-to-female ratio, 3:1 • 30–60 yr	Pelvis, ribs, proximal femur, humerus, vertebrae	• Grade determines biological behavior • Metastasizes to lungs
Osteosarcoma (see Fig. 9-1 H; Links 24-23, 24-24, and 24-25)	• Males 10–25 yr • Risk factors: Paget disease, familial retinoblastoma, irradiation, fibrous dysplasia	• Metaphysis of distal femur, proximal tibia • Most common primary bone cancer (some authors say multiple myeloma)	• Malignant osteoid. • Radiographic findings: "sunburst" appearance (spiculated pattern from calcified malignant osteoid) • "Codman triangle" (tumor lifting the periosteum) • Metastasizes to lungs
Ewing sarcoma (Links 24-26 and 24-27)	Males, 10–20 yr	Pelvic girdle, diaphysis and metaphysis of proximal femur or rib	• Small, round cell tumor • Radiographic finding: "onion skin" appearance around bone (periosteal reaction) • Possible fever and anemia

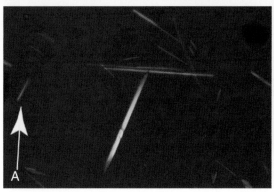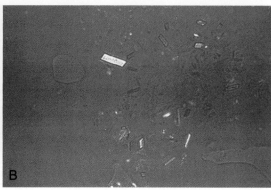

24-6: A, Synovial fluid with special polarization. Special red filter causes the background to be red. Crystals are aligned parallel to the slow ray (axis) of the compensator *(arrow)*. If the crystal is yellow when parallel to the slow ray, as in this figure, the crystal demonstrates negative birefringence indicating gout. If the crystal is blue when parallel to the slow ray, the crystal demonstrates positive birefringence. **B,** Calcium pyrophosphate crystal from a patient with pseudogout. Compensated polarized light normally shows positive birefringence in polarized light when it is parallel to the slow ray of analyzer. It is not evident in this photograph. *(A, From Henry JB: Clinical Diagnosis and Management by Laboratory Methods, 20th ed, Philadelphia, Saunders, 2001, Plate 19-7. B, from McPherson RA, Pincus MR: Henry's Clinical Diagnosis and Management by Laboratory Methods, 23rd ed, 2017, p 496, Fig. 29.14. Taken from Kjeldsberg CR, Knight JA: Body Fluids: Laboratory Examination of Amniotic, Cerebrospinal, Seminal, Serous, and Synovial Fluids, ed. 3, Chicago: © American Society for Clinical Pathology, 1993.)*

5. Swelling of the joint (effusion)
   - Caused by increased joint fluid. Examples: exudate (protein- and neutrophil-rich fluid), blood
6. Redness (rubor) and warmth (calor; "hot joint") of the joint
   - Signs of acute inflammation (see Chapter 3). Examples: septic arthritis, RA
7. Joint crepitus with motion; refers to a crackling feeling when moving a joint. Example: OA

D. Osteoarthritis (OA)
   1. **Definition:** Progressive degeneration of articular cartilage that mainly targets weight-bearing joints or joints that are used very frequently (e.g., joints in the hands and feet)
   2. Epidemiology
      a. Noninflammatory joint disease; *no* sex predilection
      b. Almost universally present in those older than 65 years of age
      c. Risk factors
         (1) Advanced age
         (2) LCP disease (see F.4.b)
         (3) Endocrine or metabolic conditions (acromegaly, chondrocalcinosis, hemochromatosis, alkaptonuria [see later])
         (4) Osteochondritis dissecans (I.G.)
         (5) Obesity, trauma, neuropathic joint, meniscus injuries

> **Ochronosis (alkaptonuria)** is an autosomal recessive disease caused by deficiency of homogentisic acid oxidase and subsequent accumulation of homogentisic acid (urine turns black when oxidized; Fig. 6-5). Homogentisic acid deposits in the intervertebral disks, causing osteoarthritis and other systemic findings.

      d. Common sites
         (1) Femoral head, knee
         (2) Cervical and lumbar vertebrae
         (3) Hands (usually genetic)
      e. Less common sites.
         (1) Shoulder, elbow
         (2) Feet with the *exception* of the first metatarsophalangeal (MTP) joint
            - MTP joint is the site for bunion formation.
   3. Pathogenesis
      a. Components of normal articular cartilage
         (1) Proteoglycans (provide elasticity)
         (2) Type II collagen (provides tensile strength)
      b. In OA, cks activate metalloproteinases that degrade proteoglycans and collagen.
      c. Joint findings (Fig. 24-7 A–C; Link 24-28)

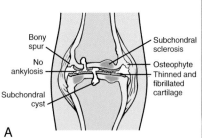 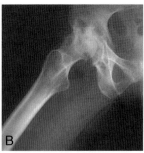 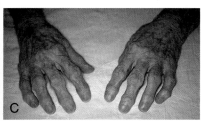

24-7: **A,** Schematic of osteoarthritis (OA) in a joint. The *blue color* represents articular cartilage. Note that the cartilage is thin and disrupted, causing narrowing of the joint space. Subchondral cysts are noted, which would appear as lucencies in a radiograph. Reactive bone formation (osteophytes) is present at the margins of the joint. The osteophytes project into the synovial tissue. **B,** Erosion of the femoral head and acetabular surfaces. Note that the joint space is narrow. Radiolucent subchondral cysts are present as well as dense sclerotic bone. **C,** OA of the hands. Both the distal interphalangeal (DIP) and proximal interphalangeal (PIP) joints in both hands show protuberances along their lateral margins representing osteophyte formation in the joints. The DIP protuberances are called Heberden nodes, and the PIP protuberances are called Bouchard nodes. *(A from Kumar V, Abbas AK, Fausto N, Mitchell RN: Robbins Basic Pathology, 8th ed, Philadelphia, Saunders Elsevier, 2007, p 820, Fig. 7-18 on the right; B from Marx J: Rosen's Emergency Medicine Concepts and Clinical Practice, 7th ed, Philadelphia, Mosby Elsevier, 2010, p 622, Fig. 53.5; C from Swartz MH: Textbook of Physical Diagnosis, 5th ed, Philadelphia, Saunders Elsevier, 2006, p 636, Fig. 20-59.)*

Erosion/clefts articular cartilage	(1) Erosion and clefts in articular cartilage
Osteophytes joint margins	(2) Reactive bone formation at the joint margins (osteophytes; Links 24-28 and 24-29)
Reactive bone formation	(a) Reactive bone formation refers to bone that is produced as a reaction to injury
Responsible for ↑serum ALP older adults	(b) Reactive bone contains bone and a cartilage matrix

Left margin keywords:

Erosion/clefts articular cartilage
Osteophytes joint margins
Reactive bone formation
Responsible for ↑serum ALP older adults
Subchondral cysts
Subchondral cysts
Sclerotic bone
No joint fusion
Joint mice: fragments articular cartilage
Clinical findings
Pain MC complaint
Irritate synovial lining
Bone on bone
Hip OA refers pain to groin
Pain with movement
2° Synovitis from ops
Joint stiffness after inactivity
Waking in AM
After sitting
Crepitus with movement; ↓ROM
Heberden nodes; enlarged DIP joint
Bouchard nodes; enlarged PIP joint
Vertebrae: DDD, neuropathy, muscle atrophy
DISH
OA variant: axial, peripheral skeletal manifestations
Radiograph findings
Calcification/ossification connecting vertebrae
IVD space preserved
No sacroiliac joint involvement
Dx osteoarthritis
Plain radiograph
MRI: synovial tissue abnormalities/effusion
ESR/CRP normal
Synovial fluid noninflammatory
Neuropathic joint
Noninflammatory; 2° neurologic disease
Loss proprioception, deep pain → recurrent trauma

    (1) Erosion and clefts in articular cartilage
    (2) Reactive bone formation at the joint margins (osteophytes; Links 24-28 and 24-29)
        (a) Reactive bone formation refers to bone that is produced as a reaction to injury
        (b) Reactive bone contains bone and a cartilage matrix
        (c) Osteophytes are responsible for the slight increase in serum ALP that is present in older adults.
    (3) Subchondral cysts (Links 24-28, 24-29, and 24-30). Degradative enzymes of the cartilage leaves the underlying bone exposed, allowing synovial fluid to be forced by the pressure of weight into the bone.
    (4) Bone eventually rubs on bone, producing dense, sclerotic bone (Link 24-30).
    (5) No ankylosis (fusion) of the joint
    (6) Joint mice: fragments of articular cartilage that break free into the joint space
4. Clinical findings
   a. Pain is the MC complaint.
    (1) Osteophytes irritate the synovial lining.
    (2) Bone rubs on bone.
    (3) Hip OA may refer pain to the groin.
    (4) Pain is aggravated with movement of the joint. Pain is caused by a secondary synovitis from osteophytes (ops).
   b. Joint stiffness occurs after inactivity, waking up in the morning, and after sitting.
   c. Crepitus of the joint with movement (crackling sound) and decreased range of motion (ROM)
   d. Hand involvement in OA (Fig. 24-7 C; Links 24-31, 24-32, and 24-33 B)
    (1) Enlargement of the distal interphalangeal (DIP) joints caused by osteophytes
    (2) Osteophytes are called Heberden nodes. Enlargement of the proximal interphalangeal (PIP) joints caused by osteophytes. Osteophytes are called Bouchard nodes.
   e. Vertebral findings in OA include degenerative disc disease (DDD) and compressive neuropathies causing pain, paresthesias (burning sensation), and atrophy of muscle.
5. Diffuse idiopathic skeletal hyperostosis (DISH)
   a. **Definition:** Variant of OA with vertebral (axial) and peripheral skeletal manifestations
   b. Radiographic finding (Link 24-33 A)
    (1) Calcification or ossification connecting the borders of at least four contiguous vertebrae
    (2) Intervertebral disk (IVD) space is preserved.
    (3) *No* sacroiliac joint involvement (unlike ankylosing spondylitis; see later)
6. Diagnosis of OA
   a. Plain radiographs (Link 24-33 B)
   b. MRI is good for synovial tissue abnormalities and effusions.
   c. ESR and CRP are usually normal.
   d. Synovial fluid is noninflammatory.
E. Neuropathic arthropathy (Charcot joint)
1. **Definition:** Noninflammatory joint disease secondary to a neurologic disease. Loss of proprioception (unconscious sense of position) and deep pain sensation (loss of pain in the joint) leads to recurrent trauma.

2. Epidemiology; causes
   a. Diabetes mellitus (DM; 15% of cases; see Chapter 23); primarily affects the tarsometatarsal joint
   b. Syringomyelia (20%–25% of cases; Link 24-34; see Chapter 26): degenerative disease of the cervical spinal cord characterized by the presence of a fluid-filled cavity; primarily affects the shoulder, elbow, and wrist joints
   c. Tabes dorsalis (10%–20% of cases; see Chapter 26): manifestation of tertiary syphilis characterized by demyelination of the nerves primarily in the dorsal columns (posterior columns) of the spinal cord causing a loss of pain sensation that primarily affects the hip, knee, and ankle joints

F. **Rheumatoid arthritis (RA)**
   1. **Definition:** Systemic disorder associated with chronic joint inflammation that most commonly affects the peripheral joints (wrists, hands, feet)
   2. Epidemiology
      a. Female-to-male ratio is 3:1; prevalence, 1% of population.
      b. In women, it typically occurs in the 30- to 50-year age bracket; MC joint disease in women.
      c. Various human leukocyte antigen (HLA) associations (HLA-DR4) that involve intracellular signaling and production of certain types of synovial citrullinated proteins
      d. ?Microbial inciting agents that initiate synovial inflammation include Epstein-Barr virus (EBV), parvovirus B19, human herpesvirus 6, and *Mycoplasma* spp.
      e. Risk factors include age, female sex, tobacco use, obesity and silicosis (Caplan syndrome with RA and intrapulmonary nodules caused by inhalation of coal dust, silica, or asbestos; see Chapter 17).
   3. Pathogenesis of joint disease may involve both type III and type IV reactions.
      a. One proposed mechanism is CD4⁺ helper T cells (cell-mediated type IV) are activated, leading to release of proinflammatory agents (e.g., TNF).
      b. Inflamed synovial cells express an antigen that triggers B cells to produce rheumatoid factor (RF). RF is an IgM autoantibody that has specificity for the Fc portion of IgG.
      c. RF and IgG join to form immunocomplexes (type III hypersensitivity; Chapter 4)
         (1) Sensitivity is ~60%, and specificity is ~80%.
         (2) RF can also form complexes with IgG or IgA.
      d. Immunocomplexes activate the complement system (C) to produce C5a, a chemotactic agent for neutrophils and other leukocytes to enter the joint space.
      e. Chronic synovitis and pannus formation eventually occur (Fig. 24-8 A; Link 24-35).
      f. Pannus is granulation tissue that is formed within the synovial tissue by fibroblasts and inflammatory cells (see Chapter 3).
      g. Pannus (P) proliferates and releases cks (e.g., ILs, TNF) that eventually destroy the articular cartilage, leading to fusion of the joint by scar tissue (called ankylosis). Bone erosions are caused by osteoclasts.
   4. Clinical findings
      a. Symmetric involvement of the metacarpophalangeal (MCP) and PIP joints (Link 24-36); notable sparing of DIP joints
      b. Causes bilateral ulnar deviation at MCP joints (Link 24-36, *arrow*) and morning stiffness >1 hour; radial deviation at the wrists (Fig. 24-8 B)
         (1) Swan neck deformity (Fig. 24-8 C; Link 24-37 A)
            (a) Flexion of the DIP joint
            (b) Extension of the PIP joint
         (2) Boutonnière deformity (Fig. 24-8 D; Link 24-37 B)
            (a) Extension of the DIP joint
            (b) Flexion of the PIP joint. Note that this is the reverse of a swan neck deformity.
         (3) Radiographs of the hands show bony erosions around involved joints and periarticular osteopenia (decrease bone density) (Link 24-38).
         (4) Other joints commonly involved in RA include the cervical spine, shoulders, elbows, hips, knees, and feet.
      c. Lung disease: chronic pleuritis with effusions (characteristic low glucose), interstitial fibrosis, and bronchiolitis obliterans (see Chapter 17)
      d. Hematologic disease
         (1) Anemia of chronic disease (ACD; see Chapter 12)
         (2) Felty syndrome (RA, splenomegaly, autoimmune neutropenia, leg ulcers)
         (3) Autoimmune hemolytic anemia (AIHA; see Chapter 12)

DM: tarsometatarsal joint

Syringomyelia: degenerative disease spinal cord

Fluid-filled cavity cervical cord → shoulder, elbow, wrist joints

Tabes dorsalis: tertiary syphilis

Demyelination dorsal columns: loss pain hip, knee, ankle joints

Rheumatoid arthritis

Systemic disorder; peripheral joints

F/M ratio 3:1

Women 30 to 50 yrs old

HLA-Dr4; intracellular signaling

?Microbial inciting agents: EBV, parvovirus

Age, female sex, tobacco use, obesity, silicosis

Activated CD4+ T cells release proinflammatory agents

Synovial cell antigen triggers B cells to produce RF

B cells produce RF; IgM antibody against Fc portion of IgG

RF forms immunocomplexes with IgG → activate complement system

Immunocomplexes activate C → C5a → neutrophils enter joint space

Chronic synovitis → pannus

Pannus (granulation tissue) formed within synovial tissue

P proliferates, produces cks destroy articular cartilage; fibrosis (ankyloses)

Clinical findings

Symmetric involvement MCP/PIP joints

Bilateral ulnar deviation; morning stiffness >1 hr

Radial deviation wrists

Swan neck deformity

Swan neck: DIP flexed, PIP extended

Boutonnière deformity

DIP extended, PIP flexed

Boney erosions, periarticular osteopenia

Cervical spine, shoulders, elbows, hips/knees/feet

Chronic pleuritis, interstitial fibrosis, effusions

Hematologic disease

ACD

Felty syndrome

AIHA

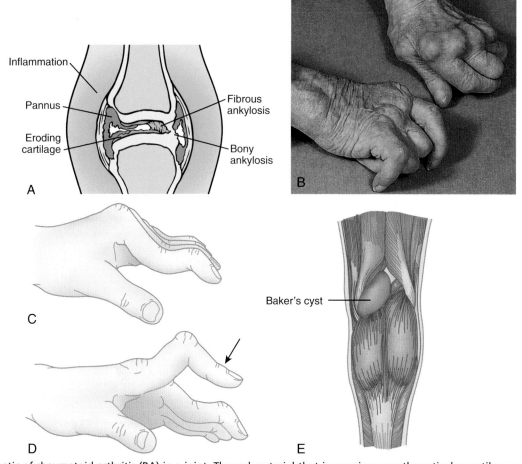

24-8: A, Schematic of rheumatoid arthritis (RA) in a joint. The red material that is growing over the articular cartilage and destroying it is pannus (granulation tissue; precursor to scar tissue). Note that fibrous ankylosis is beginning as the margin of the joint. **B,** Patient with RA showing bilateral ulnar deviation of the hands and prominent swelling of the second and third metacarpophalangeal joints. **C,** Swan neck deformity of the fingers (flexion of distal interphalangeal [DIP] joint, extension of proximal interphalangeal [PIP] joint). **D,** Boutonnière deformity of the index finger (extension of DIP joint, flexion of PIP joint; index finger), with swan neck deformity of the other fingers (third through fifth finger). **E,** Baker cyst. It is an extension of the semimembranosus bursa posteriorly. This bursa is often connected with a joint cavity. (*A from Kumar V, Abbas AK, Fausto N, Mitchell RN: Robbins Basic Pathology, 8th ed, Philadelphia, Saunders Elsevier, 2007, p 820, Fig. 7-18 on the left; B from Forbes C, Jackson W: Color Atlas and Text of Clinical Medicine, 2nd ed, London, Mosby, 2002, p 121, Fig. 3-3; C to E from Marx J: Rosen's Emergency Medicine Concepts and Clinical Practice, 7th ed, Philadelphia, Mosby Elsevier, 2010, pp 514, 664, respectively, Figs. 47-51, 47-52, 54-12, respectively.*)

e. Carpal tunnel syndrome (see Section V): entrapment of the median nerve under the transverse carpal ligament
f. Cervical spine
   (1) Entire cervical spine is frequently involved.
   (2) Subluxation of the atlantoaxial joint is particularly dangerous (Link 24-39).
      (a) Risk for compression of the spinal cord
      (b) Risk for compression of the vertebral artery, causing a stroke (see Chapter 26)
g. Rheumatoid nodules
   (1) Nodules occur on the extensor surface of the fingers, forearms, and pressure points (Achilles tendon, olecranon process) and in the lungs (Links 24-40, 24-41, and 24-42 A). They are present in 20% of patients.
      • Caplan syndrome: rheumatoid nodules in the lung plus a pneumoconiosis caused by silica, asbestos, or coal dust (see Chapter 17)
   (2) Fibrinoid necrosis is present in the center of the nodules with palisading of fibroblasts (Link 24-42 B; see Chapter 2).
   (3) Presence of rheumatoid nodules correlates with very high titers of RF.
h. Cardiovascular disease
   (1) Fibrinous pericarditis, constrictive pericarditis (see Chapter 11)
   (2) Aortitis (see Chapter 11)
   (3) Immunocomplex small-vessel vasculitis (see Chapter 10)

(a) Vasculitis is usually located around the ankles.

(b) Vasculitis correlates with high RF titers.

i. Popliteal (Baker) cyst behind the knee joint (Fig. 24-8 E)

(1) Extension of the semimembranous bursa into the posterior joint space because of increased intraarticular pressure

(2) Sometimes ruptures and dissects into the calf and is frequently misdiagnosed as deep venous thrombosis (DVT)

(3) *Not* pulsatile; a key to differentiating from a popliteal artery aneurysm (pulsatile mass). Differentiation is confirmed with ultrasonography.

j. Ocular changes include episcleritis and scleritis (see Chapter 26).

5. Laboratory findings

a. Positive serum antinuclear antibody (ANA) test is present in 30% of cases.

b. Positive serum RF is present in 70% to 90% of cases; IgM-RF, 60% to 80% sensitivity; IgG-RF, 80% to 90% specificity.

c. Anticyclic citrullinated peptide (anti-CCP) has a specificity of 95% to 98% and a sensitivity of 68% to 80%; more likely present in early RA than RF.

d. Normal to increased serum complement C3 and a decreased synovial fluid complement C3

e. ESR and CRP are both increased.

f. Total serum protein is increased.

(1) Caused by an increase in IgG γ-globulins (IgG) in chronic inflammation (CI; see Chapter 3)

(2) Polyclonal gammopathy (numerous clones of plasma cells are synthesizing IgG) is present on serum protein electrophoresis (see Fig. 3-23 B).

6. Overview of clinical findings in RA (Link 24-43). Overview of joints involved in RA versus OA (Link 24-44). Classification schemes are available for diagnosing RA.

G. Sjögren syndrome (SS)

1. **Definition:** Autoimmune disease characterized by the destruction of minor salivary glands (dry mouth) and the lacrimal glands (dry eyes)

2. Epidemiology

a. Primary and secondary subtypes (associated with other autoimmune diseases)

b. Female-dominant autoimmune disease (10:1 female-to-male ratio)

c. Associated with HLA-DQ/HLA-DR subtypes; hepatitis C (HCV) or EBV may be triggers

d. Peaks in the fourth and fifth decades of life

3. Clinical findings in SS

a. RA (secondary)

b. Keratoconjunctivitis sicca

(1) Dry eyes described by the patient as "sand in my eyes"

(2) Autoimmune destruction of the lacrimal glands

c. Xerostomia or dry mouth

(1) Autoimmune destruction of the minor salivary glands: "Doctor, I can't swallow dry crackers."

(2) Increased incidence of dental caries caused by the absence of saliva

d. Other findings: leukocytoclastic vasculitis (see Chapter 10), interstitial lung disease, esophageal dysmotility, biliary cirrhosis, malignant lymphoma (B cell type; 5%), and renal tubular acidosis (RTA)

4. Laboratory findings in SS

a. Serum ANA has a sensitivity of 80%.

b. Serum RF is positive in 90% of cases.

c. Anti–SS-A antibodies (anti-Ro; 60%–70%) and anti–SS-B (anti-La; 40%–60%)

d. Anti–SS-B antibodies (anti-La) are present in 60% to 90% of cases.

5. Confirmation of SS is secured with a lip biopsy showing lymphoid destruction of the minor salivary glands.

H. Juvenile idiopathic arthritis (JIA)

(*Some information excerpted from Ferri FF:* 2016 Ferri's Clinical Advisor, *Philadelphia, Elsevier, 2017, pp 703-704, Table 1J-2.*)

1. **Definition:** A type of arthritis in children <17 years of age that has several subgroups with different clinical characteristics, pathogenesis, and response to therapy

2. Systemic JIA (Still disease)

a. Epidemiology

(1) Accounts for ~10% of all cases of JIA

(2) Peak age of onset is 2 to 4 years of age.

(3) Male:female sex ratio is equal (1:1).

Margin notes:

Immuncomplex small vessel vasculitis around ankles

High RF titers

Popliteal cyst: behind knee joint

Sometimes rupture

Not pulsatile; confused with aneurysm

Episcleritis, scleritis

Laboratory findings

+Serum ANA 30%

+Serum IgM/IgG RF most cases

Anti-CCP ↑specificity/↓ sensitivity

N/↓Serum C3; ↓synovial fluid C3

↑ESR/CRP

↑Total serum protein

↑IgG γ-globulins; CI

Polyclonal gammopathy

Sjögren syndrome

Destruction minor salivary/ lacrimal glands

1°/2° subtypes

Female dominant

HLA-DQ/-DR subtypes; HCV/ EBV possible triggers

Peaks 4th/5th decades

Clinical findings

RA

Keratoconjunctivitis sicca

Dry eyes; "sand in my eyes"

Autoimmune destruction lacrimal glands

Xerostomia: dry mouth

Autoimmune destruction minor salivary glands

Dental caries

+Serum ANA (80%)

Serum RF (90%)

Serum anti–SS-A (>60%), anti–SS-B (40%)

Confirm with lip biopsy: destruction minor salivary glands

Juvenile idiopathic arthritis

Type arthritis children <17 yrs

Systemic JIA

10% JIA

2 to 4 yrs

M:F ratio 1:1

Clinical findings

Polyarticular; TMJ

Fever spikes

Pericarditis/pleuritic, rash, hepatosplenomegaly

Possible MAS

Triggers EBV, CMV

Neutrophil leukocytosis

ACD

Thrombocytosis

↑ESR/CRP/ferritin

Oligoarticular JIA

50% to 60% JIA

>6 yrs old

Male:female: 1:4

Knees MC, ankles/fingers

Chronic uveitis

Potential for blindness

+Serum ANA 60%

RF negative polyarthritis

30% JIA

1–4, 10–12 yrs old

Male:female 1:3

Symmetric or asymmetric arthritis

Small/large joints; cervical spine; TMJ

Chronic uveitis

+Serum ANA 40%

↑CRP > ↑ESR

Mild anemia

RF+ polyarthritis

10% JIA

9-12 yrs old

Male:female 1:9

Aggressive symmetric polyarthritis

Rheumatoid nodules 10%

Uveitis *not* key feature

Low-grade fever

+RF

↑ESR > ↑CRP

Mild anemia

Psoriatic/enthesitis JIA each 10% of cases

Gouty arthritis

Tissue deposition MSU; hyperuricemia

b. Clinical findings
  (1) Arthritis pattern is polyarticular and involves the fingers, wrists, neck, hip, knees, and temporomandibular joint (TMJ; micrognathia; Link 24-45).
  (2) Commonly presents as an "infectious disease" with fever spikes once or twice a day, sore throat, rash, polyarthritis, and generalized painful lymphadenopathy
  (3) Extraarticular features include pericarditis, pleuritis, an evanescent rash, hepatomegaly, and splenomegaly.
  (4) Most-feared life-threatening complication is the macrophage activation syndrome (MAS; 10% of patients) consisting of persistent fever, organomegaly, prolonged prothrombin time and partial thromboplastin time, cytopenias, liver dysfunction, hypertriglyceridemia, and central nervous system (CNS) signs (coma, seizures). Triggers for MAS include EBV and cytomegalovirus (CMV).
c. Laboratory findings in in systemic JIA are *not* specific for this subgroup.
  (1) Neutrophilic leukocytosis often with a leukemoid increase (see Chapter 13)
  (2) Mild to moderate anemia of chronic disease (ACD) (see Chapter 12)
  (3) Increased platelets (thrombocytosis, *not* thrombocytopenia)
  (4) Increase in acute phase reactants (ferritin, CRP, ESR; see Chapter 3)
3. Oligoarticular JIA
  a. Epidemiology
    (1) Accounts for 50% to 60% of all cases of JIA
    (2) Peak age of onset is >6 yrs old.
    (3) Male:female ratio is 1:4.
  b. Clinical findings in oligoarticular JIA
    (1) Arthritis in the knees (MC), ankles, and fingers
    (2) Chronic uveitis (inflammation of the iris, ciliary body and choroid) occurs in ~30% of patients; potential for blindness.
  c. Laboratory findings in oligoarticular JIA
    (1) Serum ANA test is positive in 60% of cases.
    (2) ESR and CRP are mildly elevated.
4. RF-negative polyarthritis
  a. Epidemiology
    (1) Accounts for 30% of cases of JIA
    (2) Peak ages of onset are 1 to 4 and 10 to 12 years of age.
    (3) Male:female ratio is 1:3.
  b. Clinical findings in RF-negative polyarthritis
    (1) Symmetric or asymmetric
    (2) Small and large joints; cervical spine; TMJ (Link 24-45)
    (3) Chronic uveitis in ~10% of cases
  c. Laboratory findings in RF-negative polyarthritis
    (1) Serum ANA test is positive in 40% of cases.
    (2) CRP is more elevated than the ESR.
    (3) Mild anemia may be present.
5. RF-positive polyarthritis
  a. Epidemiology
    (1) Accounts for >10% of JIA
    (2) Peak age of onset is 9 to 12 years old.
    (3) Male:female ratio is 1:9.
  b. Clinical findings in RF-positive polyarthritis
    (1) Aggressive symmetric polyarthritis
    (2) Rheumatoid nodules occur in 10% of cases.
    (3) Uveitis is *not* a key feature of the disease (0%–2%).
    (4) Low-grade fever
  c. Laboratory findings in RF-positive polyarthritis
    (1) RF is positive.
    (2) ESR is increased more than CRP.
    (3) Mild anemia is present.
6. Psoriatic type of JIA and enthesitis-related JIA each account for 10% of cases of JIA and will *not* be further discussed. Enthesitis is inflammation in which tendons or ligaments insert into bone.

I. Gouty arthritis
  1. **Definition:** Group of disease states caused by tissue deposition of monosodium urate (MSU) associated with prolonged hyperuricemia

2. Epidemiology
   a. Occurs more often in men >30 years of age (95% of cases). Male to female ratio is ~4:1.
   b. Uncommon in women *before* menopause (5% of cases)
   c. Primary gout arises from inborn errors of metabolism involving purine metabolism.
      - Examples: deficiency of hypoxanthine-guanine phosphoribosyltransferase (HGPRT) in Lesch-Nyhan syndrome, glycogen storage disease (see Chapter 6)
   d. Secondary causes are more common.
      (1) Underexcretion of uric acid (UA) in kidneys (80%–90% of cases)
         - Examples: lead (Pb) nephropathy, alcoholism, diets rich in red meat, seafood, beer, drugs (thiazides, low-dose aspirin, cyclosporine A), ketoacidosis (KA), and lactic acidosis (LA)
      (2) Overproduction of UA caused by increased nucleated cell turnover accounts for 10%–20% of cases of gout.
         - Examples: treating leukemia, psoriasis ($\uparrow$epithelial cell turnover), alcohol, myeloproliferative disorder (MPD), tumor lysis disorder (TLD)
   e. Clinical conditions commonly associated with gout
      (1) Urate nephropathy, renal stones (see Chapter 20)
      (2) Hypertension (HTN), coronary artery disease (CAD)
      (3) Pb poisoning (see Chapters 7, 12, and 20). Pb produces interstitial nephritis, which interferes with UA excretion.
   f. More than 75% of individuals with hyperuricemia remain asymptomatic.
   g. Common sites of deposition of UA (Link 24-46)
3. Acute gout
   a. Most commonly involves the first MTP joint (called podagra; Link 24-47)
      (1) Joint in the foot that experiences the most trauma
      (2) Polyarticular involvement occurs in 10% to 15% of cases.
      (3) Recurrent attacks of acute gout are the rule.
   b. Often precipitated by dietary indiscretions, illness, exercise, or emotional stress
   c. Free UA crystals in the synovial fluid are proinflammatory.
      (1) Activate synovial cells, neutrophils, and the complement cascade
         (a) Complement cascade releases C5a, which attracts neutrophils into the joint, producing acute inflammation (Link 24-48).
         (b) Phagocytosis of UA crystals by neutrophils results in their lysis with subsequent release of proinflammatory chemicals that enhance the inflammatory reaction (Link 24-49).
      (2) Another common site for acute gout is the extensor tenosynovium on the dorsum of the midfoot.
   d. Clinical findings in acute gout
      (1) Sudden onset of severe pain in the great toe (50% of cases)
      (2) Joint is hot, red, and swollen (Fig. 24-9 A; Link 24-47). Fever is present.
      (3) MC in postpubertal men when UA is most increased
      (4) MC in postmenopausal females when UA is highest
   e. Laboratory findings in acute gout
      (1) Hyperuricemia >80%; may be normal in a small number of cases.
      (2) Absolute neutrophilic leukocytosis (increased number neutrophils)
   f. Diagnosis of acute gout
      (1) Joint aspiration is confirmatory. Crystals are present both free and within the phagosomes of neutrophils.
      (2) Polarization reveals negatively birefringent MSU crystals (see Fig. 24-6 A).
4. Chronic gout
   a. Chronic gout is likely to occur if gout is poorly controlled.
   b. UA crystals accumulate in and around the joint and produce a tophus.
      (1) **Definition:** A deposit of MSU in a joint, skin, or cartilage that produces a granulomatous inflammation that damages the surrounding tissue
      (2) In a joint, MSU crystals leak into the soft tissue around the joint (Fig. 24-9 B and C; Links 24-49 and 24-50). Aspiration of the joint reveals crystals (Link 24-51).
      (3) PIP joints in the finger and the MTP joint are favored sites for tophi. Other sites include the pinna of the ears, overlying extensor surfaces of the forearms, and at pressures points (where the tendon inserts in the bone).
      (4) MSU crystals excite a brisk granulomatous reaction in the periarticular tissue.
      (5) Microscopic sections reveal numerous multinucleated giant cells (MGCs) within which are polarizable MSU crystals.

Male:female ratio ~4:1

1° Gout inborn errors metabolism

Deficiency HGPRT

2° Gout more common than 1°

Underexcretion UA MCC

Pb nephro, alcohol, red meat/seafood/beer, thiazides, low-dose aspirin, KA, LA

Overproduction gout uncommon

Rx leukemia, psoriasis, alcohol, MPD, TLD

Urate nephropathy, stones, HTN, CAD, Pb poisoning

>75% remain asymptomatic

Acute gout: 1st MTP joint most often involved

1st MTP; podagra

Joint with most trauma

Recurrent attacks the rule

Precipitating factors: dietary, illness, exercise, stress

Free UA crystals initiate the attack

Activate synovial cells, neutrophils, C5a

Neutrophils lyse → release proinflammatory chemicals

Extensor tenosynovium dorsum midfoot

Severe pain great toe

Hot, red, swollen

Fever

Postpubertal males

Postmenopausal females

Laboratory findings

Hyperuricemia

Absolute neutrophil leukocytosis

Diagnosis

Free crystals, neutrophil phagosomes

Acute gout: must confirm with joint aspiration; hyperuricemia does not define gout

Chronic gout

Gout poorly controlled

UA accumulates around joints → tophus

MSU in joint/skin/cartilage; granulomatous inflammation

MSU leaks into soft tissue

Tophi PIP, MTP, Achilles tendon insertion, pinna ear, extensor surfaces forearms

MGCs with MSU crystals

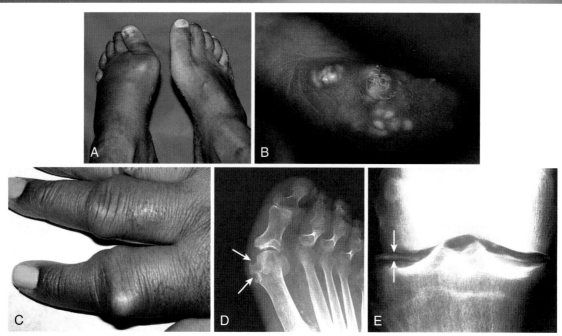

24-9: **A,** Acute gouty arthritis involving the left big toe. Note the erythema and swelling of the joint. **B,** Digit with white, tophaceous crystals beneath the skin. **C,** Tophus over the proximal interphalangeal joint. Note white discoloration beneath the skin. This may be confused with Bouchard nodes in osteoarthritis. **D,** Gout. Metatarsal-phalangeal joint of the great toe shows an erosive arthritis. The hallmark of gout is the sharply marginated, juxtaarticular erosion, which may have a sclerotic border *(solid white arrows)* and overhanging edges, as in this case. **E,** Chondrocalcinosis (CC). CC refers only to calcification of the articular cartilage *(solid white arrows)* or fibrocartilage. If this patient had acute pain, redness, swelling, and limitation of motion, the combination would be called pseudogout. *(**A** from Swartz MH: Textbook of Physical Diagnosis, 5th ed, Philadelphia, Saunders Elsevier, 2006, p 634, Fig. 20-55; **B** from Bouloux, P: Self-Assessment Picture Tests Medicine, Vol. 3, London, Mosby-Wolfe, 1997, p 13, Fig. 25; **C** from Goldman L, Schafer AI: Cecil's Medicine, 24th ed, Philadelphia, Saunders Elsevier, 2012, p 1740, Fig. 281-4D; **D** from Herring W: Learning Radiology Recognizing the Basics, 2nd ed, Philadelphia, Elsevier Saunders, 2012, p 257, Fig. 23-16; **E,** from Marx J: Rosen's Emergency Medicine Concepts and Clinical Practice, 7th ed, Philadelphia, Mosby Elsevier, 2010, p 1482, Fig. 114.8.)*

Erosive arthritis; bone breaks down leaving overhanging edges

CPPD

Deposition CPPD cartilage

Hemochromatosis, hemosiderosis

1° HPTH

Most cases idiopathic

MC in elderly

Degenerative arthritis similar to OA

Knee MC joint

Deposits in articular cartilage

Linear deposit

Called chondrocalcinosis

Called pseudogout pain, redness, swelling, joint limitation

Seronegative spondyloarthritis

Overlapping clinical features; +HLA-B27

(6) Tophi destroy subjacent bone, causing erosion of bone, leaving overhanging edges (sometimes called "rat bites"; Fig. 24-9 D; Link 24-52).

J. Calcium pyrophosphate dihydrate deposition (CPPD) disease
1. **Definition:** Deposition of calcium pyrophosphate dihydrate in cartilage and less commonly in tendons, ligaments, and synovial tissue
2. Epidemiology
   a. Factors that increase the incidence of CPPD
      (1) Hemochromatosis, hemosiderosis (see Chapter 19)
         (a) Pyrophosphate inhibitor is increased in these diseases.
         (b) Causes an increase in the inorganic pyrophosphate concentration in tissue
      (2) Primary hyperparathyroidism (HPTH): increase in calcium is responsible for CPPD.
   b. Most cases are idiopathic.
      (1) Most commonly occurs in older adults; present in 50% of patients who are >80 years old
      (2) Degenerative arthritis with symptoms similar to osteoarthritis (OA)
      (3) Knee joint is most commonly involved.
      (4) Calcium pyrophosphate crystals commonly deposit in the articular cartilage of the knee. Other sites of deposition include the wrist and symphysis pubis.
         (a) Crystals produce linear deposits in the articular cartilage (Fig. 24-9 E; Link 24-53).
         (b) Called chondrocalcinosis when it deposits in the articular cartilage; called pseudogout if the patient has acute pain, redness, swelling, and limitation of motion in the joint
      (5) Crystals that are phagocytized by neutrophils show positive birefringence (see Fig. 24-6 B; Link 24-54).

K. Seronegative spondyloarthropathies (spondyloarthritis)
1. **Definition:** Family of diseases that are grouped together by overlapping clinical features and molecular evidence of a common etiology; majority are HLA-B27 positive. Seronegative refers to the fact that rheumatoid factor is *not* present.

2. Epidemiology and characteristics
   (*Excerpted from Ashar BH, Miller RG, Sisso SD:* The Johns Hopkins Internal Medicine Board Review, *4th ed, Elsevier, 2012, pp 355-358.*)
   a. Diseases that have overlapping clinical features and evidence of a common etiology
      (1) Ankylosing spondylitis
      (2) Reactive arthritis
         (a) Reiter syndrome is associated with *Chlamydia trachomatis* urethritis.
         (b) Pathogens that are associated with gastroenteritis include *Shigella flexneri, Salmonella typhimurium, Campylobacter jejuni,* and *Yersinia enterocolitica.*
      (3) Psoriatic arthritis (see later)
      (4) Enteropathic arthritis (see later)
   b. Common clinical features
      (1) RF negative
      (2) HLA-B27 association
      (3) Inflammation at the site of ligamentous and tendinous insertions into bone (enthesitis)
      (4) Mucocutaneous manifestations
      (5) Inflammatory eye disease (anterior uveitis)
      (6) Inflammatory bowel disease (Crohn disease or ulcerative colitis)
      (7) Inflammatory back disease (sacroiliitis)
3. Ankylosing spondylitis
   a. **Definition:** Seronegative spondyloarthropathy that initially targets the sacroiliac joint in young men; presents with bilateral sacroiliitis and morning stiffness
   b. Epidemiology
      (1) Male:female ratio is 5:1.
      (2) Predominant age of onset is 15 to 35 years.
      (3) HLA-B27 is positive in 95% of patients.
   c. Clinical findings in ankylosing spondylitis
      (1) Begins as bilateral (symmetric) sacroiliitis (pain and tenderness); eventually involves the vertebral column (Link 24-55)
         (a) Fusion of the vertebrae (bamboo spine) causes forward curvature of the spine (kyphosis; Fig. 24-10 A, B; Links 24-56, 24-57, and 24-58).
         (b) Kyphosis interferes with chest wall movement.
            • Example of a nonpulmonary restrictive lung disease (RLD)
            • Schober test evaluates the degree of restriction to forward bending.
            • Compensatory hyperextension of the neck
            • Loss of lumbar lordosis (normally there is increased inward curving of the lumbar spine just above the buttocks)
      (2) Achilles tendinitis with pain and tenderness at the junction of the tendon with the plantar fascia may occur in ~25% of cases (Link 24-59); also occurs in reactive arthritis caused by Reiter syndrome (see later)
      (3) Aortitis produces aortic regurgitation.
      (4) Pulmonary fibrosis may occur in the apices of the lungs.
      (5) Anterior uveitis occurs in 25% to 40% of cases; blurry vision and a potential for blindness.
      (6) Peripheral arthritis ~25%; not as common as in other types with the exception of enteropathic arthropathy
4. Reiter syndrome
   a. **Definition:** Reactive type of seronegative spondyloarthropathy associated with urethritis, arthritis, conjunctivitis, and balanitis (inflammation of glans penis)
   b. Epidemiology
      (1) Male:female ratio is 9:1.
      (2) HLA-B27 is positive in 40% to 80% of cases.
      (3) Age at onset is 20 to 40 years.
   c. Clinical findings in Reiter syndrome
      (1) Classic triad is arthritis, conjunctivitis, and a history of urethritis.
      (2) Urethritis is usually caused by *C. trachomatis.*
      (3) Symmetric peripheral polyarthritis may involve the knee and ankle.
      (4) Asymmetric sacroiliitis or spondylitis may occur in ~40% of cases.
      (5) Heel pain is caused by Achilles tendinitis. Bone formation at the junction of the Achilles tendinitis with the plantar fascia is a confirmatory radiologic sign of Achilles tendinitis (Fig. 24-10 C; Links 24-59 and 24-60).
      (6) Swollen toe (s) (Link 24-61)

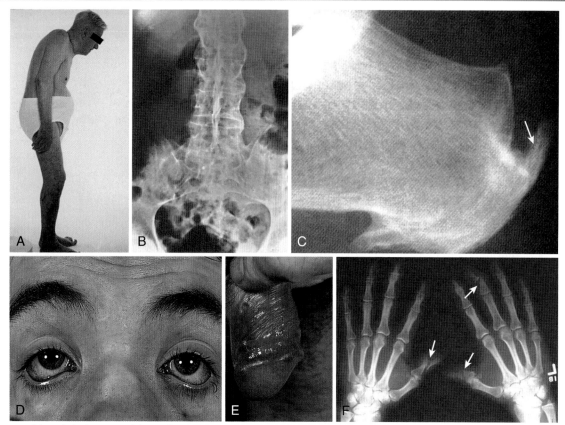

24-10: **A,** Man with ankylosing spondylitis. The patient cannot bend forward owing to fusion of the vertebrae. **B,** Radiograph showing fused vertebrae (bamboo spine) in ankylosing spondylitis. **C,** New bone formation at the junction of the Achilles tendon with the plantar fascia in a patient with Reiter syndrome. **D,** Sterile conjunctivitis (note redness of the conjunctiva) in a patient with Reiter syndrome. **E,** Circinate balanitis in Reiter syndrome. Shallow ulcerations are noted on the distal shaft and glans penis. **F,** Psoriatic arthritis of the hand. Psoriatic arthritis typically involves the small joints of the hands, especially the distal interphalangeal joints *(solid white arrows)*, leading to telescoping of one phalanx into another (pencil-in-cup deformity). (*A from Forbes C, Jackson W:* Color Atlas and Text of Clinical Medicine, *2nd ed, London, Mosby, 2002, Fig. 3-48; B from Katz D, Math K, Groskin S:* Radiology Secrets, *Philadelphia, Hanley & Belfus, 1998, p 277, Fig. 7; C from Doherty M, George E:* Self-Assessment Picture Tests In Medicine: Rheumatology, *London, Mosby-Wolfe, 1995, p 30, Fig. 42b: D and E from Bouloux P:* Self-Assessment Picture Tests Medicine, *Vol. 4, London, Mosby-Wolfe, 1997, p 3, Fig. 6, both pictures; F from Herring W:* Learning Radiology Recognizing the Basics, *2nd ed, Philadelphia, Elsevier Saunders, 2012, p 258, Fig. 23-18A.)*

Noninfectious conjunctivitis

Anterior uveitis

Circinate balanitis

Keratoderma blennorrhagica

Psoriatic arthritis

SS may occur with psoriasis skin/nails

Male to female ratio 1:1

HLA-B27+ 40% to 50%

Age onset 35–55 yrs

Psoriasis usually precedes arthritis

DIP joint disease nail changes or sacroiliitis/spondylitis

(7) Conjunctivitis is noninfectious (Fig. 24-10 D).
(8) Anterior uveitis is present in 25% of cases and may lead to blindness.
(9) Circinate balanitis is a mucocutaneous manifestation of the disease. Rash on the distal shaft and glans penis appears as vesicles, shallow ulcerations, or both (see Fig. 24-10 E; Link 24-62).
(10) Aphthous ulcers are another mucocutaneous manifestation of the disease (see Fig. 18-4).
(11) Keratoderma blennorrhagica (Link 24-63)
5. Psoriatic arthritis
a. **Definition:** SS that may occur in up to 15% of those with psoriatic skin and nail disease (see Chapter 25)
b. Epidemiology
(1) Male to female ratio is 1:1.
(2) HLA-B27 is positive in 40% to 50% of cases.
(3) Age at onset is 35 to 55 years.
(4) Psoriasis usually precedes reactive arthritis in 70% of cases.
c. Clinical and radiographic findings in psoriatic arthritis
(1) Patterns of joint involvement in psoriatic arthritis include peripheral joint disease (e.g., DIP joints with nail changes in 25% of cases) or axial disease (e.g., sacroiliitis or spondylitis) (Link 24-64).
(2) Classic radiographic finding is the pencil-in-cup deformity caused by erosion of the distal end of the interphalangeal joint with bony proliferation at the proximal end of the affected joint (Fig. 24-10 F; Link 24-65).

(3) Digit is sausage shaped and frequently has psoriatic skin disease evident on the dorsum of the fingers as well as pitting of the nails (Link 24-66 A). Nails also have onycholysis (separation of the nail from the nail bed) and an "oil drop" sign (yellow-orange discoloration of the nail; see Fig. 24-10 F; Link 24-66 B).

6. Enteropathic arthritis
   a. **Definition:** Inflammatory spondyloarthropathy associated with inflammatory bowel disease (e.g., ulcerative colitis or Crohn disease) and reactive arthritis initiated by bacterial or parasitic disease
   b. Epidemiology
      (1) Male:female ratio is 1:1.
      (2) Usually begins in young adults
      (3) HLA-B27 is present in 7% of cases.
   c. Clinical findings in enteropathic arthritis
      (1) Association with ulcerative colitis or Crohn disease in 10% to 20%
      (2) Bacteria associations include *Shigella* spp., *Salmonella* spp., *Campylobacter* spp., *Yersinia* spp., and *Clostridium difficile*.
      (3) Parasitic associations include *Strongyloides stercoralis, Giardia lamblia,* and *Ascaris lumbricoides*.
      (4) Symmetric sacroiliitis or spondylitis is present in <20% of cases.
      (5) Peripheral arthritis is present in 15% to 20% of cases; correlates with GI disease (see earlier).
      (6) Anterior uveitis with the potential for blindness occurs in 10% to 36% of cases.

L. **Septic arthritis**
   1. **Definition:** Painful infection of a joint; may occur via the bloodstream or direct inoculation (e.g., a penetrating injury of the joint)
   2. Epidemiology
      a. *S. aureus* is the MC nongonococcal cause of septic arthritis (Link 24-67). Predisposing factors include rheumatoid arthritis (RA), diabetes mellitus, corticosteroid therapy, and after surgical procedures.
      b. *Neisseria gonorrhoeae* is the MCC of septic arthritis in urban populations.
         (1) Usually occurs in adults <30 years old
         (2) May produce disseminated GC
            (a) Disseminated GC most commonly occurs in young women.
            (b) May also occur if there is a deficiency of complement components C6 to C9
               • These components are required to kill the bacteria.
         (3) Other clinical findings
            (a) Septic arthritis (knee)
            (b) Tenosynovitis (wrists and ankles)
            (c) Dermatitis (pustules on the wrists or ankles; see Chapter 22; Links 22-28 and 22-29)
      c. Other bacterial causes
         (1) *S. pneumoniae*: risk factors: sickle cell anemia, HIV, alcoholism
         (2) *Mycoplasma pneumoniae*: risk factor: primary immunoglobulin deficiency
      d. Viral arthritis: causes
         (1) Direct synovial invasion or via an immune reaction
         (2) Parvovirus B19
            (a) Usually involves the hands
            (b) Adult infections can occur without rash (see Chapter 25) or fever.
            (c) Usually self-limited, with resolution within 8 to 10 weeks
         (3) Hepatitis B virus (HBV)
            (a) Symmetrical arthritis or arthralgias (pain; no inflammation)
            (b) Often occurs *before* jaundice and resolves as jaundice develops
   3. Lyme disease (LD)
      a. **Definition:** Multisystem inflammatory disease caused by *Borrelia burgdorferi*, a spirochete that is transmitted by the bite of an *Ixodes* tick (Link 24-68 A)
      b. Epidemiology
         (1) Different ticks produce the disease in North America, Europe, and Asia.
         (2) Adult ticks acquire the spirochete by feeding on an infected white-tailed deer (reservoir for the disease).
         (3) Nymphs acquire the spirochete by feeding on an infected white-footed mouse. Nymphs are responsible for the majority of human cases (90%), particularly in the summer months.
         (4) Most cases in the United States occur in the Northeast and the Upper Midwest.
         (5) LD is the fastest growing vector-borne disease in the United States.

Marginal notes:

Psoriatic arthritis: sausage-shaped DIP joints; pencil-in-cup deformity

Enteropathic arthritis

Associated with ulcerative colitis or Crohn disease, infections

Male to female ratio 1:1

Young adults

HLA-B27+ 7%

Ulcerative colitis or Crohn disease

Bacteria associations

Parasitic associations

Symmetric sacroiliitis

Peripheral arthritis: correlates with GI disease

Anterior uveitis

Septic arthritis

Joint infection

S. aureus MCC nongonococcal septic arthritis

N. gonorrhoeae: MCC septic arthritis urban populations

Less 30 yrs old

Disseminated GC MC young women

Disseminated GC C6–C9 deficiency

Septic arthritis knee

Tenosynovitis wrists/ankles

Pustules wrists/ankles

Other bacteria

Streptococcus pneumoniae: sickle cell anemia

M. pneumoniae: immunoglobulin deficiency

Viral arthritis

Direct invasion, immune reaction

Parvovirus B19

Hands

Adults: often *no* rash/fever

Self-limited

HBV

Symmetrical arthritis, arthralgia

Occurs before jaundice, resolves when jaundice present

Lyme disease

Borrelia burgdorferi spirochete; bite *Ixodes* tick

Adult ticks acquire *Ixodes* from white-tailed deer

Nymphs acquire *Ixodes* from white-footed mouse; MCC LD

Northeast, Upper Midwest U.S.

Fastest growing vector-borne disease U.S.

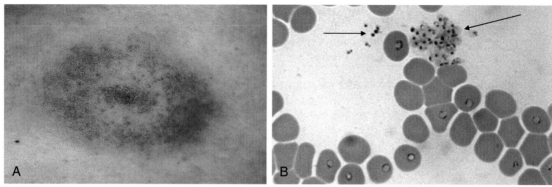

24-11: **A,** Erythema chronicum migrans in a patient with Lyme disease. Raised central area is the site of the tick bite. Concentric area of erythema surrounds the bite site. **B,** *Babesia microti.* Red blood cells in the peripheral blood show a predominance of ring forms. Clusters of extraerythrocytic parasites *(arrows)* are also seen free in the plasma. *(A from Swartz M: Textbook of Physical Diagnosis: History and Examination, 5th ed, Philadelphia, Saunders Elsevier, 2006, p 185, Fig. 8.113; B from Goldman L, Schafer AI: Cecil's Medicine, 24th ed, Philadelphia, Saunders Elsevier, 2012, p 2048, Fig. 361-1.)*

Preferred sites: skin, CNS, joints, heart, eyes

All ages/sexes

Mechanism: organism inflammation, type II/III HSR

Early localized infection

EM earliest sign

Pathognomonic for LD

Bull's eye appearance; blister center (bite site)

Single lesion MC

Empirical Rx if EM present

Fever, flulike, neck stiffness

1/3rd EM no further symptoms; 2/3rd progress

Early dissemination (wks/mths post-tick bite)

Spread skin/lymphatics

Migratory polyarticular arthritis; knee MC

Neuroborreliosis: bilateral facial nerve palsy, meningeal irritation

Chronic disease: mths to yrs post infection

Disabling arthritis; knee

Encephalopathy, -myelitis; neuropathy

Myo/pericarditis, iritis, keratitis, optic neuritis

ELISA high sensitivity (screen)

Western blot confirms

PCR

(6) Organism has a strong tropism for the skin, CNS, joints, heart, and eyes.

(7) Affects all ages and sexes but has a predilection for the white population (higher exposure rate to ticks than other races)

(8) Factors that have been implicated in the pathology of LD include inflammation related to the organism itself, cross-reacting antibodies to spirochetal proteins against human tissue (type II hypersensitivity reaction [HSR]), and immunocomplex deposition (type III HSR).

c. Clinical presentation of LD

(1) Early localized infection (first month)

(a) Erythema migrans (EM) develops on the skin 1 to 2 weeks after removal of the tick in 80% of the cases (Fig. 24-11 A).

- Pathognomonic lesion of LD; its presence alone is enough to make the diagnosis of LD

- Lesion has a bull's eye appearance with a small fluid-filled blister in the center (site of the tick bite) surrounded by a red, expanding lesion with concentric circles.

- Single lesions are MC; however, multiple lesions may also occur that are *not* caused by multiple tick bites.

- Presence of this lesion alone is enough to begin treatment of the disease without laboratory confirmation.

(b) Common complaints include fever, flulike symptoms (e.g., fever, chills, headache, arthralgia), and neck stiffness.

(c) One-third of patients with EM do *not* develop further symptoms, but two-thirds progress to further stages of the disease.

(2) Early disseminated disease (weeks to months after tick bite)

(a) Further spread to skin and lymphatics (painful lymphadenopathy)

(b) Migratory polyarticular arthritis (involving bursa, tendons, joints) that evolves into a monoarticular arthritis (e.g., knee [MC site], wrist)

(c) Neuroborreliosis is characterized by bilateral facial nerve palsy and meningeal irritation (nuchal rigidity).

(3) Chronic disease (months to years after infection)

(a) Produces a disabling arthritis (e.g., knee)

(b) Subacute encephalopathy, encephalomyelitis, and peripheral neuropathies may occur.

(c) Other systemic findings include myocarditis, pericarditis, iritis (ring-shaped membrane behind the cornea), keratitis (inflammation of the cornea), and optic neuritis (inflammation of the optic nerve).

d. Diagnosis for other stages of LD (excluding the phase with EM)

(1) Enzyme-linked immunosorbent assay (ELISA) test is a highly sensitive screening test for LD.

(2) Western blot assay is used for an equivocal or a positive ELISA test to confirm LD (specificity, 94%–96%).

(3) Polymerase chain reaction (PCR) test is also available.

e. Babesiosis
    (1) **Definition:** Intraerythrocytic (sometimes extraerythrocytic) protozoal disease caused by *Babesia microti*; transmitted by *Ixodes* tick (Link 24-68 B)
    (2) Epidemiology: may present concurrently with LD if the tick also is carrying the spirochete *Borrelia burgdorferi* (Link 24-68 B)
    (3) Clinical findings include fever, headache, and a hemolytic anemia (see Chapter 12).
    (4) Diagnostic tests
        (a) Examination of a Wright- or Giemsa-stained peripheral smear to look for organisms within red blood cells (RBCs) or free in the plasma (Fig. 24-11 B)
        (b) Serologic testing
4. Septic arthritis and tendinitis caused by a cat or dog bite; epidemiology
    a. Causal agent is *Pasteurella multocida,* a gram-negative coccobacillus with bipolar staining.
    b. MC infection secondary to animal injury
        (1) Cat bites or scratches are more likely than dog bites to cause disease.
        (2) Approximately 60% to 90% of cats normally have the organism in their mouths.
        (3) Only 5% to 15% of dogs have the organism in their mouths.
    c. Types of infection caused by a cat or dog bite
        (1) Cellulitis (MC)
        (2) Septic arthritis or tendinitis
        (3) Osteomyelitis, endocarditis, meningitis
    d. Rapid onset of infection at the bite site (usually within 24 hours)
5. Viral arthritis; epidemiology
    a. Direct synovial invasion or via an immune reaction; migratory polyarthritis
    b. Parvovirus B19
        (1) Usually involves the hands
        (2) Adult infections can occur without rash (see Chapter 25) or fever.
        (3) Usually self-limited, with resolution in 8 to 10 weeks
    c. Hepatitis B virus (HBV)
        (1) Symmetrical arthritis or arthralgias (pain; no inflammation)
        (2) Often occurs *before* jaundice and resolves when jaundice develops
    d. Rubella
        (1) May occur after immunization or infection
        (2) Predominantly occurs in women
        (3) Usually self-limited; occasionally persists for years
    e. Mumps
        (1) More common in men than women
        (2) Usually occurs within 2 weeks of parotitis (swelling of parotid glands)
    M. Miscellaneous joint disease
    • **Bunion:** Deformity of the joint that connects the great toe to the foot (Link 24-69)
III. **Muscle Disorders**
    A. Muscle fibers
        1. Normal muscle consists of fibers arranged into fascicles (Link 24-70).
        2. Innervation of the muscle determines the fiber type. Special stains determine fiber type (Link 24-71).
        3. Type 1 fiber characteristics
            a. Slow-twitch (red) fiber characteristics
                (1) Contract slowly and high fatigue resistance
                (2) Used in aerobic activities (long-distance running)
            b. Rich in mitochondria (mT), myoglobin (MG; why they are red), and oxidative enzymes; primarily use oxidative metabolism (oxidative phosphorylation [OP]) in the mitochondria for generating adenosine triphosphate (ATP)
            c. Weak in ATPase enzymes and scant in glycogen
            d. High in myoglobin content
            e. Olympic marathon runners have 80% slow-twitch fibers.
        4. Type 2 fibers
            a. Subdivided into type 2a and 2b fibers
            b. Type 2a fibers
                (1) Moderate fatigue resistance but not as much as type 1 fibers (intermediate fast-twitch fibers)
                (2) Use both aerobic and anaerobic metabolism
                (3) Large number of mT
                (4) Generates ATP by both OP in mitochondria and glycolysis in the cytoplasm

Contract quickly
Stop and go activities, weight lifting
Type 2b fibers
Decreased myoglobin (white color)
Very easily fatigued
Use anaerobic metabolism
Increased glycogen
Low number mT
Glycolysis for ATP
Very fast contraction
Great contraction power
Sprinting, heavy weights
Muscle disorders
Muscle weakness
Abnormality motor neurons; polio
Abnormality neuromuscular synapse; myasthenia
Abnormality muscle: MD
Neurogenic atrophy
Degeneration motor neuron and/or axon
Atrophy type 1, 2 muscle fibers
Trichinella spiralis
Trichinosis
Trichinella spiralis (nematode)
Transmission
Eating raw/poorly cooked pork (encysted larvae)
Pigs fed uncooked garbage
Bear/seal meat
Pork + deer meat
Larva excyst → adult worms small intestine mucosa
Eggs hatch in adult female worm
Larvae released into blood
Larvae encyst in striated muscle
Calcified larvae visible on x-ray
Larvae die if not deposited in skeletal muscle
Clinical findings
Muscle pain
Periorbital edema
Splinter hemorrhages nails
Myocarditis, encephalitis
Dx trichinosis
Pronounced eosinophilia (leukemoid reaction)
Muscle biopsy (encysted larvae)
Invasive group A streptococcus
Types of invasive infections
Necrotizing fasciitis
Myositis
STSS
Toxins produced by streptococcus
Pyrogenic exotoxin A
Superantigen
Activate all T cells → release cytokines
Exotoxin B
Protease destroys tissue; necrotizing fasciitis
Varying mortality
Clostridium tetani: tetanus
G+ anaerobic rod; soil
Spores in soil

(5) Contract quickly; moderate amount of power when contracted
(6) Most useful for stop-and-go activities such as basketball, soccer, and hockey, as well as maximum-output activities such as weight lifting
c. Type 2b fibers
(1) White color caused by decreased myoglobin
(2) Low fatigue resistance
(3) Use anaerobic metabolism
(4) Increased amount of glycogen
(5) Low number of mT; generates ATP mainly from glycolysis
(6) Very fast contraction (highest rate of contraction of all muscle fibers but the fastest rate of fatigue)
(7) Great amount of power when contracting
(8) Useful in short-term anaerobic activities such as sprinting and lifting heavy weights (activities less than a minute). Olympic sprinters have 80% fast-twitch fibers.

B. **Muscle disorders**
1. Pathogenesis of muscle weakness
   a. Abnormality in motor neuron pathways. Example: poliomyelitis
   b. Abnormality in neuromuscular synapse. Example: myasthenia gravis (MG)
   c. Abnormality in muscle. Example: muscular dystrophy (MD)
2. Neurogenic atrophy (Links 24-72 and 24-73)
   a. **Definition:** Muscle atrophy secondary to degeneration of the motor neuron or its axon
   b. Produces atrophy of type 1 and 2 muscle fibers
3. *Trichinella spiralis* infection (called trichinosis)
   a. Epidemiology
      (1) Causative agent is *T. spiralis* (nematode)
      (2) Transmission (Link 24-74)
         (a) Transmitted by eating raw or poorly cooked pork containing the encysted larvae in the muscle
         (b) Common infection on pig farms where pigs are fed uncooked garbage
         (c) Can be transmitted by eating bear and seal meat
         (d) Pork often mixed in with deer meat to make sausage
         (e) Larvae excyst and develop into adult worms within the small intestine mucosa.
            • Eggs hatch within the adult female worm.
            • Larvae are released into the bloodstream.
            • Larvae encyst in striated muscle (Fig. 24-12 A).
            • Larvae encysted in skeletal muscle commonly undergo dystrophic calcification; may be visible on radiography
         (f) Larvae die if they are deposited in other sites.
   b. Clinical findings in trichinosis
      • Muscle pain, periorbital edema (larva), and splinter hemorrhages in the nails
   c. Complications in trichinosis include myocarditis and encephalitis.
   d. Diagnosis of trichinosis
      (1) Pronounced eosinophilia in the peripheral blood that can reach leukemoid proportions (see Chapter 13)
      (2) Muscle biopsy shows the encysted larvae (Link 24-75).
4. Invasive infections caused by group A streptococcus
   a. Types of invasive infections
      (1) Necrotizing fasciitis (see Chapter 25)
      (2) Myositis
      (3) Streptococcal toxic shock syndrome (STSS)
   b. Toxins produced by the streptococcus, causing the clinical findings in the invasive infections
      (1) Pyrogenic exotoxin A
         (a) Superantigen that is associated with STSS
         (b) Superantigens are proteins that bind to and activate all of the T, cells resulting in polyclonal T-cell activation and a massive release of cks.
      (2) Exotoxin B: protease that destroys tissue associated with necrotizing fasciitis (see later)
   c. Death rates range from 20% to 100%.
5. *Clostridium tetani*: tetanus
   a. Epidemiology
      (1) Gram-positive anaerobic rod that lives in the soil
      (2) Transmission: spores in soil

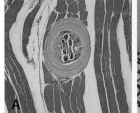
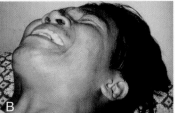
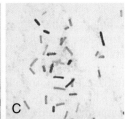
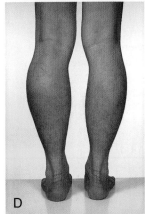
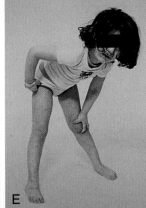
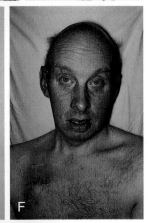
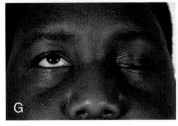
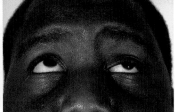

24-12: A, *Trichinella spiralis,* cross-section of a larva in gastrocnemius muscle. **B,** Risus sardonicus in a person with tetanus caused by *Clostridium tetani.* **C,** Gram stain of *Clostridium perfringens* in a wound specimen. Note the rectangular shape of the rods, the presence of many decolorized rods appearing gram negative, and the absence of blood cells. **D,** Duchenne muscular dystrophy (DMD) showing pseudohypertrophy of the calf. **E,** DMD showing a child performing the Gower maneuver to stand up. **F,** Myotonic dystrophy. The patient shows frontal balding, drooping of the eyelids, sagging of the facial muscles, and atrophy of the sternocleidomastoid muscles. **G,** Patient with myasthenia gravis showing ptosis of the left eye *(left)* followed by opening of the eye *(right)* after intravenous injection of Tensilon. *(A from McPherson R, Pincus M:* Henry's Clinical Diagnosis and Management by Laboratory Methods, *22nd ed, Philadelphia, Saunders, 2011, p 1221, Fig. 62-18E; B and C from Murray PR, Rosenthal KS, Pfaller MA:* Medical Microbiology, *6th ed, Philadelphia, Mosby Elsevier, 2009, pp 383, 379, respectively, Figs. 39.4, 39.1, respectively; D to G from Perkin GD:* Mosby's Color Atlas and Text of Neurology, *St. Louis, Mosby, 2002, pp 269, 269, 272, 263, respectively, Figs. 14-10. 14-12, 14-16, 14-5A, B, respectively.)*

(a) Closed wounds (e.g., nail puncture wound)
(b) Skin popping among intravenous drug abusers (IVDA)
(c) Umbilical cord or circumcision sites in newborns

(3) Germination of spores is enhanced if necrosis occurs in association with a poor blood supply.

(4) Organisms are rarely isolated in the wound.

(5) Bacterial proliferation in the wound releases a neurotoxin called tetanospasmin (virulence factor for *C. tetani*; Link 24-76).

(a) *No* inflammatory exudate
(b) Toxin is carried intraaxonally (retrograde) to the CNS.
(c) Toxin binds to ganglioside receptors of spinal afferent fibers; inhibits the release of the inhibitory neurotransmitters (NTs) glycine and γ-amino-butyric acid (GABA) in the spinal cord, causing sustained motor stimulation of all the voluntary muscles.

b. Clinical findings in tetanus

(1) Incubation period is a few days to 2 months.

(2) Begins with muscle stiffness in the jaw followed by:
(a) lockjaw (inability to open the mouth).
(b) risus sardonicus (perpetual, sardonic smile on the face; Fig. 24-12 B).

(3) Slightest stimulus causes generalized, painful muscle contractions.

(4) Contractions of back muscles produce opisthotonus (painful arching of the back; Link 24-77).

(5) Patients are mentally alert.

(6) The mortality rate is 10% to 30% in generalized disease. Pneumonia and cardiac failure are the MC cause of death (COD).

(7) *No* permanent sequelae are present if the patient survives.

(8) Protective antibody titers are *not* high enough to prevent the disease in the future. This underscores the reason why a tetanus toxoid shot at appropriate intervals.

Closed wounds (nail puncture)
Skin-popping IVDA
Umbilical cord/circumcision site
Spores germinate: necrosis/poor blood supply
Rarely isolated in wound
Neurotoxin tetanospasmin (virulence factor)
No inflammatory exudate
Toxin carried intraaxonally (retrograde) → CNS
Binds ganglioside receptors spinal afferent fibers
Inhibit release inhibitory NTs glycine, GABA → sustained contraction voluntary muscles
Clinical findings
Few days to 2 mths
Muscle stiffness jaw
Lockjaw
Risus sardonicus
Painful muscle contractions
Painful arching of back
Mentally alert
Mortality 10% to 30%
Pneumonia, heart failure MC COD
No permanent sequelae
Protective abs do *not* prevent disease in future
Underscores tetanus toxoid shot

6. *Clostridium perfringens*
   a. Epidemiology
      (1) Gram-positive anaerobic rod (Fig. 24-12 C); part of the normal flora in the vagina and colon
      (2) Type A *C. perfringens* is most virulent in humans. Virulence factor is alpha toxin (lecithinase and phospholipase C [PLC]), which damage cell membranes, producing lysis of RBCs (RBC hemolysis), endothelial cells (increased vascular permeability), and tissue destruction.
   b. Diseases associated with *C. perfringens*
      (1) Gas gangrene (myonecrosis)
         (a) Gas bubbles present in tissue produce skin crepitus (grating feeling under the skin) (Link 24-78). Gas is produced by the organism's anaerobic metabolism. Gas is noted on radiographs (e.g., wet gangrene in a diabetic foot; see Fig. 2-16 F).
         (b) Pain, edema, cellulitis, and a foul-smelling exudate in the wound
         (c) Clinical findings: hemolytic anemia, jaundice, shock, disseminated intravascular coagulation (DIC), and renal failure
      (2) Food poisoning
         (a) Heat-resistant spores survive cooking and germinate in food.
         (b) Organisms proliferate rapidly in reheated foods. Example: meat dishes such as beef and turkey
         (c) Enterotoxin (superantigen similar to *S. aureus*) is the virulence factor; produced during spore formation in the gut
         (d) Disease is self-limited.
      (3) Septicemia
      (4) Intraabdominal infections: peritonitis (see Chapter 18), gangrenous cholecystitis (see Chapter 19)
      (5) Pelvic inflammatory disease (PID; see Chapter 22)
      (6) "Backroom abortion" produces septic endometritis (see Chapter 22).
7. Duchenne muscular dystrophy (DMD)
   a. **Definition:** Sex-linked recessive (XR) degenerative muscle disease causing progressive weakness, loss of ambulation, and death from respiratory and cardiac failure in the second decade of life
   b. Epidemiology
      (1) Incidence is 1:3500 male births.
      (2) Pathogenesis
         (a) Absence of dystrophin caused by a frameshift mutation of the dystrophin gene on the X chromosome (Link 24-79)
            • Dystrophin normally anchors actin to the cell membrane glycoprotein in striated and cardiac muscle.
            • Becker type of muscular dystrophy (DM; XR) has reduced amounts of dystrophin or has a defective dystrophin (abnormal size); more benign course than DMD with a life expectancy twice as long as for DMD.
         (b) MC childhood MD
         (c) Progressive degeneration of type 1 and 2 muscle fibers
         (d) Fibrosis and infiltration of muscle tissue by fatty tissue; increase in fatty tissue produces pseudohypertrophy of the calf muscles (Fig. 24-12 D)
   c. Clinical findings in DMD
      (1) Clinically evident by 3 to 5 years of age
      (2) Weakness and wasting of the pelvic muscles
         (a) Child places the hands on the knees for help in standing (Gower maneuver; Fig. 24-12 E; Link 24-80).
         (b) Waddling (duck-like) gait
         (c) Loss ambulation by 9 to 12 years
         (d) Scoliosis
      (3) Cardiac involvement causes cardiomyopathy, leading to heart failure and arrhythmias.
      (4) Death from respiratory failure or cardiac failure by age 20 years
   d. Laboratory findings in DMD
      (1) Serum creatine kinase (CK) is increased at birth (20–100 times greater).
      (2) Progressively declines as the muscle degenerates over time
      (3) Female carriers have increased levels of serum creatine kinase (CK).

e. Diagnosis of DMD
   (1) Muscle biopsy
   (2) Electromyography (EMG)
   (3) DNA testing (Western blot). Using this test, prenatal diagnosis via chorionic villous (CV) sampling is possible.

8. Myotonic dystrophy
   a. **Definition:** Progressive AD disease in which the muscles are weak and are slow to relax after contraction
   b. Epidemiology
      (1) AD disease
      (2) MC adult muscular dystrophy (MD)
      (3) Trinucleotide repeat disorder involving the repeat of CTG (cytosine-thymine-adenine; see Chapter 6); genetic disorder encoded on chromosome 19
      (4) Selective atrophy of type 1 slow fibers
   c. Clinical findings in myotonic dystrophy
      (1) Facial muscle weakness (Fig. 24-12 F); sagging in the face and problems closing the mouth
      (2) Percussion (tapping the muscle) and grip myotonia. Myotonia refers to an inability to relax the voluntary muscles (sustained grip).
      (3) Frontal balding (Fig. 24-12 F), cataracts, testicular atrophy
      (4) Glucose intolerance
      (5) Cardiac involvement (conduction defects)
   d. Laboratory studies show an increase in serum CK.
   e. Diagnosis of myotonic dystrophy is made by EMG and muscle biopsy.
   f. Muscle wasting and defects in cardiac function are the MCCs of death.

9. Congenital myopathies
   a. **Definition:** Rare group of myopathies in children attributable to multiple different protein polymorphisms. Muscle hypotonia is a key feature.
   b. Epidemiology; causes
      (1) Muscle hypotonia is a state of low muscle tone (amount of tension or resistance to stretch in a muscle). It is often accompanied by decreased muscle strength.
      (2) Often called floppy baby syndrome (Link 24-81)
      (3) Some examples include central core disease and nemaline rod disease.

10. Myasthenia gravis
    a. **Definition:** Autoimmune disorder of postsynaptic neuromuscular transmission leading to muscle weakness
    b. Epidemiology
       (1) More common in females than males. Male:female ratio is 2:3.
       (2) Affects men in the sixth and seventh decades of life
       (3) Affects women in the second and third decades of life
       (4) Pathogenesis
          (a) Autoimmune disease that affects postsynaptic neuromuscular transmission
          (b) Autoantibodies directed against the acetylcholine (ACh) receptors (type II HSR; Link 24-82). Antibodies inhibit or destroy the receptors, causing a decrease in functional Ach receptors.
          (c) Antibody is synthesized in the thymus. Thymic hyperplasia is present with lymphoid follicles with germinal centers in 85% of cases.
    c. Clinical findings in myasthenia gravis
       (1) Fluctuating muscle weakness that is worsened with exercise and improved with rest
       (2) Ptosis (drooping of the eyelids) is the MC initial finding (Fig. 24-12 G, *left*). Diplopia (double vision) is also common and is caused by eye muscle weakness.
       (3) Weakness in the proximal muscles, diaphragm, and in neck extension and neck flexion in 85% of cases
       (4) Dysphagia (difficulty in swallowing) for solids and liquids (see Chapter 18). Dysphagia primarily occurs in the upper esophagus, which has striated muscle rather than smooth muscle.
       (5) Deep tendon reflexes (DTRs), skin sensation, and coordination are all normal.
       (6) Increased risk for developing a thymoma in 15% of cases
    d. Diagnosis
       (1) Tensilon (edrophonium) test
          (a) Tensilon inhibits acetylcholinesterase (normally hydrolyzes Ach).
          (b) Increase in acetylcholine reverses muscle weakness (Fig. 24-12 G, *right*).
       (2) Single-fiber EMG results are abnormal in 95% of cases.

24-13: Dupuytren contractures in the hand. The *arrows* show thickening of the palmar fascia, producing cords that cause the fingers to have a hooklike deformity. *(From Grieg JD:* Color Atlas of Surgical Diagnosis, *London, Mosby-Wolfe, 1996, p 40, Fig. 7-4.)*

Soft tissue disorders

Fibromyalgia

Musculoskeletal pain without inflammation

Female > males: M:F ratio 1:2

MCC female muscular pain

Disorder of pain regulation

Fatigue, sleep disruption, anxiety/depression

Specific tender points

Fibromatosis

Non-neoplastic proliferation connective tissue

Fibrous tissue infiltration muscle

Dupuytren contracture: fibromatosis of palmar fascia

Fibromatosis palmar fascia

Contraction single/multiple fingers; palpable cords

Ring finger MC; index finger/thumb spared

Jack hammer, hand trauma, alcoholism, smoking, DM

Desmoid tumor

Aggressive fibromatosis

M:F = 1:2

?Role of estrogen

Abdominal wall common in women

Painless lump

Often recur after surgery

Previous trauma some cases

FAP/Gardner syndrome

Liposarcoma: MC adult sarcoma

IV. Soft Tissue Disorders

  A. Fibromyalgia *(Modified from Ferri FF:* 2017 Ferri's Clinical Advisor, *Philadelphia, Elsevier, 2017, p 475.)*

    1. **Definition:** Syndrome characterized by widespread musculoskeletal pain without evidence of muscle inflammation or increase in muscle enzymes

    2. Epidemiology

      a. More common in females than males. Male:female ratio is 1:2.

      b. MCC of muscular pain in women between the ages of 20 and 55 years

      c. Disorder of pain regulation (abnormal ascending and descending pain pathways leads to central amplification of pain signals)

    3. Clinical findings in fibromyalgia

      a. Key features include fatigue and sleep disruption (easily fatigued, unrefreshed sleep), psychiatric (anxiety, depression), somatic symptoms (headache), and cognitive disturbance (learning, memory, perception, and problem solving).

      b. Specific tender points have been identified (Link 24-83).

  B. Fibromatosis

    1. **Definition:** Disorder characterized by a non-neoplastic, proliferation of connective tissue

    2. Fibrous tissue infiltration of tissue (usually muscle)

    3. Dupuytren contracture (Fig. 24-13)

      a. **Definition:** Fibromatosis of the palmar fascia

      b. Epidemiology/clinical

        (1) Causes forward contraction of single or multiple fingers (palpable cords); frequently involves MCP joints or PIP joints

        (2) Most commonly observed in persons of Northern European descent

        (3) Ring finger is most commonly involved followed by the fifth digit and then the middle finger. Index finger and the thumb are usually spared.

        (4) Risk factors include manual labor with vibration exposure (jack hammer), prior hand trauma, alcoholism, smoking, and DM.

    4. Desmoid tumor

      a. **Definition:** Aggressive fibromatosis that may involve any part of the body

      b. Epidemiology

        (1) Male:female ratio is 1:2. E may play a role in women.

        (2) Abdominal wall is a common site in women; presents as a painless lump in the tissue.

        (3) Often recur after surgical excision in 20% to 50% of cases

        (4) Frequently associated with previous trauma

        (5) Associated with familial adenomatous polyposis (FAP) syndrome and Gardner syndrome (see Chapter 18)

  C. Selected soft tissue tumors (Table 24-2; Link 24-84)

V. Selected Orthopedic Disorders (Table 24-3; Figs. 24-14 and 24-15)

  • Link 24-85 depicts different types of fractures.

TABLE 24-2   Soft Tissue Tumors

TUMOR TYPE	LOCATION	COMMENT
Lipoma (see Fig. 9-1 B)	Trunk, neck, proximal extremities	• Most common benign soft tissue tumor • Arises in subcutaneous tissue (? after trauma to tissue) • *No* clinical significance
Liposarcoma	Thigh, retroperitoneum	• Most common adult sarcoma • Lipoblasts identified with fat stains
Fibrosarcoma	Thigh, upper limb	May arise after irradiation
Malignant fibrous histiocytoma	Retroperitoneum, thigh	Associated with radiation therapy and scarring
Rhabdomyoma	Heart, tongue, and vagina	Benign heart tumor associated with tuberous sclerosis.
Embryonal rhabdomyosarcoma (see Fig. 22-3 A; Link 21-16; see Chapter 21)	Penis and vagina	• Most common sarcoma in children • Grapelike, necrotic mass protrudes from penis or vagina
Leiomyoma (see Fig. 22-11 F; Links 24-80, 24-81, and 24-82)	Uterus, stomach	• Most commonly located in uterus • Most common benign tumor in GI tract
Leiomyosarcoma	GI tract, uterus	Most common sarcoma of GI tract and uterus
Neurofibrosarcoma	Major nerve trunks	Associated with neurofibromatosis (see Chapter 26)
Synovial sarcoma (Link 24-84)	Around joints	• Does *not* arise from synovial cells in joints but from mesenchymal cells around joints • Biphasic pattern: epithelial cells forming glands + intervening spindle cells

GI, Gastrointestinal.

TABLE 24-3   Selected Orthopedic Disorders

DISORDER	COMMENTS
Types of fractures (Link 24-85)	• Simple incomplete, simple complete, compound, and comminuted.
Colles fracture (Fig. 24-14 A)	• Common fracture when falling on outstretched hand • Fracture of distal radius with or without fracture of ulnar styloid
Clavicular fracture (Link 24-86)	• Clavicular fractures are seen in neonates; often caused by a fall onto an outstretched upper extremity, a fall onto a shoulder, or a direct blow to the clavicle
Scaphoid bone fracture in wrist (Link 24-87)	• Largest of the proximal bones in the wrist and the most frequently fractured carpal bone • Has a prominent laterally located tubercle, which can be palpated in the "anatomic snuff box" (depression below the base of the thumb) • Proximal and distal ends of the bone are connected by a narrow waist, which may fracture with forced abduction and extension • The waist comes in contact with the radial styloid process and can be fractured • Proximal fragment of the bone has a diminished or no blood supply; may result in either poor healing or aseptic necrosis (infarction)
Rotator cuff and tear (see Fig. 24-14 B; Link 24-88)	• Components: tendon insertions of supraspinatus, infraspinatus, teres minor, subscapularis muscles • Rotator cuff tear: pain or weakness with active shoulder abduction • Diagnosis: arthrography, MRI
Tennis elbow	• Causes: racquet sports, repetitive use of a hammer or screwdriver, arm wrestling (top roll; pronation of forearm; palm faces down). • Pain where the extensor muscle tendons insert near the lateral epicondyle (lateral epicondylitis) of the distal radius; pain when gripping something or pronating the forearm
Golfer's elbow	• Pain where the flexor muscle tendons insert near the medial epicondyle (medial epicondylitis) of the distal radius • Pain duplicated by flexing hand muscles and supinating the arm (hook in arm wrestling movement; palm faces up)
De Quervain tenosynovitis (see Fig. 24-14 C)	• Chronic stenosing tenosynovitis of the first dorsal compartment of the wrist • Overuse of the hands and wrist • First dorsal compartment has abductor pollicis longus and extensor pollicis brevis • Excessive friction thickens tendon sheath, causing stenosis of the osseofibrous tunnel • Pain on the radial aspect of the wrist is aggravated by moving the thumb • Finkelstein test: patient puts thumb in the palm, closes fist, tilts hand toward little finger (ulnar deviation); causes pain in the first dorsal compartment
Ganglion (synovial) cyst (see Fig. 24-14 D)	• Bulge on the dorsum of the wrist when the wrist is flexed • More common in women than in men • Cyst communicates with synovial sheaths on the dorsum of the wrist
Compartment syndrome (see Fig. 24-14 E)	• Increase of pressure in a confined space (fascial compartment) • Pressure reduces perfusion, may cause ischemic contractures of the muscle(s) • Most common locations are anterior and posterior compartments in the leg and the forearm muscle compartment • 5 *Ps*: pain, paresthesias, pallor, paralysis, and pulselessness • Risk factors: fractures, injuries to arteries or soft tissue, excessive use of the muscles (cyclists; arm wrestlers) • Volkmann ischemic contracture: displaced supracondylar fracture of the distal humerus causes compression of the brachial artery and median nerve. Forearm muscles (superficial and deep flexor muscles) may undergo contracture. Although most of the muscles are innervated by the median nerve, the flexor carpi ulnaris is innervated by the ulnar nerve. Diagnosis: Measure pressures in the compartment.

Continued

TABLE 24-3   Selected Orthopedic Disorders—cont'd

DISORDER	COMMENTS
Carpal tunnel syndrome (see Fig. 24-14 F, G; (Links 24-89 and 24-90)	• Entrapment syndrome of the median nerve in the transverse carpal ligament of the wrist • Causes: rheumatoid arthritis and pregnancy most common causes. Other causes: obesity, excessive use of hands, acromegaly, amyloidosis, wrist curls in arm wrestling • Pain, numbness, or paresthesias in the thumb, index finger, second finger, third finger, and the radial side of the fourth finger • Thenar atrophy produces "ape hand" appearance • Diagnosis: nerve conduction, electromyography
Intervertebral disk disease (see Fig. 24-14 H; Links 24-91, 24-92, 24-93, 24-94, 24-95 and 24-96)	• Degeneration of fibrocartilage/nucleus pulposus. Ruptured disk material may herniate posteriorly and compress the nerve root, spinal cord, or both. • Radicular pain: depends the location of the ruptured disk • Herniation of L3–L4 disk: loss of knee jerk (femoral nerve L2–L4) • Herniation of L4–L5 disk: *no* loss of reflexes (ankle and knee reflexes intact) • Herniation of L5–S1 disk: loss of ankle reflex (tibial nerve L4–S3)
Knee joint injuries (see Fig. 24-14 I, J; (Links 24-97, 24-98, 24-99, and 24-100)	• Valgus injury: angulation away from the midline. Laterally originating force is applied to the knee (e.g., clipping injury in football). • Varus injury: angulation toward the midline. Medially originating force is applied to the knee. • McMurray test: meniscus injuries • Anterior and posterior draw test: cruciate injuries • "Unhappy triad": most common internal derangement of the knee joint. Valgus injury (acute): damage to the lateral meniscus, medial collateral ligament, anterior cruciate ligament. If chronic, the medial meniscus is more commonly injured than the lateral meniscus.
Scoliosis (see Fig. 24-14 K; Link 24-101)	• Lateral curvature of the spine (S- or C-shaped on radiographs) • Congenital, idiopathic, or related to another disease (e.g., cerebral palsy) • Idiopathic type: usually affects adolescent girls between 10 and 16 years of age. Usually a right thoracic curve. Forward bending causes a paraspinous prominence on the right from a hump in the ribs caused by a rotational component of the vertebra.
Talipes equinovarus (clubfoot; see Fig. 24-14 L) Genu varus and genu valgus	• Malalignment of the calcaneotalar–navicular complex. Entire foot is deviated toward the midline. Results in forefoot adduction, fixed inversion of the hindfoot, and fixed plantar flexion. The Achilles tendon is shortened; hence, the foot assumes the position of a horse's hoof. • Occurs in 1:1000 births. Multifactorial inheritance. More common in males than females. Bilateral in 50% of cases. Increased risk if either parent has the condition. Increased risk with smoking during pregnancy. • Associations: deformation in oligohydramnios (decreased amount of amniotic fluid in the amniotic sac) in association with juvenile polycystic kidney disease (see Chapter 6), breech presentation, spina bifida, and neuromuscular disorders • Genu varus (Links 24-102, *left*, 24-103 A, and 24-104): bowleg; common in the 1- to 3-year-old age group • Genu valgus (Links 24-102, *right* and 24-103 B): knock-knee; common in the 3- to 5-year-old age group

MRI, Magnetic resonance imaging.

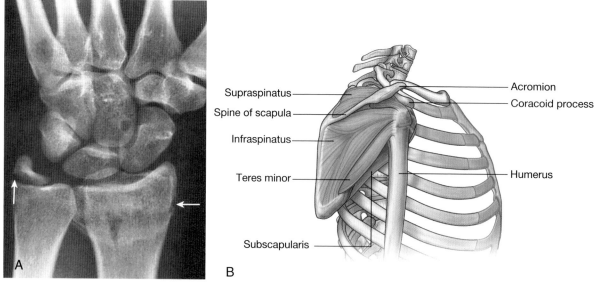

24-14: A, Radiograph showing a Colles fracture. Note the fracture lines *(arrows)* in the distal radius and the styloid process of the ulna. **B,** Rotator cuff muscles (supraspinatus, infraspinatus, teres minor, subscapularis).

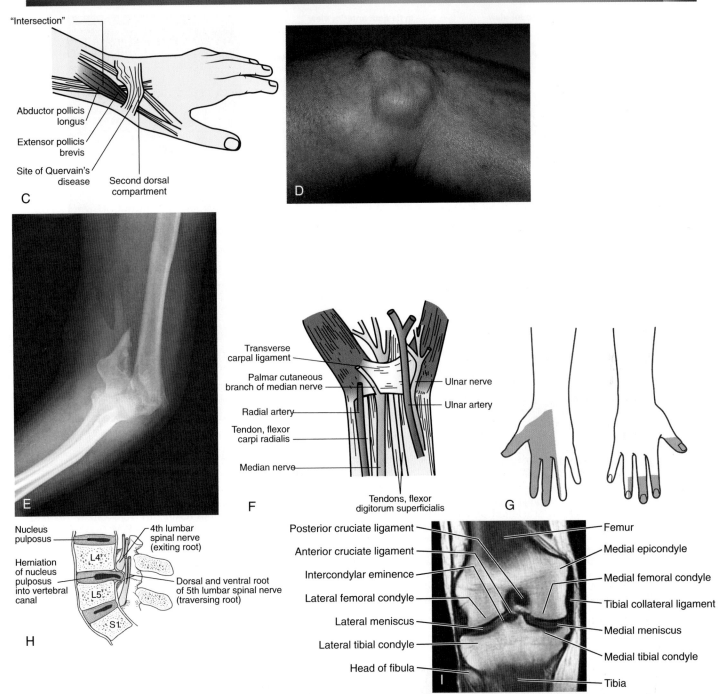

"Intersection"

Abductor pollicis
longus

Extensor pollicis
brevis

Site of Quervain's
disease

Second dorsal
compartment

C

D

E

Transverse
carpal ligament

Palmar cutaneous
branch of median nerve

Radial artery

Tendon, flexor
carpi radialis

Median nerve

Ulnar nerve

Ulnar artery

Tendons, flexor
digitorum superficialis

F

G

Nucleus
pulposus

Herniation
of nucleus
pulposus
into vertebral
canal

4th lumbar
spinal nerve
(exiting root)

Dorsal and ventral root
of 5th lumbar spinal nerve
(traversing root)

L4

L5

S1

H

Posterior cruciate ligament

Anterior cruciate ligament

Intercondylar eminence

Lateral femoral condyle

Lateral meniscus

Lateral tibial condyle

Head of fibula

Femur

Medial epicondyle

Medial femoral condyle

Tibial collateral ligament

Medial meniscus

Medial tibial condyle

Tibia

I

24-14 cont'd: C, De Quervain tenosynovitis. First dorsal compartment has the abductor pollicis longus and extensor pollicis brevis. Excessive friction thickens tendon sheath causing stenosis of the osseofibrous tunnel. **D,** Ganglion cyst on the dorsum of the wrist. **E,** Supracondylar fracture with significant displacement of the distal fragment. **F,** Carpal tunnel anatomy. **G,** Cutaneous distribution of the median nerve. **H,** Herniated lumbar intervertebral disk. Herniation usually occurs posterolaterally and affects traversing root, not exiting root (i.e., herniation at L4–L5 affects the L5 root, and herniation at L5–S1 affects the S1 root). **I,** Magnetic resonance image of a normal knee joint and its structures.

Continued

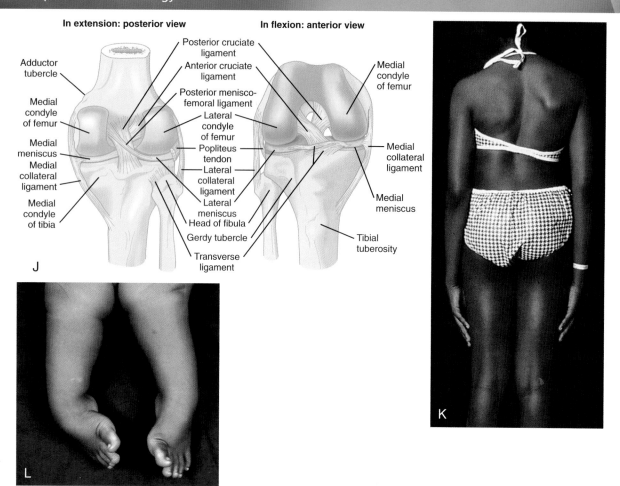

In extension: posterior view   In flexion: anterior view

24-14 cont'd: **J,** Anatomy of the knee joint. **K,** Patient with scoliosis. The patient has lateral curvature of the spine with increased convexity to the right. There is obvious scapular asymmetry in the upright position. **L,** Talipes equinovarus (clubfoot). Note the plantar flexion (cavus) and adduction of the forefoot or midfoot on the hindfoot, and the hindfoot is in varus and equinus (CAVE). *(A from Katz D, Math K, Groskin S: Radiology Secrets, Philadelphia, Hanley & Belfus, 1998, p 440, Fig. 9; B from Drake RL, Vogl AW, Mitchell AWM: Gray's Anatomy for Students, 2nd ed, Philadelphia, Churchill Livingstone Elsevier, 2010, p 656, Fig. 7-9C; C and F from Townsend C: Sabiston Textbook of Surgery, 18th ed, Philadelphia, Saunders Elsevier, 2008, pp 2185, 2187, respectively, Figs. 74-35, 74-36, respectively; D from Swartz MH: Textbook of Physical Diagnosis, 5th ed, Philadelphia, Saunders Elsevier, 2006, p 171, Fig. 8-74; E and J from Marx J: Rosen's Emergency Medicine Concepts and Clinical Practice, 7th ed, Philadelphia, Mosby Elsevier, 2010, pp 556, 646, respectively, Figs. 49-20, 54-1, respectively; G to I from Moore NA, Roy WA: Rapid Review Gross and Developmental Anatomy, 2nd ed, Philadelphia, Mosby Elsevier, 2007, pp 187, 6, 148, respectively, Figs. 6-16, 1-8, 5-6, respectively; K from Zitelli B: Atlas of Pediatric Physical Diagnosis, 3rd ed, Philadelphia, Mosby, 1997; L from Kliegman R: Nelson Textbook of Pediatrics, 19th ed, Philadelphia, Elsevier Saunders, 2011, p 2337, Fig. 666-2.)*

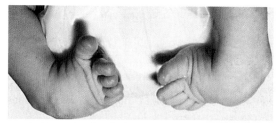

24-15: Bilateral clubfoot (talipes equinovarus). Note the fixed plantar flexion (cavus) and adduction (bent toward the midline) of the forefoot and midfoot. The hindfoot is in varus (distal part of the joint is medial) and equinus (upward bending motion of the ankle joint is limited). *(From Zitelli B, McIntire S, Nowalk A: Zitelli and Davis' Atlas of Pediatric Physical Diagnosis, Saunders Elsevier 6th ed, 2012, p 9, Fig. 1-20F.)*

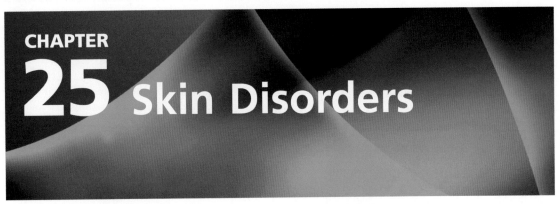

CHAPTER 25 Skin Disorders

ABBREVIATIONS

MC most common   MCC most common cause   Hx history

I. Skin Histology and Terminology
  A. Normal skin histology
   1. Epidermis layers (Fig. 25-1; Link 25-1)
      a. Stratum basalis
         (1) **Definition:** Lowermost layer of the epidermis along the BM; only layer where there are actively dividing stem cells present
         (2) Mitoses should be limited to this area.
      b. Stratum spinosum. **Definition:** Layer that contains prominent desmosome attachments.
      c. Stratum granulosum. **Definition:** Granular layer with keratohyaline granules
      d. Stratum corneum. **Definition:** Superficial layer of skin; contains anucleate cells with keratin
         • Site for superficial dermatophyte infections (see later).
   2. Dermis (Fig. 25-1)
      a. Papillary dermis
         • **Definition:** The superficial aspects of the dermis; composed of loose connective tissue; location where edema fluid collects
      b. Reticular dermis
         • **Definition:** The deeper layer of the dermis; composed of dense dermal collagen
   3. Histology of sweat gland, apocrine gland, and hair follicle with sebaceous glands (Fig. 25-2)
   4. Melanocytes
      a. **Definition:** Melanin-producing cells derived from the neural crest cells
      b. Located in the stratum basalis; dendritic processes extend between the keratinocytes
      c. Melanin pigment is synthesized in membrane-bound melanosomes.
         (1) Tyrosinase converts tyrosine to 3,4-dihydroxyphenylalanine (DOPA).
         (2) DOPA is converted to melanin.
         (3) Melanosomes are transferred by dendritic processes to the keratinocytes.
      d. Skin color
         (1) Number of melanocytes is essentially the *same* in all races.
         (2) Melanin is degraded more rapidly in whites than in blacks.
         (3) In whites, melanosomes are concentrated in the basal layer.
         (4) In blacks, melanosomes are present throughout all layers. In blacks, melanocytes are larger than those in whites and have more dendritic processes. Blacks have the same number of melanocytes as whites.
      e. Sunlight and adrenocorticotropic hormone (ACTH) from the anterior pituitary gland stimulate melanin synthesis in the melanocytes.

Stratum basalis

Basalis: stem cells for division

No mitoses beyond this layer

Stratus spinosum

Desmosome attachments

Stratus granulosum

Keratohyaline granules

Stratum corneum

Anucleate cells/keratin

Superficial dermatophyte infections

Dermis

Papillary dermis

Loose connective tissue; site for edema fluid

Reticular dermis

Dense dermal collagen

Melanocytes

Neural crest origin

Stratum basalis

Melanin synthesized in melanosomes

Tyrosinase: tyrosine → DOPA

DOPA → melanin

Melanosomes transferred by dendritic processes to keratinocytes

Skin color

Melanocytes *same* all races

Whites: melanin basal layer

Blacks: melanin all layers

Melanocytes larger in blacks

Sunlight/ACTH stimulate melanin synthesis

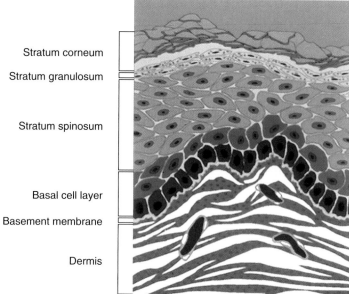

25-1: Epidermal layers and papillary dermis. *(From Fitzpatrick JE, Morelli JG: Dermatology Secrets Plus, 4th ed, Philadelphia, Elsevier Mosby, 2011, p 7, Fig. 1.2.)*

Stratum corneum
Stratum granulosum
Stratum spinosum
Basal cell layer
Basement membrane
Dermis

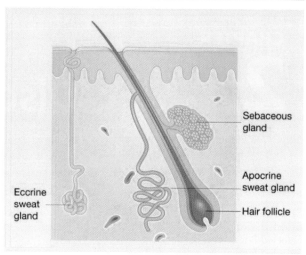

25-2: Sweat gland, apocrine gland, and hair follicle with sebaceous glands. *(From Marks JG, Miller JJ: Lookingbill and Marks' Principles of Dermatology, 5th ed, Philadelphia, Saunders Elsevier, 2013, p 7, Fig. 2.11.)*

Sebaceous gland
Apocrine sweat gland
Hair follicle
Eccrine sweat gland

5. Age-related skin changes (Table 6-7)
   a. Common sites for dermatologic lesions in older adults (Fig. 25-3)
   b. Histologic changes in older adults (Fig. 25-4)
      (1) Decreased number of hair follicles and sweat glands, the latter associated with an increased risk of heat-related injuries
      (2) Decreased thickness of the epidermis
      (3) Decreased amount of dermal collagen and elastic tissue; decreased amount of subcutaneous fat
      (4) Increase in cross-linking (X-linking) of collagen and elastic tissue makes the skin brittle and the small blood vessels fragile, leading to rupture and extravasation of blood into the subcutaneous tissue (senile purpura [SP]; Link 25-2).
      (5) Increase in flat, brown lesions in sun-exposed area (solar lentigo; Link 25-2). Colloquial term is "liver spots."
      (6) Longitudinal ridging and beading in the nails (look like teardrops; Link 25-3).
   B. **Common terms used in dermatology** (Table 25-1; Link 25-4)
II. **Selected Viral Disorders**
   A. **Common wart**
      1. **Definition:** Benign tumor caused by human papillomavirus (HPV)
      2. Epidemiology
         a. Verrucous papular lesions that are covered by scales (Fig. 25-5 A)
         b. Caused by HPV (DNA virus)
         c. Common sites are the fingers (Link 25-5) and soles of the feet (Link 25-6).
   B. **Molluscum contagiosum**
      1. **Definition:** Bowl-shaped lesion with a central depression filled with keratin (Fig. 25-5 B)
      2. Epidemiology
         a. Caused by a poxvirus (DNA virus)
         b. Central depressions contain viral particles called molluscum bodies (Links 25-7 and 25-8) that turn bright red when the immune response is initiated.
         c. Common disorder in children because their immune systems are not fully developed
         d. Usually disseminated in human immunodeficiency virus (HIV) infections because of the loss of cellular immunity
         e. Transmission
            (1) Can be sexually transmitted in adults (common in AIDS)
            (2) Self-inoculation may occur through scratching; causes translocation of the infective viral particles from the crater to another location. It commonly occurs in children because they constantly pick at the lesions.
         f. Lesions usually resolve over 2 to 3 weeks

Age-related skin changes

Histologic changes

↓Number hair follicles/ sweat glands

↓Thickness epidermis

↓ Dermal collagen/elastic tissue

↓Subcutaneous fat

↑X-linking collagen/elastic tissue → fragile vessels → SP

Solar lentigo ("liver spots")

Longitudinal ridges, nail beading

Viral disorders

Common warts

Benign tumor: HPV

Verrucous papular lesions

HPV: DNA virus

Fingers/soles feet

Molluscum contagiosum

Bowl shaped

Poxvirus (DNA)

Umbilicated; viral particles (molluscum bodies)

Common in children

Disseminated in HIV infections

Sexual transmission adults

Self-inoculation (children)

Resolve 2–3 wks

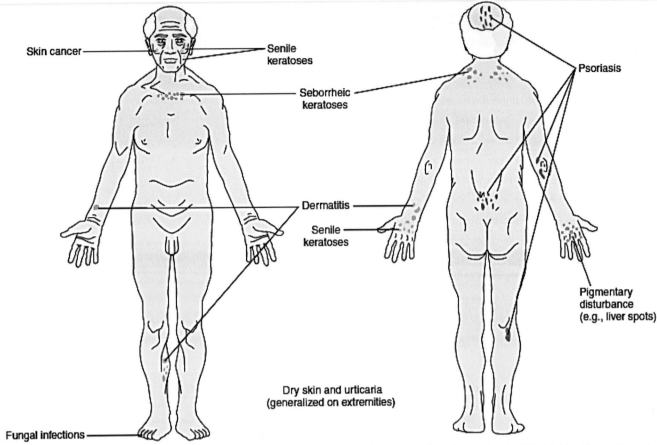

25-3: Sites of common dermatoses of older adults. *(From Copstead LE, Banasik JL:* Pathophysiology, *5th ed, Philadelphia, Elsevier Saunders, 2013, p 1087, Fig. 53-41.)*

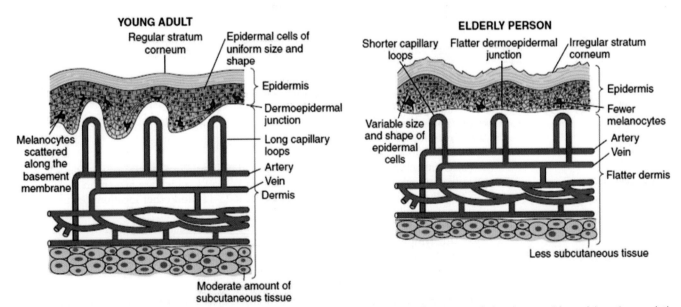

25-4: Histologic changes associated with aging in normal human skin. Note the flattening of the dermoepidermal junction and the shortening of capillary loops in older skin. Variability in size and shape of epidermal cells, irregularity of stratum corneum, and loss of melanocytes are also apparent. Age-associated loss of dermal thickness and subcutaneous fat is also illustrated. *(From Copstead LE, Banasik JL:* Pathophysiology, *5th ed, Philadelphia, Elsevier Saunders, 2013, p 1058, Fig. 53-2.)*

TABLE 25-1 Common Terms in Dermatology

TERM	DEFINITION	EXAMPLE
MACROSCOPIC		
Macule	Pigmented or erythematous flat lesion on skin	Tinea versicolor
Papule	Peaked or dome-shaped surface elevation <5 mm in diameter	Acne vulgaris
Nodule	Elevated, dome-shaped lesion >5 mm in diameter	Basal cell carcinoma
Plaque	Flattened, elevated area on epidermis >5 mm in diameter	Psoriasis
Vesicle	Fluid-filled blister <5 mm in diameter	Varicella (chickenpox)
Bulla	Fluid-filled blister >5 mm in diameter	Bullous pemphigoid
Pustule	Fluid-filled blister with inflammatory cells	Impetigo
Wheal (hive)	Edematous, transient papule or plaque caused by infiltration of dermis by fluid	Urticaria
Scales	Excessive number of dead keratinocytes produced by abnormal keratinization	Seborrheic dermatitis
Verrucous	Thickened epidermis with scales giving it a "warty" appearance	Venereal warts (condyloma acuminate)
MICROSCOPIC		
Hyperkeratosis	Increased thickness of stratum corneum produces scaly appearance of skin	Psoriasis
Parakeratosis	Persistence of nuclei within the stratum corneum layer	Psoriasis
Papillomatosis	Spire-like projections from surface of skin or downward into papillary dermis	Verruca vulgaris
Acantholysis	Loss of cohesion between keratinocytes	Pemphigus vulgaris

Rubeola

Maculopapular rash

RNA paramyxovirus

Vaccination ↓incidence

Clinical findings

Threes Cs: cough, coryza, *conjunctivitis*

Koplik spots buccal mucosa

Erythematous rash *after* Koplik spots disappear

Cytotoxic T cell damage ECs

Rash "down and out"

Head, trunk, extremities

Confluent face/trunk; discrete extremities

Complications

Giant cell pneumonia

WF MGCs, eosinophilic intranuclear inclusions

Acute appendicitis children

Lymphoid hyperplasia → ischemia → necrosis → acute inflammation

Otitis media

Encephalitis

Before immunization common COD

Not teratogenic; *no* congenital malformations

Rubella

3-Day measles; 3 Cs (cough, coryza, conjunctivitis)

C. **Rubeola (regular measles)**
1. **Definition:** Viral infectious disease characterized by a confluent erythematous maculopapular rash on the skin and Koplik spots on the buccal mucosa
2. Epidemiology
   a. Caused by an RNA paramyxovirus
   b. Vaccination has reduced the incidence of rubeola.
3. Clinical findings
   a. Prodrome consists of fever, cough, coryza (runny nose), and conjunctivitis (3 Cs).
   b. Koplik spots develop on the buccal mucosa, initially near the second molars. They appear as white spots overlying an erythematous base (Fig. 25-5 C; Link 25-9).
   c. Erythematous maculopapular rash develops *after* disappearance the Koplik spots (Fig. 25-5 D; Link 25-10).
      (1) Cytotoxic T cell damage of endothelial cells (ECs) that contain the virus
      (2) Typically, the rash begins on the head and then spreads to the trunk and extremities ("down and out" rash).
      (3) Tends to become confluent on the face and trunk but discrete (localized) on the extremities
   d. Complications
      (1) Giant cell pneumonia: Fusion of infected cells produce Warthin-Finkeldey (WF) multinucleated giant cells (MGCs). The WF cells, which are present in the inflammatory infiltrate in the lungs (Link 25-11) and other locations, exhibit eosinophilic intranuclear and intracytoplasmic inclusions.
      (2) Acute appendicitis in children: Rubeola virus stimulates lymphoid hyperplasia in the lymphoid tissue in the wall of the appendix, causing lymphoid hyperplasia. The lymphoid hyperplasia causes ischemia from compression of small vessels, leading to ischemic injury, necrosis, and acute inflammation with neutrophils.
      (3) Otitis media (infection of the middle ear)
      (4) Encephalitis (inflammation of the brain): *Before* immunization, encephalitis was a common cause of death (COD) in people with rubeola; now it is seen primarily in underdeveloped countries because of a lack of immunization.
      (5) Virus is *not* teratogenic and does *not* cause congenital malformations.
D. **Rubella (German measles)**
1. **Definition:** Rubella is characterized by a viral exanthema (rash) caused by hematogenous dissemination to the skin. The rash, which characteristically lasts for 3 days (thus the alternate name of "3-day measles"), is associated with the classic prodrome of cough, coryza (runny nose [rhinorrhea]), and conjunctivitis (the 3 Cs).

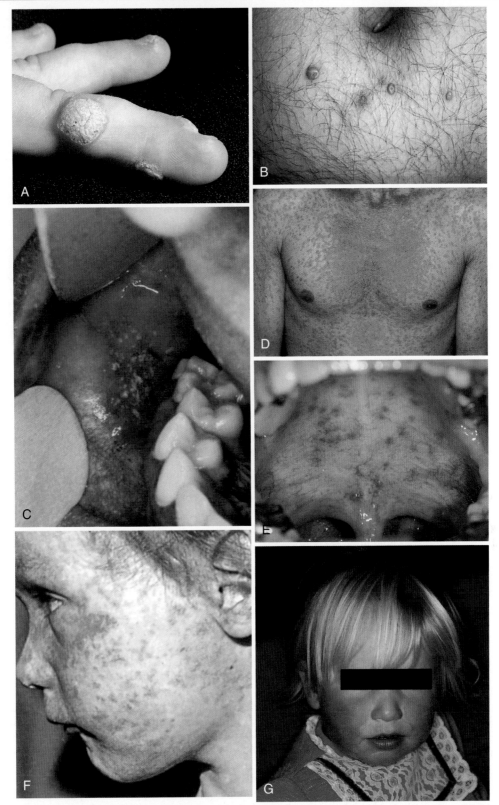

25-5: Viral infections. **A,** Verruca vulgaris (common wart) on the fingers, showing scaling, verrucous papules with interrupted skin lines. **B,** Molluscum contagiosum, showing small bowl-shaped lesions with central areas of depression (umbilication). **C,** Rubeola (regular measles). Note the white Koplik spots on the erythematous surface of the buccal mucosa. **D,** Rubeola. A macular rash begins on the face and neck and then becomes maculopapular and spreads to the trunk and extremities in irregular confluent patches. **E,** Rubella. Note the red Forchheimer spots on the soft and hard palate. **F,** Rubella. Note the fine pinkish red maculopapular rash that usually begins on the hairline and then extends cephalocaudally. **G,** Erythema infectiosum. Note the "slapped face" appearance.

Continued

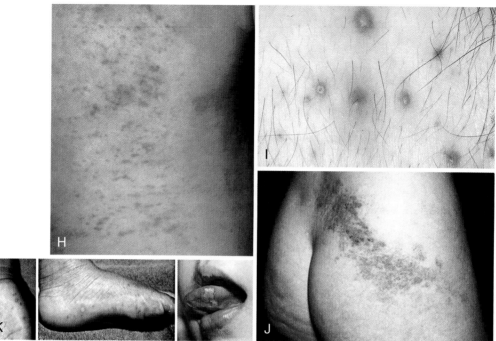

25-5 cont'd: H, Roseola infantum. Note the maculopapular rash, which normally blanches with pressure. There are subtle peripheral halos caused by vasoconstriction around some of the lesions. **I,** Varicella. Note the vesicles and pustules surrounded by an erythematous base. The lesions are at different stages of development. **J,** Herpes zoster (shingles). Note the erythematous vesicular rash with the characteristic "band" distribution, which starts from the midline and extends to the lateral trunk. **K,** Hand-foot-and-mouth disease caused by coxsackievirus. Note the vesicles on the hands and feet and in the mouth. **(A** from Lookingbill D, Marks J: Principles of Dermatology, 3rd ed, Philadelphia, Saunders, 2000, p 68, Fig. 6-1A; **B** and **G** from Savin JA, Hunter JAA, Hepburn NC: Diagnosis in Color: Skin Signs in Clinical Medicine, London, Mosby-Wolfe, 1997, pp 79, 6, respectively, Figs. 2-47, 1-10, respectively; **C** from Goldman L, Schafer AI: Cecil's Medicine, 24th ed, Philadelphia, Saunders Elsevier, 2012, p 2105, Fig. 375-1; **D** from Goldman L, Ausiello D: Cecil's Medicine, 23rd ed, Philadelphia, Saunders Elsevier, 2008, p 2476, Fig. 390.2); **E** from Eisen D, Lynch DP: The Mouth: Diagnosis and Treatment, St. Louis, Mosby, 1998; **F** and **K** from Kliegman, R: Nelson Textbook of Pediatrics, 19th ed, Philadelphia, Elsevier Saunders, 2011, pp 1076, 1090, respectively, Figs. 239-3, 242-1, respectively; **H** from Paller AS, Mancini AJ [eds]: Hurwitz Clinical Pediatric Dermatology, 3rd ed, Philadelphia, Elsevier, 2006, p 434; **I** from Bouloux P: Self-Assessment Picture Tests Medicine, Vol. 2, London, Mosby-Wolfe, 1997, p 99, Fig. 198; **J** from Forbes C, Jackson W: Color Atlas and Text of Clinical Medicine, 2nd ed, London, Mosby, 2002, p 29, Fig. 1-85.)

RNA togavirus
Vaccination reduced incidence
Clinical findings
50% asymptomatic
Forchheimer spots
Dusky red, soft/hard palate
Beginning of rash
Rash lasts 3 days
Red maculopapular rash with discrete lesions

Not confluent
Spreads head to toe
Painful postauricular lymphadenopathy
Polyarthritis (unvaccinated adult)
Rubella teratogenic
Erythema infectiosum (fifth disease)
"Slapped face" appearance
Parvovirus B19 (DNA)

Respiratory secretions
Children (5–10 yrs); late winter/early spring

Often occurs in epidemics
Clinical findings
Fever, sore throat, malaise
Confluent net-like erythematous rash

"Slapped face" appearance; "gloves + socks"

2. Epidemiology
   a. RNA togavirus
   b. Vaccination has reduced the incidence of rubella in the United States.
3. Clinical findings
   a. Up to 50% of infections are asymptomatic.
   b. Forchheimer spots (Fig. 25-5 E)
      (1) Dusky red spots that develop on the posterior soft and hard palate
      (2) Develop at the beginning of the rash
   c. Erythematous maculopapular rash lasts 3 days (Fig. 25-5 F).
      (1) Red, maculopapular eruption with discrete lesions that, unlike rubeola, do *not* become confluent
      (2) Begins at the hairline and they rapidly spreads cephalocaudally (from head to toe)
   d. Painful postauricular (behind the ear) lymphadenopathy: diagnostic finding in rubella
   e. Polyarthritis is common in unvaccinated adults.
   f. Infection during the first trimester may produce congenital anomalies (teratogen; see Chapter 6).

E. **Erythema infectiosum (fifth disease)**
   1. **Definition:** Viral disease characterized by a "slapped face" appearance
   2. Epidemiology
      a. Caused by the parvovirus B19 (DNA virus); spread by respiratory secretions
      b. Occurs in children ages 5 to 10 years during late winter or early spring; often occurs in epidemics
   3. Clinical findings
      a. Prodromal period characterized by mild fever, a sore throat, and malaise
      b. Prodrome is followed by the development of a confluent netlike erythematous rash. Rash begins on the cheeks ("slapped face" appearance; Fig. 25-5 G) and extends to the

trunk and proximal extremities; papular-purpuric "gloves [hands] and socks" syndrome (Links 25-12 and 25-13)

c. Recurrence may occur after changes in temperature, exposure to sunlight, or emotional stress.

d. Polyarthritis is common in adults.

Recurrences may occur

Polyarthritis common in adults

Other disorders caused by parvovirus B19 include pure red blood cell (RBC) aplasia and aplastic anemia in chronic hemolytic diseases (e.g., hereditary spherocytosis) and chronic arthritis. Pregnant mothers exposed to a child with the infection may abort the fetus.

Pure RBC aplasia, aplastic anemia in hemolytic anemias, chronic arthritis, aborted fetus

F. **Roseola infantum (exanthem subitum)**

1. **Definition:** Viral disease that presents in a typically healthy child <2 years old with fever followed by a rash (sixth disease)

2. Epidemiology
   a. Caused by human herpesvirus 6 (HHV6; DNA virus).
   b. MC viral exanthem in children <2 years old

3. Clinical findings
   a. Erythematous macules develop on the soft palate 48 hours *before* appearance of a rash. Maculopapular rash occurs abruptly after 3 to 7 days of high fever (Fig. 25-5 H).
   b. Tender cervical or postauricular (behind the ear) lymphadenopathy is a key feature in differentiating between roseola and rubella.
   c. High fever may precipitate a febrile convulsion.

Roseola infantum

Child <2 yrs; fever → rash

HHV6, DNA virus

MC viral exanthem children <2 yrs

Clinical findings

Red macules soft palate *before* rash

Abrupt maculopapular rash

Cervical/postauricular nodes

High fever → febrile convulsion

G. **Disorders caused by varicella-zoster virus (VZV)**

1. **Definition:** VZV is a DNA herpesvirus that produces a vesicular rash called varicella (chickenpox). VZV remains latent in the cranial and thoracic sensory ganglia.

2. Varicella (chickenpox)
   a. Epidemiology
      (1) Predominantly a childhood disease
      (2) Approximately 90% of cases occur in children <10 years of age
      (3) Incidence of varicella peaks in the spring months. Incubation period is 2 to 3 weeks.
      (4) Patient is infectious 1 week *before* the rash appears.
      (5) Patient is infectious an additional 4 to 5 days until vesicles become crusted.
   b. Clinical findings
      (1) Pruritic rash progresses from macules, to vesicles, to pustules (Fig. 25-5 I; Links 25-14 and 25-15).
         (a) All stages of development are present simultaneously (i.e., macules, papules, and pustules are present all at once).
         (b) Lesions are most prominent on the trunk.
         (c) Lesions also involve the extremities (including palms and soles), mucous membranes in the mouth, and conjunctiva.
         (d) Vesicles are often umbilicated (depressed center) and may be hemorrhagic.
      (2) Positive Tzanck test result similar to herpes simplex virus (HSV). Tzanck preparation: scrapings removed from the base of vesicle or pustule that are stained show multinucleated (MN) squamous cells (SCs) with eosinophilic intranuclear (IN) inclusions.
      (3) Complications
         (a) Reye syndrome if the child takes aspirin (see Chapter 19)
         (b) Pneumonia (severe): self-limited cerebellitis
      (4) Adults with varicella may develop hepatitis, pneumonia, and encephalitis.

3. Herpes zoster (shingles)
   a. **Definition:** Viral disease characterized by reactivation of VZV that leads to the spread of the virus from the sensory nerve to the dermatome.
   b. Epidemiology
      (1) Occurs in 10% to 20% of people in their lifetime. Incidence (I) increases with age.
      (2) It is increased in patients with cancer and AIDS because of impaired cell-mediated immunity (CMI).
   c. Clinical findings
      (1) Prodrome of radicular pain and itching occurs *before* onset of the rash.
      (2) Eruption is characterized by the presence of groups of vesicles surrounded by an erythematous base (Links 25-16 and 25-17).

Varicella-zoster virus

Latent DNA herpesvirus (varicella)

Varicella (chickenpox)

Predominantly childhood disease

Children <10 yrs

Peaks spring

Incubation 2–3 wks

Infectious *before* rash

Infectious 4–5 days until vesicles crusted

Clinical findings

Macules → vesicles → pustules

Macules, vesicles, pustules same time

Prominent on trunk

Palms/soles/mouth/ conjunctiva

Vesicles umbilicated/often hemorrhagic

+Tzanck test

Multinucleated SCs; eosinophilic IN inclusions

Complications

Reye syndrome (aspirin)

Severe pneumonia

Self-limited cerebellitis

Adult: hepatitis, pneumonia, encephalitis

Herpes zoster (shingles)

Activation VZV → sensory nerve to dermatome

10%–20% people

↑I with age

↑I with impaired CMI (AIDS)

Clinical findings

Prodrome radicular pain/ itch *before* rash

Grouped vesicles erythematous base

(3) Rash follows sensory dermatomes in the distribution of cranial nerves or spinal nerves (Fig. 25-5 J).

(4) Similar to varicella, pustules form that then rupture, causing crusting and weeping.

4. Smallpox (variola)

a. **Definition:** Poxvirus is a virus that strictly uses a human host (*no* animal reservoirs); characterized by pustules that are well synchronized and heal with permanent scarring

b. Epidemiology

(1) Only disease that has been eradicated from the earth.

(2) Eradication is attributable to vaccination.

(3) Potential use for bioterrorism. Other bioterrorism agents associated with skin manifestations include anthrax, tularemia, plague, and viral hemorrhagic fever.

(4) Transmission

(a) Respiratory droplet, fomites (objects or materials that carry infection), person to person

(b) Incubation period is 5 to 17 days.

(5) Variants of smallpox include variola major (mortality rate, 15%–40%) and variola minor (mortality rate, 1%).

(6) Unlike varicella (chickenpox), the vesicles appear at the same stage of development (i.e., are well synchronized). Vesicles develop into pustules, which rupture and produce scabs (Links 25-18 and 25-19).

(7) Vesicles cover the skin and mucous membranes. The palms and soles are involved (*not* present in varicella).

(8) Vesicles rupture and leave pock marks with permanent scarring.

H. **Herpes simplex virus (HSV)-1** (see Chapter 18; Table 18-1)

1. **Definition:** Acute, self-limiting, vesicular eruption caused by HSV-1

2. Epidemiology and clinical

a. Transmission

(1) Saliva or direct contact with virus in vesicle

(2) CMI is important in limiting the virus.

b. Gingivostomatitis (Link 25-20)

(1) **Definition:** A combination of inflammation of the oral mucosa and gingiva

(2) Often the initial presentation during the first ("primary") HSV infection

(3) Usually occurs in children <5 years of age

(4) Systemic signs of fever and painful cervical lymphadenopathy

(5) Painful vesicles usually develop on the lips, gingiva, and oropharyngeal mucosa.

c. Herpes labialis (fever blisters, cold sores; see Fig. 18-3 C; Link 25-18)

(1) Recurrent HSV-1 (latent virus)

(2) Nonsystemic involving mucocutaneous junction of the lips and nose; recurs at the same site

(3) Reactivated by stress, sunlight, and menses

(4) Tzanck prep (scrapping of the lesion: Link 25-21). MN SCs with red IN inclusions.

d. Herpetic whitlow

(1) **Definition:** Traumatic implantation of the virus into the finger or hand (Link 25-22)

(2) Painful pustular lesion

(3) Commonly occurs in dentists (contact with sharp teeth)

e. Eczema herpeticum (EH). HSV-1 infection superimposed on a previous dermatitis, usually in an immunodeficient person (Link 25-23)

I. Hand-foot-and-mouth (HFM) disease (see Table 18-1)

1. **Definition:** Viral rash that occurs on the hands, feet, and mouth

2. Epidemiology

a. Caused by coxsackievirus A16

b. Febrile disease that primarily occurs in children <10 years old

3. Clinical findings. Vesicular rash occurs on the hands, feet, and in the mouth (Fig. 25-5 K; Links 25-24 and 25-25).

III. **Selected Bacterial Disorders**

A. *Staphylococcus aureus* **skin infections**

1. **Definition:** Coagulase-positive, gram-positive coccus that occurs in clusters (Fig. 25-6 A)

2. Overview of morphology of purulent skin infections and overview of *S. aureus* infections in all sites (Links 25-26 and 25-27)

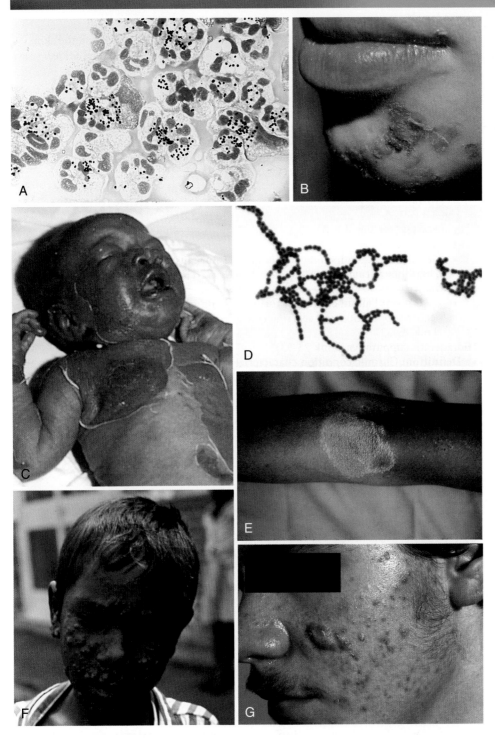

25-6: Bacterial infections. **A,** Gram stain of *Staphylococcus aureus*. Note the gram-positive cocci, some of which are forming clusters. **B,** Impetigo of the face showing honey-colored crusts overlying an erythematous base. Caused by *S. aureus*. **C,** Infant with scalded child syndrome caused by *S. aureus*. **D,** Gram stain of *Streptococcus pyogenes*. Note the gram-positive cocci in chains. **E,** Tuberculoid leprosy. Note the hypopigmented macule, an early finding in tuberculoid leprosy. **F,** Lepromatous leprosy. Note the nodular lesions on the face giving the patient a leonine facies. **G,** Acne vulgaris. Note the severe facial acne with inflamed papules and cystic lesions. (*A from McPherson R, Pincus M:* Henry's Clinical Diagnosis and Management by Laboratory Methods, *21st ed, Philadelphia, Saunders, 2007, p 1018, Fig. 56-2; B from Lookingbill D, Marks J:* Principles of Dermatology, *3rd ed, Philadelphia, Saunders, 2000, pp 217, 213, respectively, Figs. 13-9, 13-4A, respectively; C from Kliegman R:* Nelson Textbook of Pediatrics, *19th ed, Philadelphia, Elsevier Saunders, 2011, p 2303, Fig. 657-3; D from Murray PR, Shea YR:* Medical Microbiology, *2nd ed, St. Louis, Mosby, 2002, p 238, Fig. 23-1; E from Cohen J:* Infectious Disease, *2nd ed, St. Louis, Mosby, 2003; F and G from Savin JA, Hunter JAA, Hepburn NC:* Diagnosis in Color: Skin Signs in Clinical Medicine, *London, Mosby-Wolfe, 1997, pp 23, 135, Figs. 1-48, 5-20, respectively.*)

3. Toxic shock syndrome (TSS)
   a. **Definition:** Acute febrile illness characterized by multisystem organ dysfunction, most commonly caused by a bacterium-produced exotoxin (e.g., *S. aureus*)
   b. Epidemiology
      (1) *S. aureus* exotoxins are superantigens that stimulate release of cytokines (CKs, e.g., interleukins 1 and 3, tumor necrosis factor [TNF], and γ-interferon [γ-IFN]) which are important in mediating the signs and symptoms of the syndrome. Other less common causative agents include streptococci producing exotoxin B or C and exotoxin A produced by group A, β-hemolytic *Streptococcus pyogenes*.
      (2) Usually occurs in healthy menstruating white women between the ages of 10 and 30 years who use tampons, diaphragms, or vaginal sponges

Toxic shock syndrome

Multisystem; *S. aureus* exotoxin

Exotoxins (superantigens) → release IL-1/3, TNF, γ-IFN

Menstruating white females

Tampons, diaphragms, vaginal sponges

c. Clinical findings
   (1) Erythematous, desquamating, sunburn-like rash that involves involving the skin and mucous membranes as well as the palms and soles (Link 25-28). The rash blanches with pressure (Link 25-29).
   (2) Fever, orthostatic hypotension (hypotension when standing)
   (3) Strawberry tongue (white coated tongue with enlarged papillae project as red points similar to scarlet fever) (Link 25-30)
   (4) Multisystem systemic findings include vomiting and diarrhea, vaginal discharge and redness of the vaginal wall, hepatic failure, acute respiratory distress syndrome, acute renal failure, and disseminated intravascular coagulation (DIC).
4. Other infections associated with *S. aureus*
   a. Cellulitis
      • **Definition:** Acute inflammation of subcutaneous (SC) connective tissue (see Fig. 3.8 B)
   b. Skin abscesses (see Fig. 3-8 A)
      (1) Furuncle
         • **Definition:** Painful, dome-shaped skin lesion caused by a deep infection around a hair follicle caused by *S. aureus*. (Links 25-26 and 25-31)
      (2) Carbuncle
         • **Definition:** Painful clusters of furuncles connected subcutaneously, causing deeper suppuration and scarring (Link 25-26); larger than furuncles (Link 25-32)
   c. Hidradenitis suppurativa (Link 25-33)
      • **Definition:** Chronic condition characterized by an infection of the apocrine glands (e.g., axillae, groin) with swelling, pain, and the presence of draining sinus tracts to the surface of the skin (hallmark of the disease)
   d. Postsurgical wound infection (*S. aureus* MC pathogen)
   e. Impetigo
      (1) **Definition:** Superficial skin infection that is characterized by an erythematous rash, usually beginning on the face
      (2) Epidemiology
         (a) MCC is *S. aureus*.
         (b) *S. pyogenes* is the second MCC.
         (c) Highly contagious
      (3) Clinical findings
         (a) Rash consists of vesicles and pustules that rupture to form honey-colored, crusted lesions (Fig. 25-6 B; Links 25-26, 25-34, and 25-35).
         (b) Bullae commonly occur (Link 25-36)
   f. Scalded skin syndrome (Ritter disease)
      (1) **Definition:** Febrile, superficial blistering disease occurring as a cutaneous response to circulating toxins (exfoliative toxins A and B) derived from *S. aureus*
      (2) Epidemiology and clinical
         (a) MC in neonates and children; less common in adults
         (b) Exfoliative toxins A and B cause a split high in the epidermis, which leads to superficial blistering and peeling of the skin (Fig. 25-6 C).
         (c) Sloughing of the skin results in a significant loss of electrolytes. Skin blanches with pressure (Link 25-37).
         (d) Low mortality rate in children (1%–5%). High mortality rate in adults (50%–60%).
   g. Folliculitis barbae
      (1) **Definition:** Acute inflammation in the hair follicle caused by bacteria, usually *S. aureus*
      (2) Epidemiology and clinical: appears as a pustule, often with a central hair (Link 25-38)
   h. Bacterial folliculitis unrelated to shaving is most often caused by *S. aureus* (Link 25-39). Follicles can become blocked or irritated by sweat, machine oils, or makeup. Wearing tight clothes can also be a cause.
   i. Hot tube folliculitis.
      (1) **Definition:** Folliculitis arising secondary to exposure to hot tubs and swimming pools contaminated with *Pseudomonas aeruginosa*, a water-loving gram-negative rod
      (2) Clinical findings: Lesions initially are pustules that become hemorrhagic centrally with a characteristic red flare; often but *not* always occurring underneath a bathing suit (Link 25-40).

B. *S. pyogenes* skin infections

  1. **Definition of *S. pyogenes*:** Gram-positive coccus in chains (Fig. 25-6 D)

  2. Scarlet fever

    a. **Definition:** Febrile disease characterized by an erythematous rash involving the skin and tongue that complicates a group A *S. pyogenes* pharyngitis or tonsillitis

    b. Epidemiology

      (1) Caused by erythrogenic toxin-producing strains of *S. pyogenes*

      (2) Usually occurs in children between the ages of 5 and 15 years old

      (3) Usually in late fall, winter, and early spring when temperatures are cooler

      (4) Increased risk for developing poststreptococcal glomerulonephritis (see Chapter 20)

    c. Clinical findings

      (1) Rash presents as a fine, erythematous, macular and papular eruption involving the skin and tongue (Link 25-41).

      (2) Initially occurs on the face and neck before spreading to other parts of the body

      (3) Mouth is spared, producing a conspicuous circumoral pallor.

      (4) Rash feels like sandpaper.

      (5) Tongue is red and swollen (glossitis) and is covered by a white exudate studded with prominent red papillae.

      (6) Rash begins to fade after 6 days followed by desquamation (peeling) of several days (up to 10) (Link 25-42).

      (7) White exudate on the tongue disappears, and the tongue is beefy red (strawberry tongue; Link 25-43).

      (8) Increased risk for developing poststreptococcal glomerulonephritis (nephritic syndrome; see Chapter 20)

  3. Erysipelas

    a. **Definition:** Type of cellulitis caused by *S. pyogenes* involving the superficial layers of the epidermis and cutaneous lymphatics (lymphangitis; red streak)

    b. Epidemiology

      (1) Most commonly occurs in young people and older adults

      (2) Risk factors for developing erysipelas

        (a) Impaired lymphatic drainage (e.g., postmastectomy)

        (b) Harvesting saphenous veins for coronary artery bypass

        (c) Tinea pedis (athletes foot). Cracking of the skin allows entry of bacteria into the lymphatics.

    c. Clinical findings

      (1) Border of the infected skin is raised, and the surface appears like an orange peel (Link 25-44).

      (2) Skin is hot and bright red (rubor of acute inflammation).

      (3) Commonly occurs on the face and lower extremities

      (4) Patient feels ill and is febrile.

C. Leprosy

  1. **Definition:** Chronic granulomatous infection caused by *Myobacterium leprae* that primarily affects the skin and peripheral nerves

  2. Epidemiology

    a. Gram-positive obligate intracellular (IC) acid-fast (A-F) bacterium

    b. Grows in the footpads of mice and armadillos; *cannot* be cultured

    c. Genetic susceptibility for developing leprosy

    d. Primarily transmitted by coughing and sneezing

    e. India has the most number of cases worldwide.

  3. Tuberculoid type.

    a. **Definition:** Type of leprosy in which granulomas are present, indicating intact cell-mediated immunity (CMI); characterized by localized skin lesions with nerve involvement

    b. Epidemiology

      (1) Positive lepromin skin test indicating intact CMI

      (2) Granulomas are present; however, very few A-F bacteria are present in the granulomas.

    c. Clinical findings

      (1) Hypopigmented macular lesions with complete sensory loss (Fig. 25-6 E)

      (2) Very characteristic finding is the presence of palpable thickened superficial nerves.

  4. Lepromatous type

Absence granulomas, leonine facies; lack CMI

–Lepromin skin test; lack CMI

Absence granulomas

Peripheral nerves *not* palpable

Numerous acid-fast bacteria (Grenz zone)

Digital autoamputation; leonine face

Acne vulgaris

CI pilosebaceous unit

MC skin disease seen by dermatologists

Begins 9–11 yrs old

Male dominant

Sebaceous glands have ARs

Anaerobic G+ rod *P. acnes* produces lipases → FAs

ARs bind T/DHT; hyperresponsiveness

5-α-Reductase converts T to DHT

↑Severity in teenagers

Papules, pustules, nodules, cysts

Noninflamed comedones

Comedones: open (blackhead), closed (whitehead)

Outlet plugged by keratin or open

Open outlet → blackhead (oxidized melanin in sebum)

Outlet closed → whitehead

Fungal disorders

Superficial dermatophytes: live in stratum corneum/ adnexal structures

Fungi confined to stratum corneum/adnexal structures

Warm, humid climates

Scaling rash

Tinea describes superficial infection

Tinea– capitis, pedis, corporis, cruris

T. pedis MC

KOH prep first step in diagnosis. Wood lamp: detects fluorescent fungal metabolites.

a. **Definition:** Type of leprosy in which granulomas are *not* present, indicating a defect in CMI; characterized by classic nodular lesions on the face producing the leonine (lion-like) facies

b. Epidemiology
   (1) Negative lepromin skin test result indicates a lack of CMI.
   (2) Absence of granulomas
   (3) Peripheral nerves *not* palpable
   (4) Numerous A-F bacteria are present within foamy macrophages (MPs) that are located under a subepidermal zone free of organisms (called the Grenz zone).
   (5) Clinical findings in lepromatous leprosy include nodular lesions involving the face that produce a classic leonine (lion-like) facies (Fig. 25-6 F; Link 25-45). Autoamputation of the digits caused by trauma occurs secondary to loss of sensation (neurotropic atrophy; Link 25-46).
   (6) Borderline tuberculoid leprosy, midborderline leprosy, and borderline lepromatous leprosy have also been defined.

D. **Acne vulgaris**
   1. **Definition:** Chronic inflammation (CI) of the pilosebaceous glands in the skin
   2. Epidemiology
      a. MC skin disease seen by dermatologists
      b. Begins at an early age (9–11 years old); male dominant
      c. Sebaceous glands have androgen receptors (ARs).
         (1) Anaerobic Gram-positive rod *Propionibacterium acnes* produces lipases that break down sebum in the hair follicle into fatty acids. The fatty acids subsequently lead to an inflammatory reaction (Link 25-47).
         (2) Both testosterone (T) and dihydrotestosterone (DHT) bind to the ARs, although DHT binds with 10 times greater affinity. Regardless, the majority of patients with acne vulgaris do *not* overproduce androgens; rather, they have a genetic hyperresponsiveness to androgens.
            • Enzyme 5α-reductase converts T to DHT in the hair follicles and other sites.
      d. Acne vulgaris increases in severity in the teenage years because of an increase in sebum production during puberty.
   3. Clinical lesions
      • Inflammatory papules, pustules, nodules, and cysts (Fig. 25-6 G)
   4. Noninflamed comedones
      a. **Definition:** Classic skin lesions in acne vulgaris; include "whiteheads" and "blackheads"
      b. Epidemiology
         (1) Outlet of a hair follicle can be plugged by keratin debris, or it can be open for drainage of sebum.
         (2) If the outlet of a hair follicle is open, the pore opening to the skin will be dilated and filled with black keratinous material (oxidized melanin in sebum), thus the term *blackhead* (Link 25-48).
         (3) If the outlet of a hair follicle is closed, the melanin in the keratinous material is *not* oxidized into melanin, thus the term *whitehead* (Links 25-49 and 25-50).

IV. **Selected Fungal Disorders**
   A. **Superficial mycoses (dermatophytoses)**
      1. **Definition:** Group of fungal diseases confined to the stratum corneum and adnexal structures (Fig. 25-7 A; Link 25-51)
      2. Epidemiology
         a. Incidence of infection increases in warm, humid climates.
         b. Most infections present with a scaling rash.
         c. Tinea means "worm" in Latin, but it is also used to describe superficial fungal infections.
            (1) Tinea is followed by a word that qualifies its location (e.g., capitis [head], pedis [feet], corporis [body], cruris [crotch area]).
            (2) The MC superficial fungal infections in decreasing order are tinea pedis (foot), tinea unguium (nail), tinea versicolor (describes color variation rather than location), and tinea cruris (groin).

Wood lamp and potassium hydroxide (KOH)-treated skin scrapings from lesions are commonly used for diagnosis of the dermatophytoses. A Wood lamp (ultraviolet A [UVA] light; Link 25-52) detects fluorescent metabolites produced by organisms (e.g., fungi, some bacteria). KOH preparations identify yeasts and hyphae in the stratum corneum or hair shafts (Fig. 25-7 B; Link 25-53).

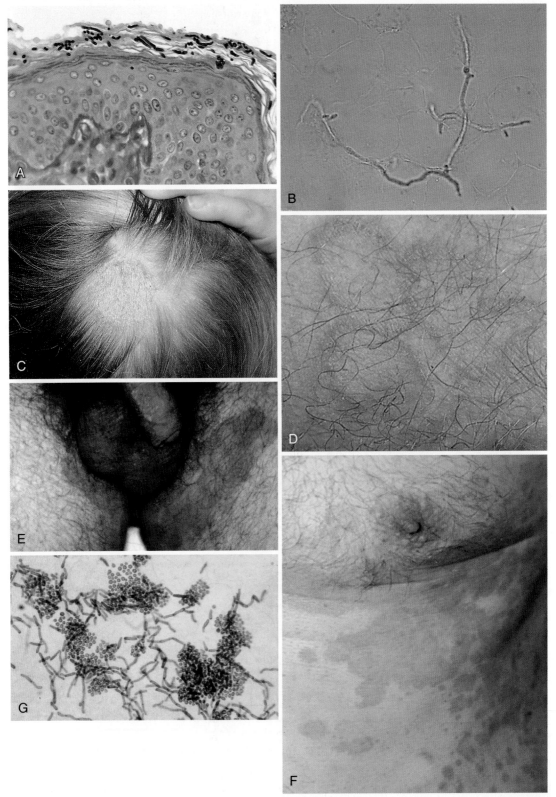

25-7: A, Dermatophytosis caused by *Trichophyton*, demonstrated by periodic acid–Schiff stain. **B,** Potassium hydroxide (KOH) preparation of skin scrapings showing hyphae and yeasts. **C,** Tinea capitis caused by *Trichophyton tonsurans*. Note the area of alopecia (hair loss) with *black dots* representing broken off hairs and scaling of the skin. **D,** Tinea corporis showing annular lesions with erythematous margins and clear centers. **E,** Tinea cruris. Note the scaly, erythematous rash in the groin. **F,** Tinea versicolor caused by *Malassezia globosa* showing skin with pink-tan patches (hyperpigmentation) intermixed with normal skin. The hyperpigmented lesions should be scraped for a KOH preparation. **G,** *Malassezia globosa*. Note the classic spaghetti (hyphae) and meatball (yeasts) morphologic appearance in this KOH preparation.

Continued

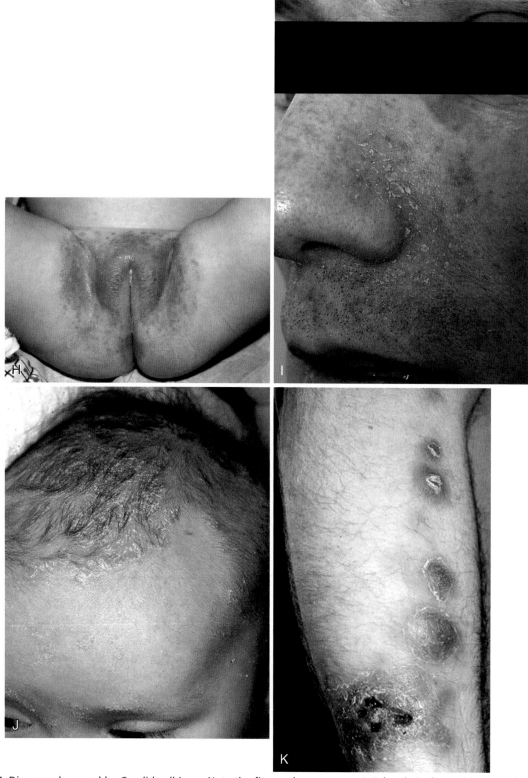

25-7 cont'd: H, Diaper rash caused by *Candida albicans*. Note the fiery red appearance. **I,** Seborrheic dermatitis. Note the erythematous, greasy scaling rash in the nasolabial fold. It is caused by *Malassezia furfur*. **J,** Seborrheic dermatitis in a newborn (cradle cap). Note the greasy, yellow, scaly rash on the scalp. **K,** Lymphocutaneous sporotrichosis showing a linear array of suppurating subcutaneous nodules. (*A from Rosai J:* Rosai and Ackerman's Surgical Pathology, *9th ed, St. Louis, Mosby, 2004, p 101, Fig. 4-13;* **B** and **C** from Goldstein BG: Practical Dermatology, *2nd ed, St. Louis, Mosby, 1997, pp 24, 97, Figs. 3-2, 10-1, respectively;* **D** from Forbes C, Jackson W: Color Atlas and Text of Clinical Medicine, *2nd ed, London, Mosby, 2002, p 97, Fig. 2-57;* **E** and **I** from Savin JA, Hunter JAA, Hepburn NC: Diagnosis in Color: Skin Signs in Clinical Medicine, *London, Mosby-Wolfe, 1997, pp 123, 9, respectively, Figs. 4.78, 1.17, respectively;* **F** from Ashar BH, Miller RG, Sisso SD: The Johns Hopkins Internal Medicine Board Review, *4th ed, Elsevier, 2012, p 540, Fig. 65-16;* **G** from Midgley G, Clayton Y, Hay RJ: Diagnosis in Color: Medical Mycology, *London, Mosby-Wolfe, 1997, p 73, Fig. 93;* **H** from Kliegman R: Nelson Textbook of Pediatrics, *19th ed, Philadelphia, Elsevier Saunders, 2011, p 2314, Fig. 658-14;* **J** and **K** from Fitzpatrick JE, Morelli JG: Dermatology Secrets Plus, *4th ed, Philadelphia, Elsevier Mosby, 2011, pp 61, 225, respectively, Figs. 8.4A, 32-1B, respectively.*)

3. Tinea capitis
   a. **Definition:** Superficial fungal infection of the scalp
   b. Epidemiology
      (1) Most often caused by *Trichophyton tonsurans*
         (a) Infects the inner hair shaft
         (b) Negative Wood lamp test result because the location in the inner hair shaft prevents detection of its fluorescent metabolites by a Wood lamp
         (c) Predominant type of infection in blacks
      (2) *Microsporum canis* (dog) and *Microsporum audouinii*
         (a) Former type is associated with exposure to dogs (canis)
         (b) Both fungi infect the outer hair shaft.
         (c) Wood lamp test result is positive.
         (d) These two species are the predominant pathogens in whites.
   c. Clinical findings in tinea capitis
      (1) Circular or ring-shaped patches of hair loss (alopecia)
      (2) Visible black dot on the scalp is where the hair breaks off (Fig. 25-7 C; Link 25-54).
4. Other superficial mycosis infections in other areas of the body are most often caused by *Trichophyton rubrum*.
   a. Tinea corporis (body surface) (Fig. 25-7 D)
      (1) Sometimes called ringworm, which is a misnomer
      (2) May be a Hx of exposure to a cat or dog
      (3) One or more lesions may be present.
      (4) Typically, they are annular lesions with an elevated red, scaly border and clear centers (Links 25-55 and 25-56).
   b. Tinea pedis (athlete's foot)
      (1) MC overall site for superficial dermatophyte infections
      (2) MC in a person with sweaty feet
      (3) Macerated scaling rash between one or more toes (Links 25-57, 25-58, and 25-59)
      (4) Older adults often have diffuse plantar scaling (bottom of the foot). The bottom of the foot has a "moccasin" appearance.
   c. Tinea cruris (groin; jock itch) (Fig. 25-7 E; Link 25-60)
      (1) Patients frequently have tinea pedis along with tinea cruris.
      (2) Both the feet and groin are areas associated with excessive sweating.
      (3) Rash is *not* annular but has elevated, scaly borders.
      (4) Scrotum is frequently involved as well.
   d. *Tinea unguium* (nail; onychomycosis)
      (1) Second MC superficial dermatophyte infection that affects the nails
      (2) *T. rubrum* (MC) and *T. mentagrophytes* are the usual pathogens.
      (3) Nail is raised, and the nail plate is white, thick, and crumbly (Link 25-61). It is frequently discolored.
5. Tinea versicolor (pityriasis rosea)
   a. **Definition:** Superficial dermatophyte infection of the stratum corneum that results in an alteration in skin pigmentation
   b. Epidemiology
      (1) Hypopigmented type is caused by a decrease in melanin synthesis.
      (2) Hyperpigmented type (MC) is caused by an enlargement of melanosomes.
      (3) Wood lamp accentuates the color variation in the skin.
      (4) Infection is caused by *Malassezia globose* (old term *furfur*). It involves the upper trunk or upper extremities and may also involve the penile shaft.
         (a) In the hypopigmented type, fungus-derived acids inhibit tyrosinase in the synthesis of melanin in melanocytes.
         (b) In the hyperpigmented type, the fungus induces enlargement of melanosomes in melanocytes along the basal cell layer (Fig. 25-7 F; Link 25-62).
   c. Clinical findings in tinea versicolor
      (1) Affected skin does *not* tan ("white spots"); however, the normal skin does tan.
      (2) Lesions become hyperpigmented and scaly in the winter months.
   d. Potassium hydroxide (KOH) findings in skin scrapings (Fig. 25-7 G)
      (1) Hypopigmented and hyperpigmented areas contain the organism.
      (2) Short hyphae have the appearance of "spaghetti."
      (3) Yeasts have the appearance of "meatballs."
6. Tinea barbae

a. **Definition:** Dermatophyte infection of the beard area most often caused *by Trichophyton mentagrophytes* or *Trichophyton verrucosum*
b. Manifests in the beard area as superficial annular lesions; deeper infection similar to folliculitis may also occur (Link 25-63)
7. Infections caused by *Candida albicans*
a. Intertrigo.
(1) **Definition:** Erythematous rash that occurs in body folds. KOH preparation shows pseudohyphae and yeast (see Fig. 22-1 A).
(2) Examples of intertrigo: rash under pendulous breasts, diaper rash (Fig. 25-7 H)
b. Onychomycosis (nail infection)
8. Seborrheic dermatitis (dandruff)
a. **Definition:** Chronic, superficial fungal infection that affects the hairy regions with skin rich in sebaceous glands, which include the scalp, eyebrows, nasal creases (Fig. 25-7 I), face, chest, and intertriginous areas (axilla, groin, buttocks, under female breasts, and groin
b. Epidemiology
(1) Affects 3% to 5% of the population
(2) Caused by *Malassezia* yeast
(3) Called "cradle cap" in newborns (NBs) (Fig. 25-7 J)
(4) Common associations
(a) Parkinson disease
(b) AIDS and AIDS-related complex
c. Clinical findings in seborrheic dermatitis
• Scaly, yellowish, greasy dermatitis (Links 25-64, 25-65, and 25-66)
B. **Sporotrichosis**
1. **Definition:** Dimorphic fungus (grows in both mold and yeast forms) caused by *Sporothrix schenckii* that produces a lymphocutaneous infection
2. Epidemiology
a. Mold in soil and a yeast in tissue
b. Usually caused by traumatic implantation of the fungus
(1) Thorns in rose gardening
(2) Sphagnum peat moss for packing material (packing lobsters) or landscaping
(3) Splinters from carpentry work; berry pickers
3. Clinical findings in sporotrichosis: produces lymphocutaneous disease characterized by a chain of suppurating lymphocutaneous nodules in the subcutaneous tissue (Fig. 25-7 K)
C. *Fusarium* **spp. infection**
1. **Definition:** Molds that are normally found in soil and the air that may result in localized infections in the nail, burn sites, surgical wounds, or in immunocompromised patients (cytotoxic chemotherapy, bone marrow transplantations)
2. Epidemiology and clinical
a. Serious opportunistic fungal infection
b. Neutropenia is the MC risk factor.
c. Immunocompromised patients may present with refractory fever, skin lesions, sinusitis, pneumonia, or infections of the eye (hematogenous spread). Multiorgan involvement may occur.
3. Diagnosis of *Fusarium* infections: skin biopsy, fungal culture of skin and blood (Link 25-67)
V. **Selected Parasitic and Arthropod Disorders**
A. **Cutaneous larva migrans**
1. **Definition:** Subcutaneous infection in humans who come in contact with infective larvae of the dog or cat hookworms (nematodes) *Ancylostoma braziliense* or *Ancylostoma caninum*
2. Epidemiology
• Transmission of cutaneous larva migrans
(1) Dogs and cats are the definitive host. Definitive host has the sexually mature hookworm that can mate and lay eggs.
(2) Larvae evolve in sand (sand boxes) or soil from eggs passed in the feces of dogs or cats. Prevention note: Cover sandboxes so dogs and cats do not use them as litter boxes.
(3) Larvae penetrate the skin in children and adults, who become the intermediate hosts for the disease (Fig. 25-8 A; Link 25-68).

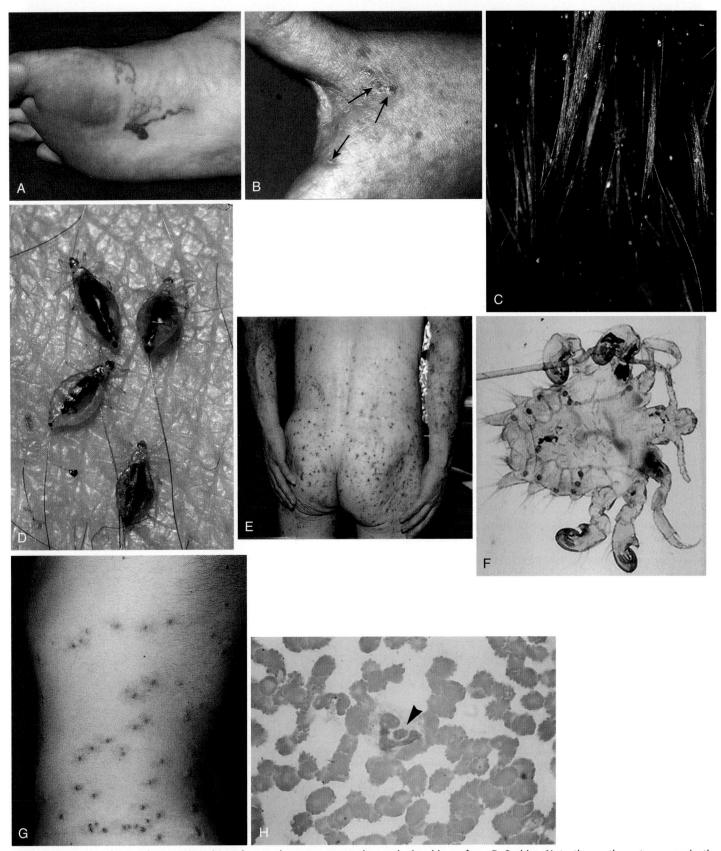

25-8: A, Cutaneous larva migrans. Note irregular, erythematous tracts beneath the skin surface. **B,** Scabies. Note the erythematous area in the web between the fingers. The *arrows* show raised burrows. **C,** *Pediculus capitis.* Note the white nits (eggs) attached to the hair shafts. **D,** *Pediculus corporis* feeding. **E,** *Pediculus corporis.* Note the numerous erythematous papules over the back of this homeless person. **F,** *Pthirus pubis.* Note the crablike appearance of the louse. **G,** Bedbug bites. Note the red papules and wheals. **H,** Morula *(arrow)* of *Anaplasma* in a granulocyte. *(A and B courtesy R.A. Marsden, MD, St. George's Hospital, London; C and H from Kliegman RM, Jenson HB, Behrman RE, Stanton BF: Nelson's Textbook of Pediatrics, 18th ed, Philadelphia, Saunders Elsevier, 2007, pp 2758, 1050, respectively, Figs. 667-6, 228-1B, respectively; D from Cohen J, Opal SM, Powderly WG: Infectious Diseases, 3rd ed, St. Louis, Mosby Elsevier, 2010, p 135, Fig. 11-10; E from Savin JA, Hunter JAA, Hepburn NC: Diagnosis in Color: Skin Signs in Clinical Medicine, London, Mosby-Wolfe, 1997, p 214, Fig. 9.3; F from Klatt E: Robbins and Cotran Atlas of Pathology, Philadelphia, Saunders, 2006, p 399, Fig. 16-90, right; G from Swartz M: Textbook of Physical Diagnosis History and Examination, 5th ed, Philadelphia, Saunders Elsevier, 2006, p 176, Fig. 8-90.)*

B. **Cutaneous leishmaniasis**
1. **Definition:** Cutaneous leishmaniasis (also known as oriental/tropical sore) is the MC form of leishmaniasis affecting humans. It is a skin infection caused *Leishmania* spp. that is transmitted by the bite of an infected *Phlebotomus* sandfly.
2. Epidemiology and clinical
   a. The disease is found in most tropical and subtropical areas of the world.
   b. Link 25-69 shows the lifecycle of *Leishmania*. Tissue protozoa that locates in MPs and dendritic cells (DCs) in the dermis.
   c. Initially a papule develops followed by ulceration of the skin with raised borders (Link 25-70). Ulcers develop a few weeks to a few months after the bite.
   d. Painful regional lymphadenopathy develops. A secondary bacterial infection of the ulcers is common.

C. **Arthropod disorders: chiggers**
1. **Definition:** Skin disease producing a pruritic dermatitis that is caused by the human itch mite
2. Epidemiology
   a. Chigger is a small red to orange mite (Link 25-71)
   b. Induces a pruritic dermatitis
      (1) Lesions are bright red papular, urticarial, or vesicular rash (Link 25-72).
      (2) Favor the legs and areas of tight-fitting clothing

D. **Arthropod disorders: scabies**
1. **Definition:** A human itch mite infection caused by *Sarcoptes scabiei* var. *hominis*
2. Epidemiology and clinical
   a. Sites of involvement by scabies (Link 25-73)
   b. Adult females bore into the stratum corneum (Link 25-74, 25-75, and 25-76)
      (1) Burrows are visible as dark lines between the fingers, at the wrists, on the nipples, or on the scrotum.
      (2) Females lay eggs at the end of the tunnel. Eggs are responsible for the intensely pruritic lesion.
   c. Adults with scabies
      (1) The disease commonly occurs in the webs between the fingers (Fig. 25-8 B) and intertriginous areas (Links 25-77 to 25-79).
      (2) Spares the face and head
   d. Infants with scabies
      (1) *No* burrows are present.
      (2) Pruritic rash occurs on the palms, soles, face, or head.

E. **Arthropod disorders: lice**
1. Pediculus humanus capitis (head louse)
   a. Adults lay eggs (nits) on hair shafts (Fig. 25-8 C; Links 25-80 and 25-81).
   b. Causes itching of the scalp
2. Pediculus humanus corporis (body louse)
   a. Adults live on the surface of the skin (*not* invasive) and breed in the clothing (Fig. 25-8 D).
   b. Skin lesions are papular and produce intense itching (Fig. 25-8 E).
   c. To eradicate the disease, treat the clothing, *not* the patient.
3. *Pthirus pubis* (pubic louse, crabs)
   a. Adults live in the pubic hairs (Fig. 25-8 F; Link 25-82).
   b. Looks like a crab; hence, the nickname "crabs" in describing the disease

F. **Arthropod disorders: bedbug**
1. Common bedbug is *Cimex lectularius* (Link 25-83).
2. Dwellings (houses, motels) are usually completely infested.
3. Bedbugs feed on human blood.
   a. Active just *before* dawn
   b. Attracted by warmth and CO_2 derived from the sleeping patient
4. Skin lesions bedbugs
   a. Intensely pruritic red papules or wheals (Fig. 25-8 G)
   b. Skin lesions are an allergic reaction to the anesthetic in the saliva of the bedbug.

G. **Arthropod: tick**
1. Rocky Mountain spotted fever (RMSF; see Fig. 10-17 J and Table 10-3)
2. Ehrlichiosis (*Ehrlichia chaffeensis*): human monocyte ehrlichiosis (HME)
   a. **Definition:** Tickborne rickettsial disease caused by *E. chaffeensis*
   b. Epidemiology

(1) Life cycles of HME (*E. chaffeensis*) and human granulocytic ehrlichiosis (HGA, with *Anaplasma phagocytophilum*) or infection with *Ehrlichia ewingii* (Link 25-84)

(2) Rickettsia infects monocytes in the peripheral blood (Link 25-85)

(3) Locations for HME infections include southeastern (SE), south-central, and mid-Atlantic United States, which are the same areas for contracting RMSF.

(4) Reservoir for the bacteria is the white-tailed deer.

(5) Rickettsia produces a mulberry-like inclusion called a morula in the cytoplasm of a monocyte. *Anaplasma*, the cause of anaplasmosis, is a closely related species that is also tick transmitted (*Ixodes* deer tick); however, it infects granulocytes (Fig. 25-8 H).

(6) Transmission of *Ehrlichia chaffeensis* is by the bite of a tick (*Amblyomma* spp.; lone star tick).

  c. Clinical findings in ehrlichiosis

    (1) Initial symptoms of fever, chills, headache (meningoencephalitis; lymphocyte predominant), and myalgia

    (2) Additional clinical findings

      (a) Rash (macular, maculopapular, or petechial; <40% of cases)

      (b) Hepatosplenomegaly (children; 50% of cases)

      (c) Edema in the face, hands, and feet (more common in children than adults)

      (d) Pneumonitis

  d. Laboratory findings include neutropenia and thrombocytopenia.

  e. Diagnostic tests include serologic testing and demonstration of the organism in tissue.

  f. Mortality rate is 3%.

H. Arthropod: fire ants

  1. **Definition:** Originally from South America, they are red ants with a severe sting that burns like fire.

  2. Epidemiology

    a. Native fire ants are located in the southeastern United States (Link 25-86).

    b. More aggressive imported fire ants occur in the southern states from Texas to Florida and north to the Carolinas.

    c. Attaches to a person by biting with its jaws, and then it pivots around in a circle to sting in multiples sites

    d. Stings are painful, resulting in flares and wheals that may reach an inch or more in diameter, followed by the formation of vesicles, which often become purulent within 24 hours (Link 25-87).

    e. Necrotizing toxin, solenamine, has been identified as the active chemical in the toxin. The bulk of the venom consists mainly of alkaloids, which are hemolytic and have been shown to cause histamine release and necrosis when injected into human skin.

    f. Approximately 15% of individuals experience systemic allergic reactions after fire ant stings. Clinical findings include fever, urticaria, localized edema, and necrosis. Fatalities have been reported.

VI. Melanocytic Disorders

  A. Overview of pigmented lesions (Link 25-88)

  B. Solar lentigo ("liver spots")

    1. **Definition:** Hyperpigmented, brown macules caused by an increase in number of melanocytes within sun-exposed areas (Fig. 25-9 A)

    2. Epidemiology

      a. Common finding in older adults

      b. In contradistinction, freckles (ephelides; Link 25-89) have a normal number of melanocytes but an increase in melanosomes.

      c. *Not* precancerous

  C. Vitiligo

    1. **Definition:** Autoimmune disorder characterized by autoimmune destruction of melanocytes causing areas of depigmentation

    2. Epidemiology

      a. Although it can occur in whites, vitiligo is more common in the black population.

      b. Causes localized to extensive areas of skin depigmentation (Fig. 25-9 B). Wood lamp accentuates the areas of depigmentation (Links 25-90 and 25-91). Vitiligo should *not* be confused with albinism, which is a genetic disease caused by a deficiency of tyrosinase that leads to absence of melanin synthesis in melanocytes (Link 25-92).

      c. Vitiligo is often associated with other autoimmune conditions. Examples include Hashimoto thyroiditis and hypoparathyroidism.

Margin notes:

Infects monocytes/granulocytes

Distribution same as RMSF

Reservoir white-tailed deer

Morula in cytoplasm

Anaplasma: morula in granulocytes

Tick transmitted (lone star tick)

Clinical findings

Fever, headache (meningoencephalitis)

Rash

Hepatosplenomegaly

Edema face, hands, feet

Pneumonitis

Neutropenia, thrombocytopenia

Serology, organism in tissue

Fire ants

Originally South America; red ants, severe stings

Native fire ants SE U.S.

Imported fire ants Texas to Florida, Carolinas

Attaches by biting with jaws; pivots/stings in circles

Painful stings

Vesicles → pustules

Necrotizing toxin solenamine

Systemic allergic reaction some cases

Fatalities reported

Melanocytic disorders

Solar lentigo

Pigmented brown macules

↑Melanocytes sun-exposed areas

Common in elderly

Freckles: normal # melanocytes with ↑melanosomes

Not precancerous

Vitiligo

Autoimmune destruction melanocytes

Black (MC)/white populations

Areas skin depigmentation

Albinism: ↓tyrosinase; absent melanin synthesis

Hashimoto thyroiditis, hypoparathyroidism

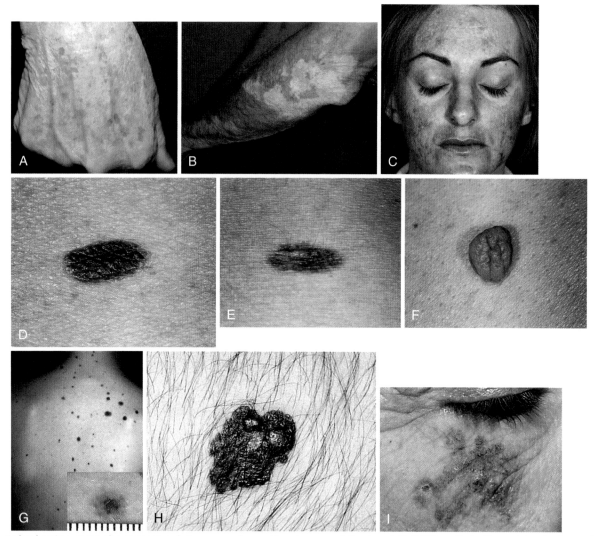

25-9: A, Solar lentigo. Note the numerous brown macules on the dorsum of the hand. **B,** Vitiligo. Note the patchy depigmentation of the skin. **C,** Melasma. Note the facial hyperpigmentation in this pregnant woman. **D,** Junctional nevus. Note the oval, uniformly pigmented macular lesion. **E,** Compound nevus. Note the pigmented lesion with the slightly papillomatous appearing surface. **F,** Intradermal nevus. Note the raised, pigmented lesion with the papillomatous appearing surface. **G,** Dysplastic nevus syndrome. Note the numerous pigmented lesions over the back and neck. The inset shows a dysplastic nevus that is larger than 6 mm in diameter and shows variable pigmentation. **H,** Superficial spreading malignant melanoma. The lesion on the patient's forearm is black, is multinodular, and has an irregular border with areas of pale gray discoloration. **I,** Lentigo maligna melanoma. Note that the facial lesion shows asymmetry, border irregularity, color variation, and a diameter larger than 6 mm.

Melasma
Macular hyperpigmented lesions forehead/cheeks women
Exacerbated pregnancy/OCP/sunlight
Nevocellular nevus
Benign neoplasm

Neural crest-derived nevus cells
Whites average 15 to 40 nevi
Frequently contain hair
Junctional nevus
Pigmented flat lesion
Nests nevus cells along basal cell layer
Junctional nevus → compound nevus
Children/adolescents
Nevus cells into superficial dermis
Junctional/intradermal

D. **Melasma**
   1. **Definition:** Macular, hyperpigmented lesions on the forehead and cheeks in women (Fig. 25-9 C)
   2. Epidemiology: exacerbated (melanocytes produce more melanin) by oral contraceptive pills (OCPs), pregnancy (mask of pregnancy), and sunlight
E. **Nevocellular nevus (mole)**
   1. **Definition:** Benign neoplastic melanocytic disorder of neural crest–derived nevus cells (modified melanocytes)
   2. Epidemiology/clinical
      a. Whites have an average of 15 to 40 nevi on their skin.
      b. Frequently contain hair
      c. Begin to develop as early as 6 months of age as a junctional nevus (Fig. 25-9 D)
         (1) Pigmented macular (flat) lesion
         (2) Nests of benign nevus cells are located along the basal cell layer of the epidermis.
      d. A junctional nevus develops into a compound nevus.
         (1) Usually develops in children and adolescents
         (2) Nevus cells extend into the superficial dermis. Both junctional and intradermal components are present, hence the term *compound*.

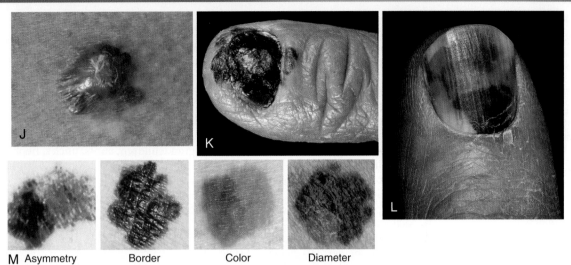

M Asymmetry   Border   Color   Diameter

25-9 cont'd: J, Nodular melanoma. Note the dark, red nodular mass in the center of the lesion and the irregular border. A biopsy would show absence of a radial growth phase and distinguish this melanoma from a superficial malignant melanoma. **K,** Acral lentiginous malignant melanoma. Note the pigmented lesion under the nail that has spread to involve the proximal nail bed. **L,** Subungual hematoma. The easiest way of differentiating this from a subungual hematoma is that the hematoma would have a history of trauma to the nail. **M,** ABCD changes in malignant melanoma. See text for discussion. (*A and I from Lookingbill D, Marks J:* Principles of Dermatology, *3rd ed, Philadelphia, Saunders, 2000, p 94, Figs. 7-2, 7-4B, respectively; **B** courtesy of The Honickman Collection of Medical Images in memory of Elaine Garfinkel and The Jefferson Clinical Images Collection [through the generosity of JMB, AKR, LKB, and DA]; **C** to **F** from Habif T:* Clinical Dermatology, *4th ed, St. Louis, Mosby, 2004; **G** from Kumar V, Abbas AK, Fausto N, Mitchell RN:* Robbins Basic Pathology, *8th ed, Philadelphia, Saunders Elsevier, 2007, p 854, Fig. 22-20C; **H** from my friend Ivan Damjanov, MD, PhD, Linder J:* Pathology: A Color Atlas, *St. Louis, Mosby, 2000, p 327, Fig. 15-57A; **J** from Townsend, C:* Sabiston Textbook of Surgery, *18th ed, Philadelphia, Saunders Elsevier, 2008, p 771, Fig. 30-5; **K** from Savin JA, Hunter JAA, Hepburn NC:* Diagnosis in Color: Skin Signs in Clinical Medicine, *London, Mosby-Wolfe, 1997, p 119, Fig. 4.63; **L** from Seidel H, Ball J, Dains, J, Benedict G:* Mosby's Guide to Physical Examination, *6th ed, St. Louis, Mosby Elsevier, 2006, p 218, Fig. 8-63; **M** reproduced with permission from the American Academy of Dermatology, Copyright © 2012. All rights reserved.*)

(3) Pigmented nevus with a papillomatous surface ("spike-like" projections; Fig. 25-9 E). Some develop a halo around the nevus (Link 25-93).

e. Intradermal nevus (ID) develops when a compound nevus loses its junctional component (Fig. 25-9 F); MC nevus in adults

f. Dysplastic nevus (atypical nevus)
  (1) **Definition:** Benign acquired melanocytic neoplasms with clinical features that are similar to a malignant melanoma, including asymmetry, irregular borders, multiple colors, and diameter of the lesion
  (2) Epidemiology
    (a) Prevalence of a dysplastic nevus in the white population is 2% to 10% of the population depending on the criteria used to define a dysplastic nevus.
    (b) Those with dysplastic nevi are at an increased risk for developing a malignant melanoma.
    (c) First appear during puberty and may develop throughout life
  (3) Characteristics
    (a) Usually >5 mm in diameter
    (b) Variegated color (pink, tan, brown, or dark brown) with an erythematous background. Dysplastic nevi do *not* have red, white, or blue colors, which are colors that are often associated with a malignant melanoma.
    (c) Irregular borders
    (d) May be associated with the dysplastic nevus syndrome (Fig. 25-9 G). Autosomal dominant syndrome associated with >100 nevi on the skin. Nearly everyone with the syndrome will ultimately develop malignant melanoma. All persons with this syndrome should have a yearly exam by a dermatologist specializing in pigmented skin lesions.

F. **Cutaneous malignant melanoma**
  1. **Definition:** Malignancy of skin melanocytes
  2. Epidemiology
    a. Most rapidly increasing cancer worldwide
    b. More common in whites than blacks

Papillomatous surface

ID nevus loses junctional cmpt: MC nevus adults

Dysplastic/atypical nevus
Benign, acquired melanocytic neoplasm

Prevalence 2%–10%

↑Risk for melanoma
First appear in puberty
Usually >5 mm diameter
Variegated colors; erythematous background
Lack red, white, blue colors
Irregular borders
Dysplastic nevus syndrome
Autosomal dominant syndrome; >100 nevi
Nearly everyone develops malignant melanoma
Yearly exam advised
Cutaneous malignant melanoma
Malignancy skin melanocytes
Most rapidly increasing cancer worldwide
Whites > blacks

Leading COD due to skin cancer
Mean age 53 yrs
Risk factors
Exposure excessive sunlight early age
Hx family member with melanoma
Excessive use tanning booths
Dysplastic nevus syndrome
Hx melanoma 1st or 2nd degree relative
Xeroderma pigmentosum
Radial growth phase
Initial phase of invasion
Melanocytes proliferate:
Laterally within epidermis
Along DE junction
Within papillary dermis
No metastatic potential in radial growth phase
Vertical growth phase
Final phase invasion
Penetration malignant cells into reticular dermis
Vertical growth phase: metastatic potential
Types of malignant melanoma
Superficial spreading melanoma
MC melanoma; 70%
Lower extremities, arms, upper back
LMM 5% to 10%
Common in elderly
Extension lentigo maligna into dermis
Long radial growth phase
Parts of face most exposed to sun
Least likely to have vertical phase
Nodular melanoma 15% to 20%
No radial growth phase
Trunk exposed to sun
Only vertical phase; poorest prognosis
ALM: 7% to 10%
Not causally related to sun exposure
Palm, sole, beneath nail
Confused with subungual hematoma
Asians/blacks
Poor prognosis
Depth invasion key factor
Prognosis in malignant melanoma: depth of invasion most important
ABCD
Asymmetry
Border irregularity
Color variation
Diameter >6 mm
Prevention
Sunscreen >15 SPF (controversial)
Prevention for UVA/UVB
Protective clothing best prevention
Sentinel lymph node Bx determines stage
Breslow system: depth of invasion for staging

  c. Leading COD from skin cancer
  d. Median age at diagnosis is 53 years.
  e. Risk factors for malignant melanoma
    (1) Excessive exposure to sunlight (UVA and ultraviolet light B [UVB]) at an early age. This is the most important risk factor for developing a malignant melanoma.
    (2) History of a family member with malignant melanoma. Risk is 8% to 10%.
    (3) Excessive use of tanning booths; dysplastic nevus syndrome
    (4) History of a malignant melanoma in a first- (person's parent, sibling, or child) or second-degree relative (grandparents, grandchildren, aunts, uncles, nephews, nieces, or half-siblings)
    (5) Xeroderma pigmentosum (see Chapter 9)
3. Radial growth phase
  a. Initial phase of invasion of a malignant melanoma
  b. Melanocytes proliferate:
    (1) laterally within the epidermis.
    (2) along the dermal–epidermal (DE) junction.
    (3) within the papillary dermis (uppermost layer of the dermis composed of loose areolar connective tissue).
  c. *No* metastatic potential in this phase
4. Vertical growth phase
  a. Final phase of invasion
  b. Penetration of malignant cells into the underlying reticular dermis
  c. Potential for metastasis in this phase
5. Types of cutaneous malignant melanoma
  a. Superficial spreading melanoma (SSM; Fig. 25-9 H; Link 25-94)
    (1) MC type of cutaneous malignant melanoma (70% of cases)
    (2) Common sites include the lower extremities, arms, and upper back.
  b. Lentigo maligna melanoma (LMM; 5%–10% of cases)
    (1) Common in older adults
    (2) Extension of lentigo maligna (intraepidermal lesion) into the dermis
    (3) Long radial growth phase
    (4) Occurs on parts of the face that are most exposed to the sun (Fig. 25-9 I; Link 25-95)
    (5) *Least* likely of all melanomas to have a vertical phase; therefore, it has a good prognosis
  c. Nodular melanoma (15%–20% of cases; Fig. 25-9 J; Link 25-96)
    (1) *No* radial growth phase
    (2) Found in any sun-exposed area; however, it is most often located on the trunk
    (3) Only has a vertical phase; therefore, the prognosis is very poor
  d. Acral lentiginous melanoma (ALM; 7% to 10% of cases)
    (1) *Not* causally related to sun exposure
    (2) Located on the palm, sole (Link 25-97), or beneath the nail (Fig. 25-9 K); most often confused with a subungual hematoma from trauma to the nail (Fig. 25-9 L)
    (3) Most often occurs in Asians and blacks
    (4) Poor prognosis
6. Biological behavior of a cutaneous malignant melanoma is best determined by the depth of invasion.
  a. Invasion of >0.76 mm corresponds with a 99% 5-year survival rate.
  b. Invasion of >4 mm invasion corresponds with a 44% 5-year survival rate.
7. ABCD criteria for malignancy include (Fig. 25-9 M)
  a. <u>A</u>symmetry of shape
  b. <u>B</u>order irregularity
  c. <u>C</u>olor variation
  d. <u>D</u>iameter >6 mm
8. Prevention of cutaneous malignant melanoma
  a. Sunscreen >15 SPF (controversial); prevention for both UVA and UVB light
  b. Protective clothing (best prevention)
  c. Sentinel lymph node biopsy to determine stage (see Chapter 9)
  d. Breslow system for measuring the depth of invasion: used for staging (Link 25-98)
  e. Link 25-99 shows the transformation of melanocytes into melanoma.

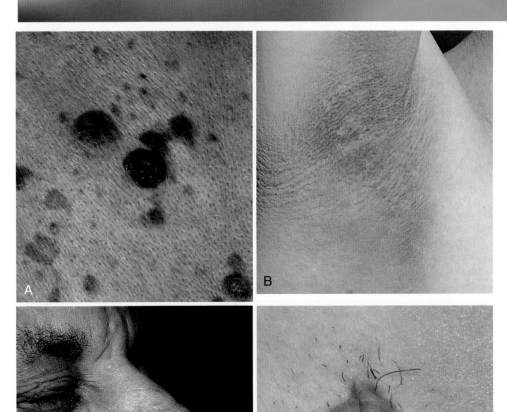

25-10: A, Seborrheic keratosis. Note the numerous raised, pigmented lesions with a verrucoid surface. These lesions appeared suddenly (Leser-Trélat sign) in this patient, indicating a possible underlying gastric adenocarcinoma. In most cases, they are a common lesion in the older adult population, in which they frequently occur on the face and axilla. **B,** Acanthosis nigricans. Note the pigmented verrucoid lesion in the axilla. Similar to the Leser-Trélat sign, these lesions may be associated with an underlying gastric adenocarcinoma or other disorders. **C,** Keratoacanthoma. Note the crateriform tumor with a central keratin plug. This looks very similar to a basal cell carcinoma (BCC); however, it appears rapidly and spontaneously resolves, unlike BCC . A biopsy settles the issue. **D,** Fibroepithelial tag. Note the flesh-colored pedunculated lesion attached to the body by a narrow stalk. These are common lesions in older adults. (*A from Kumar V, Cotran RS, Robbins SL:* Robbins Basic Pathology, *7th ed, Philadelphia, Saunders, 2003, p 799, Fig. 22-13A; B from Lookingbill D, Marks J:* Principles of Dermatology, *3rd ed, Philadelphia, Saunders, 2000, pp 350, 83, respectively, Figs. 25-5, 6-12, respectively; C from Rosai J:* Rosai and Ackerman's Surgical Pathology, *9th ed, St. Louis, Mosby, 2004, p 150, Fig. 4-88; D from Habif T:* Clinical Dermatology, *4th ed, St. Louis, Mosby, 2004.)*

VII. Benign Epithelial Tumors

A. Seborrheic keratosis

1. **Definition:** Benign, pigmented epidermal tumor that is a "coin-like," macular to raised verrucoid lesion with a "stuck-on" appearance (Link 25-100)
2. Epidemiology and clinical
   a. MC benign tumor in older adults
   b. Occurs in individuals >50 years of age
   c. Extremities, shoulders, and axilla are the MC sites.
   d. Commonly occurs on the face in the older population
3. Leser-Trélat sign (Link 25-101; see Chapter 9)
   a. Rapid increase in the number of seborrheic keratoses (Fig. 25-10 A)
   b. Phenotypic marker for gastric adenocarcinoma

B. Acanthosis nigricans (AN)

1. **Definition:** Velvety, hyperpigmented, papillomatous, "dirty-appearing" lesion on the skin
2. Epidemiology
   a. Most commonly located in the axilla (Fig. 25-10 B). Other sites include the neck, groin, and inframammary.
   b. Pathogenesis: excess insulin is noted in many cases
   c. Clinical associations of acanthosis nigricans
      (1) Metabolic syndrome (see Chapter 23). Obesity is important because of its association with insulin resistance (downregulation of insulin receptors), which produces hyperinsulinemia.
      (2) Insulin receptor deficiency (see Chapter 23)
      (3) Polycystic ovary syndrome (PCOS; see Chapter 22)
      (4) Phenotypic marker for gastric cancer (see Chapters 9 and 18)
      (5) Multiple endocrine neoplasia (MEN) type IIb (see Chapter 23)

C. **Keratoacanthoma (KA)**
   1. **Definition:** Rapidly growing, crateriform tumor with a central keratin plug (Fig. 25-10 C)
   2. Epidemiology
      a. More common in men than women
      b. Rapid growth (within 4–6 weeks) from normal-appearing skin
      c. Develops in sun-exposed areas
      d. Histologically, it looks like a well-differentiated squamous cell carcinoma (SCC), *except* for the Hx of its rapid growth within 4 to 6 weeks.
      e. Most regress spontaneously with scarring within 6 months.

D. **Fibroepithelial polyp (skin tag)**
   1. **Definition:** Flesh-colored soft tag of skin attached to the body by a narrow stalk (see Fig. 25-10 D; Link 25-102)
   2. Epidemiology
      a. Common finding in older adults
      b. Common locations include the neck, upper chest, and upper back.

E. **Syringoma**
   1. **Definition:** Benign sweat duct tumor composed of small, firm flesh-colored dermal papules that occur on the lower eyelids (Link 25-103)
   2. Epidemiology
      a. Appear during third and fourth decades of life
      b. More numerous over time; *no* malignant potential

VIII. **Premalignant and Malignant Epithelial Tumors**
   A. **Actinic (solar) keratosis** (see Chapter 9)
      1. **Definition:** Dysplasia of the epidermal keratinocytes; may be either partial- or full-thickness dysplasia (SCC in situ)
      2. Epidemiology
         a. Caused by excessive exposure to sunlight; increases one's risk of invasive SCC of the skin
         b. Hyperkeratotic, pearly gray-white appearance
         c. Occurs in sun-exposed areas such as the face (Link 25-104), back of the neck, and dorsum of the hands and forearms (Fig. 25-11 A)
         d. Commonly recurs when scraped off
         e. Increase in number with age

   B. **Basal cell carcinoma (BCC)**
      1. **Definition:** Malignant neoplasm that arises from the basal cells in the basal cell layer of the epidermis
      2. Epidemiology
         a. MC malignant tumor of skin
         b. Caused by chronic exposure to UV light
         c. Occurs in sun-exposed areas
            (1) Raised nodule with a central crater (Fig. 25-11 B; Links 25-105, 25-106, and 25-107). Sides of the crater are surfaced by telangiectatic (dilated) vessels.
            (2) Common locations include the inner canthus of the eye, upper lip, and ear lobe.
            (3) The maxim that BCCs favor the upper lip and higher, while SC carcinomas favor the lower lip and lower should *not* be relied on (biopsy the lesion!).
         d. Locally aggressive, infiltrating cancer that nearly never metastasizes
         e. Arises from the basal cell layer of the epidermis and is multifocal in origin in that large areas in the basal cell layer have carcinogenic alterations ("field effect"). This makes it difficult to get free margins after surgery, and it also explains why recurrence is common.
         f. Histologic exam reveals cords of basophilic-staining basal cells infiltrating the underlying dermis (Fig. 25-11 C).
      3. Diagnosis is made with a punch biopsy or a shave biopsy. If the biopsy result is positive for tumor, then a full excision of the cancer is performed to ensure free margins.

   C. **Squamous cell carcinoma (SCC)**
      1. **Definition:** Malignancy of keratinocytes
      2. Epidemiology and clinical
         a. Risk factors
            (1) Excessive exposure to UV light (greatest risk factor)
            (2) Actinic (solar) keratosis
            (3) History of arsenic exposure

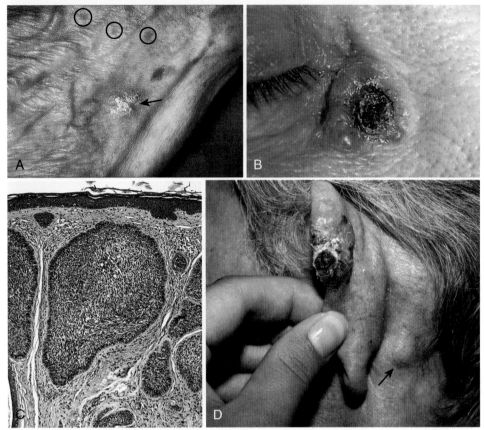

25-11: A, Actinic (solar) keratosis. Note the pearly gray-white hyperkeratotic lesion *(arrow)* on the hand. The other lesions *(circles)* are good examples of solar lentigo. Both of these types of lesions are common in the older adult population and are located in sun-exposed areas. **B,** Basal cell carcinoma (BCC). Note the ulcerated nodular mass on the inner aspect of the nose. This is a particularly common site for this cancer that invades but does not metastasize. **C,** BCC. This microscopic section shows multifocal nests of basophilic staining cells with peripheral palisading. This section does not show a connection with the basal cell layer of skin; however, these tumors arise from multifocal locations and extend into the dermis. **D,** Squamous cell carcinoma. Note the nodular, hyperkeratotic lesion occurring on the ear. This is a common site for this cancer in the older adult population. The *arrow* shows metastasis to a lymph node. *(A courtesy of R.A. Marsden, MD, St. George's Hospital, London; B from Savin JA, Hunter JAA, Hepburn NC: Diagnosis in Color: Skin Signs in Clinical Medicine, London, Mosby-Wolfe, 1997, p 104, Fig. 4-27; C from Rosai J, Ackerman LV: Surgical Pathology, 9th ed, St. Louis, Mosby, 2004, p 137, Fig. 4-60; D from Kumar V, Abbas AK, Fausto N, Mitchell RN: Robbins Basic Pathology, 8th ed, Philadelphia, Saunders Elsevier, 2007, p 851, Fig. 22-17.)*

(4) Scar tissue in a third-degree burn (see Chapter 7)

(5) Orifice of chronically draining sinus tract (see Chapter 7)

(6) Immunosuppressive therapy in renal transplant patients (see Chapter 4). Nine years after renal transplantation, patients have more than a 40% incidence of SCC.

(7) Men >60 years old

b. Scaly to nodular lesions of the skin in sun-exposed areas of the body

(1) Nodular lesions are often ulcerated.

(2) Common locations include the ears (Fig. 25-11 D), lip (see Fig. 18-6 D), and dorsum of the hands.

c. Usually very well differentiated and have numerous squamous pearls present (see Fig. 9-1E; Links 25-108, 25-109, 25-110, 25-111, and 25-112); minimal risk for metastasis

IX. Selected Skin Disorders

A. Ichthyosis vulgaris

1. **Definition:** Autosomal dominant (AD) disorder characterized by a defect in keratinization

2. Epidemiology

a. MC inherited skin disorder

b. Defect in keratinization causes increased thickness of the stratum corneum and absence of the stratum granulosum (Link 25-113).

3. Clinical findings in ichthyosis

a. Skin is hyperkeratotic and dry.

b. Primary sites of involvement include the palms, soles, and extensor areas.

Scar tissue 3rd degree burn

Orifice chronic-draining sinus

Immunosuppressive Rx renal transplant patients

Men > 60 yrs

Scaly to nodular lesions

Nodular lesions often ulcerated

Ears, lower lip, dorsum of hands

Selected skin disorders

Ichthyosis vulgaris, AD

Defect in keratinization

MC inherited skin disorder

↑Stratum corneum, absence stratum granulosum

Clinical findings

Hyperkeratotic, dry

Palms, soles, extensor areas

B. Xerosis
1. **Definition:** Condition characterized by dry skin and pruritus (itchiness)
2. Epidemiology
   a. MCC of dry skin and pruritus in older adults
   b. Caused by a decrease in skin lipids

C. Polymorphous light eruption (PML)
1. **Definition:** Common light-induced eruption of skin
2. Epidemiology
   a. MC photodermatitis
   b. Affects ~10% of the population
   c. Positive family Hx; very common in Native Americans (hereditary type PML)
   d. More common in women than men; more common in those with fair skin
3. Clinical findings in polymorphous light eruption
   a. Rapid onset after sun exposure (Fig. 25-12 A)
   b. Skin findings include erythematous macules, papules, plaques, or vesicles or bullae (Link 25-114)
   c. Pruritic rash that is sometimes painful
   d. *Not* a drug reaction

D. Eczema (see Chapter 4)
1. **Definition:** Group of inflammatory dermatoses characterized by pruritus (itchy skin)
2. Epidemiology
   a. Acute eczema. **Definition:** Weeping, erythematous, pruritic rash with vesicles
   b. Chronic eczema. **Definition**: Characterized by continual scratching of skin, which, over time, produces dry, thickened skin (hyperkeratosis)
3. Atopic dermatitis
   a. **Definition:** Chronic, pruritic, eczematous condition of the skin that is associated with a positive family Hx of atopic disease (e.g., allergic rhinitis, bronchial asthma, or atopic dermatitis)
   b. Epidemiology
      (1) Type I IgE-mediated hypersensitivity reaction (HSR; see Chapter 4)
      (2) Atopic dermatitis in children; skin is dry, and eczema is located on the cheeks and extensor and flexural surfaces (Fig. 25-12 B and C)
      (3) Atopic dermatitis in adults; characterized by dry skin and eczema on the hands, eyelids, elbows, and knees
4. Contact dermatitis (CD)
   a. **Definition:** Red, itchy rash caused by a substance that comes into contact with the skin
      • Allergic CD (see Chapter 4). Type IV HSR. Examples include poison ivy (see later) and nickel in jewelry (Link 25-115).
   b. Irritant CD: a skin reaction to an irritant (e.g., laundry detergent; Link 4-20; Chapter 4)
   c. Contact photodermatitis
      (1) UV light reacts with drugs that have a photosensitizing effect
      (2) Examples: tetracycline, sulfonamides, isotretinoin
   d. Poison ivy (rhus dermatitis) (Fig. 25-12 D; Link 25-116)
      (1) Sensitizing agent in poison ivy is urushiol, which is in the sap of the plant.
      (2) Sensitivity to poison ivy results in sensitivity to poison oak and sumac as well.
      (3) Contact with the smoke of burning plants often results in widespread, severe dermatitis of the skin that may even extend into the respiratory tract.

E. Autoimmune skin disorders
1. Chronic cutaneous lupus erythematosus (LE; see Chapter 4)
   a. Associated with atrophy of the epidermis
   b. DNA–anti-DNA immunocomplexes (ICs) deposit in the basement membrane (BM)
      (1) Degeneration of the basal cells and hair shafts (alopecia)
      (2) Positive immunofluorescent (IF) band test (Link 4-23; see Chapter 4): Immunofluorescence shows ICs deposited along the BM.
   c. Clinical findings in cutaneous LE
      (1) Erythematous maculopapular eruption; usually located over the malar eminences and bridge of the nose ("butterfly" rash; see Fig. 4-11 A)
      (2) Skin lesions are exacerbated by UV light.
2. Pemphigus vulgaris
   a. **Definition:** Autoimmune disease characterized by vesicles and bullae of the skin and mucous membranes

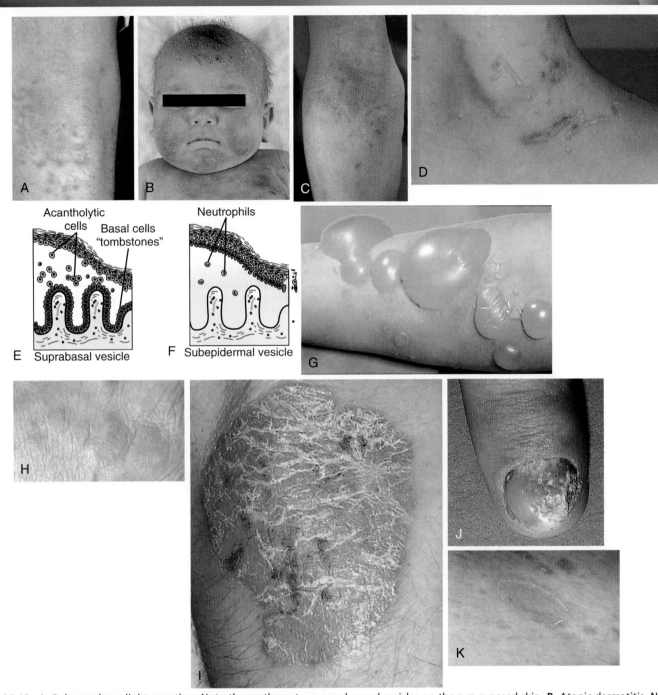

25-12: **A,** Polymorphous light eruption. Note the erythematous papules and vesicles on the sun-exposed skin. **B,** Atopic dermatitis. Note the erythematous, scaling rash on the cheeks and chin of this infant. Also note the scaling rash on the scalp, which is cradle cap (seborrheic dermatitis). **C,** Atopic dermatitis. Note the erythematous, scaling rash with thickening of the skin (lichenification) from constant scratching in the elbow flexure. **D,** Poison ivy. Note the acute eczematous rash with vesicle formation. **E,** Schematic of a suprabasal vesicle (e.g., pemphigus vulgaris). See text for discussion. **F,** Schematic of a subepidermal vesicle (e.g., bullous pemphigoid). See text for discussion. **G,** Bullous pemphigoid. Note the tense bullae. **H,** Lichen planus. Note the flat-topped violaceous papules. **I,** Psoriasis. The elbow shows a flat, salmon-colored plaque covered by white to silver-colored scales. **J,** Nail pitting in psoriasis. The nails show pitting. **K,** Pityriasis rosea. The initial oval herald patch is present in the center of the picture. Smaller erythematous patches surround the herald patch.

Continued

b. Epidemiology
   (1) IgG antibodies are directed against the intercellular attachment sites (desmosomes) between keratinocytes.
   (2) Type II HSR (see Chapter 4)
c. Clinical findings in pemphigus vulgaris
   (1) Vesicles and bullae develop on the skin (Link 25-117) and oral mucosa.
   (2) Intraepithelial vesicles are located *above* the basal layer (suprabasal; Fig. 25-12 E; Link 25-118).

IgG abs against desmosomes between keratinocytes

Type II HSR

Clinical findings

Vesicles/bullae skin, oral mucosa

Vesicles *above* basal layer

25-12 cont'd: L, Erythema multiforme. The palms show the classic target lesions with three zones of color. **M,** Erythema nodosum. Note the raised, erythematous nodular lesions on the anterior shins. This is commonly associated with coccidioidomycosis. **N,** Granuloma annulare. Note the erythematous, annular plaque on the dorsum of the hands. There is an increased association of this skin lesion with diabetes mellitus. **O,** Porphyria cutanea tarda. Wood light examination of the urine in a patient with porphyria cutanea tarda demonstrating classic coral red fluorescence with normal urine specimen exhibited for comparison. **P,** Urticaria. One of the manifestations of urticaria is dermatographism. In this case, there is swelling with the word HIVE. **Q,** Cherry angiomas. Note the red, papular lesions on the chest. These are extremely common in the older adult population. **R,** Acne rosacea. Note the pustules and papules superimposed on a background of erythema and telangiectasias (dilated vessels). There is also enlargement of the nose due to sebaceous gland hyperplasia (rhinophyma). **S,** Pyoderma gangrenosum. Note the large ulcer with the prominent red border. *(A courtesy of The Honickman Collection of Medical Images in memory of Elaine Garfinkel and The Jefferson Clinical Images Collection [through the generosity of JMB, AKR, LKB and DA]; B from Eichenfield L, Frieden I, Esterly N: Textbook of Neonatal Dermatology, Philadelphia, Saunders, 2001, p 242; C and M from Savin JA, Hunter JAA, Hepburn NC: Diagnosis in Color: Skin Signs in Clinical Medicine, London, Mosby-Wolfe, 1997, pp 9, 8, respectively, Figs. 1.16, 1.14, respectively; D and I from Forbes C, Jackson W: Color Atlas and Text of Clinical Medicine, 2nd ed, London, Mosby, 2002, pp 73, 69, respectively; E and F from Goljan EF: Star Series: Pathology, Philadelphia, Saunders, 1998, Fig 21-2BC; G from Walker BR, Colledge NR, Ralston SH, Penman ID: Davidson's Principles and Practice of Medicine, 22nd ed, Churchill Livingstone Elsevier, 2014, p 1294, Fig. 28.37A). H, P, and R from Lookingbill D, Marks J: Principles of Dermatology, 3rd ed, Philadelphia, Saunders, 2000, pp 201, 264, 213,repectively, Figs. 12-7A, 17-2, 13-4A, respectively; J, L, and S from Swartz M: Textbook of Physical Diagnosis History and Examination, 5th ed, Philadelphia, Saunders Elsevier, 2006, pp 149, 173, 175, respectively, Figs. 8-16B, 8-81, 8-88, respectively; K from Goldman L, Ausiello D: Cecil's Medicine, 23rd ed, Philadelphia, Saunders Elsevier, 2008, p 2942, Fig. 464-11; N from Goldstein BG: Practical Dermatology, 2nd ed, St. Louis, Mosby, 1997, p 312, Fig. 23-4; O and Q from Fitzpatrick JE, Morelli JG: Dermatology Secrets Plus, 4th ed, Philadelphia, Elsevier Mosby, 2011, pp 23, 303, respectively, Figs. 3.3, 42-6, respectively.)*

Basal cells resemble tombstones

Acantholysis vesicle fluid

+Nikolsky sign

Outer surface separates from basal layer

Bullous pemphigoid

Autoimmune disease with subepidermal bullae

(a) Linear row of intact basal cells resembling a row of tombstones

(b) Acantholysis of keratinocytes is present in the vesicle fluid.

(c) Positive Nikolsky sign: Outer epidermis separates from the basal layer with minimal pressure (Link 25-119).

3. Bullous pemphigoid

a. **Definition:** Autoimmune disorder characterized by subepidermal bullae

b. Epidemiology

(1) IgG antibodies are directed against the epidermis BM (Link 25-120).

(2) Type II HSR (see Chapter 4)

  c. Clinical findings

    (1) Vesicles are subepidermal (Fig. 25-12 F; Link 25-120).

      (a) Vesicles develop on the skin and oral mucosa (Fig. 25-12 G; Link 25-121).

      (b) Acantholytic cells are *not* present in the vesicle fluid.

      (c) Nikolsky sign is negative.

    (2) Disease usually subsides after months or years.

4. Dermatitis herpetiformis (DH; see Fig. 18-21 C)

  a. **Definition:** Chronic, pruritic vesicular disease characterized by symmetrical groups of vesicles on the elbows (key location), shoulders, lower back, and knees

  b. Epidemiology

    (1) IgA–anti-IgA complexes (type III HSR) deposit at the tips of the dermal papillae.

    (2) Subepidermal vesicles contain neutrophils.

    (3) DH has a strong correlation with celiac disease (see Chapter 18). Antireticulin and antiendomysial antibodies are present.

F. Lichen planus (LP)

1. **Definition:** Idiopathic inflammatory disease manifested by pruritic papules located over the flexor surfaces of the extremities, genitalia, and mucous membranes

2. Epidemiology

  a. Common skin disorder (1 in every 100 patients in dermatology clinics)

  b. Found in persons between the ages of 30 and 60 years old

  c. Association with hepatitis C virus (HCV), autoimmune diseases (e.g. primary biliary cirrhosis, inflammatory bowel disease [IBD], diabetes mellitus [DM]), and drugs (e.g., β-blockers, methyldopa, nonsteroidal antiinflammatory drugs [NSAIDs], angiotensin-converting enzyme inhibitors)

3. Clinical findings in lichen planus

  a. Rash is intensely pruritic, scaly, and violaceous and has flat-topped papules (Fig. 25-12 H; Link 25-122).

    (1) Rash has a fine white reticular pattern on the surface (called Wickham striae).

    (2) Commonly located on the wrists and ankles

  b. Nails are commonly dystrophic (Link 25-123).

    (1) Lesions develop in areas of scratching (Koebner phenomenon).

    (2) Oral mucosa is often involved (50% of cases; see Fig. 18-6 C); MC presentation

      (a) Fine, white, netlike lesions (Wickham striae) are present.

      (b) Slight risk of developing squamous cell carcinoma (SCC) in the oral cavity

G. Psoriasis

1. **Definition:** Chronic skin disorder characterized by an excessive proliferation of keratinocytes resulting in raised, salmon-colored plaques covered by silvery scales

2. Epidemiology

  a. Affects 1% to 3% of the world population

  b. Peak age at onset is bimodal (<20 years old to > 60 years old).

  c. *No* gender difference

  d. Pathogenesis

    (1) T-cell mediated disorder in which CD^{4+} and CD^{8+} memory T cells stimulate hyperproliferation of keratinocytes

    (2) Genetic factors are involved in 30% of cases; strong human leukocyte antigen (HLA) relationship.

    (3) Aggravating factors

      (a) S. pyogenes pharyngitis

      (b) HIV: Sudden onset of psoriasis is highly suspicious for HIV.

      (c) Drugs: lithium, β-blockers, NSAIDs

    (4) Microcirculatory changes are present in the superficial papillary dermis.

3. Clinical findings in psoriasis

  a. Erythematous plaques are well demarcated (Fig. 25-12 I).

  b. Erythematous plaques covered by adherent white to silver-colored scales (Links 25-124, 25-125, and 25-126). Pinpoint areas of bleeding occur when the scales are scraped off (Auspitz sign; Link 25-127).

  c. Plaques commonly develops in areas of trauma (elbows, lower back); called Koebner phenomenon.

  d. Nail pitting in 30% of cases (Fig. 25-12 J; Link 25-128)

  e. Geographic tongue is the MC mucosal manifestation (Link 25-129).

Margin notes:

IgG abs against BM

Type II HSR

Subepidermal vesicles

Skin, oral mucosa

No acantholytic cells in vesicle fluid

Negative Nikolsky sign

Subsides after months/years

Dermatitis herpetiformis

Symmetrical vesicles elbows

IgA-anti-IgA ICs; type III HSR

Subepidermal vesicles with neutrophils

Correlation with celiac disease

Antireticulin/endomysial abs

Lichen planus

Pruritic papules flexor surfaces, genitalia, mucous membranes

Common

30 to 60 yrs

HCV, autoimmune disease, drug

Clinical findings

Scaly, violaceous, flat-topped papules

Wickham striae (fine white reticular pattern)

Common on wrists, ankles

Nails dystrophic

Koebner phenomenon

Oral mucosa commonly involved

Wickham striae: fine, white, net-like

Slight risk SCC

Psoriasis

↑↑Keratinocytes; raised, salmon-colored plaques, silvery scales

1%–3% world population

Peak age bimodal: <20; >60 yrs

No gender difference

T-cell mediated hyperproliferation keratinocytes

Strong HLA relationship

Aggravating factors

Streptococcus pyogenes pharyngitis

HIV

Sudden onset psoriasis → think HIV

Drugs: lithium, NSAIDs, β-blockers

Microcirculatory changes superficial papillary dermis

Plaques well-demarcated

Erythematous plaques, silver scales

Pinpoint hemorrhages where scales scraped off (Auspitz sign)

Plaques areas trauma (e.g., elbows; Koebner phenomenon)

Nail pitting

Geographic tongue MC mucosal sign

4. Classic microscopic findings in psoriasis (Link 25-130)
   a. Hyperkeratosis and parakeratosis (retention of nuclei in the stratum corneum)
   b. Thinning of the epidermis overlying dermal papillae (i.e., extension of the papillary dermis close to the surface epithelium). Blood vessels in the dermis rupture when scales are picked off (Auspitz sign).
   c. Neutrophils collect in the stratum corneum; called Munro microabscesses.

H. Pityriasis rosea
1. **Definition:** Self-limiting eruptive dermatitis of unknown origin
2. Epidemiology and clinical
   a. Third MC papulosquamous disease seen by dermatologists
   b. Incidence is highest in the fall and spring. Mean age of the disease is 23 years old.
3. Clinical findings in pityriasis rosea
   a. Initially presents as a single, large, oval, scaly, rose-colored plaque on the trunk
      (1) Called the herald patch (Fig. 25-12 K; Link 25-131)
      (2) Frequently misdiagnosed as tinea corporis (ringworm)
   b. Days or weeks later, a pruritic papular eruption develops on the trunk.
      (1) Pruritic rash follows the lines of cleavage ("Christmas tree" distribution).
      (2) Rash remits spontaneously in 2 to 10 weeks.

I. Erythema multiforme (EM)
1. **Definition:** Cell-mediated (CM) cytotoxic reaction in the skin and mucous membranes that is triggered by infection or drugs
2. Epidemiology
   a. Triggers for developing the rash
      (1) Infection
         (a) *Mycoplasma pneumoniae* and herpes simplex virus (HSV); especially consider HSV in those with recurrent disease
         (b) Most cases follow outbreaks of HSV-1 and -2.
      (2) Drugs: sulfonamides, penicillin, barbiturates, NSAIDs, and phenytoin
   b. Occurs between 20 and 40 years of age
   c. In >50% of cases, there is *no* specific cause.
   d. Clinical findings in erythema multiforme (EM)
      (1) Vesicles and bullae have a "targetoid" appearance (Fig. 25-12 L; Link 25-132).
      (2) Lesions are located on the palms, soles, and extensor surfaces.
3. Stevens-Johnson syndrome (SJS) and toxic epidermal necrolysis (TEN)
   (Excerpted from Ferri FF: 2017 Ferri's Clinical Advisor, Philadelphia, Elsevier, 2017, pp 1206–1207.)
   a. **Definition:** Rare, severe vesiculobullous form of EM affecting the skin, mouth, eyes, and genitalia
   b. Epidemiology
      • Immune complex–mediated HSR (type III) that typically involves the skin and the mucous membranes. Classification schemes include:
         (a) SJS: A minor form of TEN (see later), with <10% body surface area (BSA) detachment.
         (b) SJS–TEN overlap syndrome: detachment of 10% to 30% of the BSA.
         (c) TEN: detachment of more than 30% of the BSA (see later).
   c. SJS predominantly affects children and young adults.
      (1) Causes
         (a) Infections (e.g., *M. pneumoniae,* HSV)
         (b) Drugs: antibiotics MC (penicillin, sulfa drugs), anticonvulsants, NSAIDs, allopurinol
      (2) Clinical findings (Links 25-133 and 25-134)
         (a) Vesiculobullous purpuric lesions on mucous membranes of mouth, nostrils, skin (targetoid lesions), and genital regions. Corneal ulcerations may result in blindness.
         (b) Can be a fatal disease
   d. TENS syndrome (TENS)
      (1) **Definition:** Life-threating mucocutaneous disease characterized by the apoptosis of keratinocytes followed by separation of the dermal-epidermal (D-E) junction over more than 30% of the body surface
      (2) Epidemiology
         (a) Most commonly drug induced (e.g., sulfonamides, NSAIDs, anticonvulsants, to name a few)
         (b) May occur alone or overlap with SJS

(3) Clinical findings in TENS
  (a) Characterized by extensive areas of erythema, necrosis, and bullous detachment of the epidermis and mucous membranes followed by exfoliation of the skin. Skin separation occurs with slight finger pressure (Nikolsky sign; Link 25-135 and 25-136).
  (b) Mucous membrane involvement can result in gastrointestinal (GI) bleeding, respiratory failure, and genitourinary (GU) complications.
  (c) Can be fatal

J. Erythema nodosum
  1. **Definition:** Acute, tender, inflammatory lesion involving the subcutaneous fat (panniculitis)
  2. Epidemiology
    a. More common in women than men (3 to 4 : 1 ratio)
    b. Common associations
      (1) Coccidioidomycosis, histoplasmosis
      (2) Tuberculosis (TB), leprosy
      (3) Streptococcal pharyngitis, *Yersinia enterocolitica* infections
      (4) Sarcoidosis, ulcerative colitis (UC)
      (5) Pregnancy, OCPs
  3. Clinical findings in erythema nodosum
    a. Red, raised painful nodules that are most commonly located on the anterior portion of the shins (Fig. 25-12 M; Link 25-137) and occasionally on the wrist (not to be confused with a ganglion cyst)
    b. Fever, painful lymphadenopathy, arthralgia, signs of underlying disease

K. Granuloma annulare
  1. **Definition:** Chronic, semi-limited, asymptomatic, dermal inflammatory disorder of unknown etiology that forms annular plaques on the dorsal aspect of the hands or feet
  2. Epidemiology
    a. Primarily occurs in children and young adults (<30 years old)
    b. Male:female ratio is 1 : 2.
    c. Possible causes include vasculitis, trauma, delayed type hypersensitivity (type IV HSR), and activation of monocytes.
    d. Usually a localized disease but can be disseminated in diabetes mellitus (DM)
    e. Recurs in 40% of affected patients
  3. Clinical findings in granuloma annulare
    a. Begins with erythematous papules that later evolve into annular plaques (Fig. 25-12 N)
    b. In the localized form, it occurs on the dorsum of the hands and feet.
    c. Spontaneously resolves within 2 years. Recurrence may occur in 40% of cases.

L. Porphyria cutanea tarda (PCT)
  1. **Definition:** Genetic or acquired disease involving porphyrin metabolism
  2. Epidemiology
    a. Caused by a deficiency of uroporphyrinogen decarboxylase (Link 25-138), the enzyme responsible for converting uroporphyrinogen III to coproporphyrinogen III
    b. Autosomal dominant in 20% of cases. Inherited mutations in the *UROD* gene (gene involved in heme synthesis) occurs in ~20% of cases. Remaining cases are sporadic.
    c. Urine is wine-red color on voiding and is coral red when viewed with a Wood lamp (Fig. 25-12 O).
    d. Uroporphyrin I is increased in the urine.
    e. Precipitating factors include sunlight, HCV infection, excessive alcohol intake, oral contraceptive pills (OCPs), and iron.
  3. Clinical findings in porphyria cutanea tarda (Links 25-139, 25-140, and 25-141)
    a. Photosensitive bullous skin lesions caused by the deposition of porphyrin metabolites in the skin. Patients commonly avoid light.
    b. Hyperpigmentation, fragile skin, and hypertrichosis (increased hair) are other findings.

M. Urticaria
  1. **Definition:** Condition characterized by pruritic, transient wheals (localized area of edema) in the skin resulting from dermal edema (Link 25-142)
  2. Epidemiology
    a. Most often caused by mast cell release of histamine
    b. Type I IgE-mediated HSRs (see Chapter 4) that are associated with a variety of exposures, including:
      (1) certain foods (e.g., peanuts).
      (2) insect bites (e.g., fire ant, mosquito).

(3) drugs (e.g., penicillin, morphine, aspirin, laxatives), emotional stress.

(4) HBV (part of serum sickness prodrome); type III HSR.

3. Clinical findings in urticaria

   a. Dermatographism is present ("skin writing"; Fig. 25-12 P).

   b. Urticaria develops in areas of mechanical pressure on the skin.

N. Cherry angiomas

1. **Definition:** Tiny bright red papules that turn brown with time (Fig. 25-12 Q; Link 25-143)

2. Epidemiology and clinical

   a. Invariably occur in all individuals >30 years old.

   b. Bleed profusely when scraped off

   c. *No* treatment is required.

O. Rosacea

1. **Definition:** Inflammatory erythematous reaction of the blood vessels and pilosebaceous units of facial skin

2. Epidemiology

   a. Occurs in 1 in 20 people between the ages of 30 and 50 years old

   b. Male:female ratio is 1:3.

   c. Causal relationship with mite *(Demodex folliculorum;* Link 25-144)

3. Clinical findings in acne rosacea

   a. Papules and pustules are present on the face (Link 25-145).

   b. Excessive redness of the face (Fig. 25-12 R; Link 25-145).

   c. Redness is exacerbated by drinking alcohol, stress, and eating spicy foods.

   d. Sebaceous gland hyperplasia causes enlargement and pitting of the nose (rhinophyma; Link 25-146).

P. Pyoderma gangrenosum

1. **Definition:** Ulcerative cutaneous condition often associated with systemic disease in >50% of cases

2. Epidemiology

   a. Probable dysregulation of the immune system. Neutrophil dysfunction is often present.

   b. May be initiated by trauma (called pathergy)

   c. Systemic disease associations.

      (1) Ulcerative colitis (UC), Crohn disease (CD)

      (2) Myeloproliferative disease (MPD)

      (3) Monoclonal gammopathy (MG)

      (4) Seronegative spondyloarthropathy, rheumatoid arthritis

3. Clinical findings in pyoderma gangrenosum

   a. Small red pustules or papules ulcerate and enlarge (Fig. 25-12 S; Link 25-147).

      (1) Reminiscent of a brown recluse spider bite

      (2) Single or multiple ulcers may be present.

   b. Violaceous border overhangs the ulcer crater.

4. Diagnosis of pyoderma gangrenosum: culture to rule out secondary infection and biopsy

Q. Necrotizing fasciitis

1. **Definition:** Rapidly progressive necrotizing infection of the skin, subcutaneous tissue, and superficial fascia frequently associated with severe systemic toxicity

2. Epidemiology and clinical

   a. Sometimes called hospital gangrene, streptococcal gangrene, or flesh-eating bacteria disease

   b. Usually caused by group A β-hemolytic *S. pyogenes;* may be polymicrobial and be associated with other streptococci, *Pseudomonas aeruginosa, S. aureus,* or other pathogens

   c. MC in individuals with decreased local resistance (skin injury, surgery, varicella), malnutrition, or chronic disease

   d. Usually occurs on an extremity. Patients often have soft tissue swelling and pain near a site of trauma with a break in the skin.

   e. Initially, pain with manipulation is often out of proportion to the skin findings. This is followed by sequential stages of ecchymosis, bullae, necrosis, gangrene with deep and extensive infection with overlying skin anesthesia. Inflammation extends deeply along fascial planes (Link 25-148).

   f. The most serious complication is streptococcal toxic shock syndrome (STSS), which is characterized by hypotension, renal failure, DIC, liver abnormalities, respiratory distress, and a diffuse erythematous cutaneous eruption. There is often a lack of a rapid response to systemic antibiotic therapy.

3. Laboratory findings in necrotizing fasciitis include neutrophilic leukocytosis, increased serum creatine kinase (CK; damage to muscle), and bacteremia (positive blood cultures).

4. Diagnosis is accomplished with a Gram stain and culture of the blister fluid. Polymerase chain reaction (PCR) analysis for pyrogenic exotoxin B on tissue biopsy specimens is very useful.

    a. Computed tomography and magnetic resonance imaging are useful in detecting gas in the subcutaneous tissue.

    b. Without prompt therapy (debridement and systemic antibiotics), there is a 100% mortality rate. Case mortality rate is ~25%.

X. Dermal and Subcutaneous Growths

A. Dermatofibroma

1. **Definition:** Nodule with focal dermal fibrosis accompanied by epidermal thickness and brown pigmentation (Link 25-149)

2. Epidemiology

    a. Most often seen in young adults

    b. Usually asymptomatic but may itch

    c. Pinching reveals central dimpling (key finding; Link 25-150).

B. Epidermal inclusion cyst (sebaceous cyst)

1. **Definition:** Freely moveable lesions that may be located anywhere on the body

2. Epidemiology

    a. Locations include the back, face, ears, chest or any surface on the body; freely moveable.

    b. Wall of the cyst is lined with keratin-producing stratified squamous epithelium.

    c. Communicates with the surface through a narrow channel; opening on the surface is keratin-filled, small, round and sometimes imperceptible (Link 25-151). The keratin often has a black color from oxidation of the keratin similar to a comedone (blackhead). They may originate from comedones and are sometimes called giant comedones, especially those located on the back.

    d. May be associated with Gardner syndrome (see Chapter 18)

C. Pilar cysts (wen)

1. **Definition:** Freely moveable cystic nodule on the scalp

2. Epidemiology

    a. Located on the scalp and may be multiple (Link 25-152)

    b. Epithelial-lined wall produces keratin of a different quality than an epidermal inclusion cyst.

    c. Cyst contains concentric layers of keratin (not stratified squamous epithelium). Over time, the keratin becomes macerated, soft, and cheesy.

XI. Selected Skin Disorders in Newborns (NBs)

A. Sites of common dermatoses in infants and children (Link 25-153)

B. Erythema toxicum neonatorum (ETN)

1. **Definition:** Self-limited benign eruption of unknown cause

2. Epidemiology

    a. *Not* present at birth

    b. Occurs in 20% to 50% of full-term NBs (*not* premature NBs)

    c. Lasts 2 to 3 weeks

3. Clinical findings

    a. Erythematous papules, macules, and pustules (Fig. 25-13 A)

    b. Present in all sites *except* the palms and soles

C. Sebaceous hyperplasia

1. **Definition:** Profuse yellow-white papules on the skin

2. Epidemiology

    a. Located on the forehead, nose (Fig. 25-13B; Link 25-154), upper lip, and cheeks

    b. Disappear in the first weeks of life

D. Milia

1. **Definition:** Superficial epidermal inclusion cysts in neonates

2. Epidemiology

    a. In neonates, they can be located on the face (Fig. 25-13 C; Links 25-155 and 25-156), gingiva, and midline of the palate and gingiva, where they are called Epstein pearls.

    b. Pearly white papules contain laminated keratin material.

3. Exfoliate spontaneously (or may be unroofed with a fine needle)

Margin notes:

Leukocytosis, ↑serum CK, bacteremia

PCR for exotoxin B

Gas in subcutaneous tissue

Very high mortality rate

Dermal/subcutaneous growths

Dermatofibroma

Nodule, fibrosis, brown pigmentation

Young adults

Usually asymptomatic

Pinching reveals central dimpling

Epidermal inclusion cyst

Nodule, central depression, opening with keratin debris

Any location; moveable

Lining stratified squamous epithelium producing keratin

Keratin-filled orifice

Giant blackhead

Gardner syndrome association

Pilar cyst (wen)

Cystic nodule scalp

May be multiple

Wall lined by keratin

Concentric layers keratin (not squamous epithelium)

Skin disorders newborns

ETN

Self-limited; cause unknown

Not present at birth

Full-term NBs

Self-limited; 2 to 3 wks

Erythematous papules, macules, pustules

All sites except palms/soles

Sebaceous hyperplasia

Yellow-white papules on skin

Forehead, nose, upper lip, cheeks

Disappear first weeks of life

Milia

Superficial epidermal inclusion cysts; neonates

Face, gingiva, midline palate/gingiva (Epstein pearls)

Pearly white papules contain laminated keratin

Exfoliate spontaneously

25-13: A, Erythema toxicum. Note the yellow-white papules and pustules with a surrounding erythematous flare over the chest and arms of this newborn. **B,** Sebaceous gland hyperplasia. Note the yellow papules on the nose of the newborn. **C,** Milia. Note the white papules on the face of this newborn. **D,** Miliaria crystallina. Note the clear vesicles on the skin of this newborn. **E,** Miliaria rubra. Note the erythematous maculopapular rash on the face of this newborn. **F,** Mongolian spot. Note the area of black discoloration above the crease of the buttocks in this newborn. *(A, B, and D from Kliegman RM, Jenson HB, Behrman RE, Stanton BF: Nelson's Textbook of Pediatrics, 18th ed, Philadelphia, Saunders Elsevier, 2007, pp 2662, 2661, 2725, respectively, Figs. 646-3, 646-1, 660-1, respectively; C from Seidel HM, Ball JW, Danis JE, Benedict GW: Mosby's Guide to Physical Examination, 6th ed, St. Louis, Mosby Elsevier, 2006, p 199, Fig. 8-25; E from Habif T: Clinical Dermatology, 4th ed, St. Louis, Mosby, 2004; F from Lemmi FO, Lemmi CAE: Physical Assessment Findings CD-ROM, Philadelphia, Saunders, 2000.)*

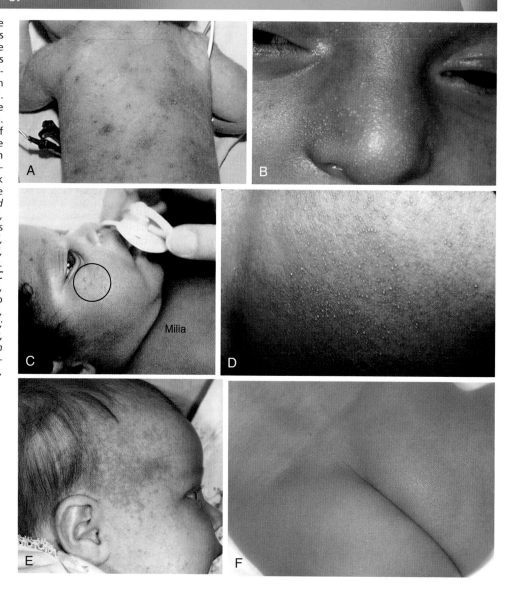

Milia

Miliaria
Miliaria crystallina
Retention sweat in occluded eccrine sweat glands
Pinpoint clear vesicles; sweat in occluded sweat glands
Sudden eruption
Warm/humid climates, fever
Cooling of neonate, remove excess clothing
Miliaria rubra ("heat rash")
Occlusion intraepidermal section eccrine sweat glands
Miliaria rubra: prickly heat; erythematous papulovesicles
Both types of miliaria respond to cooling
Salmon patch
Blanchable vascular patch of glabella/forehead
MC vascular lesion of childhood

E. **Miliaria**
   1. Miliaria crystallina
      a. **Definition:** Represent the retention of sweat *under* the stratum corneum due to occluded eccrine sweat glands
      b. Epidemiology and clinical
         (1) Appear as pinpoint, clear vesicles ("dewdrop") on the skin
         (2) May suddenly erupt in profusion over large areas of the body (Fig. 25-13 D)
         (3) May occur in warm, humid conditions or with fever
         (4) Respond dramatically to cooling of the neonate and removal of excess clothing
   2. Miliaria rubra ("heat rash")
      a. **Definition:** Occlusion of the intraepidermal section of the eccrine sweat glands causing minute erythematous papulovesicles on the skin
      b. Epidemiology and clinical
         (1) Erythematous, minute papulovesicles on the skin (Fig. 25-13E; Link 25-157)
         (2) Similar to miliaria crystallina, the lesions respond dramatically to cooling.
F. **Salmon patch** (Link 25-158)
   1. **Definition:** Blanchable vascular patch of the glabella (smooth part of the forehead above and between the eyebrows) and forehead that becomes more prominent with crying or increased body temperature
   2. Epidemiology. MC vascular lesion of childhood

G. Irritant contact dermatitis; diaper rash
1. **Definition:** Diaper dermatitis is an erythematous rash affecting the groin and buttocks.
2. Caused by moisture and feces
3. Secondary infection with bacteria or yeast may occur.

H. Seborrheic dermatitis of the scalp (cradle cap)
1. **Definition:** Skin disorder of infancy that presents as a yellow, greasy, scaling adherent rash on the scalp; may extend to the forehead, eyes, ears, eyebrows, nose, and back of the head (Link 25-159)
2. Epidemiology and clinical findings
   a. Appears in the first few months of life and generally resolves in several weeks to a few months
   b. The cause of cradle cap is unknown.
      (1) A possible contributing factor may be hormones passing from the mother to the baby *before* birth. These hormones can cause too much production of oil (sebum) in the oil glands and hair follicles.
      (2) Another possible cause may be the fungus *Malassezia furfur* that grows in the sebum along with bacteria.
   c. Itching is *not* present.
   d. Responds rapidly to topical steroid shampoo

I. Congenital dermal melanocytosis (Mongolian spots)
1. **Definition:** Congenital dermal melanocytosis characterized by a bluish black to slate gray hyperpigmented spot in the sacrococcygeal region (Fig. 25-13 F; Link 25-160)
2. Epidemiology and clinical
   a. Most frequently present in black, Asian, or Indian population, but also occurs in infants of other races
   b. Believed to represent delayed disappearance of dermal melanocytes
   c. Pigmentation often lightens spontaneously in the first 3 to 5 years of life; however, some may persist into adulthood.

J. Cutis marmorata
1. **Definition:** Reticulate (netlike) bluish mottling of the skin on the trunk and extremities (Link 25-161)
2. Epidemiology: normal physiologic response to chilling with resultant dilation of capillaries and small venules that usually disappears as the infant is rewarmed

XII. Selected Hair and Nail Disorders
A. Phases of hair growth in succession
1. Anagen phase
   a. Development of a new shaft of hair comes from the hair bulb.
   b. Hair length is determined in this stage.
   c. Growth stops at the end of this phase.
2. Telogen phase
   a. Resting phase
   b. Matrix portion shrivels, and hair within the follicle is shed.
   c. New matrix is formed at the bottom of the follicle.
   d. Cycle repeats itself.
3. Length of each phase varies in the body. In scalp hair, the anagen phase lasts 6 years, and the telogen phase lasts 4 months.
4. Hair growth is usually asynchronous.
   a. At any one time, ~80% of the scalp hair is in the anagen phase, and ~10% to 20% is in the telogen phase.
   b. Only a small percentage of scalp hair is lost at any point in time.
5. Estrogen (E) effect on hair growth
   a. E causes synchronous hair growth.
   b. All hairs enter the resting phase at once.

B. Massive hair loss; causes
1. Postpartum state (MCC)
2. Use of OCPs; stress
3. Radiation or chemotherapy: caused by inhibition of the anagen phase when cells in the hair bulb are dividing

C. Alopecia areata
1. **Definition:** Idiopathic disorder characterized by well-circumscribed patches of nonscarring hair loss
2. Epidemiology

25-14: A, Alopecia areata. Note the area of baldness and the short hairs that have the appearance of exclamation marks. **B,** Nail anatomy. See text for discussion. **C,** Mees bands. Note the transverse white lines in the nail plate that extend proximally until they are pared off. **D,** Beau lines. Note the transverse grooves or depressions that are oriented parallel to the lunula. *(A from Savin JA, Hunter JAA, Hepburn NC: Diagnosis in Color: Skin Signs in Clinical Medicine, London, Mosby-Wolfe, 1997, p 96, Fig. 4.5; B and C from Swartz MH: Textbook of Physical Diagnosis, 5th ed, Philadelphia, Saunders Elsevier, 2006, pp 140, 146, respectively, Figs. 8-3, 8-7, respectively; D from Callen JP, Paller AS, Greer KE, Swinyer LJ: Color Atlas of Dermatology, 2nd ed, Philadelphia, Saunders, 2000.)*

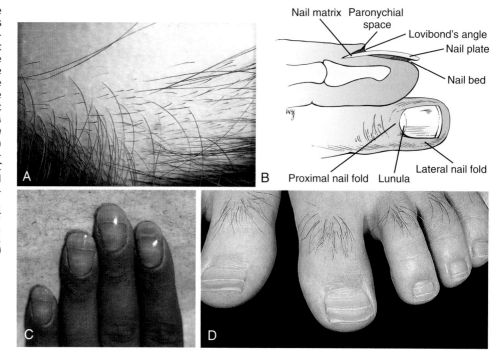

Sexes equally affected

Young adults

Hashimoto thyroiditis, pernicious anemia autoimmune association

Family Hx 20% to 25%

Clinical findings

Well-circumscribed, round/oval smooth pink/peach patches

Hair loss scalp, beard, eyebrows, eyelashes

Hairs "exclamation marks"

Hair loss over period of weeks

Hair regrowth several mths

May recur 1/3rd cases

Pitting of nails

Nail disorders

Nail anatomy

Lunula

White half-moon

Nail plate

Attached to nail bed (except distally)

Nail matrix

Underneath cuticle

Where nail plate originates

Mees lines

Transverse white lines nail plate

Arsenic poisoning; systemic illness

Beau lines

Transverse grooves parallel to lunula

Infections, nutritional disorders, hypothyroidism

a. Affects both sexes equally
b. Onset young adulthood most commonly
c. Some cases are associated with the autoimmune disorders Hashimoto thyroiditis and pernicious anemia.
d. Family Hx is present in 20% to 25% of cases.
3. Clinical findings in alopecia areata
   a. Hair is lost in well-circumscribed, round smooth to oval pink to peach-colored patches. Hair loss may occur on the scalp, beard, eyebrows, and eyelashes.
   b. Hairs have the appearance of "exclamation marks" (Fig. 25-14 A; Links 25-162 and 25-163).
   c. Hair loss occurs over a period of weeks.
   d. Regrowth of hair occurs over several months.
   e. May recur in up to one-third of cases
   f. Pitting (punctate depressions of the nails) is also present (Link 25-164).
D. Nail disorders
1. Nail anatomy (Fig. 25-14 B, Link 25-165)
   a. Lunula
      (1) **Definition:** White half-moon–shaped area proximal to the cuticle (dead skin at the base of a fingernail or toenail)
      (2) Underlying nail bed is partially keratinized, which produces the white color.
   b. Nail plate: attached to the nail bed *except* distally where it separates from the hyponychium (thickened layer of epidermis beneath the free end of a nail)
   c. Nail matrix
      (1) Underneath the cuticle
      (2) Where the nail plate originates
   d. Normal nail in the black population (Link 25-166)
2. Nail disorders (Link 25-167)
   a. Mees bands
      (1) **Definition:** Transverse white lines in the nail plate (Fig. 25-14 C; Link 25-167)
      (2) Extend proximally until they are pared off
      (3) Sign of arsenic poisoning and systemic illness of any kind
   b. Beau lines
      (1) **Definition:** Transverse grooves or depressions parallel to the lunula (Fig. 25-14 D; Links 25-167 and 25-168)
      (2) Caused by conditions that cause the nail to grow slowly. Examples: infections, nutritional disorders, hypothyroidism

c. Lindsay's nails
   (1) **Definition:** Proximal portions of the nail bed are white, but the distal portion of the nail are reddish ("half and half" nails; Links 25-167 and 25-169)
   (2) Caused by chronic renal disease with azotemia (increase in blood urea nitrogen and creatinine)
d. Terry's nails
   (1) **Definition:** White nail beds that extend to within 1 to 2 mm from the distal border of the nail (Links 25-167 and 25-170)
   (2) Most commonly associated with liver failure (e.g., cirrhosis), hypoalbuminemia (e.g., nephrotic syndrome), or chronic heart failure
e. Chronic iron deficiency; koilonychia (spoon nails; see Fig. 12-10 C; Links 25-167 and 25-171)
f. Clubbing
   (1) **Definition:** Condition in which the angle between the nail plate and the proximal nail fold straightens out to greater than 180 degrees (Links 25-167 and 25-172)
   (2) Epidemiology and clinical
      (a) Common factor in most types of clubbing is distal digital vasodilation, which results in increased blood flow to the distal portion of the digits.
      (b) Whether the vasodilation results from a circulating or local vasodilator, neural mechanism, response to hypoxemia, genetic predisposition, platelet-derived growth factor (PDGF), or a combination of these or other mediators is not agreed upon.
g. Psoriasis: More than 80% of patients exhibit pitting of the nails (Fig. 25-12 J; Link 25-167).
h. Subacute infective endocarditis and trichinosis; splinter hemorrhages in nails (see Fig. 11-20 C)
i. Subungual hematoma
   (1) **Definition:** Blood clot underneath the nail plate secondary to trauma (e.g., hammer injury; see Fig. 25-9 L)
   (2) Often confused with acral lentiginous melanoma
j. Ingrown toenail
   (1) **Definition:** The lateral portion of the nail plate grows into the lateral nail fold, causing an inflammatory response (Link 25-173)
   (2) Clinical findings ingrown toenail
      (a) Great toe most often involved.
      (b) Causes include tight footwear, infection, improperly trimmed toenails, trauma, and heredity.
      (c) Ingrown nail plate acts as a foreign body, leading to an acute inflammatory reaction.
      (d) Pain and swelling with possible secondary bacterial infection (*S. aureus*)
k. Paronychial infection
   (1) **Definition:** Acute inflammation of the lateral nail fold
   (2) Epidemiology and clinical
      (a) Most often the result of a bacterial infection caused by *S. aureus*
      (b) Trauma or maceration producing a break in the cuticle between the nail fold and the nail plate is the MCC. Pocket collects moisture, which promotes growth of bacteria.
      (c) Second and third digits of the hand are most frequently involved.
      (d) Painful, red, and swollen; often accompanied by an abscess or cellulitis (Link 25-174)
      (e) May develop into a chronic infection (usually *Candida albicans*) characterized by a loss of the cuticle, tenderness, swelling, and erythema are present; seen in people with diabetes mellitus (~10%) and children who are thumb suckers

Lindsay's nails

Proximal nail white, distal nail red ("half and half")

Chronic renal disease

Terry's nails

White nail beds extend to distal border

Liver failure, hypoalbuminemia, chronic heart failure

Chronic iron deficiency

Koilonychia (spoon nails)

Clubbing

Angle of nail straightens out to >180 degrees

Distal digital vasodilation

?Local vasodilator, neural mechanism, hypoxemia, genetic, PDGF

Psoriasis

Nail pitting

Subacute infective endocarditis; trichinosis

Splinter hemorrhages

Subungual hematoma

Blood clot under nail plate

Confused with acral lentiginous melanoma

Ingrown toenail

Lateral portion nail plate grows into lateral nail fold

Clinical findings

Great toe MC site

Tight footwear, infection, improper trimming, trauma

Ingrown nail plate foreign body

Pain, swelling, 2° bacterial infection

Paronychial infection

Acute inflammation lateral nail fold

Epidemiology/clinical

S. aureus MC pathogen

Trauma: break in cuticle between nail fold and nail plate

2nd/3rd digits MC

Painful, red, swollen; abscess/cellulitis

Chronic: *C. albicans*; diabetics, thumb suckers

CHAPTER 26
Nervous System and Special Sensory Disorders

ABBREVIATIONS

MC most common   MCC most common cause

I. **Overview of Central Nervous System** (Links 26-1, 26-2, 26-3, 26-4, 26-5, 26-6, 26-7, 26-8, 28-9, 26-10, 26-11, 26-12, 26-13, 26-14, 26-15, 26-16 and 26-17)

II. **Cerebrospinal Fluid Analysis**

A. **Overview of CSF**

1. Cerebrospinal fluid (CSF) derives from the choroid plexus in the ventricles (Links 26-18 and 26-19). The average male adult has 100 to 150 mL of CSF.
2. CSF enters the subarachnoid space.
   a. CSF cushions the brain and spinal cord.
   b. Important in autoregulation of cerebral blood flow
   c. Circulates nutrients and chemicals filtered from the blood
   d. Removes waste products derived from the brain
3. CSF is reabsorbed by arachnoid granulations (small protrusions of arachnoid through the dura matter). It drains into dural venous sinuses.
4. Route of CSF from production to clearance
   • Choroid plexus → lateral ventricle → interventricular foramen of Monro → third ventricle → cerebral aqueduct of Sylvius (AoS) → fourth ventricle → two lateral foramina of Luschka and one medial foramen of Magendie → subarachnoid space → arachnoid granulations → dural sinus → venous drainage

B. **CSF analysis**

1. Obtained by a lumbar puncture; ideal spinal level is below the conus medullaris (most distal bulbous part of the spinal cord) at approximately vertebral level L4 to L5
2. Three tubes for CSF analysis are usually collected.
   a. First tube: microbiologic studies
   b. Second tube
      (1) Chemistry: glucose, total protein
      (2) Cytology: if malignancy is suspected
      (3) Serologic tests
         (a) Syphilis serology (e.g., Venereal Disease Research Laboratory [VDRL])
         (b) Rapid plasma reagin (RPR) test *cannot* be used on CSF.
   c. Third tube: white blood cell (WBC) count and differential
3. Gross appearance
   a. Normal CSF is clear and colorless.
   b. Turbidity; causes:
      (1) increased protein (e.g., CSF infection).
      (2) increase in cellular elements (e.g., neutrophils).

774

(Margin notes:) CSF analysis; Overview CSF; CSF choroid plexus ventricles; Enters SAD space; Cushions brain/spinal cord; Autoregulation blood flow; Circulates nutrients/chemicals; Removes waste products; Reabsorbed by arachnoid granulations; Drained into dural venous sinuses; CSF analysis; Lumbar puncture; L4 to L5; 1st: microbiologic studies; 2nd: chemistry; glucose, total protein; 2nd: Cytologic test if necessary; 2nd: VDRL; 3rd: WBC count/differential; Clear/colorless; Turbidity; ↑Protein; ↑WBCs

(3) presence of microbial elements (e.g., bacteria, fungi).

(4) combinations of the previously mentioned causes.

c. Bloody CSF taps; causes:

    (1) most often caused by a traumatic tap (iatrogenic). Occurs in ~20% of lumbar taps. If traumatic, the hemorrhagic CSF fluid usually clears between the first and third collecting tubes.

    (2) pathologic hemorrhage into the subarachnoid space

      (a) Examples: ruptured berry aneurysm, intracerebral bleed close to the surface of the brain or ventricles

      (b) If the hemorrhage is pathologic (e.g., subarachnoid bleed), the CSF will be hemorrhagic in all the tubes.

    (3) CSF color changes in pathologic bleeds

      (a) Pink, yellow, or orange-tinged CSF after high-speed centrifugation

      (b) Pink color is caused by oxyhemoglobin (oxyHb) from hemolyzed red blood cells (RBCs). Color first occurs 2 to 4 hours after a bleed; peaks in 24 to 36 hours; subsides in 4 to 8 days.

      (c) Yellow to orange color (xanthochromia) is caused by oxyHb breakdown to bilirubin. It first appears in 12 hours after a bleed and peaks in 2 to 4 days and subsides in 2 to 4 weeks.

      (d) Macrophages (MPs) can phagocytize RBCs, break them down, and produce hemosiderin (Link 26-20).

4. CSF protein

  a. Normal 15 to 60 mg/dL

  b. CSF prealbumin and albumin

    (1) Normal levels derive from plasma.

    (2) Increased levels of CSF prealbumin and albumin are caused by increased capillary permeability (e.g., acute inflammation).

  c. CSF gamma (γ)-globulin

    (1) Normal levels derive from the synthesis of IgG by plasma cells within the central nervous system (CNS); represent <12% of the total protein in a CSF electrophoresis

    (2) Increased CSF IgG levels; causes:

      (a) increased synthesis of IgG from plasma cells within the CNS. Examples: demyelinating disorders (e.g., multiple sclerosis).

      (b) increased capillary permeability. Example: acute meningitis

    (3) CSF IgG index distinguishes acute inflammation from demyelinating diseases.

      (a) CSF IgG index = [CSF IgG mg/dL × Serum albumin (g/dL] ÷ [CSF albumin (mg/dL) x serum IgG (g/dL]. Normal upper limit is 0.8.

      (b) An increased CSF IgG index indicates demyelinating disease. A decreased index indicates acute inflammation.

    (4) A routine CSF electrophoresis is used to quantitate the amount of γ-globulins when CSF protein is increased (i.e., >60 mg/dL).

    (5) High-resolution (HR) CSF electrophoresis (EPS)

      (a) Most useful test in detecting demyelinating disease (see Fig. 26-17 D) Examples: Multiple sclerosis, neurosyphilis (NS), Guillain-Barré syndrome (GBS)

      (b) Detects oligoclonal bands in the γ-globulin region

        • **Definition:** Discrete discontinuous bands originating from single clones of immunocompetent B cells

  d. Myelin basic protein (MBP) in multiple sclerosis

    (1) **Definition:** The protein that is present in myelin

    (2) In multiple sclerosis, antibodies (Abs) attack MBP in myelin.

    (3) Increased CSF MBP occurs in active demyelinating diseases (e.g., multiple sclerosis). When multiple sclerosis is in remission, the CSF MBP is decreased.

    (4) Additional demyelinating diseases associated with an increase in MBP include GBS, systemic lupus erythematosus (SLE) involving the CNS, subacute sclerosing panencephalitis (SSP), various brain tumors, and after CNS irradiation and chemotherapy.

5. CSF glucose

  a. Normal CSF glucose is 50 to 80 mg/dL.

  b. Slightly less concentration than the serum glucose

  c. Should be ~66% of a serum sample of glucose obtained 30 to 90 minutes *before* lumbar puncture. Very useful if the patient has diabetes mellitus (DM) with an elevated serum

---

Bacteria/fungi

Combinations

Blood in CSF

Traumatic tap MCC

Subarachnoid hemorrhage

Ruptured aneurysm, intracerebral bleed

All tubes have blood

Pink, yellow, orange tinged

Pink oxyHb hemolyzed RBCs

2 to 4 hrs post bleed

Yellow to orange: xanthochromia (bilirubin)

12 hrs after bleed

CSF protein

Prealbumin/albumin from plasma

↑Prealbumin/albumin: ↑capillary permeability acute inflammation

CSF γ-globulin

Normal levels synthesis IgG CNS plasma cells

↑CSF IgG

↑Synthesis plasma cells in CNS

Demyelinating disorders (e.g., mutliple sclerosis)

↑Capillary permeability

Acute meningitis

CSF IgG index

CSF IgG × serum albumin ÷ CSF albumin x serum IgG

↑ CSF IgG index → demyelination

↓ CSF IgG index → acute inflammation

Routine CSF electrophoresis: quantitates amount γ-globulins

HR CSF electrophoresis: most useful

Detects demyelinating disease

Multiple sclerosis, NS, GBS

Detects oligoclonal bands

Discrete bands single clone B cells

MBP: protein in myelin

Abs attack MBP in myelin in multiple sclerosis

↑CSF MBP: active multiple sclerosis

Multiple sclerosis remission: ↓CSF MBP

GBS, SLE (CNS), SSP, brain tumors, post rad/chemo

CSF glucose

CSF glucose < serum glucose

glucose and requires a spinal tap to rule/out a CNS infection. Example: With a serum glucose level of 300 mg/dL, the CSF glucose should be ~200 mg/dL.

   d. Decrease CSF glucose is called hypoglycorrhachia.

     (1) Defined as a CSF glucose <40 mg/dL

     (2) May be caused by increased uptake of glucose by cellular elements. Examples: neutrophils (acute bacterial meningitis), CSF fungal infection, malignant cells (leukemia metastatic to the brain)

     (3) May be caused by a defective glucose carrier system. Example: frequently occurs in bacterial and fungal infections in the brain

   e. CSF glucose levels are usually normal in viral meningitis, neurosyphilis (NS), demyelinating disease, and cerebral abscesses. Exceptions include mumps (meningoencephalitis), herpes simplex virus (HSV), and lymphocytic choriomeningitis (LCM).

6. CSF WBC count

   a. Normal is 0 to 5 mononuclear cells/mm³. Neutrophils are *never* a normal finding in the CSF.

   b. Causes of an increased CSF WBC count

     (1) Bacterial meningitis, fungal meningitis, viral meningitis (normal or slightly increased in early disease, metastasis (Link 26-21) (discussed later; Table 26-1)

     (2) Multiple sclerosis (variants helper T cells)

7. Detection of microbial pathogens in CSF

   a. Gram stain (bacteria): most useful for bacteria (75%–80% sensitivity)

   b. Culture

   c. India ink for *Cryptococcus neoformans*: Sensitivity is 50%.

   d. Antigen detection

     (1) Latex agglutination and coagglutination

       (a) CSF or urine can be used.

       (b) Sensitivity depends on the pathogen.

       (c) Specificity is 96% to 100%.

     (2) Enzyme immunoassay (EIA): high sensitivity and specificity (96–100% in both)

     (3) Polymerase chain reaction (PCR): detects DNA; high sensitivity (94%) and specificity (96%)

III. Cerebral Edema, Idiopathic Intracranial Hypertension, Herniation, and Hydrocephalus

  A. Cerebral edema

    1. **Definition:** Intracellular (IC) or extracellular (EC) accumulation of excess fluid in the brain; causes an increase in intracranial pressure. Grossly, the brain swells, causing a midline shift. Widening and flattening of the gyri and narrowing of the sulci are present (Link 26-22).

    2. Epidemiology

      a. Subdivided into IC and EC types (Fig. 26-1 A)

      b. IC edema

        (1) **Definition:** Water moves into neurons and astrocytes.

        (2) Causes

          (a) Dysfunctional Na⁺/K⁺-ATPase pump (e.g., global hypoxia)

          (b) Hyponatremia causing an osmotic shift into the cells (e.g., syndrome of inappropriate antidiuretic hormone [SIADH]; see Chapter 5)

TABLE 26-1   Cerebrospinal Fluid Findings in Viral, Bacterial, and Fungal Meningitis

CSF FEATURE	BACTERIAL	VIRAL	FUNGUS
Total cell count	Increased (>1000/mm³) TB (10–500/mm³)	Usually normal or slightly increased (<100/mm³)	Usually normal or slightly increased (20–500/mm³)
Differential count	• Predominantly neutrophils • TB, usually lymphocytes	First 24–48 hr, neutrophils, followed by predominantly lymphocytes after 48 hr	Lymphocytes
CSF glucose	Decreased (<30 mg/dL)	Normal; exceptions: mumps, herpes, LCM	Decreased
CSF protein	Increased (>120 mg/dL) TB 100–500 mg/dL	Increased	Increased
Gram stain	• Frequently positive (60%–90%) • Culture positive (65%–90%)	Negative	Frequently positive

CSF, Cerebrospinal fluid; *LCM,* lymphocytic choriomeningitis; *TB,* tuberculosis.

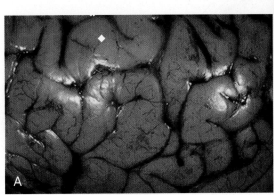
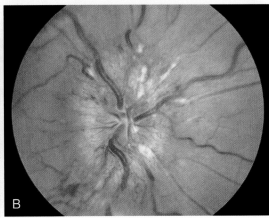

26-1: **A,** Cerebral edema. Note the widening and flattening of the gyri and the narrowing of the sulci. **B,** Optic disk with papilledema showing loss of the disk margin and hard exudates (white streaks). *(A from Klatt E:* Robbins and Cotran Atlas of Pathology, *Philadelphia, Saunders, 2006, p 449, Fig. 19-11; B from Perkin GD:* Mosby's Color Atlas and Text of Neurology, *St. Louis, Mosby, 2002, p 160, Fig. 9-4.)*

c. EC edema
  (1) **Definition:** Increased vessel permeability in acute inflammation (vasogenic; see Chapters 3 and 5)
  (2) Causes
    (a) Acute inflammation (e.g., meningitis, encephalitis)
    (b) Metastasis, trauma, and lead poisoning (see Chapters 7 and 12)

EC edema
↑Vessel permeability in acute inflammation
Meningitis, encephalitis
Metastasis, trauma, lead poisoning
Respiratory alkalosis: ↑cerebral vessel vasoconstriction

A temporizing measure in a patient with head trauma is purposely induce hyperventilation. Because elevated PCO_2 (respiratory acidosis) is associated with increased cerebral blood flow, one can purposely hyperventilate the patient to produce respiratory alkalosis. This causes cerebral vessel vasoconstriction (VC). The reduction in cerebral blood flow decreases the vascular permeability, thus decreasing cerebral edema. Respiratory acidosis and hypoxemia cause vasodilation of cerebral vessels, which increases cerebral vessel permeability, resulting in cerebral edema. Both conditions cause increased activity of the K^+ channels in smooth muscle cells → produces hyperpolarization → relaxes smooth muscle cells (↓IC calcium), producing vasodilation with increased vessel permeability.

3. Clinical findings in cerebral edema are related to intracranial pressure (intracranial hypertension [ICH]).
  a. Papilledema (swelling of the optic disk (Fig. 26-1 B; Links 26-23 and 26-24)
  b. Headache
  c. Projectile vomiting *without* nausea
  d. Sinus bradycardia (reduced heart rate); hypertension (HTN)
  e. Potential for herniation (see later)
B. **Idiopathic ICH (pseudotumor cerebri)**
  1. **Definition:** An increase in intracranial pressure without a mass lesion

Respiratory acidosis, hypoxemia: ↑cerebral vessel permeability→ ↑cerebral edema
Clinical findings
Papilledema: swelling optic disk
Headache
Projectile vomiting without nausea
Sinus bradycardia

Hypertension
Potential for herniation
Idiopathic ICH
↑Intracranial pressure without mass lesion

Normal intracranial pressure is 7.5 to 20 cm H_2O (5–15 mm Hg) in adults and 4 to 9.5 cm H_2O (3–7 mm Hg) in children. Greater than 20 cm H_2O (14.7 mm Hg) for >10 minutes is considered an increase in intracranial pressure.

2. Epidemiology
  a. Increased intracranial pressure and papilledema (swelling of optic disk present; Fig. 26-1 B)
  b. Pathogenesis
    (1) CSF reabsorption is decreased in the arachnoid villi.
    (2) Eventual equilibration occurs with inflow and outflow.
  c. Most commonly seen in obese women of childbearing age
  d. Risk factors for papilledema
    (1) Use of all-*trans*-retinoic acid (ATRA) used in treating acute promyelocytic leukemia (see Chapter 13)
    (2) Hypothyroidism, Cushing disease
    (3) Oral contraceptive pills (OCPs)
    (4) Use of isotretinoin in treatment of acne; tamoxifen (estrogen antagonist)

Epidemiology
↑IC pressure + papilledema
↓CSF reabsorption in arachnoid villi
Eventual equilibration with inflow and outflow
MC obese women childbearing age
Risk factors
ATRA
Hypothyroidism
Cushing disease
OCPs
Isotretinoin for acne
Tamoxifen

26-2: **A,** Brain herniations. See text for discussion. **B,** Cerebellar coning. Note the notching in the cerebellar tonsils *(arrows)* caused by downward displacement of the cerebellar tonsils through the foramen magnum. *(A adapted from Fishman RA: Brain edema.* N Engl J Med *1975;293:706 in Kumar V, Abbas AK, Fausto N, Mitchell RN:* Robbins Basic Pathology, *8th ed, Philadelphia, Saunders Elsevier, 2007, p 862, Fig. 23-4;* **B** *from Grieg JD:* Color Atlas of Surgical Diagnosis, *London, Mosby-Wolfe, 1996, p 312, Fig. 39-2.)*

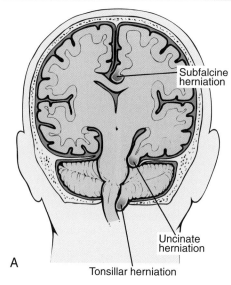
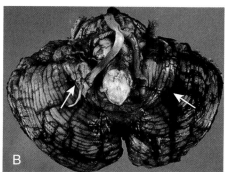

A

Subfalcine herniation

Uncinate herniation

Tonsillar herniation

B

Negative clinical findings
Absence tumor/obstruction CSF
Absence mental status alterations
Absence focal neurologic signs
Positive clinical findings
Headache
Rhythmic sound one/both ears
Diplopia
Blurry vision
DX idiopathic ICH
MRI: flattening posterior globe
↑CSF pressure
Usually >300 mm H₂O
↓CSF protein (dilutional)
Cerebral herniation
Displacement portions of brain from ↑IP
Complication ↑intracranial pressure
Openings dural partitions/skull
Subfalcine herniation
Cingulate gyrus herniates under falx cerebri
Subfalcine herniation: compresses ACA
Uncal herniation
Medial portion TL herniates thru tentorium cerebelli
Duret hemorrhages: compression midbrain
Compression of CN III
Eye deviated down/out
Pupil mydriatic (dilated)
Compression parasympathetic postganglionic fibers
Compression PCA
Hemorrhagic infarction occipital lobe
Tonsillar herniation
Cerebellar tonsils herniate into FM
Coning cerebellar tonsils
Cardiorespiratory arrest

   e. Negative clinical findings
     (1) *Absence* of tumor and obstruction to CSF flow
     (2) *Absence* of mental status alterations one would expect with cerebral edema
     (3) *Absence* of focal neurologic signs
   f. Positive clinical findings
     (1) Headache
     (2) Rhythmic sound heard in one or both ears
     (3) Diplopia (double vision)
     (4) Blurry vision (danger of complete visual loss caused by optic nerve atrophy)
 3. Diagnosis of idiopathic ICH
   a. Magnetic resonance imaging (MRI) shows flattening of the posterior globe (100% positive predictive value).
   b. CSF pressure is increased; usually >300 mm H₂O (normal, 70–180 mm H₂O)
   c. *Decrease* in CSF protein, a dilutional effect related to an increased amount of CSF

C. Cerebral herniation
 1. **Definition:** A displacement of distinct portions of the brain caused by increased intracranial pressure
 2. Epidemiology; pathogenesis
   a. Complication of increased intracranial pressure
   b. Portions of the brain become displaced through openings of dural partitions or openings in the skull (Fig. 26-2 A).
 3. Subfalcine herniation
   a. **Definition:** Cingulate gyrus herniates under the falx cerebri (Links 26-25 and 26-26).
   b. Herniation causes compression of the anterior cerebral artery (ACA).
 4. Uncal (uncinate) herniation
   a. **Definition:** Medial portion of the temporal lobe (TL; uncus and parahippocampal gyrus) herniates through the tentorial notch (Links 26-25 and 26-27).
   b. Complications
     (1) Compression of midbrain; produces Duret hemorrhages (small linear hemorrhages; Link 26-28)
     (2) Compression of the oculomotor nerve (cranial nerve [CN] III)
       (a) Eye on the affected side is deviated down and out.
       (b) Pupil on the affected side is mydriatic (dilated). This is caused by compression of the parasympathetic postganglionic fibers.
     (3) Compression of the posterior cerebral artery (PCA) causes a hemorrhagic infarction of the occipital lobe on the affected side.
 5. Tonsillar herniation
   a. **Definition:** Cerebellar tonsils herniate into the foramen magnum (FM).
   b. Causes "coning" of the cerebellar tonsils caused by increased pressure pushing the cerebellar tonsils into the smaller FM (Fig. 26-2 A, B; Link 26-25)
   c. Produces cardiorespiratory arrest

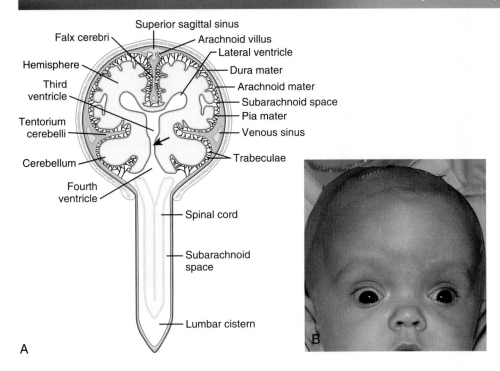

Superior sagittal sinus
Falx cerebri
Arachnoid villus
Lateral ventricle
Hemisphere
Dura mater
Third ventricle
Arachnoid mater
Subarachnoid space
Tentorium cerebelli
Pia mater
Venous sinus
Cerebellum
Trabeculae
Fourth ventricle
Spinal cord
Subarachnoid space
Lumbar cistern

A

B

26-3: **A,** Schematic of the ventricles. Cerebrospinal fluid (CSF) is synthesized by the choroid plexus in the ventricles. The aqueduct of Sylvius (AoS; *arrow*) is a narrow communication between the third and fourth ventricles. CSF exits the fourth ventricle via the foramina of Luschka and Magendie (not shown in the schematic), where it enters the subarachnoid space. CSF is reabsorbed in the arachnoid villus (parasagittal location), which empties into the dural venous sinuses. **B,** Hydrocephalus and Parinaud syndrome. Note the increased head circumference and paralysis of upward gaze in this newborn with stenosis of the AoS. (**A** *from Weyhenmeyer J, Gallman E:* Neuroscience, Rapid Review Series, *1st ed, 2007, Philadelphia, Mosby, p 20, Fig. 2.3;* **B** *courtesy of Dr. Albert Biglan, Children's Hospital of Pittsburgh.*)

D. **Hydrocephalus**
1. Normal ventricle anatomy and flow of CSF (Fig. 26-3 A; Link 26-29 A, B)
2. **Definition:** Increase in the CSF volume that causes enlargement of the ventricles (Links 26-30 and 26-31)
3. Communicating (nonobstructive) hydrocephalus
   a. **Definition:** Open communication between the ventricles and the subarachnoid space with enlargement of all of the ventricles
   b. Epidemiology and causes:
      (1) Increased production of CSF. Example: a benign choroid plexus papilloma.
      (2) Decreased reabsorption of CSF by the arachnoid villi
         • Examples: postinflammatory scarring, tumor, subarachnoid hemorrhage (SAH)
4. Noncommunicating (obstructive) hydrocephalus
   a. **Definition:** Hydrocephalus that is caused by a block in CSF flow in the ventricular system or between the ventricular system and the spinal canal
   b. Epidemiology and causes
      (1) Stricture of the AoS
         (a) MCC in newborns (NBs); causes paralysis of upward gaze (Parinaud syndrome; Fig. 26-3 B)
         (b) Pineal gland tumor can also obstruct the AoS and cause Parinaud syndrome (see Chapter 23).
      (2) Tumor in the fourth ventricle. Examples: ependymoma, medulloblastoma
      (3) Scarring at the base of the brain. Example: tuberculous meningitis
      (4) Colloid cyst in the third ventricle
      (5) Developmental disorders (see later)
5. In NBs with hydrocephalus, the ventricles dilate, and the head circumference is increased (see Fig. 26-3 B). MCC of hydrocephalus in the NB period is intraventricular hemorrhage (IVH). Other causes are blocked reabsorption of CSF by the meninges (arachnoid granulation), as occurs with inflammation associated with subarachnoid hemorrhage and meningitis. Other causes of hydrocephalus at birth are aqueductal stenosis, myelomeningocele associated with Arnold-Chiari syndrome, communicating hydrocephalus, and Dandy-Walker malformation.
6. In adults with hydrocephalus, the ventricles dilate, and the head circumference is normal.
7. Hydrocephalus ex vacuo
   a. **Definition:** A dilated appearance of the ventricles when the brain mass is decreased from cerebral atrophy
   b. Example: cerebral atrophy in Alzheimer disease
8. Normal pressure hydrocephalus

Hydrocephalus
Hydrocephalus: ↑CSF volume → enlargement ventricles
Communicating hydrocephalus
Communication ventricles with subarachnoid space
↑Production CSF
Benign choroid plexus papilloma
Obstruction reabsorption CSF arachnoid villi
Postmeningitic scarring, tumor, subarachnoid hemorrhage
Noncommunicating: obstruction CSF flow out of ventricles
Block CSF in ventricles/ ventricles and spinal canal
Stricture AoS MCC NBs
Paralysis upward gaze
Parinaud syndrome
Pineal gland tumor block AoS: Parinaud syndrome
Tumor 4th ventricle
Ependymoma, medulloblastoma
Scarring base of brain
TB meningitis
Colloid cyst 3rd ventricle
Developmental disorders
MCC hydrocephalus NB IVH
Hydrocephalus in children: ventricles dilate and increase head circumference
Hydrocephalus in adults: no increased head size
Hydrocephalus ex vacuo
Dilated appearance due to cerebral atrophy
Cerebral atrophy Alzheimer disease
Normal pressure hydrocephalus

a. **Definition:** The presence of dilated ventricles in the presence of a normal CSF pressure
b. Epidemiology
   (1) Dilated ventricles plus the following symptom complex
      • Wide-based gait, urinary incontinence, dementia
   (2) Accounts for 5% of dementia cases
   (3) Potentially reversible cause of dementia
   (4) Causes of normal-pressure hydrocephalus
      (a) Idiopathic (50% of cases)
      (b) Secondary causes include prior subarachnoid hemorrhage, intracranial surgery, and brain tumor.
   (5) Pathogenesis of symptom complex in normal pressure hydrocephalus
      (a) Ventricular dilation is out of proportion (OoP) to sulcal atrophy (ventriculomegaly).
      (b) Wide-based gait and urinary incontinence are caused by stretching of sacral motor fibers near the dilated ventricle.
      (c) Dementia is caused by stretching of limbic fibers near the dilated ventricle.
c. Diagnosis of normal pressure hydrocephalus
   (1) MRI documents ventriculomegaly and sulcal atrophy (sulcus is a grove or furrow on the surface of the brain; Link 26-32).
   (2) Large volume of CSF is removed at lumbar puncture to determine if symptoms improve with removal of the fluid.
IV. **Developmental Disorders**
   A. **Neural tube defects (NTDs)**
      1. **Definition:** A type of birth defect associated with failure of the neural tube (NT) to close. This defect, which may involve the brain, spine, and spinal cord, arises during the first month of gestation.

The neural tube (NT) is the precursor to the brain and spinal cord and is developed via a process called *neurulation*. The ectodermal cells just dorsal to the notochord increase in height to form a thickened neural plate (Link 26-33 A). The neural plate folds inward (invaginates) to form the neural groove, and the elevations at the groove's open end are called the neural folds (Link 26-33 B). As the groove deepens, the elevations fuse with each other to form the NT, which separates from the overlying surface ectoderm and appears to sink into the underlying mesoderm (Link 26-33 C). The future neural crest cells migrate out of the neural folds as they fuse to become the neural crest cells, which now lie between the ectoderm and the NT (Link 26-34 A).

(The excerpt is taken from Bogart BI, Ort FH: *Elsevier's Integrated Anatomy and Embryology*, St. Louis, Mosby Elsevier, 2007, p 8.)

---

2. Epidemiology and pathogenesis
   a. Lateral neural plate normally closes anterior to posterior on days 24 to 28 gestation.
   b. In NTDs, the lateral folds of the neural plate fail to fuse.
   c. May be caused by a rupture of a previously closed neural tube
   d. Maternal folic acid levels must be adequate *before* pregnancy to prevent an open NTD (see Chapter 8). Adequate intake of folic acid is a minimum of 0.4 mg/day.
   e. Types of open neural defects include anencephaly, spinal bifida occulta, meningocele, and myelomeningocele.
   f. Maternal finding in open NTDs is an increase in maternal α-fetoprotein (AFP) in serum or amniotic fluid (AF).
3. Anencephaly (Fig. 26-4)
   a. **Definition:** Complete absence of the brain
   b. Epidemiology
      (1) Defect in closure of the anterior neuropore on day 24 to 26 of gestation
      (2) Anterior neuropore is the opening of the embryonic NT in the anterior portion of the prosencephalon.
   c. Clinical findings in the NB include a froglike appearance and an open spinal canal.
   d. Maternal polyhydramnios (increased amniotic fluid) is present caused by craniospinal defects that allow the CSF to empty into the AF.
4. Spina bifida occulta (SBO; Fig. 26-4 C; Link 26-34 B)
   a. **Definition:** Defect in closure of the posterior vertebral arch
   b. Dimple or tuft of hair in the skin overlying L5 to S1present in the NB
5. Meningocele (Fig. 26-4 D; Link 26-34 C, E)
   a. **Definition:** Spina bifida with a cystic mass containing the meninges
   b. MC in the lumbosacral region

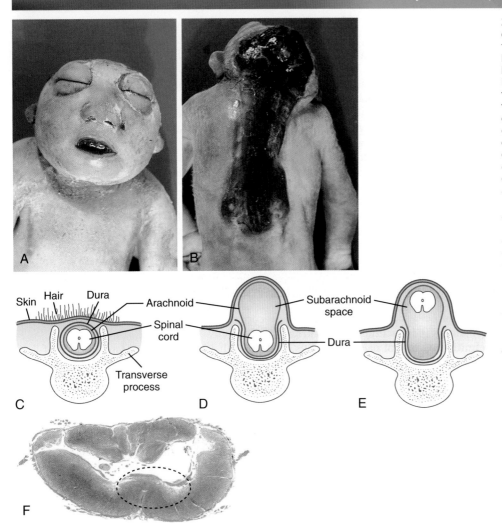

26-4: A, Anencephaly: frontal view. The entire cranium is missing, and the foreshortened face appears froglike. **B,** Anencephaly, posterior view. The brain is missing, and the spinal canal is open. **C,** Spina bifida occulta. See text for discussion. **D,** Meningocele. See text for discussion. **E,** Meningomyelocele. See text for discussion. **F,** Syringomyelia. Note the collapsed cystic cavity (syrinx) in the center of the cervical spinal cord. The *oval dashed circle* encompasses the area where the crossed spinothalamic tracts and anterior horn cells would have been located. (*A and B from my friend Ivan Damjanov, MD, PhD:* Pathology for the Health-Related Professions, *2nd ed, Philadelphia, Saunders, 2000, p 117, Fig. 5-23A and B; C to E from Moore NA, Roy WA:* Rapid Review Gross and Developmental Anatomy, *2nd ed, Philadelphia, Mosby Elsevier, 2007, p 12, Fig. 1-13; F from Burger PC, Scheithauer BW, Vogel KS:* Surgical Pathology of the Nervous System, *4th ed, London, Churchill Livingstone, 2002, p 554, Fig. 11-70.)*

6. Meningomyelocele (Fig. 26-4 E; Link 26-34 D). Sometimes called myelomeningocele
   a. **Definition:** Spina bifida with a cystic mass containing meninges and the spinal cord
   b. MC in the lumbosacral region
7. Encephalocele (Link 26-35)
   - **Definition:** NTD characterized by a cystic mass containing the brain and the membranes that cover it through openings in the skull

B. Arnold-Chiari malformation
1. **Definition:** Caudal extension of the medulla and cerebellar vermis through the foramen magnum (FM) (Links 26-36 and 26-37 A)
2. Noncommunicating hydrocephalus is present.
3. Platybasia (flattening of the base of the skull) is present.
4. Additional findings may include meningomyelocele and syringomyelia (see later).

C. Dandy-Walker malformation
1. **Definition:** A partial or complete absence of the cerebellar vermis
2. Components
   a. Cystic dilation of the fourth ventricle
   b. Partial or complete agenesis of the cerebellar vermis
   c. Enlargement of the posterior fossa (contains the brainstem and cerebellum) with a high attachment of the tentorium cerebelli
   d. Agenesis of corpus callosum or cortical migration defect coexist in many cases; if present, the patient is at an increased risk of intellectual disability.
3. Noncommunicating hydrocephalus; may *not* be present at birth but develops in the first year of life

D. Syringomyelia
1. **Definition:** Degenerative disease of the spinal cord; longitudinal cystic cavity that develops within the substance of the spinal cord

Meningomyelocele

Cystic mass with meninges/spinal cord

Usually lumbosacral area

NDT cystic mass (brain and membranes)

Arnold-Chiari malformation

Caudal extension medulla/cerebellar vermis thru FM

Noncommunicating hydrocephalus

Platybasia

Meningomyelocele; syringomyelia

Dandy-Walker malformation

Partial/complete absence cerebellar vermis

Cystic dilation 4th ventricle

Partial/complete agenesis cerebellar vermis

Enlargement posterior fossa

Agenesis corpus callosum (risk intellectual disability)

Noncommunicating hydrocephalus

Syringomyelia

Degenerative disease spinal cord; cystic cavity

2. Epidemiology
   a. Pathogenesis
      (1) Obstruction of outflow of spinal fluid from the fourth ventricle
      (2) Birth injury
   b. A fluid-filled cavity (syrinx) is present within the cervical spinal cord (Fig. 26-4 F).
   c. Produces cervical cord enlargement
   d. Cavity expands and causes degeneration of the spinal tracts.
   e. Associated with the Arnold-Chiari malformation (see earlier)
3. Clinical findings in syringomyelia
   a. Symptoms appear in the third and fourth decades of life
   b. Disruption of the crossed lateral spinothalamic tracts (Fig. 26-4 F)
      (1) Pain and temperature sensation is lost in the hands. "Cape and shawl" distribution sensory loss bilaterally. Tactile sense (proprioception) is preserved.
      (2) People can burn their hands without being aware of the burn.
   c. Destruction of the anterior horn cells (Fig. 26-4 F)
      (1) Causes atrophy of the intrinsic muscles of the hands
      (2) Often confused with amyotrophic lateral sclerosis (ALS); however, there are *no* sensory changes in ALS
   d. Charcot joint (neuropathic joint) may occur in the shoulder, elbow, or wrist (see Chapter 24).
4. Diagnosis: MRI shows an enlarged cervical cord and a cystic cavity.

E. **Phakomatoses (neurocutaneous syndromes)**
   1. **Definition:** Group of neurocutaneous syndromes that include a disordered growth of ectodermal tissue and malformations or tumors of the CNS. The term *phakomatosis* refers to patchy, circumscribed dermatologic lesions. Because skin and CNS tissue arise from the same ectodermal precursors, conditions that affect the CNS may have pathognomonic skin features. Furthermore, these syndromes have hamartomas (errors in development) that involve multiple tissues.
   2. Epidemiology: The phakomatoses include the following (in descending order of incidence): neurofibromatosis (NF), tuberous sclerosis (TS), and Sturge-Weber syndrome (SWS).
   3. Neurofibromatosis
      a. **Definition:** Genetic disease characterized by multiple benign tumors of peripheral nerves (PNs), pigmented lesions on the skin, benign and malignant tumors in the brain and optic nerves, and associations with other tumors
      b. Epidemiology (Table 26-2)
         (1) Autosomal dominant disorder with incomplete penetrance (failure of genetically susceptible individuals to exhibit a trait; see Chapter 6)
         (2) *No* gender predominance
         (3) NF type 1 (NF1; MC) and type 2 (NF2) variants
            (a) NF1 is associated with a mutation on chromosome 17 coding for neurofibromin. This is a cytoplasmic protein that is predominantly expressed in neurons, Schwann cells, and oligodendrocytes.
            (b) NF2 is associated with a mutation on chromosome 22 coding for merlin.
            (c) Both proteins act as tumor suppressors.
      c. NF1 (peripheral type) associations
         (1) Café au lait coffee-colored macules (Fig. 26-5 A; Link 26-38)
            (a) Occur in both NF1 and NF2
            (b) Occur in 100% of children *before* 2 years of age

TABLE 26-2   Comparison Between Neurofibromatosis Types 1 and 2

	TYPE 1	TYPE 2
Café au lait	Yes	Yes
Axillary freckling	Yes	No
Lisch nodules	Yes	No
Pigmented plexiform neurofibroma	Yes	No
Tumor associations	Pheochromocytoma, Wilms tumor: hypertension	Bilateral acoustic neuromas, meningioma
Scoliosis	Mild	No

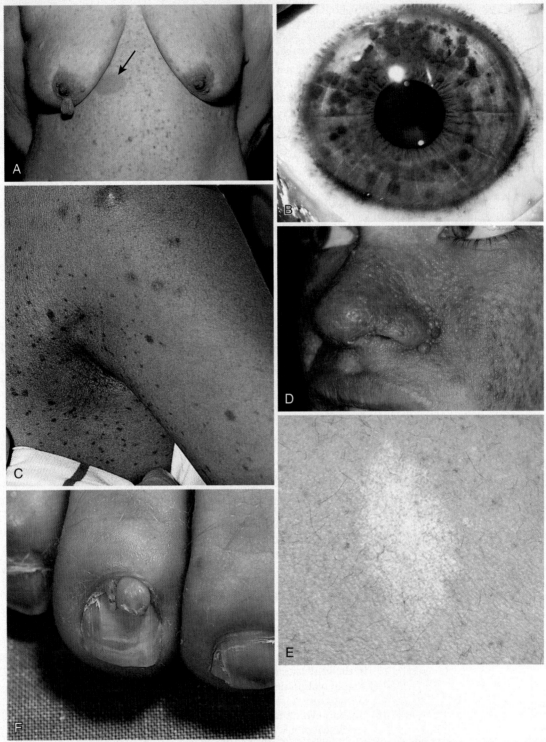

26-5: **A,** Neurofibromatosis showing café au lait macule *(arrow)* and numerous pigmented, pedunculated neurofibromas. **B,** Lisch nodules. Note the pigmented hamartomas of the iris. **C,** Axillary freckling in neurofibromatosis. **D,** Adenoma sebaceum (angiofibromas) in tuberous sclerosis. Adenoma sebaceum (angiofibromas) in tuberous sclerosis. Note the nodular lesions on the nose and cheeks. **E,** Shagreen patch ("ash leaf" spots) in tuberous sclerosis. Note the irregular area of white skin (leukoderma) with the typical ash leaf pattern of a shagreen patch. **F,** Periungual fibroma in tuberous sclerosis. *(**A** from Forbes C, Jackson W: Color Atlas and Text of Clinical Medicine, 2nd ed, London, Mosby, 2002, p 104, Fig. 2-86; **B** from Kliegman R: Nelson Textbook of Pediatrics, 19th ed, Philadelphia, Elsevier Saunders, 2011, p 2047, Fig. 589.2; taken from Zitelli BJ, Davis HW: Atlas of Pediatric Physical Diagnosis, 4th ed, Philadelphia, Mosby, 2002, p 507; **C** from Swartz M: Textbook of Physical Diagnosis History and Examination, 5th ed, Philadelphia, Saunders Elsevier, 2006, p 163, Fig. 8-47; **D** from Fitzpatrick JE, Morelli JG: Dermatology Secrets Plus, 4th ed, Philadelphia, Elsevier Mosby, 2011, p 40, Fig. 5.5; **E** from Lookingbill DP, Marks JG: Principles of Dermatology, 3rd ed, Philadelphia, Saunders, 2000, p 234, Fig. 14-7; **F** from Bouloux P: Self-Assessment Picture Tests Medicine, Vol. 4, London, Mosby-Wolfe, 1997, p 24, Fig. 47.)*

(2) Optic gliomas (2%–5% of cases) and astrocytomas

(3) Lisch nodule (>90% of cases; Fig. 26-5 B): a pigmented hamartoma of the iris

(4) Axillary and inguinal freckling (70% of cases; Fig. 26-5 C; Link 26-39)

(5) Mild scoliosis (lateral curvature of the spine)

(6) Pigmented plexiform neurofibromas at birth (Link 26-40; *not* present in NF2). May progress into neurofibrosarcoma involving large nerves.

(7) Cutaneous or subcutaneous neurofibromas (see Fig. 26-5 A; Link 26-41)

  (a) Occur in both types

  (b) Occur anywhere on the body *except* the palms and soles

  (c) Appear in late adolescence and increase in size with age

  (d) May be focal or diffuse

(8) Tumor associations

  (a) Pheochromocytoma (see Chapter 23) and Wilms tumor (see Chapter 20)

    • Both tumors produce hypertension (HTN).

    • Wilms tumor secretes renin, which activates the renin-angiotensin-aldosterone (RAA) system.

    • Pheochromocytomas release catecholamines.

  (b) Juvenile chronic myelogenous leukemia (CML)

(9) Neurodevelopment problems (30%–40% of cases)

  d. NF2 (central type) associations

    (1) Bilateral acoustic neuromas (ANs; schwannoma; >90% of cases)

      (a) Benign CN VIII tumor

      (b) Produces sensorineural hearing loss and tinnitus (see later)

    (2) Meningiomas (benign tumors arising from meningothelial cells within the arachnoid membrane; discussed later)

    (3) Spinal schwannomas (benign tumors derived from Schwann cells; discussed later)

    (4) Juvenile cataracts (opacification of the lens; ~80% of cases)

  e. Genetic testing is available for both types.

3. Tuberous sclerosis (TS)

  a. **Definition:** Genetic phakomatosis associated with mental retardation (MR), tumors and tumorlike lesions, and characteristic skin lesions

  b. Epidemiology/clinical

    (1) Autosomal dominant disorder

    (2) Second MC phakomatosis after NF

    (3) Mental retardation and seizures (infantile spasms) begin in infancy.

    (4) Angiofibromas (adenoma sebaceum; benign tumors with fibrous tissue containing vascular channels) occur on the face (Fig. 26-5 D; Link 26-42).

    (5) Hypopigmented skin lesions called shagreen patches (ash leaf spots) are present on the skin (Fig. 26-5 E; Link 26-43). They have a peau d'orange texture (analogous to dimples on an orange peel).

      (a) Best identified with a Wood lamp (black light)

      (b) Occur in >80% of cases of TS

    (6) Nail findings include subungual and periungual fibromas (Fig. 26-5 F).

    (7) Hamartomatous lesions (nontumorous overgrowths; see Chapter 9)

      (a) Astrocyte proliferations in the subependyma: look like "candlestick drippings" in the ventricles (Links 26-44 and 26-45)

      (b) Angiomyolipomas (AMLs) in the kidneys (80% of cases): contain blood vessels, smooth muscle, and adipose tissue

      (c) Rhabdomyoma in the heart (50%–60% of cases); presence is almost 100% predictive of TS

4. Sturge-Weber syndrome (SWS; see Chapter 10; see Fig. 10-14 F; Link 26-46)

  a. Vascular malformation on the face primarily occurring in distribution of the trigeminal nerve

  b. Some patients have an ipsilateral (same side) arteriovenous malformation (AVM) in the meninges.

V. Head Trauma

  A. Cerebral contusion

    1. **Definition:** Permanent damage to small blood vessels located on the surface of the brain

    2. Epidemiology

      a. Most often secondary to an acceleration-deceleration injury

      b. Coup injuries occur at the *site* of the impact (Fig. 26-6).

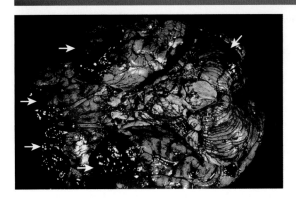

26-6: Brain contusion. The contrecoup injury involves the frontal and temporal lobes *(left arrows)*, while the coup lesion (site of impact) involves the cerebellum *(right arrow). (From my friend Ivan Damjanov, MD, PhD, Linder J:* Pathology: A Color Atlas, *St. Louis, Mosby, 2000, p 403, Fig 9-6.)*

c. Contrecoup injuries occur *opposite* the site of the impact (Links 26-47 and 26-48). Common sites are at the tips of the frontal lobe and temporal lobe.

B. Cerebral palsy (CP)

(Excerpted from Polin RA, Ditmar MF: Pediatric Secrets, *6th ed, Elsevier, 2016, pp 505–508.)*

1. **Definition:** Heterogeneous group of nonprogressive (static) motor and posture disorders of cerebral or cerebellar origin that typically manifest early in life
2. Epidemiology and clinical
   a. Primary impairment involves significant defects in motor planning and control; refers to the ability to conceive, plan, and carry out a skilled, nonhabitual motor act in the correct sequence from beginning to end.
   b. Nonprogressive clinical manifestations often change over time as the functional expression of the underlying brain is modified by brain development and maturation.
   c. Motor function that is affected results from the part of the brain that is injured
   d. Causes include cerebral malformations, metabolic and genetic causes, infection (both intrauterine and extrauterine), stroke, hypoxia-ischemia, and trauma.
   e. Brain lesions seen on MRI
      (1) Periventricular white matter lesions are the MC and can be seen in 19% to 45% of children with CP (particularly formerly premature infants).
      (2) Other common lesions include gray matter injuries of the basal ganglia and thalamus (21%), developmental cortical malformations (malf; 11%), and focal cortical infarcts (10%).
      (3) Up to 15% of cases of CP do *not* have an identifiable lesion on MRI. The varied MRI findings are believed to be emblematic of the neurodevelopmental heterogeneity of CP.
   f. Levine (POSTER) criteria for the diagnosis of CP
      (1) **P**osturing or abnormal movements
      (2) **O**ropharyngeal problems (e.g., tongue thrusts, swallowing abnormalities)
      (3) **S**trabismus (crossed eyes): condition in which the eyes do not properly align with each other when looking at an object
      (4) **T**one (hypertonia or hypotonia): Hypertonia refers to an abnormal increase in muscle tension and a reduced ability of a muscle to stretch. Hypotonia refers to a state of low muscle tone (the amount of tension or resistance to stretch in a muscle), often involving reduced muscle strength.
      (5) **E**volutional maldevelopment (primitive reflexes persist or protective or equilibrium reflexes fail to develop. An example is the parachute reflex: An infant is tested for motor nerve development by suspending him or her in the prone position and then dropping him or her a short distance onto a soft surface. If the motor nerve development is normal, the infant at 4 to 6 months will extend the arms, hands, and fingers on both sides of the body in a protective movement.
      (6) **R**eflexes (increased deep tendon reflexes [DTRs] or persistent Babinski reflex)
      (7) Abnormalities in four of these six categories strongly point to the diagnosis of CP.
   g. Types of cerebral palsy
      (1) Clinical classification is based on the nature of the movement disorder and muscle tone and anatomic distribution. A single patient may have more than one type. Spastic CP is the MC, accounting for about two-thirds of cases.
      (2) Spastic CP (pyramidal CP): characterized by neurologic signs of upper motor neuron (UMN) damage with increased "clasp knife" muscle tone, increased DTRs,

Margin notes:

Contrecoup: opposite site of impact; tips frontal/temporal lobes

Cerebral palsy

Static motor/posture disorder; cerebral or cerebellar origin

Defects motor planning/control

Clinical manifestations change over time

Motor function correlates with part or brain injure

Cerebral malformations, metabolic/genetic, stroke, hypoxia-ischemia, trauma

White matter lesions

Periventricular white matter changes

Grey matter lesions

Basal ganglia/thalamus, developmental cortical malf, focal cortical infarcts

MRI normal in some cases

Levine (POSTER) criteria

Posturing/abnormal movements

Oropharyngeal problems

Strabismus

Tone (hypo/hypertonia)

Evolutional maldevelopment

Reflexes

Spastic CP MC

UMN damage

pathologic reflexes, and spastic weakness. Spastic CP is subclassified based on distribution.

(a) Hemiplegia: primarily unilateral involvement, with the arm usually involved more than leg

(b) Quadriplegia: all limbs involved, with the legs often more involved than the arms

(c) Diplegia: legs much more involved than arms, which may show no or only minimal impairment (more common in premature infants)

(3) Dyskinetic (nonspastic or extrapyramidal) CP

(a) Characterized by prominent involuntary movements or fluctuating muscle tone, with choreoathetosis (movement disorder) the MC subtype

(b) Distribution is usually symmetric among the four limbs.

(4) Ataxic CP: primarily cerebellar signs (including ataxia, dysmetria, past pointing, nystagmus)

(5) Mixed type CP: features of multiple types of CP

C. **Acute epidural hematoma**

1. **Definition:** Arterial bleed in the brain creating a blood-filled space between the inner surface of the skull and dura (Fig. 26-7 A [left], B, C; Links 26-49 and 26-50)

2. Epidemiology

   a. Occurs in 1% to 4% of head injuries

   b. Peak incidence in adolescents and young adults; males > females; rare after 50 to 60 years of age

   c. Pathogenesis

      (1) Caused by a fracture of the temporoparietal bone

      (2) Fractures may be caused by a hammer, baseball bat, or any focused blow to the head.

      (3) Severance of the middle meningeal artery. The vessel lies between the dura and the inner table of bone.

3. Clinical findings in epidural hematoma

   a. Some patients have a lucid interval after trauma followed later by neurologic deterioration.

   b. Intracranial pressure increases, leading to herniation and death.

4. Diagnosis of epidural hematoma

   a. Computed tomography (CT) scan of the head is the imaging test of choice (Fig. 26-7 C; Link 26-51).

   b. Hematoma rarely crosses the suture line because the dura is firmly attached at these sites.

D. **Subdural hematoma**

1. **Definition:** Venous bleeding between the dura and the arachnoid membranes (Fig. 26-7 A, right; Link 26-52)

2. Epidemiology

   a. Acute or chronic

      (1) Acute common in all age groups

      (2) Chronic more common in older adults (eighth decade of life); males > females

   b. Pathogenesis

      (1) Bridging veins between brain and dural sinuses (see Fig. 26-7 A [right] and D) are torn.

      (2) Slowly enlarging blood clot covers the convexity of the brain.

   c. Causes of subdural hematoma

      (1) Most often the result of blunt trauma to the skull. Examples: car accident, baseball bat

      (2) Other causes of subdural hematoma include medical anticoagulation, hemophilia, child abuse, shaken baby syndrome, and spontaneous bleed.

      (3) Major risk factor for developing a subdural hematoma is cerebral atrophy.

         (a) Commonly present in older adults and people with chronic alcoholism

         (b) Loss of brain mass (atrophy) leads to excess traction on the inflexible bridging veins.

3. Clinical findings in subdural hematoma

   a. Consciousness level in the patient fluctuates.

   b. Herniation and death may occur if the diagnosis is not made quickly.

   c. Chronic subdural hematoma may be a cause of dementia.

4. Dx of subdural hematoma: CT is the best imaging study for detecting a subdural hematoma (Fig. 26-7 E; Link 26-53).

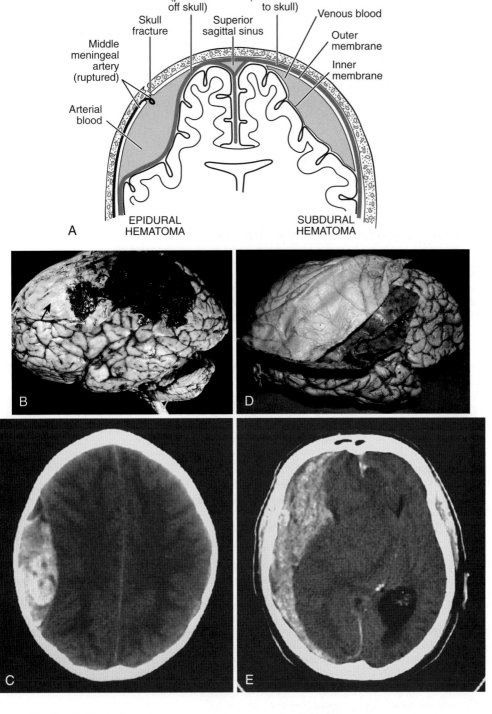

Dura
(peeled
off skull)

Dura
(still attached
to skull)

Skull
fracture

Superior
sagittal sinus

Venous blood

Middle
meningeal
artery
(ruptured)

Outer
membrane

Inner
membrane

Arterial
blood

**EPIDURAL
HEMATOMA**

**SUBDURAL
HEMATOMA**

A

B

D

C

E

26-7: A, Schematic of epidural hematoma *(left side)* and subdural hematoma *(right side).* **B,** Epidural hematoma. Note the blood is located on top of the dura *(arrow).* **C,** Non–contrast-enhanced computed tomography (CT) scan of an acute epidural hematoma at the level of the right midconvexity. There are an associated mass effect and moderate midline shift. **D,** Subdural hematoma. The reflected dura shows the outer membrane of an organized venous clot covering the convexity of the brain. **E,** Non–contrast-enhanced CT scan of an acute right temporal subdural hematoma. There is acute bleeding as well as delayed bleeding, which explains the mixed density. Mass effect is large, with a massive midline shift right to left. The right lateral ventricle has been obliterated. *(**A** from Kumar V, Abbas AK, Fausto N, Mitchell RN: Robbins Basic Pathology, 8th ed. Philadelphia, Saunders Elsevier, 2007, p 871, Fig. 23-13A; **B** courtesy of Dr. Raymond D. Adams, Massachusetts General Hospital, Boston; **C** and **E** from Marx J: Rosen's Emergency Medicine Concepts and Clinical Practice, 7th ed, Philadelphia, Mosby Elsevier, 2010, pp 306, 320, respectively, Figs. 38-7, 38-9, respectively; **D** from my friend Ivan Damjanov, MD, PhD, Linder J: Pathology: A Color Atlas, St. Louis, Mosby, 2000, p 405, Fig. 19-20.)*

E. **Cephalhematoma**
1. **Definition:** A hemorrhage in the plane between the bone and the periosteum on the surface of the skull in a newborn (NB) (Link 26-54)
2. Epidemiology and clinical
    a. Presents a well-circumscribed firm mass overlying the skull, which is confined by cranial sutures
    b. Usually increases in size after birth before resolving over a few weeks
    c. Dystrophic calcification may occur within the hematoma and may result in a hard skull protuberance that may require months of skull growth and remodeling for resolution.
    d. Most are unilateral and located over the parietal bone.
    e. Associated with forceps delivery and attributed to shearing forces that separate the periosteum from the skull bone

Cephalhematoma

Hemorrhage between bone/periosteum in NBs

Epidemiology/clinical

Mass overlying skull confined by cranial sutures

↑Size after birth

Dystrophic calcification may occur

Unilateral over parietal bone

Associated with forceps delivery

Blood loss *not* life-threatening

Underlying fracture 10% to 25%

Subgaleal hemorrhage

Hemorrhage beneath aponeurosis covering scalp

Blood may extend into posterior neck

Fluctuant mass that increases in size

Serious, life-threatening injury

Vacuum extraction

Linear skull fracture, suture diastasis, parietal bone fragmentation

Subaponeurotic space: reservoir for blood → hypovolemic shock

    f. Volume of blood lost is not life threatening because of the small size of the subperiosteal space.

    g. Cephalhematomas are associated with an underlying fracture in 10% to 25% of cases.

F. Subgaleal hemorrhage

  1. **Definition:** Hemorrhage beneath the aponeurosis (dense layer of fibrous tissue) covering the scalp and connecting the frontal and occipital components of the occipitofrontalis muscle (Link 26-54)

  2. Epidemiology and clinical

    a. Blood may spread beneath the entire scalp and into the subcutaneous tissue of the posterior neck.

    b. Typically presents in the NB as a fluctuant mass; initially increases in size over the first 24 to 48 hrs after birth and resolves over 2 to 3 weeks

    c. Often extremely serious injury and may be life-threatening in 10% to 20% of cases

    d. Hemorrhage is associated with vacuum extraction (vacuum pump) and is attributed to linear skull fracture, suture diastasis (separation), or parietal bone fragmentation that often accompanies the hemorrhage.

    e. Subaponeurotic space (potential space between the skull periosteum and the scalp galea aponeurosis) serves as a large reservoir for the accumulation of blood; may be substantial enough to cause hypovolemic shock in severe cases.

Caput succedaneum refers to the swelling, or edema, of an NB's scalp soon after delivery (Link 26-54). It appears as a lump or a bump on the head and is caused by prolonged pressure from the dilated cervix or vaginal walls during delivery. It usually resolves spontaneously within a few days. It should *not* be confused with an extradural or extracranial hemorrhage.

Caput: swelling (edema) NB scalp after delivery

Cerebrovascular diseases

Overview CVD

Thrombosis

Infarction

Hemorrhage

↓Blood supply, hypoxia, ischemia, infarction

Sites: parenchyma, subarachnoid/subdural space

Global hypoxic injury

Cardiogenic shock

Hypovolemic shock

Septic shock

CO poisoning

G. Summary of sites for extracranial and extradural hemorrhages (includes NBs; Link 26-54)

VI. Cerebrovascular Diseases

  A. Overview of cerebrovascular diseases (CVDs)

    1. CVDs are subdivided into three major categories: thrombosis (see Chapter 5), infarction (see Chapter 2), and hemorrhage.

    2. Pathophysiologic processes that produce CVDs: reduced blood supply and reduced oxygenation of cerebral tissue caused by hypoxia, ischemia, and infarction (a complication of ischemia; see Chapter 2)

    3. Sites for CNS hemorrhage include the parenchyma, subarachnoid space, and subdural space from rupture of cerebral vessels.

  B. Global hypoxic injury

    1. Causes of global hypoxic injury (see Chapter 2): cardiac arrest producing cardiogenic shock, hypovolemic shock, septic shock, and chronic carbon monoxide poisoning

---

Process of neuronal ischemia and infarction (Link 26-55). (1) Reduction of blood flow reduces supply of oxygen and hence adenosine triphosphate. H^+ is produced by anaerobic metabolism of available glucose. (2) Energy-dependent membrane ionic pumps fail, leading to cytotoxic edema and membrane depolarization, allowing calcium entry and releasing glutamate. (3) Calcium enters cells via glutamate-gated channels and (4) activates destructive intracellular enzymes (5), destroying intracellular organelles and cell membrane, with release of free radicals. Free fatty acid (FA) release activates procoagulant pathways that exacerbate local ischemia. (6) Glial cells take up H^+, can no longer take up extracellular glutamate, and suffer cell death, leading to liquefactive necrosis of whole arterial territory. Repeated episodes of **hypoglycemia** have the same effects on the brain as does global hypoxic injury. Repeated episodes of hypoglycemia, most commonly seen in type 1 DM, have the same effects on the brain.

Hypoglycemia: similar effect on brain as global hypoxia

Complications

Cerebral atrophy

Apoptosis neurons 3, 5, 6

Laminar necrosis

Neurons most susceptible cells in hypoxic injury

Red neurons: apoptotic neuron

Junctions between arterial territories

Junction ACA and MCA

Bilateral proximal weakness arms/legs

Stroke

    2. Complications in global hypoxic injury

    a. Cerebral atrophy (Fig. 2-15 A)

      (1) Atrophy is caused by apoptosis (individual cell death) of neurons in layers 3, 5, and 6 of the cerebral cortex; produces laminar necrosis (bandlike type of necrosis; Link 26-56).

      (2) Neurons are the most susceptible of all cells to hypoxic injury.

      (3) Neurons undergo apoptosis ("red" neurons; Fig. 26-8 A; Link 26-57).

    b. Watershed infarcts (see Chapter 2; see Fig. 2-6 A; Link 26-58)

      (1) Occur at the junctions of arterial territories

      (2) Example: Watershed infarcts may occur at the junction between the anterior cerebral artery (ACA) and middle cerebral artery (MCA).

      (3) Clinically present with bilateral proximal weakness of arms and legs

    c. Stroke (see later)

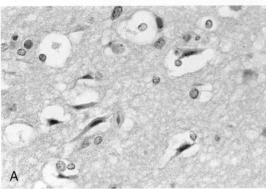

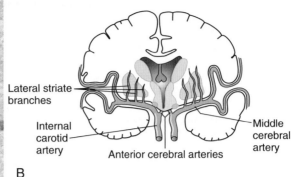

Lateral striate branches

Internal carotid artery

Anterior cerebral arteries

Middle cerebral artery

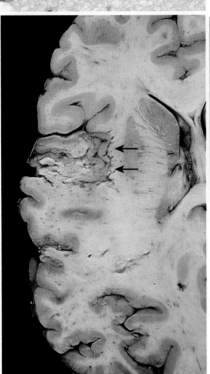

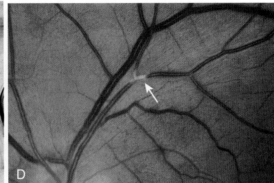

26-8: A, Red neurons. Note the brightly eosinophilic staining cells with the pyknotic nuclei within spaces representing apoptotic neurons. **B,** Distribution of the middle cerebral artery. **C,** Atherosclerotic stroke showing necrotic areas at the periphery of the cerebral cortex (pale infarction) in the distribution of the middle cerebral artery. Arrows are located at the line of demarcation between normal and infarcted tissue. **D,** Cholesterol embolus to retinal artery. Note the yellow embolus trapped at the bifurcation of the retinal artery *(arrow)*. This produces a sudden, painless loss of vision ("curtain coming down") followed in a variable period of time by restoration of vision ("curtain coming up") as the embolus dislodges. This is called amaurosis fugax. *(A from Burger PC, Scheithauer BW, Vogel KS: Surgical Pathology of the Nervous System, 4th ed. London, Churchill Livingstone, 2002, p 415, Fig. 7-34; B from Weyhenmeyer J, Gallman E: Neuroscience, Rapid Review Series, 1st ed, 2007, Philadelphia, Mosby, p 34, Fig. 3-5; C from my friend Ivan Damjanov, MD, PhD, Linder J: Pathology: A Color Atlas, St. Louis, Mosby, 2000, p 408, Fig. 19-25A; D from Swartz MH: Textbook of Physical Diagnosis, 5th ed, Philadelphia, Saunders Elsevier, 2006, p 271, Fig. 10-113.)*

C. **Stroke**
   1. **Definition:** Focal disturbance of blood flow into or out of the brain, either ischemic (87%) or hemorrhagic (13%)
   2. Epidemiology and clinical
      a. Not a single disease but the end result or many different pathologic processes leading to vascular occlusion (thrombus over atherosclerotic plaque) or rupture (rupture of lenticulostriate [LTS] vessels or berry aneurysm)
      b. Increased incidence of a stroke with age; more common in men than women
      c. Main types of strokes
         (1) Transient ischemic attack (TIA)
         (2) Ischemic stroke (MC overall stroke; 87%)
            (a) Large vessel atherosclerosis (MC). Large vessels include the carotid artery and the vertebrobasilar (VB) artery.
            (b) Cardioembolism
            (c) Small-vessel vasculopathy (called lacunar strokes)
         (3) Hemorrhagic strokes (13%)
            (a) Intracerebral hemorrhage
               • Trauma with mass contusion and laceration of the brain surface
               • Chronic HTN with small-vessel diseases (SVDs); subcortical hemorrhage after rupture of the LTS arteries)
               • Cerebral amyloid angiopathy (CAA; typically as cerebral lobar hemorrhage)

Stroke

Disturbance blood flow

Ischemic (MC), hemorrhagic

Epidemiology, clinical

Vascular occlusion/rupture

↑With age

Men > women

Types strokes

TIA

Ischemic stroke MC overall stroke

Large vessels atherosclerosis (MC)

Cardioembolism

Small vessel vasculopathy

Hemorrhagic strokes

Intracerebral hemorrhage

Trauma with massive contusion/laceration brain surface

Chronic HTN SVDs, hemorrhage/rupture lenticulostriate arteries

CAA

Tumor rupture (melanoma, GBM, metastases [RCC])

Infectious (mycotic aneurysm, angioinvasive fungal (mucor)

Reperfusion cerebral infarct

Rupture AVM

SAH

Risk factors

Hx previous stroke most important

Age next most important

HTN most important modifiable risk factor

Risk factors ischemic stroke: smoking, DM, ↓HDL, ↑TG

AF, HTN: hemorrhagic strokes

Dissection, cocaine, APL, DIC, TTP

TIA

Abrupt onset neurologic deficit

Interruption blood flow; complete resolution

TIAs last under 1 hr

Resolve 5 to 15 minutes

Ischemia to brain

TIAs serve as warning for completed stroke

Focal weakness, numbness, facial asymmetry, speech problems

Altered consciousness, vertigo, CN deficits

Posterior circulation/ cerebellar strokes

- Tumor-associated hemorrhage (most often with melanoma, glioblastoma [GBM], and metastases of highly vascular tumors [renal cell carcinoma; RCC]).
- Infectious causes (mycotic aneurysms, angioinvasive fungal infections [mucormycosis])
- Reperfusion of an ischemic cerebral infarct
- Rupture of an arteriovenous malformation (AVM)

    (b) Subarachnoid hemorrhage (SAH)

  d. Risk factors for strokes

    (1) Most important risk factor is a history of a previous stroke.

    (2) Next most important risk factor is age.

    (3) Most important modifiable risk factor is hypertension (HTN).

    (4) Risk factors for ischemic stroke include smoking, DM, low high-density lipoprotein (HDL), and high triglyceride levels. (Note: Increased low-density lipoprotein [LDL] is most closely associated with cardiac disease.)

      (a) Other risk factors include atrial fibrillation (AF; embolic stroke) and HTN (hemorrhagic strokes).

      (b) Less common risk factors include dissection of cerebral vessels, illicit drugs (cocaine), hypercoagulable states (antiphospholipid syndrome [APL], disseminated intravascular coagulation [DIC], and thrombotic thrombocytopenic purpura [TTP], to name a few).

3. Transient ischemic attack (TIA)

  a. **Definition:** An abrupt onset neurologic deficit caused by interruption of blood flow to a portion of the brain, followed by complete symptom resolution

  b. If the interruption continues long enough, an ischemic stroke will result. Historically, the classic definition for a TIA was that TIA deficits resolve within 24 hours.

  c. Contemporary definition, however, defines a TIA as lasting less than 1 hour, with most resolving within 5 to 15 minutes. Neurologic symptoms must be caused by ischemia to the brain and *not* other etiologies.

  d. TIAs serve as a warning for a completed stroke, with the first highest risk for a completed stroke occurring in the first 72 hours to 2 weeks after the TIA. Lifetime stroke risk after a TIA is 33%.

  e. Types of TIA symptoms and signs include focal weakness, numbness, facial asymmetry, or speech difficulties. Altered level of consciousness, vertigo, and cranial nerve (CN) deficits are seen with posterior circulation (cerebrovascular or brainstem) and cerebellar strokes.

4. Summary of stroke syndromes

Summary of Stroke Syndromes

SYNDROME	SYMPTOMS
Anterior cerebral artery	Contralateral leg > arm numbness and weakness; akinetic mutism or abulia (especially bilateral infarcts)
Middle cerebral artery	Ipsilateral eye deviation; contralateral face and arm > leg weakness, sensory loss, contralateral hemianopsia; aphasia (left) or neglect (right)
Posterior cerebral artery	Contralateral hemianopsia, memory loss
Top of the basilar	Coma or somnolence/inattention, cortical blindness
Brain stem infarction	Ataxia, vertigo, diplopia, "crossed" findings: contralateral weakness with ipsilateral cranial nerve deficits
Cerebellar infarction	Ataxia (unilateral appendicular or truncal), vertigo, nausea/vomiting
Lateral medullary (Wallenberg's) syndrome	Loss of pain and temperature sensation from the contralateral body and ipsilateral face; dysarthria, dysphagia, ataxia, hiccups
Pure motor*	Contralateral face, arm/leg weakness
Pure sensory*	Contralateral face, arm/sensory loss
Sensorimotor*	Contralateral face, arm/weakness and sensory loss
Ataxic hemiparesis*	Contralateral ataxia out of proportion to mild weakness

*The four classic lacunar stroke syndromes result from occlusion of a single penetrating artery, which may be caused by small-vessel vasculopathy (e.g., hyaline arteriolosclerosis), or large-vessel atherosclerosis.
(From Kass JS, Mizrahi EM: *Neurology Secrets*, 6th ed, Elsevier 2017, Table 18-1, p 223.)

5. Ischemic stroke
   a. **Definition:** Ischemic type of stroke that is caused by a platelet thrombosis that develops over a disrupted atherosclerotic plaque, leading to vessel occlusion and infarction (see Chapter 10)
   b. Epidemiology
      (1) MC overall type of stroke (87% of cases)
      (2) Common locations (Link 26-59)
         (a) Middle cerebral artery (MCA; MC location; Fig. 26-8 B)
         (b) Internal carotid artery (ICA) near the bifurcation
         (c) Basilar artery (BA)
   c. Gross and microscopic findings
      (1) Cerebral infarction with liquefactive necrosis develops at the *periphery* of the cerebral cortex (Fig. 26-8 C; Link 26-60).
         (a) Reperfusion does *not* usually occur; hence, the majority of atherosclerotic strokes are pale infarctions.
         (b) If reperfusion does occur, the area of infarction changes from a pale infarction to a hemorrhagic infarction (Link 26-61).
      (2) Cerebral edema is present.
         (a) Visual loss of demarcation between the gray and white matter
         (b) Breakdown of myelin
      (3) Gliosis is the reaction to injury (see Chapter 3; Link 26-62).
         (a) Astrocytes proliferate at the margins of the infarct.
         (b) Microglial cells (MPs) remove lipid debris.
      (4) A cystic area develops after 10 days to 3 weeks, caused by liquefactive necrosis (Link 26-63).
   d. Clinical findings in ischemic stroke
      (1) Most atherosclerotic strokes are preceded by TIAs (see earlier).
         (a) An example of a retinal TIA is amaurosis fugax (temporary or partial loss of vision in one eye).
         (b) Caused by microembolization of atherosclerotic material to a bifurcation of retinal arteries (called a Hollenhorst plaque [Fig. 26-8 D])
         (c) When the microembolic embolus resolves, the vision is restored.
      (2) Strokes involving the MCA (Fig. 26-9; see earlier table)
         (a) Contralateral hemiparesis (muscular weakness or paralysis; arm > leg) and sensory loss in the face and upper extremity
         (b) Expressive aphasia occurs if Broca's area is involved in the dominant (left) hemisphere or neglect if the lesion is in the right hemisphere.

Aphasia refers to the loss of the ability to produce language (spoken or written) or of comprehending spoken or written language. **Broca aphasia**, which is a result of injury involving the Broca area, refers to a type of aphasia characterized by impaired ability to produce language (spoken or written). **Wernicke aphasia**, a result of injury to the Wernicke area, refers to an impaired ability to comprehend language (either spoken or written). Because individuals with Wernicke aphasia cannot comprehend what is said, their language, although fluent, does not make sense.

         (c) Contralateral hemianopsia (visual field defect) is present.
         (d) The head and eyes deviate toward the side of the brain lesion.
      (3) Strokes involving the ACA (Fig. 26-10; see earlier table): contralateral hemiparesis and sensory loss in the lower extremity (leg > arm)
      (4) Strokes involving the vertebrobasilar (VB) arterial system
         (a) Ipsilateral sensory loss in the face
         (b) Contralateral hemiparesis and sensory loss in the trunk and limbs
         (c) Vertigo (sensation of spinning and loss of balance) is present.
         (d) Ataxia (loss of full control of bodily movements) is present.
6. Embolic (hemorrhagic) stroke
   a. **Definition:** Ischemic type of stroke caused by embolization from a distant site
   b. Epidemiology; source of emboli
      (1) Most emboli originate from the left side of the heart (left atrium [LA]; left ventricle [LV]; see Chapter 5; Link 26-64). Carotid artery thrombosis is a less common site for embolization (Link 26-65).
      (2) Examples
         (a) Mural thrombi in the left ventricle (Link 11-21 B) after an acute myocardial infarction (AMI; see Chapter 11), aortic or mitral valve vegetations, dilated

Site of Occlusion	Regions Affected	Signs and Symptoms
	Motor area for upper body	Paresis or paralysis of contralateral face, hand, and arm
	Somatosensory cortex for upper body	Sensory deficits involving contralateral face, hand, and arm
	Axons of coronal radiata projecting from somatic motor area for lower limb (*left arrow*)	Paresis of contralateral leg
	Axons from thalamic ventroposterolateral nucleus to somatosensory cortex for lower limb (*right arrow*)	Sensory deficit involving contralateral leg
	Frontal lobe of **dominant** hemisphere (usually left hemisphere) related to speech production (Broca area)	Expressive aphasia (nonfluent or motor aphasia)
	Superior temporal lobe areas of **dominant** hemisphere related to interpretation of speech	Receptive aphasia, fluent aphasia
	Angular gyrus and parieto-occipital cortex of **dominant** hemisphere	Acalculia, agraphia, finger agnosia, right-left disorientation (collectively referred to as Gerstmann syndrome)
	Supramarginal or angular gyrus	Loss or impairment of optokinetic reflex
	Parietal lobe of **nondominant** hemisphere	Contralateral neglect (hemi-neglect), anosognosia
	Frontal eye fields in frontal lobe	Transient loss of voluntary saccadic eye movement to contralateral side
	Optic radiation within temporal lobes (Meyer loop)	Superior quadrantanopsia
	Optic radiation within parietal and temporal lobes	Homonymous hemianopia
	Upper portion of posterior limb of internal capsule and adjacent corona radiata	Capsular (pure motor) hemiplegia

26-9: Clinical features of a stroke involving the middle cerebral artery. *(From Weyhenmeyer, J, Gallman, E: Neuroscience, Rapid Review Series, 1st edition, 2007, Philadelphia, Mosby, p 28, Table 3-1.)*

AF → stasis of blood → thrombus embolization

"Shower" emboli (fat/ amniotic fluid embolism)

G/M findings

Hemorrhagic infarction 1/ more areas

cardiomyopathy (DC), and the left atrium (LA) in atrial fibrillation (AF; breaks off emboli from clot material in the LA)
  (b) AF is particularly notable as a progenitor of embolic strokes caused by thrombus formation in the LA from stasis of blood.
  (c) "Shower" embolization refers to emboli blocking numerous small vessels (e.g., fat embolism, AF embolism; see Chapter 5).
  c. Gross and microscopic findings in embolic strokes
   (1) Embolic strokes produce a hemorrhagic infarction in one or more areas of the brain. Emboli are lysed (fibrinolytic system), resulting in restoration of blood flow.

	Regions Affected	Signs and Symptoms
	Motor area for lower body Somatosensory cortex for lower body	Paresis or paralysis of contralateral leg and foot Sensory impairment (paresthesia or anesthesia) involving contralateral foot and leg
	Fibers coursing from arm and hand area of motor cortex through corona radiata (*left arrow*) Fibers coursing to arm and hand area of somatosensory cortex through corona radiata (*right arrow*)	Mild paresis of contralateral arm Mild sensory impairment of contralateral arm
	Superior frontal gyrus (*upper*) and anterior cingulate gyrus (*lower*), bilaterally	Urinary incontinence

26-10: Clinical features of a stroke involving the anterior cerebral artery. *(From Weyhenmeyer J, Gallman E:* Neuroscience, Rapid Review Series, *1st ed, 2007, Philadelphia, Mosby, p 30, Table 3-2.)*

(2) Most embolic strokes occur in the distribution of the MCA (Fig. 26-11 A; Link 26-66). They usually get lodged at bifurcation sites.

Most in MCA distribution
Lodged bifurcation sites

(3) Vessel reperfusion after lysis of embolic material results in hemorrhage within the area of infarction.

Reperfusion occurs → hemorrhage

(4) Note that the area in the brain is the same in both atherosclerotic and embolic strokes; however, whereas the former typically result in a pale infarction (no reperfusion), the latter result in a hemorrhagic infarction (reperfusion).

d. Clinical findings in an embolic stroke are similar to those arising secondary to an atherosclerotic stroke. Headache is worse with hemorrhagic strokes than atherosclerotic strokes.

Clinical findings similar to atherosclerotic stroke
Headaches worse with hemorrhagic stroke

7. Lacunar strokes

Lacunar strokes

a. **Definition:** Ischemic stroke characterized by cystic areas of microinfarction in the brain that are <1 cm in diameter (see Fig. 26-12 C; Link 26-67)

Microinfarction <1 cm

b. Caused by hyaline arteriolosclerosis (hardening of the arterioles; see Fig. 10-7 A; Link 26-68). Hyaline arteriolosclerosis is secondary to either HTN (MC) or DM (see Chapter 10).

Hyaline arteriolosclerosis:HTN (MC)/ DM

c. Stroke syndromes associated with lacunar infarctions

Lacunar stroke syndromes

(1) Pure motor strokes with or without dysarthria (slowed or slurred speech). Occurs if the posterior limb of the internal capsule is involved.

Pure motor strokes with/ without slurred speech
Posterior limb internal capsule

(2) Pure sensory strokes; occur if the thalamus is involved

Pure sensory strokes
Thalamus

8. Intracerebral hemorrhage

Intracerebral hemorrhage

a. **Definition:** Type of stroke characterized by stress imposed on branches of the LTS vessels by HTN, causing them to rupture or less commonly by rupture of a berry aneurysm into the brain parenchyma rather than the subarachnoid space

Intracerebral bleed from HTN; stress on LTSs → rupture

b. Epidemiology

(1) Most often caused by stress imposed on vessels by HTN

Vessel stress by HTN

(a) Branches of the lenticulostriate (LTS) vessels develop Charcot-Bouchard microaneurysms (see Fig. 26-8 B) in the brain.

LTS vessels → Charcot-Bouchard microaneurysms

26-11: A, Embolic stroke showing a wedge-shaped hemorrhagic infarction *(arrow)* along the periphery of the cerebral cortex in the distribution of the middle cerebral artery. It is hemorrhagic because blood flow was reestablished when the embolus dislodged and converted a pale infarct to a hemorrhagic infarct. **B,** Intracerebral hemorrhage, showing a large blood clot within the basal ganglia area of the brain. *(A from my friend Ivan Damjanov, MD, PhD, Linder J:* Pathology: A Color Atlas, *St. Louis, Mosby, 2000, p 408, Fig. 19-25B; B from my friend Ivan Damjanov, MD, PhD:* Pathology for the Health-Related Professions, *2nd ed, Philadelphia, Saunders, 2000, p 506, Fig. 21-7.)*

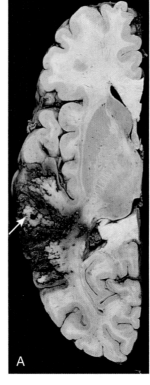
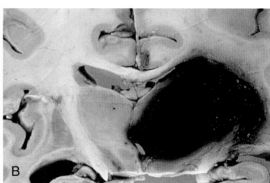

Microaneurysms rupture → intracerebral hemorrhage

Hematomas push brain parenchyma aside

Common sites

Basal ganglia MC site

Thalamus

Pons, cerebellar hemispheres

Slit hemorrhages: HTN

Rupture small caliber penetrating vessels

Clinical findings

Alterations level of consciousness

Nausea, vomiting, headache

Seizures, focal neurologic deficits (site specific)

Subarachnoid hemorrhage

Blood in subarachnoid space

Ruptured berry aneurysm/ AVM

Majority rupture of berry aneurysm

Berry aneurysm

Areas weakness; bifurcation points CoW

Not present at birth

Normal hemodynamic stress

HTN any cause

CoA

Atherosclerosis

    (b) Rupture of the microaneurysms results in an intracerebral hemorrhage (hematoma). Intracerebral hematomas push the brain parenchyma aside (space-occupying lesion; see Fig. 26-11 B).

  (2) Common sites of intracerebral hemorrhage

    (a) Basal ganglia (35%–50% of cases occur in the putamen; Link 26-69)

    (b) Thalamus (10% of cases)

    (c) Pons (Link 26-70) and cerebellar hemispheres (10% of cases)

  (3) Slit hemorrhages are associated with HTN. Rupture of small-caliber penetrating vessels produce hemorrhages that resorb blood, leaving slitlike spaces with a brownish-red pigment (hemosiderin from the breakdown of RBCs).

  c. Clinical findings in intracerebral hemorrhage

    (1) Alterations in the level of consciousness

    (2) Nausea, vomiting, and headache

    (3) Seizures and focal neurological deficits, the latter depending on the site of the intracerebral bleed

9. Subarachnoid hemorrhage (SAH)

  a. **Definition:** The presence of blood in the subarachnoid space caused by a ruptured berry aneurysm or bleeding from an arteriovenous malformation (AVM) in the brain

  b. Epidemiology

    (1) Majority are secondary to rupture of a saccular (berry) aneurysm.

    (2) Bleeding from an AVM is a less common cause.

  c. Berry (saccular) aneurysm (see Chapter 10)

    (1) **Definition:** An aneurysm that develops in areas of weakness at bifurcation points in the circle of Willis (CoW), where blood flow is most turbulent

    (2) Epidemiology

      (a) Some use the term *congenital berry aneurysm*, with the understanding that these aneurysms are *not* present at birth.

      (b) Risk factors

        • Normal hemodynamic stress

        • Presence of HTN of any cause

        • Coarctation of the aorta (CoA; increased proximal pressure on the branching vessels off the aorta)

        • Atherosclerosis (Link 26-71)

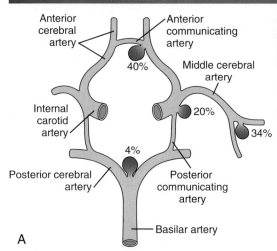

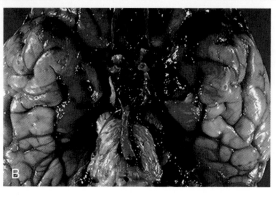

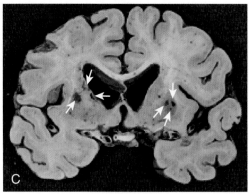

26-12: A, Schematic of locations of saccular (berry) aneurysms in the circle of Willis. **B,** Subarachnoid hemorrhage. Note the presence of blood covering the surface of the brain. **C,** Lacunar infarcts. The *arrows* show multiple small cystic spaces (liquefactive necrosis) that are most prominent in the basal ganglia. Sections under these lesions showed hyaline arteriolosclerosis. *(A from Kumar V, Abbas AK, Fausto N, Mitchell RN: Robbins Basic Pathology, 8th ed, Philadelphia, Saunders Elsevier, 2007, p 867, Fig. 23-9; B from Klatt E: Robbins and Cotran Atlas of Pathology, Philadelphia, Saunders, 2006, p 470, Fig. 19-77; C from my friend Ivan Damjanov, MD, PhD, Linder J: Pathology: A Color Atlas, St. Louis, Mosby, 2000, p 408, Fig. 19-28.)*

(c) Most berry aneurysms develop at the junctions of communicating branches of the CoW with the main cerebral artery (Fig. 26-12 A; Links 26-72 and 26-73). Less commonly, the basilar artery may be involved as well (Link 26-74).
- Junctions lack internal elastic lamina and smooth muscle.
- MC sites for a berry (saccular) aneurysm are the junction of the anterior communicating artery with the anterior cerebral artery and the MCA bifurcation.

(d) Rupture releases blood into the subarachnoid space. Blood covers the surface of the brain (Fig. 26-12 B; Links 26-75 and 26-76).

(e) Blood in the CSF is broken down into bilirubin pigment; imparts a yellow color to the CSF, called xanthochromia.

(3) Clinical findings of a berry aneurysm rupture
  (a) Classic, sudden onset of a severe occipital headache
    - Described as the "worst headache ever"
    - Nuchal rigidity is present from blood irritating the meningeal membranes.
  (b) About 50% of patients die soon after the hemorrhage.
  (c) Complications include of SAH
    - Further hemorrhage (rebleeding)
    - Hydrocephalus caused by blockage of the arachnoid villi or blockage of the egress of CSF from the foramina of Luschka (L) and Magendie (M)
    - Vasospasm causing late ischemic infarctions
    - Hyponatremia caused by release of atrial natriuretic factor (ANF)
    - Permanent neurologic deficits

(4) CT scan shows blood in the subarachnoid space (Link 26-77).

d. Arteriovenous malformation (AVM)
  (1) **Definition:** Thick-walled, aberrant vascular channels with intervening gliotic brain tissue. Some of the large vessels are arterial (Links 26-78 and 26-79).
  (2) Epidemiology and clinical
    (a) Most emerge during fetal development.
    (b) Hemorrhage into the brain (intracerebral hemorrhage). In some cases, blood may extend into the subarachnoid space.

e. Mycotic aneurysm (see Chapter 10): potential for rupture

f. Link 26-80 summarizes all intracranial hemorrhages in the brain.

10. Superior sagittal venous thrombosis (SSVT)

a. **Definition:** MC type of dural venous sinus thrombosis; is potentially devastating (Link 26-81)

b. Epidemiology and clinical

(1) Risk factors include pregnancy, volume depletion, hypercoagulable states, and pancreatitis.

(2) As with all cerebral venous thrombosis, the presentation is highly variable, ranging from asymptomatic to a rapid fulminant course with cerebral hemorrhage and death.

(3) Presentation includes headache (53%, MC); seizures (48%); hemi-, quadri-, or paraplegia (48%); visual disturbances (25%); and nuchal rigidity (18%).

11. Diagnosis of strokes

a. CT scan without contrast is best for the diagnosis of a stroke.

(1) Overall best imaging technique (Links 26-82, 26-83, and 26-84)

(2) Distinguishes hemorrhage from nonhemorrhagic strokes

b. MRI is most useful for identification of posterior fossa infarctions (small space in the skull that is near the brainstem and cerebellum).

VII. CNS Infections

A. Definition: An infection of the brain, spinal cord, or both

B. Pathogenesis.

1. Hematogenous spread (MC)

2. Traumatic implantation

3. Local extension from a nearby infection (e.g., frontal sinus, mastoid)

4. Ascent via a peripheral nerve (PN) (e.g., rabies)

5. Mechanisms for bacterial infections in the CNS (Link 26-85)

C. Meningitis

1. **Definition:** Inflammation of the pia mater covering the surface of the brain (Fig. 26-13 A; Links 26-86 and 26-87)

2. Epidemiology

a. Usually caused by hematogenous spread of a pathogen

b. Risk factors in children for meningitis

(1) Age

(a) Younger than 5 years old (infants between 6 and 12 months)

(b) Most cases occur in children between 1 month and 5 years old.

(2) Undernutrition (e.g., kwashiorkor), otitis media, pneumonia, immune deficiency, viral infection, sickle cell disease (SCD), craniofacial abnormalities

c. The primary risk factor in adults for development of meningitis is immunosuppression (ISP), etiologies of which include alcoholism, autoimmune disorders (Alzheimer disease; e.g., SLE), HIV/AIDs, cancer, DM, immunosuppressive (ISP) drugs (e.g.,

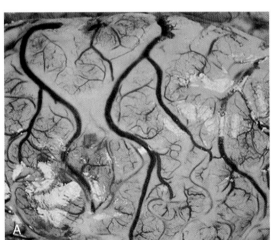
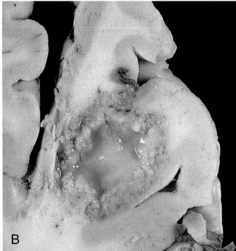

26-13: A, Bacterial meningitis showing engorged blood vessels and a creamy exudate covering the surface of the pia mater. **B,** Cerebral abscess showing a cystic mass lined by necrotic, purulent material. (**A** from Perkin GD: Mosby's Color Atlas and Text of Neurology. St. Louis, Mosby, 2002, p 196, Fig. 11-1; **B** from Burger PC, Scheithauer BW, Vogel KS: Surgical Pathology of the Nervous System, 4th ed, London, Churchill Livingstone, 2002, p 121, Fig. 3-17.)

corticosteroids, chemotherapy), intravenous drug abuse (IVDA), splenectomy or autosplenectomy in SCD, smoking, and crowded living conditions (military recruits and residents of college dorms), which specifically increases the risk of outbreaks of meningococcal meningitis.

d. Mechanisms for developing viral meningitis
   (1) Most are transmitted by the fecal–oral route. Replication in intestinal lining → viremia and seeding of CNS. Arboviruses are transmitted by mosquito bites → local replication in tissues and lymph nodes → viremia and seeding of meninges. HSV is by inoculation during time of genital infection (reactivation of genital lesions, radiculitis, meningitis).
   (2) Respiratory route is less common.

e. Mechanisms for developing bacterial meningitis (Link 26-85)
   (1) Colonization of the nasopharynx (e.g., *Neisseria meningitidis*)
   (2) Vertical transmission of infection from mother to infant shortly before or during delivery (e.g., group B streptococcus [*Streptococcus agalactiae*])
   (3) Cerebrospinal leaks that develop after penetrating trauma (e.g., *Streptococcus pneumoniae*)
   (4) Hematogenous spread from septicemia

f. Mechanisms for developing fungal meningitis
   (1) *Not* spread from person to person
   (2) Can develop after it spreads through the bloodstream from somewhere else in the body to the brain or spinal cord or from an infection adjacent to the brain or spinal cord
   (3) Can occur if introduced by lumbar puncture (e.g., contaminated preservative-free methylprednisolone acetate steroid injections)
   (4) *Cryptococcus* is thought to be acquired through inhalation of soil contaminated with pigeon droppings.
   (5) *Histoplasma* is found in environments with heavy contamination of bird or bat droppings, particularly in the Midwest near the Ohio and Mississippi Rivers.
   (6) *Blastomyces* is thought to exist in soil rich in decaying organic matter in the Midwest United States, particularly the northern Midwest.
   (7) *Coccidioides* is found in the soil of endemic areas (Southwestern United States and parts of Central and South America), and arthrospores can be inhaled in the dust, particularly after a heavy rain.
   (8) *Candida* spp. are usually acquired in a hospital setting (contaminated intravenous [IV] line).

g. Mechanisms for developing parasitic meningitis: Primary amebic meningoencephalitis (PAM) is a very rare form of parasitic meningitis that causes a brain infection that is usually fatal. PAM is caused by the microscopic ameba *Naegleria fowleri* when water containing the ameba enters the body through the nose.

h. Pathogens by age
(From Ferri FF: 2017 Ferri's Clinical Advisor, Philadelphia, Elsevier, 2017, p 779.)
   (1) Neonates (0–4 weeks): group B streptococcus (*S. agalactiae*; 40%; Guillan-Barre syndrome [GBS]; MC), *Escherichia coli* and other gram-negative rods (30%; *Klebsiella pneumoniae, Salmonella* spp., *Listeria monocytogenes*), *S. pneumoniae* (14%), *N. meningitidis* (12%).
   (2) Infants ≥3 months and <3 years: *S. pneumoniae* (45%), *N. meningitidis* (34%), *S. agalactiae* (11%), *Haemophilus influenzae, E. coli*
   (3) Ages ≥3 years and 10 years: *S. pneumoniae* (47%), *N. meningitidis* (32%)
   (4) Ages ≥10 years to <19 years: *N. meningitidis* (55%), *S. pneumoniae*
   (5) Adults: *S. pneumoniae* (MC), *N. meningitidis, L. monocytogenes* (especially after age 50–60 years with impaired cell-mediated immunity)
   (6) Older adults: *L. monocytogenes*, gram-negative Enterobacteriaceae (*E. coli*), *Pseudomonas aeruginosa, S. pneumoniae*
   (7) People with HIV/AIDS: *Cryptococcus neoformans* MC, invasive meningococcal disease

3. Key clinical findings in meningitis in infants include bulging fontanelle, paradoxic irritability (i.e., remaining quiet when stationary and crying when held), high-pitched cry, and hypotonia.

4. Key clinical findings in meningitis in adults include fever, nuchal rigidity (inflammation of the pia mater), and headache. Additional findings may include nausea, vomiting, photophobia, sleepiness, confusion, irritability, delirium, and coma. Patients with viral

Mechanisms viral

Most fecal-oral route, mosquito bites

Respiratory route

Mechanisms bacterial

Colonization NP: *N. meningitidis*

Vertical transmission: *S. agalactiae*

CSF leaks post trauma: *S. pneumoniae*

Hematogenous spread

Mechanisms fungal

Not person to person

Hematogenous/contiguous spread

Lumbar puncture

Cryptococcus: pigeon droppings; inhalation

Histoplasma: inhalation bird/bat droppings

Blastomyces: soil decaying organic matter

Coccidioides: inhaling arthrospores in dust

Candida: hospital setting (IV line)

Mechanisms parasitic (amebic)

Naegleria fowleri: contaminated water thru nose

Pathogens by age

Neonates (0–4 wks): group B streptococcus MC

Infants ≥ 3 mths–< 3 yrs: *S. pneumoniae* MC

≥ 3 yr–10 yr: *S. pneumoniae* MC

≥ 10 yr–< 19 yr: Neisseria meningitides MC

Adults *S. pneumoniae* MCC

Elderly: Listeria, E. coli, P. aeruginosa, S. pneumoniae

HIV/AIDS: Cryptococcus neoformans MC

Infants: bulging fontanelle, irritability, hypotonia

Fever, nuchal rigidity, headache

meningitis may have a history of preceding systemic symptoms (e.g., myalgias, fatigue, or anorexia).

5. Complications associated with meningitis include focal or generalized seizures, focal neurologic deficits, cranial nerve palsies (e.g., facial nerve palsy), sensorineural hearing loss, hydrocephalus (may be either communicating or noncommunicating).

6. Laboratory findings in viral meningitis (see Table 26-2)

    a. Increase in CSF protein caused by increased vessel permeability in acute inflammation and the production of an exudate (see Chapter 3)

    b. Increase in the total CSF WBC count. Initially, neutrophils are present, but this converts to lymphocytes in 24 to 48 hours.

    c. Normal CSF glucose: *Exceptions* include mumps meningoencephalitis and lymphocytic choriomeningitis (LCM), in which the CSF glucose is decreased.

7. Laboratory findings in bacterial meningitis (see Table 26-2)

    a. Increase in CSF protein

    b. Increase in the total CSF WBC count; Neutrophil-dominant leukocyte count. Lymphocytes are the dominant leukocyte in tuberculous meningitis.

    c. Decrease in the CSF glucose (used by WBCs)

8. Laboratory findings in fungal meningitis (see Table 26-2)

    a. Increase in CSF protein

    b. Increase in the total CSF WBC count. Lymphocytes are the predominant leukocytes.

    c. Decrease in the CSF glucose (used by leukocytes)

D. **Encephalitis**

1. **Definition:** Inflammation of the brain parenchyma (Link 26-88)

2. Epidemiology and clinical

3. Clinical findings

    a. Fever

    b. Headache

    c. Impaired mental status caused by inflammation of the brain

    d. Drowsiness

4. Meningoencephalitis is an overlap of meningitis and encephalitis.

E. **Cerebral abscess**

1. **Definition:** Space-occupying infection within the brain that is filled with necrotic debris

2. Epidemiology

    a. Pathogenesis

        (1) Spread from an adjacent focus of infection (e.g., sinuses, mastoiditis)

        (2) Hematogenous spread (e.g., infective endocarditis; bronchiectasis)

    b. Single or multiple lesions (Fig. 26-13 B; Links 26-89 and 26-90)

F. **Viral CNS infections and spongiform encephalopathy** (see Tables 26-2; Tables 26-3 and 26-4; Fig. 26-14)

G. **Bacterial CNS infections** (Table 26-5)

H. **Fungal and parasitic CNS infections** (Table 26-6; Fig. 26-16)

VIII. **Demyelinating Disorders**

A. **Definition of a demyelinating disorder**

1. Group of disorders characterized by the breakdown of myelin derived from Schwan cells (SCs) and oligodendrocytes (ODC) (Link 26-102)

    • Myelin is the proteolipid membrane that ensheathes and surrounds nerve axons to improve their ability to conduct electrical action potentials. When myelin is stripped away from the axon, the underlying membrane does *not* contain a high enough concentration of sodium, potassium, and other ionic channels to permit a sufficient flow of ions to cause depolarization.

2. White matter contains myelinated axons (myelinated processes are white in color).

3. Gray matter mostly contains nerve cell bodies and has a gray color (lack of myelin).

B. **Epidemiology of demyelinating disorders; pathogenesis**

1. Destruction of normal myelin. Example: multiple sclerosis

2. Production of abnormal myelin. Example: leukodystrophy

3. Destruction of oligodendrocytes. Examples: Multiple sclerosis, slow virus infections (SVIs)

4. Destruction of Schwann cells in the peripheral nervous system (PNS). Example: GBS

C. **Acquired demyelinating disorders**

1. Multiple sclerosis (MS)

    a. **Definition:** Chronic autoimmune demyelinating disease of the CNS

    b. Epidemiology

Seizures; neurologic deficits; CN palsies; sensorineural hearing loss; hydrocephalus

Lab viral meningitis

↑CSF protein

↑Vessel permeability (acute inflammation)

↑Total CSF WBC count

Initially neutrophils; switch to lymphocytes

Normal CSF glucose

Exceptions: mumps, LCM

Lab bacterial meningitis

↑CSF protein

↑CSF WBC count

Neutrophil dominant

Lymphocyte dominant TB meningitis

↓CSF glucose

Lab fungal meningitis

↑CSF protein

↑CSF WBC count

↑CSF lymphocytes

↓CSF glucose

Encephalitis

Inflammation of brain

Fever

Headache

Impaired mental status

Drowsiness

Meningoencephalitis: overlap meningitis/encephalitis

Cerebral abscess

Space occupying infection; necrotic debris

Adjacent focus infection

Hematogenous spread

Breakdown myelin (Schwann cells, oligodendrocytes)

Conduction electrical action potentials

White matter: myelinated axons

Gray matter: nerve cell bodies (lack myelin)

Destruction myelin

Multiple sclerosis

Abnormal myelin

Leukodystrophy

Destruction oligodendrocytes

Multiple sclerosis, SVI

Destruction Schwann cells (PNS)

GBS

Acquired disorders

Multiple sclerosis

Chronic acute inflammation demyelinating CNS disease

TABLE 26-3   Viral Infections of the Central Nervous System

VIRUS	DISEASE	COMMENTS
Arboviruses	Encephalitis	• Mosquitoes are the vector. • Wild birds are the reservoir for the virus. • West Nile virus: Crows and other birds have spread the disease from New York to the West Coast. • Encephalitis can be fatal.
Coxsackievirus (Link 26-87)	Meningitis, encephalitis	• Coxsackie or Echovirus groups of enteroviruses are the most common cause of viral meningitis. • Viral meningitis peaks in late summer and early autumn.
Cytomegalovirus (see Fig. 26-14 A; Link 26-91)	Encephalitis	• Most common viral CNS infection in AIDS • Primarily intranuclear eosinophilic inclusions • Periventricular calcification in newborns
Herpes simplex virus type 1 (see Fig. 26-14B; Link 26-92)	Meningitis and encephalitis	Causes hemorrhagic necrosis of the temporal lobes
HIV (Fig. 26-14 C)	Encephalitis	• Most common cause of AIDS dementia • Microglial cells fuse to form multinucleated cells, which have a perivascular orientation (very characteristic histologic finding). • Significant white matter injury with a vacuolar myelopathy. HIV-associated vacuolar myelopathy occurs during the late stages of HIV infection, when CD4+ lymphocyte counts are very low, often in conjunction with AIDS dementia complex, peripheral neuropathies, and opportunistic infections or malignancies of the central or peripheral nervous system (e.g., cytomegalovirus, progressive multifocal leukoencephalopathy, lymphoma). HIV-infected mononuclear cells secrete neurotoxic factors, including cytokines, possibly in conjunction with neurotoxic astrocyte factors. Vacuolar myelopathy typically presents as a slow progression of painless leg weakness, stiffness, sensory loss, imbalance, and sphincter dysfunction. Vacuolar myelopathy is often associated with AIDS dementia complex and peripheral neuropathy. In such cases, patients have cognitive decline and distal limb pain and numbness.
Lymphocytic choriomeningitis	Meningitis and encephalitis	• Endemic in the mouse population • Transmission: food or water contaminated with mouse urine or feces • Meningoencephalitis: combination of nuchal rigidity and mental status abnormalities (encephalitis) • CSF findings: increased protein, lymphocyte infiltrate, normal to decreased glucose
West Nile virus	Encephalitis	• Transmission by mosquito • Reservoir birds (crows and other birds). Birds often die of the disease (do not pick up). • Virus enters CNS neurons (cerebral cortex, brainstem, and spinal cord) → encephalitis (can be fatal). See microglial nodules (activated microglial cells have large rod-shaped nuclei and greatly ramified cytoplasm. They encircle degenerating neurons [neuronophagia] and form clusters around small foci of necrotic brain tissue [microglial nodules]).
Poliovirus	Encephalitis and myelitis (spinal cord)	• Destroys upper and lower motor neurons • Causes muscle paralysis • Postpolio syndrome: occurs in ~50% of people with previous poliomyelitis. Usually occurs 15–30 years after original infection. Increased muscular weakness or pain in muscle groups already affected; excessive fatigue.
Rabies virus (see Fig. 26-14 D)	Encephalitis	• Most often transmitted by dogs (WHO, 2017) • Other vectors are skunk, bat, raccoons, and coyote. • Viral receptor is acetylcholine receptor. • Initially replicates at site of the bite. Moves by axonal transport to the CNS. After CNS replication, it migrates to the saliva. • Animal transmits virus when in the agitated state (encephalitis stage). • Incubation period, 10–90 days • Prodrome: fever, paresthesias in and around the wound site • Hydrophobia: caused by spasms of throat muscles when swallowing; followed by flaccid paralysis • Encephalitis: death of neurons • Eosinophilic intracytoplasmic inclusions called Negri bodies • Seizures, coma, death • Universally fatal if not treated

CNS, Central nervous system; *CSF,* cerebrospinal fluid; *WHO,* World Health Organization.

TABLE 26-4 **Slow Viruses and Spongiform Encephalopathy of the Central Nervous System**

DISEASE	COMMENTS
Creutzfeldt-Jakob disease (CJD) (see Fig. 26-15; Links 26-93 and 26-94)	• Caused by prions (contain infectious proteins devoid of RNA or DNA) • Infective prions have misfolded proteins. PrP becomes resistant to proteases. Protease-resistant PrP promotes conversion of normal PrP to protease-resistant PrP, explaining the infectious nature of the disease. • *Cannot* be inactivated with standard sterilization techniques • Kill neurons (? apoptosis) • Brains have "bubble and holes" spongiform (spongiform encephalopathy) change in the cerebral cortex. • Transmission: corneal transplantation, contact with human brains (neurosurgeons, neuropathologists), use of improperly sterilized cortical electrodes, ingestion of tissues from cattle with bovine spongiform encephalopathy (mad cow disease) • Death occurs within 1 year.
Progressive multifocal leukoencephalopathy (PML)	• Conventional slow virus encephalitis caused by papovavirus. PML is a destructive white matter lesion that typically spares the cortex. It results from JC virus infection of oligodendroglia, resulting in the death of these cells and demyelination of the involved foci. On microscopic examination, these lesions show an alternating arrangement of reactive glial cells and histiocytes, as well as various unique glial cell types. Originally described in patients with chronic lymphocytic leukemia. • Intranuclear inclusion in oligodendrocytes • Occurs in AIDS when CD4 T_H count <50 cells/mm³; recognized as an AIDS-defining condition
Subacute sclerosing panencephalitis	• Conventional slow virus encephalitis associated with rubeola (measles) virus • Intranuclear inclusions in neurons and oligodendrocytes • Death usually occurs within 1–2 years.

JC, John Cunningham virus; *PrP,* prion protein.

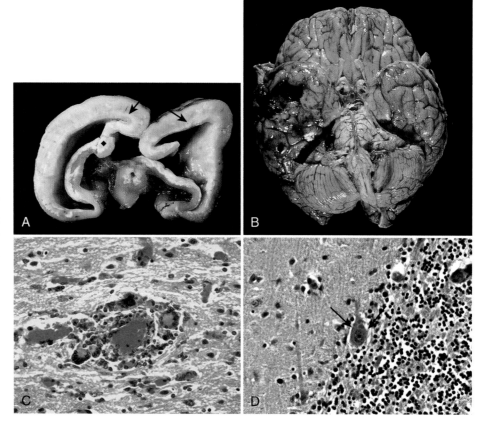

26-14: **A,** Congenital cytomegalovirus encephalitis. The *arrows* show many chalky periventricular calcifications (dystrophic calcification). **B,** Herpes simplex encephalitis. The basal view shows hemorrhagic necrosis of the right temporal lobe. Cerebral edema is also present. **C,** HIV encephalitis. Note the numerous multinucleated microglial cells, which is a characteristic finding in HIV encephalitis, the cause of AIDS dementia. **D,** Rabies. The Purkinje cells have intracytoplasmic, eosinophilic inclusions *(arrows)* called Negri bodies. *(A and C from Klatt E: Robbins and Cotran Atlas of Pathology, Philadelphia, Saunders, 2006, pp 476, 477, respectively, Figs. 19-94, 19-97, respectively; B from Perkin GD: Mosby's Color Atlas and Text of Neurology, St. Louis, Mosby, 2002, p 208, Fig. 11-15; D from Kumar V, Fausto N, Abbas A: Robbins and Cotran Pathologic Basis of Disease, 7th ed, Philadelphia, Saunders, 2004, p 1375, Fig. 28-25.)*

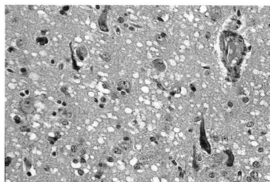

26-15: Spongiform encephalopathy in Creutzfeldt-Jakob disease showing classic "bubbles and holes" of the neuropil cell bodies. *(From my friend Ivan Damjanov, MD, PhD, Linder J: Pathology: A Color Atlas, St. Louis, Mosby, 2000.)*

TABLE 26-5   Bacterial Infections of the Central Nervous System

BACTERIUM	DISEASE	COMMENTS
Group B streptococcus (*Streptococcus agalactiae*)	Neonatal meningitis	• Gram-positive coccus • Most common cause of neonatal meningitis • Spreads from a focus of infection in the maternal vagina
Escherichia coli	Neonatal meningitis	• Gram-negative rod • Second most common cause of neonatal meningitis (18%)
Listeria monocytogenes	Neonatal meningitis	• Gram-positive rod with tumbling motility • Actin rockets help organism to move from cell to cell
Neisseria meningitidis	Meningitis	• Gram-negative diplococcus • Found in posterior nasopharynx • Most common cause of meningitis in those between 1 month and 18 years of age
Streptococcus pneumoniae	Meningitis	• Gram-positive diplococcus • Most common cause of meningitis in patients >18 years of age (some authors say *N. meningitidis* is the most common and *S. pneumoniae* the second most common)
Mycobacterium tuberculosis	Meningitis	• Complication of primary tuberculosis • Typically involves the base of brain (same location as neurosarcoidosis) • Vasculitis (infarction) and scarring (hydrocephalus)
Treponema pallidum (Link 26-95)	Meningitis, encephalitis, myelitis	• Spirochete (gram negative) • Types of neurosyphilis • **Meningovascular:** vasculitis causing stroke • **General paresis:** dementia • **Tabes dorsalis:** involves posterior root ganglia and posterior column; causes ataxia, loss of vibration sensation, absent deep tendon reflexes, and Argyll Robertson pupil (pupils accommodate [constrict with near object] but do not react to light)

TABLE 26-6   Fungal and Parasitic Infections of the Central Nervous System

FUNGUS OR PARASITE	DISEASE	COMMENTS
Cryptococcus neoformans (see Fig. 26-16 A)	Meningitis and encephalitis	• Occurs in an immunocompromised host • Most common fungal CNS infection in AIDS • Budding yeasts visible with India ink
Mucor spp. (see Fig. 26-16 B)	Frontal lobe abscess	• Occurs in DKA • Spreads from frontal sinuses into the frontal lobe
Naegleria fowleri (Link 26-96)	Meningoencephalitis	• Protozoa (amoeba) • Involves frontal lobes • Contracted by swimming in warm freshwater lakes • Organism passes through nasal cavity and across the cribriform plate into base of brain
Trypanosoma brucei gambiense and *Trypanosoma brucei rhodesiense* (Links 26-97 and 26-98)	Encephalitis	• Protozoa (hemoflagellate) • Transmission: bite of an infected tsetse fly (*Glossina*) • Trypanosomes invade the blood and lymphatics early in the disease • Initial drainage into the posterior cervical nodes produces lymphadenopathy (Winterbottom sign); encephalitis occurs in later stages • Diffuse encephalitis: somnolence (sleeping sickness) caused by the release of sleep mediators by the organisms • Trypanosomes are capable of antigen variation (cyclical fever spike) • Starvation is the most common cause of death. • Diagnosis: trypanosomes in blood, CSF. • Serologic tests with characteristic increase in IgM early in the disease
Taenia solium (see Fig. 26-16 C; Link 26-99)	Cysticercosis	• Helminth (tapeworm; cestode) • Transmitted by pigs • Patient (intermediate host) ingests food or water containing eggs. • Eggs develop into larval forms (cysticerci) that invade the brain, producing calcified cysts causing seizures and hydrocephalus.
Toxoplasma gondii (see Fig. 26-16 D, E; Links 26-100 and 26-101)	Encephalitis	• Protozoa (sporozoan); occurs in patients with compromised immune systems • Most common CNS space-occupying lesion in AIDS. Lesions have necrosis and granulomatous inflammation. Bradyzoite form is most typically seen. "Free-living" tachyzoites in brain tissue can only be detected with special techniques. • Ring-enhancing lesions on CT • Congenital toxoplasmosis produces basal ganglia dystrophic calcification

AIDS, Acquired immunodeficiency syndrome; *CNS,* central nervous system; *CT,* computed tomography; *DKA,* diabetic ketoacidosis.

26-16: A, Cryptococcus. India ink preparation showing large capsules surrounding budding yeast cells. **B,** Mucor species (zygomycosis). Note the broad, aseptate hyphae that have wide-angled branching. **C,** Neurocysticercosis. Note the multiple cysts located between the gray and white matter. **D,** Toxoplasmosis. Note the cyst *(arrow)* filled with bradyzoites. **E,** Toxoplasmosis. The computed tomography scan shows multiple enhancing lesions. Toxoplasmosis is the most common space-occupying lesion in the brain in AIDS. It can be confused with primary central nervous system lymphoma. *(A and B from Murray PR, Shea YR:* Medical Microbiology, *2nd ed, St. Louis, Mosby, 2002, pp 787, 794, Figs. 75-8, 75-18, respectively; C from my friend Ivan Damjanov, MD, PhD, Linder J:* Pathology: A Color Atlas, *St. Louis, Mosby, 2000, p 411, Fig. 19-38; D from Burger PC, Scheithauer BW, Vogel KS:* Surgical Pathology of the Nervous System, *4th ed, London, Churchill Livingstone, 2002, p 143, Fig. 3-78; E from Perkin GD:* Mosby's Color Atlas and Text of Neurology, *St. Louis, Mosby, 2002, p 216, Fig. 11-23.)*

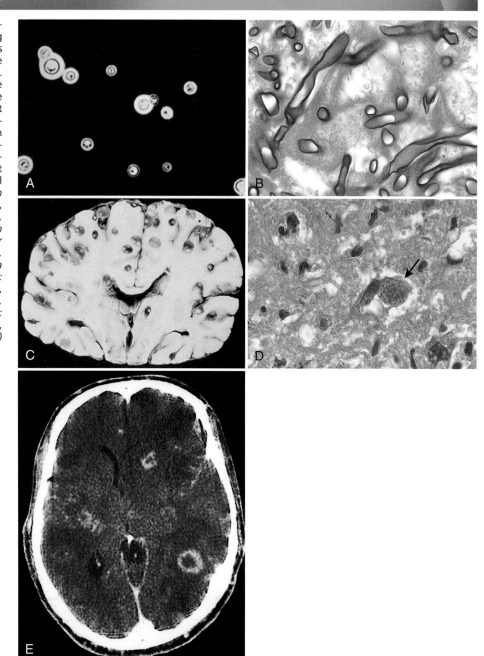

MC demyelinating disease in U.S.
MC debilitating disease young adults
M:F ratio: 1:2 to 1:3
Mean age 30 yrs
Northern latitudes
Autoimmune disease
Genetic factors: HLA-DR2
Environmental factors
EBV, HHV 6
Chlamydophila pneumoniae
Vitamin D, sun exposure

(1) MC demyelinating disease in the United States
(2) MC debilitating disease among young adults
(3) Male:female ratio is 1:2 to 1:3; most often occurs in women between 20 and 40 years of age. Mean age of onset is 30 yrs.
(4) More common in people raised in northern latitudes
(5) Autoimmune disease; initiating factors
　(a) Genetic factors (e.g., human leukocyte antigen [HLA]-DR2)
　(b) Environmental factors. Examples: microbial pathogens (e.g., Epstein-Barr virus (EBV), human herpesvirus (HHV) 6, *Chlamydophila pneumoniae*), vitamin D, and sun exposure

Possible mechanism for multiple sclerosis: CD4 TH1 cells and T-helper 17 (Th17) cells react against self-myelin antigens (e.g., MBP and other antigens; type IV hypersensitivity reaction; see Chapter 4). CD4 Th1 cells secrete interferon γ (γ-IFN), which activates macrophages (MPs; produce tumor necrosis factor-α [TNF-α]), and Th1 cells release cytokines that recruit neutrophils and monocytes. Demyelination occurs as both leukocytes and TNF-α attack the myelin sheath and oligodendrocytes. Abs produced by autoreactive B cells are directed against the myelin sheath and oligodendrocytes as well (type II hypersensitivity reaction).

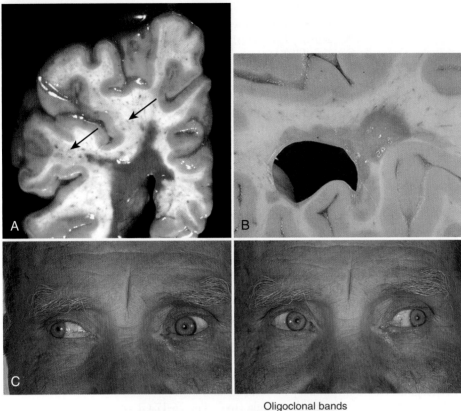

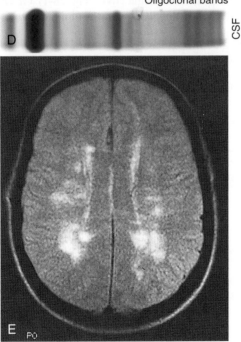

26-17: **A,** Multiple sclerosis, gross appearance. The brain shows multiple areas of demyelinated white matter (*arrows* pointing to gray-brown plaques). **B,** Multiple sclerosis, gross appearance. Note the periventricular location for the demyelinating plaques. **C,** Bilateral internuclear ophthalmoplegia in multiple sclerosis. When the patient is asked to look right, the right eye moves to the right and exhibits jerk nystagmus, and the left eye remains stationary. When the patient is asked to look left, the left eye moves to the left and shows jerk nystagmus, and the right eye remains stationary. These findings are caused by bilateral demyelination of the medial longitudinal fasciculus. **D,** High-resolution electrophoresis of spinal fluid (CSF) showing four oligoclonal bands that indicate the presence of demyelination. **E,** Magnetic resonance image showing extensive demyelination (white areas). (**A** from *Kumar V, Fausto N, Abbas A:* Robbins and Cotran Pathologic Basis of Disease, *7th ed, Philadelphia, Saunders, 2004, p 1383, Fig. 28-32;* **B** from Klatt E: Robbins and Cotran Atlas of Pathology, *Philadelphia, Saunders, 2006, p 480, Fig. 19-105;* **C, E** *from Perkin GD:* Mosby's Color Atlas and Text of Neurology, *St. Louis, Mosby, 2002, pp 183, 188, respectively.* **D** from McPherson R, Pincus M: Henry's Clinical Diagnosis and Management by Laboratory Methods, *22nd ed, St. Louis, Saunders, 2011, p 911, Fig. 46-8A.)*

c. Gross and microscopic findings in multiple sclerosis
   (1) Demyelinating plaques occur in white matter (contains myelin) of brain/spinal cord (Fig. 26-17 A and B; Links 26-103, 26-104, and 26-105). White matter looks like gray matter in the areas of demyelination.
   (2) Inflammatory infiltrate in plaques is composed predominantly of CD4 T cells, monocytes, and microglial cells with phagocytized lipid.
d. Clinical findings in mutliple sclerosis
   (1) Episodic course punctuated by acute relapses and remissions (80%–90% of cases)
   (2) MC symptoms.

Gross/microscopic

Demyelinating plaques

Inflammatory plaque: CD4 T cells, monocytes, microglial cells

Clinical findings

Episodic; acute relapses/remissions

(a) Pyramidal weakness (45%): A pattern of weakness in the extensors (upper limbs) or flexors (lower limbs), known as "pyramidal weakness"

(b) Visual loss (40%), sensory loss (35%)

(c) Brainstem dysfunction (30%), cerebellar ataxia and tremor (25%)

(d) Sphincter disturbances (20%)

(3) Sensory dysfunction signs

(a) Paresthesias ("pins and needles")

(b) Loss of pain and temperature sensation

(c) Loss of vibratory sensation (cannot feel tuning fork vibrations)

(4) Upper motor neuron (UMN) dysfunction signs

(a) Spasticity (increased muscle tone [tight and rigid] and exaggerated deep tendon reflexes [DTRs])

(b) Increased DTRs; muscle spasms

(c) Extensor plantar response (positive Babinski reflex)

(d) Weakness in shoulder abduction, finger extension, foot dorsiflexion, and hip and knee flexion

(5) Autonomic dysfunction signs

(a) Urge incontinence, hyperactive detrusor muscle (see Chapter 21)

(b) Sexual dysfunction, bowel motility problems

(6) Optic neuritis

(a) **Definition:** Inflammation of the optic nerve causing blurry vision

(b) Multiple sclerosis is the MCC of optic neuritis.

(c) Sudden loss of vision may occur.

(7) Cerebellar ataxia (failure of muscle coordination)

(8) Scanning speech (sound drunk)

(9) Intention tremor (tremors when attempting a precise movement)

(10) Nystagmus (rapid involuntary movements of the eye)

(11) Bilateral internuclear ophthalmoplegia (INO; Fig. 26-17 C): caused by demyelination of the medial longitudinal fasciculus (MLF)

(12) Flexion of the neck produces an electrical sensation down the spine.

e. Laboratory and radiologic findings

(1) Increase in CSF leukocyte count; primarily CD4 T lymphocytes and monocytes

(2) Increase in CSF protein; increase is primarily caused by an increase in γ-globulins

(3) Increase in CSF MBP: indicator of active disease

(4) Normal CSF glucose

(5) High-resolution serum electrophoresis that shows oligoclonal bands

(a) Discrete bands of protein in the γ-globulin region (Fig. 26-17 D; Link 26-106)

(b) Sign of demyelination

(6) MRI detects demyelinating plaques (Fig. 26-17 E; Links 26-107 and 26-108); highly sensitive in detecting demyelinating plaques.

(7) CT can also be used but is not the test of choice (Link 26-109).

f. Diagnosis of multiple sclerosis

(1) Lumbar spinal tap

(2) MRI with gadolinium (most sensitive test)

g. Prognosis of multiple sclerosis

(1) Varies greatly

(a) One-third of patients with multiple sclerosis do well throughout their lives without accumulating significant disability.

(b) One-third accumulate neurologic deficits sufficient to impair activities but not serious enough to prevent them from leading normal lives (e.g., holding a job, raising a family).

(c) One-third of people with multiple sclerosis become disabled, requiring a walker, wheelchair, or even total care.

(2) On the average, ~70% of patients with multiple sclerosis are alive 25 years after their diagnosis.

2. Central pontine myelinolysis (CPM; Fig. 26-18; see Chapter 5)

a. **Definition:** Demyelinating disease that affects the brainstem white matter, mostly in the central pons

b. Epidemiology (see Chapter 5)

(1) Most often occurs in alcoholics and those with malnutrition who have hyponatremia

(2) Rapid intravenous correction causes demyelination in the basis pontis. Rapid change in osmolality initiates the demyelination.

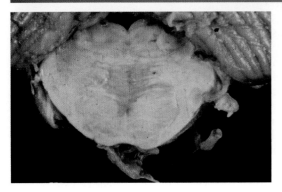

26-18: Central pontine myelinolysis. Note the central area of demyelination in the pons. *(From my friend Ivan Damjanov, MD, PhD, Linder J:* Pathology: A Color Atlas, *St. Louis, Mosby, 2000, p 413, Fig. 19-45.)*

3. Viral infections with direct infection of oligodendrocytes. Examples: subacute sclerosing panencephalitis (SSP), progressive multifocal leukoencephalopathy (PML; see later)

D. Hereditary demyelinating disorders; leukodystrophies

1. **Definition:** Inborn errors of metabolism characterized by degeneration of the white matter in the brain
2. Adrenoleukodystrophy
   a. **Definition:** Genetic disease characterized by a peroxisome defect that causes generalized loss of myelin in the brain as well as adrenal insufficiency
   b. Epidemiology
      (1) X-linked recessive (XR) disorder
      (2) Enzyme deficiency in β-oxidation of fatty acids (FAs) in peroxisomes (PXS) that results in an accumulation of long-chain FAs
      (3) Causes a generalized loss of myelin in the brain and adrenal insufficiency
      (4) Onset is between 4 and 6 years of age.
3. Metachromatic leukodystrophy
   a. **Definition:** Genetic lysosomal storage disease (LSD) characterized by the accumulation of sulfatides, resulting in the loss of myelin in the CNS
   b. Epidemiology
      (1) Autosomal recessive (AR) LSD
      (2) Caused by a deficiency of arylsulfatase A, which leads to an accumulation of sulfatides and loss of myelin in the CNS
   c. Clinical findings: ataxia, weakness, blindness, and brain atrophy
4. Krabbe disease
   a. **Definition:** Genetic LSD characterized by an accumulation of galactocerebroside
   b. Epidemiology
      (1) AR lysosomal storage disease
      (2) Caused by a deficiency of galactocerebroside β-galactocerebrosidase deficiency, which leads to an accumulation of galactocerebroside
      (3) Brain shows large, multinucleated, histiocytic cells (globoid cells).
   c. Clinical findings in Krabbe disease: hypertonicity, blindness, deafness, seizures, and atrophy of the brain

IX. Degenerative Disorders

A. Definition of degenerative disorders

- Group of unrelated diseases that are characterized by a progressive deterioration of neurons in the CNS, resulting in a variety of neurologic and psychiatric signs and symptoms

B. Alzheimer disease

1. **Definition:** Neurodegenerative disease characterized by a progressive loss of cognitive skills, including memory, thinking, and language skills, as well as changes in behavior

Marginal notes:

Viral infections direct infection oligodendrocytes: SPE, PML

Leukodystrophies

Inborn errors

Degeneration white matter brain

Adrenoleukodystrophy

Peroxisome defect → loss myelin in brain + adrenal insufficiency

XR

Enzyme deficiency β-oxidation FAs PXS

Loss myelin brain + adrenal hypofunction

Onset between 4 and 6 yrs

Metachromatic leukodystrophy

Genetic LSD

Accumulation sulfatides → loss myelin CNS

AR LSD

↓Arylsulfatase A → accumulation sulfatides → loss myelin CNS

Ataxia, weakness, blindness, brain atrophy

Krabbe disease

Genetic LSD

Accumulation galactocerebroside

AR LSD

↓ Galactocerebroside β-galactocerebrosidase → ↑galactocerebroside

Brain: multinucleated histiocytic cells (globoid cells)

Degenerative disorders

Diseases with progressive deterioration of neurons

Alzheimer disease

The term *neurodegenerative disorders* is used to describe a group of diseases of unknown etiology that are limited to the CNS (Link 26-110). These diseases, which are unrelated to one another, present with a variety of neurologic and psychiatric symptoms. For example, Parkinson disease presents with movement disorders, Huntington disease with abnormal body movements and progressive mental deterioration, and Alzheimer disease with a loss of mental capacities but *no* motor deficits.

(Excerpt modified from my friend Ivan Damjanov: *Pathology for the Health Professions*, 4th ed, Philadelphia, Saunders Elsevier, 2012, p 465.)

MCC dementia

Sporadic late-onset type MC

Sporadic early-onset (before 65 yrs)

Defect *ApoE*, allele ε4

Produced by astrocytes

Transports CH to neurons

↑Breakdown Aβ

Familial early-onset type

M APP C21

M presenilin 1 C14

M presenilin 2 C1

Prevalence ↑with age

Trisomy 21 strong association with Alzheimer disease

APP precursor for Aβ protein

APP endocytosed into endosomes in neurons

Aβ neurotoxic

Medial temporal lobes

Frontal cortex (entorhinal cortex, hippocampus)

Occipital lobes spared

Pivotal role activated GSK and Aβ neurotoxicity

Activated GSK phosphorylates Aβ

Aβ causes neuronal/ synaptic dysfunction

Aβ signals apoptosis

Phosphorylates Aβ → + feedback on GSK-3β

Activation GSK-3β → dysfunction *Wnt*

Neuronal development during embryogenesis

Norm neuronal function

Normal *Wnt* signaling: inactivates GSK-3β → prevents phosphorylation Aβ

Dysfunctional *Wnt* → GSK remains activated → phosphorylates Aβ

Aβ deposits wall cerebral vessels

Produces amyloid angiopathy

Aβ stains with Congo red → apple-green bfg

Aβ: metabolic product of APP

APP coded on C21

Defects metabolism APP by secretases → ↑Aβ → ↑neurotoxicity

α-Secretases cleave APP to harmless fragments

β-secretases followed by γ-secretases cleave APP to produce Aβ

Insulin degrading enzyme

IDE: clearance of Aβ

Insulin resistant type 2 DM: ↑insulin → ↓IDE → Aβ

2. Epidemiology
   a. MCC of dementia (50%–75% of all cases)
   b. Subdivisions
      (1) Sporadic late-onset type of Alzheimer disease (MC)
      (2) Sporadic early-onset type of Alzheimer disease (*before* age 65 years)
         (a) Related to a defect in apolipoprotein gene E (*ApoE*), allele ε4
         (b) *ApoE* is mainly produced by astrocytes.
         (c) *ApoE* transports cholesterol to neurons via *ApoE* receptors.
         (d) *ApoE* enhances the proteolytic breakdown of Aβ (see later).
      (3) Familial early-onset type of Alzheimer disease (<1% of cases)
         (a) Mutations (M) of amyloid precursor protein (APP) on chromosome (C) 21
         (b) Mutations in presenilin 1 on chromosome 14
         (c) Mutations in presenilin 2 on chromosome 1
   c. Prevalence of Alzheimer disease increases with age.
      (1) Prevalence is <1% in the 60- to 64-year-old age group.
      (2) Prevalence is 40% to 50% by the age of 95 years.
   d. Trisomy 21 (Down syndrome) has a strong association with Alzheimer disease. By 40 years of age, most people with Down syndrome have Alzheimer disease.
3. Role of β-amyloid (Aβ) protein in causing Alzheimer disease
   a. <u>A</u>myloid <u>p</u>recursor <u>p</u>rotein (APP) (see Chapter 4) is the precursor for Aβ protein.
      (1) APP is endocytosed into endosomes in neurons, where the acidic environment favors Aβ formation.
      (2) A new drug is now available (levetiracetam, an antiepileptic drug) that prevents the endocytosis of APP into endosomes.
   b. Aβ is neurotoxic and damages neurons in the following sites.
      (1) Medial temporal lobe structures
      (2) Frontal cortex, especially the entorhinal cortex and hippocampus
      (3) Occipital lobes are usually spared.
   c. Pivotal role of activated glycogen synthase kinase-3β (GSK-3β) in the neurotoxicity of Aβ
      (1) Activation of GSK-3β causes phosphorylation of Aβ, which in turn causes the following:
         (a) neuronal and synaptic dysfunction
         (b) signaling for neuronal apoptosis
      (2) Phosphorylated Aβ also has a positive feedback on GSK-3β, which maintains the cycle of neurotoxicity.
      (3) Initial activation of GSK-3β has been traced to dysfunction within the *Wnt* (<u>w</u>ingless <u>i</u>ntegration <u>p</u>athway), which is a family of genes normally involved in:
         (a) neuronal development during embryogenesis.
         (b) normal neuronal function.
      (4) Normally, the *Wnt* signaling pathway inactivates GSK-3β, which prevents phosphorylation of Aβ and its harmful effect on neurons.
      (5) However, if the *Wnt* signaling pathway is dysfunctional, GSK-3β remains activated, leading to phosphorylation of Aβ and its neurotoxic effects (e.g., apoptosis of neurons).
   d. Aβ also deposits in the wall of cerebral vessels; important in producing cerebral amyloid angiopathy (see later)
   e. Aβ stains positive with Congo red and has apple-green birefringence (bfg) with polarization (see Chapter 4).
   f. Recall that Aβ is a metabolic product of APP (Link 26-111).
      (1) APP is normally coded for on chromosome 21.
      (2) Defects in metabolism of APP by secretases cause an increase in Aβ and a corresponding increase in neurotoxicity.
      (3) α-Secretases cleave APP into fragments that *cannot* produce Aβ.
      (4) β-Secretases followed by γ-secretases (presenilin is the catalytic unit) cleave APP into fragments that are converted to Aβ.
      (5) In the sporadic early-onset type of Alzheimer disease (SeoAD), allele ε4 of apolipoprotein gene E codes for a product that *cannot* eliminate Aβ from the brain, leading to early onset of neurotoxicity.
   g. Insulin-degrading enzyme (IDE)
      (1) **Definition:** Involved in the clearance of Aβ
      (2) Insulin resistance syndromes (type 2 DM, metabolic syndrome) have an increased risk for developing Alzheimer disease because increased insulin lowers insulin degrading enzyme, which increases Aβ.

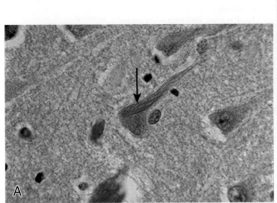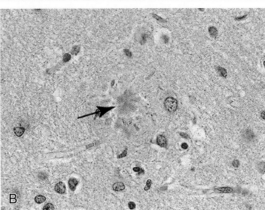

26-19: A, Neurofibrillary tangle (NFT). The stain shows a neuron with neurofilaments *(arrow)* composed of hyperphosphorylated tau protein. These are present in Alzheimer disease (AD). **B,** Senile plaque *(arrow)* shows an eosinophilic center with peripherally located distended neuronal processes (neurites). Similar to NFTs, these are present in AD. *(A from Klatt E:* Robbins and Cotran Atlas of Pathology, *Philadelphia, Saunders, 2006, p 481, Fig. 19-110; B from Burger PC, Scheithauer BW, Vogel KS:* Surgical Pathology of the Nervous System, *4th ed, London, Churchill Livingstone, 2002, p 428, Fig. 8-9.)*

4. Role of tau protein in Alzheimer disease
   a. Normal function of tau protein is to maintain microtubules in neurons. It assembles and supports the scaffolding that is important in neuron structure and function.
   b. Activated GSK enhances hyperphosphorylation of tau protein.
      (1) This process causes the protein to change shape and cluster into fibers.
      (2) Fibers appear as neurofibrillary tangles (NFTs; twisted fibers) in the cytoplasm. These are best visualized with silver stains (Fig. 26-19 A; Link 26-112).
      (3) NFTs produce neuronal dysfunction, including death of the neuron.
      (4) Pin 1 enzyme (prolyl isomerase) normally strips excess phosphate molecules from NFTs, restoring it to its original shape; however, in some cases of Alzheimer disease, this enzyme is absent or dysfunctional.
5. Gross and microscopic findings
   a. Cerebral atrophy with dilation of ventricles (hydrocephalus ex vacuo)
      (1) Atrophy is caused by loss of neurons in the temporal, frontal, and parietal lobes (Links 26-113 and 26-114).
      (2) Occipital lobe is usually spared in Alzheimer disease.
   b. Presence of NFTs in the cytoplasm of neurons (Link 26-112). NFTs may occur in other disorders; including older adult patients *without* dementia, Huntington disease, and Niemann-Pick disease (NPD).
   c. Senile (neuritic) plaques
      (1) **Definition:** Consist of a core of Aβ surrounded by neuronal cell processes containing tau protein, microglial (MG) cells, and astrocytes (Fig. 26-19 B; Link 26-115); located in the gray matter of the cerebral cortex
      (2) Aβ stains with Congo red (see Chapter 4)
      (3) Best visualized with silver stains
      (4) Although present in normal older adults, senile plaques are markedly increased in Alzheimer disease.
   d. Amyloid angiopathy (Link 26-116)
      (1) **Definition:** The presence of Aβ in cerebral vessels
      (2) Causes weakening of the vessels with an increased risk for hemorrhage
   e. Cholinergic hypothesis

Tau protein

Maintains neuron microtubules

Neuron structure/function

Activated GSK: hyperphosphorylates tau protein

Tau protein changes shape → clusters into fibers

NFT: hyperphosphorylated tau protein in neuron

NFT: neuronal dysfunction/ death neuron

PIN 1 enzyme: dephosphorylates NFTS

↓PIN1 enzyme some cases Alzheimer disease

Cerebral atrophy; dilated ventricles

Loss neurons

Occipital lobe spared

NFTs in neuron cyto

NFTs other disorders *without* dementia

Senile neuritic plaques

Core Aβ: tau protein, MG cells, astrocytes

Gray matter cerebral cortex

Aβ Congo red positive

Silver stains

Senile plaques: also in brains normal elderly people

Amyloid angiopathy

Aβ cerebral vessels

Risk cerebral hemorrhage

The cholinergic hypothesis attempts to explain many of the cognitive deficits in Alzheimer disease (particularly memory disturbance) by a deficiency of cholinergic neurotransmission. Evidence includes the fact that poor memory can be induced in normal people by anticholinergic drugs. Loss of cholinergic projection neurons in the nucleus basalis of Meynert and loss of choline acetyltransferase activity throughout the cortex of patients with Alzheimer disease correlate with the severity of memory loss.

(Extract from Kass JS, Mizrahi EM: *Neurology Secrets*, 6th ed, Elsevier, 2017, p 195, #40.)

   f. Confirmation of Alzheimer disease
      (1) Requires postmortem examination of the brain
      (2) Must show the presence of widespread NFTs and senile plaques

Confirmation

Postmortem exam of brain

Widespread NF tangles/ senile plaques

6. Clinical findings in Alzheimer disease
    a. Prominent early sign is the decline in short-term memory.
    b. Another early sign is the loss of smell. This is caused by dysfunction in the entorhinal cortex.
    c. Patients with mild to moderate disease have only cognitive defects.
    d. Additional deficits accumulate, including changes in behavior, judgment, language, and abstract thought.
    e. Eventually, the functional deficits manifest themselves as a reduced ability for self-care.
    f. *No* focal neurologic deficits are present early in the disease.
    g. Patients usually die of an infection (usually bronchopneumonia).
7. A presumptive diagnosis of Alzheimer disease is made with mental status testing, which tests for orientation (e.g., place and time), attention (selective awareness), verbal recall (recall information which was received verbally), and visual-spatial skills (e.g., complete a jigsaw puzzle).
8. Positron emission tomography (PET) is useful for the differential diagnosis of dementia. Florbetapir-PET imaging of the brain correlates with the presence and density of Aβ.

C. **Parkinsonism**
1. **Definition:** A group of progressive neurodegenerative disorders that alter dopaminergic pathways involved in voluntary muscle movement
2. Epidemiology
    a. Involves the dopaminergic pathways that are involved in voluntary muscle movement (Links 26-117 and 26-118)
        (1) Striatal system that is involved in voluntary muscle movement includes the following: substantia nigra (SN), caudate, putamen, globus pallidus (GP), subthalamus, and thalamus (Link 26-119)
        (2) Dopamine is the principal neurotransmitter in the nigrostriatal tract. This tract connects the SN with the caudate and putamen.
    b. The incidence of parkinsonism increases with age.
    c. Idiopathic Parkinson disease is the MC type of parkinsonism (see later).
    d. Other causes of parkinsonism
        (1) Encephalitis (inflammation of the brain)
        (2) Ischemia (decreased blood flow to the brain)
        (3) Chronic carbon monoxide (CO) poisoning; causes necrosis of the GP
        (4) Wilson disease
        (5) Addiction to MPTP (1-methyl-4-phenyl-1,2,3,6-tetrahydropyridine), a derivative of meperidine
        (6) Antipsychotic drugs (e.g., phenothiazines)
3. Idiopathic Parkinson disease
    a. **Definition:** Progressive neurodegenerative disorder characterized clinically by rigidity, resting tremor, impaired postural reflexes, and slowness of movement (bradykinesia)
    b. Epidemiology
        (1) MC type of parkinsonism (78%)
        (2) Sporadic (MC) and familial form
        (3) Onset occurs between 45 and 65 years of age.
        (4) Distribution is equal in men and women.
        (5) Highest incidence is in whites; the lowest incidence is in Asians and African Americans.
        (6) Pathophysiology
            (a) Degeneration and depigmentation of neurons in the substantia nigra (Fig. 26-20 A; Links 26-120 and 26-121)
            (b) Causes a deficiency of dopamine in the neurons
            (c) Example of a protein misfolding disease that contains aggregates of amyloid β, tau protein, and α-synuclein in neurons (see Chapter 4)
            (d) Neurons contain intracytoplasmic, eosinophilic bodies called Lewy bodies (Link 26-122). Lewy bodies contain ubiquitinated (damaged) neurofilaments as well as aggregates of misfolded proteins containing α-synuclein, tau protein, and amyloid β.
    c. Clinical findings in idiopathic Parkinson disease
        (1) Muscle rigidity
            (a) Slowness of voluntary muscle movement (bradykinesia)
            (b) Cogwheel rigidity (jerky muscle resistance to movement) is present on physical examination.

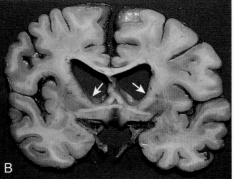

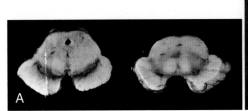

26-20: A, Substantia nigra in Parkinson disease. The normal amount of pigmentation in the substantia nigra in shown in the midbrain on the left. The midbrain on the right shows markedly diminished pigmentation in the substantia nigra. **B,** Huntington disease with atrophy of caudate nuclei *(white arrows)* on their lateral sides. *(A and B from my friend Ivan Damjanov, MD, PhD, Linder J: Pathology: A Color Atlas, St. Louis, Mosby, 2000, p 419, Figs. 19-67, 19-65, respectively.)*

    (2) Resting tremor
       (a) "Pill rolling" occurs between the thumb and index fingers (Link 26-123).
       (b) Handwriting is illegible.
    (3) Expressionless face ("poker face"; Link 26-124). Stooped posture (Link 26-125)
    (4) Difficulty in initiating the first step; shuffling gait
    (5) Blepharospasm (fine tremor of the eyelids); postural instability (responsible for falls)
    (6) Severe seborrheic dermatitis (scaly rash; see Chapter 25)
    (7) Dementia in some cases
  d. Diagnosis of idiopathic Parkinson disease. DaTscan (Ioflupane I 123 injection) is a radiopharmaceutical agent that is injected into a patient's veins in a procedure referred to as single-photon emission computed tomography (SPECT) imaging (Link 26-126).

D. Huntington's disease
  1. **Definition:** Autosomal dominant neurodegenerative disease characterized by a decline in cognitive activity, involuntary movements, and psychiatric disturbances
  2. Epidemiology
    a. Trinucleotide repeat disorder (CAG) involving chromosome 4 (see Chapter 6)
    b. Delayed appearance of symptoms until late 30 to 40 years of age; *no* gender dominance
    c. Atrophy or loss of striatal neurons, which include the caudate, putamen, and GP (Fig. 26-20 B; Link 26-127)
  3. Clinical findings in Huntington's disease
    a. Chorea
      (1) **Definition:** Irregular, rapid, nonstereotyped involuntary movements
      (2) Called choreoathetosis if it has a writhing quality (like a snake)
    b. Oculomotor abnormalities (rapid eye movements known as saccades)
    c. Parkinsonism in later stages; depression
  4. Diagnosis of Huntington's disease
    a. Genetic testing is available.
    b. Imaging studies (CT, MRI) show atrophy of the caudate and putamen.

E. Friedreich ataxia
  1. **Definition:** Genetic disease characterized by gait ataxia and involvement of the cerebellum, spinal cord, peripheral nerves, and heart
  2. Epidemiology
    a. Autosomal recessive trinucleotide repeat disorder (GAA) of the frataxin gene. Frataxin deficiency leads to impaired mitochondrial iron homeostasis, causing apoptosis of dorsal root ganglia (DRG) and degeneration in spinal cord tracts.
    b. MC neurodegenerative hereditary ataxic disorder
    c. Affects ~1:20,000 persons of European descent
    d. Manifests *before* age 25 years (usually in adolescence)
    e. Sites of degeneration
      (1) Dorsal root ganglia, posterior columns
      (2) Spinocerebellar tract, lateral corticospinal tracts
      (3) Large sensory peripheral neurons
  3. Clinical findings in Friedreich ataxia
    a. Progressive gait ataxia
    b. Loss of DTRs (initially at the ankles)
    c. Loss of vibratory sensation and proprioception

d. Muscle weakness in the legs

e. Hypertrophic cardiomyopathy (symmetric concentric type; see Chapter 11)

f. DM in 10% of cases as a result of both insulin resistance as well as impaired insulin release.

g. Progressive scoliosis

4. Diagnosis of Friedreich ataxia

a. Gene testing is available.

b. MRI shows spinal cord atrophy.

F. **Lou Gehrig disease (ALS)**

1. **Definition:** Progressive degenerative neuromuscular disease characterized by the loss of upper and lower motor neurons (LMNs); *no* sensory deficits

2. Epidemiology

a. Symptoms usually appear between 50 and 70 years of age.

b. Most cases are sporadic (90%–95% of cases). Male:female ratio is 2:1.

c. About 10% to 20% of cases are caused by mutated superoxide dismutase (SOD) 1 (neuron destruction by superoxide free radicals) or misfolded SOD 1, leading to apoptosis of neurons.

3. Clinical findings in ALS

a. UMN signs include spasticity and a positive Babinski sign.

b. LMN signs are predominantly those of muscle weakness that begins with atrophy of intrinsic muscles of the hands. Eventually, there is paralysis of the respiratory muscles.

c. Preservation of bowel and urinary bladder function

4. Diagnosis by electromyography (EMG) and nerve conduction studies (NCS). DNA studies are also available.

5. Average survival time is 3 to 5 years.

G. **Werdnig-Hoffmann disease (WHD)**

- LMN disease that occurs in children

X. **Toxic and Metabolic Disorders**

A. **Wilson disease** (see Chapter 19); brief summary

1. AR disease

a. Defect in copper excretion into bile

b. Defect in the incorporation of copper into ceruloplasmin (binding protein for copper; decreased)

c. Leads to liver cirrhosis and excess copper in hepatocytes

2. CNS findings in Wilson disease; atrophy and cavitation of the basal ganglia, particularly the globus pallidus (GP) and putamen (Fig. 26-21 A)

B. **Acute intermittent porphyria**

1. **Definition:** Genetic disease in porphyrin metabolism that produces neurologic dysfunction, peripheral neuropathy, and dementia

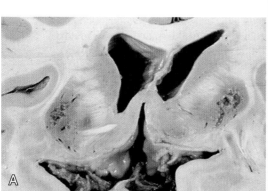
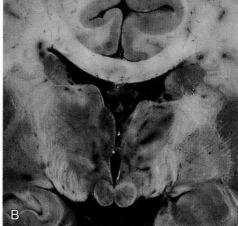

26-21: A, Wilson disease. Note cavitary necrosis of the putamen on both sides of the brain. **B,** Wernicke encephalopathy showing hemorrhage and discoloration of mammillary bodies and the wall of the third ventricle. *(A and B from my friend Ivan Damjanov, MD, PhD, Linder J: Pathology: A Color Atlas, St. Louis, Mosby, 2000, pp 414, 413, respectively, Figs.19-48, 19-43, respectively.)*

2. Epidemiology
   a. Autosomal dominant disorder
   b. Enzyme defect in porphyrin metabolism
      (1) Deficiency of uroporphyrinogen synthase (porphobilinogen [PBG] deaminase) leads to a proximal increase in PBG and δ-aminolevulinic acid (ALA) (Link 25-138; see Chapter 25).
      (2) Urine is *colorless* when first voided. Exposure to light ("window sill test") oxidizes PBG to porphobilin, producing a port-wine color of the urine sample.
      (3) Heme has a negative feedback relationship with ALA synthase, the rate-limiting enzyme of porphyrin metabolism.
      (4) Decrease in heme (distal to uroporphyrinogen synthase) precipitates porphyric attacks by increasing porphyrin synthesis proximal to the enzyme block. ALA synthase activity is increased, causing ALA to be increased. Example: drugs enhancing the liver cytochrome P450 system decrease heme (e.g., alcohol; see Chapter 2)
3. Clinical findings in acute intermittent porphyria
   a. Neurologic dysfunction
      (1) Recurrent bouts of severe abdominal pain simulating an acute abdomen
      (2) Often mistaken for a surgical abdomen (e.g., acute appendicitis). The patient has a "bellyful of scars."
   b. Psychosis, peripheral neuropathy, and dementia
4. Diagnosis of acute intermittent porphyria is made by enzyme assay in RBCs
C. **Vitamin B$_{12}$ deficiency; neurologic findings include** (see Chapter 12):
   1. subacute combined degeneration of the spinal cord (see Fig. 12-18 C); posterior column (PC) and lateral corticospinal tract demyelination.
   2. dementia and PN.
D. **CNS findings associated with alcohol abuse** (Link 26-128)
   1. Cortical and cerebellar atrophy (Link 26-129)
   2. Central pontine myelinolysis (CPM) (see Fig. 26-18; Link 26-130; see Chapter 5)
   3. Wernicke-Korsakoff syndrome (WKS)
      a. **Definition:** Syndrome caused by a deficiency of thiamine; characterized by a triad of ophthalmoplegia (eye muscle weakness), gait ataxia, and disturbances in mental function
      b. Epidemiology
         (1) Most often caused by thiamine deficiency (see Chapter 8)
         (2) Gross and microscopic
            (a) Hemorrhages of small vessels with hemosiderin deposits occur in the mammillary bodies and wall of the third and fourth ventricles (Fig. 26-21 B; Link 26-131).
            (b) Neuronal loss, gliosis (astrocyte proliferation), and small-vessel hemorrhage
      c. Wernicke encephalopathy; reversible findings; confusion, ataxia, nystagmus, and ophthalmoplegia (eye muscle weakness)
      d. Korsakoff psychosis
         (1) **Definition:** Advanced irreversible stage of Wernicke encephalopathy that targets the limbic system in the brain
         (2) Epidemiology and clinical
            (a) Anterograde amnesia (inability to form new memories)
            (b) Retrograde amnesia (inability to recall old memories)
            (c) Confabulation (fabricated or distorted memories that are *not* meant to deceive)
            (d) Hallucinations (perception of something that is *not* present)
XI. **Central Nervous System Tumors**
   A. **Definition:** Group of primary benign or malignant tumors or secondary tumors that are the result of metastasis from a primary site located outside the brain
   B. **Epidemiology**
      1. In most patients, the cause is unknown.
      2. Primary brain tumors in adults
         a. Approximately 70% occur above the tentorium cerebelli.
         b. In order of decreasing frequency in adults: glioblastoma (50%), meningioma (17%), and astrocytoma (10%)
      3. Primary brain tumors in children
         a. Second MC cancer in children
         b. Approximately 70% occur *below* the tentorium cerebelli (infratentorial).

c. In order of decreasing frequency in children: medulloblastoma (24%; more common in males), pilocytic astrocytoma (20%), and glioblastoma (20%)

4. Genetics
   a. Most primary CNS tumors are sporadic.
   b. Five percent are associated with hereditary syndromes.

5. Risk factors for the development of CNS tumors include:
   - Turcot syndrome, neurofibromatosis (NF), von Hippel-Lippau syndrome, Li-Fraumeni syndrome, retinoblastoma, tuberous sclerosis (TS), Gorlin syndrome, exposure to ionizing radiation (meningiomas, gliomas, nerve sheath tumors), oil refining, rubber manufacturing, age >65 years old (certain types of brain tumors), and illicit drugs.

6. General clinical findings in benign or malignant CNS tumors
   a. Headache (20% initially, 60% later)
      (1) Tend to be worse during the night and often wake the person up
      (2) Accompanied by nausea and vomiting (N/V)
   b. Seizures (>30% of cases)
      (1) Type of seizure depends on location.
      (2) More common in low- rather than high-grade tumors
   c. Symptoms and signs of intracranial hypertension (see Section I)
   d. Focal neurologic signs: sensory changes, muscle weakness, visual disturbances, cognitive dysfunction (memory or personality changes)

7. Imaging studies used to diagnose CNS tumors
   a. MRI with gadolinium enhancement
   b. CT is useful if calcium or hemorrhage is present.
   c. Functional MRI for lesions in vital areas measures brain activity by detecting changes associated with cerebral blood flow.
   d. Positron emission tomography (PET)

8. Gliomas are the MC types of tumor in both the CNS and PNS.
   a. Occur in the brain, spinal cord, and PNs
   b. Three types of glial cells can produce tumors
      (*Excerpted from Weyhenmeyer JA, Gallman EA: Rapid Review Neuroscience, St. Louis, Mosby Elsevier, 2007, pp 50–52.*)
      (1) Astrocytes; functions
         (a) Structural support of brain
         (b) Help transport nutrients to neurons
         (c) Buffer ions in extracellular space, particularly K⁺
         (d) Help remove chemical transmitters released by active neurons
         (e) End-feet surround brain capillaries, take up glucose, and promote formation of blood–brain barrier (BBB)
         (f) During neuronal damage, can proliferate and phagocytose dying neurons
         (g) Radial glia: guide migration of neurons, direct outgrowth of axons during brain development
         (h) Fibrous astrocytes: found in white matter
         (i) Protoplasmic astrocytes: found in gray matter
      (2) Oligodendrocytes; functions
         (a) Synthesize myelin. Single oligodendrocytes myelinates segments of many CNS axons.
      (3) Schwann cells; function
         (a) A single Schwann cell myelinates one segment of a single axon in the peripheral nervous system (PNS) at a time.
         (b) Secrete growth factors (GFs; critical to regeneration of damaged PNS axons)
      (4) Microglial cells; function
         (a) Arise from monocytes derived from bone marrow (BM)
         (b) Migrate into brain during development and become resident microglia; act as macrophages (MPs) of the CNS
         (c) Transformed into activated microglia to phagocytize dying cells after CNS damage
      (5) Ependymal cells; function
         (a) Non-neuronal cells within the CNS
         (b) Choroid epithelial cells (CECs): specialized ependymal cells that produce CSF
         (c) Most ependymal cells have cilia or microvilli at apical processes that beat to move CSF.
   c. Three types of glial tumors in the CNS are astrocytomas, ependymomas, and oligodendrogliomas. Schwannomas occur in the PNS.

C. **Locations of intracranial tumors** (Link 26-132)

D. **Astrocytoma**

1. **Definition:** Tumors that originate from a progenitor cell with differentiation down the astrocytic lineage; range from low to high grade

2. Epidemiology
   a. Account for ~70% of all neuroglial tumors (cells that support the nervous system)
   b. Tumor usually involves the frontal lobe in adults and the cerebellum in children.
   c. Grades I and II are low-grade tumors and are considered benign (Link 26-133; see Chapter 8).
   d. Grades III and IV are high-grade astrocytomas (see Chapter 9)

3. Glioblastoma
   a. **Definition:** Grade IV (high-grade) astrocytoma; may arise de novo (MC) or from dedifferentiation of a low-grade astrocytoma
   b. Epidemiology
      (1) Hemorrhagic tumor (Fig. 26-22 A; Link 26-134)
      (2) Characterized by multifocal areas of necrosis, cystic degeneration, and vascular proliferation

Progenitor cell → differentiation down astrocyte lineage

Astrocytoma: MC neuroglial tumor

Frontal lobe adults, cerebellum children

Grades I/II: low-grade benign

Grades III/IV: high-grade

Glioblastoma

Grade IV

De novo MC; dedifferentiation low grade astrocytoma

Hemorrhagic

Necrosis/cystic degeneration, vascular proliferation

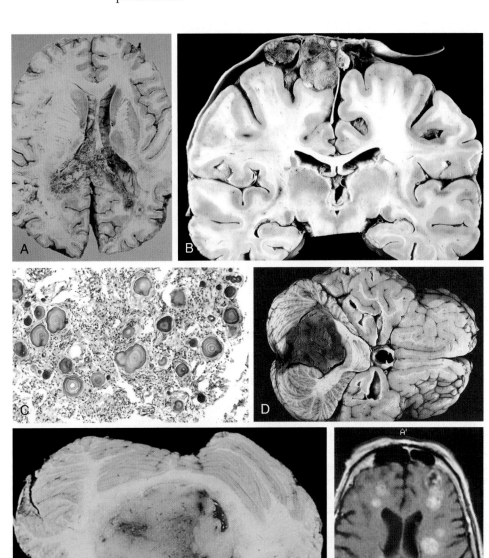

26-22: **A,** Glioblastoma multiforme showing hemorrhage and necrosis in the brain parenchyma and spreading into the adjacent hemisphere via the corpus callosum. **B,** Meningioma. Note the parasagittal multilobular tumor that is attached to the overlying dura. The tumor compresses the underlying surface of the brain. **C,** Meningioma. Note the swirling meningothelial cells and numerous basophilic staining psammoma bodies. **D,** Ependymoma of fourth ventricle. Note the hemorrhagic mass filling and expanding the fourth ventricle. **E,** Medulloblastoma. In the cerebellum, there is a centrally located hemorrhagic tumor with necrosis that has almost compressed shut the fourth ventricle. **F,** Brain metastasis. The magnetic resonance image shows multiple nodular enhancing masses of varying sizes representing metastases from a breast cancer. (*A from my friend Ivan Damjanov, MD, PhD, Linder J:* Anderson's Pathology, *10th ed, St. Louis, Mosby, 1996, p 2750, Fig. 77-120; **B** and **C** from Kumar V, Fausto N, Abbas A:* Robbins and Cotran Pathologic Basis of Disease, *7th ed, Philadelphia, Saunders, 2004, p 1409, Figs. 28-48A and B, respectively; **D** from Klatt E:* Robbins and Cotran Atlas of Pathology, *Philadelphia, Saunders, 2006, p 487, Fig. 19-127; **E** from my friend Ivan Damjanov, MD, PhD, Linder J:* Pathology: A Color Atlas, *St. Louis, Mosby, 2000, p 424, Fig. 19-82; **F** from Katz D, Math K, Groskin S:* Radiology Secrets, *Philadelphia, Hanley & Belfus, 1998, p 349, Fig. 1.*)

(3) May cross the corpus callosum and spread into the adjacent hemisphere (called "butterfly" glioblastoma; see Fig. 26-22 A; Link 26-135)

(4) May seed the neuraxis via the CSF

(5) Rarely metastasize outside the CNS

c. Poor prognosis. Even with removal of the tumor, there are microscopic cells that are infiltrative and intermixed with the normal brain.

E. **Meningioma**
1. **Definition:** Tumor that arises from meningothelial cells within the arachnoid membrane; usually benign
2. Epidemiology
   a. MC benign brain tumor in adults
   b. Benign in 90% of cases
   c. Male:female ratios are 1:3 in the brain and 1:6 in the spinal cord. Tumors usually have estrogen (E) and progesterone (P) receptors; however, some tumors have androgen (A) receptors.
   d. In children, the male:female ratio is the same.
   e. Peak incidence in men is in the sixth decade of life; slightly older (seventh decade) in women.
   f. Derived from the meningothelial cell (MC) within the arachnoid membrane that lines but is *not* adherent to the dura
   g. Most commonly have a parasagittal location, close to the midline. Other common sites are the olfactory groove and lesser wing of the sphenoid.
   h. Associated with NF 2 (see earlier)
   i. In some cases, there is a history of previous radiation to the brain.
   j. Common cause of new-onset focal seizures in an adult
3. Gross and microscopic findings of meningiomas (Fig. 26-22 B, C; Links 26-136 and 26-137)
   a. Meningiomas are firm tumors that may indent (*not* invade) the surface of the brain, hence the association with new-onset focal seizures.
   b. Often infiltrate the overlying bone, causing an increase in bone density
   c. Histologically, they are composed of swirling masses of meningothelial cells that encompass psammoma bodies (calcified bodies) (Link 26-138).
   d. MRI shows increased density and a "dural tail" sign caused by thickening of the dura related to the tumor (Link 26-139).

F. **Ependymoma**
1. **Definition:** Tumors that differentiate down the ependymal cell lineage (Fig. 26-22 D; Link 26-140)
2. Epidemiology
   a. MC spinal cord tumor in adults
   b. Arise in the cauda equina in adults
   c. In children, they arise in the fourth ventricle, where they may produce a noncommunicating hydrocephalus.

G. **Medulloblastoma**
1. **Definition:** High-grade (malignant) small cell tumor of the cerebellum; primarily seen in children
2. Epidemiology
   a. Arise from the external granular cell layer of the cerebellum (Fig. 26-22 E)
   b. Often seed the neuraxis and invade the fourth ventricle
3. Gross and microscopic
   a. Arise in the cerebellum, often in the vermis (Link 26-141)
   b. Classically appears as sheets of hyperchromatic, round cells with a monotonous appearance. Medulloblastomas may present with neuronal differentiation in the form of rosettes that lack a central canal or capillary (called Homer-Wright rosettes; Link 26-142).

H. **Oligodendroglioma**
1. **Definition:** Low-grade tumor derived from a progenitor cell with differentiation down the oligodendrocytic lineage. These tumors are slow growing with a usual survival time of several years.
2. Epidemiology
   a. Frontal lobe tumor primarily of middle-aged adults (Link 26-143)
   b. Frequently calcify, with a "fried egg" appearance histologically (Link 26-144)

I. **CNS malignant lymphoma**
1. **Definition:** Primary CNS lymphomas (PCNSLs) are most commonly EBV related and typically arise in immunosuppressed patients (e.g., AIDS). Although the incidence

in AIDS-related cases has peaked, the incidence in older adults (>65 years) continues to rise.

2. PCNSLs are most commonly EBV-related lymphomas. They are rapidly increasing due to the rapid increase in AIDS. PCNSL is an AIDS-defining criterion (Link 26-145).

J. Metastasis to the CNS; epidemiology

    1. MC CNS malignancy (Fig. 26-22 F)

    2. In order of decreasing frequency, the primary sites are the lung, breast, skin (melanoma), kidney, and gastrointestinal tract.

    3. Brain metastasis from prostate cancer is rare unless it is widely disseminated to bone and soft tissue.

    4. Skull metastasis from distant tumors occur in 4% of patients with cancer.

        a. Most are secondary to breast, lung, and prostate cancers

        b. Prostate cancer is the MCC of skull base metastases in men.

XII. Peripheral Nervous System Disorders

  A. Peripheral neuropathy

    1. **Definition:** A group of disorders that may produce focal (mononeuropathy) or generalized (polyneuropathy) nerve dysfunction

    2. Epidemiology

        a. Mononeuropathies

        (From Andreoli TE, Benjamin IJ, Griggs RC, Wing EJ: Andreoli and Carpenter's Cecil Essentials of Medicine, 8th ed, Philadelphia, Saunders Elsevier, 2010, Table 130-6, p 1174.)

          (1) Compressive (carpal tunnel syndrome [CTS], ulnar nerve neuropathy [UNN])

          (2) Inflammatory (e.g., Bell palsy; CN VII)

          (3) Multiple mononeuropathies (e.g., leprosy, DM, sarcoidosis, amyloidosis)

        b. Polyneuropathies

        (From Andreoli TE, Benjamin IJ, Griggs RC, Wing EJ: Andreoli and Carpenter's Cecil Essentials of Medicine, 8th ed, Philadelphia, Saunders Elsevier, 2010, Table 130-6, p 1174.)

          (1) Hereditary (e.g., Charcot-Marie-Tooth [CMT])

          (2) Endocrine (e.g., DM, hypothyroidism; see Chapter 23)

          (3) Metabolic (e.g., liver failure, uremia; see Chapter 19 and 20)

          (4) Infections: e.g., leprosy (see Chapter 25), Lyme disease (see Chapter 25), HIV (see Chapter 4), diphtheria

          (5) Immune mediated

          (6) Toxic (e.g., lead, arsenic, alcohol, drugs; see Chapter 7)

          (7) Paraneoplastic (e.g., lung cancer; see Chapter 9)

          (8) Nutritional deficiencies (e.g., thiamine deficiency, vitamin B_{12} deficiency; see Chapter 8)

        c. Associated with demyelination or axonal degeneration

          (1) Demyelination is often segmental. Sensory changes (e.g., paresthesias [numbness and tingling]), are often in a "glove and stocking" distribution.

          (2) Axonal degeneration is associated with muscle fasciculations (feeling of "worms beneath the skin"). This indicates that muscle atrophy is occurring.

    3. Charcot-Marie-Tooth (CMT) disease

        a. **Definition:** Hereditary polyneuropathy that involves the lower extremities

        b. Epidemiology

          (1) MC hereditary neuropathy

          (2) Autosomal dominant disease

         c. Clinical findings

          (1) Peroneal nerve neuropathy that causes atrophy of muscles of the lower legs

          (2) Legs have an "inverted bottle" appearance.

    4. Guillan-Barre syndrome (GBS)

        a. **Definition:** Immune-mediated (IM) disease that usually follows an infectious disorder; characterized by rapidly progressive ascending motor weakness

        b. Epidemiology

          (1) MC acute peripheral neuropathy

          (2) MCC of acute flaccid muscle paralysis

          (3) Involves nerve roots and peripheral nerves (PNs)

          (4) Common preceding infections include *Mycoplasma pneumoniae* pneumonia, *Campylobacter jejuni* enteritis, viral infection (HIV), EBV, cytomegalovirus (CMV), and influenza.

   c. Clinical findings in GBS
  (1) Initial symptoms are usually tingling and paresthesias in the feet and dull low-back pain (LBP).
  (2) Followed by rapidly progressive ascending motor weakness
   (a) Motor weakness usually starts in the proximal muscles; however, the distal muscles are eventually involved as well.
   (b) Danger of respiratory muscle paralysis and death
  (3) DTRs are depressed or absent in the arms and legs.
  (4) Cutaneous sensory deficits such as loss of pain and temperature sensation are mild.
  (5) Vibratory sensation with a tuning fork and proprioception (movement and position of the limbs) are more severely impaired.
  (6) Facial weakness occurs in 50% of cases.
  (7) Respiratory failure occurs in 25% of cases.
  (8) Eye muscle weakness occurs in 9% of cases.
  (9) Pain occurs in 20% of cases.

   d. Laboratory findings in GBS
  (1) Increased CSF protein (caused by the presence of oligoclonal bands [cloned or derived from one or a few cells]). Oligoclonal bands are present on high-resolution electrophoresis (small group of proteins that migrate close together; Fig. 26-17 D; Link 26-106).
  (2) Normal CSF glucose
  (3) Normal CSF WBC count

   e. Diagnosis of GBS
  (1) Spinal tap shows increased CSF protein (presence of oligoclonal bands).
  (2) Electromyography (EMG) and nerve conduction studies are also useful.

   f. Prognosis
  (1) Death occurs in 5% to 10% of cases.
  (2) Full motor recovery occurs in 60% of cases.
  (3) Residual weakness is present in 15% of cases.

5. Diabetes mellitus (DM); epidemiology
   a. MCC of peripheral neuropathy
   b. Caused by osmotic damage of Schwann cells (see Chapter 23)

6. Toxin-associated neuropathies: alcohol, heavy metals, and diphtheria

7. Idiopathic Bell palsy
   a. **Definition:** Lower motor neuron (LMN) palsy involving CN VII causing unilateral facial paralysis
   b. Epidemiology.
  (1) Inflammatory reaction of the facial nerve (CN VII). Inflammation is near the stylomastoid foramen or in the bony facial canal.
  (2) Peak incidence people <70 years old, pregnant women, especially during the third trimester or 1 week postpartum
  (3) May be associated with HSV (MC), HIV, EBV, CMV, adenovirus, rubella, mumps, or Lyme disease; often bilateral when associated with Lyme disease (caused by *Borrelia burgdorferi* a spirochete transmitted by a tick)
  (4) Can also be associated with sarcoidosis or trauma to the nerve
   c. Clinical findings in LMN disease (Fig. 26-23 A and B, at point *B* in the schematic; Links 26-146 and 26-147)
  (1) Ipsilateral upper and lower face involvement
  (2) Drooping of the corner of the mouth; difficulty speaking
  (3) Inability to close the eye; inability to wrinkle the forehead muscles
  (4) Hyperacusis (increased sensitivity to certain frequency and volume ranges of sound) in some cases
   d. Clinical findings in upper motor neuron (UMN) disease (see Fig. 26-23 B, at point *A* in the schematic)
  (1) Contralateral lower face is involved.
  (2) Contralateral upper face is spared.

8. Drugs producing peripheral neuropathy. Examples: vincristine, hydralazine, phenytoin

9. Vitamin deficiencies producing peripheral neuropathy. Examples: deficiency of thiamine, vitamin B$_{12}$, and pyridoxine

B. Schwannoma (neurilemoma)
1. **Definition:** Benign tumor derived from Schwann cells; may involve CN V (trigeminal nerve) or CN VIII (vestibulocochlear nerve; sense of hearing and pertinent to

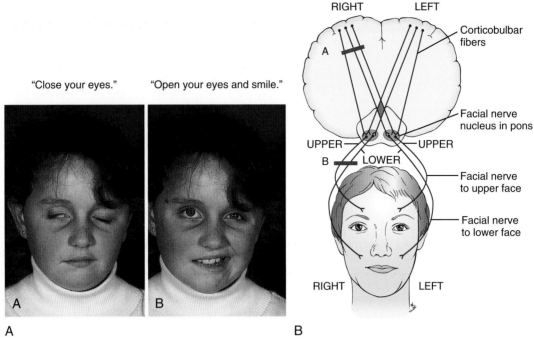

"Close your eyes."   "Open your eyes and smile."

RIGHT   LEFT

Corticobulbar fibers

A

Facial nerve nucleus in pons

UPPER   UPPER

B   LOWER

Facial nerve to upper face

Facial nerve to lower face

RIGHT   LEFT

A   B

26-23: A, Right-sided Bell palsy showing inability to fully close the right eye *(left)* and drooping of the right corner of the mouth *(right)*. **B,** Schematic of lower and upper motor neuron Bell palsy. Lower motor neuron *(point B)* is ipsilateral and involves the upper and lower face. Upper motor neuron *(point A)* involves the contralateral lower face, and there is contralateral sparing of the upper face. *(**A** from Perkin GD: Mosby's Color Atlas and Text of Neurology, St. Louis, Mosby, 2002, p 77, Fig. 4-24A and B; **B** from Swartz MH: Textbook of Physical Diagnosis, 5th ed, Philadelphia, Saunders Elsevier, 2006, p 677, Fig. 21-16.)*

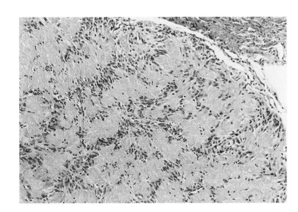

26-24: Acoustic neuroma showing spindle-shaped cells with alternating dark and light areas (similar to a zebra). *(From my friend Ivan Damjanov, MD, PhD, Linder J: Pathology: A Color Atlas, St. Louis, Mosby, 2000, p 432, Fig. 19-107.)*

balance and to body position sense). Spinal nerve roots and peripheral nerves may be involved.

2. Acoustic neuroma (AN)
   a. **Definition:** Benign neoplasm of Schwann cells involving CN VIII
   b. Epidemiology
      (1) Majority are located in the cerebellopontine angle.
      (2) Usually unilateral, encapsulated tumors. Microscopic exam shows alternating dark and light areas resembling a zebra (Fig. 26-24).
      (3) Those associated with NF2, in which they are usually bilateral; histologic difference in nerve involvement in a neurofibroma versus a schwannoma (Link 26-148)
   c. Clinical findings
      (1) Tinnitus (ringing in the ears), sensorineural deafness
      (2) Sensory changes in a CN V distribution secondary to tumor impingement on CN V by the CN VIII tumor. These two CN nerves are close to each other.
   d. Imaging (Link 26-149)
C. **Selected nerve injuries** (Table 26-7)
   • Nerve abnormalities and possible differential diagnoses (Link 26-152)

Acoustic neuroma

Schwannoma of CN VIII

Cerebellopontine angle

Unilateral, encapsulated tumor

NF2 association

Clinical findings

Tinnitus

Sensorineural deafness

CN V sensory: impingement on CN V from CN VIII tumor

TABLE 26-7   Selected Nerve Injuries

INJURY	COMMENTS
Ulnar nerve (C8–T1) (see Fig. 26-25 A)	• Fracture of medial epicondyle of the humerus • Injury produces a "claw hand" (loss of interosseous muscles)
Radial nerve (C5–T1) (see Fig. 26-25 B)	• Midshaft fractures of humerus • Draping the arm over a park bench (called "Saturday night palsy") • Injury produces wrist drop
Axillary nerve (C5–C6)	• Fracture of surgical neck of humerus • Anterior dislocation of the shoulder joint (may also injure the axillary artery) • Cannot abduct the arm to horizontal position or hold the horizontal position when a downward force is applied to the arm (paralysis of deltoid muscle)
Median nerve (C6–T1) (see Fig. 26-25C and D; Fig. 24-14 F and G)	• Most commonly caused by entrapment of the median nerve in the transverse carpal ligament of the wrist (carpal tunnel syndrome) or between the bellies of the pronator teres muscle (see Chapter 24) • Rheumatoid arthritis and pregnancy are the two most common causes. • Also caused by overuse of the hands and wrist (e.g., in barbers), amyloidosis, hypothyroidism, and a supracondylar fracture of the humerus • Clinical: nocturnal pain; pain, numbness, or paresthesias in the thumb, index finger, third finger, and radial side of fourth finger; thenar atrophy produces an "ape hand" appearance and difficulty in opposing the thumb with the fifth finger • Tinel sign: pain reproduced by tapping over the median nerve • Phalen sign: pain reproduced with forced flexion of the wrist for 1 minute • Diagnosis: NCS; EMG to rule out muscle degeneration related to nerve compression

Common peroneal nerve (L4–S2) (see Fig. 26-25 E)	• Common peripheral neuropathy
	• Causes: lead poisoning, fractured neck of the fibula, cast tightness
	• Motor deficits
	  • Loss of foot eversion caused by weakening of the peroneus longus and brevis muscles
	  • Loss of foot dorsiflexion caused by weakening of the tibialis anterior muscle; produces "slapping gait" or "high-stepping gait" like a horse
	  • Loss of toe extension caused by weakening of the extensor digitorum longus and hallucis longus muscles
	  • Combined effect of all the previous produces an equinovarus deformity, in which there is plantar flexion with foot drop and inversion of the foot.
	• Sensory deficits involve the anterolateral aspect of the leg and dorsum of the foot.
	• Loss of the ankle jerk reflex

Erb-Duchenne palsy (see Fig. 26-25 F; Link 26-150)	• Brachial plexus lesion involving the upper plexus (C5 and C6) • In 50% of cases, C7 is also affected. • Arm is held adducted, internally rotated, and pronated with wrist flexed and fingers flexed ("waiter's tip position"; Link 26-150). • Bicep reflex is absent; Moro reflex with hand movement but no shoulder abduction; palmar grasp present (flexion of the fingers caused by stimulation of the palm of the hand) • Ipsilateral diaphragmatic involvement in a small percentage of cases
Klumpke paralysis (Link 26-151)	• Brachial plexus palsy involving injury to the lower plexus (C8, T1) • Associated with weakness of the flexor muscles of the wrist and the small muscles of the hand ("claw hand"; Link 26-151) • Up to one-third of these patients have an associated Horner syndrome. Horner syndrome is marked by sinking in of the eyeball, contraction of the pupil, drooping of the upper eyelid, and vasodilation and anhidrosis (lack of sweating) of the face caused by paralysis of the cervical sympathetic nerve fibers on the affected side).

EMG, Electromyography; *NCS,* nerve conduction study.

XIII. **Spinal Cord Trauma** (Link 26-153)
XIV. **Selected Eye Disorders** (Tables 26-8 and 26-9)
  • **Overview of eye infections** (Link 26-154)
XV. **Selected Ear Disorders** (Table 26-10)
  A. **Anatomy of the ear** (Link 26-180)
  B. **Overview of infections in the ear** (Link 26-181)
  C. **Causes of deafness** (Link 26-182)

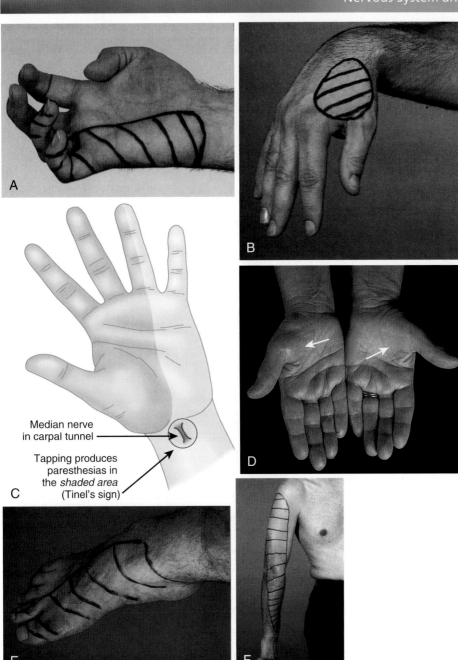

26-25: A, Ulnar nerve injury. Note the claw hand caused by an opposed action of the long flexors and extensors of the fingers. The ink markings show the distribution of impaired sensation. **B,** Radial nerve injury. Note the wrist drop. The ink markings show the distribution of impaired sensation. **C,** Effect of carpal tunnel syndrome on the median nerve. See text for discussion. **D,** *Arrows* show atrophy of thenar eminence. **E,** Common peroneal nerve injury. Note the foot drop. The ink markings show the distribution of impaired sensation. **F,** Erb-Duchenne palsy. Note how the arm is internally rotated and the forearm pronated, producing a "waiter's tip" deformity. The ink markings show the distribution of impaired sensation of the outer side of the upper arm. *(A, B, E, and F from Grieg JD:* Color Atlas of Surgical Diagnosis, *London, Mosby-Wolfe, 1996, pp 337, 334, 338, 332, respectively, Figs. 42.8, 42.4, 42.9, 42.2, respectively;* **C** *from Goldman L, Ausiello D:* Cecil's Textbook of Medicine, *23rd ed, Philadelphia, Saunders Elsevier, 2008, p 2008, Fig. 285-5;* **D** *from Perkin GD:* Mosby's Color Atlas and Text of Neurology, *St. Louis, Mosby, 2002, p 224, Fig. 12.10A.)*

Median nerve in carpal tunnel

Tapping produces paresthesias in the *shaded area* (Tinel's sign)

TABLE 26-8   Functions of the Major Parts of the Eye

STRUCTURE	FUNCTION
Sclera	External protection
Cornea	Light refraction
Choroid	Blood supply
Iris	Light absorption and regulation of pupillary diameter
Ciliary body	Secretion of vitreous fluid. Its smooth muscles change the shape of the lens.
Lens	Light refraction
Retinal layer	Light receptor that transforms optic signals into nerve impulses
Rods	Means of distinguishing light from dark and perceiving shape and movement
Cones	Color vision
Central fovea	Area of sharpest vision

Continued

TABLE 26-8 Functions of the Major Parts of the Eye—cont'd

STRUCTURE	FUNCTION
Macula lutea	Blind spot
External ocular muscles	Movement of the globe
Optic nerve (cranial nerve II)	Transmission of visual information to the brain
Lacrimal glands	Secretion of tears to lubricate the eye
Eyelids	Eye protection

From my friend Ivan Damjanov, MD, PhD: *Pathology for the Health Professions,* 4th ed, Philadelphia, Saunders Elsevier, 2012, p 476, Table 22-1.

TABLE 26-9 Selected Eye Disorders

EYE DISORDER	COMMENTS
Arcus senilis (see Fig. 26-26 A)	• Most often occurs older adults • Gray-opaque ring at the corneal margin (periphery of cornea). • Cholesterol deposits in corneal stroma; may indicate hypercholesterolemia if the patient is <50 years old and a smoker
Ophthalmia neonatorum	• Conjunctivitis in newborn • Chemical conjunctivitis (90% of treated newborns): Silver nitrate drops are no longer used and have been replaced by antibiotic drops. Irritation is noticed within hours after instillation and resolves by 48 hr in most cases. Typically bilateral. Exudate shows epithelial desquamation and neutrophils. Culture is negative. • Pathogen: *Neisseria gonorrhoeae* (2–5 days after birth; Link 26-155). Severe edema of eyelids, chemosis (edema of conjunctiva), progressive profuse purulent conjunctival exudates. Can result in perforation and loss of vision or loss of the globe. Infection can spread systemically resulting in death. Diagnosis confirmed with culture. Gram stain shows gram-negative diplococci phagocytosed by neutrophils. • Pathogen: *Chlamydia trachomatis* (usually develops between 10 and 14 days. Inflammation may be mild or severe, with primary involvement of the tarsal conjunctiva (lines the eyelids). Exudate is composed of a mixed neutrophil and mononuclear leukocytic infiltrate. Pseudomembranes may be evident. Inclusion bodies in leukocytes are located within the epithelial cells of the conjunctival surface.
"Red eye" (Link 26-156)	Causes include conjunctivitis (inflammation of conjunctiva; Link 26-157), episcleritis (episclera is a thin layer of tissue that lies between the conjunctiva and the connective tissue layer that forms the white of the eye [sclera]; Links 26-158 and 26-159), subconjunctival hemorrhage (bleeding underneath the conjunctiva. Conjunctiva contains small, fragile blood vessels that are easily ruptured.), scleritis (inflammation of the white of the eye), corneal disease (transparent anterior part of the external coat of the eye covering the iris and the pupil and continuous with the sclera. Inflammation of the cornea is called keratitis; see later), dry eye (tears are *not* able to provide adequate lubrication for the eyes. Common in elderly. May have excess tears running down the cheeks (called "reflex tearing"). Tears that are produced are mostly water and do *not* have the lubricating qualities or the rich composition of normal tears.), anterior uveitis (inflammation of the middle layer of the eye (Link 26-160). This layer includes the iris [colored part of the eye] and the adjacent tissue, known as the ciliary body), acute glaucoma (see later), blepharitis (inflammation of eyelid caused by clogging of the tiny oil glands located near the base of the eyelashes [Link 26-161]. Dandruff-like scales form on the eyelashes.)
Dacryocystitis	Refers to infection of the lacrimal sac secondary to obstruction of the nasolacrimal duct at the junction of lacrimal sac. Presents with a sudden onset of pain and redness in the medial canthal region (corner of the eye where the upper and lower eyelids meet near the nose; Link 26-162).
Bacterial conjunctivitis ("red eye"; Fig. 26-26 B)	• Purulent conjunctivitis; pain but *no* blurry vision • Pathogens: *Staphylococcus aureus* (most common), *Streptococcus pneumoniae, Haemophilus influenzae* (*Haemophilus aegyptius,* pinkeye)
Viral conjunctivitis (see Fig. 26-26 C)	• Watery exudates • Adenovirus: viral cause of pinkeye, painful preauricular lymphadenopathy • HSV-1: keratoconjunctivitis with dendritic ulcers (root-like) noted with fluorescein staining (Link 26-163)
Allergic conjunctivitis	Seasonal itching of eyes with allergic shiners and cobblestoning of the conjunctiva (Link 4-10; see Chapter 4)
Acanthamoeba infection	• Free-living ameba that causes severe infections of the eye, skin, and CNS • The ameba is found worldwide in the environment in water and soil. • Severe keratoconjunctivitis may also occur in patients who do not clean their contact lenses properly.
Stye (see Fig. 26-26 D)	Infection of the eyelid most commonly caused by *S. aureus*
Chalazion (see Fig. 26-26 E)	• Granulomatous inflammation involving the meibomian gland in the eyelid (Link 26-164) • Usually resolve spontaneously within 2 months • If they persist, they are surgically removed.
Orbital cellulitis	• Periorbital redness and swelling that is often secondary to sinusitis (e.g., ethmoiditis in children; Links 26-165 and 26-166) • Pathogens: *S. pneumoniae, H. influenza* type B, *S. aureus.* Less common pathogens include *Pseudomonas, Klebsiella, Eikenella,* and *Enterococcus* spp. • Fever, proptosis (eye bulges out), periorbital swelling, ophthalmoplegia (eye movement impaired), normal retinal examination

TABLE 26-9   Selected Eye Disorders—cont'd

EYE DISORDER	COMMENTS
Hordeolum (stye)	Refers to inflammation of one or more sebaceous glands (glands of Zeis and Moll) of the eyelid, forming an abscess on the eyelid margin (Link 26-167)
Orbital fracture (see Fig. 26-26 F)	• Most often associated with blunt trauma to the eye that produces an orbital floor fracture (Link 26-168) • Often associated with edema and ecchymoses of the eyelids and periorbital region ("raccoon" eyes) • Vertical diplopia, prolapse of orbital contents into the maxillary sinus (sunken eye), damage to infraorbital nerve may occur in severe fractures
Pterygium	• Raised, triangular encroachment of thickened conjunctiva on the nasal side of the conjunctiva (Link 26-169) • May grow onto the cornea • Caused by excessive exposure to wind, sun, and sand
Pinguecula (see Fig. 26-26 G)	• Yellow-white conjunctival degeneration at the junction of cornea and sclera on the temporal side of the conjunctiva (Link 26-170) • Does *not* grow onto the cornea like a pterygium does
Optic neuritis	• Inflammation of optic nerve (Link 26-171) • Causes: multiple sclerosis (most common), methanol poisoning • Blurry vision or loss of vision; may cause optic atrophy (Link 26-172)
Central retinal artery occlusion (see Fig. 26-26 H)	• Causes: embolization of plaque material from ipsilateral carotid or ophthalmic artery; giant cell arteritis involving the ophthalmic artery • Sudden, painless, complete loss of vision in one eye, pallor of optic disk caused by vascular occlusion; "boxcar" segmentation of blood in retinal veins, and cherry red macula.
Central retinal vein occlusion see (Fig. 26-26 I)	• Causes: hypercoagulable state (e.g., polycythemia vera) • Sudden, painless, unilateral loss of vision, swelling of optic disk, and engorged retinal veins with hemorrhage ("blood and thunder" appearance)
Glaucoma (see Fig. 26-26 J)	• Increased intraocular pressure Chronic open-angle type: • Decreased rate of aqueous outflow into the canal of Schlemm trabecular meshwork (circular canal lying in the substance of the sclerocorneal junction of the eye and draining the aqueous humor from the anterior chamber into the veins draining the eyeball; Link 26-173 A) • Common in those with severe myopia (near-sightedness) • Bilateral aching eyes • Pathologic cupping of the optic disks (Link 26-174) • Night blindness and gradual loss of peripheral vision leading to tunnel vision and blindness Acute angle-closure type: • Narrowing of anterior chamber angle (Link 26-173 B) • Medical emergency precipitated by a mydriatic agent, uveitis, or lens dislocation • Severe pain associated with photophobia and blurry vision • "Red eye" with a steamy cornea • Pupil fixed and nonreactive to light
Optic nerve atrophy (see Fig. 26-26 K)	• Pale optic disk (Link 26-172) • Most commonly caused by optic neuritis or glaucoma • *No* effective treatment
Uveitis	• Inflammation of the uveal tract (iris, ciliary body, choroid; Link 26-160) • Causes: sarcoidosis, ulcerative colitis, ankylosing spondylitis • Pain with blurry vision, miotic pupil, circumcorneal ciliary body vascular congestion, normal intraocular pressure, adhesions between iris and anterior lens capsule
Macular degeneration (see Fig. 26-26 L)	• Most common cause of permanent visual loss in older adults • Disruption of Bruch membrane in the retina (Link 26-175) • Amsler grid shows distortion of vision in macular degeneration (Link 26-176) • Dry type: thinning of the retina and formation of yellowish white deposits called drusen • Wet type: extension of the dry type; vessels under the retina hemorrhage causing retinal cells to die, creating blind spots or distorted central vision • Antioxidants may decrease risk
CMV retinitis (see Fig. 26-26 M)	• Most common cause of blindness in AIDS • Usually occurs when the CD4 T helper cell count is <50 cells/μL • Usually painless • Varicella zoster virus retinitis is usually painful. • Cotton-wool exudates and retinal hemorrhages
Cataracts (see Fig. 26-26 N)	• Opacity in the lens • Causes: advanced age (most common), diabetes mellitus (osmotic damage), infection (e.g., rubella), corticosteroids • Common in congenital infections (e.g., CMV, rubella)
Malignant tumors (see Fig. 26-26 O)	• Malignant melanoma in adults: arise from pigmented cells in the choroid (Link 26-177) • Retinoblastoma in children ("white eye reflex"); contain Homer Wright rosettes (rosette with no lumen) and Flexner-Wintersteiner rosettes (rosette with lumen) (Links 26-178 and 26-179)

CMV, Cytomegalovirus; *CNS,* central nervous system; *HSV,* herpes simplex virus.

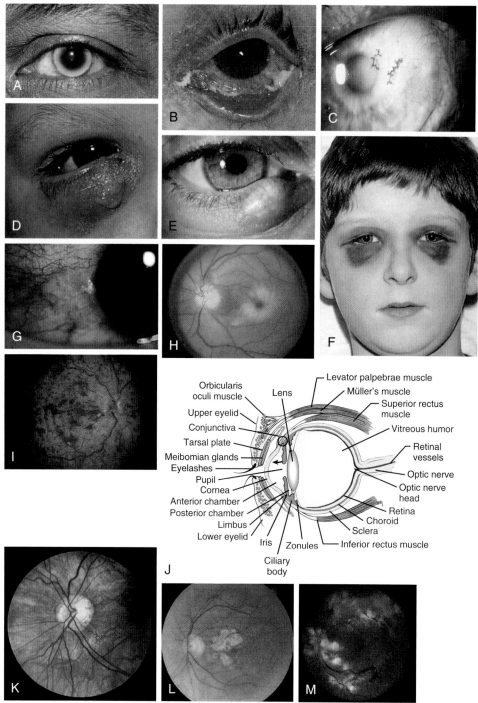

26-26: **A,** Arcus senilis. Note the gray-white ring around the perimeter of the cornea. **B,** Bacterial conjunctivitis. Note the conjunctival hemorrhage and pus. **C,** Herpes simplex virus keratoconjunctivitis. The special stain highlights the dendritic ulcers associated with this infection. **D,** Stye. Note the swelling, erythema, and pus from this infection of the lower eyelid. **E,** Chalazion. Note the swelling of the eyelid and absence of pus and conjunctival irritation, which distinguishes a chalazion from a stye. **F,** Orbital fractures. Note the periorbital swelling and ecchymoses giving the appearance of "raccoon" eyes. **G,** Pinguecula. Note the yellow-white conjunctival tissue on the temporal side of the conjunctiva. It extends to the junction of the cornea and sclera but it does not extend onto the cornea, unlike a pterygium. **H,** Central retinal artery occlusion. Note the generalized pallor of the optic disk and narrowed arteries. There is a cherry red spot on the macula, which is to the right of the optic disk. There is no boxcar segmentation in the retinal veins. **I,** Central retinal vein occlusion. Note the numerous flame hemorrhages in the retina as well as swelling of the optic disk. **J,** Schematic of the eye. Aqueous humor is produced by the ciliary body from which it flows into the anterior chamber and then out through a spongy tissue at the front of the eye called the trabecular meshwork into a drainage canal *(circle).* Glaucoma is an increase in aqueous pressure. In open-angle glaucoma, fluid cannot flow effectively through the trabecular meshwork. In acute angle-closure glaucoma there is narrowing of the anterior chamber caused by forward displacement of the ciliary body *(arrow).* **K,** Optic nerve atrophy showing a pale optic disk. **L,** Macular degeneration. Note the yellow-white deposits (drusen) in the macula. **M,** Cytomegalovirus retinitis in AIDS. Note the numerous cotton-wool exudates in the retina.

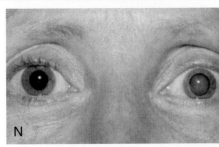
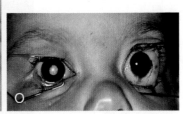

26-26 cont'd: **N,** Cataract. Note the opacity in the left eye. **O,** Retinoblastoma in the right eye of a child showing a white eye reflex. *(A, D, E, and G from Kanski JJ, Nischal KK: Ophthalmology: Clinical Signs and Differential Diagnosis, St. Louis, Mosby, 2000; B from Newell F: Ophthalmology: Principles and Concepts, 8th ed. St. Louis, Mosby, 1996; C, H, I, J, and N from Swartz MH: Textbook of Physical Diagnosis, 5th ed, Philadelphia, Saunders Elsevier, 2006, Figs. 10-57, 10-110, 10-116, 10-2, 10-67A, respectively; F from Mir MA: Atlas of Clinical Diagnosis, London, Saunders, 1995; K from Perkin GD: Mosby's Color Atlas and Text of Neurology, St. Louis, Mosby, 2002, p 64, Fig. 4-3; L from Goldman L, Ausiello D: Cecil's Medicine, 23rd ed, Philadelphia, Saunders Elsevier, 2008, p 2855, Fig. 449-12; M courtesy of Douglas A. Jobs, MD, The Wilmer Ophthalmological Institute, The Johns Hopkins University and Hospital, Baltimore; O from my friend Ivan Damjanov, MD, PhD, Linder J: Pathology: A Color Atlas, St. Louis, Mosby, 2000, p 445, Fig. 20-39.)*

TABLE 26-10   Selected Ear Disorders

EAR DISORDER	DESCRIPTION AND COMMENTS

Ménière disease	• Condition of unknown etiology that affects adults
	• Peak incidence is in those 30–60 yr of age
	• Overall prevalence of this disease is not known, but estimates indicate a prevalence of up to 5% of all adults.
	• Associated with hydrops (excess fluid) of the endolymphatic system of the cochlea and loss of cochlear hairs; cause of increased endolymphatic pressure is *not* known
	• Clinically presents with the following triad:
	  • Episodic vertigo that lasts 1 hr to several hours, typically subsiding but then recurring after a few hours or days
	  • Sensorineural hearing loss for low-frequency sound.
	  • Tinnitus, or ringing in the ears.

Sensorineural defect (see Fig. 26-27 A)	• Weber test: lateralizes to normal ear (contralateral ear is affected) • Sensory hearing loss results from cochlear abnormalities. • Noise trauma (e.g., at the workplace or very loud music) is an important cause of sensorineural hearing loss. • Ototoxic drugs, such as streptomycin, antimalarial drugs, and certain diuretics, may also cause deafness. • Presbycusis, hearing loss of unknown etiology that affects older adults, is also classified as a sensorineural defect. • Neural hearing loss results from lesions of CN VIII or of the central nervous system. This is the least common form of hearing loss. Typical causes include acoustic neuromas of CN VIII, multiple sclerosis, and cerebrovascular accidents.
Conduction defect (see Fig. 26-27 A)	• Weber test: lateralizes to affected ear • Caused by degeneration of cochlear hairs • Conductive hearing loss is caused by lesions of the external or middle ear. • In the external canal, the cause of hearing loss may be obstruction (cerumen impaction) such as with impacted cerumen. • Loss of the tympanic membrane or its perforation by trauma or infection (otitis media) also causes conductive hearing loss. • Effusion in the middle ear, cholesteatoma, or hemorrhage into the middle ear cavity can all lead to conductive hearing loss. • Otosclerosis causes deafness by impeding the transmission of signals from the tympanic membrane to the oval window.
Otosclerosis	• Most common cause of conduction deafness in older adults • Caused by fusion of middle ear ossicles
Otitis media (see Fig. 26-27 B)	• Most common cause of ear pain in young children • Most common cause of conduction deafness in children • Most common pathogens: *Streptococcus pneumoniae*, nontypeable *Haemophilus influenza*, and *Moraxella catarrhalis* • Other causes: *Staphylococcus aureus, Mycoplasma pneumoniae*, and gram-negative bacilli may also be seen.
External otitis (see Fig. 26-27 C)	• Inflammation of outer ear canal (Link 26-183) • "Swimmer's ear": caused by *Pseudomonas aeruginosa, Staphylococcus aureus, Aspergillus* spp. • Malignant external otitis: severe infection of outer ear canal in patients with diabetes mellitus. *P. aeruginosa* is the most common cause (Link 26-184)
Basilar skull fracture	• Refers to a fracture of the base of the skull (Link 26-185) • Typically involving the temporal bone, occipital bone, sphenoid bone, or ethmoid bone • Occurs in 4% of severe head injury patients • Can cause tears in the membranes surrounding the brain, or meninges, with resultant leakage of the CSF. Leaking fluid may accumulate in the middle ear space and exit via a perforated eardrum (CSF otorrhea) or into the nasopharynx via the eustachian tube, causing CSF rhinorrhea (fluid coming out of the nose).

CN, Cranial nerve; *CSF,* cerebrospinal fluid.

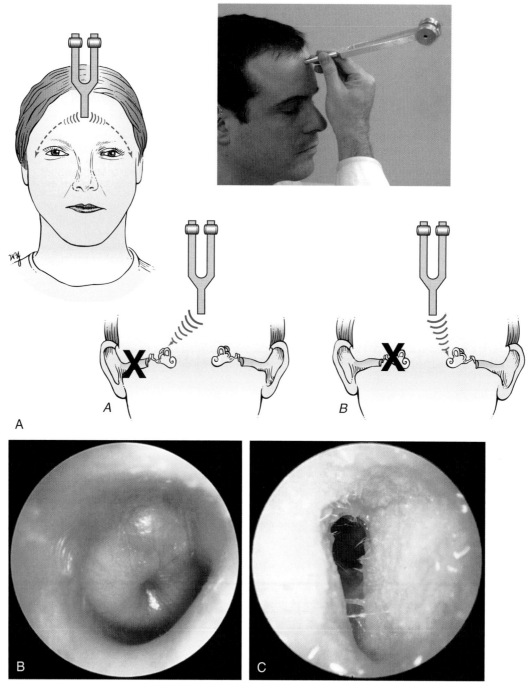

26-27: **A,** Weber test (affected ear is marked with an X). When a vibrating tuning fork is placed on the center of the forehead, the normal response is for the sound to be heard in the center without lateralization to either side. **A,** In the presence of a conductive hearing loss, the sound is heard on the side of the conductive loss. **B,** In the presence of a sensorineural loss, the sound is heard better on the opposite (unaffected) side. **B,** Otitis media. Note the bulging, erythematous tympanic membrane. **C,** Otitis externa. Note the inflammatory exudate in the external canal. *(A to C from Swartz MH: Textbook of Physical Diagnosis, 5th ed, Philadelphia, Saunders Elsevier, 2006, pp 305, 314, 314, respectively, Figs. 11-13, 11-29, 11-26, respectively.)*

Appendix: Formulas for Calculations of Acid-Base Disorders

A. **Note: Other authors use different formulas; however, they should roughly approximate each other and correctly distinguish single versus mixed acid-base disorders.**

B. **Calculation of expected compensation in acute respiratory acidosis**
   1. Sometimes calculations help in identifying whether there is more than one primary acid-base disorder in a patient (called a mixed disorder; see later).
   2. If the calculated expected compensation closely approximates the measured compensation, a single primary disorder is present.
   3. If there is an obvious disparity between calculated expected compensation and measured compensation, another primary disorder is also present.
   4. In acute respiratory acidosis, expected HCO_3^- compensation $= 0.10 \times \Delta PCO_2$ (difference from normal of 40 mm Hg)
      - Recall (refer to Chapter 5) that the expected compensation in respiratory acidosis is metabolic alkalosis ($\uparrow HCO_3^-$)
   5. Example: pH 7.20, PCO_2 74 mm Hg, HCO_3^- 27 mEq/L
      a. Expected HCO_3^- compensation $= 0.10 \times (74 - 40) = 3.4$ mEq/L increase above normal
      b. Expected HCO_3^- compensation $= 24$ mEq/L (mean HCO_3^-) $+ 3.4 = 27.4$ mEq/L
         - Note that measured and expected calculated HCO_3^- are similar; therefore, a single disorder is present.

C. **Calculation of expected compensation in chronic respiratory acidosis**
   1. Expected HCO_3^- compensation $= 0.40 \times \Delta PCO_2$
   2. Example: pH 7.34, PCO_2 60 mm Hg, HCO_3^- 32 mEq/L
      a. Expected HCO_3^- compensation $= 0.40 \times (60 - 40) = 8$ mEq/L increase above normal
      b. Expected HCO_3^- compensation $= 24 + 8 = 32$ mEq/L
         - Note that measured and expected calculated HCO_3^- are similar; therefore, a single disorder is present.

D. **Calculation of expected compensation in acute respiratory alkalosis**
   1. Expected HCO_3^- compensation $= 0.20 \times \Delta PaCO_2$ (difference from normal of 40 mm Hg)
      - Recall that the expected compensation in respiratory alkalosis is metabolic acidosis ($\downarrow HCO_3^-$)
   2. Example: pH 7.56, $PaCO_2$ 24 mm Hg, HCO_3^- 21 mEq/L
      a. Expected HCO_3^- compensation $= 0.20 \times (40 - 24) = 3.2$ mEq/L less than the normal
      b. Expected HCO_3^- compensation $= 24$ mEq/L (mean HCO_3^-) $- 3.2 = 20.8$ mEq/L
         - Note that measured and expected calculated HCO_3^- are similar; therefore, a single disorder is present.

E. **Calculation of expected compensation in chronic respiratory alkalosis**
   1. Expected $HCO_3^- = 0.50 \times \Delta PaCO_2$
   2. Example: pH 7.47, $PaCO_2$ 18 mm Hg, HCO_3^- 13 mEq/L
      a. Expected HCO_3^- compensation $= 0.50 \times (40 - 18) = 11$ mEq/L less than the normal
      b. Expected HCO_3^- compensation $= 24 - 11 = 13$ mEq/L
         - Note that measured and expected calculated HCO_3^- are similar; therefore a single disorder is present.

F. **Calculation of expected compensation in metabolic acidosis (either type)**
   1. Expected $PaCO_2 = 1.2 \times \Delta HCO_3^- \pm 2$
      a. ΔHCO_3^- is measured HCO_3^- subtracted from the mean HCO_3^- of 24 mEq/L.
      b. Recall that the expected compensation in metabolic acidosis is respiratory alkalosis ($\downarrow PaCO_2$).

2. Example: pH 7.27, $Paco_2$ 27 mm Hg, HCO_3^- 12 mEq/L
   a. Expected $Paco_2$ compensation = $1.2 \times (24 - 12) = 14.4$ mm Hg less than the normal
   b. Expected $Paco_2$ = 40 (mean $Paco_2$) − 14.4 = 25.6 mm Hg (23.6–27.6)
      • Note that measured $Paco_2$ is within the calculated range; therefore only a single disorder is present.

G. Calculation of expected compensation in metabolic alkalosis
   1. Expected $Paco_2 = 0.7 \times \Delta HCO_3^- \pm 2$
      • Recall that the expected compensation in metabolic alkalosis is respiratory acidosis ($\uparrow Paco_2$).
   2. Example: pH 7.58, $Paco_2$ 49 mm Hg, HCO_3^- 39 mEq/L
      a. Expected $Paco_2$ compensation = $0.7 \times (39 - 24) = 10.5$ greater than the normal
      b. Expected $Paco_2$ compensation = 40 + 10.5 = 50.5 mm Hg (48.5–52.5)
         • Note that measured $Paco_2$ is within the calculated range; therefore, only a single disorder is present.

H. Examples of how formulas help identify a mixed disorder
   1. pH 7.26, $Paco_2$ 38 mm Hg, HCO_3^- 17 mEq/L
      a. Presumptive diagnosis: metabolic acidosis (HCO_3^- <22 mEq/L) without compensation ($Paco_2$ in normal range)
      b. Formula for calculating expected compensation in metabolic acidosis:
         (1) Expected $Paco_2 = 1.2 \times \Delta HCO_3^- \pm 2$
         (2) Expected $Paco_2 = 1.2 \times (24 - 17) = 8.4$ mm Hg less than the normal value
         (3) Expected $Paco_2$ = 40 (mean $Paco_2$) − 8.4 = 31.6 (29.6–33.6)
         (4) The measured $Paco_2$ is 38 mm Hg, which is higher than it should be, indicating that a respiratory acidosis (retention of CO_2) must also be present as a primary disorder.
   2. pH 7.38, $Paco_2$ 70 mm Hg, HCO_3^- 41 mEq/L
      a. Presumptive diagnosis: mixed disorder (because the pH is normal) with chronic respiratory acidosis ($Paco_2$ >45 mm Hg, HCO_3^- >30 mEq/L) and primary metabolic alkalosis (HCO_3^- >28 mEq/L)
      b. Using either the formula for metabolic alkalosis or chronic respiratory acidosis will prove the presence of a mixed disorder.
      c. Using the chronic respiratory acidosis formula (expected $HCO_3^- = 0.40 \times \Delta Paco_2$)
         (1) Expected HCO_3^- compensation = $0.40 \times (70 - 40) = 12$ mEq/L increase above normal
         (2) Expected HCO_3^- compensation = 24 + 12 = 36 mEq/L
         (3) Measured HCO_3^- is 41 mEq/L, which is higher than the expected compensation indicating the presence of an additional primary metabolic alkalosis (more HCO_3^- than there should be for compensation).
      d. Using the metabolic alkalosis formula (expected $Paco_2 = 0.7 \times \Delta HCO_3^- \pm 2$)
         (1) Expected $Paco_2 = 0.7 \times (41 - 24) = 11.9$ mm Hg increase from the normal
         (2) Expected $Paco_2$ = 40 + 11.9 = 51.9 mm Hg (49.9–53.9)
         (3) The measured $Paco_2$ is 70 mm Hg, which is much higher than it should be indicating the presence of an additional primary respiratory acidosis.

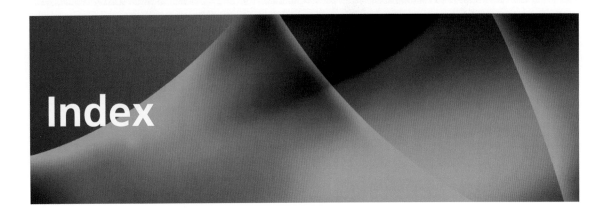

Index

Page numbers followed by "*f*" indicate figures, "*t*" indicate tables, and "*b*" indicate boxes.

A

A-a gradient. *see* Alveolar-arterial (a-a) gradient
AAT deficiency, 547–548
Abdominal aortic aneurysm (AAA), 257–258
  aorta, aneurysmal dilation of, 258*f*
Abnormal bleeding
  causes of, 633*t*
  uterine, 632, 632*t*
ABO blood group
  antigens, 408–417
    definition of, 408
    back type, 409
      identification of, 409*f*
    determination of, 409
    forward type, 409
      identification of, 409*f*
    phenotypes, 409*f*
ABO HDN, 413–414, 413*f*, 417*t*
  clinical and laboratory findings of, 414
  epidemiology of, 414
  pathogenesis of, 414
ABO hemolytic disease, Rh hemolytic disease (comparison), 417*t*
ABO incompatibility, maternal protection and, 416
Abrasion, 195
Abruptio placenta, 647*f*, 648
  clinical findings of, 648
  diagnosis of, 648
  epidemiology of, 648
Absolute leukocytosis, with left shift, 64*f*
Absolute neutrophilic leukocytosis, 63, 64*f*
Absolute polycythemia, 364, 364*f*
ACA. *see* Anterior cerebral artery
Acanthosis nigricans (AN), 759
  pigmented verrucoid lesion in, 759*f*
Accentuated A₂, 276–277
Accumulations, types of, 30
Accuracy, of test results, 7, 7*f*
Acetaminophen
  overdose of, 193
  poisoning, 24*f*, 26–27
    treatment for, *N*-acetylcysteine (usage), 27
Acetylcholine (ACh) receptors, autoantibodies (impact), 731
Achalasia, 481–482
  barium study for, 482*f*
  clinical findings of, 482
  diagnosis of, 482
  epidemiology of, 481
  pathogenesis of, 482
Achilles deep tendon reflex (DTR), delayed recovery of, 672
Achilles tendon xanthoma, 253*f*
Achondroplasia, 705
Acid-base disorders, 129–135, 193
Acid-base homeostasis, maintenance of, 562
Acne (treatment), retinoic acid (treatment avoidance), 179
Acne rosacea, 768
  pustules/papules, superimposition of, 763*f*–764*f*
Acne vulgaris, 748
  facial acne, presence of, 745*f*
Acoustic neuroma, 817, 817*f*
Acquired diverticula, 596
Acquired (adaptive) immunity, 70

Acquired immunodeficiency syndrome (AIDS), 95–103
  epidemiology of, 95–98
  immunologic abnormalities in, 102
  intravenous drug abuse (IVDA) of, 98
  laboratory tests for, 100*t*
  modes of transmission of, 98
  pathogenesis of, 98–99
  pathologic changes and clinical findings associated with, 102*f*
  pregnant women with, 103
  virus characteristics of, 97–98
Acquired preneoplastic disorders, 239*t*
Acquired thrombosis syndromes, 405–406
Acquired valvular heart disease, 297–307
Acral lentiginous malignant melanoma, 756*f*–757*f*
Acral lentiginous melanoma (ALM), 758
Acromegaly, 667
  tumor development and, 667*f*
Actin, 29
Actinic (solar) keratosis, 760
  hyperkeratotic lesion in, 761*f*
Actinomyces, sulfur granule of, 468*f*
Actinomyces israelii, 429*t*–432*t*
Activated alveolar macrophages, appearance (change) of, 79
Activated glycogen synthase kinase-3β (GSK-3β), role of, 806
Activated partial thromboplastin time (aPTT), 397–398, 397*f*
Acute adrenocortical insufficiency, 686–690
Acute anterior myocardial infarction, electrocardiogram for, 290*f*
Acute appendicitis, 520–521
  serosal surface of appendix in, erythema and vascular congestion of, 520*f*
Acute bacterial endocarditis, vegetation (presence) of, 306*f*
Acute blood loss, 337–338
Acute cerebral edema, 204
Acute cervicitis, 621–622
Acute chest syndrome (ACS), 344, 346
Acute cholecystitis, 555–556
Acute coronary artery syndromes (ACASs), 285
Acute cystitis, 594–595
  causes of, 594
Acute drug-induced TIN, 582–583
Acute endocarditis, 305
Acute endometritis, 635
Acute epidural hematoma, 786
  non-contrast-enhanced computed tomography (CT) scan for, 787*f*
Acute fatty liver, of pregnancy, 534
Acute gastritis, 486
Acute gout, 721
Acute gouty arthritis, 721, 722*f*
Acute graft-*versus*-host (GVH) reaction, 84*f*
Acute hemolytic transfusion reaction (HTR), 412–413
Acute immune thrombocytopenia, 399*t*
Acute inflammation (AI), 45–67
  cardinal sign of, 45, 46*f*
  chemical mediators of, 50–53, 51*t*–52*t*, 52*f*
  chronic inflammation, comparison of, 58*t*
  consequences of, 56, 56*f*
  definition of, 45
  fever in, pathogenesis and role of, 54–55
  fibrinous, 53*f*, 54
  granulomatous, 54, 57–58
  pseudomembranous, 53*f*, 54
  purulent (suppurative), 53, 53*f*
  sequential cellular events in, 46–50
  sequential vascular events in, 45–46, 46*f*